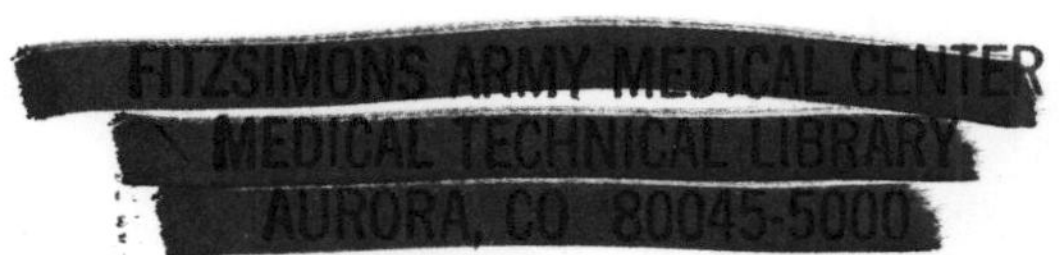

PEDIATRIC PLASTIC SURGERY

Pediatric Plastic Surgery

DONALD SERAFIN, M.D., F.A.C.S.

Professor,
Division of Plastic, Maxillofacial, and Reconstructive Surgery,
Duke University Medical Center,
Durham, North Carolina

NICHOLAS G. GEORGIADE, D.D.S., M.D., F.A.C.S.

Professor and Chairman,
Division of Plastic, Maxillofacial, Oral, and Reconstructive Surgery,
Duke University Medical Center,
Durham, North Carolina

With 2288 illustrations

The C. V. Mosby Company

St. Louis   Toronto   Princeton   1984

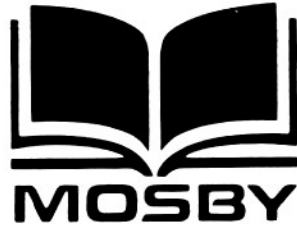

MOSBY

A TRADITION OF PUBLISHING EXCELLENCE

Editor: Karen Berger
Assistant editor: Terry Van Schaik
Manuscript editor: Sandra L. Gilfillan
Book design: Jeanne Bush
Production: Linda R. Stalnaker

TWO VOLUMES

Printed in the United States of America

The C. V. Mosby Company
11830 Westline Industrial Drive, St. Louis, Missouri 63146

Library of Congress Cataloging in Publication Data

Main entry under title:

Pediatric plastic surgery.

    Bibliography: p.
    Includes index.
    1. Surgery, Plastic. 2. Children—Surgery.
I. Serafin, Donald, 1938-   . II. Georgiade,
Nicholas G., 1918-   . [DNLM: 1. Surgery, Plastic—
In infancy and childhood. WO 600 P371]
RD118.P35   1984   617′.95′088054   83-22098
ISBN 0-8016-4491-7

GW/MV/MV 9 8 7 6 5 4 3 2 1   03/D/329

CONTRIBUTORS

W. Allen Addison, M.D.
Associate Professor; Director, Division of Gynecology, Department of Obstetrics and Gynecology, Duke University Medical Center, Durham, North Carolina

John C. Angelillo, D.D.S., M.D.
Associate Professor and Chief, Clinical Oral Surgery, Department of Surgery, Duke University Medical Center; Consultant, Section of Oral and Maxillofacial Surgery, Veterans Administration Hospital; Attending Staff, Department of Surgery, Durham County General Hospital, Durham, North Carolina

Daniel C. Baker, M.D.
Assistant Professor of Surgery (Plastic Surgery), New York University Medical School; Assistant Attending Surgeon, Institute of Reconstructive Plastic Surgery, New York University Medical Center; Attending Surgeon, Manhattan Eye, Ear, and Throat Hospital and St. Vincent's Hospital and Medical Center, New York, New York

Robert C. Bartlett, M.S., P.T.
Professor and Chairman, Department of Physical Therapy, Duke University, Medical Center, Durham, North Carolina

William J. Barwick, M.D.
Assistant Professor of Surgery, Division of Plastic, Maxillofacial, and Reconstructive Surgery, Duke University Medical Center, Durham, North Carolina

Edmond C. Bloch, M.B., F.F.A.R.C.S., F.A.A.P.
Associate Professor, Department of Anesthesiology, Duke University Medical Center, Durham, North Carolina

Warren C. Breidenbach III, M.D., F.R.C.S.(C)
Microsurgery Fellow, Department of Plastic Surgery, Microsurgery Research Laboratory, Eastern Virginia Medical School, Norfolk, Virginia

Burton D. Brent, M.D.
Assistant Clinical Professor and Research Advisor in Plastic Surgery, Stanford University, Stanford, California

Bruce Brewer, M.D.
Attending Plastic Surgeon, Department of Plastic Surgery, North Shore University Hospital, Manhasset, New York; Assistant Attending Plastic Surgeon, Department of Plastic Surgery, Nassau County Medical Center, East Meadow, New York

Prof. Dr. Med. Dieter Buck-Gramcko
Associate Professor of Hand Surgery and Plastic Surgery, University of Hamburg; Chief of Hand Surgery and Plastic Surgery, Accident Hospital for Workmen's Compensation; Consultant Hand Surgeon, Children's Hospital Wilhelmsstift, Hamburg, Germany

Harry J. Buncke, Jr., M.D.
Associate Clinical Professor, Department of Surgery, University of California School of Medicine, San Francisco, California

Arthur C. Chandler, Jr., M.S., M.D., F.A.C.S.
Clinical Associate Professor of Ophthalmology, Associate Professor of Anatomy, Duke University Medical Center, Durham, North Carolina

Wallace H.J. Chang, M.D., F.A.C.S.
Clinical Associate Professor of Plastic Surgery, Department of Surgery, University of Washington School of Medicine; Plastic and Reconstructive Surgeon, Active Staff, Children's Orthopedic Hospital Medical Center, Highline Community Hospital, Riverton General Hospital, and Valley General Hospital, Seattle, Washington

Edward Clifford, Ph.D.
Professor of Medical Psychology, Division of Plastic, Maxillofacial, and Oral Surgery, Department of Surgery; Professor of Medical Psychology, Division of Medical Psychology, Department of Psychiatry; Co-director, Facial Rehabilitation Center, Duke University Medical Center, Durham, North Carolina

Leo Clodius, M.D.
Head, Division of Plastic and Reconstructive Surgery, Second Surgical Clinic, University of Zurich Medical School, Zurich, Switzerland

Peter J. Coccaro, D.D.S., M.S., F.A.C.D.
Formerly Research Professor of Clinical Surgery (Orthodontics), Department of Plastic Surgery, New York University School of Medicine, New York University Medical Center, New York, New York

Joel J. Feldman, M.D.
Instructor in Surgery (Plastic), Harvard Medical School; Consultant Plastic Surgeon, Shriners Burns Institute, Boston, Massachusetts; Active Staff, Mount Auburn Hospital, Cambridge, Massachusetts; Associate in Surgery, Massachusetts General Hospital, Boston, Massachusetts

Marcus Castro Ferreira, M.D.
Associate Professor, Department of Plastic Surgery, University of São Paulo Medical School; Surgeon in Charge, Microsurgery Unit, University of São Paulo Hospital, São Paulo, Brazil

Howard C. Filston, M.D., F.A.C.S., F.A.A.P.
Professor of Pediatric Surgery and Pediatrics, Chief of Pediatric Surgical Service, Department of Surgery, Duke University Medical Center, Durham, North Carolina

J. William Futrell, M.D.
Professor and Chief, Division of Plastic Surgery, University of Pittsburgh School of Medicine; Chief of Plastic Surgery, Children's Hospital of Pittsburgh and Presbyterian University-Hospital, University of Pittsburgh, Pittsburgh, Pennsylvania

Gregory S. Georgiade, M.D.
Assistant Professor of General Surgery, Duke University School of Medicine; Assistant Professor of Plastic Surgery, Division of Plastic, Maxillofacial, and Reconstructive Surgery, Duke University Medical Center, Durham, North Carolina

Nicholas G. Georgiade, D.D.S., M.D., F.A.C.S.
Professor and Chairman, Division of Plastic, Maxillofacial, Oral, and Reconstructive Surgery, Duke University Medical Center, Durham, North Carolina

Kimberly S. Gibson, B.S., P.T.
Formerly Senior Physical Therapist, Division of Plastic, Maxillofacial, and Reconstructive Surgery, Department of Physical Therapy, Duke University Medical Center, Durham, North Carolina; Currently Hand Therapist, Catalina Orthopaedic Surgery, P.C., Tucson, Arizona

James F. Glenn, B.A., M.D.
President, Mt. Sinai Medical Center, New York, New York

J. Leonard Goldner, M.D.
James B. Duke Professor and Chief, Division of Orthopaedic Surgery, Duke University Medical Center, Durham, North Carolina

David J. Goodkind, M.D.
Attending in Plastic and Reconstructive Surgery, Yale–New Haven Hospital, Hospital of St. Raphael's, New Haven, Milford Hospital, Milford, Griffin Hospital, Darby, Connecticut

William P. Graham III, M.D.
Professor of Surgery and Chief, Division of Plastic and Reconstructive Surgery, Pennsylvania State University; Professor, Department of Surgery, Division of Plastic and Reconstructive Surgery, M.S. Hershey Medical Center, Hershey, Pennsylvania

Charles B. Hammond, M.D.
E.C. Hamblen Professor and Chairman, Department of Obstetrics and Gynecology, Duke University Medical Center, Durham, North Carolina

Reid H. Hansen, M.D.
Assistant Professor, Division of Plastic and Reconstructive Surgery, Southern Illinois University School of Medicine, Springfield, Illinois

Kiyonori Harii, M.D.
Associate Professor, Department of Plastic Surgery, Faculty of Medicine, The University of Tokyo, Tokyo, Japan

Gerald D. Harris, M.D.
Assistant Professor, Department of Surgery, Northwestern University; Assistant Professor, Department of Surgery, Northwestern Memorial Hospital, Children's Memorial Hospital, Shriners Hospital for Crippled Children, and Lakeside Veterans Administration Hospital, Chicago, Illinois

Dennis J. Hurwitz, M.D., F.A.C.S.
Clinical Associate Professor of Surgery (Plastic), Department of Surgery, Division of Plastic Surgery, University of Pittsburgh; Chief, Division of Plastic Surgery, Montefiore Hospital, Pittsburgh, Pennsylvania

Yoshikazu Ikuta, M.D.
Associate Professor, Department of Orthopedic Surgery, Hiroshima University School of Medicine, Hiroshima, Japan

Ian T. Jackson, M.B., CH.B, F.R.C.S.
Head, Section of Plastic and Reconstructive Surgery, Mayo Clinic; Professor, Mayo Medical School, Rochester, Minnesota

Malcolm C. Johnston, D.D.S., Ph.D.
Professor of Orthodontics and Anatomy, School of Dentistry and Medicine, Senior Scientist, Dental Research Center, University of North Carolina, Chapel Hill, North Carolina

Howard W. Klein, M.D., F.R.C.S.(C)
Instructor, Plastic, Maxillofacial, and Reconstructive Surgery, Division of Plastic, Maxillofacial, and Reconstructive Surgery, Duke University Medical Center, Durham, North Carolina

Stephen A. Kramer, M.D.
Instructor, Department of Urology, Mayo Medical School, Mayo Clinic; Consultant, Department of Urology, St. Mary's Hospital, Rochester, Minnesota

Thomas J. Krizek, M.D.
Professor of Surgery (Plastic), Chief of Plastic and Reconstructive Surgery, University of Southern California, Los Angeles, California

Ronald P. Krueger, M.D.
Associate Professor of Surgery (Urology), Assistant Professor of Pediatrics (Nephrology), Department of Surgery and Pediatrics, University of Mississippi Medical Center; Attending Physician, Department of Surgery, University Hospital, Jackson, Mississippi

Luvern H. Kunze, Ph.D.
Professor of Speech and Language Pathology, Department of Surgery, Duke University Medical Center; Director, Center for Speech and Hearing Disorders, Duke University Medical Center, Durham, North Carolina

Verne C. Lanier, Jr., M.D.
Clinical Assistant Professor of Plastic Surgery, Division of Plastic, Maxillofacial, and Reconstructive Surgery, Duke University Medical Center; Attending Plastic Surgeon, Division of Plastic Surgery, Durham County General Hospital and Durham Veterans Administration Hospital, Durham, North Carolina

Ralph A. Latham, B.SC., B.D.S., M.C.L.D., Ph.D.
Clinical Lecturer in Paediatric and Community Dentistry, Department of Paediatric and Community Dentistry, University of Western Ontario; Orthodontist, Department of Dentistry, Victoria Hospital Corporation, London, Ontario, Canada

Graham D. Lister, M.D., F.A.C.S., F.R.C.S.
Clinical Professor of Surgery (Hand), University of Louisville School of Medicine; Active Member, Jewish Hospital, Louisville, Kentucky

Guido Lozada, M.D.
Resident in Plastic Surgery, St. Francis Memorial Hospital, San Francisco, California

Charles J. MacDonald, M.D.
Metropolitan Hand Surgery Associates, P.A.; Clinical Assistant Professor, Department of Family Practice, University of Minnesota, St. Paul, Minnesota

Judith G. Mann, M.S.C.
Speech/Language Pathologist, Speech and Hearing Center, The Children's Hospital, Birmingham, Alabama

Robert M. Mason, Ph.D., D.M.D.
Associate Professor of Orthodontics, Division of Plastic, Maxillofacial, and Oral Surgery, Department of Surgery, Duke University Medical Center, Durham, North Carolina

Stephen J. Mathes, M.D., F.A.C.S.
Associate Professor, Department of Surgery, Division of Plastic and Reconstructive Surgery, University of California, San Francisco, California

James W. May, Jr., M.D.
Associate Clinical Professor, Department of Surgery, Harvard Medical School, Cambridge, Massachusetts; Chief, Division of Plastic Surgery, Department of General Surgery, Massachusetts General Hospital, Boston, Massachusetts

Joseph G. McCarthy, M.D.
Lawrence D. Bell Professor of Plastic Surgery; Director, Institute of Reconstructive Plastic Surgery, New York University Medical Center; Attending Plastic Surgeon, University Hospital; Attending Surgeon, Manhatten Eye, Ear, and Throat Hospital; Visiting Plastic Surgeon, Bellevue Hospital; Associate Attending Surgeon, Veterans Administration Hospital, Department of Surgery (Plastic Surgery), New York, New York

D. Ralph Millard, Jr., M.D., F.A.C.S.
Light-Millard Professor of Plastic Surgery and Chief, Division of Plastic Surgery, University of Miami School of Medicine, Miami, Florida

Stephen H. Miller, M.D.
Professor of Surgery, Chief of Plastic and Reconstructive Surgery, University of Oregon Health Sciences Center, Portland, Oregon

Joseph A. Moylan, M.D.
Professor, Department of Surgery, Duke University Medical Center, Durham, North Carolina

John B. Mulliken, M.D.
Associate Professor of Surgery, Harvard Medical School; Associate in Surgery, Division of Plastic and Maxillofacial Surgery, Children's Hospital Medical Center and Brigham and Women's Hospital, Boston, Massachusetts

Foad Nahai, M.D.
Assistant Professor, Department of Surgery, Division of Plastic and Reconstructive Surgery; Director of Microvascular Surgery, Emory University School of Medicine, Atlanta, Georgia

Karen R. Nailling, M.S.
Clinical Speech Pathologist, Speech and Hearing Disorders, Department of Surgery, Duke University Medical Center, Durham, North Carolina

James A. Nunley II, M.D.
Assistant Professor, Division of Orthopaedic Surgery, Duke University Medical Center, Durham, North Carolina

W. Jerry Oakes, M.D.
Assistant Professor, Division of Neurosurgery, Department of Surgery; Associate Professor, Department of Pediatrics, Duke University Medical Center, Durham, North Carolina

Dennis R. Osborne, M.D., F.R.C.R., F.R.A.C.P.
Associate Professor of Radiology, Department of Radiology, Duke University Medical Center, Durham, North Carolina

Erle E. Peacock, Jr., M.D.
Formerly Professor and Chairman, Department of Surgery, University of Arizona School of Medicine, Tucson, Arizona; Courtesy Staff, Department of Surgery, North Carolina Memorial Hospital, Chapel Hill, North Carolina

Samuel W. Parry, M.D.
Assistant Professor, Department of Surgery, Plastic Surgery Division, University of Texas Medical Branch, Galveston, Texas

Peter Randall, M.D., F.A.C.S.
Professor of Plastic Surgery and Chairman, Division of Plastic Surgery, University of Pennsylvania; Chief of Plastic Surgery, Hospital of the University of Pennsylvania; Senior Surgeon, Children's Hospital of Philadelphia, Philadelphia, Pennsylvania

Scott L. Replogle, M.D.
Clinical Instructor, University of Colorado; Attending Surgeon, Rose Medical Center; Attending, Denver General Hospital, Denver, Colorado

Ronald Riefkohl, M.D., F.A.C.S.
Assistant Professor, Department of Plastic Surgery, Division of Plastic, Maxillofacial, and Reconstructive Surgery, Duke University Medical Center, Durham, North Carolina

John E. Riski, Ph.D.
Assistant Professor, Department of Plastic Surgery, Division of Plastic, Maxillofacial, and Reconstructive Surgery, Duke University Medical Center, Durham, North Carolina

David C. Sabiston, Jr., M.D.
James B. Duke Professor of Surgery and Chairman, Department of Surgery, Duke University Medical Center, Durham, North Carolina

Donald Serafin, M.D., F.A.C.S.
Professor, Division of Plastic, Maxillofacial, and Reconstructive Surgery, Duke University Medical Center, Durham, North Carolina

Paul J. Smith, F.R.C.S.
Consultant Plastic and Hand Surgeon, Department of Plastic Surgery, Mount Vernon Hospital, London, England

Melvin Spira, M.D., D.D.S.
Professor and Head, Division of Plastic Surgery, Cora and Webb Mading Department of Surgery, Baylor College of Medicine; Chief of Plastic Surgery, Texas Children's Hospital and Methodist Hospital, Houston, Texas

Richard S. Stahl, M.D.
Assistant Professor, Section of Plastic and Reconstructive Surgery, Department of Surgery, Yale University School of Medicine, New Haven; Attending Physician, Department of Plastic and Reconstructive Surgery, Yale–New Haven Hospital and West Haven Veterans Administration Medical Center, West Haven, Connecticut

Samuel Stal, M.D.
Assistant Professor, Department of Plastic Surgery, Baylor College of Medicine; Chief of Plastic Surgery, The Institute of Research and Rehabilitation, Houston, Texas

Kathleen K. Sulik, Ph.D.
Assistant Professor of Anatomy and Ophthalmology, University of North Carolina School of Medicine, Chapel Hill, North Carolina

Julia K. Terzis, M.D., Ph.D., F.R.C.S.(C)
Associate Professor, Department of Plastic Surgery, Eastern Virginia Medical School; Associate Surgeon, Department of Plastic Surgery and Microsurgery, Norfolk General Hospital and DePaul Hospital, Norfolk, Virginia

Vernon T. Tolo, M.D.
Associate Professor, Department of Orthopaedic Surgery, The Johns Hopkins University School of Medicine; Director, Department of Pediatric Orthopaedics, The Johns Hopkins Hospital, Baltimore, Maryland

Chris P. Tountas, M.D.
Metropolitan Hand Surgery Associates, P.A.; Clinical Assistant Professor, Department of Family Practice, University of Minnesota, St. Paul, Minnesota

William C. Trier, M.D.
Professor of Surgery, University of North Carolina School of Medicine; Professor of Dentistry, University of North Carolina School of Dentistry; Attending Surgeon, Department of Surgery, North Carolina Memorial Hospital, Chapel Hill, North Carolina

James R. Urbaniak, M.D.
Professor, Division of Orthopaedic Surgery, Department of Surgery, Duke University Medical Center, Durham, North Carolina

Luis O. Vasconez, M.D.
Professor of Surgery, Chief of Plastic and Reconstructive Surgery, Department of Surgery, Division of Plastic Surgery, University of California, San Francisco, California

John L. Weinerth, B.S., M.D.
Associate Professor, Division of Urology, Department of Surgery, Duke University Medical Center, Durham, North Carolina

Robert H. Wilkins, M.D.
Professor and Chief, Division of Neurosurgery, Department of Surgery, Duke University Medical Center, Durham, North Carolina

Thomas W. Wolff, M.D.
Clinical Associate Professor of Orthopaedics, University of Louisville School of Medicine, Louisville, Kentucky

Barry M. Zide, D.M.D., M.D.
Assistant Professor of Plastic Surgery, New York University Medical Center; Assistant Professor of Plastic Surgery, Bellevue Hospital Center, New York, New York

Arnoldo V. Zumiotti, M.D.
Assistant, Department of Orthopedics, University of São Paulo Medical School, São Paulo, Brazil

To our wives

Patricia Serafin
and
Ruth Georgiade

FOREWORD

Pediatric Plastic Surgery, by Drs. Serafin and Georgiade, will undoubtedly become the landmark text in the field. The editors have prepared a text that encompasses the entire subject of pediatric plastic surgery and have sought the most authoritative contributors available to prepare each section. It is an all-inclusive undertaking, with 70 chapters and 65 primary authors. The thoroughness with which the editors have prepared this book is emphasized in the initial sections on special diagnostic considerations in infants and children, including radiographic imaging. The unique fluid and electrolyte requirements in this age group are described in detail, as are the unique problems relative to pediatric anesthesia. Special emphasis is placed on disorders of hemostasis in children and their appropriate management. Of growing significance are the psychologic aspects of various surgical disorders, and these are commendably covered in one chapter.

This is an invaluable reference. The editors have not only included classic topics in the field of plastic and maxillofacial reconstructive surgery, but have also wisely included problems in the fields of general and thoracic pediatric surgery, neurosurgery, orthopedics, otolaryngology, gynecology, and urology.

The breadth and scope of coverage in this new text are further underscored by attentive detail in the embryologic, epidemiologic, and genetic considerations in the pediatric age group. The many recent advances are presented, including the pioneering and now established composite tissue transplantation by microsurgical techniques. Drs. Serafin and Georgiade have made many basic contributions to the development of tissue transplantation in the microsurgical research laboratory in the Division of Plastic, Maxillofacial, and Reconstructive Surgery at Duke University. Moreover, this laboratory has been a resource for many others who have worked there and have applied the techniques of modern microvascular surgery. The Duke University Medical Center is fortunate to have such a strong program in this field under the direction of Dr. Nicholas G. Georgiade, representing as it does an extremely large and varied clinical service with an outstanding residency training program and research effort. These features are emphasized in the chapters prepared by the members of the current faculty, as well as former Duke University residents now in academic positions elsewhere.

Finally the editors are to be highly commended for seeking the most outstanding authorities in the field to prepare the appropriate chapters. It can be confidently predicted that this text will become the gold standard in the field, and it will be a must for all those engaged in pediatric plastic surgery.

David C. Sabiston, Jr.

PREFACE

YESTERDAY AND TODAY

The impetus for preparation of this text, begun several years ago, was provided by new developments during the past decade in plastic, reconstructive, and maxillofacial surgery that had specific applicability to children. Ralph Millard and Peter Randall's contributions to the surgical management of cleft lip and palate deformities and Miguel Orticochea's pharyngoplasty to correct velopharyngeal incompetence, to name only a few, stimulated renewed interest in the treatment of these complex problems. The improvement of surgical technique alone was only a small part of the total contribution. Cleft palate teams were organized with contributions from speech therapists, clinical psychologists, and orthodontists. Paul Tessier, the pioneer and founder of craniofacial surgery, excited the medical world with his revolutionary in-depth assessment and surgical management of these complex anomalies. Craniofacial centers developed throughout the world, and teams of individuals responsible for total patient care developed, structured in a similar manner to cleft palate teams.

Also during the last decade, techniques in microsurgery and the musculocutaneous flap concept revolutionized the reconstruction of extensive defects. Musculocutaneous flap closure in infants with spinal dysraphism and abdominal wall abnormalities became possible. The replantation of amputated digits and parts of infants and children was also accomplished with predicted viability. Microsurgical techniques were employed to treat peripheral nerve injuries and brachial plexus injuries related to birth accidents or trauma. Microsurgical composite tissue transplantation also became an acceptable treatment modality. Portions of digits and hands, amputated in utero or the result of adverse environmental conditions affecting the developing embryo, could now be successfully reconstructed using vascularized autogenic donor tissue. Thus a toe became a thumb, a fibula replaced a congenitally absent radius, and an intraabdominal testicle was transplanted to the scrotum and revascularized.

Directors of plastic surgery training programs throughout the world became concerned and also quite anxious by the rapidly increasing amount of information and new techniques that had to be translated to the resident experience. Operating on children at a younger age made a precise understanding of nutrition and fluid and electrolyte balance imperative. The importance of a strong surgical background before entering a plastic surgery residency was again emphasized. Postresidency fellowships that refined specific skills were created to augment training deficiencies. Thus as the burgeoning wealth of experience and information became available, it was evident that a compilation of this information would be useful. It was also apparent that such an accumulation of information transcended any single specialty interest.

Although this text has specific applicability to the experienced plastic surgeon operating on pediatric patients, it has applicability to other specialties as well. Because of the variety of problems that occur in this age group and, at times, the infrequency of occurrence, experiences from other specialties were often consolidated. Thus the neurosurgeon, gynecologist, urologist, and plastic surgeon may work together on a specific problem, each member of the team contributing specific expertise. The text has been prepared so that it deliberately crosses the previous guidelines defining the limits of any given surgical specialty. Any individual or member of a team contributing specific expertise to the treatment of any given problem must understand, as well, the contributions of other members of the team. Interest, knowledge, and experience dictate the relative contribution of each team member.

The text is divided into six major sections. *Section I*, Homeostasis, Disequilibrium, and Stress, consists of information essential to the surgical management of the pediatric age group. Emphasis is placed on factors affecting coagulation, fluid and electrolyte balance, and the assessment and management of the acutely ill and injured child.

Section II, Head and Neck, consists of chapters written by a variety of specialists whose different backgrounds and training exemplify the concept of the team approach in the treatment of the total patient. Thus speech therapists, orthodontists, clinical psychologists, plastic surgeons, and neurosurgeons combine their various disciplines in the treatment of these extensive congenital defects. An in-depth discussion is not possible without important contributions from the basic sciences. This is no better exemplified than in the chapters dealing with embryology of the head and neck and growth alterations of the craniofacial skeleton.

Section III is primarily devoted to problems in the pediatric age group involving the trunk. Again, the various contributions from neurosurgery, pediatric surgery, thoracic surgery, and plastic surgery are combined in a comprehensive treatment approach.

Section IV, Genitalia, describes the diagnosis and treatment of ambiguous genitalia with contributions from gynecologists, urologists, and plastic surgeons. This combined approach underlines the concept that the surgical exercise alone is merely that, an exercise, without an in-depth understanding of the genetic basis and pathophysiologic process of the various abnormalities. Management of hypospadias and epispadias without a thorough familiarity with problems related to the upper urinary tract is no longer consistent with good medical care. The efforts of urologists and plastic surgeons working together ensure an optimal result.

Section V, Upper Extremity, also represents the contributions of specialists both in orthopedics and plastic surgery. The management, evaluation, and surgical treatment of a child with congenital limb anomalies or extensive injuries of the upper extremity are detailed.

Section VI is devoted to problems of the lower extremity. Congenital problems, as well as those related to extensive trauma, are detailed and the surgical management is outlined.

During the present decade, the geometric increase of scientific information and escalating frequency of medical litigation have necessitated a multidisciplinary approach in total patient care. Consequently, any book whose objective is to provide the most complete compilation of material available on any given subject must, by necessity, contain multispecialty and multinational contributions. This text represents the combined efforts of more than 100 authors residing in six countries. In preparing the text, the editors' tasks were to define special problems of interest to pediatric plastic surgeons and to select those authors who would best provide their singular experience and expertise. A successful, integrated text therefore depends on the proper selection of subject matter and authors and the manner in which divergent subjects are blended in the construction of the whole. Thus isolated notes and bars are assimilated to form a musical score. Then talented musicians with their diverse musical instruments are selected, coordinated, and integrated. The editors, merely enthusiastic conductors, await the audience's reaction as the orchestra performs the completed symphony.

TOMORROW

Pediatric Plastic Surgery is the first comprehensive textbook published that coordinates the experiences of different specialties toward the surgical solution of both common and complex problems seen in infants and children. Total patient care managed by the team approach is emphasized throughout the text.

Both the strengths and weaknesses of plastic surgery as a specialty reside in the treatment of multiple problems involving different age groups and sexes. It requires a wide perspective, a broad training base, and the constant reassessment of the ever-changing medical horizon. A pediatric plastic surgeon must also have that broad base of specialization, but yet specific refinements in skills that make his or her contribution to the total care of the pediatric patient distinctive and unique. Preservation of plastic surgery as a specialty or pediatric plastic surgery as a discipline of that specialty will be possible in the future only if well-qualified individuals with a broad training base and specific expertise continue to make the vast number of contributions so well demonstrated during the past decade. Excellence in treatment and leadership is not a static process but a continuum. The weaknesses of a broad specialty become apparent only if the contribution is casual or superficial. Progress ceases when creativity is stifled, and the in-depth assessment of challenging problems is avoided.

The accomplishments of the past decade are now history. Future accomplishments will use this past experience, accommodating emerging technology and new discoveries. Surgical techniques for treatment of the cleft lip and palate deformity are now standardized. No doubt further refinements in technique will be forthcoming, particularly with regard to treatment of the cleft lip nasal deformity. Future investigations will also be directed toward the orthodontic and surgical treatment of maxillary hypoplasia and related alterations in growth of adjacent soft tissue. Previous experiments have demonstrated that an alteration of mesodermal migration contributes to cleft formation. It is anticipated that further research will be directed toward the prevention of cleft formation in utero and on the identification of those factors which result in its formation. Concurrently, the genetic basis and environmental influences that adversely influence normal development will be better defined. In the not too far distant future, complex genetic codes on chromosomes will be isolated and altered, perhaps removing the stimulus for cleft formation. The complex combinations and permutations of genetic coding will be simplified with computer technology. Treatment will be directed at a cellular or biochemical level. Similarly, the growth alterations of craniofacial abnormalities will be better understood. Premature suture closure will be prevented, and cells of the cranial base will be stimulated to prevent developmental hypoplasia of adjacent bony structures. Recent investigations in the etiology of hemifacial microsomia, outlined in this text, reflect the current interest and future direction of investigation toward the prevention of this and related anomalies.

It is well demonstrated both clinically and experimentally that axon regeneration proceeds more rapidly in children than in adults. Factors contributing to this accelerated growth, however, are poorly understood. Growth factors and the effects of changing electrical potential on precursor cells have been postulated. The cerebral cortex, an uncharted topographic map of hills and valleys still undisturbed by outside environmental influence, is fertile territory in children awaiting incoming messages. Sensory reeducation after peripheral nerve injury and repair is facilitated in the child. In the future, differences in nerve regeneration between children and adults will be better understood. This information will be used to regulate and accelerate axon regeneration after peripheral nerve and brachial plexus injuries. The advent of neuromicrosurgery in the past decade has expanded treatment modalities and understanding of these problems. One could anticipate that in the future infinite magnification will be employed at a cellular or biochemical level.

The immature organism, in contrast to a mature adult, has an enhanced capacity for cell dedifferentiation and regeneration. This is well demonstrated in lower phyla. In immature amphibians, amputation of a segment or part will result in the restoration of that missing part by regeneration. One can anticipate that in the future, amputated parts or segments of tissue in children will be replaced by autogenous tissue whose growth and development will be controlled by individuals skilled in genetics and cellular biology.

In the not too distant future immunosuppression will be replaced by specific immunoregulation. The recent discovery of cyclosporin A and its effect on helper T cells and suppressor cells has provided considerable information toward the controlled manipulation of the immune system. Allogeneic renal and liver transplantation in children is currently an accepted treatment modality. One can anticipate that in the future other allogeneic sources of tissue will be used to replace diseased or congenitally deficient autogenous tissues. Allogeneic islet cell transplantation is also possible in the near future.

The plastic surgeon will become more of a basic scientist in the next two decades. Treatment will be directed at a cellular level. Specialized training in areas other than surgical skills will be emphasized in postgraduate studies.

In the distant future, with the advent of new technology and an increased interest in the biochemical and cellular bases for disease, the pediatric plastic surgeon of today will be extinct. Treatment modalities will be directed at a cellular or biochemical level by individuals skilled in immunology, genetics, biochemistry, and cellular physiology. The skilled surgical technician will be replaced by the scientist. Treatment modalities will be infinitely more specific, refined, and sophisticated. Lasers will replace scalpels. Genetic information will be rearranged, and immature stem cells will be guided electronically toward organ and part replacement.

Donald Serafin
Nicholas G. Georgiade

ACKNOWLEDGMENTS

As work on a major text is completed, editors often reflect on the countless hours and numbers of people that have made completion of such a task possible. Certainly an inclusive multiauthored text is successful only if its content and direction fulfill the basic goals and criteria responsible for its preparation. Writing a chapter for a textbook is an arduous task and is frequently an act of love and dedication. Textbook chapters, although they enhance an individual's bibliography, are frequently not considered in the same category as original articles in refereed journals. Yet such a chapter may be more inclusive and actually represent an individual's total professional experience, unequaled by any other contributor. We wish to sincerely thank all the contributing authors who have given their time and shared their knowledge to make completion of such a task possible. Approximately half of the contributing authors are members of the full-time and part-time attending staff at Duke University Medical Center. Many are members of the Department of Surgery. We wish to thank these colleagues and the Chairman of the Department, David C. Sabiston, Jr., for continued support and encouragement. Significant contributions also came locally from the faculty of Medicine and Dentistry of the University of North Carolina at Chapel Hill. Heartfelt thanks are also offered to more distant colleagues both nationally and internationally who responded when their specific expertise and contributions were requested.

The task of day-to-day editing is often a difficult one, requiring intelligence, perserverance, and organization. Manuscripts must be reviewed, permissions obtained, and countless letters typed and distributed. A great deal of appreciation is extended to Ms. Patricia M. Dettmer, Editorial Assistant, for her conscientious effort and many hours spent in organization and editing.

A medical text is useful only if the illustrations and photographs clearly depict the author's intent. We are also grateful to Mr. Michael Leonard, Medical Illustrator. The cover of the text, depicting the staged treatment of a child with a bilateral cleft lip deformity, represents just one of Mr. Leonard's fine efforts. The editors also wish to express their thanks to Mr. Lewis Parrish and Mr. Charles Lewis and members of the Medical Photography Department.

Our appreciation is also extended to Mr. Scott Johnson for his diligent library research, punctuated with capital letters, semicolons, periods, and foreign abbreviations.

The publisher, The C.V. Mosby Company, and its entire editorial staff are commended for their continued support, indulgence, and encouragement.

Finally, a great deal of thanks are extended to Ms. Jacquelyn Brooks, Mrs. Mary Ewing, and Mrs. Cheryl Rogers for their help in typing and retyping the manuscripts.

Donald Serafin
Nicholas G. Georgiade

CONTENTS

HOMEOSTASIS, DISEQUILIBRIUM, AND STRESS

CHAPTER 1

Who shall live?

THOMAS J. KRIZEK

The very concept that plastic surgery might be applied to infants and children is a modern one. The long struggle of humans to bridge the gap between the animal and the rational—the instinctive and the intellectual—and to finally develop a concept of the moral and the spiritual has been studied and recorded from many aspects. Nowhere is this struggle better exemplified than in the evolution of attitudes toward offspring, particularly deformed or disabled offspring.

No deformity of infancy more typifies our interests, the evolution of our attitudes and skills, and sums up who we are, than clefts of the lip. The deformity has been with us since antiquity; mummies from thousands of years before Christ have been found with clefts. The deformity has been identified worldwide. It is not a lethal deformity and it is not one easily overlooked. What then did the early surgeons say about this obvious, disfiguring, but not totally disabling, deformity? Nothing. From the Temple of Asklepios to the lighthouse of Alexandria, the golden ages of medicine came and went with no mention of the deformity. From Hippocrates, silence; from Celsus not a word. In the second century AD, Galen referred to ''colobomata,'' which were clefts, but suggested no treatment. In about 390 AD, not exactly yesterday, but not so ancient either, clefts were being repaired in China (Tsin Dynasty). In about 950 AD, the Leech-Book of Bald described a method of cutting to freshen the edges, sew them fast with silk, and smear the deformity within and without with salve. Albucasis in 1000 AD improved clefts using cautery and Yperman in the fourteenth century used needle and thread. From then on each of our plastic surgery giants made a contribution. Paré illustrated, Tagliacozzi used interrupted sutures, and Hieronymus Fabricius used mucosa and adhesive bandages. These refinements increased the vertical length of the repaired cleft lip, used adjacent tissue to augment the deficiency, and attempted to break up the straight line. It has culminated in

Millard's resolution of the problem using a rotation-advancement cleft lip repair. It is hard even to imagine what the next step forward will be until wounds can be made to heal without scarring, and cartilage, muscle, dermis, and mucosa can be made to develop without retardation whenever they are accurately placed in infancy. Freshening two edges and fixing them together does not seem so difficult a concept; why was it so long in developing?

Like all unwanted offspring, since the beginning of time, children with cleft lips and other deformities were either abandoned or destroyed. Among many mammals there are examples of not only steadfast parental care but durable marriages as well, notably in whales, seals, hippopotami, and apes. In many species, however, the parents, particularly the father, not only disregard the deformed young, but represent a real danger to their continued existence. Humans are prominent among these.

Within the last two centuries, cultures have been identified with stages of development corresponding to the Neolithic period of the Stone Age. Tribes in this period had no knowledge of metals or fire; and their only tools derived from bone or stone. Cannibalism and infanticide were common; the method of infanticide was burial alive.[6] Included in their beliefs was life after death. An infant was killed whenever an adult died to provide company for the trip into the afterlife. In the more advanced of these cultures, more elaborate reasons for disposing of burdensome offspring had been developed. In Central Australia twins were killed immediately as something unnatural; in others, only the weaker of the twins was killed. In some territories both the twins and the mother were killed, although provisions were sometimes made to buy off the life of the mother by sacrificing a slave.[11] In one village the wife of a priest gave birth to twins. When a year later the mother again gave birth to twins, she paid for her fecundity with her life at the hand of her own husband.

The driving force behind primitive infanticide was, of course, fear of starvation. It was only natural that any infant with blemishes or who was in any way malformed was destroyed. Among the tribes of Africa children who did not enter the world in an orthodox fashion were thrown into the brush to die. These included all breech babies, those born with teeth, those born in stormy weather, and those who were born on unlucky days. Unlucky days were the months of April and March, the last week of each month, and Wednesdays and Fridays. Among the Basuto tribe all children who were born feet first were strangled, but all children of the Bondei tribe who were born head first were strangled.[9]

In most of the tribes there was some provision to make sure of limiting the size of families. On Radack Island in the Pacific a woman was allowed three children. She was expected to bury alive every succeeding child. Commonly, any child that appeared weak or sickly was destroyed. Among some of the Australian tribes, the mother killed and ate has firstborn to strengthen her for future pregnancies. Sometimes a young healthy child was killed and fed to an older but sickly child in the hope that some of the strength of the younger would be transferred. Among nomadic tribes of South America, families were limited to two children because it was difficult to handle more than two children, one to be carried by each parent. In times of starvation, all children were eaten to keep up the strength of the parent. Nature's methods are stern and progress was slow. When we see the customs of these peoples, which have remained stationary during the millenia of human progress, perhaps we have a true glimpse into the lives of earliest humans. Time passed these peoples by, just as surely as it brought progress to other humans and the great civilizations developed. A brief but revealing stop made at each of these civilizations and a glance taken at their family life perhaps reflects why surgery for cleft lip and other deformities was slow to develop.

From the writings of Confucius in 484 BC, much can be learned of the Chinese culture. It is apparent that Confucius shared the opinion of most of the Chinese that the father was the sovereign of the house and the child was the subject. At that time infanticide was not practiced, and it was not until the great famine of 232 BC that the practice of abandoning children developed. The famine eventually passed, but abandonment of children continued until the reign of Chen Teche when an attempt was made to stop it. An edict was sent forth in 1659 AD forbidding parents from drowning their daughters. Some provinces continued the practice, however, and it is recorded that midwives could not become Christians because part of their job was drowning the infant if the parents did not have the courage. As late as 1875 the practice flourished, although the children were allowed to die rather than be killed. Outside the walls of Peking there was a "baby house" into which the children were placed when dead to be eaten by dogs. That Wei Yang-Chi, the

Chinese farmer's son, born with a cleft lip in the Tsin Dynasty (fourth century AD) should have been recorded is a surprise.

Millard[8] reviewed cleft lip repair during the Ching Dynasty, and in the Tang Dynasty (600 to 900 AD) found "doctors of lips." Wei and his "lip doctors" were the exception, not the rule. It was not a golden age for development. In Japan, influenced by the Shinto religion, the practice of human sacrifice was less common. According to one source, such sacrifice was abandoned in the year 3 AD. However, during a great famine in 1783, the practice of cannibalism became rampant. There is the interesting story of a father who, having lost his wife and two daughters by starvation, went to his neighbor and requested that the neighbor kill his only son, who was also going to die within a few days, so that he might have his son while there was eatable flesh on his bones. The neighbor obliged, whereupon the father immediately took the opportunity of killing the neighbor to avenge his son's death, thereby doubling his available food supply.[10] As late as 1905, after the Russo-Japanese war, the people were unable to bear the weight of heavy taxes and resorted to female infanticide to lighten the financial burden.

The most commonly considered site of the earliest civilization was the Tigris-Euphrates valley, or Mesopotamia. Although only fragmentary evidence is available, it appears that sacrifice of the first born was practiced, but abandoned rather early. In the earliest known code of laws, the code of Hammurabi (King of Babylon in about the eighteenth century BC), provision is made for the adoption of abandoned children. Although little more than a slave under the code, at least some consideration is made for preservation of the child's life. The Babylonians are truly remarkable in that no example of human sacrifice is recorded. The same is true of the Egyptians, whose culture can be traced back to about 11,500 BC. Their attitude toward children had already been settled, seemingly in favor of the child. Except for certain sacrificial offerings and occasionally burying a child or two alive along with a dead nobleman, the child was cared for quite well. The Egyptians of this time were quite stable economically; food was not a problem, and the climate was such that the children were never clothed. The financial burden of raising a child was less significant. Despite the favorable circumstances and documentation of cleft lip deformity at the time, no specific recognition of it, either pro or con, is available.

Moving across the Mediterranean into Central Europe, however, conditions were quite different. Among the Aryan primitives, who are commonly considered to be the ancestors of the Celts, Teutons, Hellenes, Goths, and Italians, there was a constant struggle against nature and also the problem of intertribal warfare. Under such unfavorable circumstances it is not surprising that human sacrifice and infanticide were common. There is good evidence that cannibalism was common in Britain. The practice of breaking a champagne bottle over the bow of a new ship can be traced back to the Vikings who tied a child to the prow of their war galley so that the keel would be sprinkled with sacrificial blood.

Farther to the east, in India, a much more practical approach was followed. All newly born children were publically examined for defects or weaknesses of constitution, and a vote was taken as to whether the child met the standards of beauty and strength set down in their laws. If they failed, they were destroyed immediately. In 1789 the British governmment was still trying to do away with the Hindu practice, supposedly of divine origin, of putting female children to death. Some of their methods of infanticide are particularly interesting. One of the favorites about 1800 was that of the mother coating the nipple of her breast with opium so that the child would be quietly disposed of when sucking the milk. Another cruder method was that of putting the umbilical cord down the female child's throat until it smothered. To show the Hindu sense of values, it was considered that to kill 100 cows was equal to killing 1 Brahmin; to kill 100 Brahmins was equal to killing 1 woman; to kill 100 women was equal to killing 1 child; and to kill 100 children was equal to telling one lie.[7] Among one group in India it was common to bury an infant up to the shoulders in the ground in the middle of a road. Then as the men rode their carts out of the village, they would crush the child as an omen that this would be a successful business trip. Finally in 1891 infanticide in India came to an end by order of the British government.

In Peru the Indians would either drown unwanted children, or, for a sacrifice, they would decapitate the child and anoint themselves and the temple with the blood. It was customary to sacrifice the firstborn to the chief of the tribe. With much ceremony and dancing, the ritual was carried out, reaching a climax when the mother would dash the head of the infant on a tree stump. Barren women in these tribes often made a vow to the gods that they would sacrifice their firstborn. If a son were born, he would be allowed to live until puberty. With great ceremony the child would be taken to the top of a cliff and then, at his mother's order, would throw himself off to be killed on the rocks below. The Central and South American Indians indeed represent a cultural anomaly. Despite infanticide and ritual sacrifice, the child with a cleft lip was almost uniquely spared. A sculpture from the year 12 AD shows an Indian chief with a cleft lip. Pottery and artwork from Peruvian and other cultures of almost 200 years ago similarly confirm the presence of the anomaly and its distinct recognition apparently in adults. Clearly infanticide for this cause was not uniform.

Among the Semitic tribes, Judaism, Christianity, and Islamism, sacrifice of the firstborn was common. In Palestine it was common practice to bury living infants in the cornerstones of new buildings. Evidence for similar practice has been found among the people of India, New Zealand, China, Mexico, and Germany. In 1843 in Germany a child was buried in the foundation of a bridge. In 1867 in Alaska a chief was building a new house and had four infants placed in the corners. Young saplings were placed across the infants' necks and at the chief's signal, relatives of the infants jumped on the ends of the saplings, thus choking the children.[10]

In Arabia the sacrifice of life consisted of slaughtering the child and boiling it till the flesh came off the bones. The flesh was then kneaded with flour, oil, and spices and made into small cakes that were baked and eaten. Women, slaves, and idiots were not allowed to eat the cakes. Another Arabian practice was to deliver the mother at the edge of a deep pit in the ground so that if she delivered a female it could be disposed of without further ado.[10]

The Greeks, with all their humanity, art, and morality, extended none of these feelings either to the enemy, slaves, or children. In Athens infanticide was particularly common, and the father had complete rights over the life of his children. The Greek method of disposal was quite humane and consisted of abandonment, often in a place where the child might be found and cared for. To this end they often included gifts along with the infant as an added incentive to the finder of the child to raise it. The chief reason for disposing of children was the expense, since the Greeks required that all boys be educated to age 16 and girls be provided with a large dowry. If a Greek were to be asked why he disposed of a child, he would tell you that it was because he loved the child he had.

In Rome, Romulus pledged his people to raise all male children with a view toward building a powerful nation. However, the father had complete right over life and death, except for the lame or malformed, who were killed immediately. The father was the judge as to who was to live. It was not until the time of Augustus, in 31 BC, that any efforts were made to spare children who were abandoned. At this time, rewards were offered for raising an orphan. However, the practice continued and special sites were established in which the child could be conveniently disposed.

Religion has had a profound but slow effect on these cultural dispositions. It was centuries after Christianity arrived before the Irish were weened from cannibalism, the Germans from drowning, and the especially prevalent practice of disposing of illicit children down sewers.[2] Although cannibalism and sacrifice were over in Europe by the end of the fifteenth century, it was years before institutions were established to actually care for children. It is only in the last 150 years or less that children have been emancipated from forced labor in factories to the present state. Looking back now, it is easy to see the rationale of these primitive peoples. Cannibalism was first born of necessity, infanticide of poverty. Later the sacrifice of humans developed, probably, from a belief that human food was most agreeable to the gods. In the cannibalistic stage of sacrifice the child was eaten to establish a connecting link between humans and the invisible gods they hoped to appease. These sacrifices were born of fear, and only when economic conditions were improved was sacrifice of a substitute object attempted. The child was supposedly freer from sin and therefore a more suitable sacrifice. It is interesting that when infanticide sprung from economic need, it was the female who suffered, but when it sprung from the spirit of sacrifice, then the male suffered.

This review of attitudes toward offspring would easily explain the slow development of surgery for children or specific identification of their problems. It does not emphasize an equally important dimension of the problem—in addition to being children, they were also deformed. They were "different." They were "oddities, abnormalities, anomalies, mutants, mistakes of nature, monsters, monstrosities . . . they were in a word, freaks."[3] Fiedler[3] has pointed out that the oldest word in our tongue for anomalies is *monster* and until rather recently the standard medical term was *monstrosity.* His treatise on the subject takes a most thoughtful, sympathetic and insightful look at the world of freaks. Efforts to rename them "very special people" or "prodigies" fall woefully short of the truth that there always have been people who are different, people whom we label freaks. They have been and are a source of some amusement and the "freak" concept derives from *lusus naturae,* a Latin term for "play of nature." Normal persons laugh in the presence of freaks—do we not need this to identify and confirm our own normalcy and acceptance? "How's the air up there?" to the giant fulfills our need to titter at and separate ourselves from those who are different. Freaks represent to us the ultimate threat of being different and for being shown up as such. The word monster is from *monstrum,* evil omen, or the French *monère,* to warn—the implications being the same, a frightening possibility that this work, this freak, is no mere accident but rather part of Divine Providence put here to "show us." Among the ancients, the signs were deciphered by experts in fetomancy (prophecy from fetuses) and teratoscopy (divination based on examination of abnormal births).

The oldest documents dealing with monsters date to 2800 BC in a Babylonian lexicon of monsterology.[3] There were three classes of monsters. (1) those with "too much," such as six toes on each foot, which always portended ill; (2) those with "too little," for example, a child without a penis and nose suggested that the "army of the king will be strong," whereas one without a penis and an umbilicus augured "ill will in the house"; (3) those with "double parts" or other duplications, for example, a "head upon a head" was a good omen. The Romans, interpreting the same signs and observing the same classes concluded that they *all* portended ill wind. All these cultures had priestly executioners who dispatched monstrous children at birth by exposure or ritual sacrifice.

Fiedler[3] pointed out that the true freak stirs in all of us both supernatural terror and natural sympathy, since unlike the monsters of antiquity, the freak of today is recognized as the human child of human parents. It could have been us! The true freak "challenges our conventional boundaries between male and female, large and small, animal and human, self and other and consequently between reality and illusion, experience and fantasy, fact and myth."[3] If there were no freaks, we probably would invent them, if only to confirm our normalcy. A small group locked in a room as the last survivors on earth would probably find it necessary to sort from the group the "different," and therefore the less worthy. Any distortion, congenital, traumatic, surgical, or medical, may turn any of us into that most terrifying of prospects, to be a freak. It is totally appropriate that this is the word used so frequently by women who have had mastectomies.

The line drawn between freak and normal is not all that clear. Nor does it have a necessary "humanity" that would allow the differences to transcend time, distance, and cultural variation. There are no true absolutes for defining freakishness. The changes from normality to abnormality may be subtle and appear insidiously, but also dramatically, and all within a generation or two. Which are more normal, large or small breasts, long or short hair, noses with or without bumps? That most insightful social philosopher, Dr. Seuss, recorded these subtleties in his book about Sneetches.[5]

Sneetches, all of whom lived together on the beaches, were divided into two nonintermingling social groups, depending on whether or not the individual Sneetch had a small star on its belly. Since the star-studded group was egregiously self-important and the starless group deprived, they were natural candidates for Sylvester McMonkey McBean and his "star-on machine." When all Sneetches became star bellied, the need for difference appeared and many flocked to McBean's "star-off machine." "In again, on again, out again, off again" went the Sneetches into the star machines. The happy insightful recognition that all were equal and beautiful, with or without stars, was Dr. Seuss' resolution of the story. Would that the world so easily accept those of us who were born without a star on the belly or whose star was lost from injury or disease or merely faded with age. Is it not something so intangible as the figurative star on the belly that separates normal persons from the freaks among us and our offspring?

"Who shall live and who shall die, who shall fulfill his days and who shall die before his time . . ." are words from the Yom Kippur prayer book and formed the theme for Victor Fuchs' masterful analysis of societal choices in the economy of health and medical care.[4] He predicted a decade ago the problems and decisions facing those in health fields. His economics have a basic threefold thrust: (1) resources are scarce in relation to human wants, (2) all resources have alternative potential uses, and (3) there is tremendous variation among the wants of people and the relative importance attached to these wants. Although it is often said, that "health is the most important goal," he observed that this is really profound nonsense, since people regularly choose other activities which are more important than health, such as smoking, overeating, or driving fast. The basic problem is how to allocate scarce resources to best satisfy human wants. He states that romantics often fail to recognize the scarcity of resources relative to wants and that they tend to blame the need to make choices on other factors, like capitalism, communism, unions, war, unemployment, or some other scapegoat. When confronted by the obvious imbalance between wants and resources, it is alternately sufficient to then label some of the wants as ''unnecessary'' or ''inappropriate,'' thus protecting the illusion that no scarcity really exists. That operation for microtia may become ''unnecessary'' because it is ''esthetic'' and not ''functional.'' All cleft lip surgery in California, supported by state funds, must now be done on an outpatient basis because in 1983, hospitalization is ''no longer necessary.'' The state Crippled Children's Program ran out of money 6 months into the fiscal year and *all* cleft lip and palate surgery became ''inappropriate'' and ''unnecessary'' until further notice. Fuchs observed further that ''economics is the science of the means, not of ends.'' It can explain how market prices are determined but not how basic values are formed. Economics can tell us the consequences of various alternatives, but cannot make the choices for us.

Historical cycles are repeating themselves. Associated Press reports from China (February 1983) indicate that the murder of female babies is on the rise again. There is a fine of $2000 for an extra child, and female babies do not have good prospects. Girl babies are drowned, strangled, tossed down public toilets and left to die in the wilderness. Even now and closer to home, a court order has allowed a child with Down's syndrome to die while a presidential commission struggles with ''guidelines'' for managing deformed infants.

This book on pediatric plastic surgery is a tribute not only to the surgeons who write it but to all our predecessors in reconstructive surgery. They are, however, with a few notable exceptions persons of the last century—no more usually than two professional generations from us. Their contributions are almost more of a tribute to the kind of cultural times that the last century allowed us.

The history of the world has not been distinguished by kindness to its children, much less to its deformed children. It was not merely economics that led to infanticide and sacrifice, but profound concern for the providential hand in monstrosities; the freaks made and make us frightened and in awe. These past injustices are not necessarily forever abandoned, but are more likely to reappear in hard times in the future.

Difficult economic times are again demanding choices between wants and resources. When these choices have been made in the past, the care of the deformed has always been a less necessary cause than other societal wants. The decisions still seem obvious and the emotional concerns are less when the deformity is profound, the infant monstrous, and the outlook grim—repair becomes ''inappropriate.'' The decisions are less clear when the deformity is less and the disability is less likely to be profound. It is then that correction becomes, not inappropriate, but ''unnecessary.'' What will happen when the deformity becomes subtle, like being a female baby in China. The difference runs the historical risk of being no more than whether we have a small star on our belly.

REFERENCES
1. Brinton, D.G.: Religions of primitive peoples, New York, 1897, The Putnam Publishing Group.
2. Brinton, D.G.: Races and peoples: lectures on the science of ethnology, New York, 1890, The Putnam Publishing Group.
3. Fiedler, L.: Freaks: myths and image of the secret self, New York, 1978, Simon & Schuster.
4. Fuchs, V.R.: Who shall live? Health economics and social change, New York, 1974, Basic Books, Inc., Publishers.
5. Geisel, T. Seuss: Sneetches and other stories, New York, 1961, Random House, Inc.
6. Krizek, T.J.: Infanticide, Marquette Med. **22**(3):143, 1957.
7. Lyon, D.G., and More, G.F., editors: Studies in the history of religions, New York, 1912, Macmillan Publishing Co., Inc.
8. Millard, D.R., Jr.: Cleft craft—the evolution of its surgery, Boston, 1976, Little, Brown & Co.
9. Murray, J.H.P.: Papua, or British New Guinea, New York, 1912, Charles Scribner's Sons.
10. Payne, G.H.: The child in human progress, New York, 1916, The Putnam Publishing Group.
11. Spencer, B., and Gillen, F.J.: Native tribes of Central Australia, London, 1899, Macmillan Publishing Co., Inc.

CHAPTER 2

The physical therapist's role in rehabilitation of the pediatric patient

KIMBERLY S. GIBSON and ROBERT C. BARTLETT

The physical therapist must be prepared to deal with wound problems and attempt to minimize scarring whenever possible. Early after trauma or surgery the physical therapist is an active participant in the entire rehabilitation process, which consists of wound care, mobility of the injured part, function, cosmesis, and self-image. The child presents a special problem because injury interferes with the normal developmental and family processes. This chapter deals with concepts and methods for the management of pediatric patients.

SCAR FORMATION

We refer the reader to the literature for an in-depth discussion of wound healing.[22-24,34,36] To facilitate discussion, a brief summary of collagen deposition and maturation is provided.

Collagen fibers are responsible for the physical properties of a scar. During the early phases of wound healing, dead space in a wound is filled completely with cells and randomly oriented collagen fibers. At this time the scar is a single unit. All injured tissues of varying histologic types are bound together in the newly synthesized scar (one wound–one scar concept).[32] The scar remains metabolically active for years, slowly changing in size, shape, color, texture, and strength.[23,24]

To understand the changing physical properties of a scar, it is necessary to discuss the properties of the collagen fibril. Collagen is structurally insoluble and aggregates quickly, forming a random mat of fibrils. Initially, aggregated collagen molecules are held together by hydrogen bonds and other weak physical forces, allowing new fibrils to be easily ruptured under stress. Stronger covalent bonds form as the fibrils mature, causing a notable increase in fibril strength. A strong flexible fibril is produced that can be woven into a variety of tissue patterns. Therefore physical properties of the injured tissues are altered by collagen synthesis, aggregation, and cross bonding. Physical characteristics of the scar are thus determined by the quantity of collagen, anatomic configuration of the fibers, and density of covalent bonding.[23,24]

Collagen synthesis begins on the third day and increases rapidly during the first 3 weeks. Synthesis stabilizes at about the second to fourth week, remaining constant for long intervals.[16] Studies have shown that collagen remains metabolically active for prolonged periods despite a stable collagen content.[15,19] New collagen is deposited at a substantially higher rate in a scar at 4 months after wounding than in normal skin.[23] Total scar content consists of a balance between the degradation and removal of old collagen molecules and the synthesis and deposition of new molecules.[23,24]

Large amounts of glucosamine, found in mucopolysaccharides and most likely synthesized by the fibroblasts, are found in scar tissue.[21] It is believed that it assists in the organization of collagen molecules in normal and scarred tissues.

As mentioned previously, all wounds are dynamic and constantly undergo metabolic remodeling. Biologic events influencing scar remodeling include physical forces, surfaces against which the scar is deposited, age, the total quantity of the scar deposited, the presence of an old scar, and the condition of the tissues at the time of injury.[24] The effects of stress applied to a remodeling scar have been demonstrated experimentally; however, the influences of rate, frequency, duration, and direction of stress application are unknown.[3] It is also unknown how adjacent structures produce architectural changes on scar tissue. It has been hypothesized that an increase in the rate of metabolic turnover is responsible for the rapid and effective remodeling rate found in children.[24] The quantity of scar deposited is directly proportional to the amount of tissue injured. The ability to change the structure of a scar is lost with time, even though scars remain metabolically active for years.[23,24]

Open wounds, with or without tissue loss, exhibit the same morphologic and chemical processes as closed and sharply incised wounds.[22] Open wounds, however, are characterized by wound contraction and epithelialization. After 2 or 3 days wound margins begin to move actively toward each other, trying to stretch the surrounding skin to close the defect.[23,24] At 2 or 3 weeks the wound area is less than 20% of the original area. Collagen does not influence wound contraction because it is not composed of contractile proteins. Myofibroblasts, cells in granulation tissue, are believed to have contractile properties and appear to supply the force for wound contraction.[23,24,36] These forces of contraction act to close the wound until they are opposed by the resisting tension of the surrounding skin. A wound contracts until fixed tissues prevent further contraction.

The physical therapist must consider these principles of scar formation in developing a plan of care to minimize the potentially deforming consequences of scarring and maximize function of the injured part.[37] Guidelines and specific techniques for intervention will be discussed elsewhere in the chapter.

PATIENT EVALUATION

A thorough evaluation of the child is critical to the development of an appropriate physical therapy treatment program. The purpose of the evaluation is to (1) define problems and their characteristics in one or more areas of function and behavior and (2) establish a baseline of the child's performance from which a treatment program is to be developed and changes measured.

To obtain a total picture of the child's physical and behavioral status, an evaluation consisting of a history and a selective review of systems must be performed. The history contains pertinent information obtained from the patient's chart and the interview, at right. The review of systems consists of observations and tests carried out by the therapist that are designed to provide information needed to focus on the child's specific problems. Table 2-1 describes four systems considered essential to the physical therapist in understanding the child's problem. A graded scale of measurement and observation is provided for each system. It should be recognized that these criteria are not all inclusive and should be modified or expanded to meet any specific requirement. The initial screening process should

identify those systems which need more detailed investigation.

It is not the intent of the physical therapist to duplicate the physician's examination. Some tests, however, should be repeated to familiarize the therapist with specific problems and establish appropriate goals for treatment. In the evaluation period the therapist establishes an initial relationship with the child, observing and exploring a variety of behaviors and attitudes, such as the child's response to firmness and supportiveness and ability to select within limited choices. An ongoing process of reevaluating the child is required throughout physical therapy in order to readjust goals and the treatment regimen because of alterations in function and behavior. A final evaluation is performed on

---

PATIENT'S HISTORY

Individual
Name ______________________________
Sex ______________________________
Age ______________________________
Date of birth ______________________________

Family
Interview with family ______________________________
____
Interview with patient ______________________________
____
Interview with social worker ______________________________
____
Home visit ______________________________
____

Past medical history
Operative procedures ______________________________
____
Medications ______________________________
____
Injuries applicable to present problems ______________________________
____

Nature of injury
Date of injury ______________________________
Description of incident ______________________________
____
Environment of incident ______________________________
____
Operative procedures this hospitalization ______________________________

Table 2-1. Systems for evaluation

Review of systems	Measurements and observations
Neurologic system	
Mental status	Orientation to person, place, and time; appropriateness of language and type of communication; level of consciousness: pupillary reactions, ocular motion, ability to track
Cranial nerves	Standard neurologic testing
Tone and reflexes	"Decerebrate" or "decorticate" posture; quick stretch: clonus, hypertonia, hypotonia, ataxia, rigidity, alternating tone; primitive reflexes: asymmetric, tonic, labryinthine, Moro's
Sensation	Pinprick; vibration; light touch; Tinel's sign; ninhydrin test; Weber's test; stereognosis; graphesthesia; joint position sense; position of limb in space; pain: protective postures, splinting, patient's description of discomfort
Coordination	Placement tests: finger to nose, finger to finger, heel to toe walking, timed test, rapid alternating movements
Postural reflex mechanism	Equilibrium: protective reactions, ability to recover of maintain position
Development	Appropriate motor, psychological, and social functions; Denver Developmental Screening Test (0 to 6 years); oral-motor behavior; level of speech
Musculoskeletal system	
Soft tissue	Skin quality: color, hair; wounds: size, color, drainage, odor, necrotic tissue, epithelialization, granulation; scar: location, visual and palpable characteristics; nodules
Mobility	Joint congruity: hypermobility, hypomobility, capsular patterns; range of motion: active, passive; muscle-tendon glide: pull of scar with motion
Strength	Graded muscle testing, grip and pinch tests
Performance	Activities of daily living, gait, endurance
Cardiovascular system	Pulse; temperature; capillary refill, Allen test; edema: volumetric, circumferential, pitting color
Pulmonary system	Auscultation; respiration rate: use of accessory muscles, wheezing; chest expansion: symmetric, asymmetric; chest-girth measurement; cough: effective, productive, sputum measurement

discharge from the hospital or physical therapy. If the child is referred to another facility for follow-up treatment, results of this final evaluation will provide a baseline for the physical therapist and other health care personnel.

DETERMINING GOALS AND PRIORITIES

The ultimate purpose of any rehabilitation program is to restore as much normal function as possible with minimal deformity, to the individual. This can be achieved only through sharing information and cooperation of all members of the team responsible for the child's care. The following treatment goals are applicable to most young patients:

1. Wound care
2. Reduction of edema
3. Range of motion—contracture prevention
4. Maintaining or increasing strengths
5. Reduction of pain
6. Promotion of human maturation
7. Pulmonary hygiene
8. Remodeling of scar
9. Restoration of sensibility

The process of recovery and healing in the young child differs significantly from the adult with regard to time and quality of repair. Secondary disabilities of joint stiffness and contracture in children are not as great as in adults after prolonged periods of immobilization. The child establishes early mobility through the need to be active; problems do occur, however, in the child who experiences pain with movement and tends to hold the body in a position of comfort. In these situations it is imperative that early mobility be instituted through a supervised activity program, oftentimes play, by the therapist or family. General muscle strengthening and progression of normal developmental skills are given increased priority after the patient moves through the period of critical care.

RATIONALE

The treatment program should consist of a variety of age- and developmentally appropriate activities. Attention spans vary in children, and a mixture of play activities and specific exercises is crucial to maintain the child's interest. The treatment may need to be carried out in a structured environment using behavior modification and limit-setting techniques. When appropriate, the program should provide limited choices that are attainable and allow for a positive reward system. When at all possible, the family should be asked to actively participate in the child's treatment program.

When the problem is congenital or a result of trauma to the central nervous system, additional considerations must be given to long-term neurodevelopmental status. The neurodevelopmental prognosis will have direct implication on the ranking of goals in nonneurologic areas.

WOUND CARE

Meticulous wound care facilitates the closure of partial-thickness wounds by primary healing and prepares the full-thickness wounds for surgical coverage. The wound must be free of devitalized tissue before surgical closure can be attempted. Hydrotherapy, aggressive debridement, and dressing changes are used to accomplish this.

Wound cleansing with hydrotherapy is performed in an isotonic saline solution at a temperature between 34.5° and 38° C (94° and 100° F).[10] The saline solution prevents loss of electrolytes and protects the granulation tissue. A detergent additive provides a gentle cleansing action at the wound site. A variety of detergent additives is available, and one is chosen based on the patient's skin sensitivity and the topical agent to be used on the wound after cleansing. These include a povidone-iodine complex (Betadine), acetic acid, and chlorine bleach. Detergents with soap bases are avoided because of their cytotoxicity.

In addition to its soothing effects, agitated water serves as a mechanical debrider and promotes increasing circulation, which supports formation of granulation tissue. In recent years, use of a galvanic current during hydrotherapy to promote granulation has increased. Some machines now on the market safely permit placement of the electrode pads in the water. It is necessary to maintain a warm environment to prevent chilling of the patient. Strict adherence to sterile technique is most important.

Debridement of the wound is initiated with removal of the dressing. Wet-to-dry dressings are the most effective. Debridement continues with the agitation of the whirlpool. The water softens the devitalized tissue, making removal with gauze sponges easier and more comfortable to the patient, and also removes the old topical agent from the wound. The physical therapist may also sharply debride the wound with either a scalpel, forceps, or scissors. Debridement should be performed with care, avoiding injury to viable tissue. Preserving vital tissues prevents additional scarring.[23]

After hydrotherapy, appropriate dressings are applied using topical agents chosen by the surgeon. Silver sulfadiazine (Silvadene), silver nitrate, acetic acid, sodium chloride, Betadine, bismuth tribromophenate (Zeroform) gauze, and nitrofurazone (Furacin) gauze are but a few of the wound preparations available.

The surgeon usually decides which dressing will be most beneficial. The semiopen method of wound care is most often used after hydrotherapy, debridement, and the application of a dressing over a topical agent. If further debridement is desired, wet-to-dry dressings may be preferred. Strict sterile technique must be followed to prevent contamination. Dressings should be applied with care because newly formed tissues are easily injured. Dressings also should be applied to suit the needs of the patient. If motion is desired, the dressing should permit mobility. If a splint is to be applied over the dressing, bulk should be kept to a minimum to allow for a proper fit.

Simple explanations should be given before the procedure to decrease the patient's anxiety and promote cooperation. If at all possible, the child should be given a chance to assist in the procedure, such as removing dressings or helping to clean wounds and tearing tape for dressing changes. this will enhance cooperation, give the child some control, and decrease fear of pain.

REDUCTION OF EDEMA

An acute inflammatory response always occurs after trauma. An increase in capillary permeability occurs initially with a subsequent loss of fluid from the vascular compartment.[23,24] Edema is formed in the surrounding tissues, the amount being proportional to the extent of the tissue injury. A ballooning of the surrounding tissues results, creating vascular compromise and inhibiting the normal return of fluids through both lymphatic and venous channels. Ischemia also may result from vascular compression. The presence of this protein-rich fluid within the tissues potentiates fibrosis. The amount of fibrosis is directly proportional to the amount of edema fluid present and the period of time it persists.[17] All tissues, including vessels, nerves, joints, and muscles, become involved in a state of reduced nutrition and inelasticity.[17] Once the edema becomes chronic, a certain amount is reversible, but soft tissue fibrosis is not. This problem will be addressed in the discussion on remodeling of scars. The most pronounced edema will be seen in the distal portions of the extremities and around joints that are consistently gravity dependent. Prevention is the key to management. The sooner edema can be minimized, the less the potential for tissue scarring.

Young children show more rapid reduction in edema than older children. This might be explained by the more rapid repair rate of tissues in younger children and the greater pliability of joint structures.[29]

Therapy is directed toward enhancing the return of fluid through the venous and lymphatic systems. Muscle action through joint motion and compression of fascial compartments is required to enhance venous and lymphatic flow.[17] Active muscle contraction, combined with elevation of the edematous part, is the most effective mode of treatment. If active motion is contraindicated, such as immediately after surgical repair or before repair of ruptured structures, elevation can still be instituted. Active motion, however, should be initiated as soon as possible. With children this activity can be accomplished by choosing age-appropriate play activities or goal-oriented tasks.

Massage also assists venous and lymphatic return. Hunter and Mackin[17] describe techniques for distal-to-proximal string wrapping and use of surgical gloves and various elasticized gloves to mobilize edema of the hand. Distal-to-proximal elastic bandage wrapping is also helpful in reducing edema in both upper and lower extremities, especially during activities requiring dependent positioning.

Modalities are rarely used to treat edema in young children because cooperation is a large factor in their successful application. In the adolescent, modalities such as the Jobst Intermittent Compression unit or electrical stimulation may be effective.

Splinting the edematous extremity also can be effective in decreasing or controlling edema. Immediate compressive splinting of burned extremities is considered one of the keys to controlling acute edema. Dynamic splinting of an edematous hand places the part in an antideformity position but allows active muscle action in a desired plane, helping to decrease edema. The subject of splinting will be discussed later in this chapter.

RANGE OF MOTION—CONTRACTURE PREVENTION

Full, unlimited joint motion is a prerequisite for maximal muscle funciton. The surrounding soft tissue must be freely mobile to allow for quick adaptability in movement. In examining a particular joint or body part, it is important to recognize the following factors:
1. Motion takes place in more than one plane.
2. Motion involves varying types of movement at an articulation, such as rotation, sliding, or gliding (as seen in a joint).
3. Movement at a joint is one component of a subset of a larger pattern of motion.
4. Movement has intraarticular, capsular, ligamentous, muscular, and soft tissue components.

Disruption of any of these factors may interfere with normal activity. Localization of the problem allows specific therapeutic intervention to restore the components necessary for full range of motion.

A therapeutic program to restore range of motion often involves a balance of modalities such as joint mobilization, exercise, activity, and splinting. Techniques to decrease pain and edema and promote wound healing and scar remodeling are often prerequisites to treating mobility problems. These techniques prepare the soft tissues and joint for elongation. Tight joint capsules and ligaments and development of adhesions within the joint space are problems most commonly associated with adults and older adolescents, as a result of prolonged immobilization of a body part. This is only occasionally seen in the young child and adolescent. Passive exercise techniques directed at soft tissue and muscles cannot be maximized unless full articulation of the joint surfaces is available. Therapeutic techniques to restore capsular length or reduce adhesions in the joint space must be addressed at the outset of treatment.

Before discussing the various techniques to restore mobility, it is important to review the timetable for mobilizing repaired structures. The principles of wound healing serve as a guide to the therapist as to when stress forces can be applied to individual tissues. The following timetable is a general guideline for mobilizing repaired structures[37]:
1. Skin: 10 to 14 days
2. Subcutaneous tissues and blood vessels: 14 to 21 days, depending on the joints traversed
3. Tendons: $3^{1}/_{2}$ to 5 weeks; stress forces across certain joints must be considered and flexor muscles are stronger than extensor muscles, imposing an imbalance
4. Ligamentous structures and joint capsules: unstable for at least 3 months; may take 6 to 10 months for complete healing and comfort after trauma
5. Bone structures: closed reduction, 4 weeks; open reduction, 8 weeks; severe fracture with internal fixation, 12 weeks; immobilization depends on the individual situation and radiologic evidence of healing
6. Nerves: 14 days for outer epineural sheath strength; axon regeneration responds negatively to stretch forces; mobilization is geared to the available length of the nerve as it traverses a particular joint

This timetable is modified in young children, since healing rates are more rapid. Often immobilization is prolonged to protect the repaired structure from premature and excessive stress induced by the child's activities. Initiation of mobilization will depend on the surgical repair, age of the child, and decision of the surgeon.

Before discussion joint mobilization, certain terminology must be expressed. All joints have physiologic movements and accessory movements. Maitland[25] has defined physiologic movements as those which the patient carried out actively, such as shoulder flexion. Accessory movements are those movements which cannot be performed alone but which can be performed on the patient by someone else, such as moving the head of the humerous up and down in the glenoid cavity. Accessory motions are essential to normal full range of motion and painless function of joints. Joint mobilization is directed at restoring this component of joint mobility as well. Mobilizations are defined by Maitland as " . . . passive movements performed in such a way that at all times they are within the control of the patient so that he can prevent the movement if he so chooses."[25] This is not to be confused with passive range of motion or stretching. The goals of joint mobilization are to (1) restore structures in a joint to their normal position or pain-free positions to allow full range of painless movement, (2) stretch stiff painless joints to restore range, and (3) relieve pain by using special techniques.[25] Cyriax,[7] Maitland,[25] and Kaltenbourn[20] are considered authorities in this area and have written extensively on the subject of evaluation and proper application of mobilization techniques. Older adolescents are more capable of voluntary relaxation, which is a necessary prerequisite to joint mobilization. One of the authors, (K.S.G.), has used these techniques effectively in small children with congenital deformities of the hand with good results. Parents can be instructed to perform carefully a few of these techniques. It is important to combine joint mobilization techniques with an appropriate program of active and passive exercises.

Having addressed joint movement, it is important to consider other factors of normal motion. Passive and active exercises are necessary to restore elongation of soft tissue and muscle structures and can be performedin sagittal planes or functional patterns. It is necessary to exercise body parts in the directions they are to be used and to involve parts proximal and distal to the problem area. Normal movement is performed in diagonal and rotational patterns. Proprioceptive neuromuscular facilitation (PNF) is a technique frequently used to accomplish the desired movement patterns. Large muscle groups of the extremities and trunk are exercised in these diagonal patterns. Children who cannot perform active exercises should have a full program of passive exercises.

Age-appropriate play activities and gross motor skills are an integral part of every exercise program. They are an excellent way to supplement other therapeutic measures, since these activities are quite familiar. It also takes the child's mind off the idea of being exercised. Such activities may include dressing skills, eating with utensils, toothbrushing, and other personal care activities appropriate for the child's age and skill level.[13] There is the possibility of deterioration of developmental milestones in the injured infant and toddler. The infant with burns to the popliteal fossa may be unwilling to progress to crawling. The toddler with injuries to the feet may avoid weight-bearing activities. Age-appropriate developmental activities may be used to achieve the desired range of motion in one or more joints. The discussion on promotion of human maturation provides additional information.

Splinting is an excellent adjunct to the treatment program currently discussed and should be considered an integral part of the program of protecting the affected area or attaining more normal joint mobility. The function of a splint is to maintain the correct position during rest, alignment, or controlled activity. There are two basic types of splints: static and dynamic. A static splint has no movable parts and is generally used to provide protection, support, or correction to the involved body part (Fig. 2-1). A dynamic splint has movable parts, and a force may be applied to assist the moving parts (Fig. 2-2). excellent in-depth discussions of the principles, forces, and construction of splints are given in the literature.[4,11,26,27] Splinting should begin as soon as possible after injury. Deformity of a body part occurs rapidly, making timing of application of the splint a crucial factor.

It has been our experience that the splint with the fewest movable parts is the most durable and causes the fewest complications. The splints should be constructed from materials that are durable, washable, removable, lightweight, and easily applied. Low-temperature thermoplastic materials seem best suited (Orthoplast, Polyform, K splint, and Aquaplast). These are not only strong, lightweight, and washable, but are also easily moldable and can be adjusted. Serial plaster casts also may be appropriate, especially in the treatment of preexisting joint contractures. These casts cannot be removed or adjusted by the child, allowing the tissues involved to slowly elongate.[5] Splints must be fabricated individually to conform to the specific needs of each patient. It is important to choose a splint type and design carefully with regard to the child's problem, age, developmental level, and amount of family support.

Young children and infants are often placed in static splints to protect them against undesired motion or to reinforce the position of preference. They respond extremely well to prolonged periods of static splinting. Joint mobility is quickly restored when the splint is removed for periods of supervised exercised. Dynamic splinting is particularly effective in older children because they can be expected to

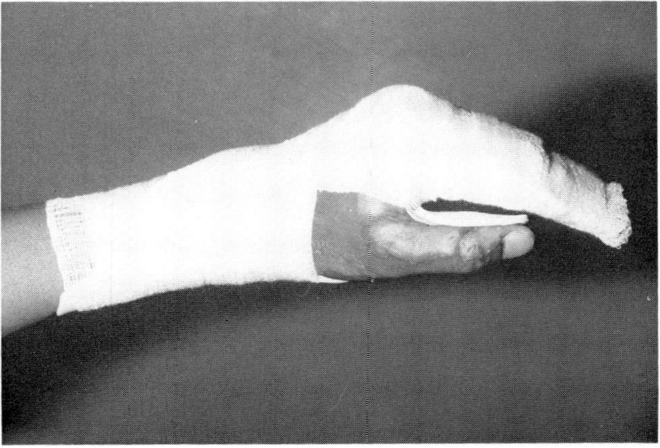

Fig. 2-1. Static splint in neutral position.

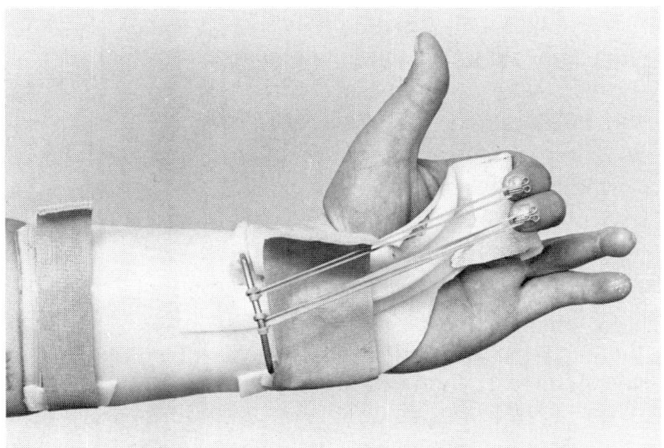

Fig. 2-2. Dynamic splint with finger flexion assist and extension resistance.

comply more adequately with the therapeutic regimen. Young children may also be good candidates for dynamic splinting if the family is cooperative. When applying traction to a joint it must be remembered that a child's periarticular structures are more easily stretched, and forces must not be too great. Joint laxity may result from overstretching. Light, slow traction over a long period of time is more effective than a lot of traction over a short period of time.[5]

All patients undergoing an intensive therapeutic program to increase or maintain mobility should have nighttime splints to maintain daily gains. The injured part should be taken out of the splint as long as possible without sacrificing any range of motion. Often the weaning process takes place over a long period of time, with increasing periods of activity and decreasing periods of splinting.

Splinting the pediatric patient presents a few challenges not encountered with adults. The child may be less cooperative and less responsible for maintaining or preventing mobility. In the hospital, allied health professional are responsible for frequent removal and reapplications of splints. In outpatient management demands are made on the family for proper application and monitoring the child's splinting program. In either case, the cooperation of the family and allied health personnel is critical for a child's splinting program to be a success. All must understand the purpose of the splint and how to properly apply and care for it and be aware of pressure areas of any other signs of an ill-fitting splint.

Splinting is not the panacea for restoring or preserving joint mobility. It is merely an adjunct to therapy. One of the worst abuses of splinting is its use without a program of therapeutic exercise. No patient should be sent home with a splint alone, and no adjunct therapy, unless the goal is to totally immobilize the joint. If this is the case, arrangements should be made to observe the child once mobility is permitted.

MAINTAINING OR INCREASING STRENGTHS

The following general principles apply to increasing, restoring, and maintaining strength:

1. It is important for the muscles to perform shortening, lengthening, and stabilizing patterns during exercise.
2. A muscle functions in a group, so exercise should incorporate all muscles in the group.
3. The desired motor response needs to be consistent with the child's neurologic age.
4. Loss of muscle strength and loss of muscle endurance must be differentiated.
5. Fatigue can damage a muscle that is less than a fair-grade strength.
6. Sensation plays an important role in the development of strength, specifically when muscles are transferred to another area to perform a different activity from their previous action.

It is crucial that an immobilized patient receive an active program of exercise. If disuse atrophy can be minimized during periods of immobility, subsequent recovery can be expected to be accomplished in a shorter time. A patient immobilized by traction or undergoing pedical flap coverage who is confined to bed will lose strength rapidly if not provided with some sort of maintenance exercise program. A daily program using weights or manual resistance by the therapist to the parts not requiring immobilization is necessary to maintain muscle tone and some endurance. Isometric exercises, which will not cause too much stress to the healing structures, are employed to the immobilized part to increase circulation and preserve muscle contractility. When the patient is able to resume out-of-bed activities, normal strength and endurance will be achieved much more rapidly if strength deterioration is prevented. An exercise program is important for any patient confined to bed for a long period of time, since prolonged bed rest can result in depression. This is especially true for children because they are accustomed to a high level of daily physical activity.

If strength in a particular muscle or body part is diminished to less than a fair grade, precautions must be taken to prevent overfatigue and overstretch of these weakened muscles. For example, when an antigravity muscle is unable to contract against gravity (less than a fair grade according to manual muscle testing[8]) care must be taken to protect this muscle from stretch when forces of gravity are acting on it. An example of this is the patient with a deltoid muscle of less than fair grade strength. The weight of the forces of gravity is acting on it, resulting in irreversible lengthening of the muscle and subluxation of the humerus. If muscle length is not preserved during this period of vulnerability, shoulder mobility will be severely impaired when the muscle does regain fair-grade strength because the mechanical relationship between the humerus and scapula will have been lost. A sling can provide appropriate support to the humerus and maintain the humeral-scapular relationship when the arm is in the gravity-dependent position. Exercises should be isometric or active assistive in nature until the muscle has achieved a fair-grade strength. Frequent, short exercise sessions only to the point where the muscle is minimally fatigued, followed by adequate rest periods, are necessary to prevent muscle damage due to overuse. Once a fair grade is reached, standard principles of exercise provide appropriate guidelines for increasing strength and endurance.

During adolescence, exercise programs should be formulated around play activities that call for muscle activities within desired groups. Activity should be carried out with a full understanding of an appropriate attention span. When the child reaches an age to accept formal direction, therapeutic techniques such as PNF, conventional therapeutic exercise, or isokinetic activities with the Cybex and Kinetron or other resistive equipment may be used. Gym and equipment are appealing. Group activities can provide peer reinforcement, encouragement, competition, and challenge.

A muscle that has been surgically transferred needs reeducation and strengthening. The cortical connection has to be reestablished for the muscle in its new role. This concept is described in the discussion on restoration of sensibility. The younger the child, the easier the muscle adapts to the new role. The reason for this is that patterns of movement have not been totally established, and the central nervous system is plastic enough to accept new and varying sensory input with great ease. Older children and adolescents have more difficulty reestablishing the cortical connection. Electric stimulation is effective in helping to teach the muscle its new function. Biofeedback is also effective and enjoyed by children because it provides a reward system for a properly performed activity with an audible or visual cue from the machine. Both provide appropriate sensory feedback to develop a new cortical reference and establish memory patterns for function. The assumption in this discussion is that cutaneous sensation is intact. If abnormal sensibility is present, the cortex will receive altered input that may make muscle reeducation difficult. If this is the case, sensibility retraining must be combined with muscle reeducation to regain functional activity. It also must be remembered that a surgically transferred muscle loses one grade of muscle strength. The transferred muscle must be strengthened to its maximal potential to preserve agonist and antagonist balance. PNF is an excellent way to promote muscle strengthening in functional patterns, using normal proximal and distal muscles to facilitate strength. It also encourages increased sensory input to the cortex through the automatic responses in functional patterns. Play activities and age-appropriate developmental activities are excellent ways of promoting increased sensory feedback and muscle strength.

Dynamic splinting can be useful both as a strengthening tool and as an orthosis to protect weak muscles from damage. To increase strength, rubber band traction can be applied to act as a resistive force for the specific muscles. An example of a protective orthosis is well demonstrated in a patient with radial nerve palsy. A dynamic splint can be constructed supporting the wrist, metacarpophalangeal joints, and thumb in extension, with rubber band traction. This not only protects and provides support for the denervated muscles, but also permits active finger, wrist, and thumb flexion to maintain joint mobility and strength of the functioning muscles.

REDUCTION OF PAIN

It is a normal response in both children and adults to demonstrate regressive behavior when experiencing pain. Pain has both physical and psychologic components that overlap and are frequently difficult to separate. Physical pain results from specific activities such as wound care and exercise. Psychologic pain evolves from anxiety or anticipated procedures, fear of outcome, and loneliness. The resultant muscle tension and loss of sleep further reinforce the level of discomfort. Children have a lower level of communication skills, which means they must depend on more overt expressions of these needs and feelings. Examples are withdrawal, hostility, combative behavior, crying, and verbal abuse. The ability of children to use these reactions to manipulate the environment must be recognized. Children in distress often look for support rather than conflict, and this support must be provided in a manner that enhances the treatment.

Many of the necessary treatment procedures induce pain; unfortunately there are no specific therapeutic methods of alleviating pain. Treatment that elicits pain in the child causes the greatest concern on the part of most adults involved in the delivery of care. The child also may come to view the therapist as a "deliverer of pain" and become frightened, thereby heightening pain perception. A simple explanation of treatment procedures before touching the patient is important; however, gentleness, tone of voice, positive facial expressions, and touch are also effective in easing the child's anxieties. Pretreatment medications can reduce the intensity of pain and should be used to make the child as comfortable as possible during treatment.

Activities that divert the child's attention away from the painful area, while accomplishing the desired movement, are effective treatment measures. When elbow flexion and extension are desired, two-handed passing of a ball will enable the child to focus on the goal of the ball reaching the partner rather than on the dysfunction and pain at the elbow. When neck extension is required, having the child move around prone on a scooter board will require head, neck, and trunk extension.

Equally important in caring for children is their ability to exert "control" over their own care, control that is limited by the hospitalization. The ability to participate in treatment helps to ease the fear of pain elicited by movement and direct care. Examples would be allowing the child to remove dressings or assist in wound cleansing. This role enables the child to control the speed of care and the intensity of discomfort.

The use of physical modalities to support the child's care is less acceptable than with the adult. Hydrotherapy may be effective as a form of diversion to enable the child to move in a pleasant, gravity-free environment in order to achieve movement with reduced pain. Modalities such as ice, heat, galvanic stimulation, and vibration are rarely used to relieve pain in young children, since they are not able to cooperate during the treatment.

PROMOTION OF HUMAN MATURATION

Earlier in this chapter attention was given to the wound, healing process, and therapeutic procedures specific to the wound. In caring for the child attention also must be given to the dynamic process of development and maturation. The physical therapist and other caregivers must be concerned with the child's total integration of function and behavior related to chronologic age. In addition, the therapist must be aware of the influence of the child's situation on long-

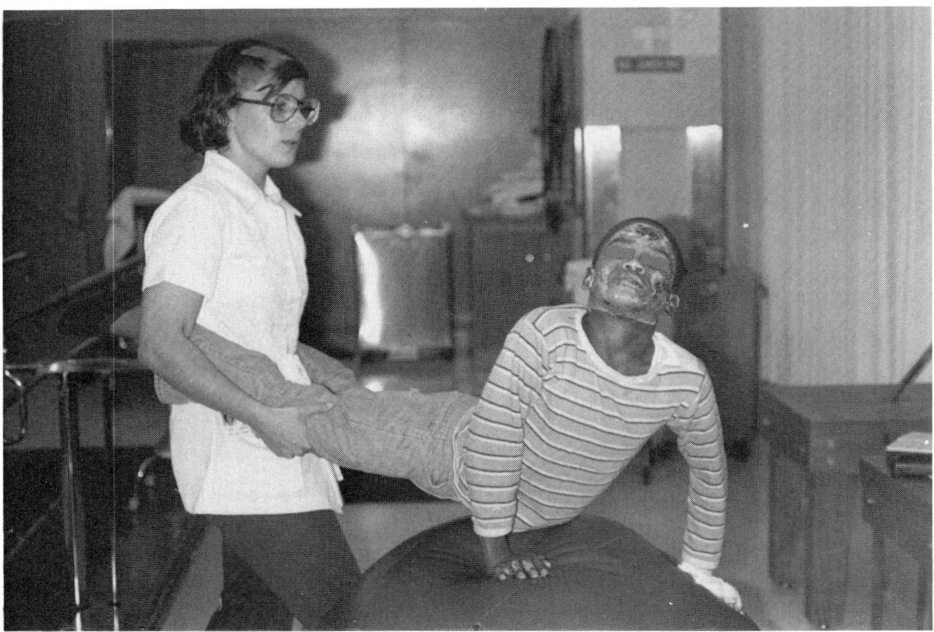

Fig. 2-3. Total trunk and lower extremity extension of therapy ball.

term growth and development. Gesell stated that "the behavioral end products of the total developmental process are a consequence of continuing reciprocal interaction between the genetic endowment and the environment."[13] The physical therapist must have a primary concern for the influence the injury has on gross and fine motor behavior, as well as personal-social behavior. In dealing with these factors, consideration should also be given to the child's adaptive behavior.

Systematic studies of healthy children have provided a framework that clearly delineates the relationship of various behavioral components of development in relationship to one another at specific levels of chronologic age.[13,14,18] The physical therapist and other caregivers should use these characteristics and their relationships in formulating an age-appropriate program of care to not only meet the needs of the child's trauma but also for developmental advances.

Children are not miniature adults and their responses to hospitalization will be particularly influenced by factors such as age, previous hospitalizations, the circumstances of admission, preparation for hospitalization, and the security of family life.[40] Responses to hospitalization may be significantly different when the admission is required by sudden accidental trauma. The reaction of the family may be influenced by the reason for hospitalization and can also have an impact on the child's response. Regardless of the circumstances, the hospital environment is one in which children may be unable to grasp what is going to happen, even though they may have been well prepared. They are separated from their parents at a time when they need them most and are being handled by strangers and involved in a routine

that is unfamiliar. Adding the element of potential pain leads to even greater unhappiness. Children react differently to their surroundings. Some demonstrate introverted behavior, whereas others are quite overt in their response.

Awareness and use of principles of neuromotor development are primary to the physical therapist in fostering continuing gross and fine motor behavior, as well as accomplishing desired movement goals identified in the previous discussion on stretching. The development of movements is described by many authors,[13] and it is not our intent to replicate all of this information. In caring for the newborn and infant, understanding the nature and mechanisms of neurologic reflex activity is primary in modifying and directing the child's gross motor behavior. As the nervous sytem continues its development, many of the early reflexes are inhibited and others are modified and incorporated into more complex actions. After progressing through a stage where movement is random and related to reflex activity, the child acquires more appropriate motor function oriented around equilibrium and postural attitudes. As an example, the 6- or 7-month-old child can sit unsupported and exhibit righting of the head, with protective extension of the arm when body weight is shifted laterally. At 1 year, the child pulls to standing, cruises, and walks with assistance. The continuing neuromotor development that requires a highly interactive central and peripheral nervous system progresses the child to a level of coordinated, variable, and selective movement.[6]

The pain and scarring associated with many injuries cause the child to regress in gross motor behavior and avoid many desired normal movements. This may result in shortening

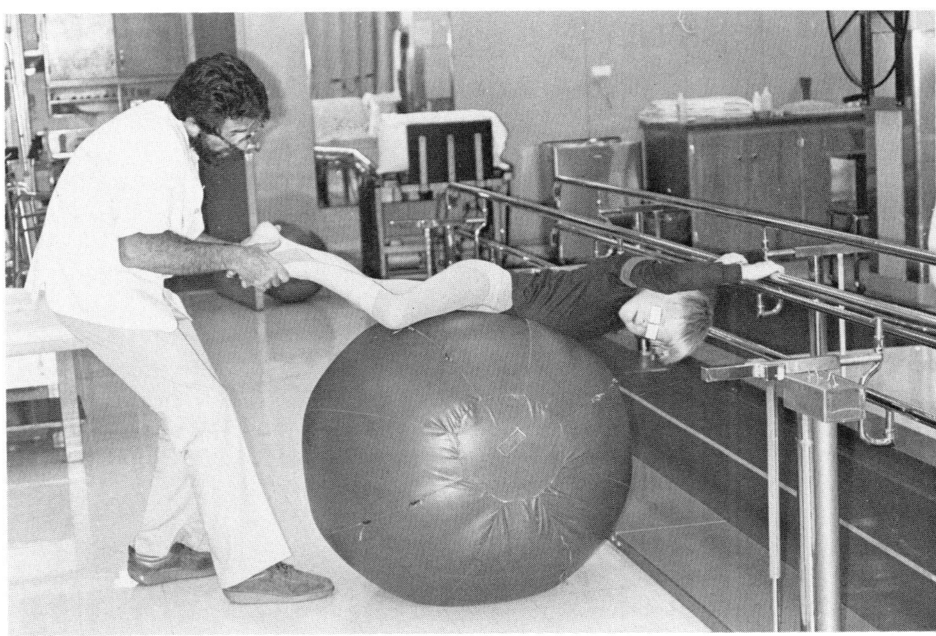

Fig. 2-4. Facilitating right leg flexion with trunk in extension.

of some tissues and weakening of selective muscle groups. No amount of passive assistance or verbal reinforcement will enable the child to overcome fear and carry out the desired motor activity. However, since numerous motor behaviors are based on reflex activity, postural responses, or predetermined motor patterns, the use of techniques based on these factors will often achieve the desired motor outcomes without the child's conscious awareness. An example of this approach would be the use of equilibrium reaction to the side when in sitting to achieve elbow extension with a child who has the tendency to continually hold the arm in flexion. Attainment of total body and lower limb extension in the prone position on a "therapy ball" will overcome flexion attitudes of the lower extremity and trunk (Fig. 2-3). Likewise, asymmetric activity incorporating rotation of the trunk with flexion of one leg can be accomplished with total cooperation of the child (Fig. 2-4).

PULMONARY HYGIENE

Children sustaining thermal injuries to the chest, face, and trachea must be aggressively treated to prevent pulmonary complications. Those children who have undergone plastic surgery procedures to the face or chest may also develop pulmonary complications. In some instances children may have preexisting pulmonary disease, which increases the probability of postoperative respiratory difficulties. In these instances the physical therapist needs to assist in removing excess secretions and maximizing ventilation of the lungs.

The principles of respiratory management for children are similar to those for adults, with some modifications in techniques for the infant and small child. Breathing exercises emphasizing lower costal and diaphragmatic expansion are desirable and best performed in the sitting position. When treating the infant, crying and spontaneous coughing provide adequate ventilation of the lung. Games with the therapist are appealing ways to facilitate good breathing techniques in young children.

Mobilization of secretions can be achieved by regular breathing exercises, coughing, and techniques of postural drainage, percussion, and vibration.[12] It is important to provide pulmonary hygiene to patients who are receiving mechanical ventilation. Children with postoperative congestion usually develop it in the lower lobes because of reduced costal expansion secondary to decreased activity, pain, and supine positioning. Drainage positions and breathing techniques are directed to these areas using a reverse Trendelenburg's position. Contraindications for tipping include vascular procedures and a rise in blood or intracranial pressure that may be detrimental. Postural drainage positions are modified for children with thermal injuries, but other manual techniques to improve pulmonary hygiene are the same.

Suctioning should never be used as a substitute for coughing. A suction catheter or the "trachea tickle" can be used to facilitate a cough when the techniques just mentioned fail to do so.[6] Children in intermaxillary fixation can have secretions removed from the mouth by a suction catheter. Very young children will swallow their secretions.

Movement is essential to any program that attempts to restore function to normal. Generally, assistance with appropriate exercises is provided until the child is able to move independently. Once a child is moving independently in bed, respiratory recovery is spontaneous and quick.

If pulmonary complications are expected postoperatively, meeting with the child and family postoperatively to explain techniques of good postoperative respiratory care and practice breathing and coughing techniques is advisable. This greatly aids in quick postoperative recovery of respiratory function.

REMODELING OF SCAR

As discussed earlier, there are two types of wounds: simple closed wounds and open wounds with or without tissue loss. Scarring results during healing from both.

The one wound–one scar concept states that the scar is a single unit and all injured tissues are bound together.[34,35] Scar tissue ties gliding surfaces firmly to fixed surrounding structures, creating adhesions. Dysfunction is most prevalent in those body parts where multiple structures move freely relative to fixed units, such as in the hand. In body parts such as the knee, where there are layers of connective tissue between movement planes, the scar does not create such extensive mobility dysfunction. In the hand, where movement planes are in close approximation, scar fixation can severely limit mobility. In the case of severed tendons that are subsequently repaired, the scar formed both at the repair site and at surrounding incised tissues results in a diminution of movement by limiting the excursion of tissue planes and gliding surfaces. Limited tendon excursion can also result from injury to adjacent structures without any actual injury to the tendon itself. Nerves entrapped by scar can undergo degeneration. Similarly, blood vessels can become constricted by scar tissue with diminished tissue perfusion and necrosis.[31]

Wound contraction occurs in open wounds with or without tissue loss.[23,24,36] A wound will contract until it meets an equal and opposing force.[23,24] If healing continues without an opposing force, joints will assume abnormal positions. If this position remains unchanged for a prolonged period of time, secondary changes in the periarticular structures will take place, leading to permanent joint stiffness.[22] This is most graphically seen in the burned patient in whom large areas of tissue destruction often result in the rapid formation of contractures. If healing is permitted to continue without opposing the forces of wound contraction, joint contractures occur. This is reflected by a patient in a fetal position. The centripetal forces of wound healing are continuous and unrelenting until wound closure occurs. Even then the patient is not out of danger. Larson[22] states that this process of wound contraction can continue for 3 months to 3 years after healing, depending on the patient's rate of scar maturation. Sometimes healed wounds for hypertrophic scars that are highly vascular and metabolically active.

In both wound types it is important to remember that scars undergo a period of maturation characterized by continued contractility until the process is complete.[23,24] As long as the scar remains active, there is a potential for deformity and dysfunction, and no therapeutic measures can physiologically alter the quantity of scar. Therapeutic intervention is most effective, however, in influencing the movement of adjacent bound structures, minimizing the deformity secondary to wound contraction, and improving the appearance by limiting hypertrophic scar formation. Therapy is best instituted when the scar is still metabolically active. Once the scar has fully matured, little can be done to influence remodeling.

Adolescents present a greater treatment challenge than young children, since their response to scarring is more like that seen in adults, with greater potential for deformity and dysfunction. More extensive therapeutic intervention is required. Once again, active motion and deep-friction scar massage are key in promoting change in the scar tissue. With extensive scarring, modalities such as galvanic stimulation, heat, or paraffin may be used. Galvanic current stimulates adherent muscle tendon units and encourages motion and glide. This modality seems to work more effectively in the upper extremity, which is more rapidly available to stimulation than the lower extremity. A heat modality such as paraffin helps promote softening of the external tissues. Paraffin temperatures are often quite warm. This treatment modality is not recommended for parts with altered sensibility. When applying moist heat, adequate toweling should be used between the body part and the hot pack to prevent tissue burns. This is especially important when the part has altered sensibility, since the patient may not have protective sensation. Heat modalities should not be used longer than 20 minutes. Such treatment modalities are especially useful when an old scar is present.

Exercises in which the scar is immobilized by the therapist and the patient moves the part in the opposite direction can be effective in loosening a bound tendon by actively stretching the scar so that it glides with the tendon. Blocked muscle exercise is especially useful in promoting tendon glide by blocking the undesired joint motions, allowing the particular muscle to be moved in an isolated fashion. This also helps to promote scar remodeling and restore individual structure mobility.

Splinting effectively promotes glide of scarred structures in the hand, using the same principles as in blocked tendon exercises. Blocking the undesired joint motions forces isolated mobility of the adherent structure with every movement attempt. For example, to promote flexor digitorum superficialis muscle activity, a splint immobilizing the metacarpophalangeal joint but leaving the proximal interphalangeal joints free, forces muscle glide with every attempt at finger flexion. In severe cases of scar binding, a program of dynamic splinting may be required to assist the remodeling process. Extensive splinting is rarely needed to improve structural glide in the young child. If splinting is required, a static splint is generally employed because it immobilizes the extremity in the desired position, which enlarges applied force to enhance change.

The treatment of scar associated with open wounds is begun before complete wound healing. The treatment program is fourfold, consisting of splinting, exercise, bed positioning, and compression. Splints are used to place the involved part in a position where the tissues are maximally elongated. With burn injuries, splinting is begun immediately after the child is medically resuscitated. Static splinting is used and the child is maintained in these splints combined with proper bed positioning, which also places the body parts in positions of soft tissue elongation at all times, except for periods of supervised exercise, play activities, activities of daily living, and ambulation. If grafting is required, the grafted part is splinted in much the same way. The patient is not allowed to move the grafted part until the graft "take" is successful. Exercise is then resumed in combination with static splinting. Splinting is continued after complete wound healing has been achieved and throughout the entire period of scar maturation.[22] The balance between splinting and exercise is determined by the physical therapist, based on the child's prognosis, age, and ability to cooperate and the extent of the child's injuries and scarring. When the child can adequately maintain joint mobility independent of the splints for a period of time, the splints are used intermittently, for example, 2 hours on and 2 hours off or a schedule that corresponds with functional and play activities. With young children, this is often unrealistic. Prolonged splinting is not harmful and in most cases is necessary to prevent contractures. Night splinting is continued throughout the period of scar maturation.

Splinting and "distal-to-proximal" elastic bandage wrapping are used to apply constant external pressure to healing wounds (Fig. 2-5). This is believed by many researchers to significantly alter the scarring process. Larson,[22] in his extensive research, found that the application of external pressure to maturing burn scars greatly decreases the incidence of contractures and reduces the frequency and necessity for contracture release procedures. He believes that the continuous application of pressure above normal capillary pressure (25 mm Hg) to hypertrophic scars resulted in the gradual opening of compact collagen in the underlying dermis, allowing the fibers to assume a more parallel pattern characteristic of normal skin and nonhypertrophic scars.*[22] All patients exhibiting the potential for hypertrophic scarring are measured for a scar elastic pressure-garment, which is custom made and engineered to apply the physiologically correct pressure to the burned area. This is worn throughout the period of scar maturation for 24 hours a day. Disfigurement and dysfunction are believed to be retarded. These garments have to be remeasured periodically to allow for the child's growth and to ensure continued proper pressure. Often compressive splints are required in addition to elastic garments to provide additional pressure to difficult areas, such as face conformers worn under the face mask and neck conformers worn over the top of the garment.[22]

RESTORATION OF SENSIBILITY

Over the past decade increased attention and emphasis have been placed on quality of sensory return after peripheral nerve repair. Both surgeons and physical therapists are no longer willing to accept mediocre postoperative functional recovery. Most rehabilitation facilities are employing organized sensory reeducation programs for their patients. The importance of sensory restoration in the hand needs no emphasis. Touch is one's connection with the environment.

Axon regeneration occurs at a rate of approximately 1 mm per day or 2.5 cm (1 inch) per month.[38,39] It is also known that sensory recovery continues to improve slowly for many years after nerve repair. Dellon[9] has suggested that continued sensory recovery is due in part to the maturation of the newly reunited fiber-receptor systems. Much later return, however, is due to subliminal reeducation obtained with daily guarded use of the injured hand. Sensory reeducation permits a patient to achieve the potential for functional recovery after nerve repair.

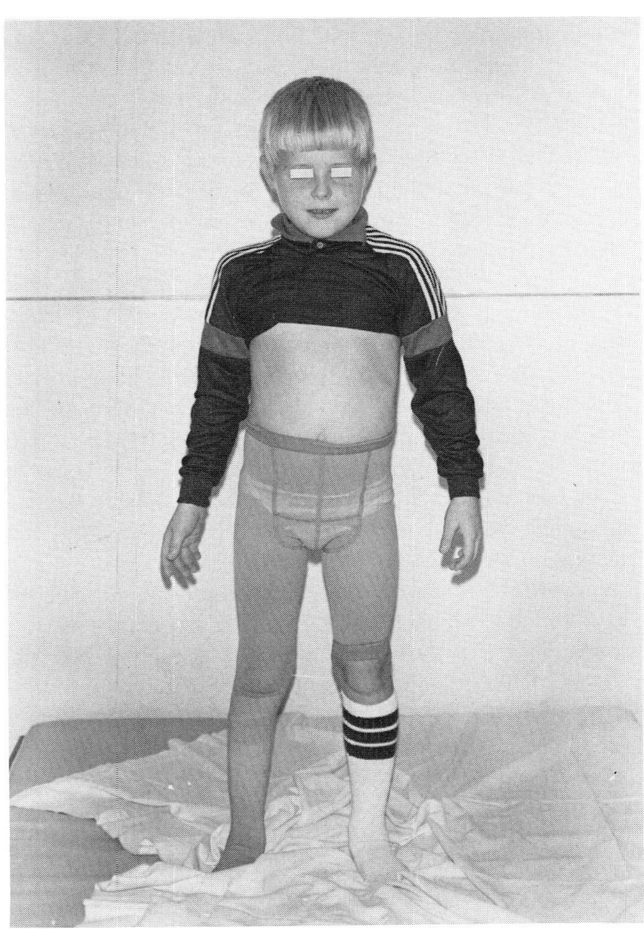

Fig. 2-5. Pressure gradient garment for lower trunk and leg.

---

*The efficacy of pressure in the structural modification of wound collagen remains controversial.

Sensory receptors are stimulated when the hand contacts an object, eliciting a profile of neural impulses impacting on the sensory cortex.[9] These impulses are associated in the cortex with previous memory and experiences leading to a perception of the object. After nerve division and repair, the same contact with the object elicits a different profile of neural impulses, making no association in the sensory cortex. This leads to altered peripheral sensibility. Almquist's studies[1] found that poor sensory function after peripheral nerve injury was a failure of cortical function rather than a failure of the regenerated axons alone. Therefore the goal of sensory reeducation is to "... help the patient with sensory impairment learn to reinterpret the altered profile of neural impulses reaching his conscious level after his injured hand has been stimulated."[9]

It is well known that children regain excellent sensibility after peripheral nerve repair. It has been believed that this is primarily because of their superior abilities to reorganize central connections. Studies on blind persons and persons recovering from upper motor neuron lesions, however, indicate that young and old individuals can improve their cerebral reorganization using a tactile visual substitution retraining process. Almquist's studies[2] comparing children to adults also support the effectiveness of retraining to improve sensory recovery. Dellon[9] has hypothesized that the success in sensory recovery in children may be due partly to their continuous tactile investigation of their surroundings. Studies by Önne[33] showed that after 12 years of age, two-point discrimination equals a person's age in millimeters. Evaluation of sensory reeducation programs has indicated that all patients receiving sensory reeducation did better than the result predicted for their age.[9] Although children and adolescents seem to make a better functional recovery than adults, their recovery can be hastened and maximized with sensibility reeducation.

An appropriate evaluation is necessary to determine if the patient is ready for sensibility retraining. Until the appropriate fiber-receptor system has been united, attempts at retraining are fruitless.[9] There are several documented methods for specific sensory testing. Remembering that there is a considerable amount of subjectivity present in testing, the age of the child must be strongly considered when choosing the type of test. The younger the child, the more difficult it will be to determine the extent of sensory deprivation and the exact point at which reeducation should be initiated. Observing the child in play activities and attempts at handling objects can be most helpful in determining the child's readiness for sensory retraining. Testing is considerably more reliable in older children and adolescents, because they are better able to comply with the testing procedures.

The two most specific methods of sensory reeducation are those designed by Wynn-Parry[42] and Dellon.[9] Both are used extensively and have been proven successful. Different techniques of assessment before use are required; however, sensibility retraining in both methods is not initiated until

moving touch is perceived at the fingertips. Both authors concur that if hyperesthesia or dysesthesia is present, retraining activities should be discontinued and specific desensitization should be begun until the period of excess response is considerably lessened.[9,28,42] Effective techniques are gentle stroking with different fabrics, tapping, vibration, transcutaneous nerve stimulation, and bombardment of the area with different textures, such as beans, corn, and oats. Until this situation is alleviated, perception of the reeducation exercises will be blocked.[28]

The pattern theory is the basis of Wynn-Parry's sensibility reeducation program. This theory states that the skin is reinnervated at random and the patient must learn this new pattern.[42] Sensory retraining is initiated when the patient can perceive moving touch at the fingertips. All training is done with the patient blindfolded and is begun with large wooden blocks of different shapes, progressing to recognition of different textures, for example, sandpaper, wool, canvas, carpet, and leather.[41,42] When this is achieved tha patient is asked to differentiate between large and small objects. The time taken and number of objects recognized correctly is recorded. The patient never knows whether the objects have been identified correctly so that a "training effect" can be avoided. The patient is asked to compare the abnormal sensation with what is felt with the normal hand and make comparisons with the eyes open and closed, trying to relate what is felt to what is seen. Localization of touch is also tested.[41,42]

The Dellon technique[9,28] is based on Mountcastle's work of 1966 and 1967, which showed that the beta nerve fibers responsible for the perception of touch are reinnervated in a specific pattern. Mountcastle[30] divided these fibers into two groups based on their response to stimulus of their cutaneous receptors. Slow-adapting fibers (10% of the fibers) respond to stimulus and then fire continuously until the stimulus stops.[9,28] Quick-adapting fibers (90% of the fibers) respond to stimulus with a short burst of firing and then stop firing even if the stimulus continues. The quick-adapting fibers are then further divided into two groups based on their response to vibratory stimulus. One group is maximally responsive to stimulus frequencies of 30 cps, and the other group is maximally responsive at 256 cps. Dellon states that an evaluation for the presence of these fibers can be accomplished using tuning forks. Recovering sensory modalities are identified in the following manner: pain, vibration of 30 cps; and moving and constant touch, vibration of 256 cps.

The patient is ready for reeducation when vibratory stimuli of 30 or 256 cps are perceived.[9,25] All retraining is stimulated with vision and duplicated with vision eliminated. Moving touch is relearned by stroking from the palm outward, proximal to distal; heavy moving touch is learned first and then progresses to light touch.[9,28] Constant touch is learned in the same fashion, depending on the intensity and location of the stimulus. Direction of movement can be learned by outlining familiar numbers on the volar surface of the patient's fingertips. Retraining of combined vibratory sense and moving touch is then started using hexagonal nuts and large washers. Progressively smaller sizes are used until the patient can recognize them with vision eliminated. Bilateral exercises are important to learn important tactile cues such as pain, temperature, shape, and weight of objects. Functional objects such as coins are then added, learning first with vision and then without.

Other techniques of retraining can be used by themselves or more frequently are incorporated with the previously discussed techniques. Papers with braille on them in various designs, shapes, and pattern irregularities are excellent for practicing identification. Burying objects in a medium such as sand, beans, or corn is helpful for training recognition of objects out of the visual field.[9]

Objects must be chosen that are recognizable for the child's age level, regardless of what sensibility retraining method is used. Sensibility retraining requires considerable concentration in a distraction-free environment, and training sessions should be adjusted to consider the child's wavering attention span. Children generally do not require reinforcement through a home program because they are still inquisitive and explore their environment employing their tactile sensibilities. The younger the child, the less cortical "old learning" needs to be replaced by "new learning."[28] Older adolescents should be treated as adults, but their level of reinforcement will not need to be as extensive as with young children. Adults require long-term reinforcement in the form of a home program. If previous work and home activities are resumed, however, then formal reinforcement is not required.[9]

It should be remembered that perception of sensory stimuli requires motor control, since an object needs to be manipulated before sensory identification. Movement of an object in the hand stimulates the moving touch receptors.[9,28] Incorporation of motor function in conjunction with sensibility reeducation is necessary for successful rehabilitation. Intelligence and previous learning also affect the patient's behavior and response to stimuli. In any event, creativity should be used in making the program interesting and pertinent for the child's age level.

SUMMARY AND CONCLUSIONS

Care of the child undergoing plastic surgical procedures must be a team effort that takes into consideration the multiple elements affecting the child's normal maturation and injury. A thorough evaluation of the child and the problem is key to the development of an appropriate physical therapy treatment program. Certain treatment goals are applicable to most young patients. These include wound care, reduction of edema, range of motion, maintenance of or increase in strengths, reduction of pain, promotion of human maturation, pulmonary hygiene, remodeling of scars, and restoration of sensibility. The treatment program should consist of a variety of age- and developmentally appropriate activities. Care should also be taken to involve the family, since their understanding and support are primary to the child's long-term care. A background in human maturation combined with competence in wound management, exercise, and application of various physical modalities makes the physical therapist an important member of the team.

REFERENCES

1. Almquist, E., and Eeg-Olofsson, O.: Sensory-nerve-conduction velocity and two-point discrimination in sutured nerves, J. Bone Joint Surg. **52A:**791, 1970.
2. Almquist, E., Smith, O., and Fry, L.: Nerve conduction velocity: microscopic studies comparing repaired adult and baby monkey median nerves, Presented at the twenty-eighth annual meeting of the American Society for Surgery of the Hand, Las Vegas, 1973.
3. Arem, A.J., and Madden, J.W.: Effects of stress on healing wounds. 1. Intermittent non-cyclical tension, J. Surg. Res. **20:**93, 1976.
4. Barr, N.R.: The hand: principles and techniques of simple splintmaking in rehabilitation, Boston, 1975, Butterworth Publishers.
5. Bell, J.A., and Harkrider, A.: Splinting and the stiff hand—use and misuse. In Hunter, J.M., Schneider, L.H., Mackin, E.J., and Bell, J., editors: Rehabilitation of the hand, St. Louis, 1978, The C.V. Mosby Co.
6. Cash, J.E., editor: Chest, heart and vascular disorders for physiotherapists, London, 1975, Faber & Faber, Ltd.
7. Cyriax, J.: Textbook of orthopaedic medicine, ed. 6, vol. 1, Baltimore, 1975, The Williams & Wilkins Co.
8. Daniels, L., and Worthingham, C.: Muscle testing: techniques of manual examination, ed. 3, Philadelphia, 1972, W.B. Saunders Co.
9. Dellon, A.L.: Evaluation of sensibility and reeducation of sensation in the hand, Baltimore, 1981, The Williams & Wilkins Co.
10. Feller, I., and Jones, A.C.: Nursing the burned patient, Ann Arbor, Mich., 1973, Institute for Burn Medicine.
11. Fess, E.E., Gettle, K.S., and Strickland, J.W.: Hand splinting: principles and methods, St. Louis, 1981, The C.V. Mosby Co.
12. Gaskell, D.V., and Webber, B.A.: The Brompton Hospital guide to chest physiotherapy, ed. 2, Oxford, 1974, Blackwell Scientific Publications.
13. Gesell, A.L., and Amatruda, C.S.: Developmental diagnosis, Hagerstown, Md., 1974, Harper & Row, Publishers, Inc.
14. Holt, K.S.: Developmental paediatrics: perspectives and practice, Boston, 1977, Butterworth Publishers.
15. Howes, E.L., Harvey, S.C., and Hewitt, C.: Rate of fibroplasia and differentiation in the healing of cutaneous wounds in different species of animals, Arch. Surg. **38:**934, 1939.
16. Howes, E.L., Sooy, J.W., and Harvey, S.C.: The healing of wounds as determined by their tensile strength, J.A.M.A. **92:**42, 1929.
17. Hunter, J.M., and Mackin, E.J.: Edema and bandaging. In Hunter, J.M., Schneider, L.H., Mackin, E.J., and Bell, J., editors: Rehabilitation of the hand, St. Louis, 1978, The C.V. Mosby Co.
18. Illingworth, R.S.: The development of the infant and young child: normal and abnormal, Edinburgh, 1960, E. & S. Livingstone.
19. Jacques, J.: Wound contraction in experimental lathyrism, Br. J. Exp. Pathol. **50:**486, 1969.
20. Kaltenborn, F.M.: Manual therapy for the extremity joints, ed. 2, Oslo, 1976, Olaf Norlis Bokhandel.
21. Kefalides, N.A.: Isolation of a collagen from basement membranes containing three identical α-chains, Biochem. Biophys. Res. Commun. **45:**226, 1971.
22. Larson, D., Huang, T., and Linares, H.: Prevention and treatment of scar contracture. In Artz, C.P., Moncrief, J.A., and Pruitt, B.A., Jr., editors: Burns: a team approach, Philadelphia, 1979, W.B. Saunders Co.
23. Madden, J.W.: Wound healing: biologic and clinical features. In Sabiston, D.C., Jr., editor: Davis-Christopher textbook of surgery: the biological basis of modern surgical practice, ed. 11, vol. 1, Philadelphia, 1977, W.B. Saunders Co.
24. Madden, J.W.: Wound healing: the biological basis of hand surgery. In Hunter, J.M., Schneider, L.H., Mackin, E.J., and Bell, J., editors: Rehabilitation of the hand, St. Louis, 1978, The C.V. Mosby Co.

25. Maitland, G.D.: Vertebral manipulation, ed. 2, Boston, 1977, Butterworth Publishers.
26. Malick, M.H.: Manual on static splinting, Pittsburgh, 1973, Harmarville Rehabilitation Center.
27. Malick, M.H.: Manual and dynamic hand splinting with thermoplastic materials, Pittsburgh, 1974, Harmarville Rehabilitation Center.
28. Maynard, C.J.: Sensory reeducation following peripheral nerve injury. In Hunter, J.M., Schneider, L.H., Mackin, E.J., and Bell, J., editors: Rehabilitation of the hand, St. Louis, 1978, The C.V. Mosby Co.
29. McMinn, R.M.H.: Tissue repair, New York, 1969, Academic Press, Inc.
30. Mountcastle, V.B.: Medical physiology, ed. 14, vol. 2, St. Louis, 1980, The C.V. Mosby Co.
31. Newmeyer, W.L.: Primary care of hand injuries, Philadelphia, 1979, Lea & Febiger.
32. Northwestern University Special Therapeutic Exercise Project (NUSTEP): an exploratory and analytical survey of therapeutic exercise, Am. J. Phys. Med. **46:**3, 1967.
33. Önne, L.: Recovery of sensibility and sudomotor activity in the hand after nerve suture, Acta Chir. Scand. **300:**1, 1962.
34. Peacock, E.E., Jr.: Fundamental aspects of wound healing relating to the restoration of gliding function after tendon repair, Surg. Gynecol. Obstet. **119:**241, 1964.
35. Peacock, E.E., Jr.: Dynamic aspects of collagen biology. I. Synthesis and assembly, J. Surg. Res. **7:**433, 1967.
36. Peacock, E.E., Jr., and Van Winkle, W.: Wound repair, ed. 2, Philadelphia, 1976, W.B. Saunders Co.
37. Prendergast, K.H.: Therapists management of a mutilated hand. In Hunter, J.M., Schneider, L.H., Mackin, E.J., and Bell, J., editors: Rehabilitation of the hand, St. Louis, 1978, The C.V. Mosby Co.
38. Seddon, H.J., Medawar, P.B., and Smith, H.: Rate of regeneration of peripheral nerves in man, J. Physiol. **102:**191, 1943.
39. Sunderland, S.: Rate of regeneration in human peripheral nerves, Arch. Neurol. Psychiatry **58:**251, 1947.
40. Thompson, E.D.: Pediatric nursing: an introductory text, ed. 4, Philadelphia, 1981, W.B. Saunders Co.
41. Wynn-Parry, C.B.: Rehabilitation of the hand, ed. 3, Boston, 1973, Butterworth Publishers.
42. Wynn-Parry, C.B.: Sensory rehabilitation of the hand, Aust. N.Z. J. Surg. **50:**224, 1980.

CHAPTER 3

Diagnostic imaging in pediatric plastic surgery practice

DENNIS R. OSBORNE

Diagnostic imaging methods can be used to evaluate the structural nature and extent of a lesion and to clarify its relationship to surrounding structures. They can establish or confirm a diagnosis or evaluate unusual manifestations and associated disease entities. Serial imaging studies can document the natural history and progression of a disease, and a special skeletal series can indicate the probable physical growth potential of a child. Important functional information may be provided by fluoroscopic and cineradiographic techniques, as is well illustrated in pediatric plastic surgical practice by their use in the assessment of velopharyngeal competence.

The purpose of this chapter is to discuss the imaging techniques available,[19,54,69] when they are useful, and some of the findings in diseases that will be encountered in a pediatric plastic surgical practice.

TECHNIQUES
Plain film examination

Plain film examination remains the most commonly used imaging method and is usually the first examination performed when an imaging evaluation is required. At least two projections taken at approximately right angles are necessary for integrated three-dimensional reconstruction of anatomic structures. The method's advantage is that it is simple, readily available, and relatively inexpensive. It adequately images the skeletal system and, with appropriate modifications in technique, can provide important information on soft tissues structures. Local radiologic examination of a potential or known lesion is usually undertaken to establish or confirm a diagnosis or evaluate the structure, extent, and anatomic relations of the lesion.

Tomography is of considerable value in the assessment of any complex anatomic structure, especially where overlying structures obscure detail. It also is useful in confirming an abnormality suspected on a routine radiograph or in the detailed analysis of the architecture and extent of a lesion. It is especially helpful in assessing complex developmental abnormalities of the skull. The limitations of tomography in pediatric practice relate to the long exposure time (1 to 5 seconds), a frequent requirement for sedation, and additional patient radiation.

Fluoroscopy or cineradiography have special advantages in that they allow dynamic and functional assessment of anatomic structures. The techniques are simple and readily available. They are especially useful in evaluating the airways, deglutition, and gastrointestinal action. In pediatric plastic surgery they are of proven value in the functional evaluation of the upper airway and swallowing mechanism. The techniques are often combined with a positive contrast agent to enhance the examined structure, be it a hollow organ or tube, cavity, or blood vessel.

Contrast-enhanced studies

Contrast-enhanced studies are routinely used in the detailed examination of soft tissues, hollow organs, and vascular structures. Although they do not have widespread use in pediatric plastic surgical practice, they can provide invaluable information in certain preoperative and postoperative situations.

Excretory urography is the most common method of examining the renal tract. It is performed after an intravenous injection of a water-soluble iodine salt. Its most important indications in pediatric practice include assessment of repeated urinary tract infection, evaluation of abdominal masses and congenital anomalies of the renal tract, the intersex states, neonatal ascites, trauma, hypertension, and occasionally abdominal pain. The examination has few complications, but it should not be performed when a child is severely dehydrated or in shock. Contrast medium reactions during and after intravenous urography are very uncommon in children.[4] If a history of allergy exists, especially to seafood, eggs, milk, or chocolate, an open intravenous line is useful so that intravenous access is available should any reaction develop. It is rare for an examination to be deferred or cancelled because of a reaction in children.

The renal tract also may be evaluated by direct invasion techniques, namely, percutaneous translumbar pyelography, retrograde pyelography, and voiding or retrograde cystoure-thrography.[18,54,63] Discussion of these techniques is beyond the scope of this chapter, since they are only rarely used in pediatric plastic surgical practice.

The genital tract is often imaged in the diagnostic or preoperative evaluation of patients with genital abnormalities or intersex states. The examination technique largely depends on the number of external orifices present. In general, a separate tube is inserted into as many of the external orifices as is possible. The purpose of the examination is to define the internal genital anatomic structures before any possible corrective surgery.

Angiography has only a limited place in pediatric plastic surgery at present.[26] Its most important indications in children are in the assessment of renal or extrarenal retroperitoneal masses, hepatic tumors, trauma, hypertension, and peripheral arteriovenous malformations.[11] In the cranial cavity, it is still generally indicated in the assessment of tumors or vascular malformations, and it has a special place in the pretreatment evaluation of nasopharyngeal tumors. The studies are usually performed under general anesthesia or heavy sedation and are only rarely associated with complications.[26,31]

Iodinated contrast material may also be used to opacify the lymphatic system. The technique is tedious for both the operator and child and at present has only a limited place in pediatric plastic surgical practice. In children with lymphedema, lymphatic channels may be aplastic, hypoplastic, or hyperplastic. This information is of only limited value today but improving surgical techniques may render it an important preoperative investigative modality. When lymphohemangiomas, lymphangiomas, or lymphoceles are present a direct injection of contrast medium into the lesion may help determine its nature, drainage, and size.

The gastrointestinal tract is infrequently examined in pediatric plastic surgery but is routine in a pediatric radiology department. The technique employs a positive contrast agent, usually barium, to opacify the tract. As mentioned previously, it is often combined with fluoroscopy or cineradiography to enable a functional, as well as anatomic, evaluation of the gastrointestinal tract to be made.

Computed tomography

Computed tomography (CT) is a recently developed imaging modality that greatly enhances tissue discrimination. Its tissue-discriminating capacity is at least 100 times that of conventional radiographic techniques. It provides a unique display of anatomic structures in thin cross sections with negligible artifact from tissues above and below the selected level. It is useful in determining the extent and nature of a structural abnormality.[13,33] In the acutely injured child it is invaluable in documenting and assessing head trauma,[21,34] and its place in determining the local and distant spread of tumors, especially to soft tissue, is well established.[13] The final role of CT in diagnosis is not established, but it is increasingly used in the evaluation of complex anatomic and pathologic problems, and, in this context, it may well have a role in pediatric plastic surgical practice.

Radioisotopic scintigraphy

Radioisotopic scintigraphy[41] uses a radiopharmaceutical or radioactively labeled complex whose chemical, physical, and biologic properties allow it to concentrate in a target organ or system being studied. In most instances, the radiopharmaceutical concentrates in normally functioning tissue, diseased areas being represented by decreased or absent activity. In a few organs the abnormal tissue concentrates the radiopharmaceutical to a greater degree than adjacent normal tissue. Tissue or organ localization may be due to active transport, phagocytosis, cell sequestration, capillary blockade, simple or exchange diffusion, and compartmental localization.

These techniques have only a limited role in pediatric plastic surgical practice, but they can be valuable in determining the extent of local and distant spread of tumor or in the identification of a presumed thyroid mass. Radionuclide techniques are also useful in evaluating bone function, and in this sense they are useful in determining the incorporation of bone grafts.[68]

The current limits of radionuclide studies are largely related to nonspecificity of the radiopharmaceuticals. There is a major possibility for advances in diagnosis as the specificity of these studies improve.

Ancillary imaging methods

Diagnostic ultrasound examinations are finding an increasingly large place in the pediatric practice. They are particularly useful in the evaluation or confirmation of cystic structures.[65] The easy accessibility of soft tissues to the ultrasound scanning head make it a useful modality in plastic surgery. A great advantage of the technique is that it does not require ionizing radiation.

Xeroradiography features a sensitized paper rather than film for recording images and is used in the examination of soft tissues. Its capacity to edge enhance structures makes it valuable in the assessment of the internal architecture of a soft tissue lesion. The radiation dose, although still low with this technique, is greater than with conventional plain film examination and therefore must be used with discretion.

RADIATION DOSE

Radiation dose depends on the technique and equipment used. Appropriate modifications of technique and equipment can materially reduce the patient dose, and this is a primary function of the radiologist and radiologic technician. Although generalization is difficult, most plain film radiographic examinations requiring two to five films deliver less than a rad to the skin, and the mean whole body doses in children for conventional studies range from 0.01 to 0.1 rad.[2,29,72] Radionuclide imaging and function tests in children are usually associated with a dose of less than 3 rad to the critical organ, and many tests deliver less than 1 rad. CT should be considered separately because the dose depends on the machine, technique, and body section examined.[12,71,73]

Precise information on the effects of this low-dose radiation is meager and inferential. Fabrikant[24] believes that it ''appears best for conservative planning to assume a linear relationship without a threshold between dose and affect in the region of low dose.'' If it is assumed that there is no threshold dose, each examination must be carefully weighed according to risk versus benefit.[45,48] The overall risk of leukemia from radiation is estimated to be one to two cases per million persons exposed per year per rad.[24] This is a minute risk for the individual. Genetic risks are similarly poorly defined at low-dose levels in humans. The usual gonadal mutation rate has been estimated not to double under 50 rad,[51] a gonadal dose much below that from most radiologic examinations. This implies that each examination be justified as potentially beneficial to the child.

GENERAL PRINCIPLES OF RADIOLOGIC INTERPRETATION

Radiologic methods basically display anatomy. Interpretation requires a thorough familiarity with the normal anatomic structures and their display by the appropriate imaging method. The continuing growth of the child complicates the issue, and what appears normal in a 5-year-old may not be normal in a 2-year-old. Detailed evaluation of normal radiologic anatomic structures is beyond the scope of this chapter and is well covered in the appropriate pediatric radiologic texts.[18] Radiologic abnormalities are recognized as departures from the normal. There may be deformity of or a deficiency in a normal structure or there may be additional tissue. Imaging methods may also evaluate function. Angiography and scintigraphy assess blood flow and distribution, fluoroscopy and cineradiography show respiratory and gastrointestinal movements, and serial plain films show skeletal growth and development.

In any diagnostic evaluation, it is important to know the common pitfalls. Projection, patient motion or rotation, and radiologic technique must be taken into account, especially when comparing structures on opposite sides of the body (Fig. 3-1).

X-ray beam penetration is determined largely by the incident kilovoltage; contrast and film blackening are determined by the milliamperage used for the exposure. Soft tissues are best examined with low kilovoltage, although enhancement of the difference between soft tissue and air-containing structures, such as the tracheal or nasal airway, is best done with a high-kilovoltage examination. The more sophisticated imaging methods require at least some knowledge of the mechanism or generation of the image. Thus CT cannot be sensibly interpreted without some knowledge of the window width and attenuation mean used to generate the image. Radionuclide studies must not be interpreted without some knowledge of the radiopharmaceutical used, timing of the images, and target organ.

HEAD AND NECK

The basic technique for examining the head and neck remains the plain film examination. This should include a posteroanterior (PA) projection inclined 15 degrees toward the orbitomeatal baseline (Fig. 3-2), a half-axial anteroposterior (AP) projection inclined 25 degrees to the orbitomeatal baseline (Fig. 3-3), a lateral examination centered over the region of the pituitary fossa, and an axial or submentovertex projection inclined at 90 degrees to the orbitomeatal baseline (Fig. 3-4). There are numerous modifications of this basic technique and specialized projections available when examination of the facial bones, sinuses, orbits, mastoid process, sella turcia, mandible, nasal bones, and palate are required.[19,54,69]

Radiologic examination is indicated in the evaluation of trauma, growth failure, and the presence of craniofacial developmental anomalies. It is also indicated in the assessment of diseases involving the mastoid process, sinuses, teeth, orbits, and optic canals.

Cephalometry is valuable with craniofacial anomalies. It uses a device which holds the head in a fixed position so that consistently reproducible radiographs of the skull and face can be obtained. Cephalometry can be used to assess facial bone growth and the progress of facial reconstruction. It requires a cooperative child who is prepared to sit still for the film, although some success has been achieved in infants with a modified supine cephalometer.[56] Tomography is useful in the skull, face, and petromastoid region. It can display complex bony anatomic structures clearly without superimposition of adjacent structures. The ocular radiation dose may be significantly reduced by performing the examination with the patient in a PA position or using eye shields.[9]

CT has revolutionized intracranial imaging and is of great value in the current assessment of head trauma. It appears likely that it will have an important place in the assessment of complex craniofacial anomalies, although this has not yet been firmly established.[15,16,42]

All of these methods require that the skull be immobilized during the examination. In the uncooperative young patient this may be difficult, and sedation may be necessary. To

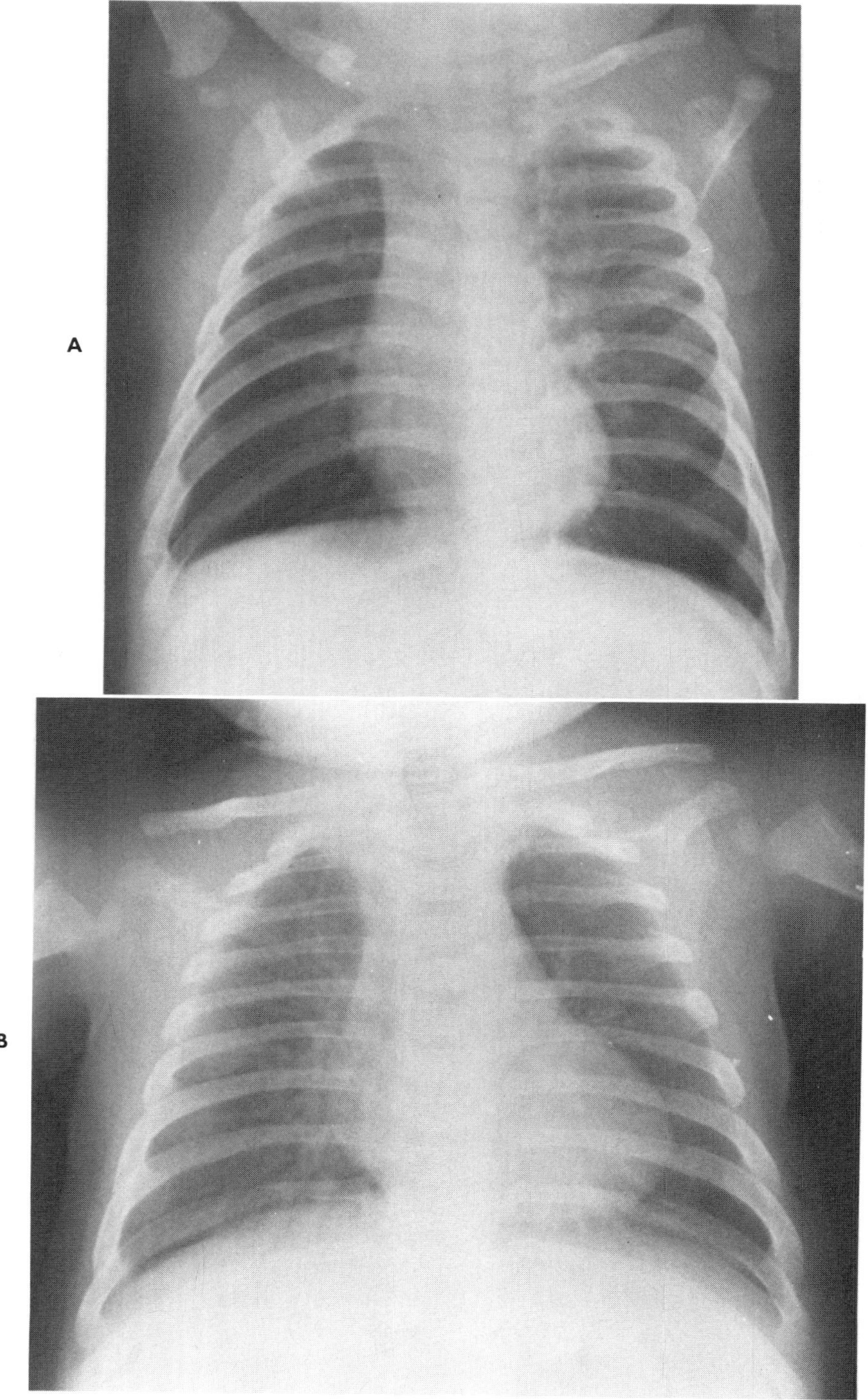

Fig. 3-1. A, Radiograph of child with chest rotated to right side. Note hypertransradiant right-sided hemithorax and configuration of heart, hilum, and mediastinum. **B,** Radiograph of same child with correct centering and absence of rotation.

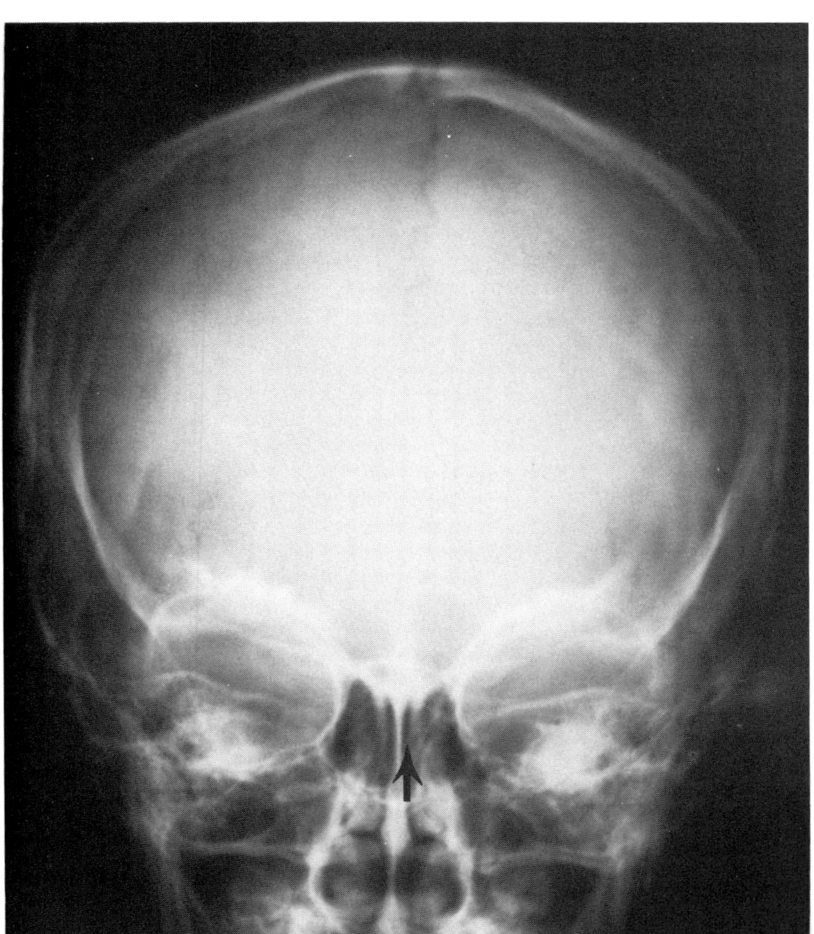

Fig. 3-3. Skull radiograph showing half-axial AP projection inclined 25 degrees to orbitomeatal baseline. This view demonstrates occipital bone, petrous bone, and pineal gland if calcified.

Fig. 3-2. Skull radiograph. PA projection midline 15 degrees toward orbitomeatal baseline demonstrates the frontal bone, orbits, ethmoid bone, and floor of pituitary fossa *(arrow)*.

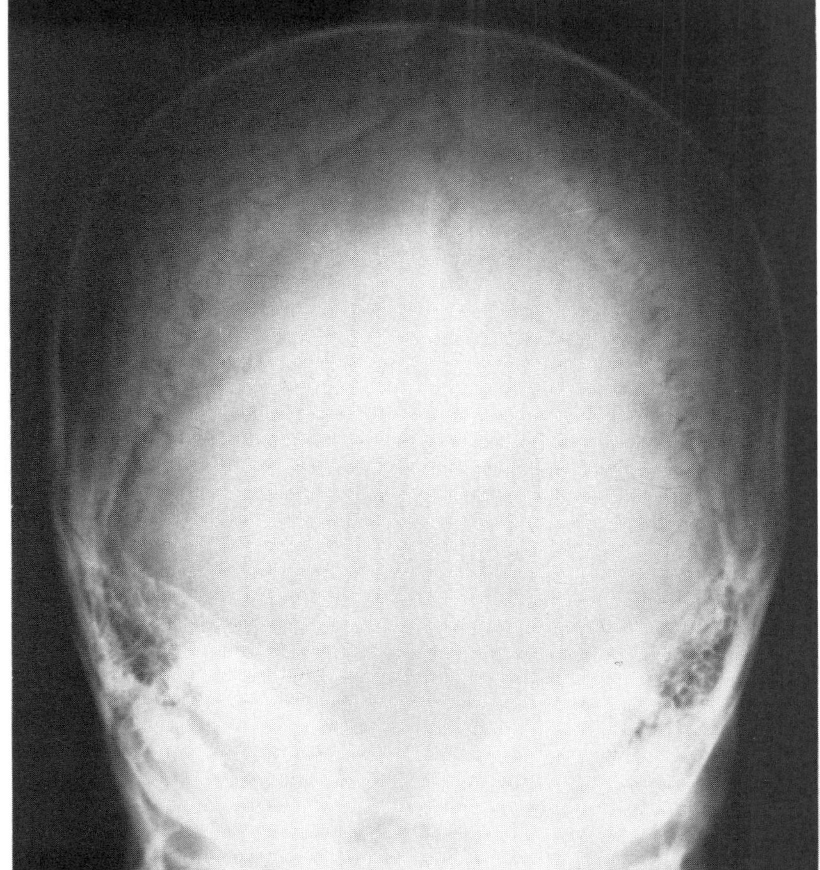

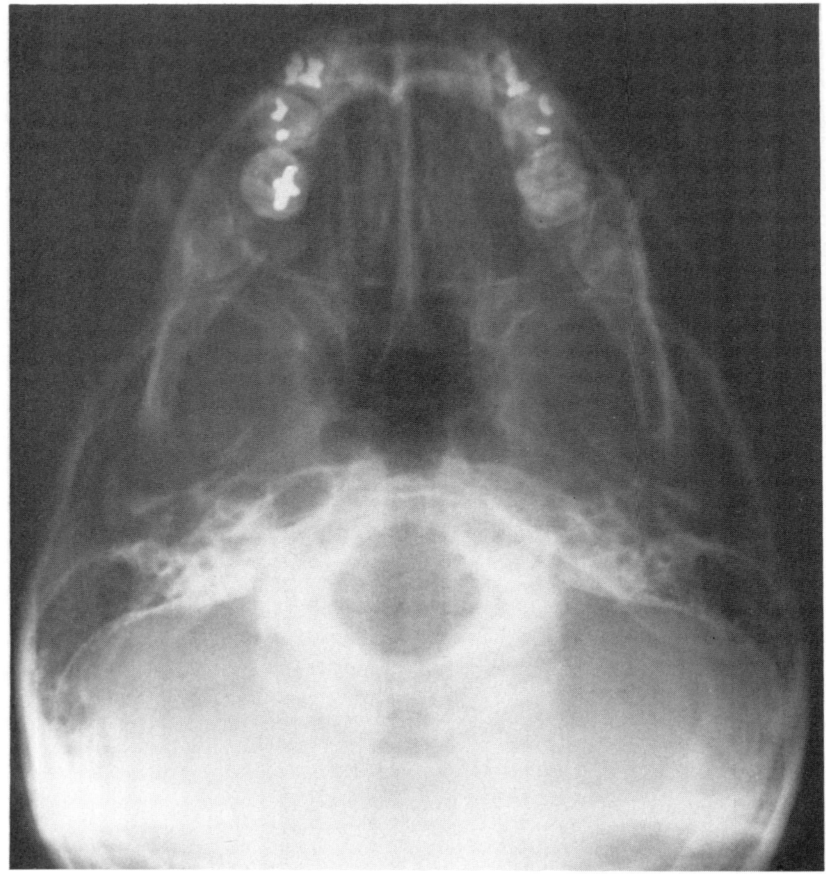

Fig. 3-4. Skull radiograph of axial or submentovertex basal projection inclined 90 degrees to orbitomeatal baseline. This projection demonstrates petromastoid bones including middle ear, nasopharynx, and middle cranial fossa floor.

make examination times as short as possible, high-milliamperage generators should be available.

Trauma

A routine skull examination is not indicated for every trivial injury. Classification of patients according to high or low risk allows a more rational use of skull radiography. Patients in the high-risk group include those with loss of consciousness, amnesia, stupor and semicoma, abnormal neurologic findings, palpable bony misalignments, discharges from the ear and nose, bilateral black eyes, and breathing difficulties. When Bell and Loop[5] divided their patients into these groups, they found 92 fractures in 1065 radiographic examinations in the high-risk group, and only one fracture in 435 examinations in the low-risk group. Fractures correlate poorly with cerebral complications. Harwood-Nash, Hendrick and Hudson[35] evaluated 4465 children with head trauma and found that fractures occurred in less than half the children with extradural hematomas. They also found that subdural hematomas occurred twice as frequently in children without fractures as in those with fractures. Roberts and Schopfner[59] reviewed 570 cases of head trauma in children and found 49 fractures. The presence of a fracture affected treatment in only two cases. In one of these it was depressed, and in the other it was associated with a foreign body.

CT is much more valuable in the high-risk group of patients with head injuries than plain film radiography. It is the best imaging method available for all major intracranial traumatic lesions.[21,40,74] It may demonstrate contusion or edema (Fig. 3-5), cerebral hemorrhage, and subdural or extradural fluid collections (Figs. 3-6 and 3-7). Intracranial air and air-fluid levels in the paranasal sinuses should raise the question of a possible fracture of the skull base. The detection of these fractures is difficult and may require detailed polytomography. This is, of course, impractical in acute injuries and is best left until the patient is improved clinically.

Facial fractures are an important subgroup that may necessitate detailed radiographic assessment. Apart from those

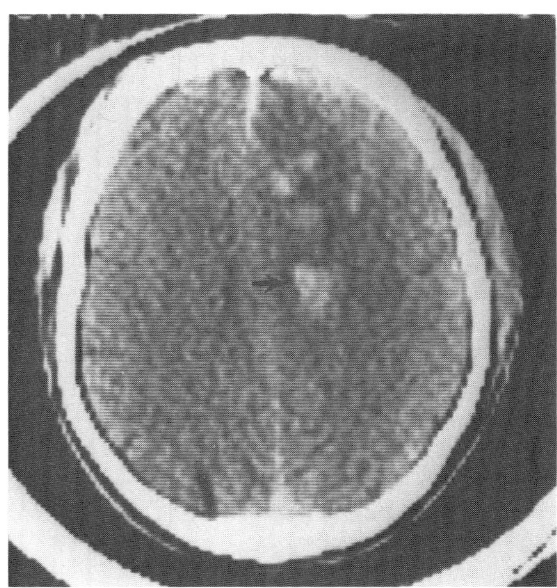

Fig. 3-5. Cranial CT scan of traumatic cerebral contusion and edema. High-density lesions in right cerebral hemisphere characteristic of hemorrhage *(arrow)*. Surrounding low density is consistent with cerebral edema.

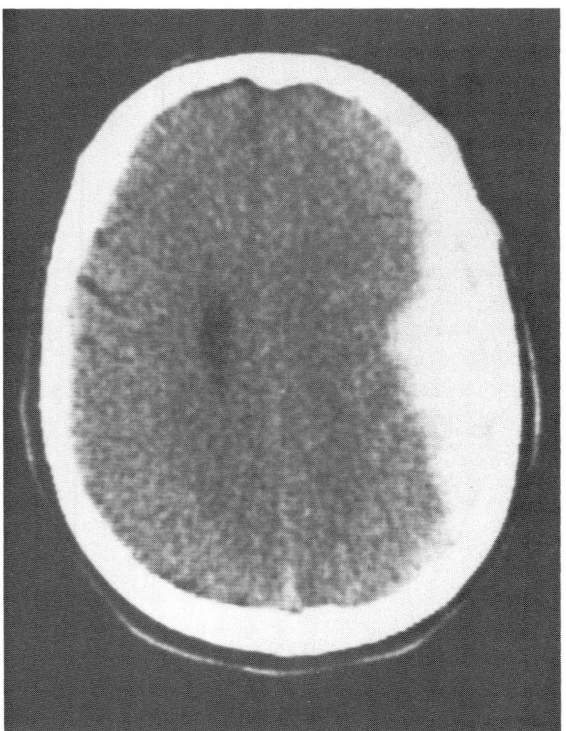

Fig. 3-6. Cranial CT scan demonstrating acute extradural hematoma. High-density rim around right cerebral hemisphere is characteristic of acute extracerebral hematoma.

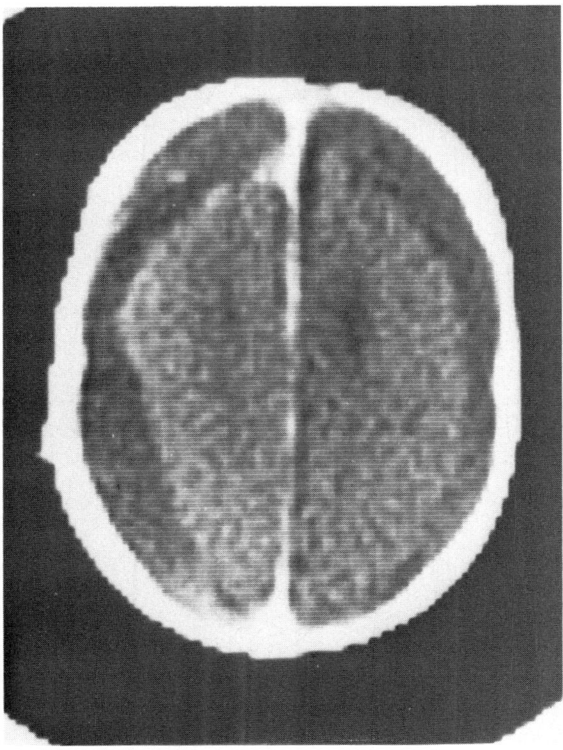

Fig. 3-7. Cranial CT scan demonstrating chronic extracerebral hematoma. Low-density rim about both cerebral hemispheres is characteristic of extracerebral collections.

involving the nasal apparatus facial fractures are relatively uncommon in children. This is probably because of the large cartilaginous component of the face, which provides greater resilience to trauma. Plain radiographic examination of the facial bones should include a standard AP-inclined projection, an occipitomental projection inclined 25 to 35 degrees to the orbitomeatal baseline (Fig. 3-8, *A*), a lateral projection centered on the outer canthus of the eye (Fig. 3-8, *B*), and a soft tissue technique submentovertical zygomatic arch view (Fig. 3-8, *C*).[19,69] These may not always demonstrate the extent and site of trauma accurately, and tomography is often necessary when a fracture is suspected or the lesion is complex and involves more than one facial bone. Tomographic examination is usually performed in the coronal plane, although the ethmoid bones are better assessed in a lateral section. When orbital fractures are present or suspected, tomography is the most effective way of establishing a diagnosis and determining bony displacement (Fig. 3-9).

Nasal fractures may be difficult to diagnose radiologically. Axial and soft tissue low-kilovoltage profile views of the nose represent the minimal examination that should be performed. The axial view demonstrates the relationship of the nasal bones to the nasal septum and maxilla and as such is essential in the assessment of unilateral nasal bone fractures. Even then unilateral fractures may not be seen, and a history of trauma, bleeding, and localized tenderness is more reliable. The profile examination, although useful in demonstrating fractures of the anterior nasal bridge, may be of little value in unilateral nasal bone fractures. When nasal bone fractures are complicated and there is maxillary involvement, tomography may be required.

Mandibular fractures in children occur most frequently about the bicuspids. Fractures of the condylar processes are relatively common and may be associated with rotary displacement. This can be indicated on the half-axial examination of the skull, which often shows the condylar heads. However, the diagnosis may require tomography in coronal and lateral planes. Lateral section tomography, after the place of the temporomandibular joint has been determined, should be performed with mouth opened and closed. Radiologic examination by this method gives a good anatomic assessment of joint function.

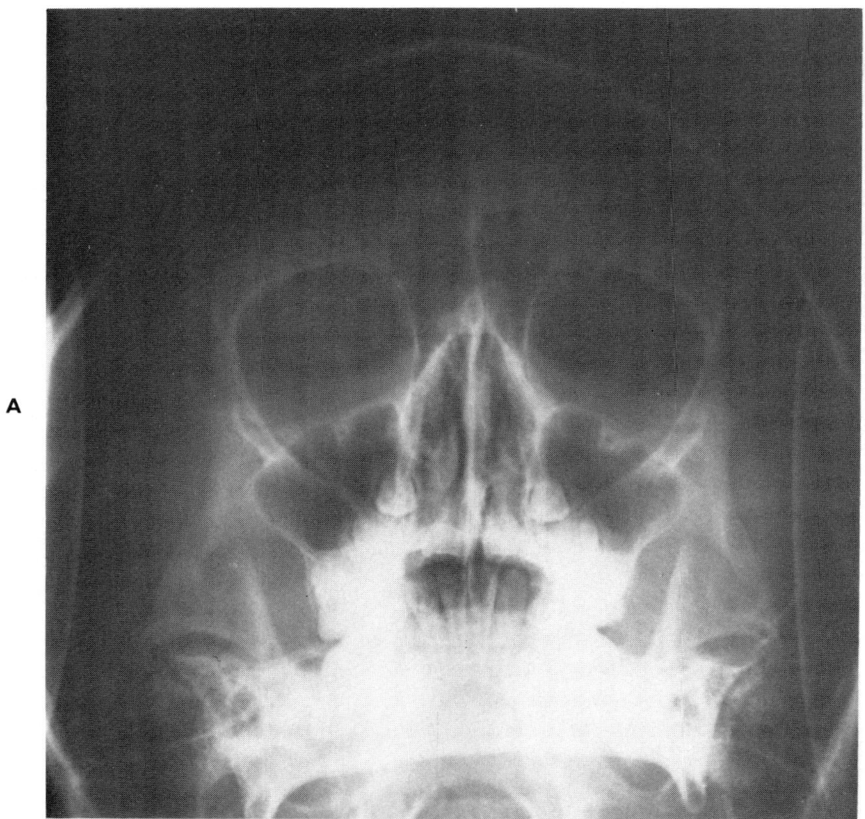

Fig. 3-8. Facial bone radiographic series. **A,** Occipitomental projection inclined 30 degrees to orbitomeatal baseline. **B,** Lateral projection. **C,** Soft tissue technique submentovertical zygomatic arch view. Occipitomental projection demonstrates maxillary antra and orbital floors particularly well.

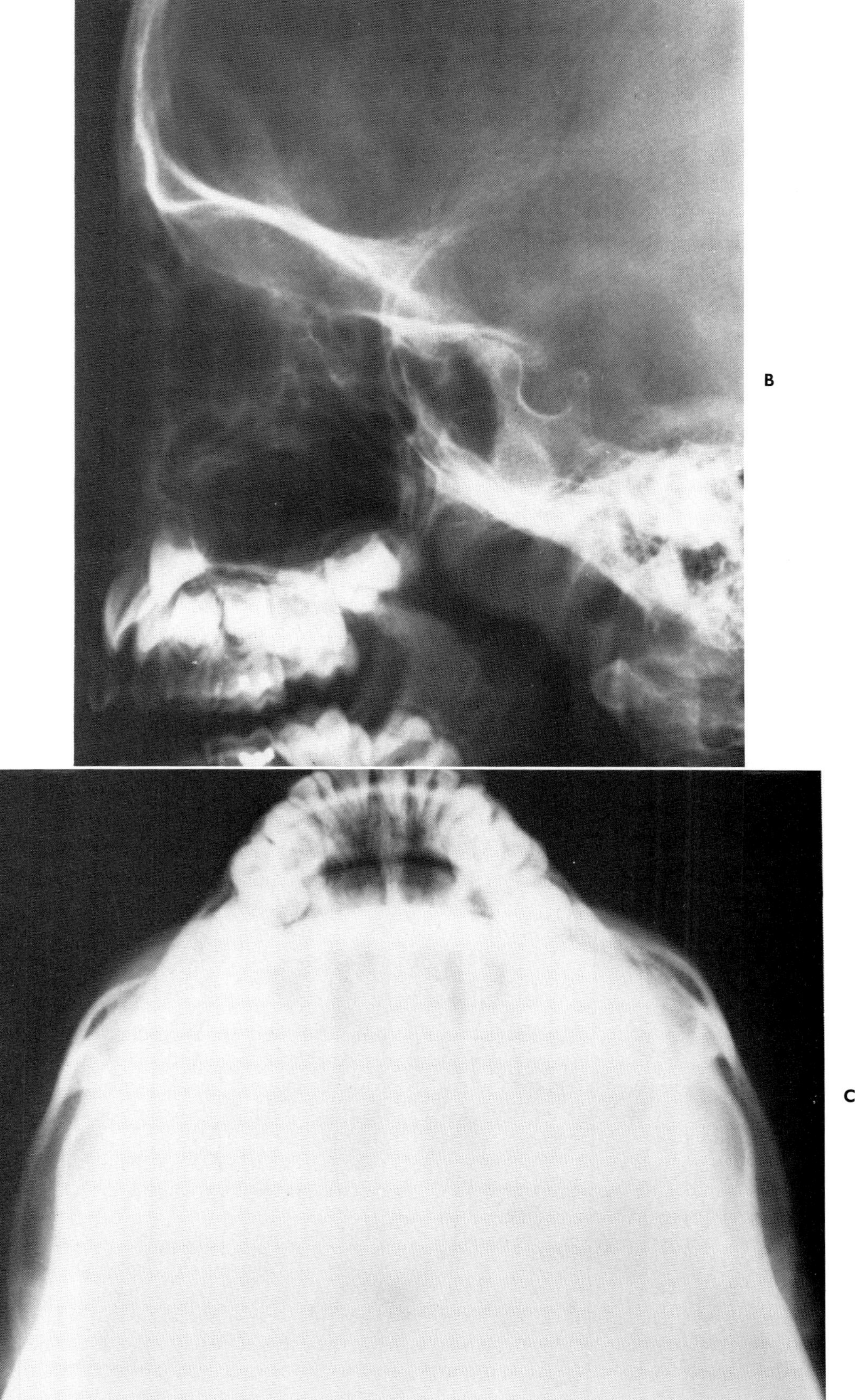

Fig. 3-8, cont'd. For legend see opposite page.

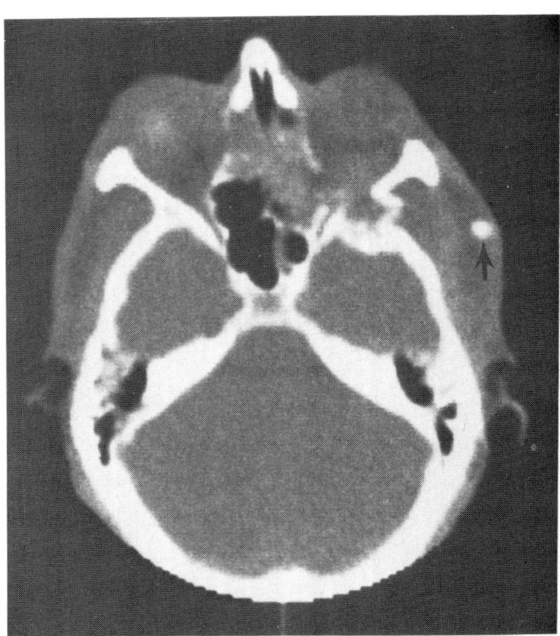

Fig. 3-9. Cranial CT scan showing fractures of ethmoid bones and right lateral orbital wall. Spent bullet fragment is seen *(arrow)* in soft tissues of temporal fossa.

Craniofacial anomalies

The role of the imaging method for craniofacial anomalies[62] is to define the anatomic abnormality and observe its progress both before and after treatment. Routine projections are frequently combined with cephalometric examinations and in recent years a CT examination. When the anomaly is midline there may be associated intracranial maldevelopment and cranial CT should be performed (Fig. 3-10). Cranial CT, angiography, gas encephalography, or metrizamide computed cisternography may be required to evaluate patients with hydrocephalus, meningoceles, and cranial encephaloceles, especially when operative treatment is considered (Fig. 3-11).[17,50]

Orbital hypertelorism may develop as an isolated phenomenon or coexist with craniosynostosis, craniofacial dysraphism, or a frontal encephalocele. The principal finding in hypertelorism is widening of the ethmoidal sinuses anteriorly with inferior displacement of the cribriform plate. There is widening of the interorbital distance as measured between the medial wall of the orbits at the junction of the angular process of the frontal bone with the maxillary and lacrimal bones. Standards for this have been determined by Currarino and Silverman[20] and Hansman.[32]

Craniostenosis is the most common craniofacial developmental anomaly. The configuration of the skull depends upon the sutures involved. Sagittal stenosis is associated with a long narrow skull (Fig. 3-12), coronal stenosis with a tall foreshortened skull when bilateral (Fig. 3-13), and an asymmetric skull when unilateral (Fig. 3-14). Both sagittal and coronal sutures may be obliterated, in which case the skull has a long vertical diameter and a short AP and lateral

diameter. If the lambdoidal suture is synostosed it can produce elongation of the vertical diameter of the skull. Lambdoidal synostosis may be unilateral or bilateral. In some cases generalized synostosis of all sutures may occur, microcephaly is present, and there is often increased intracranial pressure, exophthalmos, and optic atrophy. Radiographic examination of these patients needs to be precise, and careful attention to patient positioning is required. Projections taken tangential to an involved suture may reveal local hyperostosis and ridging.

A common concomitant of the craniostenoses is midface hypoplasia. In Crouzon's disease, in addition to the scaphocephalic and trigoncephalic calvarial deformities mandibular prognathism, shallow orbits, and exophthalmos are present (Fig. 3-15). In Apert's syndrome the midface hypoplasia is associated with oxycephaly from coronal synostosis, a high incidence of cleft palate, and a complex syndactyly of the hands and feet (Fig. 3-16). Treacher Collins' syndrome is characterized by hypoplasia of the zygomatic bone, short mandibular rami, small maxillae, significant deformity of the external ear, and an antimongoloid slant to the eyes.[25,47] These and other facial dysostoses need to be carefully examined radiologically and clinically before surgical correction is attempted.

Cleft palate

A high incidence of associated anomalies occurs with cleft lip and palate.[44] These include the Pierre Robin syndrome, Klippel-Feil syndrome, orofaciodigital syndrome,[22,28] Ellis–van Creveld syndrome, and congenital heart disease.

Radiologic examination may do no more than document

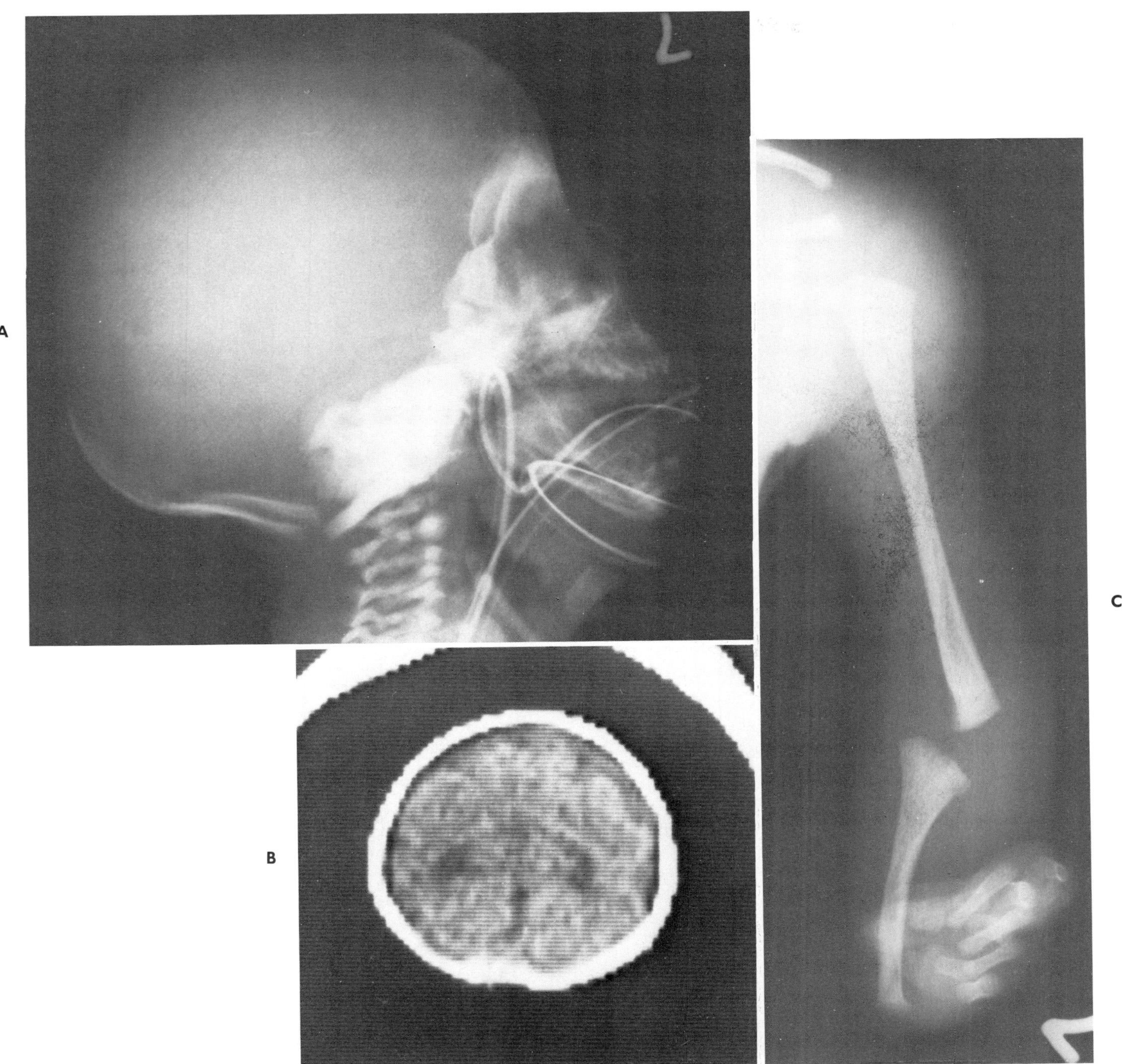

Fig. 3-10. Midline facial abnormalities. **A,** Lateral view of skull demonstrating facial abnormality and microcephaly. **B,** Cranial CT scan. Same patient as **A** with absence of frontal horns. **C,** Radiograph of upper limb shows absent radius and dislocated wrist.

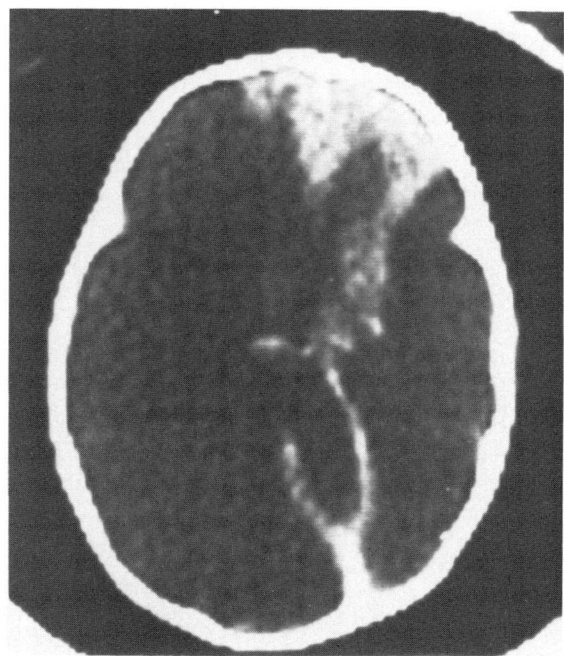

Fig. 3-11. Cranial CT scan demonstrating gross hydranencephaly. Cerebral remnants of frontal lobes are visualized anteriorly. Asymmetric tentorium is present.

the cleft palate, but it does have a valuable role in the assessment of associated anomalies. Imaging methods also may be important in the progress assessment of treatment. Cephalometric methods generally are used but these can be combined with cineradiography of the nasopharynx and oropharynx to document velopharyngeal function when its competence is in question after palatal repair.[44]

Auricular deformities

Since auricular deformities may be associated with anomalies of the middle and inner ear, the morphologic assessment should include a polytomographic radiologic examination. A urographic examination also should be performed because of the increased incidence of developmental anomalies associated with auricular deformities.[10,67]

Tumors

Tumors[18] characteristically deform the tissue in which they are localized and as such may be recognized radiographically. Tumors of bone are usually readily appreciated with conventional techniques, although they may require special projections and tomographic examination to clarify their nature. When tumor growth is slow and involves bone, a characteristic sclerotic margin of the lesion is recognizable radiologically. This represents a reparative bony response to the tumor and suggests that the underlying tumor is grow-

ing slowly or not at all. It contrasts with the rather irregular ragged appearance of the margin of a malignant lesion. CT is useful in determining tumor extent, particularly in the nasopharyngeal and paranasal sinus regions.

When a tumor involves the soft tissues it may be difficult to image by conventional methods. If it has a cystic component, such as in a developmental or remnant cyst of the head and neck, diagnostic ultrasound may be of value.

TRUNK AND SPINE

In practical terms lesions of the trunk that are treated by the plastic surgeon only occasionally require an imaging evaluation. However, techniques are available to define the site, extent, and possible internal architecture. The spine needs special consideration, and many imaging methods are available to assess the vertebral column and its canal and contents.[34,43] A plain film series is always the preliminary procedure. This should include at least an AP and lateral examination. Measurements of the interpediculate distances and sagittal diameter are important in determining the presence or absence of spinal rachischisis.[18,36-38,66] When diastematomyelia is suspected, the examination should be combined with tomography. Clinically silent anomalies of the vertebrae and vertebral laminae frequently are seen without any significant associated sequelae. In infancy evaluation

Text continued on p. 40.

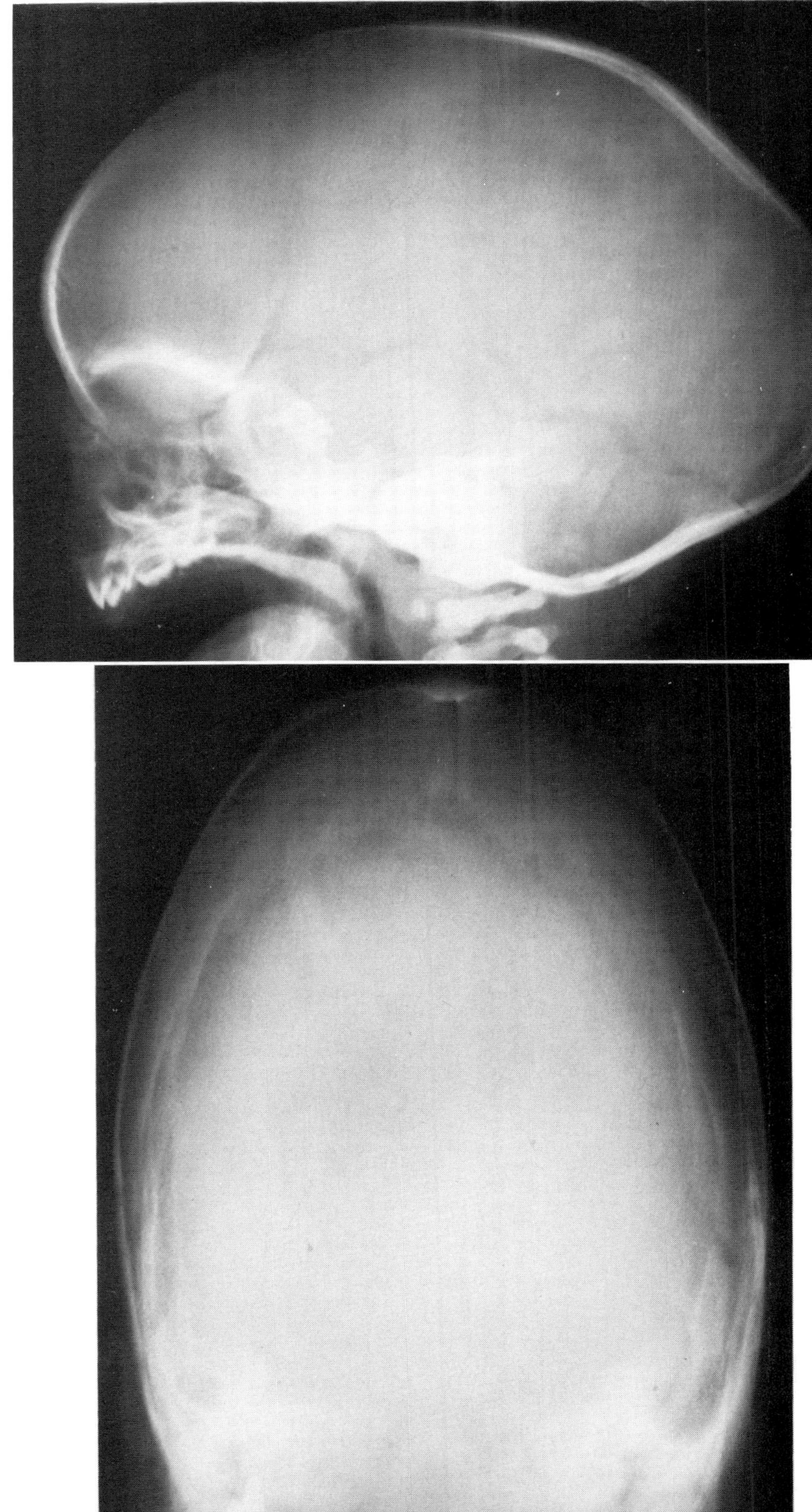

Fig. 3-12. Sagittal synostosis.

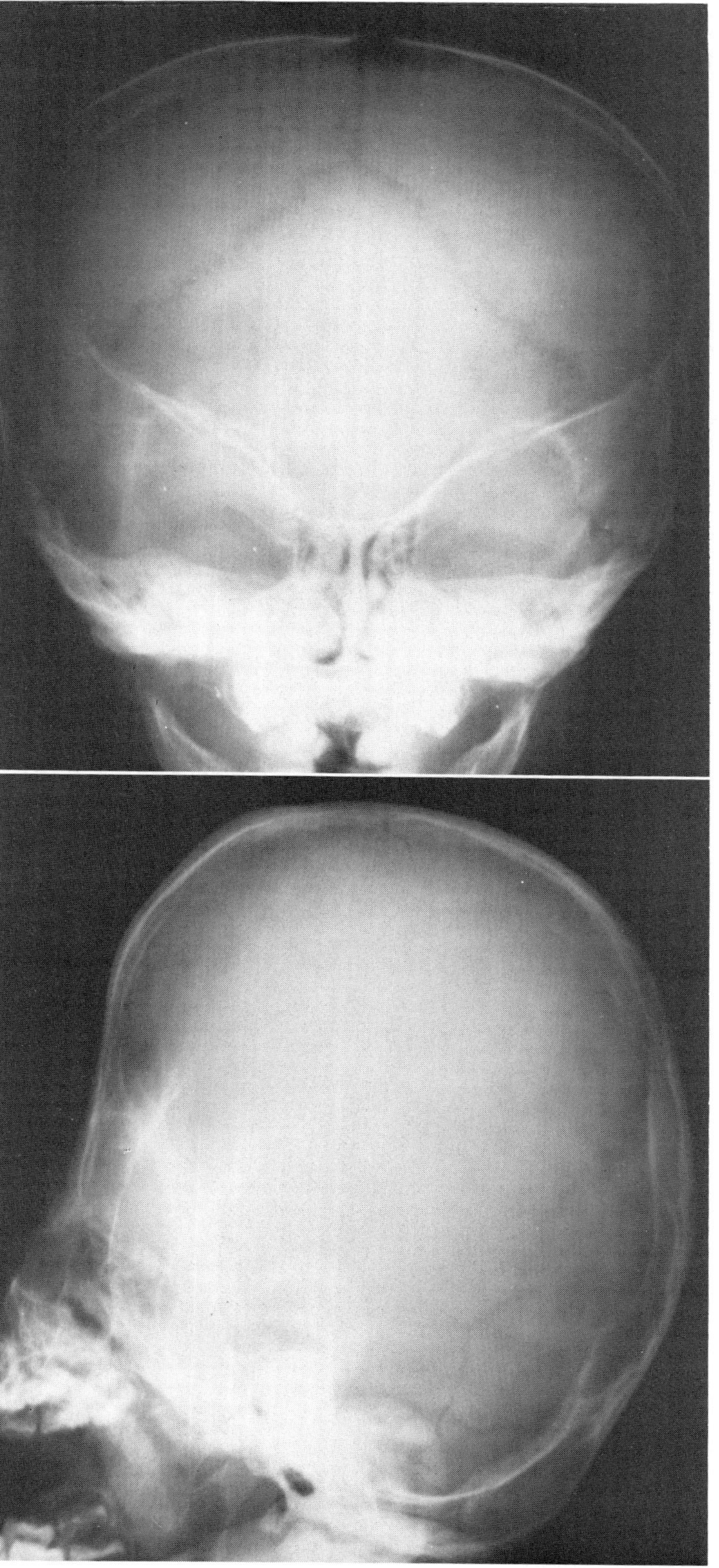

Fig. 3-13. Coronal synostosis.

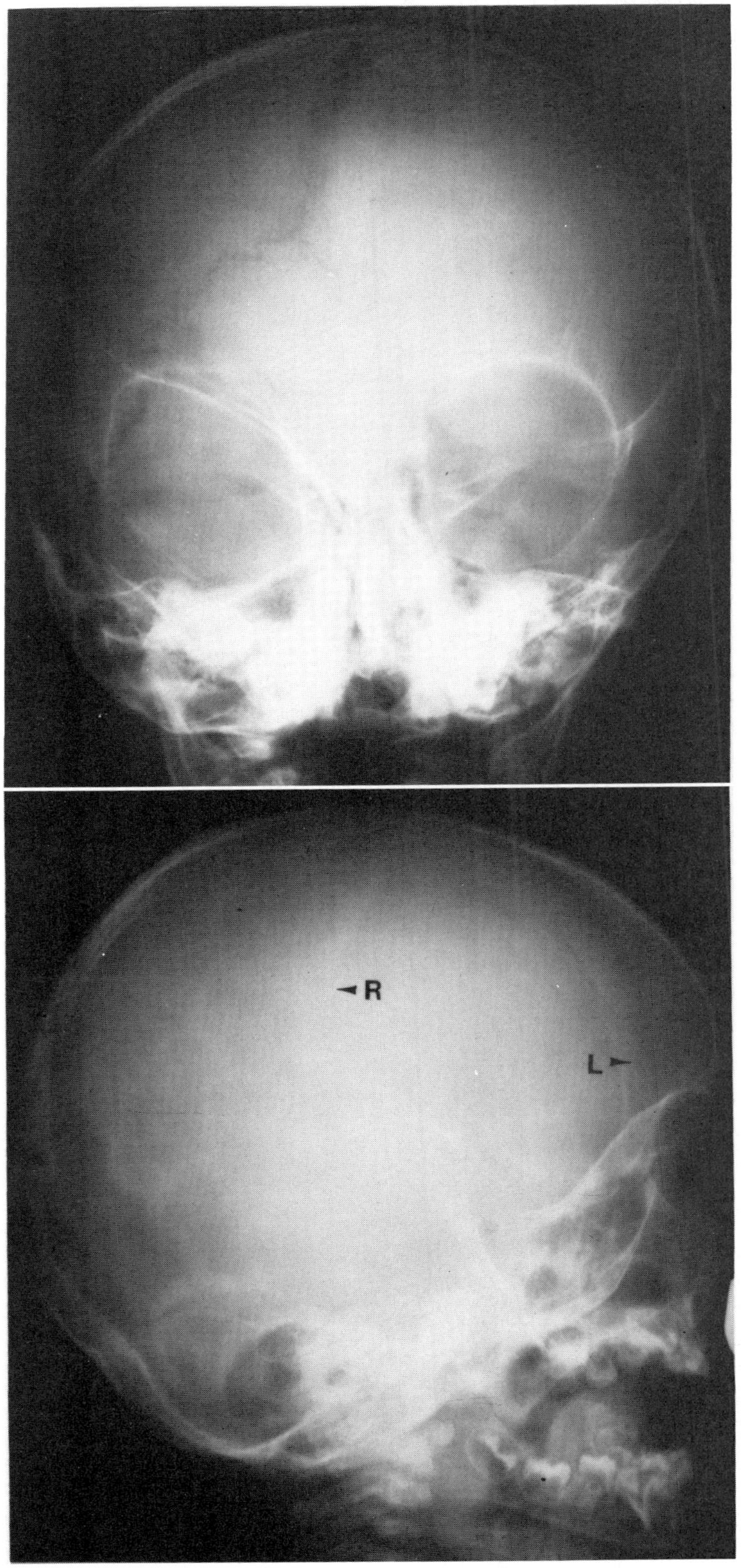

Fig. 3-14. Right-sided coronal synostosis.

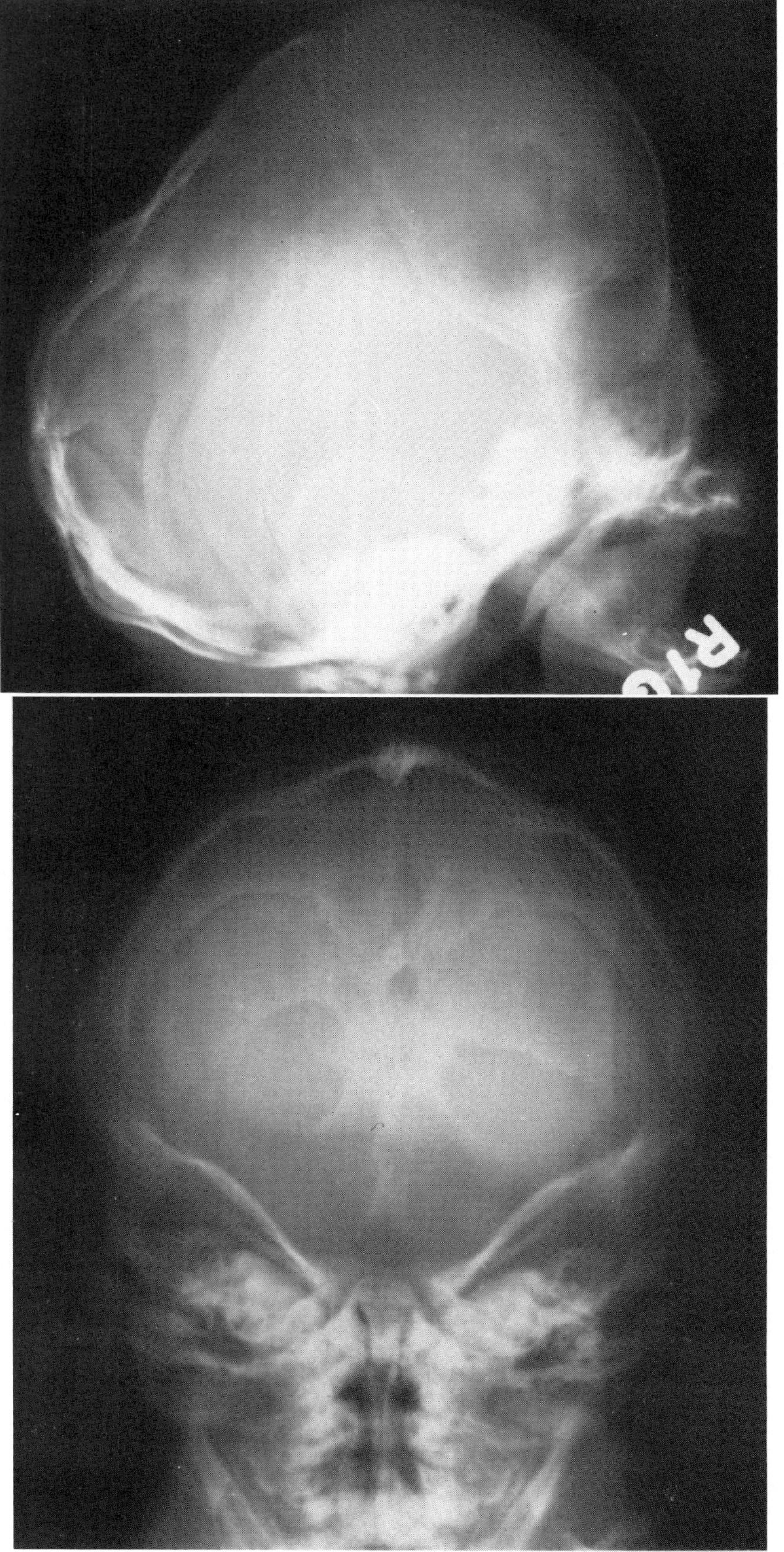

Fig. 3-15. Crouzon's disease showing midface hypoplasia, shallow orbits, and extensive cranio-synostosis.

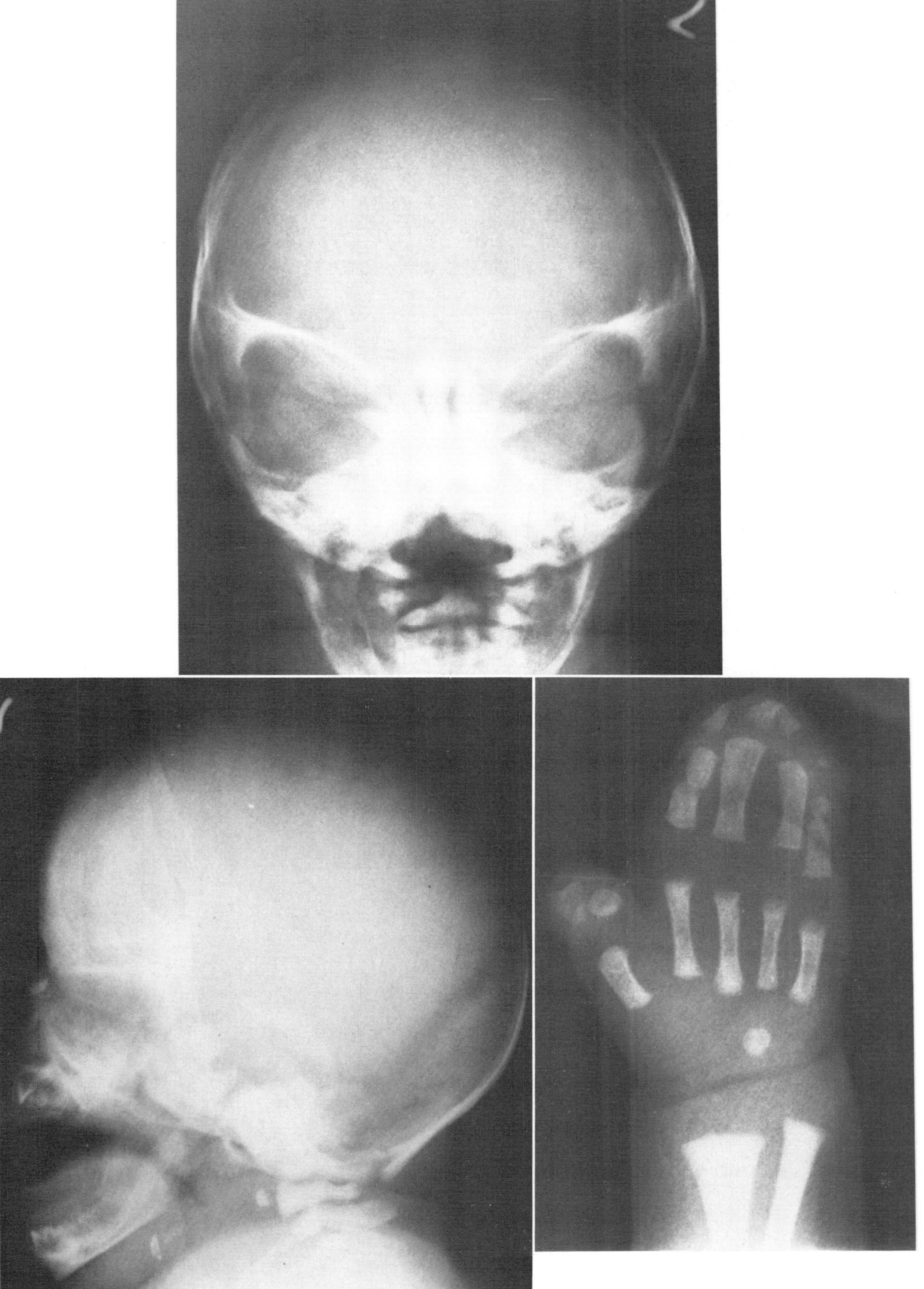

Fig. 3-16. Apert's syndrome.

may be difficult because the laminal ossification centers, although present, do not fuse until ages 6 to 24 months. In the upper cervical region and lower lumbar region, laminal fusion is further delayed until the second or third year in the former and the fifth in the latter. Measurements of interpediculate distances may be difficult in the young because the pedicles exist partly in cartilage; however, tables of interpediculate distances are available for use in children. In the occult situation, developmental anomalies of the vertebral column do not justify invasive examination unless symptoms or signs of neurologic dysfunction are present. If these symptoms and signs are present, myelography with metrizamide or oxygen and occasionally CT are indicated.

Meningoceles or meningomyeloceles appear radiologically as fusiform dilatations of the spinal canal. There is failure of laminal development, widening of the interpediculate distances, sloping pedicles, and anomalies of segmentation. Although these defects are usually obvious, if they are small or present anteriorly, they may require myelography and CT for diagnosis.[34]

EXTREMITIES

Radiologic evaluation of developmental defects of the limbs is important to their understanding; when surgical correction is contemplated, radiologic evaluation is mandatory (Fig. 3-17). Since unossified epiphyses cannot be visualized in the newborn, accurate evaluation using conventional radiologic methods may not be possible. If developmental anomalies are present, comparison views from both sides of the body should be performed. When bone age assessment is required,* it is important to realize that the most useful and accurate radiologic techniques are different at different ages. From birth to 2 years, the examination should include a PA view of the hands, including the wrists; and AP and lateral examination of the knees; and an AP and lateral examination of the feet. Beyond the age of 2 years a PA examination of the hands, including the wrists, is required, and this is sometimes supplemented with a PA and lateral examination of the knees. Bone age examination should be obtained in children who are too small or tall and those have congenital malformations. The method has some value in the prediction of final height.[3,58] Disharmonic maturation of the carpal bones and long bones is often present in congenital disorders and can be an important factor in diagnosis.[55] The individual lenghts of the metacarpal bones and phalanges and carpal angles similarly can be useful in

---

*References, 1, 30, 39, 57, and 58.

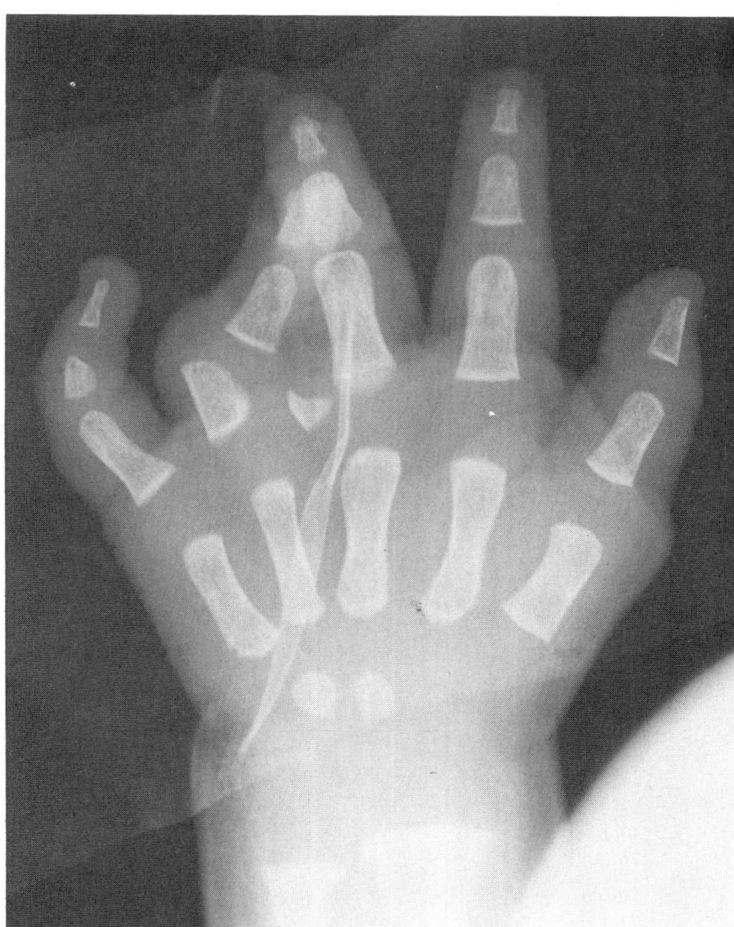

Fig. 3-17. Left hand with congenital webbing of third and fourth digits and accessory bone.

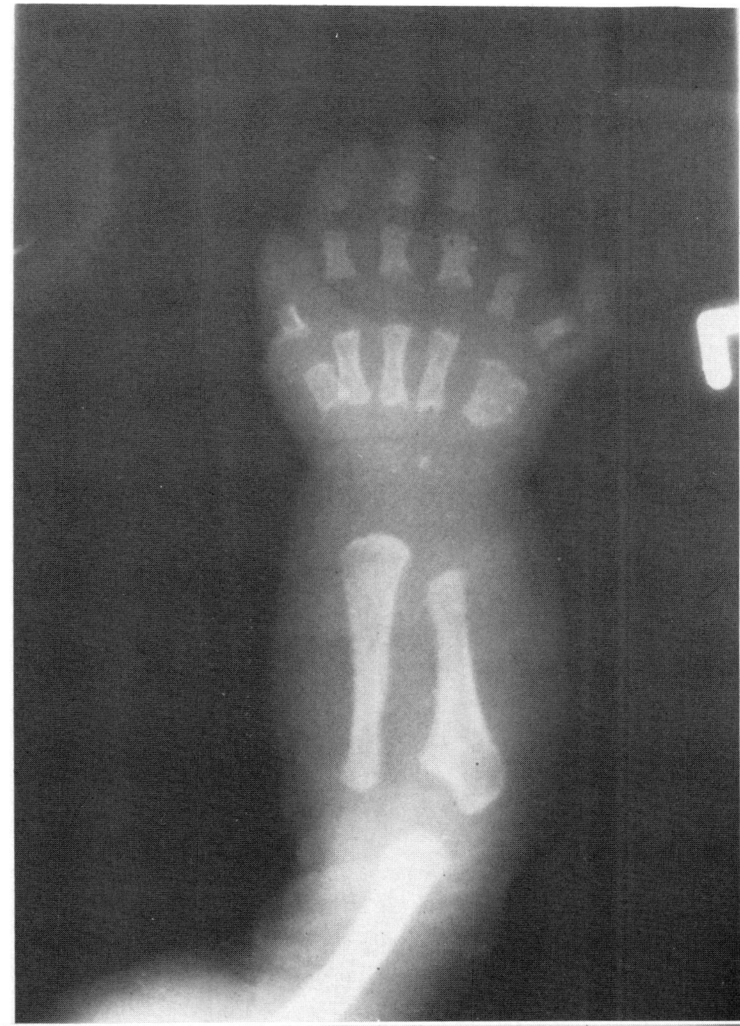

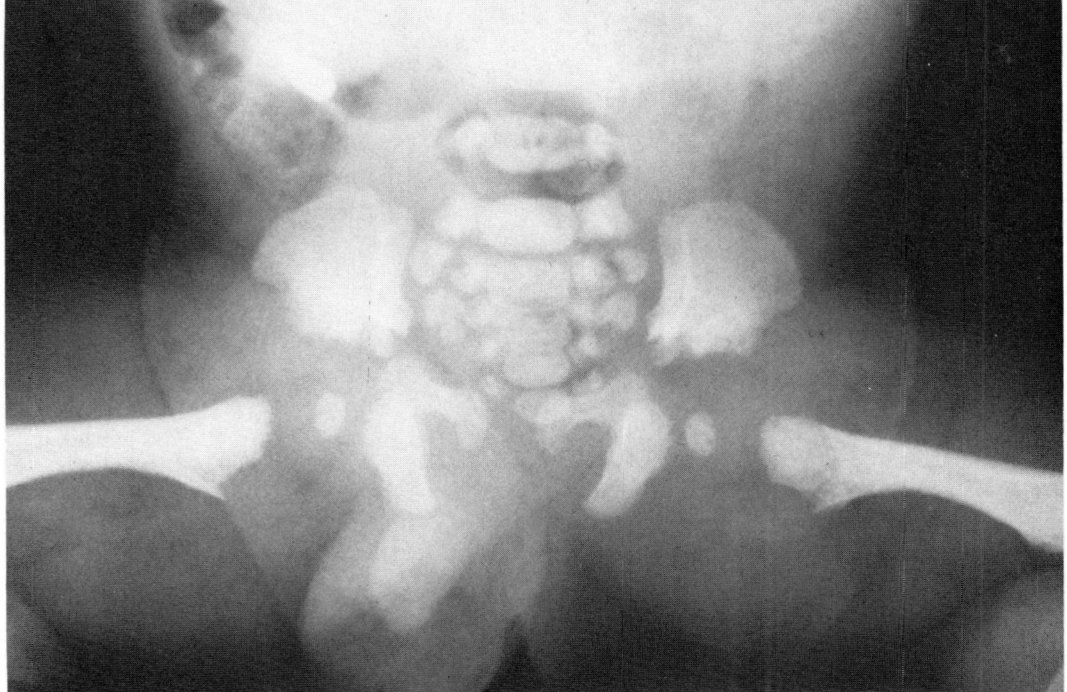

Fig. 3-18. Ellis–van Creveld syndrome showing polydactyly, flared hypoplastic iliac wings, small sciatic notches, and bowed femur.

the elucidation of developmental anomalies.[53] Where an underlying skeletal dysplasia or dysostosis is suspected, a general skeletal radiologic examination should be undertaken (Fig. 3-18). This usually comprises an AP and lateral examination of the lumbar spine, including an AP examination of the pelvis; an AP and lateral examination of the dorsal spine, including the thoracic cage; an AP examination of both the right and left femur; an AP examination of the right and left tibia and fibula; an AP examination of the right and left humerus; an AP examination of the right and left radius and ulna; a PA examination of the hands; an AP examination of the feet; and a PA and lateral examination of the skull. A developmental problem should be suspected when multiple bones and joints are involved or multiple clinical abnormalities are present. Acquired abnormalities

may locally destroy, expand, deform, or otherwise alter normal tissues at least as judged radiologically. Thus benign tumors typically expand or deform and malignant tumors typically destroy bone (Fig. 3-19).

Examination of the soft tissues of the extremities can be enhanced by low-kilovoltage techniques or xerography. This will probably be superseded by CT in areas where the anatomy is complex. Vascular abnormalities, although partly visualized sometimes on plain film examination, are much better analyzed with an added contrast medium. Thus venography in venous, arteriography in arterial, and lymphography in lymphatic abnormalities are indicated when these structures are implicated and therapy planned. Arteriovenous malformations or fistulae need detailed angiographic examination before any primary resection is at-

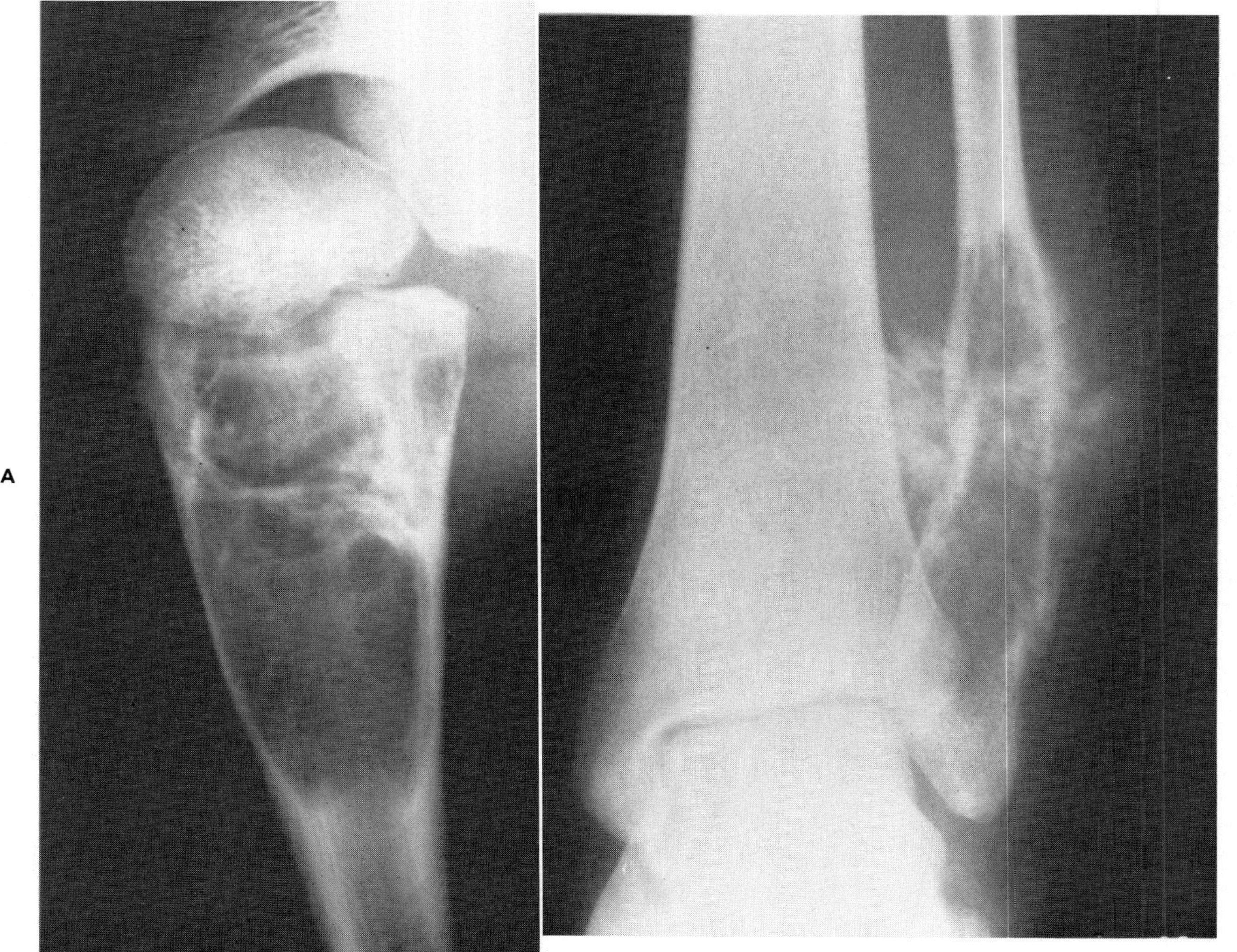

Fig. 3-19. A, Radiograph of benign cystic lesions of upper end of humerus that caused compensatory bone expansion and marginal bone sclerosis. **B,** Radiograph of malignant tumor of lower end of fibula. Destructive lesion of bone induced florid periosteal response.

tempted. Lymphangiography may document the presence and nature of a congenital or acquired lymphatic abnormality, and, although this was largely of academic interest until recently, advances in surgical techniques may see it routinely used in the preoperative evaluation of lymphatic disorders.

GENITOURINARY ABNORMALITIES

Among many other indications, urography is usually performed in children with an imperforate anus[6,8]; developmental anomalies of the ear, trunk, and face[20,37,52,67]; prune belly syndrome[7,23]; most genital anomalies and intersex problems[46]; congenital scoliosis of kyphosis[49,70]; or myelomeningoceles or myelodysplasia because of the frequent association of renal tract abnormalities.[27] Intravenous urography is the examination of first choice in the evaluation of the structure of the upper renal tracts and bladder. Preliminary dehydration of a child is not usually required and in fact is contraindicated in the infant. Complications are very

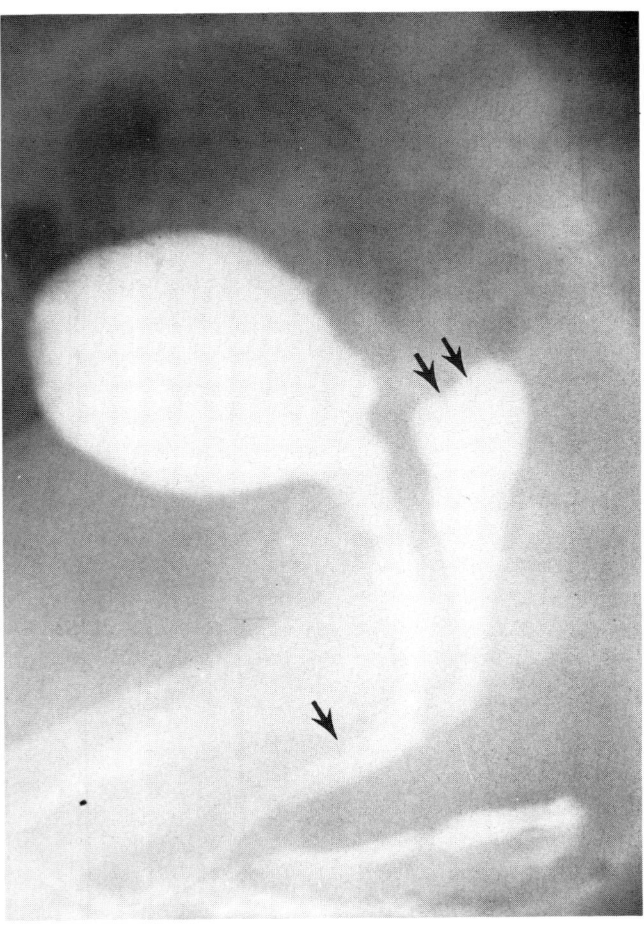

Fig. 3-20. Genitogram of 2-month-old virilized girl with adrenogenital syndrome. Genitogram demonstrates large urogenital sinus indented by cervix *(arrows)* and penile urethra *(arrow).*

rare in children undergoing intravenous urography.[4] Voiding cystourethrography[63] is an importtant technique to evaluate the lower renal tract, especially when genital anomalies are present. After retrograde filling of the bladder with a diluted contrast medium, spot films are taking during voiding.

Genitography[64] is similarly useful in children with genital anomalies, particularly those which are complex. Its object is to determine the internal structures of the urogenital tracts. The examination is performed by either a flushing or multiple catheter technique combined with fluoroscopy and sometimes cineradiography to document any flash filling of the internal genital passages (Fig. 3-20). Ultrasound is useful in these children to demonstrate a uterus and ovaries.

PREOPERATIVE CHEST RADIOGRAPHY

The value of a routine preoperative chest radiography in children remains controversial. Brill, Ewing, and Dunn[14]reviewed the chest radiographs of 1000 healthy children in a preventive clinic in a low-income area in New York City. Six percent of the children had minor radiographic abnormalities, none of which required treatment. Sagel et al.[60] similarly found no significant abnormality in 521 patients under 20 years of age who had routine preoperative chest radiography. These studies are countered by that from the Minneapolis Children's Health Center. Sane et al.[61] prospectively studied the routine radiographs of 1500 pediatric patients and found that 7.5% demonstrated at least one abnormality. In 4.7% of the patients the abnormality was totally unsuspected, and in 3.8% it led to surgery being postponed or canceled or an alteration in the anesthetic technique used.

Drawing conclusions from these conflicting data is difficult; however, in many centers routine preoperative chest radiography in children has been abandoned. In practice it seems reasonable to only undertake a preoperative chest radiographic examination when the patient's condition warrants. This should be when there is a clinical evidence of underlying chest or cardiac disease processes. In some centers many children having major surgery undergo preoperative chest radiography; the younger the child the more frequently this occurs.

POSTOPERATIVE CHEST RADIOGRAPHY

Although complications are uncommon after pediatric plastic surgical procedures, pulmonary collapse, aspiration, pulmonary edema, and pneumonia occur. Often these can be differentiated radiologically. Pulmonary collapse is characterized by fissure shift, increased pulmonary density, and secondary compensatory movement of the mediastinum or diaphragm to the side of the pulmonary collapse (Fig. 3-21). Aspiration characteristically occurs in the dependent portions of the lungs. Pulmonary collapse is often bilateral and may be widespread. It typically produces a patchy opacification of the posterior and basal lung parenchyma. Postoperative pulmonary edema (Fig. 3-22) is typically as-

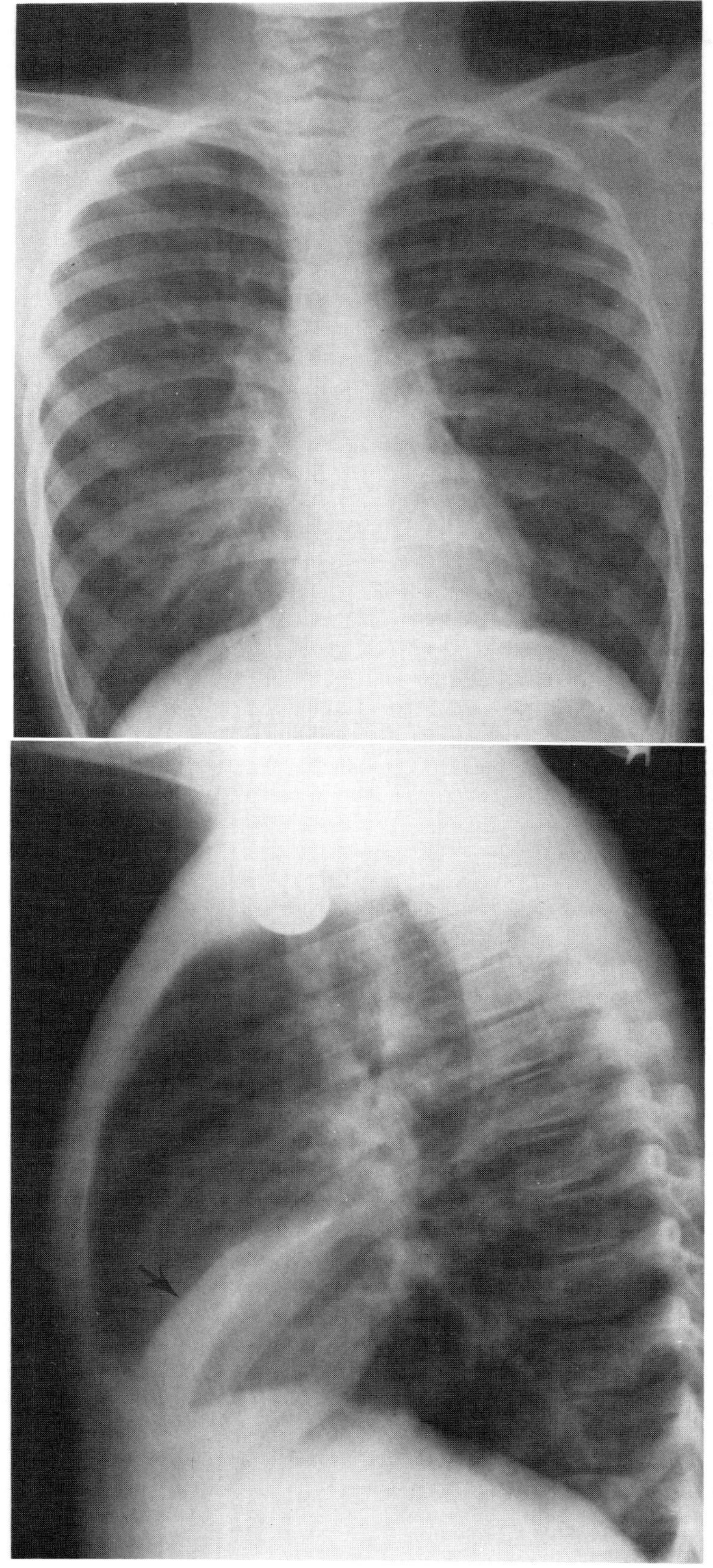

Fig. 3-21. Radiographs demonstrating collapse of right middle lobe. Note reduction in volume of middle lobe *(arrow)*, which is best demonstrated on lateral examination of chest.

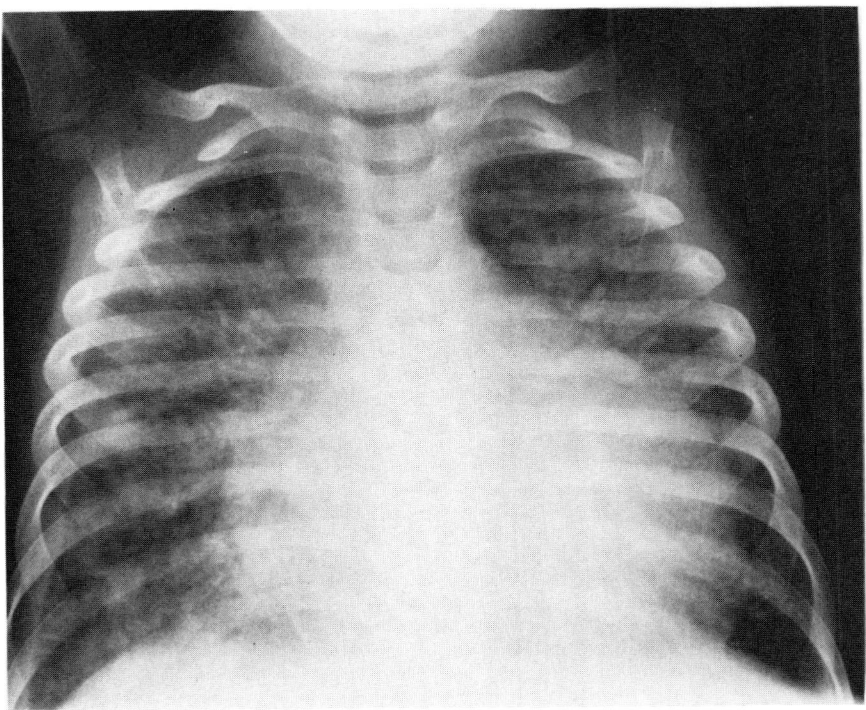

Fig. 3-22. Radiograph of pulmonary edema. Note cardiac enlargement, indistinct perihilar and hilar anatomy, and right-sided basal pleural effusion.

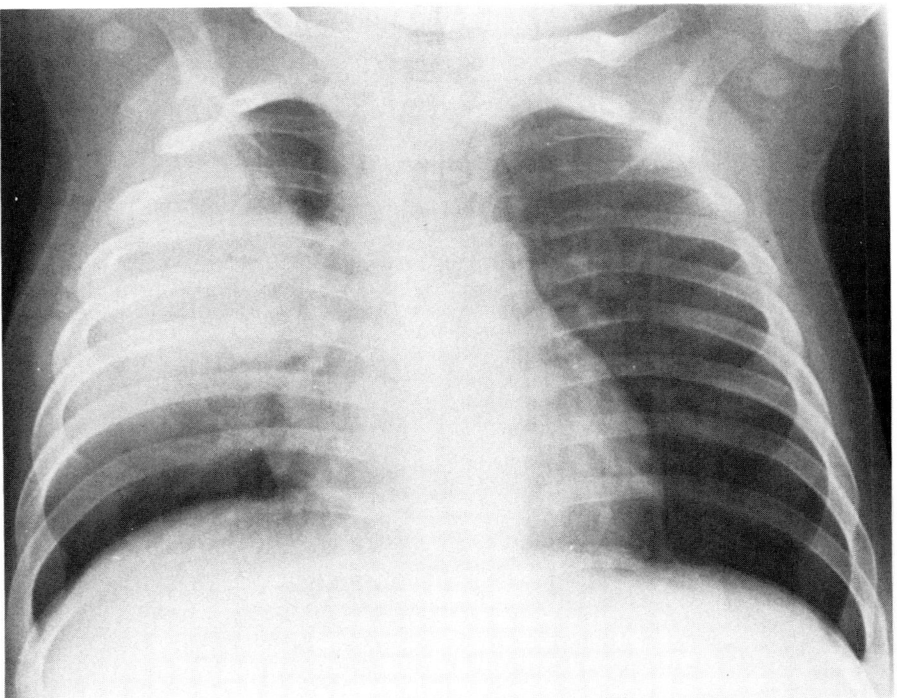

Fig. 3-23. Radiograph of right upper lobe pneumonia characterized by focal air-space opacification.

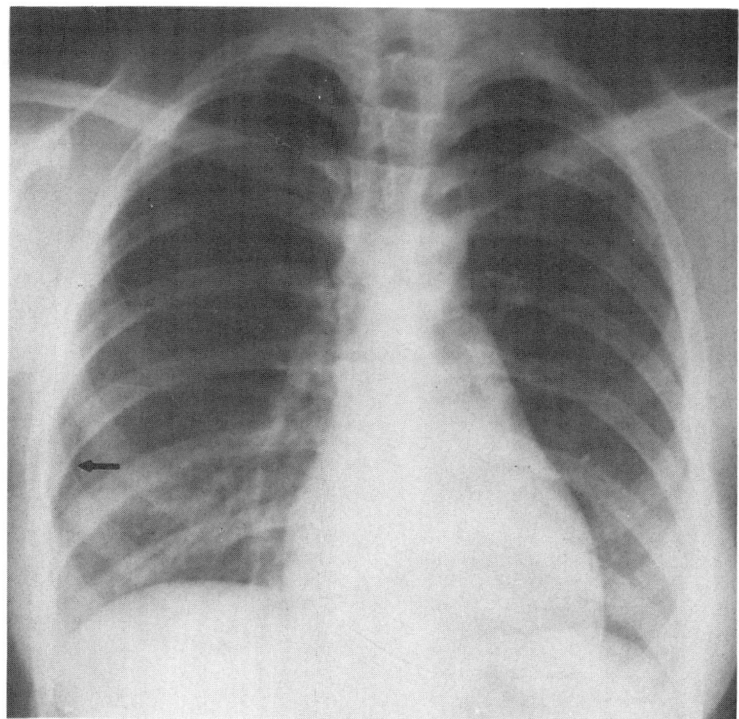

Fig. 3-24. Radiograph of right-sided pneumothorax *(arrow)*. Film taken in expiratory phase of respiration will accentuate radiographic appearance of pneumothorax.

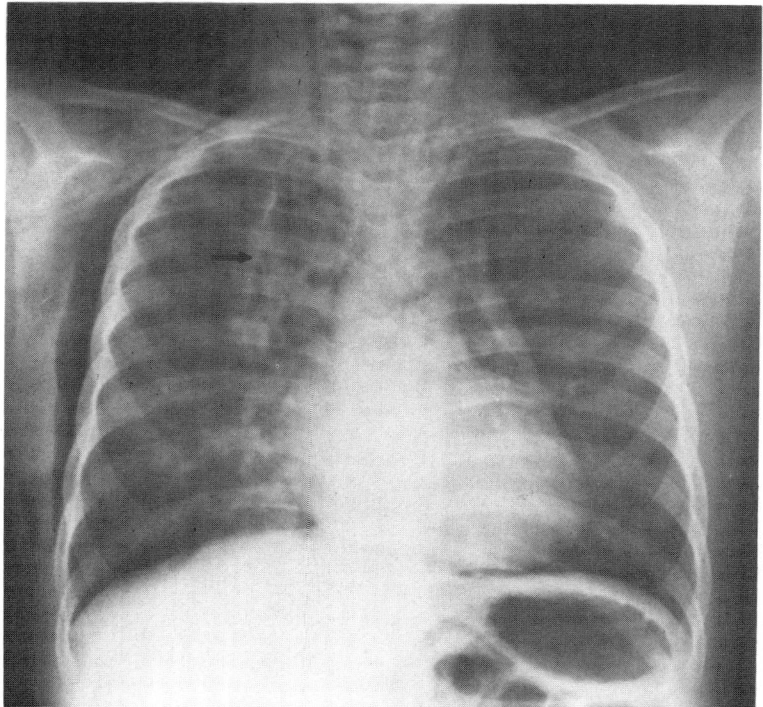

Fig. 3-25. Radiograph of pneumomediastinum. Arrow defines right side of air-displaced mediastinal pleura.

sociated with cardiac enlargement, bilateral widespread parenchymal pulmonary opacification, and often a pleural effusion. Postoperative pneumonia commonly is associated with a more localized parenchymal process, usually pleural effusion, and occasionally with pulmonary cavitation. Radiographic signs are usually not seen early in the postoperative period, but may be present later in the week after surgery (Fig. 3-23). A postoperative pneumothorax or pneumomediastinum is occasionally seen and can be easily demonstrated radiographically (Figs. 3-24 and 3-25).

SUMMARY AND CONCLUSIONS

Throughout this chapter the imaging techniques available, application, and some of the findings in diseases that are encountered frequently in a pediatric plastic surgery practice are discussed. Plain film radiography in both the AP and lateral projection remains the most commonly used imaging method. Tomography is especially useful in assessing complex developmental abnormalities of the skull. Its limitations in pediatric practice relate to long exposures (1 to 5 seconds). Fluoroscopy or cineradiography allow dynamic and functional assessment of examined structures. Contrast enhanced studies are routinely used in the detailed examination of soft tissues, hollow organs, and vascular structures. CT is invaluable in documenting and assessing head trauma in the acutely injured child. It also is extremely useful in determining the local and distant spread of tumor, especially to soft tissue.

Although generalization is difficult, most plain film radiographic examinations requiring, for example, two to five films, deliver less than 1 rad to the skin. The mean whole body doses for conventional studies in children range from 0.01 to 0.1 rad. With these low doses, risk of leukemia and genetic risks are minimal. Each examination, however, must be justified as potentially beneficial to the child.

During a routine evaluation of the structures in the head and neck, the following radiographs should be obtained:
1. A PA projection inclined 15 degrees toward the orbitomeatal baseline
2. A half-axial AP projection inclined 25 degrees to the orbitomeatal baseline
3. A lateral examination centered over the region of the pituitary fossa
4. An axial or submentovertex projection inclined at 90 degrees to the orbitomeatal baseline

Cephalometry is essential during the radiographic evaluation of craniofacial abnormalities. It can be employed to assess facial bone growth and is useful in the progressive evaluation after reconstructive procedures.

Radiographs of trivial injuries to the skull should be avoided. These radiographs should be obtained in high-risk patients, such as those with loss of consciousness, amnesia, stupor and semicoma, abnormal neurologic findings, palpable bony misalignments, discharges from the ear and nose, bilateral black eyes, and breathing difficulties. CT is of much greater value in this high-risk group than plain film radiography. Facial films should always be obtained when facial fractures are suspected. The following radiographs are usually obtained when a facial series is requested:
1. A standard AP, inclined projection
2. An occipitomental projection inclined 25 to 35 degrees to the orbitomeatal baseline
3. A lateral projection centered on the outer canthus of the eye
4. A soft tissue technique submentovertical zygomatic arch view

Mandibular views are important when mandibular fractures are evident. Tomography, however, may be required in both coronal and lateral plains to demonstrate condylar neck fractures.

Radiographic evaluation of the extremities is most important after trauma and is useful to the plastic surgeon in determining bone age and evaluating bone tumors. Benign tumors typically expand or deform surrounding bone, whereas malignant tumors typically destroy the bone.

A thorough genitourinary radiographic assessment is most important in the evaluation and treatment of children with genitourinary anomalies. The object of genitography is to determine the internal anatomy of the urogenital tracts.

The value of routine preoperative chest radiography remains controversial. In practice it seems reasonable to only undertake preoperative chest radiography when the patient's condition warrants it.

REFERENCES

1. Acheson, R.M., Vicinus, J.H., and Fowler, G.B.: Studies on the reliability of assessing skeletal maturity from x-rays, Hum. Biol. **38**:204, 1966.
2. Aspin, N.: The gonadal x-ray dose to children from diagnostic radiographic techniques, Radiology **85**:946, 1965.
3. Baker, D.H., and Berdon, W.E.: The use and safety of "high" dosage in pediatric urography: a survey of the Society of Pediatric Radiology, Radiology **103**:371, 1972.
4. Bayley, N., and Pinneau, S.R.: Tables for predicting adult height from skeletal age: revised for use with Greulich and Pyle hand standards, J. Pediatr. **40**:423, 1952.
5. Bell, R.S., and Loop, J.W.: The utility and futility of radiographic skull examination for trauma, N. Engl. J. Med. **284**:236, 1971.
6. Belman, A.B., and King, L.R.: Urinary tract abnormalities associated with imperforate anus, J. Urol. **108**:823, 1972.
7. Berdon, W.E., Baker, D.H., Wigger, H.J., and Blanc, W.A.: The radiologic and pathologic spectrum of prune belly syndrome, Radiol. Clin. North Am. **15**:83, 1977.
8. Berdon, W.K., Hochberg, B., Baker, D.H., et al.: The association of lumbosacral spine and genitourinary anomalies with imperforate anus, A.J.R. **98**:181, 1966.
9. Berger, P., Gildersleeve, S., and Poznanski, A.: The feasibility of the PA projection for tomography of the petrous bone: a significant reduction in radiation dose to the lens of the eye, Am. J. Roentgenol. Radium Ther. Nucl. Med. **122**:67, 1974.
10. Blanc, W.A., and Baens, G.: Ear malformation, abnormal facies and genitourinary tract anomalies, Am. J. Dis. Child. **100**:781, 1960.
11. Bliznak, J., and Staple, T.W.: Radiology of angiodysplasia of the limb, Radiology **110**:35, 1974.
12. Brasch, R.C., Boyd, P.B., and Gooding, C.: Computed tomographic

scanning in children: comparison of radiation dose and resolving power of commercial CT scanners, A.J.R. **131**:95, 1978.

13. Brasch, R.C., Korobkin, M., and Gooding, C.: Computed tomography in children: evaluation of 45 patients, A.J.R. **131**:21, 1978.

14. Brill, P.W., Ewing, M.L., and Dunn, A.A.: The value (?) of routine chest radiography in children and adolescents, Pediatrics **52**:125, 1973.

15. Byrd, S.E., Harwood-Nash, D., Barry, J.F., et al.: Coronal computed tomography of the skull and brain in infants and children. I. Technique and results, Radiology **124**:705, 1977.

16. Byrd, S.E., Harwood-Nash, D.C., Barry, J.F., et al.: Coronal computer tomography of the skull and brain in infants and children. II. Clinical value, Radiology **124**:710, 1977.

17. Byrd, S.E., Harwood-Nash, D.C., Fitz, C.R., Rogovitz, D.M.: Computed tomography in the evaluation of encephaloceles in infants and children, J. Can. Assoc. Radiol. **29**:108, 1978.

18. Caffey, J.: Pediatric x-ray diagnosis, ed. 7, Chicago, 1978, Year Book Medical Publishers, Inc.

19. Clark, K.C.: Positioning in radiography, ed. 9, vol 1, London, 1973, Williams Heinemann Medical Books, Ltd.

20. Currarino, G., and Silverman, F.N.: Orbital hypotelorism, arhinencephaly, and trigonocephaly, Radiology **74**:206, 1960.

21. Dublin, A.B., French, B.N., and Rennick, J.M.: Computed tomography in head trauma, Radiology **122**:365, 1977.

22. Dudding, B.A., Gorlin, R.J., and Langaer, L.O.: The otopalatal digital syndrome, Am. J. Dis. Child. **113**:214, 1967.

23. Eagle, J.F., Jr., and Barret, G.S.: Congenital deficiency of abdominal musculature with associated genitourinary tract abnormalities: a syndrome report of nine cases, Pediatrics **6**:721, 1950.

24. Fabrikant, J.I.: Public health considerations of the biological effects of small doses of radiation: health physics in the healing arts, Pub. No. 78-029, Washington, D.C., Department of Health, Education, and Welfare, 1978.

25. Fazer, L.E., Elmore, J., and Nadler, H.C.: Mandibulofacial dysostosis (Treacher-Collins syndrome), Am. J. Dis. Child. **113**:405, 1967.

26. Fellows, K.E.: The uses and abuses of abdominal and peripheral angiography in children, Radiol. Clin. North Am. **10**:349, 1972.

27. Fleisher, D.S.: Lateral displacement of the nipples: a sign of bilateral renal hypoplasia, J. Pediatr. **69**:806, 1966.

28. Gall, J.C., Stem, A.M., Poznanski, A.K., et al.: Oto-palatal-digital syndrome: comparison of clinical and radiographic manifestations in males and females, Am. J. Hum. Genet. **24**:24, 1972.

29. Gray, J.E.: The radiation hazard—let's put it in perspective, Mayo Clin. Proc. **54**:809, 1979.

30. Greulich, W.W., and Pyle, S.I.: Radiographic atlas of skeletal development of the hand and wrist, ed. 2, Stanford, Calif., 1959, Stanford University Press.

31. Gyepes, M.T.: Angiography in infants and children, New York, 1974, Grune & Stratton, Inc.

32. Hansman, C.F.: Growth of interorbital distance and skull thickness as observed in roentgenographic measurements, Radiology **86**:87, 1966.

33. Harwood-Nash, D.C., and Breckbill, D.L.: Computed tomography in children: a diagnostic technique, J. Pediatr. **89**:343, 1976.

34. Harwood-Nash, D.C., and Fitz, C.R.: Neuroradiology in infants and children, St. Louis, 1976, The C.V. Mosby Co.

35. Harwood-Nash, D.C., Hendrick, E.B., and Hudson, A.R.: The significance of skull fractures in children: a study of 1187 patients, Radiology **101**:151, 1971.

36. Hinck, V.C., Hopkins, C.E., and Clark, W.M.: Sagittal diameter of lumbar spinal canal in children and adults, Radiology **85**:929, 1965.

37. Hinck, V.C., Hopkins, C.E., and Clark, W.M.: Normal interpediculate distances (minimum and maximum) in children and adults, A.J.R. **97**:141, 1966.

38. Hinck, V.C., Hopkins, C.E., Clark, W.M., and Savara, B.S.: Sagittal diameter of the cervical canal in children, Radiology **79**:97, 1962.

39. Hoerr, N.L., and Pyle, S.I.: Radiographic atlas of skeletal development of the foot and ankle, Springfield, Ill., 1962, Charles C Thomas, Publisher.

40. Houser, O.W., Smith, J.B., Gomez, M.R., Baker, H.L., Jr.: Evaluation of intracranial disorders in children by computerized axial tomography: a preliminary report, Neuroradiology **25**:607, 1975.

41. James, A.E., Wagner, H.N., and Cooke, R.E.: Pediatric nuclear medicine, Philadelphia, 1974, W.B. Saunders Co.

42. Kendall, B.E., and Kingsley, D.: The value of computerized axial tomography (CAT) in craniocerebral malformations, Br. J. Radiol. **51**:171, 1978.

43. Kittleson, A.C., and Lim, L.W.: Measurement of scoliosis, Am. J. Roentgenol. Radium Ther. Nucl. Med. **198**:775, 1970.

44. Lindsay, W.K.: Cleft palate. In Ravitch, M.M., Welch, K.J., Benson, C.D., et al., editors: Pediatric surgery, ed. 2, vol. 1, Chicago, 1969, Year Book Medical Publishers, Inc.

45. MacMahon, B.: Prenatal x-ray exposure and childhood cancer, J. Natl. Cancer Inst. **28**:1173, 1962.

46. McArdle, R., and Lebowitz, R.L.: Uncomplicated hypospadias and anomalies of upper renal tract: need for screening? Urology **5**:712, 1975.

47. McKenzie, J., and Craig, L.: Mandibular facial dysostosis (Treacher-Collins syndrome), Arch. Dis. Child. **30**:371, 1953.

48. Merriam, G.R., and Focht, E.F.: A clinical study of radiation cataracts and the relationship to dose, Am. J. Roentgenol. Radium Ther. Nucl. Med. **77**:759, 1957.

49. Moore, W.B., Mathews, T.J., and Rabinowitz, R.: Genitourinary anomalies associated with Klippel-Feil syndrome, J. Bone Joint Surg. **57**:355, 1975.

50. Naidich, T.P., Epstein, F., Lin, J.P., et al.: Evaluation of pediatric hydrocephalus by computed tomography, Radiology **119**:337, 1976.

51. Neel, J.V.: Atomic bombs, inbreeding and Japanese genes. The Russel Lecture for 1966, Univ. Mich. Med. Center J. **32**:107, 1966.

52. Potter, E.L.: Facial characteristics of infants with bilateral renal agenesis, Am. J. Obstet. Gynecol. **51**:885, 1946.

53. Poznanski, A.K.: The hand in radiologic diagnosis, Philadelphia, 1974, W.B. Saunders Co.

54. Poznanski, A.K.: Practical approaches to pediatric radiology, Chicago, 1975, Year Book Medical Publishers, Inc.

55. Poznanski, A.K., Garn, S.M., Kuhns, L.R., and Sandusky, S.T.: Dysharmonic maturation of the hand in the congenital malformation syndromes, Am. J. Phys. Anthropol. **35**:417, 1971.

56. Pruzansky, S., and Lis, E.F.: Cephalometric roentgenography in infants: sedation, instrumentation, and research, Am. J. Orthod. **44**:159, 1958.

57. Pyle, S.I., and Hoerr, N.L.: A radiographic standard of reference for the growing knee, Springfield, Ill., 1969, Charles C Thomas, Publisher.

58. Pyle, S.I., Waterhouse, A.M., and Greulich, W.W.: A radiographic standard of reference for the growing hand and wrist, Cleveland, 1971, Case Western Reserve University Press.

59. Roberts, F., and Shopfner, C.E.: Plain skull roentgenograms in children with head trauma, Am. J. Roentgenol. Radium Ther. Nucl. Med. **114**:23, 1972.

60. Sagel, S.S., Evens, R.G., Forrest, J.V., et al.: Efficacy of routine screening and lateral chest radiographs in a hospital based population, N. Engl. J. Med. **291**:1001, 1974.

61. Sane, S.M., Worsing, R.A., Wiens, C.W., and Sharma, R.K.: The value of preoperative chest x-ray examinations in children, Pediatrics **60**:669, 1977.

62. Shillito, J., Jr., and Matson, D.D.: Craniosynostosis: a review of 519 surgical patients, Pediatrics **41**:829, 1968.

63. Shkolnik, A.: Gray scale ultrasound of the pediatric abdomen and pelvis: current problems in diagnostic radiology, **7**:3, 1977.

64. Shopfner, C.E.: Cystourethrography: methodology, normal anatomy and pathology, J. Urol. **103**:92, 1970.

65. Shopfner, C.E.: Genitography in intersexual states, Radiology **82**:664, 1964.

66. Simril, W.A., and Thurston, D.: Normal interpediculate space in the spines of infants and children, Radiology **64**:340, 1955.

67. Taylor, W.C.: Deformity of ears and kidneys, Can. Med. Assoc. J. **93**:107, 1965.

68. Triplett, R.G., Kelly, J.F., Mendenhall, K.G., and Vieras, F.: Quantitative radionuclide imaging for early determination of fate of bone grafts, J. Nucl. Med. **20**:297, 1979.

69. Vinita, M.: Atlas of roentgenographic positions and standard radiologic procedures, St. Louis, 1975, The C.V. Mosby Co.

70. Vitko, R.J., Cass, A.S., and Winter, R.B.: Anomalies of the genitourinary tract associated with congenital scoliosis and kyphosis, J. Urol. **108:**655, 1972.
71. Wall, B.R., and Green, D.A.C.: The radiation dose to patients from EMI brain and body scanners, Br. J. Radiol. **52:**189, 1979.
72. Webster, E.W., Alpert, N.M., and Brownell, G.L.: Radiation doses in pediatric nuclear medicine and diagnostic x-ray procedures. In James, A.E., Wagner, H.N., Jr., and Cooke, R.E., editors: Pediatric nuclear medicine, Philadelphia, 1974, W.B. Saunders Co.
73. Whitmore, R.C., Bushong, S.C., Archer, B.A.S., and Glaze, S.A.: Radiation dose in neurologic computed tomographic scanning, Radiol. Technol. **51:**21, 1979.
74. Zimmerman, R.A., Bilaniuk, E.T., Gennarelli, T., et al.: Cranial computed tomography in diagnosis and management of head trauma, A.J.R. **131:**27, 1978.

CHAPTER 4

Anesthesia for the pediatric patient undergoing plastic surgery

EDMOND C. BLOCH

The use of anesthesia for the surgical correction of disfiguring lesions in infants and children dates back to the time of the early Egyptians. The methods used were varied, often consisting of exhaustion by starvation, physical restraint, a crude narcotic, an overdose of alcohol, deliberate cerebral concussion, or even partial asphyxia by strangulation. Needless to say, the chances of survival were better without "anesthesia," and the efficacy of these methods is left to the imagination. After its introduction in 1846,[6] ether, often supplemented by nitrous oxide, remained the agent of choice for over a century. It was administered by open mask, various inhalers, or insufflation, commonly through an unprotected airway with spontaneous ventilation. Aspiration was common, and the attendant mortality and morbidity were unacceptable by present-day standards.

THE RISK OF ANESTHESIA

The risk to the child undergoing anesthesia and surgery is determined by many factors. Among these are the patient's physical status, the skill and experience of the anesthesiologist and surgeon, the availability of expert pediatric consultants and nurses, and facilities within the hospital's operating suite, recovery rooms, intensive care units, and laboratories.[132] In 1964 the anesthetic-related death rate in infants and children was reported to be 3.3 per 10,000 general anesthetics, and half of these occurred in apparently healthy patients.[69] In 1966 this rate at the Children's Hospital Medical Center of Boston was reported as 1.4 per 10,000. More recent studies indicate that the rate has fallen and that it is considerably lower in major pediatric centers. A rate of 0.2 per 10,000 is reported from the Children's Hospital of Philadelphia, all in critically ill patients.[52] The major causes of anesthesia-related morbidity and mortality are hypoxia and hypovolemia.[119]

PREOPERATIVE PREPARATION

Preoperative preparation should commence when the decision to operate is made. Hospitalization can be a stressful and traumatic experience for children. Unfamiliar people, environment, and routines provoke anxiety, and painful procedures and separation from family make the acceptance of hospital experiences difficult. Children may return home surgically corrected yet suffer lasting psychologic scars. Many hospitals today offer preadmission programs for pediatric patients and their parents in the form of a tour of the pediatric facility and operating suite, introduction to the nursing and medical staff, parent handouts, and question and answer sessions. There are many excellent books for children dealing with this aspect of their hospitalization.*

The preoperative visit provides an opportunity for the anesthesiologist to establish rapport with the patient and parents, reassure them, and explain the procedures and events that occur before and after surgery. This aspect is most important, especially in plastic surgery because the patient often is exposed to multiple types of anesthetics. The knowledge and understanding of what lies ahead, together with rapport and confidence in the anesthesiologist, will result in less emotional trauma to the patient and a smoother procedure.

Preanesthetic evaluation is made on the basis of the history, physical examination, and laboratory data. Of particular importance is a history of respiratory illnesses, possible recent contact with infectious diseases, medicine currently being taken, steroid therapy, allergies, untoward reactions to drugs, blood transfusions and previous anesthetics, and the family history relating to anesthesia. The question of upper respiratory tract infection in small children has re-

---

*References 13, 31, 59, 62, 86, 111, 128, 137, 142, and 144.

cently been discussed.[96] Symptoms of note are a stuffy nose, rhinorrhea, a fever, and coughing or croup with coarse upper airway sounds on examination. It is recommended that when a patient has a history of upper respiratory tract illness during the preceding month or has physical signs in the chest on examination, radiographs of the chest should be obtained. Atelectasis or pneumonitis may be present and not clinically detectable. Before any emergency procedure, the time of recent intake of food and fluids should be noted. It is advisable to regard ambulatory patients and those who have suffered acute trauma as having a full stomach. The physical examination is directed in particular to the cardiorespiratory system. After sedation or induction of anesthesia, upper airway obstruction may occur in the presence of allergic rhinitis, enlarged tonsils and adenoids, or in patients with a hypoplastic mandible with protruding maxillae. The mouth should be examined for loose teeth and the larynx palpated. An elevated larynx is an indication of possible difficulty with laryngoscopy. Cleft palate is sometimes associated with severe macroglossia and retrognathia (e.g., the Pierre Robin syndrome). Minimal laboratory data required in an apparently healthy child for routine surgery are hemoglobin or hematocrit values, a white blood cell count, and urinalysis. Because of high hemoglobin levels at birth, hematopoiesis is not active after birth, but is resumed when hemoglobin levels fall to 11 or 12 g/dL, by which time the infant is 6 to 12 weeks old, and supplemental iron is advisable. The response to iron therapy is reflected in a rise in reticulocyte count within a few days and normal hemoglobin levels within a month. Even though this anemia is regarded as physiologic, it is an inescapable fact that the oxygen-carrying capacity of the red cell is reduced. Further investigations, such as electrocardiography (ECG); chest radiography; serum electrolytes, bilirubin, creatinine, and enzyme studies; arterial blood gas studies; and pulmonary function tests, will be dictated by abnormal findings. The physical status of the child is determined on the basis of all these findings and may be documented according to the following scale of the American Society of Anesthesiologists[118]:

Classification of physical status*

Class I	No organic, physiologic, biochemical, or psychiatric disturbance
Class II	Mild to moderate systemic abnormalities caused either by the disease to be treated surgically or by another pathophysiologic process
Class III	Severe systemic abnormality from any cause
Class IV	Immediately life-threatening, severe systemic disorder
Class V	Moribund patient who is submitted to operation in desperation
Emergency	The letter E is added to the classification number for any patient undergoing emergency surgery

Pharmacologic premedication (Table 4-1) may not be needed in many patients. Sedation in particular should be minimized or avoided when an airway problem is antici-

*From Saklad, M.: Anesthesiology 2:281, 1941.

pated. If medication is deemed necessary for nocturnal sedation, triclofos sodium or diazepam is effective. Preoperatively, it is our practice to give a vagolytic agent to all children for whom ketamine or an inhalation induction is planned, because excessive secretions increase the incidence of laryngospasm during induction. Intramuscular atropine sulfate or glycopyrrolate is given 1 hour before the scheduled time of operation. When given orally atropine has its peak effect in 2 hours, but glycopyrrolate is poorly absorbed.[98] Most anesthesiologists do not use narcotics for children under 10 kg of body weight or 1 year of age, but children who are restless or afraid and who weigh over 6 kg may be given morphine 1 hour before they are taken to the operating

Table 4-1. Pediatric drug doses

Drug	Routes of administration*		
	Intravenous	Intra-muscular	Oral
Premedication			
Atropine	0.01	0.01	0.02
Glycopyrrolate	0.004	0.008	
Scopolamine	0.01	0.01	0.05
Morphine sulfate	0.1	0.2	
Meperidine	0.5 to 1	1	
Diazepam	0.1	0.2	0.2
Droperidol	0.1	0.15	0.2
Promethazine	0.25 to 0.5	0.75	
Pentobarbital		2	4
Secobarbital		2	
Triclofos			50 to 70
Diphenhydramine	1	1	1
Chlorpromazine	0.5	0.5	0.5
Induction			
Thiopental	4		
Methohexital	1.5		8 to 10
Ketamine	2		8 to 10
Diazepam	0.1 to 0.2		
Fentanyl	0.001 to 0.002		
Droperidol	0.15 to 0.2		
Fentanyl-droperidol (Innovar)	0.1 ml/kg		
Relaxants			
Succinylcholine			
Under 1 year	2	4	
Over 1 year	1	2	
d-Tubocurarine	0.5		
Pancuronium	0.10		
Gallamine	0.125		
Dimethyl tubo-curarine	0.25		

For the newborn, use one third of these doses in the first week of life and two thirds of these doses in the second week of life; thereafter use full doses.

Increments: one fourth of first dose; reduce all doses of nondepolarizing relaxants by one third in presence of halothane, enflurane, shock, acidosis, dehydration, antibiotics and prematurity

*All doses are in mg/kg unless otherwise stated.   *Continued.*

Table 4-1. Pediatric drug doses—cont'd

	Intravenous	Intra-muscular		Intravenous	Intra-muscular
Reversal			**Other drugs**		
Atropine	0.025		Aminophylline	Loading dose: up to 5.6 mg/kg over 15 minutes; infusion 0.85 mg/kg/hour	
Glycopyrrolate	0.2 for each milligram of neostigmine or 4 mg of pyridostigmine		Calcium chloride	10 to 20 mg/kg for cardiac arrest	
Neostigmine	0.06 to 0.08		Calcium gluconate	10 mg/kg for hypocalcemia; 50 mg/100 ml of blood for massive transfusion	
Pyridostigmine	0.25				
Physostigmine	0.015; repeat in 15 minutes if needed		Dantrolene	1 mg/kg initially; total dose, 10 mg; oral prophylaxis, 2 mg/kg, three times daily for 1 day preoperatively	
Naloxone	0.005; repeat in 15 minutes if needed				
Doxapram	0.5 to 1		Dopamine	3 μg/kg/min (range 1 to 10)	
Narcotics			Epinephrine*	Subcutaneous route, 0.01 mg/kg at 15-minute intervals; infiltration, maximal dose, 1.5 μg/kg, maximum of three doses/hour; topical administration, 2 to 4 μg/kg; intravenous route, 1 to 10 μg/kg; infusion, 0.1 to 1 μg/kg/min; 5 to 10 μg/kg for cardiac arrest	
Morphine sulfate	0.1	0.2			
Fentanyl	1 μg/kg				
Meperidine	0.5 to 1	1			
Steroids					
Hydrocortisone	Up to 50				
Methylprednisolone	Up to 30		Furosemide	0.5 to 1	
Dexamethasone	0.25 (maximum, 10 mg total)		Heparin	3 mg/kg intravenously	
Local anesthetics			Isoproterenol	0.1 to 3.5 μg/kg/min (average 0.8)	
Maximal doses for infiltration or nerve blocks[34,41,99]; expected duration of effect is indicated in parentheses			Lidocaine	1 mg/kg	
Lidocaine	5 mg/kg/hour		Mannitol	1 g/kg	
Bupivacaine	4 mg/kg (2 to 8 hours)		Propranolol	5 to 10 μg/kg intravenously	
Procaine	14 mg/kg/hour		Racemic epinephrine (2.25%)	0.1 to 0.5 ml in 2.5 ml saline nebulized for 5 minutes every 1 or 2 hours	
Mepivacaine	7 mg/kg (1.5 hour)				
Tetracaine	1 mg/kg (4 to 6 hours)		Sodium nitroprusside	Infusion: maximal dosage of 10 μg/kg/min; total maximal dose, 1.5 mg/kg	
Cocaine, 5% solution	1 mg/kg (2 to 3 hours)				

*One ml of a 1/1000 solution contains 1000 μg.

room. It provides consistently good sedation with good analgesia during and after anesthesia. For those patients having an operation involving the upper airways, we prefer meperidine, since it produces less depression of the pharyngeal, laryngeal, and cough reflexes, an important consideration in the immediate postoperative period. Diazepam, barbiturates, and phenothiazines are not analgesics; since the latter two may even be antalgesic and may increase laryngeal sensitivity and anesthetic requirements, they are not agents of choice. If injections have to be avoided, diazepam, promethazine, or pentobarbital may be given by mouth with a sip of water 2 hours before induction. The rectal administration of drugs is best avoided, since absorption is erratic and the effect may be delayed.

INDUCTION OF ANESTHESIA

The intramuscular route is useful in patients who are totally unmanageable, and induction may be commenced in the anesthetic room or even in the hallway, provided the necessary supportive equipment is at hand. If there is no specific reason for using ketamine, then methohexital is preferred, since postoperatively its effects are of shorter duration and more acceptable to the patient and physician. The intravenous route using a vein on the dorsum of the hand is usually best, and injection here can be almost painless, given a sharp 25- or 27-gauge needle and a skilled operator. Other sites are the volar aspect of the wrist and the dorsum of the foot. Inhalational induction can, with skill and patience, be pleasant for both the patient and physician.

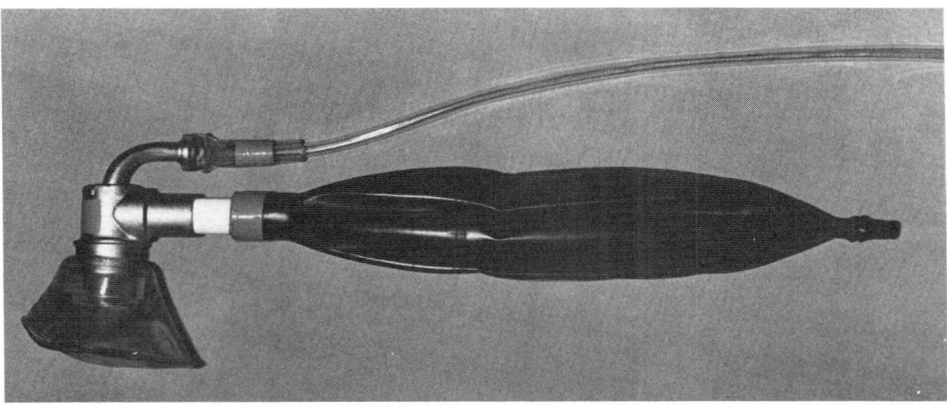

Fig. 4-1. Norman mask elbow with Rendell-Baker-Soucek mask.

A Rendell-Baker-Soucek mask with a Nesi or Norman mask elbow (Fig. 4-1) and a high, fresh gas flow rate is best suited to this. This combination is lightweight and has virtually no apparatus dead space, no valves, and all the advantages of the Mapleson D system. It is well suited to the maintenance of anesthesia by mask with spontaneous ventilation for long periods.

INTUBATION

Endotracheal intubation is mandatory when there is any doubt about maintaining the patency and integrity of the upper airway and when ventilation is to be controlled in the following situations:

1. Where there is a risk of aspiration of stomach contents, such as after recent intake of food and fluids or in trauma patients when gastric stasis is almost always present.
2. Most infants under 12 months of age.
3. When controlled ventilation is required for any reasons, such as intraabdominal, intrathoracic, or intracranial procedures or for operations carried out with the patient in the prone position.
4. All head and neck operations, since access to the patient's head is not always possible during surgery.
5. Intraoral and pharyngeal procedures in which blood and other foreign material must be kept out of the trachea.

Intubation may be achieved after an inhalation induction. However, the abolition of tracheal and carinal reflexes requires a greater depth of anesthesia than that needed for routine operations; in fact, the minimal alveolar concentration for intubation with halothane[146] and enflurane[147] is almost double that required for surgical anesthesia. This may produce unwarranted cardiovascular depression, and conditions for intubation may not be optimal, making it more difficult and more traumatic. Intubation after neuromuscular blockade is preferred, provided that control of ventilation is adequate after induction.

Laryngoscope blades are distinguished by a multiplicity of designs and sizes. The best blade to use is the one with which the operator is familiar. In our hospital we use the Robertshaw size 1 or 2 blade (Figs. 4-2 and 4-3) for smaller patients, and the Macintosh size 1 or 2 blade for larger patients. The Robertshaw blade is used in the same manner as a Miller or Magill blade, but because it is wider it allows binocular vision, a distinct advantage in the limited area provided by these small patients. Intubation before induction of anesthesia is preferred in the neonate and in weak or debilitated infants. This ensures continued ventilation during the procedure and provides for a safe situation in the event any difficulties are encountered. The larynx is elevated and often obscured by the large tongue and may be difficult to see.[53] Neonates do not tolerate even short periods of apnea and despite preoxygenation readily exhibit cyanosis. This is because the neonate uses 50% more oxygen than adults and has a high cardiac output and small functional residual capacity.[79] The small quantity of oxygen in the apneic lung is rapidly taken up and used. A small towel is placed under the shoulders, and an assistant holds the head in the "sniffing" position (Fig. 4-4). The anesthetist preoxygenates the patient, then slowly and gently inserts the laryngoscope blade until the epiglottis can be seen; the tip of the blade is now placed on the inferior (caudad) surface of the epiglottis. Under no circumstances should the operator attempt to expose the larynx at this stage by pronation of the forearm. This maneuver elevates the larynx out of view behind the tongue and brings the proximal part of the blade against the upper gum, frequently injuring it. The wrist must be held absolutely rigid and pressure exerted in the long axis of the laryngoscope handle. This will bring the larynx into view, whereupon the endotracheal tube is inserted with a slight rotary motion. The blade should be a straight one such as a No. 1 Robertshaw or Miller blade. If difficulty is encountered, the blade can be advanced into the esophagus and then slowly withdrawn; the first structure to come into view will be the larynx. Guidelines for selecting the internal

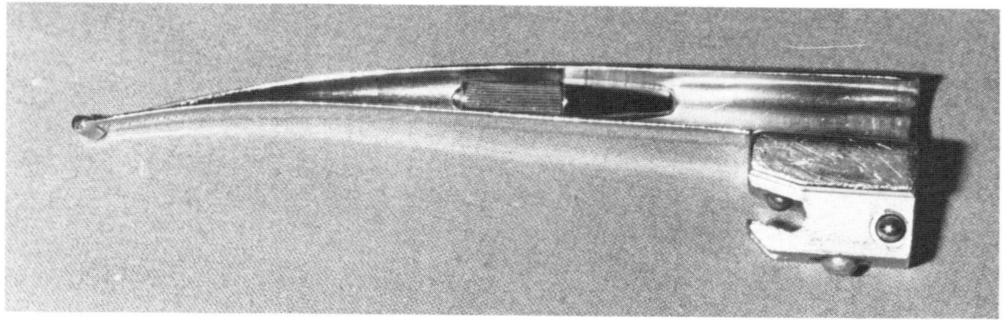

Fig. 4-2. Side view of Robertshaw laryngoscope blade.

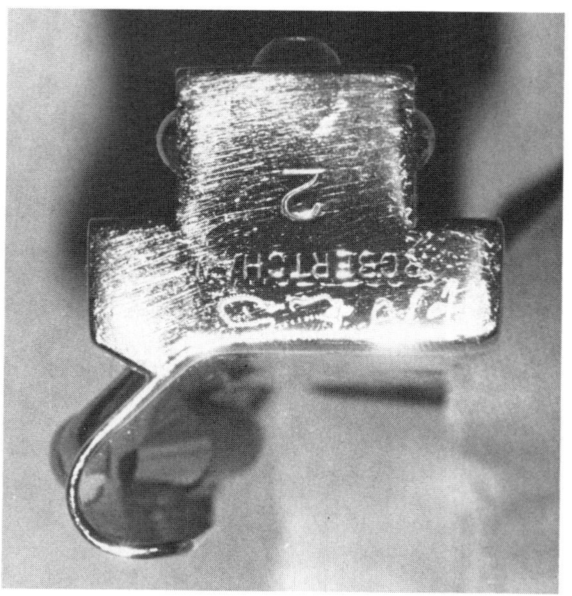

Fig. 4-3. Anesthesiologist's view of Robertshaw laryngoscope blade.

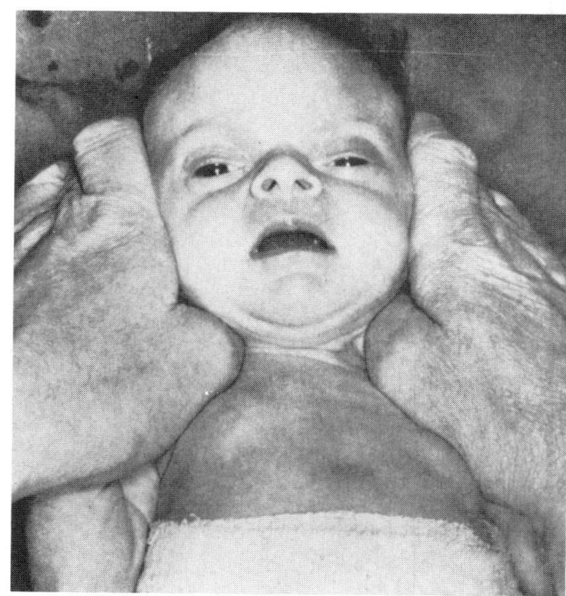

Fig. 4-4. Awake intubation. Assistant holds patient's head in sniffing position. (From Wilton, T.N.P., and Wilson, F.: Neonatal anaesthesia, Oxford, 1965, Blackwell Scientific Publications.)

Table 4-2. Average orotracheal tube dimensions

Age	Internal diameter (mm)	Minimal length (cm)*
Premature neonate	2.5 to 3	10 to 11
Term neonate	3 to 3.5	11 to 12
6 months	4	13
12 months	4.5	14
18 to 24 months	5	15
4 years	5.5	16
6 years	6	18
8 years	6.5	20
10 years	7	21
12 years	7.5	22
14 years	8	23

*Add 2 to 3 cm to the length for nasotracheal tubes.

diameter and length of the endotracheal tube are indicated in Table 4-2.

Two additional tubes, one a size larger and the other a size smaller, should be immediately available for use if the size of the selected tube proves to be unsuitable. The aim is to obtain a good fit within the trachea with a slight leak when positive pressure is applied. A cuffed tube is unnecessary up to the age of 8 years, since a well-selected tube will fit snugly in the cricoid ring, which is the narrowest part of the upper airway in children. Because tracheal dimensions in patients over 8 years vary widely, a cuffed tube should be used for them, selecting one that is smaller by 0.5 mm. Always preoxygenate the patient for at least 60 seconds before and after intubation, and always check air entry by inspection of the chest and auscultation of the lungs both before and after fixation of the endotracheal tube and final positioning of the head. When indicated, pass an oro-gastric tube to deflate the stomach after intubation.

MAINTENANCE OF ANESTHESIA

Nitrous oxide is a widely used agent for maintenance of anesthesia. It provides good analgesia, and supplements volatile agents like halothane and enflurane, reducing their dose requirements by 50%. Halothane is probably the most popular volatile agent in use in pediatric anesthesia today. So-called hepatotoxicity after administration of halothane in children is rarely reported, and many centers use it without reservation for repeated anesthesia in children.[67] Halothane, despite its widespread acceptance and many advantages, has some drawbacks. The minimal alveolar concentration required for surgical anesthesia is higher in infants under 6 months of age[73] as is the median effective dose (ED_{50}).[101] This results in more cardiovascular depression for a given degree of anesthesia. Because of this and the more rapid uptake of halothane in children, sudden alarming falls in blood pressure[67] are liable to occur in children under 6 months old, so that great care and close monitoring are required. As experience with enflurane increases, it is being used more often despite the possibility of seizures occurring at deeper levels of anesthesia.[100] Studies have shown no evidence of cerebral hypoxia during these seizures in healthy young volunteers,[145] and no sequelae have been noted.[67] They can be terminated by decreasing the level of anesthesia.[100] There seems to be no special advantage in using enflurane, although induction and recovery may be faster than with halothane (an advantage for outpatient anesthesia). Methoxyflurane is rapidly falling into disuse because of its nephrotoxic effect,[94] and it has been suggested that it be completely abandoned.[47] Irrespective of the agent selected it should be remembered that inhalational agents tend to depress the bone marrow and leukocyte phagocytosis, arrest cell division, activate the microsomal enzyme systems concerned with drug metabolism, and alter the body's responses to exogenous drugs and radiation therapy. Most inhalational agents are actively metabolized, and the metabolic product itself may be harmful.*

Narcotics may be used to supplement nitrous oxide. After morphine or meperidine, prolonged respiratory depression may be troublesome.[141] Fentanyl will provide comparable analgesia with return to spontaneous ventilation after approximately 2 hours, provided the total dose does not exceed 2 μ/kg. There appear to be no additional adverse effects on the infant other than respiratory depression as observed in adults.[51] Initial enthusiasm for ketamine has waned as its disadvantages have become apparent. Ketamine may be given intramuscularly, and the patency of the upper airway tends to be maintained because jaw muscle tone is increased, and it causes little central depression of ventilation. It is also sympathomimetic; the blood pressure and heart rate are

increased so that cardiovascular function appears to be maintained. However, it depresses the myocardium[50] and should not be used in patients who are hypertensive. It causes significant salivation in patients who have not received adequate doses of antisialagogues, and in this situation laryngospasm is prone to occur.[148] It depresses protective reflexes,[138] and pulmonary aspiration may occur.[106] By increasing cerebral blood flow ketamine causes a threefold increase in intracranial pressure.[63] Administration of ketamine produces catatonic stupor; the patient becomes immobile and unresponsive to painful stimuli.[81] Recovery from anesthesia is not rapid and may be accompanied by unpleasant dreams for up to 24 hours, and prolonged psychosis has been reported.[84] Because of all these effects and the deceptive ease of administration, ketamine should only be administered under the supervision of a trained anesthetist with all the necessary supportive equipment at hand. Currently ketamine has limited uses; however, it is useful when repeated anesthetics are necessary, such as for burn dressings or radiotherapy when intravenous sites are difficult to find, radiological procedures, and ophthalmic examination. It should be remembered that infants under 6 months of age may require up to four times the dose needed for older children.[90]

Muscle relaxants (Table 4-1) have greatly facilitated anesthesia for the pediatric patient. They enable volatile agents to be used in lower concentrations, thereby facilitating recovery and also reducing the side effects of these agents. Moreover, volatile agents such as halothane and enflurane potentiate neuromuscular blockade, enabling lower doses of the relaxants to be employed. Succinylcholine may produce nodal dysrhythmia, bradycardia, or atrial or ventricular bigeminy, more commonly after repeat administration. These dysrhythmias are usually transient and their incidence is reduced by giving the drug intramuscularly or by prior administration of atropine, 0.01 mg/kg, intravenously. Myoglobinemia occurs in 20% of children, and if halothane is given concurrently, this incidence rises to 40%.[117] Fatal rhabdomyolysis has been reported.[125] Children under 3 years of age seldom have fasciculations after succinylcholine. The increase in intraabdominal pressure that may occur after fasciculations and may result in regurgitation does not tend to occur in this age group,[122] so that pretreatment with a nondepolarizing drug is not needed. Prolonged apnea may occur in patients with genetically abnormal pseudocholinesterase or low serum levels of the enzyme, but this is readily managed by efficient ventilation and the infusion of fresh frozen plasma. A precipitious increase in serum potassium with resulting dysrhythmias or cardiac arrest may occur in patients who have suffered burns, renal failure, muscle trauma,[18] and denervation or even disuse of muscle groups[33] during the preceding 6 months.[83] Succinylcholine also causes profuse salivation and may rarely cause histamine release. Muscle pain in the postoperative period may occur. On the basis of body weight, children under a year require

---

*References 35, 36, 71, 72, 116, and 136.

twice the intravenous dose needed by older children[32,134]; when succinylcholine is given by the intramuscular or intralingual[95] route the intravenous dose should be doubled.

Pancuronium[68] and *d*-tubocurarine[65] are presently the two commonly used nondepolarizing neuromuscular blocking drugs. They resemble each other with respect to their actions, but pancuronium has a slightly shorter duration of action,[68] may cause a mild increase in heart rate and arterial pressure, and seldom cause histamine release. The controversial question of increased sensitivity to these drugs during the first month of life[27] has been much discussed. In the newborn it would appear prudent to use lower initial doses of nondepolarizing muscle relaxants when calculated on a body weight basis (Table 4-1). Because of the inefficiency of the respiratory system in meeting abnormal demands, all children should receive atropine or glycopyrrolate and neostigmine at the conclusion of the procedure to restore neuromuscular transmission. Inadequate reversal may be caused by relative overdose, respiratory acidosis, hypokalemia, hypocalcemia, hypermagnesemia, and the effect of antibiotics, especially the aminoglycosides. A peripheral nerve stimulator is essential to the safe and intelligent use of drugs that block neuromuscular transmission.

ANESTHESIA SYSTEMS

Of the many circuits devised for pediatric anesthesia,[49] the circle system is commonly used for children weighing over 25 to 30 kg. For smaller children the Mapleson D system is used either in the form of the Bain coaxial system[9] or as the Ayres T-piece[8] as modified by Rees.[110] It is much lighter, less bulky, has no valves, and provides for good control of $Paco_2$ levels without the use of soda lime. In the form of a coaxial system, it consists of a single tube to the patient, permits easy scavenging of waste gases, provides some warming and humidification of inspired gases,[107,143] and is suitable for all age groups and all procedures. The coaxial system has been called a universal breathing system. Many studies have been conducted to determine optimal usage of these systems.* Both the coaxial and T-piece systems can be used as either nonrebreathing or partial rebreathing systems, depending on the fresh gas flow rate delivered from the anesthesia machine. Minute ventilation should be 120 to 150 ml/kg, and fresh gas flow rates delivered from the anesthesia machine should be those indicated in Table 4-3.

The physiologic importance of the nasal passages in providing a means of filtering, warming, and humidifying inspired air is well known. This is bypassed by an endotracheal tube. The adverse effects of dry cool gases entering the tracheobronchial tree include hypothermia,[127] depression or arrest of ciliary activity and mucus flow,[92] hyperemia of the tracheobronchial mucosa,[92] and desiccation of mucus with resulting increased viscosity.[30] Inspired anesthetic mixtures

Table 4-3. Fresh gas flow rates for pediatric systems

System	Spontaneous ventilation	Controlled ventilation
T-piece	2½ × minute ventilation[91]	220 ml/kg/min[102]
Bain circuit	Over 24 kg: 150 ml/kg/min[12]	Over 35 kg: 100 ml/kg/min[11]
	Under 25 kg: 200 ml/kg/min[133]	Under 35 kg: 3.5 L/min[12]
		Under 10 kg: 2 L/min[12]

for children should therefore be warmed and humidified when delivered through an endotracheal tube. An electrically heated thermostatically controlled apparatus is available for this purpose and should be used for all pediatric patients who are intubated when anesthesia is anticipated to last longer than 10 to 15 minutes. The temperature of the gases thus delivered to the patient's trachea should be at least 32° C.

MONITORING DURING ANESTHESIA

The four minimal monitoring requirements for pediatric anesthesia are (1) a precordial or esophageal stethoscope for observing heart and breath sounds; (2) measurement of blood pressure by a conventional cuff and stethoscope, oscillotonometer, Doppler transducer, oscillometric apparatus, or an indwelling peripheral arterial cannula when arterial blood gases and the acid-base status need to be monitored; (3) temperature monitoring, preferably by means of an electric thermometer with the probe placed in the esophagus, nasopharynx, or rectum, since the axillary temperature is less reliable in the operating room; and (4) electrocardiography.

The Doppler transducer will accurately transmit sounds with systolic pressures as low as 40 mm Hg.[97] It has to be used with earphones, which are cumbersome, or a loudspeaker, which is noisy. The oscillometric apparatus, although more costly, is convenient to use, is noninvasive, and automatically provides digital readouts of systolic/diastolic and mean arterial pressures, as well as heart rate, as often as every 60 seconds. Correlation with intraarterial pressure is good in all age groups. An arterial cannula should only be inserted in the radial artery, dorsal artery of the foot, or posterior tibial artery after ensuring the adequacy of the collateral circulation by performing a modified Allen test.[4,108] A digital pulse monitor attached to a finger or toe has been found useful for this purpose[25] and also for monitoring the peripheral circulation, especially in older children. Cannulation of the temporal artery[64] is more difficult, and the vessel is tortuous so that results are erratic. The cannula should be no bigger than 22 gauge, and clotting within its lumen must be prevented by a constant pressurized infusion of heparinized saline (1 unit/ml) at a rate of 1.5 ml/hour, through a small-bore flush system.* A central ve-

---

*References, 8-10, 78, 91, 102, 110, and 113.

*IntraFlow system, Sorenson Research Co., Salt Lake City, Utah.

Table 4-4. Blood loss measurement

Method	Comment
Visual estimation	Unreliable, involve guesswork[28,140]
Vital signs	Affected by other factors; changes often occur late
Central venous pressure	An indication of blood volume, but also affected by right ventricular function and venous capacitance
Serial hematocrit values	A measure of hemoconcentration or dilution in the acute situation, not of blood loss[28]
Gravimetric (sponges)	Technically easy; impaired by evaporation,[139] body fluids, irrigating solutions
Gravimetric (patient)	Cannot be used intraoperatively; many potential errors; cumbersome
Electrolyte conductivity	Irrigating solutions, body fluids, anemia, and serum protein changes impair accuracy[89]
Blood volume	Not continuous; time consuming; of no value during hemorrhage[28]
Colorimetric	Practical, simple, and acceptably accurate[139]
Red blood cell volume studies	Not suited to rapid, repetitive intraoperative measurements

nous line inserted via the basilic, external jugular, or internal jugular vein provides useful information when large fluctuations in circulating blood volume are anticipated. In patients who have serious cardiopulmonary disorders, a Swan-Ganz catheter directed into the pulmonary artery will provide vital hemodynamic information. Organ perfusion, intravenous fluid therapy, and renal function are monitored by an indwelling urinary catheter or a bag applied over the genitalia and connected to a graduated container. Blood loss can be evaluated by various means, some more accurate than others (Table 4-4). We have found the colorimetric method to be particularly suited to the measurement of small volume losses encountered during pediatric surgery. It can be carried out with an inexpensive colorimeter,* although a more costly automated apparatus[105] is available.† A graduated container with a small surface area may be placed in the suction line to trap and measure aspirated blood, although allowances must be made for body fluids and irrigating solutions.

POSITIONING FOR ANESTHESIA AND SURGERY

Injuries to the unconscious patient are most distressing to patient and physician alike. Inadequate padding of pressure points may result in tissue ischemia with loss of tissue viability and necrosis. This type of injury is most likely to occur over bony prominences, especially in patients with poor tissue perfusion because of hypotension. The resulting painful ulcerated areas are prone to infection and delayed healing. Injuries to nerves occur as a result of direct pressure, stretching, or tourniquet compression and have been divided into three histopathologic categories according to severity[46]: neuropraxia, axonotmesis, and neurotmesis. The functional effects of pressure on a nerve have been graded[126] as nil, paralysis with complete recovery on release of pres-

sure, paralysis with delayed recovery but without degeneration, and paralysis with degeneration.

In the supine position the radial and ulnar nerves may be compressed by the edge of the operating table if the arm is not completely positioned on the table. Even then, no traction must be applied to the arm as is sometimes done to stop the patient from slipping when in the head-down position, since this may stretch the upper roots of the brachial plexus. Nor should the hand be placed under the buttock; I have seen gangrene of the thumb and index finger resulting from this. If the arm is to be abducted, it should be placed on an arm board that is padded so that the surface on which the arm rests is not lower or higher than that of the operating table mattress. Abduction beyond 90 degrees must not be permitted to avoid stretching of the lower roots of the brachial plexus. The foot should be supported at 90 degrees to the leg, especially when heavy drapes weigh down on it over long periods.

In the prone position the radial and ulnar nerves again need to be protected from pressure and the brachial plexus from stretching. The facial nerve may be compressed in the region of the mandible and the lateral femoral cutaneous nerve may be injured by the pressure from padding placed to support the pelvis. A pad under the ankles will avoid pressure on the toes, tendons and nerves of the dorsum of the foot, and common peroneal nerve as it rounds the head of the fibula. The eyes, ears, and male genitalia must be protected, and the head must be positioned to avoid pressure on the carotid sinus and extreme rotation and extension of the cervical spine. An improperly positioned nasotracheal tube may produce pressure on the nasal cartilage or on the skin of the ala nasi with subsequent painful and troublesome ulceration. In the prone position the abdomen should be free of pressure, which will restrict ventilation and may compress the inferior vena cava and thereby not only impede venous return to the heart, but also cause venous congestion in surgical fields in the lower half of the body.

In the sitting position, the sciatic nerve may be stretched

---

*Colorimeter Model LRTK-284; Markson Science, Phoenix, Ariz.

†Perometer monitor, Particle Data, Inc., Elmhurst, Ill.

because of hip flexion and knee joint extension over a prolonged period; the hips and knees should be comfortably flexed and the feet secured at right angles to the legs to prevent foot drop.

When moving an anesthetized patient from one position to another, the two major concerns are avoidance of injury and cardiovascular changes. All moves must be planned and executed without haste and with sufficient personnel to assist. The move that seems to receive the least attention takes place when the patient is moved from the operating table at the conclusion of the procedure. There is a tendency toward haste because the room has to be cleared or personnel wish to go off duty. Again, as many people as needed to safely move the patient must be available; care must be taken to protect flail limbs, the spine, and the head and neck. The temptation to scoop up small patients must be resisted. The hazard of carrying an infant or child in the arms from the operating table to the bed or cart is great because flexion of the lumbar spine causes an increase in intraabdominal pressure that can result in regurgitation and pulmonary aspiration of stomach contents. In turning a patient from the supine to the prone position and vice versa the shoulders and hips must be kept in the same plane throughout to avoid spinal injury[130] and rotation or extension of the cervical spine must be controlled by the anesthesiologist. The brachial plexus may be stretched, and joints may be injured. These remarks are even more pertinent to the deeply anesthetized patient or one who has received muscle relaxant drugs. For some unintelligible reason children seem to be turned with less care than adults by the average operating room team, probably because they are small and weigh less and appear easier to handle. This attitude is deplorable, and the same standards and precautions must be applied to children as to adults.

Cardiovascular parameters are not significantly affected by changes in posture in healthy nonanesthetized patients, since autonomic reflexes initiated by baroreceptors rapidly compensate for changes in blood volume distribution. This is not the case in the patient who is anesthetized. The autonomic system (and especially the sympathetic system) is suppressed by anesthetic agents in a dose-dependent fashion, so that compensating mechanisms which normally maintain cardiovascular homeostasis are incompetent. Changes in blood pressure and heart rate can be alarming in these circumstances, and careful management is required to minimize them. Significant postural changes should be made under light anesthesia and in the presence of an adequate blood volume. Any change in position should be made slowly, and frequent blood pressure measurements should be taken to monitor whether the change is well tolerated. If hypotension occurs, the patient should be returned to the original position, an intravenous fluid bolus administered, the concentration of the anesthetic agent reduced, and, if necessary, a vasopressor administered. The operation must not proceed until an acceptable arterial pressure is established and maintained. Inadequate ventilation during anesthesia or, more accurately, anything that reduces the functional residual capacity of the lungs, frequently results in atelectasis. This is the most common cause of postoperative pyrexia, and pneumonia is often the result. Even though ventilatory depression during anesthesia is not always clinically evident, the insidious development of atelectasis is reflected intraoperatively in falling arterial oxygen saturations, which are a consequence of intrapulmonary shunting. For this reason anesthesiologists prefer to assist or control ventilation in those patients who are positioned in the prone, Trendelenburg, lithotomy, lateral decubitus, and kidney positions and, of course, also when muscle relaxants have been used, even in small doses.

A detailed description of positions required for various operations with a comprehensive discussion of their effects on body systems, hazards, and prudent management has been published.[93]

THERMOREGULATION

The temperature in modern air-conditioned operating rooms will usually be around 20° C with a relative humidity of 60%. Anesthetized infants readily become hypothermic,[112] even during short procedures,[66] as do older children undergoing longer procedures. Hypothermia is especially a risk when a body cavity has been opened or large surface areas are exposed, such as during extensive skin grafting or in the patient with burns. In infants, shivering only appears after 3 to 6 months of age.[1] Oxygen consumption is increased in infants anesthetized with halothane when their temperature falls below 36.8° C.[67] The greatest heat loss occurs during induction of anesthesia and preparation for surgery. Measures taken to control heat loss include (1) elevation of room temperature to 24° C; (2) a mattress through which water, warmed at 40° C, is circulated, although the value of this measure in children over 10 kg in weight has been questioned[66]; (3) an overhead radiant heater, especially during induction of anesthesia and surgical preparation of infants; (4) covering the infant's limbs and trunk with a plastic drape[15]; (5) delivery to the trachea of humidified gases heated to a temperature of 36° C[109]; and (6) warming to body temperature of all intravenous solutions and blood products. Ambient temperature and that of the patient (esophageal, rectal, or nasopharyngeal), the water in the warming mattress, and the warmed anesthetic gases delivered to the patient should be monitored and recorded at 15-minute intervals throughout the procedure. The application of all these measures sometimes results in an increase in the infant's body temperature so that the provision of exogenous heat requires careful monitoring.

FLUID MANAGEMENT

The belief that the kidney of the premature and newborn infant is unable to secrete sodium adequately still seems to be widely held. In fact, it has been known for some time[29] that the inability to retain sodium is a feature of the renal system in immature newborns. Their ability to vary the concentration of urinary solutes is moderately impaired, since urinary osmolalities varying from 85 to 600 mOsm/kg are attainable.[34] After the first few weeks of life the newborn should have normal renal function.

All intravenous fluids should be given through a graduated burette-type infusion set, and the burette should contain no more than 25% of the patient's estimated blood volume at any time. This will avoid the possibility of fluid overload resulting from failure or mismanagement of the infusion control device. In infants and small children, infusion rates should be controlled by means of a calibrated infusion apparatus, such as a Holter or an IVAC pump.

The three considerations that apply to the calculation of intraoperative fluid volume therapy are the hourly maintenance requirements, the fluid deficit accumulated since the patient's last intake of fluid, and provision for any translocation of fluid to the extravascular compartment (also referred to as the shift, or third-space, loss). We use 5% dextrose in one-fourth strength saline to manage routine maintenance requirements and to replace the deficit due to preoperative withholding of oral fluids. This solution provides the patient with the normal daily requirements in terms of electrolytes and volume. Translocated fluids are replaced as follows with lactated Ringer's solution[14]:

Hourly maintenance volumes

0 to 10 kg body weight	4 ml/kg/hour
10 to 20 kg body weight	40 ml + 2 ml/kg/hour for each kg over 10
Over 20 kg body weight	60 ml + 1 ml/kg/hour for each kg over 20

Preoperative deficit

Hourly maintenance volume ×
        number of hours since last intake =
                the total deficit volume

Plan to give one half this volume during the first hour of anesthesia and one quarter during each of the second and third hours. As an example, a 7.5 kg child who has had no oral intake for 6 hours preoperatively would have a deficit of 7.5 (kg) × 4 (ml/kg/hour) × 6 (hours) = 180 ml. During the first hour of anesthesia, one would, in addition to hourly maintenance volumes, give 90 ml of 5% dextrose in one-fourth strength saline during the first hour of anesthesia and 45 ml during each of the second and third hours.

Translocation (shifts to "third space")

Translocation is very much a judgment decision. Lactated Ringer's solution, 3 to 10 ml/kg/hour, is added to the calculated maintenance volumes, depending on the nature and extent of the procedure. Translocation of fluid does not go on indefinitely and usually can be discounted after the first 2 or 3 hours of surgery. It should also be remembered that pyrexia increases basic fluid requirements by 7% for each 1° C. The urine is an invaluable indication of the efficacy of fluid therapy and replacement of losses. Urine output should be 0.5 to 1 ml/kg/hour, and the specific gravity should not fall below 1.014.

BLOOD LOSS REPLACEMENT

The average normal blood volume is generally assumed to be 90 ml/kg in the newborn, 80 ml/kg in the infant, and 70 to 75 ml/kg in the child. Blood loss is replaced on the following basis[14]: (1) if blood loss is under 10% of the estimated blood volume, it is replaced with an equal volume of warmed 5% dextrose in lactated Ringer's solution; (2) if blood loss is over 20% of estimated blood volume, it is replaced with whole blood or packed cells depending on the patient's hematocrit value, and (3) blood losses between 10% and 20% of estimated blood volume are usually replaced with 5% albumin in lactated Ringer's solution. Discretion must be used here. If the patient's hematocrit value was low to begin with, it would be wiser to replace losses of this magnitude with packed cells or whole blood. The transfusion of blood should be only undertaken after due consideration of the hazards involved and in the belief that they are outweighed by benefits of the transfusion. All blood should be filtered and warmed to body temperature before administration. The most convenient and accurate method of administration is a 10 or 20 ml syringe with a three-way stopcock in the infusion line.

RECOVERY FROM ANESTHESIA

Vital signs must be observed and recorded regularly. In the small patient the narrow upper airway means that otherwise minor degrees of obstruction are of major importance, especially since ventilatory reserve is reduced by adult standards. Ventilatory depression in the recovery room may be caused by the persistent effects of anesthetic agents, narcotics, or muscle relaxant drugs or by hypoxia, acidosis, hypothermia, or hypoglycemia. Intravenous naloxone rapidly and effectively reverses the respiratory and analgesic effects of narcotics. Since this effect only lasts approximately 20 minutes when the drug is given intravenously, an additional and equivalent intramuscular dose should be given, and the patient kept in the recovery room for 2 hours thereafter. Inadequate reversal of neuromuscular blockade is diagnosed with the aid of a nerve stimulator.[85] Possible causes such as respiratory acidosis, electrolyte imbalance, hypocalcemia, or antibiotics should receive attention, and neostigmine with atropine is, if deemed necessary, repeated in half the original dose. Stridor after extubation is especially likely to occur in children who have upper respiratory tract infections when the head has been moved frequently during the procedure or when the endotracheal tube fit has been too tight. Treatment consists of warmed humidified oxygen inhalation, nebulized racemic epinephrine inhalations and adequate hydration. Occasionally reintubation or a tracheostomy may be necessary. Steroids such as dexamethasone have been shown to be of no value.[82]

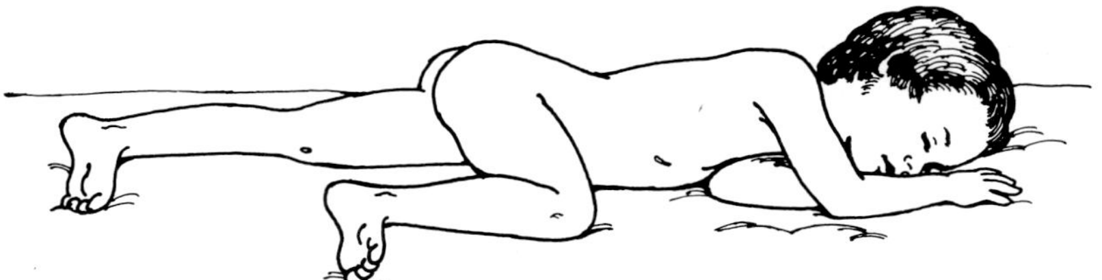

Fig. 4-5. Posttonsillectomy position.

After operations involving the nose, mouth, or throat, secretions and oozing are a potentially lethal hazard. The patient should be placed in the so-called posttonsillectomy position (Fig. 4-5). The patient lies on the side, the upper arm is flexed with the hand near the head, and the lower arm is comfortably positioned. This position allows forward rotation of the shoulders. The head is extended to facilitate airway maintenance and is somewhat rotated toward the mattress to promote pharyngeal drainage. A small pillow is placed between the legs with the lower leg extended, and the upper leg is well flexed at the knee and hip so that the upper femur acts as a strut to stabilize the pelvis in the lateral position. A large pillow is positioned behind the patient and a strap applied across the hips. Attention to detail is important.

Excitement and delirium during recovery are not uncommon, especially in the 3- to 9-year age group and in those who have undergone a tonsillectomy or have been given barbiturates or scopolamine as premedication.[54,88] This could be detrimental to the surgical result, especially when reconstructive repair has been performed. The incidence may be reduced by premedication with morphine[61] and adequate postoperative analgesia. Pharmacologic control may be considered, but only after hypoxia has been excluded as a possible cause. Diazepam given intravenously and physostigmine salicylate given intramuscularly 20 minutes before the end of the surgery have been advocated as a prophylactic measure.[124] They should not be used in patients who have asthma or who have received nondepolarizing muscle relaxants. Delay in the return of consciousness may be due to many factors. High concentrations of halothane or enflurane taken up during long surgical procedures will require time for elimination, and this process will be prolonged by ventilatory depression. Consideration should be given to hypothermia in particular, but also to the persistent effects of the premedication to osmolar disturbances, hypercapnia, hypoglycemia, and prolonged hypoxia or hypotension that may have occurred during anesthesia. Examination of the cardiorespiratory and nervous systems (including an EEG)[103] is supplemented by laboratory evaluation of arterial pH levels, blood gases, acid-base status, serum electrolytes and osmolality, and blood glucose levels.

LOCAL ANESTHESIA

The use of local anesthesia in pediatric surgery is limited for obvious reasons. Nevertheless, it is frequently possible to carry out procedures under local anesthesia when the surgeon succeeds in establishing mutual confidence and good rapport with an amenable young patient. Premedication may not be needed but, if desired, oral diazepam (Table 4-1) is recommended. It has good antianxiety properties and offers the best protection against the consequences of an inadvertently administered overdose of the local anesthetic agent. The drugs most commonly used and their maximal doses are listed in Table 4-1, and a detailed description of techniques is presented by Moore.[99]

Central nervous system signs of drug toxicity are usually seen 5 to 10 minutes after injection (unless accidental intravenous injection has occurred). They are manifested as amnesia and drowsiness, although cocaine and procaine tend to produce excitement and euphoria. The patient may complain of headache, lightheadedness, numbness or tingling of the lips and tongue, tinnitus, nausea, diplopia, and a flushed or chilly feeling. Slurred speech, confusion, nystagmus, and muscle tremors or twitching may be seen. These symptoms and signs are indicative of a rising serum level of the drug and may be followed by generalized convulsions that are indistinguishable from grand mal seizures. To avoid these manifestations, the maximal dose of local anesthetic agent that can be safely used (Table 4-1) should be determined; only the amount needed for the procedure should be used, and a vasoconstrictor such as epinephrine should be included, especially when the solution is to be injected into highly vascular areas or applied topically to mucous membranes. Care should be taken to avoid intravenous injection by frequent aspiration during infiltration, and it is wise to administer a test dose before proceeding with the full intended dose. There is much evidence[42,60] that diazepam is superior to any other drug used for the prevention and treatment of seizures induced by local anesthetic agents. Its prophylactic efficiency is, of course, dose related, but 0.1 to 0.15 mg/kg[41] given intramuscularly or orally an hour before administration of the local anesthetic will significantly raise the seizure threshold. If seizures do occur, they are usually of short duration, and important aspects of management include prevention of injury to the patient, maintenance of the airway and ventilation, and oxygen administration; thiopental in small incremental doses (1 to 2 mg/kg intravenously) has been used for many years, but diazepam in doses of 0.1 mg/kg intravenously may be equally effective, with few untoward effects on the cardiovascular system.[43] Even after therapeutic doses, local anesthetic agents may depress the cardiovascular system. The well-known signs of pallor, sweating, hypotension, and dysrhythmias (usually bradycardia) may be accompanied by clouding or loss of consciousness. There may be a skin wheal at the injection site or generalized urticaria with angioneurotic edema and bronchospasm, indicating an allergic reaction. Therapeutic measures include lowering of the head; support of ventilation; administration of oxygen, vasopressors (ephedrine or methoxamine), intravenous fluids, and steroids (hydrocortisone); and, if necessary, cardiopulmonary resuscitation.

The preceding discussion emphasizes the importance of having the necessary expertise and equipment at hand and close patient surveillance during procedures carried out under local anesthesia. Basic monitoring should comprise an ECG, a chest stethoscope, and blood pressure and body temperature measurements. An intravenous infusion should be in situ, through which incremental doses of diazepam are given for sedation as indicated, and supplemental oxygen should be given by mask if the patient will tolerate it. Thoughtful attention to posture and comfort in these awake patients minimizes the need for intraoperative sedation, since restlessness is often due to discomfort generated by having to lie still in an awkward position for long periods of time.

MALIGNANT HYPERTHERMIA

Malignant hyperthermia, first described in 1960,[44] is considered to be a pharmacogenetic myopathy of humans and swine.[21] It usually appears as a drug-induced pyrexic crisis,[24] but it also may be precipitated by emotional or physical stress or a high environmental temperature.[19] Malignant hyperthermia occurs in all age groups, with an overall incidence of approximately 1:20,000 of the anesthetized population, but, as with most genetic conditions, the incidence is greater and is about 1:12,000 in the pediatric age group.[24] The mortality is as high as 65%.[87] The inherited gene is autosomal dominant, and families with this gene have a greater incidence of musculoskeletal defects[56] such as strabismus, inguinal hernia, kyphoscoliosis, pes cavus, patellar subluxation, and cardiomyopathy[80] (idiopathic hypertrophic subaortic stenosis). Patients with acrocyanosis should be suspect, and there is a positive correlation between athletic activity and the disease. Not everyone who is susceptible to malignant hyperthermia responds every time to exposure to a precipitating factor. Persons have responded with an attack only at a second or third exposure or even later.

Almost all the drugs and agents used in general anesthesia have been incriminated as precipitating agents, although succinylcholine and halothane are the two most commonly reported.[120] Other drugs in this category include local anesthetics of the amide type, the phenothiazines, monoamine oxidase inhibitors, and some drugs used in psychiatric practice. Reactions may be aggravated by sympathomimetics, parasympatholytics, cardiac glycosides, and calcium salts.[21] Identification of susceptible persons is not easy. Since inheritance is dominant, approximately half the close relatives of a patient with an established diagnosis will be affected. Raised serum creatine phosphokinase (CPK) levels are not reliable predictors. The best diagnostic test currently available is done in vitro,[57,76] wherein a muscle specimen is exposed to halothane or caffeine. Tension in muscle from a susceptible person increases, whereas tension decreases in muscle taken from a normal subject.

The disorder manifests itself clinically a few minutes to 5 hours after commencement of anesthesia. The earliest sign is unexplained tachycardia.[22] Tachypnea and cyanosis appear, but the former may not be evident as an early sign in patients who have received paralyzing doses of muscle relaxants. Dysrhythmias occur as an early manifestation, usually as premature ventricular contractions, which increase in frequency as the serum potassium level rises. These early signs may arise from other causes and, if no immediate reason can be found for them, arterial blood gases must be determined without delay. Body temperature rises rapidly and in fulminating cases may ascend to 46° C, during which the increase may be greater than 6° C each hour. Any increase of more than 0.5° C must be explained. Muscle rigidity or spasm, especially of the masseter muscles, occurs early in 75% of cases but is not invariable and may develop several hours later.[56] Biochemical disturbances include severe hyperglycemia and a significant increase in CPK (in only two thirds of patients), lactic dehydrogenase, and transaminases. Depletion of platelets, fibrinogen, and clotting factors may result in generalized bleeding,[23] and myoglobinuria from massive muscle breakdown during the episode may be serious enough to result in acute renal failure.[22] All these clinical and biochemical changes are evidence of an acute hypermetabolic storm, and unless prompt active treatment (p. 62) is instituted the patient will die. For the acute episode, dantrolene sodium given intravenously in doses ranging from 1 to 10 mg/kg appears to be the most effective drug currently available. If circumstances permit, 2 mg/kg can be given three times daily for 1 day before the operation and again early on the day of the operation.[104] When given prophylactically by mouth, side effects such as weakness with incoordination of voluntary muscles, dizziness, diplopia, and drowsiness may occur. Procainamide given intravenously is of use during the episode, mainly to control ventricular dysrhythmias; it must be given slowly, since it may produce severe hypotension, necessitating the use of

---

TREATMENT OF MALIGNANT HYPERTHERMIA

Prevention

1. Constant awareness of the possibility of the syndrome
2. Obtain a careful history of patient and family
3. Look for musculoskeletal deformities
4. Obtain a CPK estimation (not conclusive)
5. Consider use of ester group of local anesthetics
6. Consider in vitro test on muscle specimen taken under appropriate local anesthesia

Pretreatment

Dantrolene sodium, 2 mg/kg, three times daily for 1 day before the operation

Immediate treatment

1. Discontinue anesthesia
2. Hyperventilate with 100% oxygen by nonrebreathing system
3. Cool patient: immerse in ice; administer cold intravenous saline, 25 ml/kg; administer intracavity cold fluids.
4. Correct acidosis: 2 to 4 mEq/kg sodium bicarbonate intravenously
5. Give dantrolene sodium: 1 to 10 mg intravenously
6. Give vasodilators to aid cooling: chlorpromazine, 1 mg/kg
7. Provide renal support: mannitol, 1 g/kg; furosemide, 1 mg/kg
8. Correct hyperkalemia: insulin and glucose
9. Give procainamide for dysrhythmias: 3 mg/kg intravenously, slowly; repeat if necessary

Later measures

1. Arterial line for blood gases and blood pressure
2. Monitoring central venous pressure; calcium, potassium, and glucose levels; disseminated intravascular coagulation
3. Urinary catheter for output and myoglobin
4. Control intracranial pressure if necessary
5. Continue dantrolene orally

---

vasopressors. Procaine may be used in attempts to reduce the muscle rigidity, but the high doses needed for this introduce the danger of severe cardiovascular depression.[7] It should be realized that, after an episode has been controlled, relapse may occur; muscle pain and swelling may persist for days or weeks and weakness and wasting for months. Anesthetic agents and drugs currently favored for use in susceptible patients are oral diazepam for premedication, thiopental or neuroleptanalgesia for induction, and fentanyl and nitrous oxide and oxygen with or without droperidol for maintenance. If muscle relaxation is required, pancuronium may be used. For local analgesia procaine, tetracaine, or chloroprocaine should be used, since bupivacaine, mepivacaine, etidocaine, prilocaine, and lidocaine have all been suspected of initiating the disorder.

THE DRY SURGICAL FIELD

Control of perfusion pressure is only one of a number of factors needed to produce a dry surgical field. Venous congestion is avoided by appropriate positioning of the patient, and local hyperemia is minimized by avoiding hypercapnia, tachycardia, and hypoxia, while the surgeon may choose to infiltrate the area with drugs to produce vasoconstriction. The maximal doses indicated in Table 4-1 should be adhered to to minimize the likelihood of dysrhythmias that may occur, especially in the presence of halothane and, to a lesser extent, with enflurane. These measures will reduce blood flow to the area concerned and provide the desired operating conditions. Controlled hypotension is commonly achieved by specific drugs supplemented by halothane. The use of ganglion blocking drugs such as trimethaphan and pentolinium[121] has generally been superseded by sodium nitroprusside.[16,39] It must be administered as an intravenous infusion via a controlled-rate infusion device, and intraarterial pressure monitoring is essential to safety. Care should be taken not to exceed the permissable dose of sodium nitroprusside, which is 10 µg/kg/min with a total maximum of 1.5 mg/kg.[16] Other important aspects are adequate ventilation and oxygenation, adequate hydration, careful replacement of blood loss, and frequent monitoring of arterial blood gases and acid-base status. Satisfactory control of arterial pressure is possible and results are good; but the technique should only be employed by someone conversant with the problems and hazards associated with its use.

CLEFT LIP AND CLEFT PALATE

Repair of cleft lip is usually undertaken when the infant is 4 to 6 weeks old, but sometimes sooner if they have feeding problems. The anesthesiologist should be aware of the possibility of chronic dehydration because of poor fluid intake and the hemoglobin level and white blood cell count should be checked preoperatively. Children with cleft palate may have coexisting anomalies such as congenital heart disease, Treacher Collins' syndrome, or Pierre Robin syndrome,[38,45,115] and middle ear infections and nasopharyngeal discharge are common. An abnormal nasal humidification system and copious nasopharyngeal secretions are a natural consequence of the anomaly and are no contraindication to anesthesia; but in the presence of acute upper respiratory tract infection elective surgery should be postponed. The major anesthetic consideration is the establishment of an airway and its maintenance throughout anesthesia and during the postoperative period. For this reason preoperative sedation is omitted, but atropine or glycopyrrolate is given to minimize secretions.

Induction is by inhalation of nitrous oxide and halothane, and an intravenous infusion is established. When satisfactory control of the airway is established, succinylcholine may be given for intubation. This assists smooth introduc-

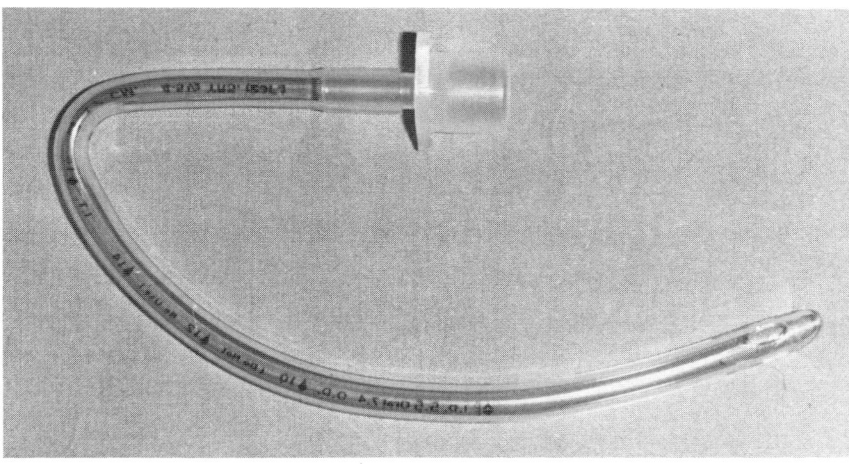

Fig. 4-6. Rae endotracheal tube.

tion of a correctly fitting endotracheal tube and minimizes trauma to the upper airway. It also obviates the need for deep halothane anesthesia, which may be hazardous in these infants. Left-sided clefts, which more commonly occur, do not interfere much with intubation. Right-sided clefts do, however, because of the folds of the lip structures and the fact that the laryngoscope blade tends to fall into the cleft. A prerolled gauze pack can be fitted into the cleft to prevent this. A No. 1 Miller or Robertshaw laryngoscope blade is usually best, although sometimes a Macintosh blade may be better. A preformed right-angled Rae endotracheal tube (Fig. 4-6) is better than either a standard tube or a nylon-reinforced armored tube. It should be securely taped to the center of the lower lip, and a firm gauze pack placed in the hypopharynx to seal the airway and to stabilize the tube and minimize the possibility of it being dislodged by forward and downward rotation. Anesthesia is maintained with 0.5% halothane in nitrous oxide and oxygen, and ventilation is controlled with the aid of a nondepolarizing relaxant such as pancuronium. Alternatively one may use higher concentrations of halothane in nitrous oxide and oxygen, without a relaxant, and ventilation can be assisted intermittently. However, the former technique allows better control of ventilation (an important consideration in view of the steep Trendelenburg position required for surgical access) and prompt return of laryngeal reflexes and function at the termination of the operation, provided the effect of the relaxant is reversed at that time. Extubation must always be performed with the patient almost awake. This is because laryngospasm is much more likely to occur during emergence from anesthesia, especially in the presence of secretions and blood oozing from the surgical field, and attempts at overcoming this may result in disruption of the repair. If there is concern about the airway at the end of surgery, a silk suture should be placed deeply in the tongue so that forward traction is available to help control the airway. This is par-

ticularly important after pharyngeal flap surgery during which a flap of pharyngeal mucosa is rotated forward to close off the incompetent soft palate, leaving small orifices bilaterally for nasal breathing. Extensive dissection results in more tissue edema postoperatively and the possibility of upper respiratory tract obstruction. A tongue suture and light anesthesia are especially important for extubation after anesthesia for this procedure.

Postoperative supervision by trained and experienced personnel is essential. Patients with clefts are accustomed to breathing through the cleft; therefore repair of the defect, operative edema, and the ever-present nasopharyngeal secretions readily produce obstruction of the narrow airway. Postoperative oozing often poses a most difficult problem. The extent of the bleeding may be concealed by the fact that the patient swallows a good deal of the blood; clots, blood, and secretions tend to obstruct the limited airway, resulting in hypoxia, which in turn causes restlessness and increases the bleeding. Heavy sedation must be avoided. The patient is placed in an oxygen tent lying in the posttonsillectomy position (Fig. 4-5), and intravenous diazepam in small divided doses is administered until the desired degree of sedation is obtained. The patient must be kept in the posttonsillectomy position and be constantly under the supervision of a trained observer. It is important to maintain an adequate blood volume and body temperature, especially since losses may be concealed and the patient may have to be anesthetized again to control the bleeding. Laryngeal edema may occur and is usually effectively managed by mist therapy and inhalation of racemic epinephrine (Table 4-1). Reintubation or tracheostomy rarely are required. Patients are discharged from the operating room when the surgeon is satisfied that there is no bleeding, the anesthesiologist is satisfied that the airway is in no way compromised, the laryngeal reflexes and the ability to cough are present, secretions are not troublesome, and cardiovascular and respiratory functions are normal. These patients often stay in the recovery room for a longer time than most, but this is an eminently worthwhile precaution.

CRANIOFACIAL SURGERY

In approaching anesthesia for craniofacial deformities, the anesthesiologist should have a clear understanding of the proposed procedure and its complications and of any coexisting medical problems. The essential anesthesia problems are those of airway management, large blood losses, the control of brain volume, and the prolonged duration of surgery. The possibility of problems associated with the airway is indicated by a history of chronic airway obstruction (commonly due to adenoid hypertrophy) or by the presence of gross disturbances of maxillary-mandibular relationships. Hypoplasia of the mandible, decreased mandibular excursion, microstomia, a high-arched palate, and prominent central incisors all make exposure of the larynx difficult or impossible.[48,114] The problems associated with the difficult airway have been reviewed.[74,120] No preoperative sedatives are ordered for these patients, and, since tachycardia is undesirable when controlled hypotension is planned, anticholinergics are omitted. Induction is by inhalational agents such as halothane, and no muscle relaxants are given until the anesthesiologist is satisfied that the patient can be ventilated. Oral intubation, using a Rae tube (Fig. 4-6) is performed for procedures above the lower third of the maxilla; nasotracheal intubation is used when maxillary advancement is planned, the tube being placed with its tip near the carina to allow for as much as 3 cm of cephalad advancement without extubation during surgery.[40] The tube must be secured by a suture, and a pharyngeal pack inserted to stabilize it. A tracheostomy is performed when intubation is impossible or when intermaxillary fixation is combined with a posterior pharyngeal flap or other extensive intraoral surgery. Anesthesia is maintained with nitrous oxide and oxygen supplemented by intermittent doses of fentanyl (0.002 mg/kg/hour), and controlled ventilation is facilitated by neuromusclar blockade. Postoperatively when the airway is in doubt, the endotracheal tube is left in situ for 48 hours or longer, whereupon extubation is performed, in the operating room if necessary. In anticipation of large blood losses, which may occur especially during a mandibular osteotomy or during a craniectomy from a torn sagittal sinus, an intraarterial line, a central venous catheter, and two large-bore peripheral infusion lines should be set up. The blood loss should be measured, urine output monitored, and attention paid to thermal homeostasis. All pressure points should be well protected. For intracranial procedures brain volume is controlled by reducing the $Paco_2$ to 25 mm Hg,[70,75] administering mannitol and dexamethasone,[129] or draining spinal fluid via a malleable needle positioned in the lumbar subarachnoid space. Ketamine is contraindicated. Controlled hypotension will minimize blood loss; however, blood should be replaced using lactated Ringer's solution, with or without 5% albumin, or whole blood. Clotting factors and platelets should receive attention, and calcium is given as indicated by serial ionized calcium estimations. Anesthetic complications include those of massive blood replacement and pulmonary edema from excess fluid therapy. Deaths have occurred as a result of inadequate volume replacement, excessive volume replacement, cerebral edema, and postoperative airway obstruction.

SICKLE CELL DISEASE

Sickle cell hemoglobin (Hb S) results from the replacement of glutamine by valine in the hemoglobin molecule, with an alteration in the electrical charge of the molecule; this results in the formation of crystals and tactoids in the presence of hypoxia or acidosis. The erythrocytes become deformed and irregular and may assume a sickle shape, resulting in obstruction of the microcirculation. The incidence of sickle cell anemia in blacks is about 4/1000, and these patients ahve a pathologic condition that is of great importance to the surgeon and anesthesiologist. They exhibit varying degrees of anemia because of excessive hemolysis and the sequestration by the spleen of the abnormally shaped erythrocytes. On the average the hemoglobin level is around 7 g/dL. Incessant hemopoiesis results in high reticulocyte counts and expanded bone marrow spaces in the long bones and skull. Microthrombi in the pulmonary circulation cause infarcts, which in turn result in pulmonary hypertension and ventilation/perfusion defects. A large proportion of patients have cardiomegaly caused by the high cardiac output of anemia, increased plasma volume, and pulmonary hypertension. The concentrating ability of the kidneys may be impaired by repeated cortical infarctions, so that dehydration occurs rapidly, and urinary specific gravity is not a reliable parameter. Resistance to infection is low because of immune suppression, which results from the functional splenectomy and reticuloendothelial incompetence caused by red blood cell debris. Crises are precipitated by hypoxia, acidosis, or infections.

Patients scheduled for an elective operation[17] should receive transfusions with fresh packed cells at weekly intervals until the level of Hb S falls below 30% and normal hemoglobin values are achieved, if time permits. The rate of transfusion should not be in excess of 10 ml/kg over a 12-hour period because of the risk of volume overload in a chronically anemic patient. Transfusion reactions are more likely to occur because the patient in all probability will have received a previous transfusion. In an emergency, a transfusion with fresh packed cells should be commenced as soon as possible and continued throughout the operation and postoperatively to maintain a hemoglobin level of at least 10 g/dL. However, when it is possible to delay an operation for a few hours, an exchange transfusion should be considered. Dehydration, hypothermia, acidosis, and hypoxia must be corrected, and any infection must be treated vigorously. Anesthesia is conducted with a view to avoiding hypoxia, acidosis, hypothermia, and hypotension. Crystalloid fluid therapy must be aggressive, and dextran should be avoided. Spinal anesthesia and tourniquets are contraindicated.[17] Browne[26] has presented a comprehensive review of the anesthetic problems and management of these patients.

HEMOPHILIA

Hemophilia A or B is not considered a contraindication to operation and anesthesia, provided the patient is well prepared. Commercial preparations of factor VIII or IX are preferred to cryoprecipitates, since the latter have a large amount of fibrinogen, which may interfere with proper clot formation.[77] The aim should be to raise serum levels to at least 50% of normal,[123] although levels of 80% to 100% may be preferable. Levels above 30% of normal have been shown to be necessary for surgical hemostasis,[58] but in any event a normal activated partial thromboplastin time after infusion will indicate a satisfactory response. The infusion should be given 2 hours before surgery and again immediately after, followed by 8 hourly infusions for the next 3 to 5 days and 12 hourly transfusions thereafter until the patient leaves the hospital. In these circumstances laryngoscopy and intubation may be performed, and any of the currently available anesthetic agents may be used, but drugs such as aspirin, indomethacin, phenylbutazone, clofibrate, and sulfisoxazole must be avoided.[55]

OUTPATIENT ANESTHESIA

There are several advantages to pediatric outpatient surgery. More hospital beds are conserved for those who need them and the cost of medical care is reduced by about 50%. Separation from family minimizes psychologic problems,[131] and family expenses in terms of repeated trips to the hospital, meals away from home, and time away from work are reduced. The risk of cross infection is also greatly reduced. However, although there may be minor operations, there is no such thing as a minor anesthetic; these patients require the same clinical care, supervision, and monitoring that is provided for inpatient surgery.[5] Simple complications such as aspiration, overdose, and undetected blood loss are the commonest causes of anesthetic mortality.[119] The patient should be in good health or have a systemic disease that is well controlled (American Society of Anesthesiologists classes I or II, see p. 51). Surgical procedures best suited to outpatient anesthesia are those of short duration with minimal bleeding; infected patients are not considered suitable unless separate facilities in the recovery areas can be provided. Certain patients require minimal preoperative preparation, but do need postoperative hospitalization. They may be dealt with in the same way as outpatients, thus saving a night in the hospital.[2] Preoperative assessment by the anesthesiologist may be carried out either at the time of the initial surgical consultation or on the day of the procedure. It consists of a history and examination, and discussion with the parents and the patient, including an explanation of the anesthetic procedure. Routine laboratory data consist of a determination of the hemoglobin levels, white blood cell count, and urinalysis; more extensvie investigations are only undertaken when indications for them exist. Before the patient is taken to the operating room, the anesthesiologist must document the time of the last ingestion of fluids or food and check the consent form. At this point admission may be turned down if any doubts exist as to recent intake of food or fluids, pyrexia, or a respiratory tract infection. If all is well, no premedication is given and the child is taken to the operating room area where anesthesia is induced by mask, using a mixture of nitrous oxide with halothane or enflurane. There is no contraindication to the use of an intravenous induction agent such as thiopental or methohexital, muscle relaxants, or endotracheal intubation, but drugs with prolonged effects, such as ketamine or droperidol, are best avoided.

When the operation is complete, a small dose of fentanyl may be given or an appropriate nerve block performed if the procedure has been a painful one, and the child is taken to the recovery area. The mother is called in when the patient is sufficiently recovered. After a check by the anesthesiologist the child is discharged, with instructions to the parent concerning feeding and follow-up care. Some institutions have guidelines regarding the discharge time, which may vary from 2 to 4 hours; those children who have been intubated should be detained for up to 4 hours. Patients requiring admission postoperatively include those with unexplained fever, croup, bleeding, drowsiness, or repeated vomiting[135] but this occurs in less than 2% of cases.[3]

The American Society of Anesthesiologists has laid down guidelines[5] that detail the recommendations for a facility dealing with outpatient anesthesia. These are recommended to anyone interested in establishing such a facility or updating an existing one.

SUMMARY AND CONCLUSIONS

The risk to the child undergoing anesthesia is determined by many factors. The mortality has fallen significantly during the past decade; a major study revealed the mortality of critically ill pediatric patients undergoing surgery to be approximately 0.2/10,000 patients. The major causes of anesthesia-related morbidity and mortality in pediatric patients are hypoxia and hypovolemia.

Anesthetized infants readily become hypothermic even during short procedures, as do older children undergoing longer procedures, especially when a body cavity has been opened or large surface areas are exposed, such as during skin grafting of burns. The greatest degree of heat loss occurs during induction of anesthesia and preparation for surgery. Measures to control heat loss include the following:

1. Elevation of room temperature to 24° C
2. A warmed mattress
3. An overhead radiant heater

4. Covering the infant's limbs and trunk with a plastic drape
5. Delivery to the trachea of humidified gases heated to a temperature of 36° C
6. Warming to body temperature all intravenous solutions and blood products

During the first few weeks of life, the kidney of the newborn infant is unable to secrete sodium adequately, and the ability to vary the concentration of urinary solutes is therefore moderately impaired. After the first few weeks of life, the newborn should achieve normal renal function. Dextrose (5%) in one-fourth strength saline is used to provide maintenance fluid requirements and to replace the deficit due to preoperative withholding of oral fluids. Hourly maintenance and blood loss replacement formulas, depending on the patient's weight, are detailed in the text.

Delayed return of consciousness after anesthesia may be due to many factors, among which are delayed elimination of the anesthetic agents (e.g., hypoventilation), hypothermia, electrolyte and osmolar disturbances, hypoglycemia, hyperglycemia, and prolonged hypoxia or hypotension, which may have occurred intraoperatively.

After the administration of local anesthetic agents, central nervous system signs of drug toxicity are usually seen within 10 minutes. These are manifested as amnesia and drowsiness, although procaine and cocaine tend to produce excitement and euphoria. The patient may complain of headache, lightheadedness, numbness and tingling of the lips and tongue, tinnitus, nausea, diplopia, and a flushed or chilly feeling. These signs and symptoms are indicative of a rising serum level of the drug and may be followed by generalized convulsions. To avoid these manifestions, the maximal safe level of local anesthetic agent should not be exceeded. Pediatric drug doses according to weight are indicated in Table 4-1.

Malignant hyperthermia is considered to be a pharmacogenetic myopathy. It usually appears as a drug-induced pyrexic crisis, but it may also be precipitated by emotional or physical stress or a high environmental temperature. The incidence in the pediatric age group is approximately 1/12,000. Mortality may be as high as 65%. This disorder is inherited as an autosomal dominant trait. Succinylcholine and halothane are the two most commonly reported drugs incriminated as precipitating agents. Dantrolene sodiumn given intravenously in doses ranging from 1 to 10 mg/kg appears to be the most effective drug currently available for treatment of this condition.

Patients born with clefts of the lip or palate become accustomed to breathing through the cleft. After repair of the defect, as a result of the operative trauma and ever-present nasopharyngeal secretions, airway obstruction may readily occur. This may be further complicated by postoperative oozing from the operative site. After surgery the patient should be placed in an oxygen tent, in a posttonsillectomy position. Heavy sedation must be avoided.

Essential anesthesia problems that arise during craniofacial surgery are those of airway management, large blood losses, control of brain volume, and prolonged duration of the surgery. An adequate airway must be maintained postoperatively for 48 hours or longer. This may be accomplished by leaving the endotracheal tube in situ or by a tracheostomy.

Patients with sickle cell disease have erythrocytes that become deformed and irregular in the presence of hypoxia or acidosis, thus obstructing the microcirculation. Multiple microthrombi may form in all organ systems. For this reason, the concentrating ability of the kidneys may be impaired by repeated cortical infarctions, and resistance to infection may be low due to immune suppression that results from the functional splenectomy and reticuloendothelial incompetence caused by red blood cell debris. When scheduled for elective surgery these patients should be given transfusions with fresh packed cells at weekly intervals until the level of Hb S falls below 30%. Patients with hemophilia A or B should receive commercial preparations of factor VIII or IX so that serum levels rise to at least 50% of normal.

There are many advantages to pediatric outpatient surgery. There is no such thing as a minor anesthetic, and patients undergoing this type of surgery require the same clinical care, supervision, and monitoring that is provided for inpatient surgery. Surgical procedures best suited to outpatient anesthesia are those of short duration with minimal bleeding. Certain guidelines and recommendations for a facility dealing with outpatient anesthesia are given.

REFERENCES

1. Adamsons, K., Jr., Gandy, G.M., and James, L.S.: The influence of thermal factors upon oxygen consumption of the newborn infant, J. Pediatr. **66:**495, 1965.
2. Ahlgren, E.W.: Pediatric outpatient anesthesia: a four-year review, Am. J. Dis. Child. **126:**36, 1973.
3. Ahlgren, E.W., Bennett, E.J., and Stephen, C.R.: Outpatient pediatric anesthesiology: a case series, Anesth. Analg. **50:**402, 1971.
4. Allen, E.V.: Thromboangiitis obliterans: methods of diagnosis of chronic occlusive arterial lesions distal to the wrist with illustrative cases, Am. J. Med. Sci. **178:**237, 1929.
5. American Society of Anesthesiologists: Guidelines for ambulatory services, Park Ridge, Ill., 1977, The Society.
6. Atkinson, R.S., Rushman, G.B., and Lee, J.A.: A synopsis of anesthesia, ed. 8, Bristol, 1977, John Wright & Sons, Ltd.
7. Austin, K.L., and Denborough, M.A.: Drug treatment of malignant hyperpyrexia, Anaesth. Intensive Care **5:**207, 1977.
8. Ayre, P.: Endotracheal anesthesia for babies: with special reference to hare-lip and cleft palate operations, Curr. Res. Anesth. Analg. **16:**330, 1937.
9. Bain, J.A., and Spoerel, W.E.: A streamlined anesthetic system, Can. Anaesth. Soc. J. **19:**426, 1972.
10. Bain, J.A., and Spoerel, W.E.: Flow requirements for a modified Mapleson D system during controlled ventilation, Can. Anaesth. Soc. J. **20:**629, 1973.
11. Bain, J.A., and Spoerel, W.E.: Prediction of arterial carbon dioxide tension during controlled ventilation with a modified Mapleson D system, Can. Anaesth. Soc. J. **22:**34, 1975.
12. Bain, J.A., and Spoerel, W.E.: Carbon dioxide output and elimination in children under anesthesia, Can. Anaesth. Soc. J. **24:**533, 1977.
13. Bemelmans, L.: Madeline, New York, 1939, The Viking Press.

14. Bennett, E.J.: Fluids for anesthesia and surgery in the newborn and the infant, Springfield, Ill., 1975, Charles C Thomas, Publisher.

15. Bennett, E.J., Patel, K.P., and Grundy, E.M.: Neonatal temperature and surgery, Anesthesiology **46:**303, 1977.

16. Bennett, N.R., and Abbott, T.R.: The use of sodium nitroprusside in children, Anaesthesia **32:**456, 1977.

17. Bently, P.G., and Howard, E.R.: Surgery in children with homozygous sickle cell anaemia, Ann. R. Coll. Surg. Engl. **61:**55, 1979.

18. Birch, A.A., Jr., Mitchell, G.D., Playford, G.A., and Lang, C.A.: Changes in serum potassium response to succinylcholine following trauma, J.A.M.A. **210:**490, 1969.

19. Britt, B.A.: Malignant hyperthermia: a pharmacogenetic disease of skeletal and cardiac muscle, N. Engl. J. Med. **290:**1140, 1974.

20. Britt, B.A.: Malignant hyperthermia, Mod. Med. Canada **31:**511, 1976.

21. Britt, B.A.: Etiology and pathophysiology of malignant hyperthermia, Fed. Proc. **38:**44, 1979.

22. Britt, B.A., and Kalow, W.: Malignant hyperthermia: a statistical review, Can. Anaesth. Soc. J. **17:**293, 1970.

23. Britt, B.A., Kwong, F.H-F., and Endrenyi, I.: The clinical and laboratory features of malignant hyperthermia management—a review. In Henschel, E.O., editor: Malignant hyperthermia: current concepts, New York, 1977, Appleton-Century-Crofts.

24. Britt, B.A., Locher, W.G., and Kalow, W.: Hereditary aspects of malignant hyperthermia, Can. Anaesth. Soc. J. **16:**89, 1969.

25. Brodsky, J.B.: A simple method to determine patency of the ulnar artery intraoperatively prior to radial-artery cannulation, Anesthesiology **42:**626, 1975.

26. Browne, R.A.: Anaesthesia in patients with sickle-cell anaemia, Br. J. Anaesth. **37:**181, 1965.

27. Bush, G.H., and Stead, A.L.: The use of *d*-tubocurarine in neonatal anaesthesia, Br. J. Anaesth. **34:**721, 1962.

28. Caceres, E., and Whittembury, G.: Evaluation of blood losses during surgical operations, comparison of the gravimetric method with the blood volume determination, Surgery **45:**681, 1959.

29. Calcagno, P.L., Rubin, M.I., Weintraub, D.H., et al.: Studies on the renal concentrating and diluting mechanisms in the premature infant, J. Clin. Invest. **33:**91, 1954.

30. Chamney, A.R.: Humidification requirements and techniques, including a review of the performance of equipment in current use, Anaesthesia **24:**602, 1969.

31. Clark, B., and Coleman, L.L.: Pop-up going to the hospital, New York, 1971, Random House, Inc.

32. Cook, D.R., and Fischer, C.G.: Neuromuscular blocking effects of succinylcholine in infants and children, Anesthesiology **42:**662, 1975.

33. Cooperman, L.H.: Succinylcholine-induced hyperkalemia in neuromuscular disease, J.A.M.A. **213:**1867, 1970.

34. Coran, A.G., Das, J.B., and Eraklis, A.J.: Use of osmometry in the preoperative and postoperative management of the newborn, J. Pediatr. Surg. **6:**529, 1971.

35. Cousins, M.J.: Halothane and the liver: "firm ground" at last? Anaesth. Intensive Care **7:**5, 1979.

36. Cousins, M.J., Sharp, J.H., Gourlay, G.K., et al.: Hepatotoxicity and halothane metabolism in an animal model with application for human toxicity, Anaesth. Intensive Care **7:**9, 1979.

37. Cullen, S.C., and Larson, C.P.: Essentials of anesthetic practice, Chicago, 1974, Year Book Medical Publishers, Inc.

38. Davies, D.W., Chappell, C., Whiting, D.H., and Adendorff, D.J.: An approach to the management of children with cleft lip or palate, S. Afr. Med. J. **54:**1001, 1978.

39. Davies, D.W., Greiss, L., Kadar, D., and Steward, D.J.: Sodium nitroprusside in children: observations on metabolism during normal and abnormal responses, Can. Anaesth. Soc. J. **22:**553, 1975.

40. Davies, D.W., and Munro, I.R.: The anesthetic management and intraoperative care of patients undergoing major facial osteotomies, Plast. Reconstr. Surg. **55:**50, 1975.

41. De Jong, R.H.: Local anesthetics, ed. 2, Springfield, Ill., 1977, Charles C Thomas, Publisher.

42. De Jong, R.H., and Heavner, J.E.: Diazepam prevents local anesthetic seizures, Anesthesiology **34:**523, 1971.

43. De Jong, R.H., and Heavner, J.E.: Local anesthetic seizure prevention: diazepam versus pentobarbital, Anesthesiology **36:**449, 1972.

44. Denborough, M.A., and Lovell, R.R.H.: Anaesthetic deaths in a family, Lancet **2:**45, 1960.

45. Dennison, W.M.: The Pierre Robin syndrome, Pediatrics **36:**336, 1965.

46. Denny-Brown, D., and Brenner, C.: Paralysis of nerve induced by direct pressure and by tourniquet, Arch. Neurol. Psychiatr. **51:**1, 1944.

47. Desmond, J.W.: Methoxyflurane nephrotoxicity, Can. Anaesth. Soc. J. **21:**294, 1974.

48. Divekab, V.M., and Sircar, B.N.: Anesthetic management in Treacher Collins' syndrome, Anesthesiology **26:**692, 1965.

49. Dorsch, J.A., and Dorsch, S.E.: Understanding anesthesia equipment: construction, care and complications, Baltimore, 1975, The Williams & Wilkins Co.

50. Dowdy, E.G., and Kaya, K.: Studies of the mechanism of cardiovascular responses to CI-581, Anesthesiology **29:**931, 1968.

51. Downes, J.J., Kemp, R.A., and Lambersten, C.J.: The magnitude and duration of respiratory depression due to fentanyl and meperidine in man, J. Pharmacol. Exp. Ther. **158:**416, 1967.

52. Downes, J.J., and Raphaely, R.C.: Anesthesia and intensive care. In Ravitch, M.D., editor: Pediatric surgery, ed. 3, Chicago, 1979, Year Book Medical Publishers, Inc.

53. Eckenhoff, J.E.: Some anatomic considerations of the infant larynx influencing endotracheal anesthesia, Anesthesiology **12:**401, 1951.

54. Eckenhoff, J.E., Kneale, D.H., and Dripps, R.D.: The incidence and etiology of postanesthetic excitement, Anesthesiology **22:**667, 1961.

55. Eipe, J.: Drugs affecting therapy with anticoagulants, Med. Clin. North Am. **56:**255, 1972.

56. Ellis, F.R.: Malignant hyperthermia. In Vickers, M.D., editor: Medicine for anaesthetists, Oxford, 1977, Blackwell Scientific Publications.

57. Ellis, F.R., Keaney, N.P., and Harriman, D.G.: Screening for malignant hyperpyrexia, Br. Med. J. **3:**559, 1972.

58. Ellison, N.: Diagnosis and management of bleeding disorders, Anesthesiology **47:**171, 1977.

59. Falk, A.M.: The ambulance, Toronto, 1972, Burke Publishing (Canada), Ltd.

60. Feinstein, M.B., Lenard, W., and Mathias, J.: The antagonism of local anesthetic induced convulsions by the benzodiazepine derivative diazepam, Arch. Int. Pharmacodyn. Ther. **187:**144, 1970.

61. Freeman, A., and Bachman, L.: Pediatric anesthesia: an evaluation of preoperative medication, Anesth. Analg. **38:**429, 1959.

62. Fromen, R.: Let's find out about the clinic, New York, 1969, Franklin Watts, Inc.

63. Gardner, A.E., Olson, B.E., and Lichtiger, M.: Cerebrospinal fluid pressure during dissociative anesthesia and ketamine, Anesthesiology **35:**226, 1971.

64. Gauderer, M., and Holgersen, L.O.: Peripheral arterial line insertion in neonates and infants: a simplified method of temporal artery cannulation, J. Pediatr. Surg. **9:**875, 1974.

65. Goudsouzian, N.G., Donlon, J.V., Savarese, J.J., and Ryan, J.F.: Reevaluation of dosage and duration of action of *d*-tubocurarine in the pediatric age group, Anesthesiology **43:**416, 1975.

66. Goudsouzian, N.G., Morris, R.H., and Ryan, J.F.: The effects of a warming blanket on the maintenance of body temperatures in anesthetised infants and children, Anesthesiology **39:**351, 1973.

67. Goudsouzian, N.G., and Ryan, J.F.: Recent advances in pediatric anesthesia, Pediatr. Clin. North Am. **23:**345, 1976.

68. Goudsouzian, N.G., Ryan, J.F., and Savarese, J.J.: The neuromuscular effects of pancuronium in infants and children, Anesthesiology **41:**95, 1974.

69. Graff, T.D., Phillips, O.C., Benson, D.W., and Kelley, E.: Baltimore anesthesia study committee: factors in pediatric anesthesia mortality, Anesth. Analg. **43:**407, 1964.

70. Granholm, L.: Cerebral effects of hyperventilation, Acta Anaesthesiol. Scand. **34:**115, 1971.

71. Grant, C.J., Powell, J.N., and Radford, S.G.: Effects of halothane on DNA synthesis and mitosis in root tip meristems of *Vicia faba*, Br. J. Anaesth. **46:**653, 1974.

72. Grant, C.J., Powell, J.N., and Radford, S.G.: The induction of chromosomal abnormalities by inhalation anesthetics, Mutat. Res. **46:**177, 1977.

73. Gregory, G.A., Eger, E.I., II, and Munson, E.S.: The relationship between age and halothane requirements in man, Anesthesiology **30:**488, 1969.

74. Handler, S.E., Beaugard, M.E., Whitaker, L.A., and Potsic, W.P.: Airway management in the repair of craniofacial defects, Cleft Palate J. **16:**16, 1979.

75. Harp, J.R., and Wollman, H.: Cerebral metabolic effects of hyperventilation and deliberate hypotension, Br. J. Anaesth. **45:**256, 1973.

76. Harriman, D.G.F., Sumner, D.W., and Ellis, F.R.: Malignant hyperpyrexia myopathy, Q.J. Med. **42:**639, 1973.

77. Hathaway, W.E., Mahasandana, C., Clarke, S., and Humbert, J.R.: Paradoxical bleeding in intensively transfused hemophiliacs: alteration of platelet function, Transfusion **13:**6, 1973.

78. Henville, J.D., and Adams, A.P.: The Bain anaesthetic system: an assessment during controlled ventilation, Anaesthesia **31:**247, 1976.

79. Hey, E.: Physiological principles involved in the care of the preterm human infant. In Austin, C.R.: The mammalian fetus in vitro, New York, 1973, Halstead Press.

80. Huckell, V.F., Staniloff, H.M., Britt, B.A., et al.: Cardiac manifestations of malignant hyperthermia susceptibility, Circulation **58:**919, 1978.

81. Hunter, A.R.: Drugs for producing dissociative states, Int. Anesthesiol. Clin. **11:**1, 1973.

82. James, J.A.: Dexamethasone in croup: a controlled study, Am. J. Dis. Child. **117:**511, 1969.

83. John, D.A., Tobey, R.E., Homer, L.D., and Rice, C.L.: Onset of succinylcholine-induced hyperkalemia following denervation, Anesthesiology **45:**294, 1976.

84. Johnson, B.D.: Psychosis and ketamine, Br. Med. J. **4:**428, 1971.

85. Katz, R.L.: Comparison of electrical and mechanical recording of spontaneous and evoked muscle activity, Anesthesiology **26:**204, 1965.

86. Kay, E.: The operating room, New York, 1970, Franklin Watts, Inc.

87. King, J.O., and Denborough, M.A.: Anesthetic-induced malignant hyperpyrexia in children, J. Pediatr. **83:**37, 1973.

88. Korsch, B.M.: The child and the operating room, Anesthesiology **43:**251, 1975.

89. LeVeen, H.H., and Rubricius, J.L.: Continuous, automatic, electronic determinations of operative blood loss, Surg. Gynecol. Obstet. **106:**368, 1958.

90. Lockhart, C.H., and Nelson, W.L.: The relationship of ketamine requirement to age in pediatric patients, Anesthesiology **40:**507, 1974.

91. Mapleson, W.W.: The elimination of rebreathing in various semiclosed anaesthetic systems, Br. J. Anaesth. **26:**323, 1954.

92. Marfatia, S., Donahoe, P.K., and Hendren, W.H.: Effect of dry and humidified gases on the respiratory epithelium in rabbits, J. Pediatr. Surg. **10:**583, 1975.

93. Martin, J.T.: Positioning in anesthesia and surgery, Philadelphia, 1978, W.B. Saunders Co.

94. Mazze, R.I., and Cousins, M.J.: Renal toxicity of anaesthetics with specific reference to the nephrotoxicity of methoxyflurane, Can. Anaesth. Soc. J. **20:**64, 1973.

95. Mazze, R.I., and Dunbar, R.W.: Intralingual succinylcholine administration in children: an alternative to intravenous and intramuscular routes? Anesth. Analg. **47:**605, 1968.

96. McGill, W.A., Coveler, L.A., and Epstein, B.S.: Subacute upper respiratory infection in small children, Anesth. Analg. **58:**331, 1979.

97. McLaughlin, G.W., Kirby, R.R., and Kemmerer, W.T.: Indirect measurement of blood pressure in infants utilizing Doppler ultrasound, J. Pediatr. **79:**300, 1971.

98. Mirakhur, R.K.: Comparative study of the effects of oral and I.M. atropine and hyoscine in volunteers, B. J. Anaesth. **50:**591, 1978.

99. Moore, D.C.: Regional block, ed. 4, Springfield, Ill., 1965, Charles C Thomas, Publisher.

100. Neigh, J.L., Garman, J.K., and Harp, J.R.: The electroencephalographic pattern during anesthesia with Ethrane: effects of depth of anesthesia, $Paco_2$, and nitrous oxide, Anesthesiology **35:**482, 1971.

101. Nicodemus, H.F., Massiri-Rahimi, C., Bachman, L., and Smith, T.C.: Median effective doses (ED_{50}) of halothane in adults and children, Anesthesiology **31:**344, 1969.

102. Nightingale, D.A., Richards, C.C., and Glass, A.: An evaluation of rebreathing in a modified t-piece system during controlled ventilation of anaesthetised children, Br. J. Anaesth. **37:**762, 1965.

103. Pampiglione, G., and Harden, A.: Resuscitation after cardiocirculatory arrest: prognostic evaluation of early electroencephalographic findings, Lancet **1:**1261, 1968.

104. Pandit, S.K., Kothary, S.P., and Cohen, P.J.: Orally administered dantrolene for prophylaxis of malignant hyperthermia, Anesthesiology **50:**156, 1979.

105. Paton, J.S., Cunningham, A.D., Shaw, A., and Gregory, N.L.: An improved blood-loss monitor, Lancet **2:**744, 1977.

106. Penrose, B.H.: Aspiration pneumonitis following ketamine induction for general anesthesia, Anesth. Analg. **51:**41, 1972.

107. Ramanathan, S., Chalon, J., Capan, L., et al.: Rebreathing characteristics of the Bain anesthesia circuit, Anesth. Analg. **56:**822, 1977.

108. Ramanathan, S., Chalon, J., and Turndorf, H.: Determining patency of palmar arches by retrograde radial pulsation, Anesthesiology **42:**756, 1975.

109. Rashad, K.F., and Benson, D.W.: Role of humidity in prevention of hypothermia in infants and children, Anesth. Analg. **46:**712, 1967.

110. Rees, G.J.: Anaesthesia in the newborn, Br. Med. J. **2:**1419, 1950.

111. Rey, M., and Rey, H.A.: Curious George goes to hospital, Boston, 1966, Houghton Mifflin Co.

112. Roe, C.F., Santulli, T.V., and Blair, C.S.: Heat loss in infants during general anesthesia and operations, J. Pediatr. Surg. **1:**266, 1966.

113. Rose, D.K., and Froese, A.B.: The regulation of $Paco_2$ during controlled ventilation of children with a t-piece, Can. Anaesth. Soc. J. **26:**104, 1979.

114. Ross, E.D.T.: Treacher Collins' syndrome: an anaesthetic hazard, Anaesthesia **18:**350, 1963.

115. Ross, R.B., and Johnston, M.C.: Cleft lip and palate, Baltimore, 1972, The Williams and Wilkins Co.

116. Ross, W.T., and Cardell, R.R.: Proliferation of smooth endoplasmic reticulum and induction of microsomal drug-metabolizing enzymes after ether or halothane, Anesthesiology **48:**325, 1978.

117. Ryan, J.F., Kagan, L.J., and Hyman, A.I.: Myoglobinemia after a single dose of succinylcholine, N. Engl. J. Med. **285:**824, 1971.

118. Saklad, M.: Grading of patients for surgical procedures, Anesthesiology **2:**281, 1941.

119. Salem, M.R., Bennett, E.J., Schweiss, J.F., et al.: Cardiac arrest related to anesthesia: contributing factors in infants and children, J.A.M.A. **233:**238, 1975.

120. Salem, M.R., Mathrubhutham, M., and Bennett, E.J.: Difficult intubation, N. Engl. J. Med. **295:**879, 1976.

121. Salem, M.R., Toyama, T., Wong, A.Y., et al.: Haemodynamic responses to induced arterial hypotension in children, Br. J. Anaesth. **50:**489, 1978.

122. Salem, M.R., Wong, A.Y., and Lin, Y.H.: The effect of suxamethonium on the intragastric pressure in infants and children, Br. J. Anaesth. **44:**166, 1972.

123. Sampson, J.F., Hamstra, R., and Aldrete, J.A.: Management of hemophilic patients undergoing surgical procedures, Anesth. Analg. **58:**133, 1979.

124. Savage, G.J., and Metzger, J.T.: The prevention of postanesthetic delirium, Plast. Reconstr. Surg. **62:**81, 1978.

125. Schaer, H., Steinmann, B., Jerusalem, S., and Maier, C. Rhabdomyolysis induced by anaesthesia with intraoperative cardiac arrest, Br. J. Anaesth. **49:**495, 1977.

126. Seddon, H.J.: Three types of nerve injury, Brain **66:**238, 1943.

127. Shanks, C.A.: Humidification and loss of body heat during anesthesia. I. Quantification and correlation in the dog, Br. J. Anaesth. **46:**859, 1974.

128. Shay, A.: What happens when you go to the hospital, Chicago, 1969, Reilly & Lee.

129. Shenkin, H.A., and Bouzarth, W.F.: Clinical methods of reducing intracranial pressure: role of the cerebral circulation, N. Engl. J. Med. **282:**1465, 1970.

130. Smith, R.H.: The prone position. In Martin, J.T., editor: Positioning in anesthesia and surgery, Philadelphia, 1978, W.B. Saunders Co.

131. Smith, R.M.: Children, hospitals and parents, Anesthesiology **25:**461, 1964.

132. Smith, R.M.: Anesthesia for infants and children, ed. 4, St. Louis, 1979, The C.V. Mosby Co.

133. Soliman, M.G., and Laberge, R.: The use of the Bain circuit in spontaneously breathing paediatric patients, Can. Anaesth. Soc. J. **25:**276, 1978.

134. Stead, A.L.: The response of the newborn infant to muscle relaxants, Br. J. Anaesth. **27:**124, 1955.

135. Steward, D.J.: Outpatient pediatric anesthesia, Anesthesiology **43:**268, 1975.

136. Sturrock, J.E., and Nunn, J.F.: Mitosis in mammalian cells during exposure to anesthetics, Anesthesiology **43:**21, 1975.

137. Tambourine, J.: I think I will go to the hospital, Nashville, Tenn., 1965, Abingdon Press.

138. Taylor, P.A., and Towey, R.M.: Depression of layrngeal reflexes during ketamine anaesthesia, Br. Med. J. **2:**688, 1971.

139. Thornton, J.A., Saynor, R., Schroeder, H.G., et al.: Estimation of blood loss with particular reference to cardiac surgery, Br. J. Anaesth. **35:**91, 1963.

140. Tsueda, K., Bizzarri, D., Giuffrida, J., and Fierro, F.E.: Operative blood loss: its measurement and replacement, Int. Surg. **45:**117, 1966.

141. Way, W.L., Costley, E.C., and Way, E.L.: Respiratory sensitivity of the newborn infant to meperidine and morphine, Clin. Pharmacol. Ther. **6:**454, 1965.

142. Weber, A.: Elizabeth gets well, New York, 1969, Thomas Y. Crowell Co.

143. Weeks, D.B.: Provision of endogenous and exogenous humidity for the Bain breathing circuit, Can. Anaesth. Soc. J. **23:**185, 1976.

144. Welzenbach, J.F., and Welzenbach, N.: A "millyun" hospital questions, Chicago, 1970, Medical Educator, Inc.

145. Wolman, H., Smith, A.L., and Hoffman, J.C.: Cerebral blood flow and oxygen consumption in man during electroencephalographic seizure patterns induced by anesthesia with ethrane, Fed. Proc. **28:**356, 1969.

146. Yakaitis, R.W., Blitt, C.D., and Angiulo, J.P.: End-tidal halothane concentration for endotracheal intubation, Anesthesiology **47:**386, 1977.

147. Yakaitis, R.W., Blitt, C.D., and Angiulo, J.P.: End-tidal enflurane concentration for endotracheal intubation, Anesthesiology **50:**59, 1979.

148. Yeung, M.L., and Lin, R.S.H.: Laryngeal reflexes in children under ketamine anaesthesia, Br. J. Anaesth. **44:**1089, 1972.

CHAPTER 5

Parenteral fluid and nutritional maintenance of the pediatric surgical patient

HOWARD C. FILSTON

Before embarking on a detailed discussion of parenteral fluid and nutritional maintenance, a brief discussion of the care and feeding of the normal infant with an intact gastrointestinal tract is in order. Few surgeons have any idea how to feed a baby or young infant. Understanding normal nutritional requirements will serve as a background for understanding the needs of the child whose gastrointestinal tract is insufficient.

An infant needs approximately 120 calories/kg of body weight for normal growth and weight gain. These calories must come from a balanced diet that includes carbohydrates, protein, and fat to provide substrates for normal growth and development. The newborn and young infant need approximately 100 ml of fluid for each kilogram of body weight. Standard infant formulas attempt to supply the child's caloric and electrolyte requirements in a composition that somewhat approximates human breast milk. The protein source in formulas is casein as in cow's milk, and the osmolality is often considerably higher than that of breast milk. Other common formulas, used when milk intolerance is suspected, use a soybean source of protein rather than casein.

The standard concentration of infant formulas provides 20 calories/ounce of fluid. The baby must be given 150 to 180 ml/kg of a standard formula to supply the 100 to 120 calories/kg requirement for growth and weight gain. This volume is divided into six to eight feedings a day, depending on the infant's size and tolerance. Since many infants will progress rapidly and demand more volume, it is generally advisable to offer a small amount more than was provided at the last feeding.

Standard formulas provide adequate nourishment until the infant is approximately 5 months old. After that time additional foods should be introduced into the diet gradually, one at a time. Foods that usually are introduced first are individual nonwheat cereals and noncitrus fruits and juices. The timing for introduction of these foods remains controversial, however.[24] Iron is an additional requirement and usually can be provided by choosing an infant formula that contains iron.[24] Baby foods may inhibit iron absorption from the intestine.[38]

By 6 months most infants eat a variety of baby foods, and by 1 year most infants either eat junior foods or mashed or pureed table foods. By the end of the first year of life, most children are on a regular three-meal-a-day schedule with perhaps a nighttime bottle supplement. This, too, can be eliminated in the second year.

With this brief and superficial discussion of routine infant feeding, we can now turn to the more challenging problems of maintaining homeostasis for the infant whose gastrointestinal tract cannot be used as a means of conveying needed fluids and nutrients to the body. An article by Dwyer[20] provides a more detailed discussion of recent oral feeding recommendations for children.

GENERAL BODY FLUID BALANCE

Total body water makes up 60% to 70% of body weight[33] and is distributed among various compartments, including the intravascular space, interstitial space, and intracellular space. Ordinarily these fluid volumes are in diffusional and osmotic equilibrium with one another, and fluids can flow back and forth between and among these spaces freely to balance any gains or losses in a particular area. However, rapid acute losses may occur from the vascular space, and the rate of diffusion from the interstitial and intracellular spaces may be inadequate to maintain vascular volume at an adequate functional level. Therefore, although fluid losses from the body will be shared among the various spaces, our major concern as surgeons will be with vascular volume.

Maintenance of vascular volume is one of the most important parts of maintaining the homeostasis of the individual. An adequate vascular volume is essential for proper tissue perfusion. When losses from the vascular volume are sustained, compensatory vasoconstriction occurs at the arteriolar level, and the body selectively shunts blood from less important tissues to maintain perfusion of the important organs, primarily the heart, lungs, and brain. When perfusion failure occurs, the tissues from which blood flow is shunted are deprived of oxygen and needed nutrients. Waste products of metabolism build up because lack of blood flow prevents them from being carried to the lungs and kidneys for disposal. Cells deprived of normal oxygenation shift from the aerobic metabolic system to the anaerobic glycolytic system. This is a far less efficient system that provides only about one seventeenth of the energy of the Krebs cycle and builds up keto acid waste products.[2] The hypoxic insult to the tissues may lead to direct damage to enzyme systems and cause loss of capillary membrane function with resultant net loss of fluid through the capillary walls. The increasing local acidosis may also interfere with enzyme functioning because the delicate acid-base balance is upset.

Not only can severe local damage in the form of hypoxic and acidotic insult result from poor perfusion, but when vascular volume and perfusion are restored, the accumulated acid waste products may be transported to the systemic circuit where a generalized metabolic acidosis may interfere with cardiac and pulmonary functioning. These effects are particularly profound in the premature newborn whose pulmonary vascular resistance may be significantly increased in the face of hypoxia, acidosis, or hypercapnia,[16,40] with resultant shunting of the pulmonary outflow from the heart through either the arterial duct or the oval foramen. The older child will not sustain this degree of abnormal shunting, but may have a considerable degree of myocardial dysfunction due to the systemic acidosis.

Of equal consequence is the damage caused to capillary membrane integrity by hypoxia. When the capillary membrane is changed from a semipermeable membrane to a "leaky" one, the restoration of perfusion to the tissues by correction of vascular volume deficits may lead to secondary losses of fluid from the capillary membranes. Albumin, the prime factor in maintenance of intravascular protein oncotic pressure, may also be lost into the surrounding extravascular fluid. This secondary loss may reestablish the vascular volume deficiency.

MECHANISMS OF NORMAL VASCULAR VOLUME MAINTENANCE

The vascular volume of a newborn is approximately 8% to 8.5% of body weight.[11,39] The adult vascular volume is 5% of body weight. Other childhood volumes can be extrapolated on a curve between these two points. The vascular volume exerts intravascular hydrostatic pressure, tending to push fluid out through the capillary wall, but this is generally balanced by the surrounding tissue hydrostatic pressure. There is, in addition, a crystalloid oncotic pressure, due mainly to the common electrolytes of sodium, chloride, and potassium, and a colloid oncotic pressure, primarily due to albumin (Fig. 5-1). Normal values for these substances are as follows: sodium, 140 mEq/L; chloride, 105 mEq/L; potassium, 4.5 mEq/L; and albumin, 5 g/100 ml.

Osmoreceptors monitor the vascular osmolality and through the renin-angiotensin-aldosterone mechanism maintain osmotic equilibrium by altering excretion or resorption of electrolytes by the kidney tubules.[13] This system maintains the normal minute-to-minute, hour-to-hour equilibrium within the body, but if acute volume depletion occurs, the osmoreceptors are overridden by volume receptors that maintain an adequate volume for perfusion even in the face of osmotic disequilibrium.[13,44,53,57,58] These receptors act through the pituitary gland to cause secretion of antidiuretic hormone (ADH), which in turn makes the collecting duct of the renal tubule permeable to fluid, so that almost mandatory reabsorption of the majority of the renal effluent occurs along the gradient from the collecting duct to the hypertonic medullary area of the loop of Henle (Fig. 5-2).[13,36,58] Because of this mechanism, the body's handling of various fluids differs considerably when ADH is being secreted compared to when it is not. Understanding these differences is essential to proper management of fluids and electrolytes in the face of volume deficiencies.

Historical background

Our present understanding of vascular volume and the importance of perfusion is of relatively recent duration. Most present-day clinical thinking about shock evolved during the 1960s. Before that, attempts to understand shock mechanisms focused primarily on blood pressure as an indicator of vascular volume. The fallacy that blood pressure is a good indicator of vascular volume sufficiency is discussed in Chapter 9.

In the 1940s, Wiggers[54] at the Case Western Reserve University School of Medicine performed an extensive series of experiments in which he developed a replicable shock model for experimental manipulation. Dogs were bled down to blood pressures of 50 mm Hg from their normal levels of 100 mm Hg (systolic), maintained there for periods up to 90 minutes, and then bled again to blood pressures of 30 mm Hg (systolic). They were maintained at 30 mm Hg for periods of 45 minutes, after which all of the shed blood was restored to the dog. This provided a model of irrevers-

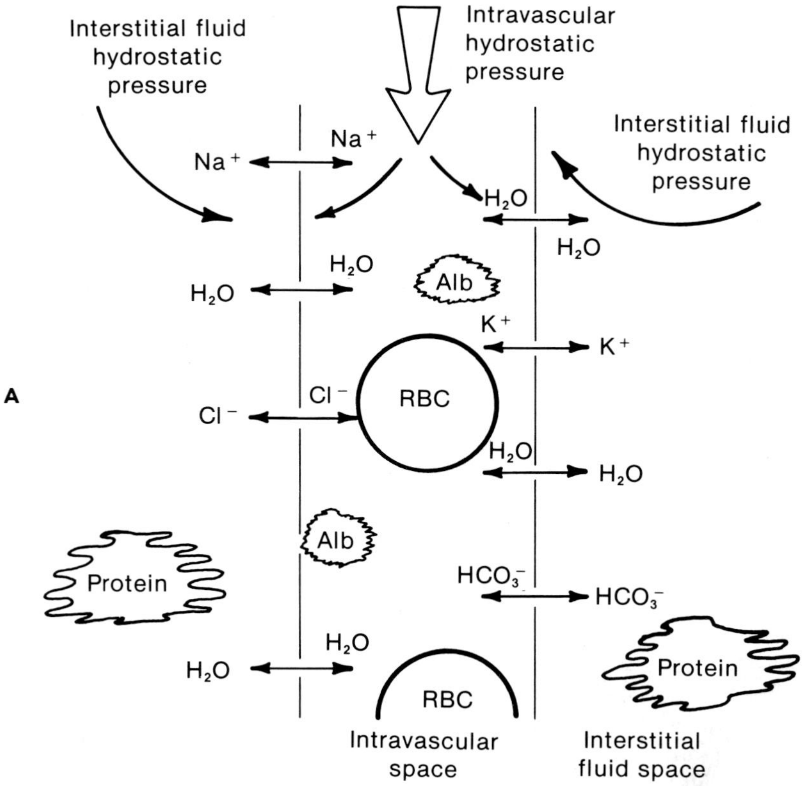

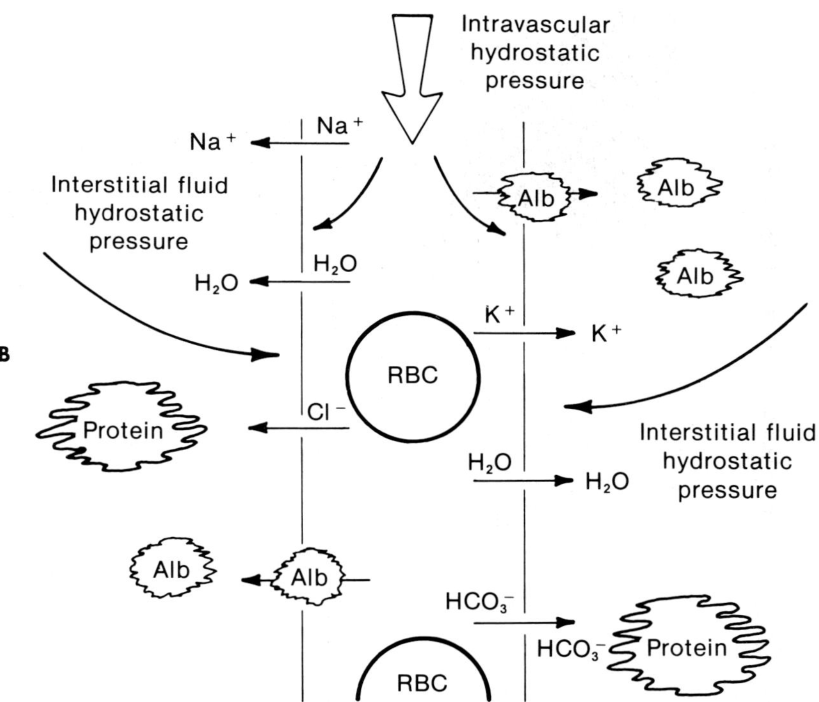

Fig. 5-1. A, Normal balance of hydrostatic and oncotic forces across semipermeable membrane results in no net gain or loss from vascular space. **B,** "Leaky" capillary resulting from membrane damage after hypoxia or endotoxin allows albumin to pass through to interstitial fluid and upsets the normal oncotic relationships. Vascular depletion and interstitial edema result.

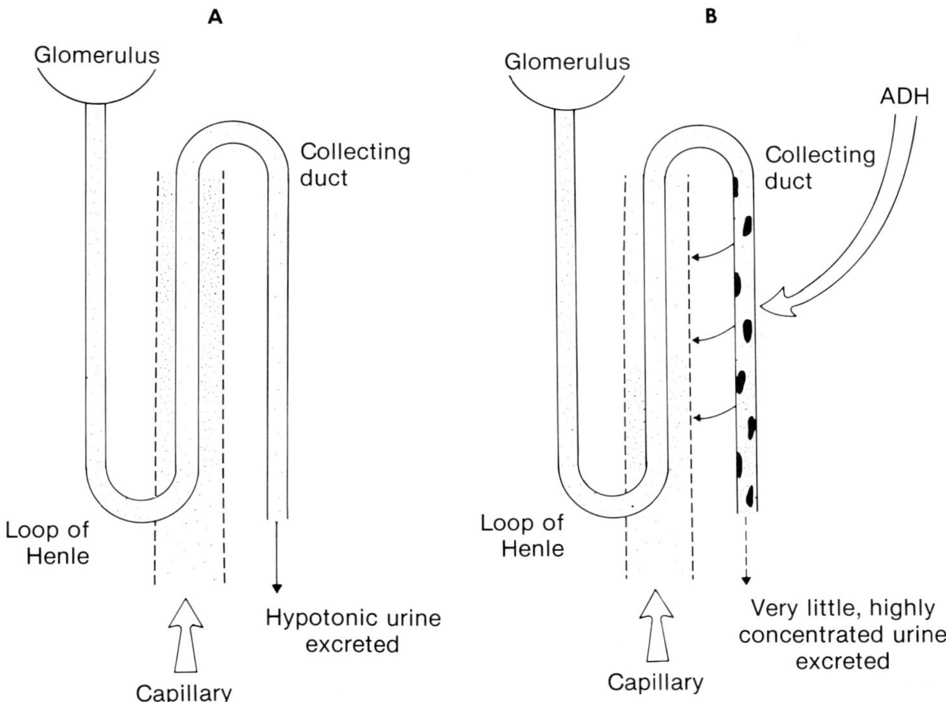

Fig. 5-2. A, Normal handling of water load. Countercurrent mechanism in loop absorbs electrolytes against concentration gradient, and diffusion into capillary leaves hypotonic urine to pass down impermeable collecting duct for excretion. **B,** ADH makes collecting duct permeable. Water is passively absorbed into the concentrated capillary, reducing urine flow and concentrating the urine.

ible shock, since an average of 82% of the dogs died. Subsequently, reserach focused on attempts to find the mechanism responsible for the irreversibility of the shock.

In the 1950s, primarily in Moore's laboratory at Harvard Medical School, a series of carefully performed experiments demonstrated the high level of circulating aldosterone and ADH in patients after trauma and major surgery.[36] Since ADH was believed to be secreted primarily in response to increases in osmolarity, it was considered by many investigators and clinicians to be "inappropriate." Consequently, salt and water restriction in the postoperative period became a common clinical dictum.[36,41,42]

Finally, in the 1960s, Share[44] demonstrated in animals and Wright and Gann[57] confirmed in humans that volume depletion was the significant stimulus to ADH release. Numerous researchers, including Weil and Shubin[53] and Wright, Gann, and Drucker,[57,58] contributed to a renewed understanding of the hypovolemic character of surgical and traumatic shock and demonstrated that the ADH was an *appropriate* response to the volume deficit and perfusion inadequacy in these patients. In addition, it was shown that the ADH effect could be overcome by rapid infusion of electrolyte solutions.[44,57,58] By the mid-1960s, Shires[46] was able to repeat Wiggers' experiments creating the irreversible shock model and salvage most of the dogs by infusing volumes of balanced saline solution (Ringer's lactace) in addition to restoring the shed blood.

Major past errors about volume depletion included the following assumptions: that blood pressure was a good indicator of organ perfusion, which it is not; that ADH release after major surgery or trauma is "inappropriate" when it is an appropriate response for maintaining vascular volume; that there is an unknown cause of irreversible shock, even though it is caused by secondary loss of the fluid phase of the vascular volume through the leaky capillary membranes produced during the hypoperfusion hypoxic phase of shock; and that low urine output represents renal failure rather than volume depletion and consequent renal hypoperfusion.

Summary of vascular volume principles

With significant losses of vascular volume, either through frank blood loss internally or externally or major fluid losses or shifts, volume receptors stimulate secretion of ADH from the pituitary gland and lead to obligatory reabsorption of the majority of urine from the collecting duct. Vasoconstrictive mechanisms are brought into action to shunt blood from less vital tissues and maintain perfusion of the more important core organs. For a time, this vasoconstriction can maintain blood pressure at normal levels, making blood pressure a poor gauge of vascular volume sufficiency. Those tissues from which the blood is shunted by the vasoconstrictive responses maintain themselves for a time on anaerobic glycolytic mechanisms, but the energy generated by these systems is insufficient and, in addition, severe hypoxic

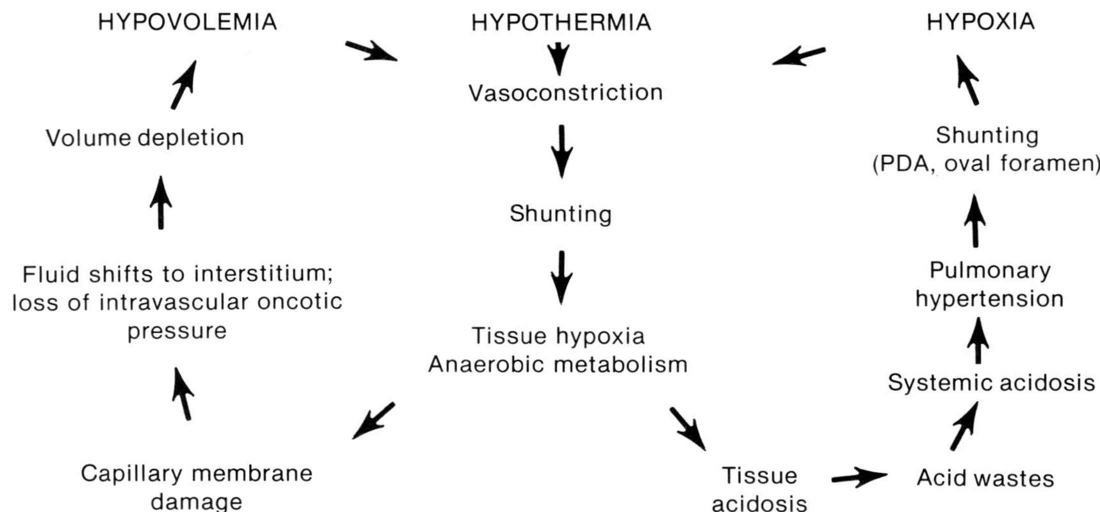

Fig. 5-3. The low-flow syndrome. (Modified from Filston, H.C., and Izant, R.: The surgical neonate, East Norwalk, Conn., 1978, Appleton-Century-Crofts.)

injury to membranes and enzymes may occur. Additional injury may result from the acid waste products that build up during hypoperfusion. Severe ongoing shock may lead to persistent vasoconstriction, hypoperfusion, and hypoxia, so that actual tissue death and necrosis may occur.

If volume is restored before cell death occurs, restoration of flow to the previously hypoxic and hypoperfused tissues may result in secondary fluid losses through the leaky capillary membranes, producing a "third-space" sequestration of fluid within the body. Until capillary membrane integrity is restored and oncotic relationships return to normal, these sequestered fluids are truly lost and unrecoverable to the vascular space. In addition, the acid waste products that have accumulated are carried into the systemic circuit where they may have profound effects on myocardial functioning and, in the infant, may produce pulmonary vascular resistance with resultant reopening of the ductal and atrial shunts. Thus shock may lead to a double vicious circle in which ongoing hypoxic and hypovolemic insults are maintained (Fig. 5-3).

With this background we can now direct our attention to an understanding of the types of fluids required for maintenance of homeostasis after major surgery.

FLUID REQUIREMENTS FOR PARENTERAL MAINTENANCE OF HOMEOSTASIS

Certain fluids are lost from the body in normal respiration, ventilation, and metabolism each 24 hours regardless of whether or not any pathologic processes are taking place. Insensible losses take place through the skin by evaporation, a process that does not require energy and therefore can be differentiated from perspiration. Insensible losses from the lungs are due to the need to hydrate the inspired air to a partial pressure of water vapor of 47 mm Hg to adequately

moisten the inspired gases for diffusion across the alveolar membranes. Sizable amounts of water vapor are then exhaled with each breath. In adults these insensible losses range from 800 to 1000 ml/m^2/day, and in children they are between 50 and 60 ml/kg/day.

The other loss requiring daily replacement is that of obligatory urine production. This must be differentiated from total urine production, which will be directly related to the amount of fluid ingested. Obligatory urine is the volume of urine required to dissolve the solutes produced as waste products of the body's daily metabolism. In adults this amounts to approximately 800 to 1000 ml/day, and for children it is approximately 40 ml/kg/day.[52]

Fluids replacing these insensible and urinary losses are known as maintenance fluids. Since the patient receiving parenteral feedings usually has less than full metabolism, maintenance fluids should be kept to minimal levels to ensure that an excess of dilute fluid is not given to the patient who may have ADH circulating after surgery or trauma. The adult minimums of 1500 ml/day of maintenance fluid and 1200 ml/day of urine output serve as maximal volumes for children when the formula calculations exceed these amounts.

There are several standard formulas for calculating maintenance fluid requirements in infants and children. The most widely used probably are 100 ml/kg up to 10 kg, then 50 ml/kg up to 20 kg, and 20 ml/kg over 20 kg. We have preferred a single formula described by Wallace[52] in 1953, which represents the infant and child maintenance fluid and caloric requirements (M) as follows:

$$M = 100 \text{ ml} - (3 \times \text{age} \times \text{weight in kilograms})$$

The maximal amount of maintenance fluid is 1500 ml. Furthermore, once the child reaches 30 kg of body weight, the 40 ml/kg urine volume requirement will have reached the adult minimal level of 1200 ml/day, the maximal level for children in the early postoperative period.

This maintenance requirement is for free water and therefore should be supplied as 5% dextrose and water. However, the child also has a requirement for some electrolytes because of electrolyte losses in the urine and stool. This amounts to 2 to 3 mEq/kg of sodium and chloride and 2 to 3 mEq/kg of potassium.[56] An adult requires approximately 45 to 60 mEq of sodium and chloride and 40 mEq of potassium for maintenance daily. Since normal saline contains 154 mEq/L of sodium and chloride or 15 mEq/100 ml, one-fifth normal saline would contain 3 mEq/100 ml of sodium and chloride and would therefore supply the infant's daily maintenance when roughly 100 ml/kg of fluids are given. Adding 2 or 3 mEq/100 ml of potassium chloride or potassium phosphate would satisfy the child's maintenance requirements for potassium. One-fourth normal saline is used in many institutions because it is more readily available.

It is important to recognize that this maintenance fluid is calculated by weight and that there are few indications for giving additional amounts to the postoperative patient. When amounts above the maintenance level are given to patients who are in the postoperative, posttraumatic, or septic shock state, hypotonic fluids may be retained because of circulating ADH. This results in a lower intravascular oncotic pressure and a shift of the maintenance fluids into the extravascular space. The resultant interstitial edema is of little consequence in most tissues, but in the myocardium or pulmonary interstitial space it may lead to myocardial inefficiency or difficulty in diffusion of gases across the increased alveolar capillary distance. We believe, therefore, that maintenance fluids should be held to a minimum when ADH may be circulating.

Measurable losses

The next category is perhaps the easiest to understand and represents fluid that is lost outside the body and can be measured directly. It is replaced volume for volume with the type of fluid lost; most often it is gastric juice from a nasogastric tube. Gastric juice is made up of acid, sodium, chloride, and potassium, with approximately 60 mEq/L of sodium, 105 to 150 mEq/L of chloride, 5 to 30 mEq/L of potassium, and the rest hydrogen ions.[17] It can be replaced by half normal saline with 30 mEq/L of added potassium chloride, resulting in a solution containing 75 mEq/L of sodium, 105 mEq/L of chloride, and 30 mEq/L of potassium. If concern for renal function mitigates against the use of potassium in the solution, normal saline should be used to replace the gastric juice.

Gastrointestinal juices beyond the pylorus approximate extracellular fluid in their composition and are best replaced with a balanced salt solution such as Ringer's lactate.[17] If large volumes of specific fluid, such as bile, pancreatic juice, or ileostomy drainage, are being lost over a long period of time, aliquots should be sent to the laboratory to define their exact composition.

Internal fluid shifts or third-space losses

Internal fluid shifts are losses that occur *within* the body from the vascular space into the interstitial fluid space and somewhat into the intracellular fluid space as well. Malfunction of cellular membranes, including those of the capillaries, can result in significant fluid shifts to interstitial and intracellular spaces, thus depleting vascular volume.[3,6,45] Hypoperfusion of tissues can result from volume depletion, hypoxia, and sepsis, the latter probably causing volume depletion by injury to capillary membranes and bypass shunting of flow to tissues.[43] Endotoxin circulating during sepsis can probably damage the capillary membranes directly. Fluid that leaks out through the damaged capillaries is not immediately recoverable to the vascular space along the usual osmotic gradient due to the membrane malfunction and loss of oncotic particles such as albumin into the interstitial space. Eventually the capillary membranes will heal, the albumin level will be restored in the vascular space, and this fluid will be recoverable, but in the acute septic, postoperative, posttraumatic, or postshock state the fluid is temporarily lost to the *functional* vascular space. All third-space, or internal shifts, are not due to damaged capillaries. Fluid that accumulates in the lumen of the bowel during a postoperative ileus, ascites fluid in the peritoneal cavity, and any accumulation of edema fluid all represent internal fluid shifts that are not immediately recoverable to the vascular space. These acute losses are as significant in their effect on perfusion as are more obvious losses that occur externally. They must be replaced immediately to maintain vascular volume and adequate perfusion even though subsequently these fluids will be reabsorbed into the vascular space. It is imperative that the septic, postoperative, posttraumatic, or postshock patient *gain weight* if adequate fluid replacement is given into the vascular space to make up for third-space shifts. Because these shifts are essentially extracellular fluid shifts, the fluid should be replaced with a balanced saline solution such as Ringer's lactate.

In summary, the calculated maintenance fluids replacing insensible losses and obligatory urine volumes are given in a hypotonic salt solution that represents essentially free water and a minimal amount of required electrolytes. Measured losses, which are often those of gastric juice, are given in a half normal saline solution with added potassium that approximates the makeup of gastric juice without acid. All other losses of fluid, whether external, gastrointestinal losses from beyond the pylorus, or major wounds or internal shifts that represent losses from the vascular space, are given in a balanced saline solution such as Ringer's lactate. Only when severe liver disease or malfunction exists will the use of lactate cause acidosis. In most instances it is metabolized normally and provides needed base.

The volume of fluid required for maintenance is calculated as follows:

$$M = 100 \text{ ml} - (3 \times \text{age} \times \text{weight in kilograms})$$

The volume of measured loss is directly measured. The volume required to replace prior losses or internal fluid shifts cannot be determined exactly and demands a guess as to the volume required. In the septic, postoperative, posttraumatic, or postshock state the vascular space can be represented by an opaque beaker. It is recognized from the formula that a certain amount of maintenance fluid is a requirement, and this amount is poured into the beaker. Certain fluids leak out of the beaker and are measured. This amount is restored exactly, volume for volume. The beaker is now partially filled, and it contains the correct amount of maintenance fluid and replacement for measured losses. There is still a volume deficiency in the beaker, and, if there is no urine output at this point, increased levels of ADH are probably circulating. Additional amounts of Ringer's lactate must now be added to the beaker until the fluid level reaches a normal volume for the vascular space, at which point the ADH level should be reduced and a normal urine output should result. If, however, hypotonic maintenance fluid is put into the vascular space while an *increased* amount of ADH is present, it will not be excreted normally. In addition, the electrolytes and colloids will be diluted, resulting in a fluid shift to the interstitial space along the osmotic pressure gradient, the vascular space should be refilled *first* with balanced saline solution so that vascular volume is restored and ADH levels are reduced. The hypotonic fluids will then be handled appropriately.

This discussion implies that Ringer's lactate is used for all fluid replacement, but obviously when significant blood loss has occurred, the initial replacement should be with blood until adequate levels of oxygen-carrying cells are restored to the vascular space. In addition, if significant losses of plasma proteins have occurred, these too should be restored with whole blood, plasma, or albumin in Ringer's lactate solution. Albumin must be given cautiously during the first 24 hours after any trauma or sepsis that has resulted in hypovolemic shock. The albumin may leak out of the vascular space and enhance oncotic gradients into the interstitial tissues.[15,37,51] This is of particular significance if pulmonary capillary damage is suspected, since the resulting interstitial pulmonary edema may interfere with alveolar capillary gas diffusion and prolong pulmonary dysfunction. Sepsis is the most likely cause of pulmonary capillary membrane damage.[26]

In summary, balanced saline or colloid-containing solutions will be required for replacement when fluids are shifted internally into the lumen of the bowel, edema is forming, or fluids are shifted into the peritoneal cavity as ascites. They also will be required when profound hypoxia, hypoperfusion, or gram-negative sepsis has resulted in capillary membrane damage with subsequent capillary membrane dysfunction after restoration of flow. Because these volumes cannot be measured directly, a sufficient replacement solution must be given at a rapid enough rate to fill the vascular space and restore perfusion to the kidney. Refilling the vascular space will "shut off" the ADH, and once renal blood flow is restored, urine output should result. Thus urine output is the end point, representing successful refilling of the vascular space. Once urine output is established, it can be used as a direct monitor of fluid administration, maintaining urine output at the level of 40 ml/kg/day or approximately 1 or 2 ml/kg/hr. Although most children will tolerate a significant degree of fluid overload, this should be avoided by holding the urine output down to 40 ml/kg/day, as well as striving to achieve this level. Remember that 1200 ml/day is adequate for adults and therefore is the usual maximum for older children regardless of the formula calculation.

IDEAL FLUID MANAGEMENT

For elective surgery, much of the difficulty in managing fluids can be avoided by adhering to a carefully planned program. The child's hydration is maintained either by continuing oral intake up to 4 to 5 hours before surgery or, if this is not possible or sufficient, by beginning intravenous administration of maintenance fluid at an appropriate rate when a child must be deprived of oral intake before surgery. Intraoperatively, attention should be directed toward maintaining blood volume by replacing any significant blood loss and avoiding vasoconstriction and hypoperfusion, which can result in tissue damage and capillary membrane dysfunction. Fluid losses occurring intraoperatively should be replaced as well using balanced saline solutions. Continuing a careful fluid management program postoperatively will maintain good hydration, a good vascular volume, and adequate urine output. The urine output can then be used in monitoring future fluid requirements.

ADDITIONAL MONITORING WHEN URINE OUTPUT FAILS

In using urine output as a monitor of vascular volume replacement, certain assumptions are made. It is assumed that the myocardium is functioning normally and providing a normal cardiac output. It is assumed that pulmonary vascular resistance is normal, liver function is normal, and renal function is unimpaired and will respond appropriately to an adequate volume perfusing the kidney. It also is assumed that the patient is not septic and that no abnormal toxins are interfering with normal physiologic functioning. It is further assumed that there is no inappropriate ADH circulating. This assumption may not be valid when the patient has a cerebral tumor, severe head injury, gram-negative sepsis, or is being given ADH in the form of vasopressin (such as the treatment for severe hemorrhage from eosphageal varices due to portal hypertension). Whenever these assumptions cannot be relied on or urine output fails to occur in response to seemingly adequate fluid administration, further steps must be taken. The step to be avoided is giving a diuretic such as furosemide to the patient who has no urine output based on the assumption that failure of urine output represents fluid retention, overload, and kidney malfunction. This assumption is not valid in most instances, and it is incumbent on the surgeon to be sure that the vascular space is filled before prescribing a diuretic. If urine output is not an accurate monitor of fluid administration, a central venous pressure catheter or, in some instances, a Swan-Ganz[49] catheter for measuring pulmonary artery wedge pressure to monitor the function of the left ventricle of the heart is essential. Knowledge of venous pressure is mandatory before diuretics are given to a patient who may have an inadequately filled vascular space, or else profound losses of needed vascular volume may occur with resulting shock. If central venous pressure monitoring indicates that the vascular volume has been restored and central venous pressure is elevated, then either a diuretic (furosemide) or preferably in most instances an inotropic agent such as dopamine should be given. Dopamine will increase renal blood flow and improve myocardial contractility, thus achieving with one drug the desired effects on both the myocardium and the renal blood flow. Management of complex problems of this sort obviously requires someone familiar with critical care management in infants and children.

AVOIDING RECREATION OF THE SHOCK MODEL

Certain situations in surgery may recreate in the pediatric patient the pathophysiologic process that created the shock model in Wiggers' dogs.[54] If the child sustains moderate to severe blood losses during an operative procedure, particularly when the blood loss is not common or expected, significant hypovolemia may persist for prolonged periods of time before replacement is achieved. This was the condition used by Wiggers to create the irreversible shock model. When significant blood loss occurs and hypovolemia persists for a long period, a generalized vasoconstriction occurs. As a result, the core circulation is protected, but damage resulting from hypoperfusion and hypoxia occurs to other tissues. This may result in capillary membrane damage during the period of anaerobic metabolism. When the severity of the blood loss is identified later in the operative procedure or in the early postoperative period, the surgeon must be aware that the child may have sustained capillary membrane injury. The surgeon must be prepared to replace not only the volume of shed blood, but a sizable volume of balanced saline solution, as in Shires' reenactment of Wiggers' experiment,[46] to replace the volume of fluid that will be lost subsequently through the leaky capillary membranes. Again, careful monitoring of urine output with continuous administration of a balanced saline solution will achieve the necessary replacement. Delay in the replacement of lost blood may result in failure to maintain

vascular volume normality. An example is the child who, after a procedure such as a cleft palate repair, may bleed significantly throughout the night, swallow the blood, and show no external sign of a loss. In the morning the child is discovered to have hypotension and tachycardia and may vomit a large amount of blood that was previously swallowed. Blood replacement alone may be inadequate to correct the volume losses that will occur when resumption of circulation to hypoxic damaged tissues results in subsequent loss of the fluid phase of the blood volume. Careful maintenance of urine output by supplying adequate volumes of Ringer's lactate again will restore the needed volume to the vascular space and maintain continued adequate perfusion.

It is important to realize that the volume losses discussed here are acute short-term losses due to internal shifts that will be readily corrected if adequate volume is maintained in the vascular space to achieve needed perfusion of the tissues. Capillary membrane function will be restored, the ileus will subside, the ascitic fluid will be resorbed, and 24 to 48 hours after the surgery or trauma, the fluid shifts will reverse, and the fluid will reenter the vascular space. At this point, it is essential to reduce intravenous fluid therapy back to calculated maintenance volumes and provide replacement of ongoing measured losses. The continued infusion of high volumes of balanced saline solution at the levels required in the immediate postoperative period may result in significant volume overload when fluids are being resorbed into the vascular space; it is at this point that heart failure and pulmonary edema may occur if attention is not paid to this reversal. Basically all problems of fluid management become easy ones if the surgeon gives some thought to the possibility of fluid shifts occurring and provides for careful monitoring of urine output with additional central venous pressure monitoring when needed. The proper response to the urine volume, maintaining it in the normal range, will ensure that the child's fluid administration is optimal.

Throughout this discussion various fluids such as one-fifth normal saline, Ringer's lactate, half normal saline, and normal saline are mentioned. Generally, all fluids administered should contain at least 5% dextrose to provide the child with a minimal level of glucose needed to avoid hypoglycemia. Only when extremely rapid infusions of balanced saline solutions are required for patients in profound hypovolemia should consideration be given to eliminating the dextrose from the solution temporarily to avoid an inappropriate diuretic effect from the rapid increase in blood glucose levels. The usual rates of fluid administration required for the program outlined will not overload the ability of cellular metabolism to handle the glucose loads nor exceed the renal threshold for glucose unless the patient is severely septic.

This amount of dextrose provides minimal calories. Nutritional maintenance requires 100 to 120 calories/kg/day for positive nitrogen balance and normal growth. Even greater caloric levels are needed to sustain patients with severe sepsis or extensive burns. These levels usually can best be achieved by central total parenteral nutrition.

PARENTERAL NUTRITION REQUIREMENTS OF INFANTS AND CHILDREN

Ideally any patient who can use the gastrointestinal tract for nutritional maintenance in some way should have nutrition provided by that route. Even children who cannot tolerate normal feeding regimens can sometimes be maintained with special formulas. Some formulas have partial digestion of the complex foodstuffs in the form of protein hydrolysates and simple sugars, and some are from single substances such as protein, carbohydrates, or fat.[1] Elemental formulas that can provide all of the daily requirements of calories, essential fatty acids and amino acids, and minerals and vitamins are available, but often their high osmolality makes them intolerable to the infant's gastrointestinal tract. However, if the proximal gastrointestinal tract is useful, the child usually can be made to adapt to the formulas by initially feeding them in dilute concentrations and gradually increasing the concentration and osmolality of the formula as adaptation occurs. The inability to use the proximal gastrointestinal tract because of swallowing difficulties or esophageal problems can be overcome by the use of gastric, duodenal, or jejunal tube feedings with constant infusions. All of these modalities should be considered before resorting to total parenteral alimentation. Nevertheless, there are children who must realy on total parenteral nutrition for significant periods of time if they are to survive and grow. Managing total parenteral nutrition in an infant or young child is a complex procedure and involves risk of significant complications. It is accomplished best in a setting where a well thought out program of total parenteral nutrition has been established in the hospital, including direction by physicians knowledgeable in the field, pharmacy personnel with knowledge and experience in the production of parenteral nutritional fluids, and a nursing staff familiar with an established program for catheter care.[19,21,28]

For short-term parenteral nutritional supplementation and short-term total parenteral nutrition maintenance, peripheral hyperalimentation using dilute solutions in high volume may be the safest and most acceptable when personnel and facilities for central total parenteral nutrition are not available.[10] At Duke University Medical Center, we prefer to use total central parenteral nutrition in our programs, but we have years of experience in the administration of these substances and placement of the catheters. The surgeon must choose a method that can be managed safely and knowledgeably. Central catheter placement in infants and children can be easily achieved by anyone who has *extensive* experience in peripheral cannulation of infants and children and central cannulation of adults.[23] In the hands of an inexperienced operator, it can become a highly dangerous undertaking. We have long preferred the subclavian route for vascular access for central venous catheter placement and have a large series with a most acceptable complication

rate.[22] For the inexperienced operator, direct incisional access to the external jugular veins in the neck or antecubital veins in the arm is a safer approach. Subclavian access in the older child can be easily achieved by anyone experienced in subclavian access in adults.

Major complications of subclavian access procedures include a pneumothorax, arterial injury with severe hemorrhage, hematoma formation, and injuries to the thoracic duct and trachea. Extravascular positioning of the catheter may lead to infusion of the solution into the mediastinum or pleural pace with a tension hydrothorax and ventilatory and cardiovascular impairment. The major complication of catheter maintenance is sepsis,[5,27] which can only be kept at acceptable levels if well thought out programs of initial catheter placement and maintenance are developed and the proper instruction given to all personnel concerned.

A nutritional solution should be prepared under sterile conditions in a laminar flow hood by experienced pharmacy personnel. These individuals should assure the sterility of the solution and compatibility of the ingredients.

Daily requirements for parenteral nutritional maintenance

The requirements for maintaining parenteral nutritional maintenance include adequate calories, appropriate replacement and maintenance electrolytes, required minerals in the form of trace elements, an appropriate source of nitrogen, and essential fatty acids and vitamins.[31]

Calories can be provided from either carbohydrates, fats, or proteins, but if insufficient calories are provided a negative nitrogen balance results despite the provision of amino acids.[4,14,31] Although Blackburn et al.[4] have shown that amino acid solutions can be used without glucose, thus forcing the body to use endogenous fats as calories, the usual formulation for total parenteral nutrition is a 20% to 22% dextrose solution in a 5% protein base, either a protein hydrolysate or more commonly crystalline amino acids. This basic solution is supplemented with infusions of a fat emulsion (Intralipid),[8,9] and this is of particular importance in the growing infant who must have a daily source of essential fatty acids.[7,31] The younger the infant, the more important this requirement, because the rapid myelinization of nerve sheaths that is taking place requires a source of essential fatty acids for formation of sphingomyelin. Lipids should be used with caution in infants with liver disease or pulmonary problems, however, because of potential detrimental effects on these organs from lipid deposits.[12,25]

The major electrolytes, sodium, potassium, and chloride, are given in maintenance amounts approximating one-fifth normal saline or 3 mEq/kg/day sodium, chloride, and potassium. Other major ion requirements are for calcium, magnesium, and phosphorus in the following amounts[31,55]:

Calcium	0.5 to 1 mEq/kg/day
Phosphate	1 to 2 mEq/kg/day
Magnesium	0.25 mEq/kg/day

Trace elements known to be required are zinc, copper, chromium, and manganese.[32,47,48] The amounts of these elements required are given in Table 5-1.[29]

Vitamins are required and the amounts are based on recommended daily requirements, taking care to avoid excesses of the toxic vitamins, particularly vitamins A and D. Generally, an addition of 1 ml of multivitamin injection to the daily parenteral volume will provide the needed level, but care must be taken that this is not excessive for the premature infant. Recommended dosages for premature infants are 500 to 1000 units of vitamin A and 100 to 200 units of vitamin D each day.

Recent evidence shows that infants receiving long-term total parenteral nutrition therapy have an increased need for calcium and vitamin D, suggesting that the role of the latter may be more complex than simply to augment calcium absorption from the intestinal tract.[34,35] Extra high levels of calcium and phosphate may have to be provided in the daily infusate.

METABOLIC COMPLICATIONS OF TOTAL PARENTERAL NUTRITION

Most patients tolerate total parenteral nutrition well and can be advanced rapidly to full carbohydrate and nitrogen levels that provide approximately 120 calories/kg and 2.5 g/kg of protein.[31] However, some patients who are extremely ill and some premature infants will not tolerate high levels of glucose administration and become severely hyperglycemic resulting in osmotic dehydration and diuresis. Serum and urine glucose levels should be carefully monitored. Major electrolytes should be monitored frequently to ensure that adequate amounts are being provided.

Intolerance of the nitrogen load or specific deficiencies in enzymes required to handle amino acids may lead to interference in the functioning of the urea cycle with buildup of ammonia. Ammonia may be present in the protein hydrolysate or result from imbalances or deficiencies of essential amino acids in the crystalline preparation. Ammonia

levels should be carefully monitored throughout total parenteral nutrition, since the buildup of ammonia may lead to severe cerebral toxicity and death.[18,30,31]

Finally, liver enzyme functioning should be carefully monitored through total parenteral nutrition because direct injury to the liver cells may lead to fatty metamorphosis, and cholestasis may lead to severe hepatic malfunction and considerable hepatic damage.[50] Most of these effects are reversible on stopping the total parenteral nutrition, but some of them may linger for prolonged periods of time. The exact causes of these widely recognized hepatic dysfunctions are not well defined.

The exact requirements for maintaining prolonged parenteral nutrition are far from clear and probably vary widely from individual to individual.[31] A greater understanding of the nutritional needs of the patient will be forthcoming as more sophisticated research into nutritional requirements is completed. For the present, although most patients will tolerate the formulas that are being used, careful monitoring is needed throughout the period of total parenteral nutrition to identify those patients who have either deficiencies or malfunctions of organ systems during the therapy. Nevertheless, total parenteral nutrition has made a tremendous contribution to the management of the severely ill surgical patient and has allowed successful treatment of many entities that previously resulted in death. Pediatric surgery particularly has benefited by gaining time to correct gastrointestinal anomalies and dysfunction in a stepwise fashion over a prolonged period of time while maintaining the patient's growth, development, and health. However, total parenteral nutrition is a complex program that will be most successful when handled by experienced personnel, especially with a health care team that consists of a knowledgeable directing physician and experienced pharmacy and nursing personnel. When this type of program is available, it can be expected that most patients will benefit immensely from the procedure with a low incidence of metabolic and mechanical complications.

Table 5-1. Suggested daily intravenous intake of essential trace elements

	Pediatric patients (μg/kg)*	Stable adult	Adult in acute catabolic state	Stable adult with intestinal losses
Zinc	300† 100‡	2.5 to 4 mg	Additional 2 mg	Add 12.2 mg/L small-bowel fluid lost; 17.1 mg/kg of stool or ileostomy output
Copper	20	0.5 to 1.5 mg	—	—
Chromium	0.14 to 0.2	10 to 15 μg	—	20 μg
Manganese	2 to 10	0.15 to 0.8 mg	—	—

Modified from Shils, M.E.: Guidelines for essential trace element preparation for parenteral use: a statement by an expert panel, J.A.M.A. **241:**2051. Copyright 1979, American Medical Association.

*Limited data are available for infants weighing less than 1500 g. Their requirements may be more than the recommendations because of their low body reserves and increased requirements for growth.

†Applies to premature infants (weighing less than 1500 g) until they reach 3 kg of body weight. Thereafter the recommendations for full-term infants apply.

‡Applies to full-term infants and children up to 5 years old. Thereafter the recommendations for adults apply, up to a maximal dosage of 4 mg/day.

SUMMARY AND CONCLUSION

A growing normal infant requires approximately 120 kcal/kg of body weight. The newborn or young infant requires approximately 100 ml of fluids for each kilogram of body weight. The standard infant formulas are adequate to nourish the infant until approximately 5 months of age. After that time additional foods should be introduced into the diet gradually, one at a time.

The vascular volume of a newborn infant is approximately 8 to 8½% of total body weight. In the case of an acute volume depletion, volume receptors override the osmoreceptors to maintain an adequate volume for perfusion even in the face of an osmotic disequilibrium. The insensible loss in a child is approximately 50 to 60 ml/kg/day. Obligatory urinary loss of water is approximately 40 ml/kg/day. A convenient standard formula for calculating maintenance fluid requirements is indicated by the following: (100/ml − three times the age) × wieght in kilograms = M to a maximum of 1500 ml. A 3 mEq supplement of sodium and chloride should be provided each day. The child should also receive 2 or 3 mEq/100 ml of potassium.

The calculated maintenance fluids replacing insensible losses and obligatory urine volumes are given in a hypotonic saline solution that represents essentially a minimal amount of required electrolytes in free water. Measured losses, which are often those of gastric juices, are given in a half normal saline solution with added potassium. This approximates the makeup of gastric juices without acid. All other fluid losses are replaced with a balanced saline solution such as lactated Ringer's solution.

Balanced saline or colloid-containing solutions will be required for replacement when fluids are shifted internally into the lumen of the bowel, in tissues where edema is forming, or when there is ascites fluid the peritoneal cavity. They will also be required when profound hypoxia, hypoperfusion, or gram-negative sepsis has resulted in capillary membrane damage with subsequent capillary membrane dysfunction after restoration of flow. After stabilization, urine output of approximately 40 ml/kg/day should be the goal in management. Nutritional maintenance whenever possible should be provided by the enteral route. Some children, however, must rely on total parenteral nutrition for significant periods of time. This is a complex procedure involving significant risk and complications. It is accomplished best with a health care team consisting of physicians, nurses, and pharmacy personnel. Knowledge and experience must be available for the production of parenteral nutritional fluid. The nursing staff must also be familiar with an established program for catheter care.

REFERENCES

1. Andrassy, R.S., and Woolley, M.M.: Progress in the use of elemental diets in infants and children, Surg. Gynecol. Obstet. **147:**701, 1978.
2. Baldwin, E.: Dynamic aspects of biochemistry, ed. 3, Cambridge, Mass. 1957, Harvard University Press.
3. Baue, A.E., Wurth, M.A., Chaudry, I.H., and Sayeed, M.M.: Impairment of cell membrane transport during shock and after treatment, Ann. Surg. **178:**412, 1973.
4. Blackburn, G.L., Flatt, J.P., Clowes, G.H., and O'Donnell, T.E.: Peripheral intravenous feeding with isotonic amino acid solutions, Am. J. Surg. **125:**447, 1973.
5. Boeckman, C.R., and Krill, C.E.: Bacterial and fungal infections complicating parenteral alimentation in infants and children, J. Pediatr. Surg. **5:**117, 1970.
6. Bredenberg, C.E., Nomoto, S., and Webb, W.R.: Pulmonary and systemic hemodynamics during hemorrhagic shock in baboons, Ann. Surg. **192:**86, 1980.
7. Caldwell, M.D., Jonsson, H.T., and Othersen, H.B.: Essential fatty acid deficiency in an infant receiving prolonged parenteral alimentation, J. Pediatr. **81:**894, 1972.
8. Cohen, I.T., Dahms, B., and Hays, D.M.: Peripheral total parenteral nutrition employing a lipid emulsion (Intralipid): complications encountered in pediatric patients, J. Pediatr. Surg. **12:**837, 1977.
9. Coran, A.G.: The intravenous use of fat for the total parenteral nutrition of the infant, Lipids **7:**455, 1972.
10. Coran, A.G.: Total intravenous feeding of infants and children without the use of a central venous catheter, Ann. Surg. **179:**455, 1974.
11. Crumrine, R.S.: Postoperative hypoxia in infants and children, Int. Anesthesiol. Clin. **9**(4):83, 1971.
12. Dahms, B.B., and Halpin, T.C.: Preliminary arterial lipid deposit in newborn infants receiving intravenous lipid infusion, J. Pediatr. **97:**800, 1980.
13. Danielson, R.A.: Differential diagnosis and treatment of oliguria in post-traumatic and postoperative patients, Surg. Clin. North Am. **55:**697, 1975.
14. Das, J.B., and Filler, R.M.: Amino acid utilization during total parenteral nutrition in the surgical neonate, J. Pediatr. Surg. **8:**739, 1973.
15. Derks, C.M., and Peters, R.M.: The role of shock and fat embolus in leakage from pulmonary capillaries, Surg. Gynecol. Obstet. **137:**945, 1973.
16. Dibbins, A.W.: Neonatal diaphragmatic hernia: a physiologic challenge, Am. J. Surg. **131:**408, 1976.
17. Drucker, W.R., and Wright, H.K.: Physiology and pathophysiology of gastrointestinal fluids, Curr. Probl. Surg., May, 1964, p. 9.
18. Dudrick, S.J., MacFadyen, B.V., Jr., Van Buren, C.T., et al.: Parenteral hyperalimentation: metabolic problems and solutions, Ann. Surg. **176:**259, 1972.
19. Dudrick, S.J., Wilmore, D.W., Vars, H.M., and Rhoads, J.E.: Can intravenous feedings as the sole means of nutrition support growth in the child and restorew weight in the adults? An affirmative answer, Ann. Surg. **169:**974, 1969.
20. Dwyer, J.: Diets for children and adolescents that meet dietary goals, Am. J. Dis. Child. **134:**1073, 1980.
21. Filler, R.M., Eraklis, A.J., Rubin, V.G., and Das, J.B.: Long-term parenteral nutrition in infants, N. Engl. J. Med. **281:**589, 1969.
22. Filston, H.C., and Grant, J.P.: A safer system for percutaneous subclavian catheterization in newborn infants, J. Pediatr. Surg. **14:**564, 1979.
23. Filston, H.C., and Johnson, D.G.: Percutaneous venous cannulation in neonates and infants: a method for catheter insertion without "cutdown," Pediatrics **48:**896, 1971.
24. Fomon, S.J., Filer, L.J., Jr., Anderson, T.A., and Ziegler E.E.: Recommendations for feeding normal infants, Pediatrics **63:**52, 1979.
25. Friedman, Z., Marks, K.H., Maisels, M.J., et al.: Parenteral fat emulsion on the pulmonary and reticuloendothelial systems in the newborn infant, Pediatrics **61:**694, 1978.
26. Fulton, R.L., and Jones, C.E.: The cause of post-traumatic pulmonary insufficiency in man, Surg. Gynecol. Obstet. **140:**179, 1975.
27. Goldmann, D.A., Martin, W.T., and Worhington, J.W.: Growth of bacteria and fungi in total parenteral nutrition solutions, Am. J. Surg. **126:**314, 1973.
28. Grant, J.P.: Handbook of total parenteral nutrition, Philadelphia, 1980, W.B. Saunders Co.
29. Guidelines for essential trace element preparations for parenteral use: a statement by an expert panel (American Medical Association, Department of Foods and Nutrition), J.A.M.A. **241:**2051, 1979
30. Heird, W.C., Nicholson, J.F., Driscoll, J.M., Jr., et al.: Hyperammonemia resulting from intravenous alimentation using a mixture of synthetic L-amino acids: a preliminary report, J. Pediatr. **81:**162, 1972.

31. Heird, W.C., and Winters, R.W.: Total parenteral nutrition: the state of the art, J. Pediatr. **86:**2, 1975.
32. Heller, R.M., Kirchner, S.G., O'Neill, J.A., Jr., et al.: Skeletal changes of copper deficiency in infants receiving prolonged total parenteral nutrition, J. Pediatr. **92:**947, 1978.
33. Hernandez-Peon, R.: Physiology of body fluids. In Ruch, T.C., and Fulton, J.F., editors: Medical physiology and biophysics, Philadelphia, 1960, W.B. Saunders Co.
34. Knight, P.J., Buchanan, S., and Clatworthy, H.W., Jr.: Calcium and phosphate requirements of preterm infants who require prolonged hyperalimentation, J.A.M.A. **243:**1244, 1980.
35. Leape, L.L., and Valaes, T.: Rickets in low birth weight infants receiving total parenteral nutrition, J. Pediatr. Surg. **11:**665, 1975.
36. Moore, F.D.: Metabolic care of the surgical patient, Philadelphia, 1959, W.B. Saunders Co.
37. Moss, G.S., Gupta, T.K.D., Brinkman, R., et al.: Changes in lung ultrastructure following heterologous serum albumin infusion in the treatment of hemorrhagic shock, Ann. Surg. **189:**236, 1979.
38. Oski, F.A., and Landaw, S.A.: Inhibition of iron absorption from human milk by baby food, Am. J. Dis. Child. **134:**459, 1980.
39. Oski, F.A., and Naiman, J.L.: Hematologic problems in the newborn, ed. 2, Philadelphia, 1972, W.B. Saunders Co.
40. Peckham, G.J., and Fox, W.W.: Physiologic factors affecting pulmonary artery pressure in infants with persistent pulmonary hypertension, J. Pediatr. **93:**1005, 1978.
41. Rickham, P.P.: The metabolic response to neonatal surgery, Cambridge, Mass., 1957, Harvard University Press.
42. Rickham, P.P.: Preoperative and postoperative care: neonates. In Ravitch, M.M., editor: Pediatric surgery, Chicago, 1969, Year Book Medical Publishers, Inc.
43. Seyfer, A.E., Zajtchuk, R., Hazlett, D.R., and Mologne, L.A.: Systemic vascular performance in endotoxic shock, Surg. Gynecol. Obstet. **145:**401, 1977.
44. Share, L.: Acute reduction in extracellular fluid volume and concentration of antidiuretic hormone in blood, Endocrinology **69:**925, 1961.
45. Shires, G.T., Cunningham, J.N., Baker, C.R.F., et al.: Alterations in cellular membrane function during hemorrhagic shock in primates, Ann. Surg. **176:**288, 1972.
46. Shires, T.: The role of sodium-containing solutions in the treatment of oligemic shock, Surg. Clin. North Am. **45:**365, 1965.
47. Srouji, M.N., Balistreri, W.F., Caleb, M.H., et al.: Zinc deficiency during parenteral nutrition: skin manifestations and immune incompetence in a premature infant, J. Pediatr. Surg. **13:**570, 1978.
48. Suita, S., Ikeda, K., Nagasaki, A., and Hayashida, Y.: Zinc deficiency during total parenteral nutrition in childhood, J. Pediatr. Surg. **13:**5, 1978.
49. Swan, H.J., Ganz, W.F., Forrester, J., et al.: Catheterization of the heart in man with use of a flow-directed balloon-tipped catheter, N. Engl. J. Med. **283:**447, 1970.
50. Touloukian, R.J., and Seashore, J.H.: Hepatic secretory obstruction with total parenteral nutrition in the infant, J. Pediatr. Surg. **10:**353, 1975.
51. Virgilio, R.W., Rice, C.L., Smith, D.E., et al.: Crystalloid vs. colloid resuscitation: is one better? A randomized clinical study, Surgery **85:**129, 1979.
52. Wallace, W.M.: Quantitative requirements of the infant and child for water and electrolytes under varying conditions, Am. J. Clin. Pathol. **23:**1133, 1953.
53. Weil, M.H., and Shubin, H., editors: Diagnosis and treatment of shock, Baltimore, 1967, The Williams & Wilkins Co.
54. Wiggers, C.J.: The physiology of shock, New York, 1950, Harvard University Press.
55. Wilmore, D.W., Groff, D.B., Bishop, H.C., and Dudrick, S.J.: Total parenteral nutrition in infants with catastrophic gastrointestinal anomalies, J. Pediatr. Surg. **4:**181, 1969.
56. Winters, R.W., editor: The body fluids in pediatrics: medical, surgical, and neonatal disorders of acid-base status, hydration, and oxygenation, Boston, 1973, Little, Brown & Co.
57. Wright, H.K., and Gann, D.S.: Correction of defect in free water excretion in postoperative patients by extracellular fluid volume expansion, Ann. Surg. **158:**70, 1963.
58. Wright, H.K., Gann, D.S., and Drucker, W.R.: Current concepts of therapy for derangements of extracellular fluid, In Davis, J.H., editor: Current concepts in surgery: a clinical interpretation of basic knowledge, New York, 1965, McGraw-Hill Book Co.

CHAPTER 6

Management of the acutely injured pediatric patient

HOWARD C. FILSTON and JOSEPH A. MOYLAN, Jr.

Trauma is the most important illness of childhood and is the primary cause of death.[17] Once the problems of perinatal death, prematurity, and congenital anomalies have taken their toll in the first month of life, trauma moves to the forefront and leads all other illnesses as the chief cause of mortality during the childhood years. Trauma in childhood ranges from lacerations and falls sustained at play to sports injuries, ingestions, and insect, snake, and animal bites. Abuse and battering by parents are particularly malignant forms of trauma for the child. However, the leading cause of injury and mortality is blunt trauma from motor vehicle accidents sustained either as an occupant or pedestrian.[29]

The number of children involved is monumental. Varying estimates have placed the total of seriously injured children at 100,000 per year, resulting in mortalities and significant lifetime morbidity.[17] A major urban university emergency service estimates that 15 million children sustain some form of trauma each year in the United States.[20] In the state of North Carolina alone[28] 150 children a year are killed as passengers in automobile accidents.

The injuries typically associated with vehicular accidents are severe intracranial injury, contusion, rupture and lacerations of intrathoracic and intraabdominal organs, and major fractures with concomitant soft tissue injury.

As with all pathologic processes, prevention is the best remedy for the illness and injury and should be the pervading goal. Despite the statistics on morbidity and mortality, 98% of children do not use restraints in vehicles when they are available.[28] Even when parents wear restraints their children are restrained only 30% of the time. It is estimated that over 50% of the children who died in automobile accidents could have been saved had they worn the existing restraints. Only recently have efforts been made to identify toys and other equipment with which the child interacts that have hazardous potential.

Until greater efforts are put forth to prevent children from being injured, every surgeon who cares for children must have an extensive knowledge of childhood trauma and be able to deal with the many aspects of it. Obviously, the fact that trauma can affect any area of the body makes it difficult for any one specialist to maintain expertise at dealing with injuries in every area. Nevertheless, surgeons should be able to resuscitate acutely injured patients and should be aware of the range of injuries and probabilities of injuries for any given trauma source. In addition, they should be able to help guide the overall management of children. Surgeons should understand the effects of trauma on children emotionally and should be child advocates by strongly supporting and encouraging efforts to prevent trauma of all kinds and to protect children by decreasing the possibilities of trauma in the daily environment.

This chapter will be primarily directed toward giving the plastic surgeon, who so often deals with various aspects of trauma in the child. a basic knowledge of the fundamentals required to resuscitate the acutely injured patient.

INITIAL EVALUATION

Ideally the standard medical approach of obtaining a complete history and an orderly physical examination with carefully considered laboratory and radiologic evaluations, as in any other disease entity, is the optimal approach to the trauma victim. In reality the arrival of a traumatized child is as much of an intrusion into the orderly life of the surgeon as is the trauma to the patient. The severely injured child commonly has an acute life-threatening event that requires instantaneous action based on rapid minimal evaluation. Therefore the important life-maintaining functions must be assessed rapidly and thoroughly and action taken immediately. The presence, quality, and rate of the pulse should be ascertained; if these are unobtainable, heart sounds should be listened for and preparations made for external massage if necessary. At the same time, the patency of the airway must be assessed and any injuries to it rapidly noted. Adequacy of ventilation should be determined by noting the presence of respiratory efforts and the ease with which air enters and leaves the chest. If the patient is not ventilating adequately when first encountered, either mouth-to-mouth resuscitation or bag-and-mask ventilation, with oxygen if this is available, should be provided immediately. It can be generally assumed that a child with an inadequate cardiac mechanism has either a severe insult to the ventilatory function or is in overwhelming hypovolemic shock. The exceedingly low incidence of primary myocardial or coronary artery disease in this age group makes cardiac arrest as a result of cardiac disease highly unlikely. Thus reestablishing ventilation and oxygenation and refilling vascular volume immediately are primary concerns on encountering inadequate cardiac function. A possible exception would be a child struck by lightning in whom the electrical effect on the heart might cause fibrillation or standstill.

In dealing with the airway in the young child, several points are cogent. First, it is a rare child who has not ingested some form of food shortly before sustaining an injury. Thus vomiting, aspiration, and obstruction of the airway by foreign material are likely causes of pulmonary embarrassment in a child. Patency of the airway must be reestablished by manual removal of particles from the hypopharynx and by suctioning the tracheobronchial tree if necessary. A Heimlich maneuver of rapid, sharp compression of the epigastrium may be required to dislodge aspirated material. Care should be taken to ensure that a cervical fracture is not present before performing this maneuver, since the resulting

jolt may lacerate the cord if an unstable fracture is present. Early passage of a nasogastric tube will help to avoid subsequent regurgitation and aspiration, a frequent cause of additional morbidity in children once they have reached a medical facility. Regardless of the specific injury, every child with major trauma to the head, airway, chest, or abdomen and severe blood loss or shock should have a nasogastric tube placed to prevent vomiting and aspiration. This should always be accomplished before transportation.

Once the airway is clear, initial resuscitation should be provided by bag-and-mask ventilation and oxygenation. The mask should fit snugly about the child's nose and mouth, and the head should not be extended as severely as is usually done in adults. The infant's airway is maintained best in the ''sniffing position'' with the head pressed somewhat forward and the face straight ahead (Fig. 6-1).[21] Extreme extension of the head and neck will force the infant's larynx behind the base of the tongue and make it difficult to ventilate the child. Usually in the smaller infant the occiput is prominent enough that it alone will thrust the head forward relative to the body. If this is not the case, a folded towel placed behind the occiput will help elevate the head. The jaw must be pulled somewhat forward up into the mask to maintain patency of the airway. An oral airway may be helpful, but occasionally it will force the tongue down into the hypopharynx and increase rather than alleviate the obstruction.

If adequate ventilation cannot be maintained by mask or if prolonged ventilation is obviously needed, endotracheal intubation should be considered. This maneuver obviously requires skill and experience, and many individuals who are highly competent at intubating adults will find intubation of

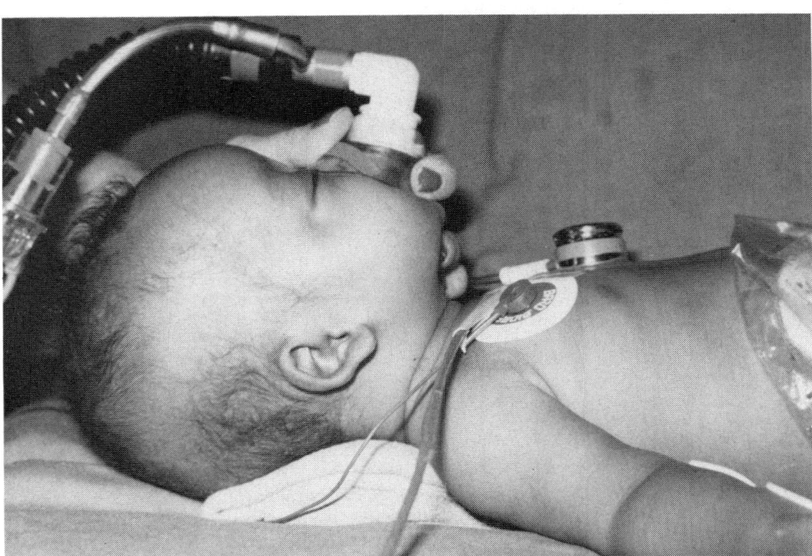

Fig. 6-1. Infant in the proper position for mask ventilation. The head is in the ''sniffing position'' and not in extension. The folded towel behind the head accentuates the forward position of the head.

the infant and younger child difficult. This is due to the differing anatomy of the infant's larynx, hypopharynx, jaw, and tongue relative to one another. The maneuver commonly used for adults of extreme extension of the head and neck during intubation will obscure the larynx behind the base of the tongue and make exposure impossible in infants. Intubation of the child is accomplished as follows:

1. Place the head in a "sniffing position."
2. Preoxygenate with 100% oxygen by mask if the situation permits.
3. Suction the pharynx.
4. Open the mouth, insert a straight-blade laryngoscope, and push the tongue to the left.
5. Touch the tip of the laryngoscope blade to the uvula, then *push* the handle of the laryngoscope toward the feet, parallel to the floor (do not "cock" wirst).
6. The epiglottis should be visible; push farther or lift the epiglottis with the blade to expose the larynx.
7. Insert a straight, uncuffed, wetted plastic tube by gentle pressure against the cords.

For children up to 8 or 9 years of age a noncuffed straight endotracheal tube with an appropriate size adapter should be chosen. The child should be well oxygenated before attempted intubation if possible. The intubation should be accomplished as atraumatically as possible. In the infant and younger child, a straight-blade laryngoscope is usually preferable. Intubation usually can be achieved if the head is placed in the "sniffing position" (Fig. 6-2), the mouth is opened as widely as possible, the tongue is pushed to the left as the laryngoscope is passed into the mouth, and the tip of the laryngoscope is passed in until it touches the uvula.

At this point the handle of the laryngoscope should be pushed toward the patient's feet, parallel to the floor. This should be a *pushing* motion, which moves the tongue and jaw forward and exposes the tip of the epiglottis. If this maneuver is done as described with the tip of the laryngoscope initially touching the uvula and then a pushing motion applied to the handle of the laryngoscope, the tip of the laryngoscope will move directly to the epiglottis. The operator's wrist should be kept fixed in full extension, with no "cocking" or flexing the wrist. The latter motion tends to push the larynx up behind the base of the tongue, making it invisible. Typically, the inexperienced operator will extend the head too much or flex or cock the wrist too much, and the combination pushes the epiglottis out of sight behind the base of the tongue. In the frustration of being unable to visualize what must be seen, the operator increases all of these mistakes and often ends up elevating the child off the table with the hypopharynx impaled on the tip of the laryngoscope blade.

The size of the child's little finger will provide a rough guide to the correct diameter of the endotracheal tube. Tubes spanning this general size should be available. Once the epiglottis is visualized, further pushing with the laryngoscope may open the epiglottis and expose the cords, or if necessary the tip of the laryngoscope blade can be gently abutted against the epiglottis and the epiglottis itself pushed forward, exposing the cords. The straight plastic endotracheal tube should then be gently inserted by placing the tip of the tube into the larynx and maintaining mild pressure against the cords. A slight twisting motion may help to pass the tube through the cords and into the trachea. If the tube

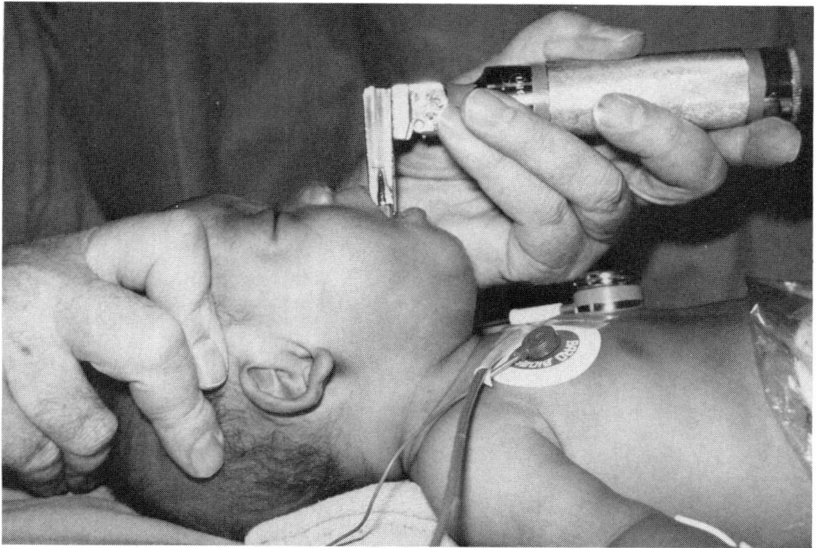

Fig. 6-2. Proper position and technique for intubation of an infant. Again the head is in the "sniffing position." Note that the laryngoscope blade does not abut the child's upper alveolar ridge and that the laryngoscope handle is maintained parallel to the table. Exposure is accomplished by a pushing force of the handle toward the infant's feet rather than a "cocking," or leverage, force.

is the correct size, persistent mild pressure will result in passage. Wetting the tube with saline or a very small amount of lubricant before insertion will facilitate its passage. The tube should not be jammed in and out of the larynx as the cords open and close. Once the tube passes the cords, it should be inserted a short distance farther. Typically the young infant is intubated too far and the tube passed well into the right main stem bronchus, resulting in occlusion of the left airway and atelectasis.

Adequate ventilation can always be provided for a child without a cuffed endotracheal tube, and some air leakage around the tube should be of no concern as long as adequate ventilatory motion is present in the chest and good aeration can be verified with the stethoscope. The adequacy of the breath sounds throughout both sides of the thorax should then be assessed and the tube taped in place.

The younger the infant, the more rapid the respiratory rate should be. Newborns and very young infants have respiratory rates two or three times that of the adult or older child, with rates of 40 to 60 breaths/min being necessary. For the infant and young child beyond the newborn period, rates of approximately 30 breaths/min should be adequate. The tidal volume required is approximately 10 cc/kg. Ventilation can best be provided by a bag system with a pop-off pressure regulator, and the correct volume can be assessed by adequate motion of the child's chest. Excess pressure should be avoided, especially in the very young infant.

The complications of air-block syndrome, a pneumothorax, a pneumomediastinum, and a pneumopericardium are real risks with excessive ventilation.[16,22] Although it has taken considerable space to describe these resuscitation maneuvers, they must be accomplished expeditiously to prevent neurologic damage.

If ventilation is established and the child still appears poorly oxygenated despite an apparently adequate cardiac mechanism, a tension pneumothorax should be considered immediately. Clues to the presence of a tension pneumothorax can sometimes be obtained by palpation of a deviated trachea at the suprasternal notch or by auscultation of the chest. Chest radiographs will invariably confirm its presence. However, if the child is in severe respiratory embarrassment, time for such confirmation may not be available, and the physician should proceed with needle aspiration of the pleural space without hesitation. This is best accomplished by using a No. 16 needle and syringe or a needle with a plastic outer sheath. In tiny infants a smaller needle may be required and may give the false impression that no pneumothorax is present. If needle aspiration fails to confirm a suspected pneumothorax and the child is in severe respiratory distress, a formal tube thoracostomy should be accomplished. If the tension pneumothorax is relieved by needle aspiration, a tube thoracostomy can be performed through a small incision in the anterior axillary line in the fourth intercostal space. Once the incision is made through the skin and subcutaneous tissue, a hemostat can be used

to dissect bluntly through the muscles into the intercostal space, puncture the intercostal space, and pass into the pleural cavity. This will create a pneumothorax, but will protect the underlying pulmonary parenchyma from injury when the chest tube is subsequently passed into the pleural space using the trocar. We prefer a polyvinyl chloride tube that has its own stylet-type trocar. This can be passed between the open blades of the hemostat, and if the tube is wet with saline, it will slide easily into the chest. The hemostat is then removed, the trocar is removed from the tube, and the tube is passed farther into the pleural space and attached to underwater seal drainage. The pleural cavity should be intubated in this fashion if satisfactory ventilation cannot be accomplished. If these maneuvers still fail to stabilize the ventilatory state, a severe injury to the airway with ongoing massive air leak into the pleural space should be suspected. At this point an immediate chest radiograph should be obtained, additional tubes placed as necessary and attached to high-pressure continuous negative suction, and preparations for emergency surgery completed.

In summary, rapid establishment of adequate respiratory function is mandatory and involves clearing of the airway; passage of a nasogastric tube to prevent emesis and aspiration; establishment of adequate ventilation either spontaneously, by bag-and-mask ventilation, or by direct endotracheal intubation; rapid assessment of ventilatory sufficiency after adequate ventilation is established; and rapid assessment and treatment of any pneumothorax or direct tracheobronchial injury.

ASSESSMENT AND EMERGENCY RESUSCITATION OF VASCULAR VOLUME DEFICIENCY

Major hemorrhage, whether external or internal, causes a blood volume deficiency that results in inadequate perfusion of the tissues. Ultimately the integrity of the vascular volume can only be confirmed by demonstrating adequate circulation to the skin and soft tissues and adequate perfusion of the kidney as assessed by urine output. Initially, however, the gross functioning of the cardiovascular system can be assessed by the rate and quality of the pulse and by the blood pressure. In addition, the color of the skin and mucous membranes and the temperature of the skin of the extremities can be used in the assessment. The pulse should be strong and of adequate rate. In the small infant rates well over a 100 should be present. A normal heart rate for the newborn and early infancy period ranges between 100 and 188 beats/min.[18] Toward the end of the first year of life, it comes down to a mean of 130 beats/min and then gradually tapers toward the adult rates of 60 to 80 beats/min. Heart rates under 100 beats/min in infants under 3 months of age should be considered bradycardia, and hypoxia due to inadequate oxygenation or perfusion should be suspected. The young infant does not respond to shock with tachycardia and a gradual fall in blood pressure as does the older child or adult. Rather, the infant becomes rapidly depressed, with bradycardia ensuing early in the course of the shock state despite the maintenance of adequate blood pressure. Blood pressures in infants, on the other hand, are well below 100 mm Hg, with the newborn having a blood pressure between 60 to 80 mm Hg systolic. Premature infants may have normal blood pressures as low as 40 to 50 mm Hg systolic. Morse's rule of thumb for systolic blood pressure in children is 80 mm Hg plus twice the age in years.

Assessment of the injury will give some clue as to whether major blood loss exists, remembering that significant blood loss can occur internally in the chest, abdomen, or even into soft tissues adjacent to a major fracture. On the other hand, many of the signs of hypovolemia such as bradycardia, hypotension, cyanosis, and poor perfusion may be due to hypoxia on a ventilatory basis as well. The considerations outlined previously for assessing and correcting deficiencies in ventilatory function and oxygenation must be kept in mind.

If hypovolemia is judged to be a significant probability, rapid restoration of blood volume should be accomplished. A dependable line for vascular access should be established as rapidly as possible, using the method with which the surgeon has the most facility. This may require incisional cutdown with isolation of the vein directly, or it may involve a percutaneous puncture with a needle-stylet plastic cannula system. All of the veins available in the adult are present in the child and can be cannulated readily with a little experience. Although the saphenous vein at the ankle has been the standard vessel used for emergency vascular access, any vein can be isolated by a small incision placed over it and minimal dissection through the subcutaneous tissue with a fine-point mosquito hemostat to elevate the vein for cannulation. If incisional cutdown is used, a ligature is passed beneath the vein to provide traction. The same catheter, needle-stylet system described for percutaneous access should be used to penetrate the vein directly while it is distended with blood rather than ligating it proximally and incising into it for access in the time-honored fashion. Direct puncture with the needle-stylet plastic cannula system will allow the placement of a larger bore cannula and may even preserve the vein for subsequent use.

PERCUTANEOUS VENIPUNCTURE TECHNIQUE

Percutaneous venipuncture[13] has been highly successful in achieving vascular access in infants and children. It should be rapidly abandoned, however, and incisional access achieved if the child is in such severe hypovolemic shock that the vessels cannot be filled and identified.

The essential points of this technique are as follows:

1. Use a soft proper sized tourniquet and place it just above the cannulation site. A rubber band serves well for newborns and a small Penrose drain for larger infants and children.
2. Choose a cannulation system consisting of a metal needle-stylet with outer plastic catheter sheath and attached syringe.

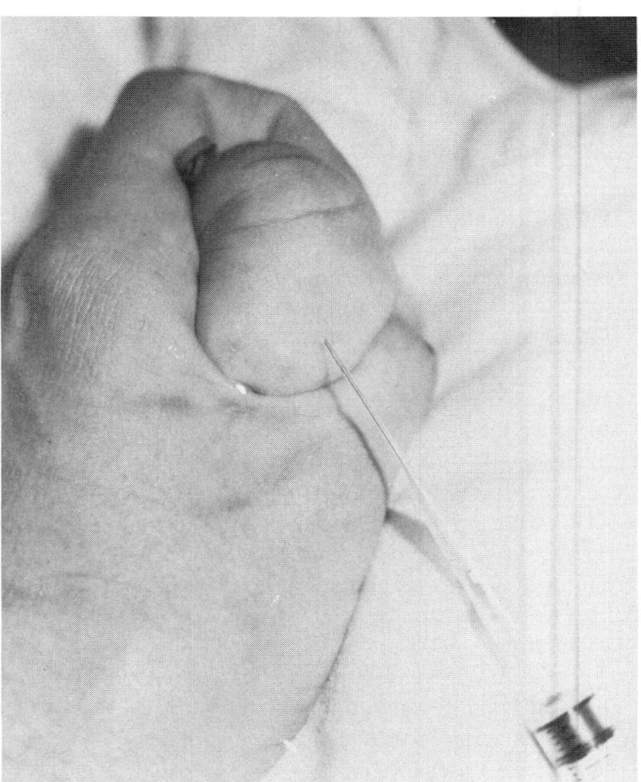

Fig. 6-3. Cannulation of the vein on the dorsum of the infant's hand is facilitated by wrapping the entire hand in the operator's hand beneath the wrist of the infant, the usual position for cannulation in older children and adults. This position allows stretching out of the vein, which prevents "buckling" of the vein when the needle and cannula pass into it. (From Filston, H.C., and Izant, R.: The surgical neonate: evaluation and care, New York, 1978, Appleton-Century-Crofts.)

We prefer the clear, plastic tapered hub of the Argyle Medicut system.
3. Make an initial skin puncture with a separate slightly larger needle approximately 1 cm proximal to the point chosen for entry into the vein.
4. When cannulating an antecubital vein, place the arm on a padded arm board with a gauze roll behind the elbow to hyperextend it. Tape the arm to the board and the board to the table for secure immobilization.
5. When cannulating a vein on the dorsum of the hand, flex the wrist to its extreme position so that the palm of the hand is pressed against the volar surface of the forearm, a position usually possible only in infants and young children. Do not place your hand between the child's forearm and palm. Rather, wrap the entire hand and arm as depicted in Fig. 6-3.
6. Keep any vein stretched out as straight as possible. If the vein buckles, the metal needle may enter it, but the plastic cannula probably will not.
7. Insert the cannula *bevel down*. The advantage of this is shown in Fig. 6-4.
8. Advance the cannula slowly with gentle suction applied to the syringe plunger until the needle enters the vein. This is confirmed by the return of blood into the syringe. Aspirate 0.5 ml of blood if possible, line up the cannula with the direction of the vein, maximize the stretch on the vein, and while

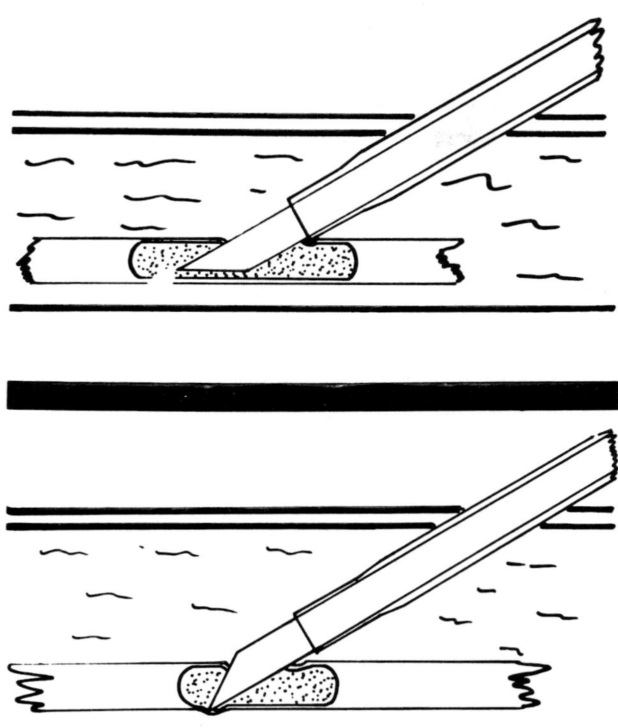

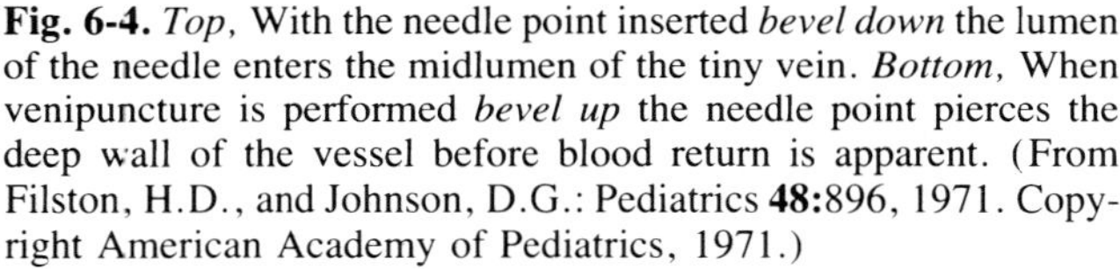

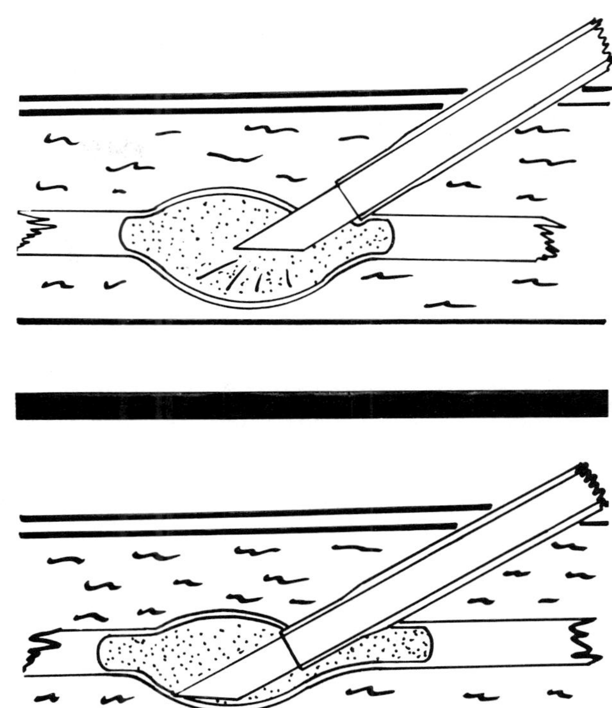

Fig. 6-4. *Top,* With the needle point inserted *bevel down* the lumen of the needle enters the midlumen of the tiny vein. *Bottom,* When venipuncture is performed *bevel up* the needle point pierces the deep wall of the vessel before blood return is apparent. (From Filston, H.D., and Johnson, D.G.: Pediatrics **48:**896, 1971. Copyright American Academy of Pediatrics, 1971.)

Fig. 6-5. *Top,* Reinjection of the aspirated blood expands the vessel, leaving room for further advancement of the needle. *Bottom,* The plastic catheter lip can then enter the lumen of the vessel without the needle perforating the deep wall. (From Filston, H.C., and Johnson, D.G.: Pediatrics **48:**896, 1971. Copyright American Academy of Pediatrics, 1971.)

reinjecting the blood, advance *the entire* cannula (needle, catheter, and syringe) a few millimeters farther into the vein. This expands the vein (Fig. 6-5) and allows the catheter to enter the lumen of the vessel.

9. Now remove the needle-stylet and syringe from the catheter. Blood should return freely from the open catheter. If it does not, the catheter may have traversed the back wall of the vein. Slowly back the catheter out until free flow of blood occurs. Then twist it and push it forward again. If the catheter entered and traversed the vein, it will usually seat itself in the lumen successfully with this technique. If one or two such attempts fail to achieve free blood return, the catheter probably never entered the vessel at all and the blood return is coming from a hole made by the needle in the side wall of the vessel.
10. Careful taping and splinting complete the procedure.

Percutaneous subclavian or internal jugular venipuncture is a useful route of vascular access if the surgeon has facility and experience with it.[10] Both are hazardous in the hands of the inexperienced operator and may lead to more complications than are acceptable. They require careful positioning and immobilization of the patient, and this may be difficult to achieve under emergency conditions.

Once vascular access is established, a rapid infusion of one fourth of the patient's blood volume will provide temporary restoration of circulatory volume. This push of fluid should be accomplished within seconds to minutes, as rapidly as the fluid can be pushed in with a syringe. This is a reasonable test of volume status, and the volume infused will be tolerated by patients with normal cardiovascular dynamics even if their volume status is normal at the time of the push infusion. Since a newborn has a blood volume of 8% to 8½%, a push of one fourth of the blood volume would amount to about 20 ml/kg.[7] This volume is useful and safe for children at any age.

Unless obvious severe hypovolemia exists and the risk of using uncross-matched blood is outweighed by the risk of continued inadequate perfusion, Ringer's lactate solution may be administered for this initial push and may stabilize the patient until type-specific cross-matched blood is available. As discussed by Morse,[25] the restoration of volume in discrete pushes of the type previously described will give a better idea of any continuing blood loss than will a constant infusion over time. It the patient continually returns to an unstable volume status after responding to volume restoration, ongoing blood loss is probable.

Sufficient volume restoration should take place initially to reestablish a normal pulse rate and quality of the pulse and a normal blood pressure for age. Once this is accomplished, ongoing monitoring of peripheral perfusion and accurate monitoring of urine volume output should be used to guide additional fluid and blood restoration.

Before delving further into the theory behind the management of volume restoration in the acutely injured patient, an appreciation of some of the techniques used in the management of cardiac arrest in the infant is essential. Almost all infants in cardiac arrest can be managed adequately by closed-chest cardiac massage. Sufficient compressive force should be applied to achieve a significant cardiac output. This should be followed by an adequate release period to allow refilling of the cardiac chambers. The respirations must be interspersed into the pattern so that the lungs can fill when the compression force of the massage has been released. A young infant can be massaged adequately by the operator placing both hands around the child's entire thorax with the thumbs close together over the sternum. The thumbs are used to compress the chest, with the fingers and palms behind the chest providing the firm support for the massage (Fig. 6-6). In the infant and younger child, the adult technique of sitting astride the patient and using the palms of the hands to compress the chest against a board or table should not be used. This technique become applicable when the child is too large for the operator's hands to enwrap the chest. A rate of between 40 to 60 beats/min is adequate for the older child, but a rate of at least 80 beats/min is necessary for the infant, remembering that the infant's normal heart rate ranges from 100 to 160 beats/min.

If severe hypoxia, hypoperfusion, or frank cardiac arrest has been sustained, pharmacologic correction of the acid-base imbalances that result will be necessary before the myocardium can be expected to resume normal function. Correction can await the results of these determinations if an arterial puncture can be accomplished easily and blood gases and the pH level can be assessed rapidly. On the other hand, it can be assumed that any near arrest, severe hypoxia, or frank arrest will result in increased acidosis and require the provision of sodium bicarbonate. This should be given at the rate of 2 mEq/kg initially, remembering a rough guideline that the average baby weighs 3 kg at birth, 10 kg at 1 year, 12 kg at 2 years, 18 kg at 5 years, 36 kg at 10 years, and 54 kg at 15 years. These are easily recalled numbers rather than true averages.

Once adequate ventilation and closed-chest cardiac massage have been established, accurate assessment of cardiac function must be achieved by electrocardiographic monitoring (ECG). Further resuscitation involves pharmacologic manipulation of the function of the myocardium combined with the appropriate electric shock therapy to overcome ventricular fibrillation or restart a heart in asystole. During these manipulations continued ventilation and effective closed-chest massage must be provided.

It is essential to restore the chemical milieu of the myocardium to as near normal as possible in order to achieve a return to efficient myocardial functioning. Correction of acidosis is the first step, and after the initial bolus of sodium bicarbonate, blood gases should be obtained if at all possible to assess the acid-base status and guide subsequent therapy. When cardiac arrest results from hypoxia or severe hypovolemia, reestablishment of adequate ventilation and correction of hypovolemia and acidosis will usually result in resumption of normal myocardial functioning. If fibrillation

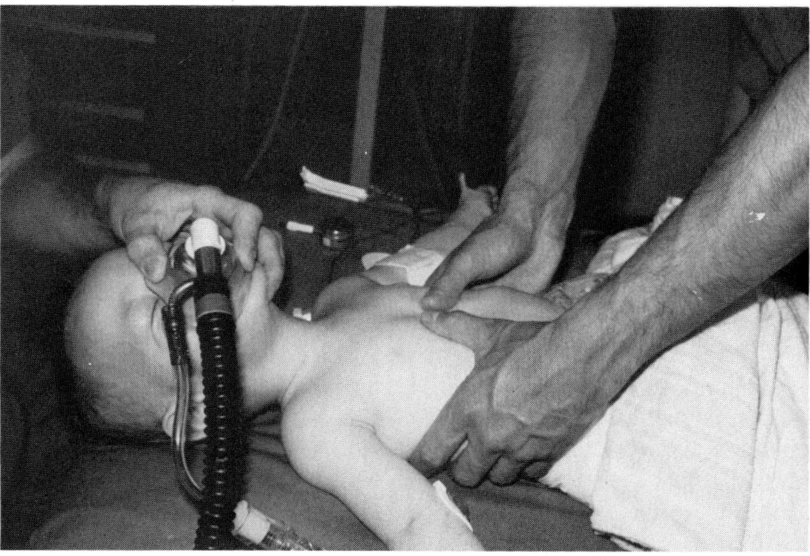

Fig. 6-6. Closed-chest cardiac massage in an infant is accomplished by using the hands as support for the dorsum of the infant's chest with the thumbs positioned over the sternum for the actual compression. This provides better control and less trauma than placing the infant on a board and using the "heel" of the palm as in adults.

or asystole persists, however, electric shock through the chest applied by shock paddles should be provided. Fibrillation usually can be arrested and a normal beat restored in this manner, but it will be unsuccessful if severe acidosis persists. Closed-chest massage should be reinstituted after the shock therapy is applied until the function of the myocardium can be assessed. If the normal cardiac rhythm cannot be established after these corrective mechanisms and after proven correction of the acidosis, some electrolyte imbalance such as hyperkalemia or hypocalcemia should be suspected. There are unusual occurrences in acute trauma, but hypocalcemia may result if excessive amounts of sodium bicarbonate have been administered. Severe hyperkalemia may require prolonged mechanical massage before myocardial function will resume, but it can be overcome by the provision of glucose and insulin. The latter agents will help to drive potassium back into the cells and normalize the serum potassium levels. Once again, this type of myocardial dysfunction is unusual in acute trauma, and myocardial dysfunction in the acute trauma patient should be considered a result of hypoxia and acidosis until proven otherwise. Thus the main thrust of resuscitation should be toward providing adequate ventilation and oxygenation and correcting the acidosis. Obviously, any sources of ongoing blood loss that can be controlled should be controlled with pressure dressings or, if necessary, a tourniquet.

TEMPERATURE CONTROL

In the severely injured patient in a hypoxic, hypovolemic state at any age, maintenance of normal body temperature may be compromised. The infant, however, is extremely susceptible to hypothermia, which may produce profound effects on respiratory and cardiovascular mechanisms. The infant has a huge surface area relative to body weight and may have inadequate thermoregulatory mechanisms, particularly within the newborn period. Hypothermia leads to compensatory vasoconstriction and increased metabolic demands with concomitant increases in demand for oxygen. In the face of acute severe injury, the child may not be able to maintain thermoregulatory mechanisms, and the resulting hypothermic state may depress the respiratory center and increase the degree of hypoxia. At the same time, the increased vasoconstriction may lead to hypoperfusion, hypoxia, and anaerobic glycolytic mechanisms that build up acid waste products in the tissues. These products may be flooded into the systemic circuit when perfusion is restored, worsening systemic acidosis. This may increase the acidosis that resulted from the initial hypoxia, and impair attempts to correct acid-base deficiencies (Fig. 6-3).[11] In the press of activities in caring for a major accident victim, the problems of temperature regulation may be ignored and severe impairment may result. An overhead warming device should be immediately available in the emergency room and po-

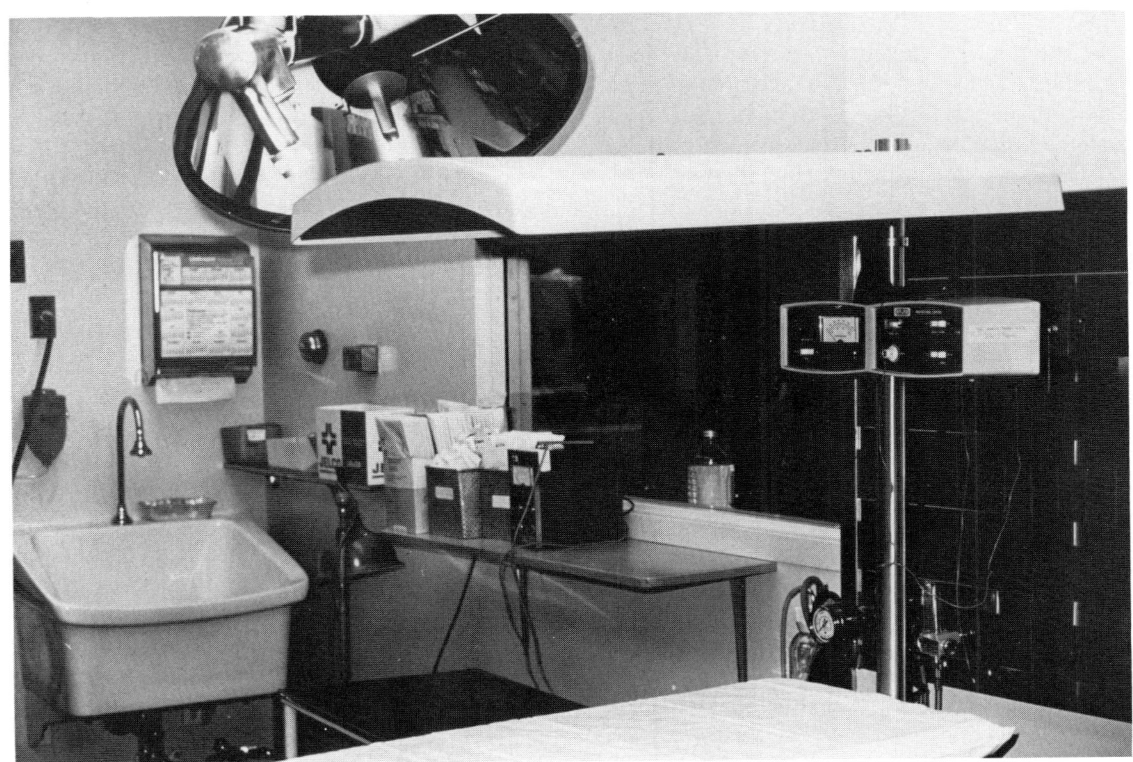

Fig. 6-7. An overhead warmer positioned above the emergency room table will maintain the infant's temperature reasonably well during prolonged evaluation and treatment in the emergency situation.

sitioned over the child during resuscitative efforts (Fig. 6-7). Body core temperature should be monitored by rectal probes or intermittent rectal temperatures, and ongoing attention given to maintaining body temperature. If successful maintenance of thermal normality is not achieved, the resulting respiratory depression and vasoconstriction may confuse the assessment of respiratory, cardiovascular, and even neurologic functioning.

HISTORY

Once cardiorespiratory function is reestablished and a stable state achieved, as much history of the cause of the injury, specific forces applied, and areas of the body involved should be obtained. Occasionally, no significant history is available, but any details that can be secured will help in the assessment of potential injuries to internal organs. In addition to obtaining the history of the injury, a history of the child's past health, particularly of drug allergies and chronic medical illness that may affect the assessment and resuscitation, is essential. The fact that most children are basically healthy, thriving individuals before injury is a boon to management, but the child with diabetes, sickle cell anemia, adrenal insufficiency, or other chronic states of malfunction must be identified. An important part of the history of the traumatic event is that of the child's state of consciousness immediately after the injury and during the period between the injury and arrival at the medical facility.

NEUROLOGIC EVALUATION

Early in the resuscitative program a careful neurologic evaluation should be accomplished. As noted before, this involves a history of the child's state of consciousness, since the initial state of consciousness and subsequent changes therein are the most significant factors in evaluating intracranial injury. If the child was conscious immediately after the injury and has remained conscious throughout the period subsequent to it, the likelihood of a severe intracranial injury is low. If the child is not conscious but was previously conscious immediately after the injury, the level of responses must be assessed as a baseline, and continued monitoring of that state of consciousness is essential. This assessment should be in terms of specific responses and not simply a statement of generalized coma. Thus response to verbal commands would be one level, and response to manipulations would be a more depressed level. Response only to deep pain is indicative of more severe injury. Total unresponsiveness or pathologic responses such as mass withdrawal or Babinski's reflex represent severest injury.

Regardless of the initial state of consciousness, it is the change from that level that must be assessed, and this requires repeated evaluation of the patient's responses. These should be recorded at regular intervals, at least every 15 minutes. A careful record of the resuscitative activities should be maintained, with one individual being assigned the task of recording both the resuscitative manipulations and the responses of the patient.

VOLUME MONITORING

At this point a Foley catheter should be passed into the bladder to monitor urine output for a continuing assessment of the adequacy of volume replacement. A brief discussion of the theory behind volume management is essential if proper considerations are to be given to restoring vascular volume. Until relatively recent years, the major focus in evaluating volume status was blood pressure. This is a highly indirect measurement of volume adequacy and may lead to significant errors in management. A moment's reflection will show that blood pressure simply reveals the pressure exerted by the pumping of the blood by the heart in a specific monitored blood vessel. If the cardiovascular system were adynamic, with fixed-caliber vessels and no elasticity or responsiveness, blood pressure would be an adequate gauge of volume. However, this is not the case, and changes in tone modify the capacity of the peripheral vascular bed. Changes in myocardial volume and force can modify the pressure, and in response to volume deprivation, the cardiovascular system can be greatly contracted in capacity by shunting blood from arteriole to venule, bypassing the capillary bed and thereby significantly reducing the volume required to fill the vascular system. Thus for a considerable period of time during which vascular contraction may be taking place, the volume of blood may remain adequate to maintain a normal blood pressure in the contracted vascular bed. An extreme example would be one in which the contracted state was so extensive that the heart was pumping into the aorta, short-circuiting to the vena cava, and returning to the heart. Under these circumstances no flow whatsoever to any other vessels would be occurring; yet if the depleted volume were adequate to fill this contracted vascular system, the pressure recorded from the aorta could be normal. Obviously, other changes in overall body functioning would make maintenance of normal blood pressure under these circumstances impossible, but it does illustrate that extreme vasoconstriction and reduction in vascular capacity can compensate for extensive losses of blood without a fall in blood pressure. Thus accurate monitoring of volume status depends on urine output as an indicator of satisfactory organ perfusion, specifically perfusion of the kidney. The assumption that an adequate urine output represents adequate renal perfusion and thereby reflects a state of adequate total body vascular volume repletion is a valid one. Urine output is an excellent gauge of vascular volume repletion if the following assumptions are valid:

1. The myocardium must be functioning at a level adequate to perfuse the kidney.
2. The kidney must be functioning normally, specifically, there must be no underlying renal disease or direct injury impairing renal function itself.
3. The urinary drainage tract must be intact, and the Foley catheter must be properly placed and patent.
4. There must be no inappropriate ADH. Note that ADH is an appropriate response to volume depletion, and its presence in the hypovolemic state is to be ex-

pected.[8,39] When volume is adequately restored, the ADH response will be suppressed and the kidney will function normally.[41]

5. No pharmacologic agents must be used that will alter renal function in an inappropriate or unexpected manner. An appropriate urine output for a child is 40 ml/kg/day or about 1 to 2 ml/kg/hr.[38]

In assessing the volume status and estimating fluid restoration needs, further understanding of shock mechanisms and the resultant physiologic malfunction is essential. Wiggers showed in the 1940s that dogs subjected to shock by severe blood volume loss and maintained at shock levels for relatively brief periods of time failed to achieve a stable state after restoration of the entire volume of shed blood.[40] This model, known as the *irreversible shock model,* led to a reproducible and predictably high mortality among the animals despite seemingly adequate volume restoration. Because volume status in that era was based on blood pressure, therapeutic interventions were directed at raising the blood pressure by providing pharmacologic agents which caused vasoconstriction and artificially restored blood pressure. These agents provided no volume replacement or increased perfusion of vital structures. As the hypovolemic nature of shock came to be understood, it soon became apparent that physiologic changes secondary to hypoxic injury to the underperfused tissues were causing sequestration of fluid within the body spaces that was not obvious to external assessment. The normal vasoconstrictive protective mechanism that comes into play in response to hypovolemia leads to low perfusion of peripheral tissues and then increasingly to more central tissues with resultant hypoxia and anaerobic metabolism. This leads to injury to the cellular mechanisms, particularly those of the capillary membrane. With injury, the capillary membrane becomes ''leaky'' and no longer acts in concert with Starling's hypothesis as a semipermeable membrane in an osmotically balanced milieu.[2,32] As a result of this damage, when blood flow is reestablished by restoring the lost blood volume, the leaky membrane allows fluid and oncotic particles to pass through into the surrounding interstitial tissue with a resultant loss of the fluid phase of the blood from the vascular space (Fig. 6-1). Thus the volume restoration that was assumed to have taken place by restoration of the externally lost blood is in fact *relost* into a sequestered space within the body. Persistent hypovolemia results with resumption of the vasoconstrictive responses and reversion back to the hypoperfused, hypoxic state. It is this secondary and ongoing hypoperfusion and hypoxia that lead to continuing severe tissue damage and ultimately to death.

During the early 1960s many people contributed to a better understanding of the shock state and its resuscitation,[33,39,41,42] but it was Shires[35] who showed that the dogs in the shock model of Wiggers could be resuscitated successfully by providing them with a volume of balanced saline solution in the form of Ringer's lactate equal to the volume of shed blood that was restored. With this modification of the resuscitative efforts, Shires was able to achieve almost total survival of the dogs in his experimental model.

Subsequent efforts to measure the exact volumes of the internal fluid shifts or sequestrations, the so-called third-space shifts, have generally met with little success, and it is far better to appreciate the dynamic state of these fluid shifts and concentrate on restoring adequate vascular volume as monitored by adequate urine output. Thus blood fluid volumes should be restored in volume pushes until a urine output is established and maintained. The continual falling off of urine output in the face of seemingly adequate volume restoration is an indication that internal bleeding may be taking place.

Fluids chosen for restoration of volume losses should be those likely to remain in the vascular space. The more osmotically active the fluid chosen, the more likely it is to remain in the vascular compartment. Water is at one extreme end of the spectrum, because it will move directly across the semipermeable membrane along an osmotic gradient, and most of it will end up in the interstitial space. At the other end of the spectrum is whole blood, which, with its cells and protein, provides an intravascular oncotic force that tends to keep it in the vascular space and even attracts additional fluid from the interstitial space. Colloid-containing solutions such as plasma and albumin in a balanced saline solution also provide an oncotic activity that tends to keep them in the vascular compartment. A balanced saline solution alone in the form of Ringer's lactate may be adequate for resuscitation once enough cells are provided by blood restoration to provide adequate oxygen-carrying capacity.[37] Nevertheless, in the face of severe blood loss, even balanced saline solution will have some tendency to shift into the interstitial compartment, since the loss of intravascular protein oncotic pressure will allow such a shift to take place. If adequate volumes of Ringer's lactate are provided to compensate for the shift, most patients will tolerate such a resuscitation program. Experimentally it has been shown that the volume of the balanced saline solution required for resuscitation from shock due to blood loss approximates eight times the volume of shed blood.[5] A 3:1 replacement of balanced saline solution to shed blood was not as effective as colloid-containing solutions.

On the other hand, patients with impaired pulmonary function may not tolerate the increased interstitial fluid resulting from these volume shifts. Pulmonary interstitial edema may interfere with oxygen transport across the alveolar capillary membrane. Much of this tendency for fluid to shift into the pulmonary interstitium can be countered by applying low levels of positive end expiratory pressure (PEEP) or continuous positive airway pressure (CPAP) by means of an endotracheal tube.

In no case should any solution less concentrated than Ringer's lactate be used for volume restoration. Such solutions as half normal saline, half lactated Ringer's solution, and maintenance type solutions as one-fourth or one-fifth normal saline solution have no place in volume restoration because the water component has a great inefficiency for refilling the vascular space, and huge volumes of water will shift across the membrane into the interstitial space, resulting in significant edema. In addition, flooding of the vascular space with hypotonic fluids will result in a further fall in oncotic pressure and a hypoelectrolyte state.

In summary, the plan for volume restoration should include provision of adequate whole blood to restore a reasonable part of the estimated whole blood lost. Once this is accomplished additional fluid restoration in the form of balanced saline solution should be provided so that perfusion is maintained, and this perfusion should be monitored by an ongoing measurement of the urinary output. Bolus blood and fluid administration at the rate of one fourth of the patient's blood volume will give the best means of assessing the adequacy of volume restoration. It will also provide a clue to ongoing internal hemorrhage.

Usually all solutions given should contain 5% dextrose so that minimal substrate for energy requirements is provided at the same time. This is particularly important in the small infant who may become severely hypoglycemic if continuous glucose is not provided in the intravenous fluid. However, if rapid infusion of a solution containing 5% dextrose is required, the possibility of a diuretic response to the rapid glucose load must be considered.

A word about hematocrit and hemoglobin determinations as a means of assessing volume restoration is important here. These determinations are of little use in assessing acute blood loss. If the vascular compartment is considered to be a beaker containing 40% cells, if even 90% of the volume in the beaker is emptied and the percentage of cells in the remaining 10% is assessed, it will remain 40%. Thus the initial hematocrit value tells nothing about the volume of blood shed. Since the normal vascular compartment is not a beaker but rather a physiologically active compartment in balance across a semipermeable membrane with another space containing interstitial fluid, the fall in vascular volume and resultant fall in pressure will lead to some shift of fluid from the interstitial space and intracellular space back into the vascular space. This volume shift will lower the percentage of blood cells and the hematocrit value subsequently *will* reflect the blood loss.

However, the usual problem is not to confirm initial blood loss, but rather to assess ongoing hemorrhage. If blood loss were restored exclusively with whole blood, ongoing hemorrhage might be assessable by the dilution factor provided by the interstitial fluid shift to the vascular compartment with the resultant dilution of hematocrit value. However, remembering the effects of hypoperfusion and hypoxia on the integrity of the semipermeable membrane, the fluid shifts *into* the interstitial space caused by the leaky capillary membranes would artificially raise the hematocrit value under these circumstances. On the other hand, once vascular volume is restored and adequate perfusion is indicated by an established and stable urinary output, any continued internal

blood loss would be reflected by an erosion of the baseline hematocrit value obtained at that point. Thus it is only relatively late in the course of the injury that the hematocrit value becomes a useful gauge of ongoing hemorrhage.

Once this general resuscitative effort is accomplished, a thorough assessment of specific organ injuries becomes essential, and attention will now be directed to the major injuries that occur in each organ system and to their initial stabilization.

MAJOR INJURIES AND THEIR INITIAL THERAPY

Although plastic surgeons may not often be responsible for the management of major internal organ injuries, they may be extensively involved with the patient because of external injuries. Therefore it is essential that plastic surgeons have a thorough knowledge of the types of injuries that the child is most likely to sustain from various trauma sources and be aware of the evaluation that should be undertaken and results to be looked for. Furthermore, recognition of the late presenting signs of certain internal injuries will help in recognizing when these injuries are present, especially when they were not identified on the initial evaluation. The remainder of the chapter will therefore present a system-by-system discussion of common major injuries, their initial evaluation, and pitfalls in diagnosis.

Neurologic injuries
Cranial injuries

Since blunt trauma, especially from vehicular accidents, is the major source of trauma to the child, head injuries are a common finding. Of utmost importance in the evaluation is the history of unconsciousness. If the child was always conscious, the likelihood of a serious intracranial injury is remote. Classically, subdural hematomas result in immediate and sustained loss of consciousness. Epidural hematomas are associated with a lucid interval of varying length followed by progressive unconsciousness. Intracerebral hemorrhage may be associated with immediate unconsciousness followed by a deepening level of coma.

Initial examination should establish a baseline neurologic level with a specifically described level of responsiveness, such as to normal conversation, direct commands, light stimulation, moderate pain, deep pain, and no response to any stimuli. The cranium should be carefully examined for obvious fractures, especially depressed skull fractures, and the ears and nose should be examined for signs of hemorrhage into the middle ear or leaking of cerebrospinal fluid (CSF) from the nose. A complete physical examination, including a careful neurologic examination, should then follow. Subsequent to this, the best means of evaluating an intracranial injury is the computerized tomographic (CT) examination of the skull.[23] This will indicate the presence of hematomas and mass lesions impinging on the ventricles. If CT scanning is unavailable, plain radiographs may identify a calcified corpus pineale, but this is an unusual finding in children. Consequently, if progressive neurologic dysfunction is identified, arteriography may be needed for proper evaluation in the absence of a CT scan.

Finally, if the patient is showing signs of progressive neurologic deterioration, exploratory subdural taps may be necessary through bur holes, especially if any localizing neurologic signs are identifiable.

Most commonly children sustain severe contusions of the brain or intracerebral hemorrhages, and these are not amenable to direct surgical correction. When severe intracranial injury is likely to lead to increasing intracranial pressure, the placement of a subdural bolt or other device for continuous monitoring of intracranial pressure has been a most useful adjunct to the ongoing management of these patients.[4] It has allowed a more direct measure of intracranial pressure and more intelligent management of fluids and diuretic therapy directed at minimizing increases in intracranial pressure. Obviously direct destruction of the brain by the injury is irreparable, but the secondary effects of increasing pressure and edema within a closed bony space can be offset when careful monitoring allows intelligent management of fluids and direct decompressive efforts when indicated.

Axial skeleton injuries

Concern for injuries to the spine with attendant damage to the spinal cord should begin at the time of initial first aid and should continue until injury to the axial skeleton is ruled out. Too often inappropriate therapeutic maneuvers or unthinking transport efforts will lead to spinal cord damage that was not present at the time of the initial injury. Whenever possible, an injured patient should be moved as though a vertebral injury is present. If proper immobilization is impossible at the scene of an accident, the patient should be dragged from the accident in a linear fashion so that no flexion or torsion is placed on the axial skeleton. Once in a stable environment, the head and neck should be immobilized by sandbags, and the patient should be supported on a firm support and moved without motion of the spine. Initial neurologic evaluation should identify any motor or sensory deficits, and if none are present and the possibility of a spinal fracture exists, early radiographs should be obtained to confirm or eliminate this possibility. Before moving the patient from the emergecy room and undertaking other therapeutic administrations, the surgeon must make certain that neurologic injuries have been identified and the patient is protected against additional injury due to manipulation of the axial skeleton.

The most important point in managing all neurologic injuries is initial and ongoing evaluation of the level of neurologic functioning, both cerebral and peripheral.

Thoracic injuries

The three most common injuries to the chest are fractured ribs with or without underlying pulmonary parenchymal injury, lung contusions with resulting functional deficiencies of varying amounts of pulmonary parenchyma, and lacerations leading to a pneumothorax or hemopneumothorax. Occasionally, pericardial injuries will lead to intrapericardial hemorrhage and tamponade. A screening chest radiograph should be part of the evaluation of every patient with blunt trauma even though no external signs of injury are present. Although a pneumothorax and often a hemopneumothorax become evident early in the postinjury period, severe pulmonary contusions and cardiac tamponade may develop later on in the course. The initial physical examination may be extremely unrevealing, but occasionally crepitus will reveal the presence of rib fractures, and subcutaneous emphysema will indicate the presence of underlying parenchymal injury.

Initial therapy for a pneumothorax or hemothorax should consist of the placement of a well-functioning tube thoracostomy placed to underwater seal drainage. If this does not expand the lung adequately, negative-pressure vacuum suction may be added. Additional chest tubes may be required. Ongoing concern for the possibility of pericardial tamponade must be maintained, and frequent reevaluation of vital signs and the quality of the pulse and the strength of the heart sounds is essential. The watchword here is continued observation and reevaluation for the presence of severe parenchymal contusion or pericardial tamponade with the realization that the obvious injuries such as rib fractures and hemopneumothorax will be easily identified on the chest radiographs. Additionally be aware of the probability that multiple rib fractures will lead to a flail chest with paradoxical respirations. Ongoing evaluation of pulmonary function through arterial blood gas determinations will demonstrate any evolving pulmonary insufficiency.

Blunt abdominal trauma

Blunt trauma to the abdomen usually leads to injury of the solid organs rather than the hollow viscera. Thus the liver, spleen, pancreas, and kidneys are the most likely organs to be injured. There may be no external evidence of injury. Physical examination in the conscious child usually is helpful in identifying serious intraabdominal trauma. The initial evaluation must be followed by repeated reevaluations, since these injuries often have ongoing hemorrhage. Once the child's hemodynamic state is restored to normal, careful examination of the abdomen with frequent reevaluation will usually identify the trauma. The presence or absence of bowel sounds should be noted, but this determination alone will not identify intraperitoneal hemorrhage. Usually the bowel sounds are hypoactive, but are rarely absent. The abdominal examination should not begin until a nasogastric tube has been passed into the stomach for decompression. An overdistended stomach will often lead to tenderness and guarding on direct examination. Adequate time should be taken to examine the abdomen thoroughly but gently; the abdominal examination of the child is one of the last remaining arts of medicine. Often in the younger child, examination by palpation while listening with the stethoscope will be fruitful in that the child may not realize pressure is being applied. Pressure should always be applied gently, and any resistance on the part of the child should result in relaxation on the part of the examiner. Easing up the pressure and then applying it again more slowly and gently will often allow the child to relax for a deeper evaluation of the abdomen. It is unusual to have a significant intraperitoneal injury with major hemorrhage and have a totally benign abdominal examination. On the other hand, minor to moderate amounts of hemorrhage may not be accompanied by spasm or guarding. Nevertheless, the purpose of the examination is not to identify all bleeding but only serious and continuing hemorrhage from a major organ injury. Once again reevaluation over the course of several hours is essential in the management of suspected blunt abdominal trauma.

Plain abdominal radiographs should be obtained, primarily to look for spine and pelvic fractures. A pneumoperitoneum as an indication of rupture of a hollow viscus is unusual on the initial screening films, and its absence must not be relied on to rule out significant intraabdominal injury.

The two major organs that result in severe hemorrhage are the liver and the spleen. Minor lacerations of these organs may result in initial hemorrhage, which then ceases but leaves a moderate amount of intraperitoneal blood. Such lesions usually heal without significant sequelae, and it is for this reason that we tend to discourage routine use of paracentesis in the conscious patient whose other injuries are not so serious that ongoing reevaluation of the abdomen becomes impossible. We insist on abdominal paracentesis for the child who is unconscious or has a major head injury, needs immediate anesthesia and extensive surgery for other major injuries, and has significant hypovolemic shock not readily explainable by obvious injuries. If the level of consciousness is such that the abdominal examination can be depended upon and the child will be available for ongoing reevaluation, paracentesis may be deferred and such continuous monitoring by physical examination achieved. Physical evaluation of the child can be difficult for the surgeon who has not had extensive experience in this regard. If faced with a questionable intraperitoneal injury and no readily available source of experienced consultation, the surgeon should err on the side of using paracentesis as a diagnostic aid and should unhesitatingly explore the child's abdomen if the tap is positive. This is preferable to missing a major liver laceration or intestinal tear. Routine paracentesis, on the other hand, may lead to unnecessary exploratory laparotomies and too often removal of a spleen whose degree of injury might not have necessitated removal. If physical examination is not suggestive of intraperitoneal injury, but major blood loss has occurred that is not explained by other injuries, paracentesis may confirm an intraperitoneal source for the bleeding. A liver-spleen scan can then be obtained and may indicate an injury to one or both of these organs. Although the literature supports nonoperative treatment of some splenic lacerations,[1,9] the inexperienced surgeon is probably wiser to explore the child's abdomen with the intention of dealing with the injured spleen as outlined in the subsequent discussion. If the paracentesis is positive[26] and the liver-spleen scan shows no injuries, careful evaluation of the child's abdomen by an experienced pediatric surgeon or traumatologist is required if nonoperative treatment is elected to ensure that a major vascular or intestinal injury has not been sustained. Any nonoperative treatment is acceptable only when the physical examination of the alert child's abdomen remains clearly benign and the child remains hemodynamically stable after initial volume resuscitation. Furthermore, nonoperative treatment demands continuous vigilence on the part of the surgeon in reevaluating the child's status over a period of time.

An important point to remember in this regard is the fact that a child can tolerate *recurrent* hemorrhage from a known source far better than an adult as long as proper *resuscitation* is carried out after each bleeding episode and there is no major head injury or pulmonary injury. Obviously, the effects of hypovolemia on the child's cardiocirculatory dynamics are the same as those of the adult, but the child is unlikely to sustain coronary or cerebrovascular occlusions as the result of such hypotension. Thus, although a serious hepatic or splenic injury may be missed on the initial evaluation and lead to subsequent hemorrhage, careful monitoring of the child and preparation for resuscitation from such hemorrhage will avoid any serious complications from this event. Too often children are subjected to major organ removal to prevent a potential hemorrhage that the child could have tolerated better than the removal of the organ. This is true not only in the treatment of trauma, but in the treatment of gastric hemorrhage from such events as stress gastritis and the occasional ulcers seen in childhood.[12]

The spleen is a frequently injured organ in blunt trauma in childhood, and if ongoing intraperitoneal hemorrhage is identified, an exploratory laparotomy should be performed. If the spleen is injured, partial splenectomy with splenorrhaphies is becoming more and more the preferred method of management with the realization that overwhelming postsplenectomy sepsis may occur.[36] It is possible to control splenic hemorrhage by selective ligation of hilar vessels, mattress suture control of the bleeding splenic surface, and hemostatic agents such as collagen (Avitene). If there is no bleeding at the time of exploration or if bleeding can be controlled by the previously described means, a splenectomy should not be performed simply because of the risk of subsequent hemorrhage. The carefully monitored child will tolerate such hemorrhage, and a secondary exploration and splenectomy can always be accomplished. Increasing numbers of sizable series of splenic injuries in children handled by these methods have shown a very low incidence of rebleeding.[30,34]

Lacerations of the liver may be minor or deep and major. A typical injury to the liver is avulsion of the diaphragmatic attachments. Remember that these attachments are more posterior or dorsal than usually recognized. Blunt trauma will cause the liver to be avulsed from the diaphragm, and the triangular ligament will tear major portions of hepatic parenchyma, often leading to deep stellate lacerations. These areas should be probed by finger dissection until their depth is verified and any hemorrhage controlled by suture ligation or electrocoagulation as seems appropriate. Adequate suction drainage should be provided. Major hepatic resections should be avoided if hemorrhage can be controlled by direct methods, and T-tube drainage of the child's normal small-caliber biliary duct system is not indicated.

Trauma to the pancreas and duodenum may result from blows to the epigastrium. They should be suspected in falls on bicycle handlebars and blows to the epigastrium when the child's hands slip off shovel or lawnmower handles. Although pancreatic trauma may present no initial serious findings, subsequent monitoring over the course of 2 to 3 weeks may show an evolving pseudocyst.[6] If no obvious injury is present on initial evaluation, but the wounding agent suggests a strong possibility of pancreatic injury, a baseline ultrasonogram should be obtained, and the child should be reevaluated over the next several weeks by ultrasound.

Rupture of the duodenum will usually be indicated by the presence of a pneumoperitoneum, but direct contusion of the duodenum may lead to a slowly evolving duodenal hematoma. The typical history of this injury is that of minimal findings in the first 24 to 48 hours after injury and then the development of progressive upper gastrointestinal obstruction with vomiting, usually becoming bile stained. The history of the onset of vomiting the day or so after epigastric trauma should immediately suggest the possibility of a duodenal hematoma.[19] An upper gastrointestinal tract radiographic series will show partial or complete obstruction of the distal duodenum with either "fingerprinting" or a

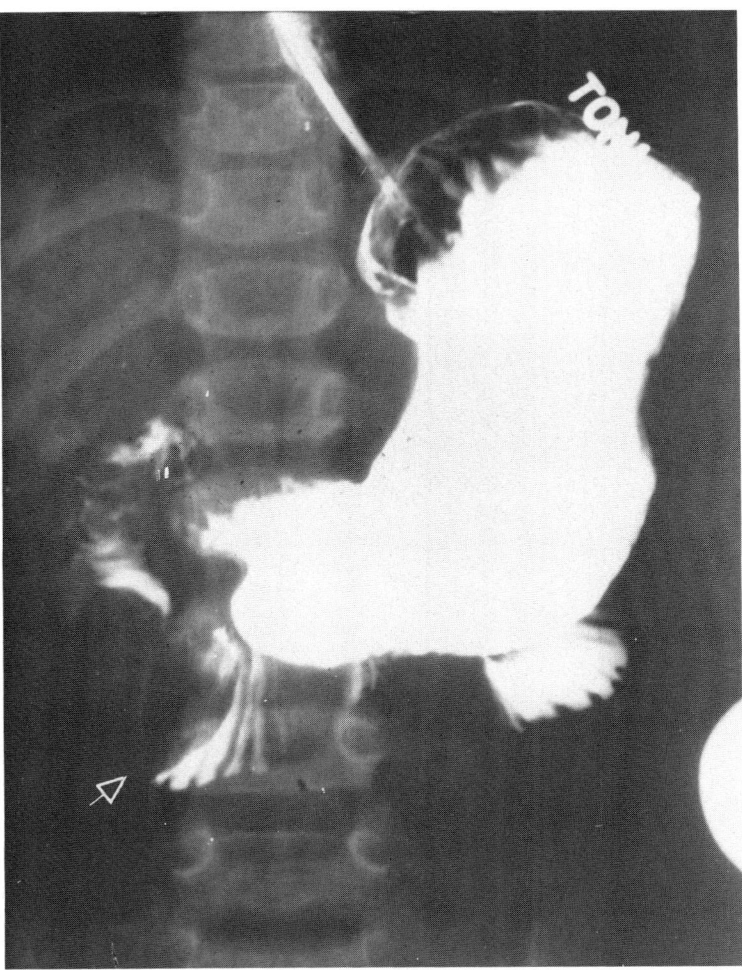

Fig. 6-8. Upper gastrointestinal tract contrast radiograph shows the typical coiled-spring obstructive appearance of a duodenal hematoma *(arrow)*. (Courtesy Donald R. Kirks, M.D., Durham, N.C.)

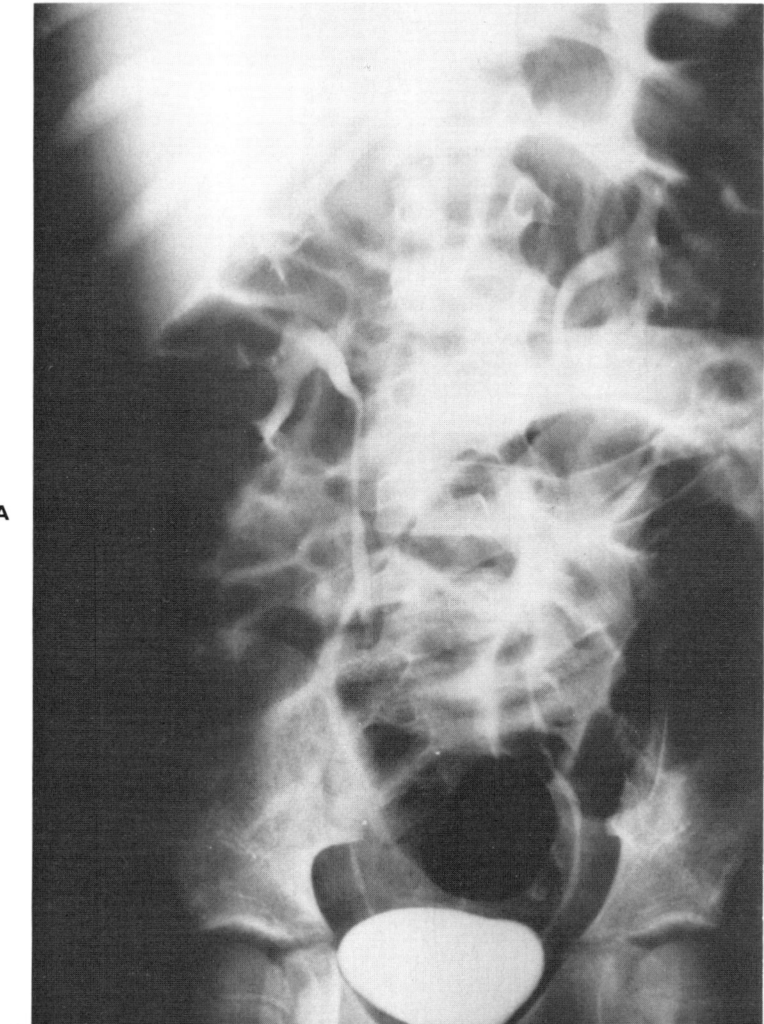

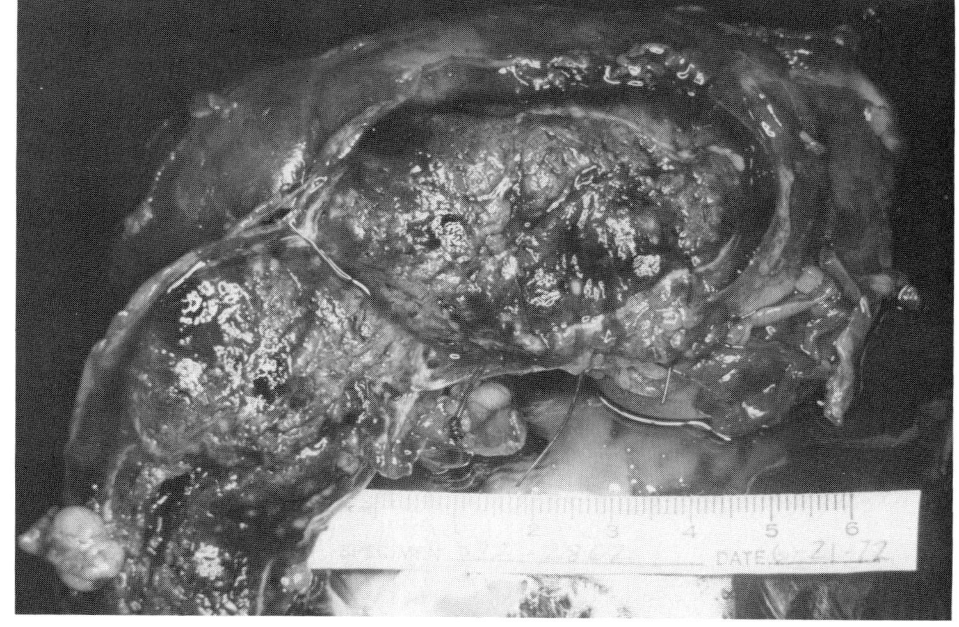

Fig. 6-9. A, Intravenous pyelogram of a child with mild trauma who was found to have a renal cell carcinoma underlying the hematoma that formed in the kidney. As is frequently the case, the intravenous pyelogram is normal except for slight disjunction of the upper pole calix on the right. **B,** The renal cell tumor occupies most of the middle portion of the kidney. A large flap of capsule has been elevated by the hematoma that resulted from mild trauma. (From Futrell, J.W., Filston, H.C., and Reid, J.D.: Cancer **41:**1565, 1978.)

"coiled-spring" effect as barium trickles through the partially obstructed lumen (Fig. 6-8). Surgery is infrequently required for this injury, since upper gastrointestinal tract decompression and volume maintenance with intravenous fluids will usually allow time for clearing the obstruction within a week.

Finally, a late sequel to pancreatic trauma may be the development of pancreatic ascites.[3] This probably results from a minor duct rupture leading to leakage and the formation of an inadequate pseudocyst with resultant dissection of the leaking pancreatic secretions through the tissue planes of the lesser omental bursa or directly into the peritoneal cavity. The posterior dissection may course up into the pleural space and appear as a pleural effusion. The presence of high amylase levels in either a pleural effusion or in ascites coming on several weeks after blunt abdominal trauma should suggest such a lesion. Albumin levels in the fluid approaching serum levels confirm the diagnosis.[31] Evaluation by endoscopic retrograde cholangiopancreatography followed by a drainage procedure usually with a Roux-en-Y jejunal limb anastomosed to the area of pancreatic leakage will correct the problem.[14]

Renal injuries resulting from blunt trauma should be suspected whenever an obvious injury to the flanks has occurred. Nevertheless, serious renal injury may result from injuries that do not leave external manifestations. Gross or microscopic hematuria may call immediate attention to the kidney, but this sign may be absent. As part of the evaluation of blunt trauma, infusion excretory urography should be performed. Serious injury will usually result in delayed or absent functioning on one side, and extravasation of contrast medium may be visible. On the other hand, significant injury may occur with minimal signs on the initial excretory urogram. If there is no function whatsoever, arteriography is indicated to rule out an avulsion of the vascular pedicle. Otherwise, most renal injuries can be observed over time, and initial exploration is rarely indicated. Earlier in this decade, interest in aggressive approaches to renal injuries flourished, resulting in more kidneys lost than with more conservative expectant treatment. The occasional late-developing hematoma or perinephric abscess can be subsequently drained. Exploration of the retroperitoneum too often leads to the finding of a severely macerated kidney that must be removed for hemostasis, whereas tamponade would have controlled hemorrhage had the kidney been left unexplored and at least part of the renal parenchyma would have been salvaged. This subject is controversial, however, and some centers prefer early exploration of renal injuries.

When renal injury is suspected or identified, ongoing evaluation of the function of the kidney is essential over the course of the next several days to weeks. Renal scans are helpful in observing the progress of the kidney and its recovery. Ultrasound may help identify fluid collections around the kidney, and the onset of fever and other signs of infection should lead to exploration of any such fluid-containing area for drainage of a perinephric abscess.

Although most renal injuries are associated with trauma severe enough to explain their occurrence, occasionally a renal injury is discovered in a patient who has seemingly minimal trauma. Since the kidney is fairly well protected by its retroperitoneal location and its covering bony cage, kidneys that are injured by seemingly minimal trauma may have either a tumor or a congenital anomaly.[24] Approximately 15% of kidneys injured by minimal trauma do have such underlying lesions (Fig. 6-9).

SOFT TISSUE INJURIES ASSOCIATED WITH MAJOR PELVIC TRAUMA

Although the urinary drainage system is rarely injured by blunt trauma, it is frequently injured in association with major pelvic fractures. The recognition of a pelvic fracture by physical examination or radiographic evaluation should lead immediately to evaluation of the urinary drainage system. A urethrogram should be obtained, and any obstruction to early flow into the bladder or extravasation should lead to urologic consultation. A catheter should then be advanced into the bladder and a cystogram obtained if possible using voiding cystourethrography. Many minor injuries to the urethra can be managed simply by catheter drainage, but experienced urologic consultation should be obtained early in the course of management of the injury.

A rectal examination also should be a part of any evaluation of major pelvic trauma, since the rectum may be lacerated by the pelvic fracture. The degree of initial displacement of the bony fragments may far exceed what is apparent on the subsequent radiograph. If palpation reveals no injury, but a significant injury is suggested, a contrast-enhanced radiograph of the rectum should be obtained. Direct injuries to the perineum should always be evaluated under anesthesia so that careful evaluation of the rectum can be accomplished. In girls vaginoscopy should be performed to ensure that no laceration between the vagina and rectum exists. Such a laceration will result in a subsequent recto-vaginal fistula. Minor lacerations that are identified in the acute situation usually can be sutured without the need for a proximal diverting colostomy, whereas few established rectovaginal fistulas will heal without such diversion.

MAJOR SKELETAL FRACTURES

All potential long bone injuries must be evaluated by careful palpation and radiographic examination. Initial management consists of adequate splinting followed by appropriate realignment and holding with either traction or casting or both. The plastic surgeon's major concern is with ongoing evaluation of neurovascular integrity. Serious injuries to the vascular supply to the extremity may occur and yet initial pulses may be present. Fractures of long bones in areas associated with injuries to vascular structures should be evaluated with arteriography if any suggestion of vascular injury exists. This is particularly true of compound fractures of the lower extremities. Subsequent to initial therapy, continuous monitoring of neurovascular integrity is essential, especially after the patient receives the cast. Edema within the solid plaster cast may lead to compression of the vascular supply with loss of perfusion and neurologic deficiency. While other injuries are being attended to, the integrity of the vascular supply to the injured extremity must be guaranteed.

PENETRATING INJURIES

The management of stab wounds is open to some debate. Some centers believe that every stab wound should be explored, whereas others individualize the treatment and use superficial explorations and sinograms to determine the depth of injury.[27] Ongoing reevaluation of any stab wound injury that is not explored is essential.

Most centers agree that all missile wounds should be explored because their tracts within the hollow cavities of the body are unpredictable.[15] Thus gunshot wounds to the neck and abdomen are usually explored, but such injuries to the thoracic cavity can be treated with tube thoracostomy and ongoing evaluation for pericardial hemorrhage. Arteriography may be necessary to evaluate potential injuries to the aorta. High-velocity missiles may cause considerable damage to structures lateral to their tracts, and the patient should be continuously monitored for late-appearing vascular injuries resulting from such lateral forces.

MONITORING FOR INJURIES SUBSEQUENT TO INITIAL EVALUATION

As noted in the previous sections, several potential injuries resulting from blunt trauma may not show themselves until late in the course. In becoming more and more involved in the reconstructive procedures, the plastic surgeon must be continually aware of the possibility of late appearances of such injuries as pulmonary contusions, pericardial tamponade, and intraabdominal hemorrhage. Reevaluation of the patient's chest by radiography before commencing surgical reconstructive procedures is essential whenever intrathoracic trauma is a strong probability. The patient's abdominal examination must be repeated over the course of several hours to days to rule out continuing hemorrhage. Obviously, continuous careful monitoring of vital signs and preparations for transfusion in the event of late-appearing serious intraabdominal injury are essential. Again it must be pointed out that children do receive serious life-threatening injuries to the intraabdominal solid organs, but if carefully resuscitated, they can tolerate the risk of a subsequent hemorrhage with the gain of possibly salvaging a nonexpendable organ.

EMOTIONAL SUPPORT OF THE INJURED CHILD

Trauma often leads to acute personality changes in the child. The medical personnel may find the child difficult to deal with, and the parents are befuddled by the change in behavior of a once cooperative, pleasant, and happy child.

Recognition of the child's view of the trauma will help in understanding the situation and lead to earlier recovery of the child's emotional equilibrium. Most children are reared to believe that traumatic events are the result of their own misbehavior. As parents we tell our children that running into the street, inappropriate activities on their bicycles, climbing on dangerous objects, and failure to wear their seat belts will lead to injury. When children then sustain an injury, they immediately believe it is the result of their own misbehavior, and their fear and anxiety over the injury are mixed with guilt over some unknown misbehavior. This often results in withdrawal and hostility and fear of punishment. Early recognition of the guilt component of the emotional upset can lead to reassurance that the accident was not of their own making or, if it was, that they are forgiven, and that love and concern for their well being are the only thoughts of their parents and the attending medical personnel. Although such reassurance will not always result in immediate change in behavior and the emotional state, recognition of this aspect of the problem will help the physician and nursing staff deal with the uncooperative and hostile activities. Explanation of these emotional factors to the parents will help them weather this period and support the child's emotional state.

Overall, children tolerate overwhelming trauma remarkably well because they have highly resilient tissues. If they are properly resuscitated with good control of the airway, adequate ventilation and oxygenation, and adequate volume replacement, they will tolerate even major injuries to organs remarkably well and recover. This is not to say that children do not sustain life-threatening or permanently disabling injuries, however. The best protection for the child is the continuing monitoring and reevaluation for serious injury with appropriate therapy. The plastic surgeon may frequently be in a position to play a role in recognizing the late appearance of such serious injuries and to help avoid complications from delay in providing appropriate therapy.

SUMMARY AND CONCLUSIONS

The leading cause of injury and mortality in the pediatric age group is blunt trauma from motor vehicle accidents sustained either as an occupant or pedestrian. One study indicates that 15 million children have some form of trauma each year in the United States.

The rapid establishment of adequate respiratory function is mandatory and involves clearing the airway; passing a nasogastric tube to prevent emesis and aspiration; establishing adequate ventilation either spontaneously, by bag-and-mask ventilation or direct endotracheal intubation; rapidly assessing ventilatory sufficiency after adequate ventilation is established; and rapidly assessing and treating any pneumothorax and direct tracheobronchial injury. The infant's airway is maintained best with the head pressed somewhat forward and the face straight ahead. Extreme extension of the head and neck is to be avoided. Once the laryngoscope is at the level of the uvula it should be pushed forward, exposing the tip of the epiglottis. No cocking or flexing of the wrist should occur because this motion tends to push up the larynx behind the base of the tongue, making it invisible. Newborns and very young infants have respiratory rates two or three times greater than those of adults or older children. Respiratory rates of 40 to 60 breaths/min are normal for this age.

A normal heart rate for the newborn in early infancy ranges between 100 and 188 beats/min. Heart rates under 100 beats/min in infants under 3 months of age should be considered bradycardia, and hypoxia due either to inadequate oxygenation or inadequate perfusion should be suspected. Blood pressure in the newborn averages between 60 to 80 mm Hg systolic. Premature infants may have normal blood pressure as low as 40 to 50 mm Hg. The normal systolic blood pressure in children can be calculated as 80 mm Hg plus twice the age in years.

The newborn has a blood volume of 8 to 8.5%. The plan for volume restoration when the patient is hypovolemic should include provision of adequate whole blood to restore a reasonable part of the estimated whole blood loss. Once this is accomplished additional fluid restoration in the form of balanced saline solution should be provided so that perfusion is maintained; perfusion should be monitored by ongoing measurement of the urinary output. Bolus blood and fluid administration at the rate of one fourth of the patient's blood volume will give the best means of assessing the adequacy of volume restoration. It will also provide a clue to ongoing internal hemorrhage.

The infant is extremely susceptible to hypothermia, which may produce profound effects on both respiratory and cardiovascular mechanisms. In the face of acute severe injury the child may not be able to maintain thermoregulatory mechanisms, and the resulting hypothermic state may depress the respiratory center and increase the degree of hypoxia. At the same time the increased vasoconstriction will lead to hypoperfusion, hypoxia, and anaerobic glycolytic mechanisms that build up acid waste products in the tissues.

Classically, a subdural hematoma results in immediate and sustained loss of consciousness. Epidural hematomas are associated with a lucid interval of varying lengths followed by progressive unconsciousness. Intracerebral hemorrhage may be associated with immediate unconsciousness followed by a deepening level of coma. When a head injury is suspected, the level of consciousness should be determined at 15-minute intervals.

Whenever possible an injured patient should be moved as though a vertebral injury is present.

The three common injuries to the chest are fractured ribs with or without underlying pulmonary parenchymal injury, lung contusions with resulting functional deficiencies of varying amounts, and lacerations leading to a pneumothorax or hemothorax. Therapy for a pneumothorax or hemothorax consists of the placement of a well-functioning tube thoracostomy attached to underwater seal drainage. Continued monitoring and reevaluation for severe parenchymal contusion or pericardial tamponade makes repeated examination mandatory.

Blunt trauma to the abdomen usually leads to injury of the solid organs rather than the hollow viscera. Abdominal paracentesis should be performed on any child who is unconscious or has a major head injury, will have to face immediate anesthesia and extensive surgery for other major injuries, and has significant hypovolemic shock not readily explainable by obvious injuries.

Children can tolerate recurrent hemorrhage from a known source far better than adults, as long as they are properly resuscitated from each bleeding episode and do not have a major head or pulmonary injury. If signs, symptoms, and studies dictate, an exploratory laparotomy is performed. Minor lacerations of the liver and spleen are best treated by selective control of bleeding, rather than by organ extirpation as in the past. Infusion excretory urography should be performed as part of the evaluation of blunt trauma. Serious injury will usually result in delayed or absent functioning on the affected side. Extravasation of the contrast medium may be visible. Most renal injuries can be observed over time, and initial exploration is rarely indicated.

The recognition of a pelvic fracture by physical examination or radiographic evaluation should lead immediately to evaluation of the urinary drainage system. A urethrogram should be obtained.

Most centers agree that all missile wounds should be explored because their tracts within the hollow cavities of the body are unpredictable. Ongoing reevaluation of any stab wound injury that is not explored is essential.

Several potential injuries resulting from blunt trauma may not appear until late in the course of the hospitalization, thus as the reconstructive procedures progress, the plastic surgeon must be continually aware of the possibility of the late appearance of such injuries as pulmonary contusions, pericardial tamponade, and intraabdominal hemorrhage.

REFERENCES

1. Aronson, D.Z., Scherz, A.W., Einhorn, A.H., et al.: Nonoperative management of splenic trauma in children: a report of six consecutive cases, Pediatrics **60**:482, 1977.
2. Baue, A.E., Wurth, M.A., Chaudry, I.H., and Sayeed, M.M.: Impairment of cell membrane transport during shock and after treatment, Ann. Surg. **178**:412, 1973.
3. Cameron, J.L., Kieffer, R.S., Anderson, W.J., and Zuidema, G.D.: Internal pancreatic fistulas: pancreatic ascites and pleural effusions, Ann. Surg. **184**:587, 1976.
4. Caniano, D.A., Nugent, S.K., Rogers, M.C., and Haller, J.A.: Intracranial pressure monitoring in the management of the pediatric trauma patient, J. Pediatr. Surg. **15**:537, 1980.
5. Cervera, A.L., and Moss, G.: Progressive hypovolemia leading to shock after continuous hemorrhage and 3:1 crystalloid replacement, Am. J. Surg. **129**:670, 1975.
6. Cooney, D.R., and Grosfeld, J.L.: Operative management of pancreatic pseudocysts in infants and children: a review of 75 cases, Ann. Surg. **182**:590, 1975.
7. Crumrine, R.S.: Postoperative hypoxia in infants and children, Int. Anesthesiol. Clin. **9**(4):83, 1971.

8. Danielson, R.A.: Differential diagnosis and treatment of oliguria in post-traumatic and postoperative patients, Surg. Clin. North Am. **55:**697, 1975.

9. Douglas, G.J., and Simpson, J.S.: The conservative management of splenic trauma, J. Pediatr. Surg. **6:**565, 1971.

10. Filston, H.C., and Grant, J.P.: A safer system for percutaneous subclavian venous catheterization in newborn infants, J. Pediatr. Surg. **14:**564, 1979.

11. Filston, H.C., and Izant, R.J., Jr.: The surgical neonate: evaluation and care, New York, 1978, Appleton-Century-Crofts.

12. Filston, H.C., Jackson, D.C., and Johnsrude, I.S.: Arteriographic embolization for control of recurrent severe gastric hemorrhage in a 10-year-old boy, J. Pediatr. Surg. **14:**276, 1979.

13. Filston, H.C., and Johnson, D.G.: Percutaneous venous cannulation in neonates and infants: a method for catheter insertion without "cutdown," Pediatrics **48:**896, 1971.

14. Filston, H.C., McLeod, M.E., Bolman, R.M., III, and Jones, R.S.: Improved management of pancreatic lesions in children aided by ERCP, J. Pediatr. Surg. **15:**121, 1980.

15. Freeark, R.J.: Penetrating wounds of the abdomen, N. Engl. J. Med. **291:**185, 1974.

16. Grosfeld, J.L., Boger, D., and Clatworthy, H.W., Jr.: Hemodynamic and manometric observations in experimental air-block syndrome, J. Pediatr. Surg. **6:**339, 1971.

17. Haller, J.A., Jr.: An overview of pediatric trauma. In Touloukian, R.J., editor: Pediatric trauma, New York, 1978, John Wiley & Sons, Inc.

18. Headings, D.L.: The Harriett Lane handbook: a manual for pediatric house officers, ed. 7, Chicago, 1975, Year Book Medical Publishers, Inc.

19. Izant, R.J., Jr., and Drucker, W.R.: Duodenal obstruction due to intramural hematoma in children, J. Trauma **4:**797, 1964.

20. Izant, R.J., Jr., and Hubay, C.A.: The annual injury of 15,000,000 children: a limited study of childhood accidental injury and death, J. Trauma **6:**65, 1966.

21. Johnson, D.G., and Jones, R.: Surgical aspects of airway management in infants and children, Surg. Clin. North Am. **56:**263, 1976.

22. Mansfield, P.B., Graham, C.B., Beckwith, J.B., et al.: Pneumopericardium and pneumomediastinum in infants and children, J. Pediatr. Surg. **8:**691, 1973.

23. McQueen, J.D.: Trauma to the central nervous system. In Randolph, J.G., Ravitch, M.M., and Welch, K.J., editors: The injured child: surgical management, Chicago, 1979, Year Book Medical Publishers, Inc.

24. Miller, R.C., Sterioff, S., Jr., Drucker, W.R., et al.: The incidental discovery of occult abdominal tumors in children following blunt abdominal trauma, J. Trauma **6:**99, 1966.

25. Morse, T.S.: Evaluation and initial management. In Touloukian, R.J., editor: Pediatric trauma, New York, 1978, John Wiley & Sons, Inc.

26. Moylan, J.A.: Office evaluation of blunt abdominal trauma, Postgrad. Med. **68:**50, Aug. 1980.

27. Nance, F.C., and Cohn, I., Jr.: Surgical judgment in the management of stab wounds of the abdomen: a retrospective and prospective analysis based on a study of 600 stabbed patients, Ann. Surg. **170:**569, 1969.

28. North Carolina Highway Safety Research Center, Reported in North Carolina Auto Club News, Raleigh, N.C., 1977.

29. Randolph, J.: Children as accident victims. In Randolph, J.G., Ravitch, M.M., Welch, K.J., et al., editors: The injured child, Chicago, 1979, Year Book Medical Publishers, Inc.

30. Ratner, M.H., Garrow, E., Valda, V., et al.: Surgical repair of the injured spleen, J. Pediatr. Surg. **12:**1019, 1977.

31. Sankaran, S., and Walt, A.J.: Pancreatic ascites: recognition and management, Arch. Surg. **111:**530, 1976.

32. Seyfer, A.E., Zajtchuk, R., Hazlett, D.R., and Mologne, L.A.: Systemic vascular performance in endotoxic shock, Surg. Gynecol. Obstet. **145:**401, 1977.

33. Share, L.: Acute reduction in extracellular fluid volume and the concentration of antidiuretic hormone in blood, Endocrinology **69:**925, 1961.

34. Sherman, N.J., and Asch, M.J.: Conservative surgery for splenic injuries, Pediatrics **61:**267, 1978.

35. Shires, T.: The role of sodium-containing solutions in the treatment of oligemic shock, Surg. Clin. North Am. **45:**365, 1965.

36. Singer, D.B.: Postsplenectomy sepsis, Perspect. Pediatr. Pathol. **1:**285, 1973.

37. Virgilio, R.W., Rice, C.L., Smith, D.E., et al.: Crystalloid vs. colloid resuscitation: Is one better? A randomized clinical study, Surgery **85:**129, 1979.

38. Wallace, W.M.: Quantitative requirements of the infant and child for water and electrolytes under varying conditions, Am. J. Clin. Pathol. **23:**1133, 1953.

39. Weil, M.H., and Shubin, H.: Diagnosis and treatment of shock, Baltimore, 1967, The Williams & Wilkins Co.

40. Wiggers, C.J.: The physiology of shock, New York, 1950, Harvard University Press.

41. Wright, H.K., and Gann, D.S.: Correction of defect in free water excretion in postoperative patients by extracellular fluid volume expansion, Ann. Surg. **158:**70, 1963.

42. Wright, H.K., Gann, D.S., and Drucker, W.R.: Current concepts of therapy for derangements of extracellular fluid. In Davis, J.H., editor: Current concepts in surgery: a clinical interpretation of basic knowledge, New York, 1965, McGraw Hill Book Co.

CHAPTER 7

Neurosurgical aspects of craniofacial trauma

ROBERT H. WILKINS

INCIDENCE OF CRANIOFACIAL TRAUMA

Accidents are the fourth most common cause of death in the United States and are the leading cause of death of individuals between 1 and 44 years of age.[23,24] Between one and two thirds of these fatal accidents involve motor vehicles. In the United States, approximately 3 million head injuries occur annually, 30,000 of them fatal.[14]

Since many head injuries, especially those occurring in vehicular accidents, involve both the face and the cranial contents, they are treated by both plastic surgeons and neurosurgeons.[3,14,17,19] Among 37,613 patients who sustained head injuries in automobile accidents and whose data were studied at the Automotive Crash Injury Research program of the Cornell Aeronautical Laboratory in Ithaca, New York, the head injury involved only external soft tissues in 61%.[14] In 86% of the head-injured patients, surgical treatment was limited to facial and cranial soft tissue repair. However, cerebral concussion occurred in 18% and brain injuries in 5%. If ejection from the automobile occurred, both the frequency and severity of head injury were increased; the case fatality rate rose from 3% to 14%.

In a series of 4465 head injuries in children under the age of 15 years who were hospitalized in Toronto, there were 270 cases of birth injury, 40 cases of extradural hematoma, 235 cases of subdural hematoma, 142 cases of brain damage, and 243 deaths (of which 121 were due to birth injuries).[9] Of these patients, 68.2% were boys and 31.8% were girls. The majority of the injuries (52.8%) were sustained in falls. Automobile accidents accounted for 31.8% (6.6% as passengers and 25.2% as pedestrians).

INITIAL CLINICAL EVALUATION

When the head-injured patient is first seen, a patent airway must be established. An unconscious patient in the supine position may have partial respiratory obstruction by the tongue, which may be relieved by manually holding the mandible forward, inserting an airway or endotracheal tube, or rolling the patient like a log into a three-quarter prone position. The attendant or physician must keep in mind that the patient also may have an injury of the cervical spine and should avoid extending, flexing, or rotating the neck. The unconscious supine patient is also likely to aspirate vomitus or blood. Aspiration should be prevented, if possible, by a position change or by the insertion of a cuffed endotracheal tube. If aspiration does occur, it should be treated appropriately.

The patient's circulatory status should be evaluated next. Except under the unusual circumstances of an infant with a large subdural hematoma or a patient in extremis, low blood pressure cannot be ascribed to intracranial injuries. If shock is present, the sources of external of internal (thorax, peritoneal cavity, retroperitoneal space, thigh) blood loss should be sought. If it is present, shock should be managed appropriately. At times the level of consciousness and degree of neurologic deficit will improve with the restitution of a normal blood pressure.

Examination of the central nervous system begins with an assessment of its coverings. The type and location of direct injuries to the scalp, face, neck, and back are noted, with a careful search of the hair-containing portions of the scalp. Scalp lacerations should be inspected and palpated, using a sterile glove, for evidence of foreign material (e.g., glass) and underlying skull fractures. These conditions are much easier to identify by inspection and palpation than by radiography.

Basilar skull fractures are ordinarily diagnosed on clinical grounds; they may be difficult to demonstrate radiographically. The presence of bilateral orbital ecchymoses (raccoon sign) may indicate a fracture of the floor of the anterior cranial fossa. Similarly, the development of an ecchymosis over the mastoid process (Battle's sign) or blood behind the tympanic membrane (hemotympanum) usually indicate a fracture of the base of the skull at the petrous pyramid. The leakage of CSF into the nose, throat, or ear also indicates a basilar skull fracture, with an additional laceration of the dura mater and arachnoid. In such cases of rhinorrhea or otorrhea the fluid can be established to be CSF (rather than tears, mucus, or saliva) is a specimen of it that has not been contaminated by blood is shown to contain an appreciable amount of glucose.

Significant craniofacial injuries may be accompanied by spinal injuries (especially involving the cervical spine), and it is imperative that the coexisting spinal lesion not be overlooked. The danger is that an undiagnosed spinal injury with no neurologic deficit might be converted to one with such a deficit while the patient is moved from one position to another during the diagnosis or treatment of craniofacial injuries; similarly, a partial spinal cord lesion might be converted to a complete lesion.

In an unconscious head-injured patient there may be clues on physical examination that the spinal cord also has been injured. The patient may not respond to pinpricks below a certain level and may have reduced or absent muscle movements and deep tendon reflexes below that level. If the lesion involves the lower cervical spinal cord the patient may lose intercostal movement and exhibit diaphragmatic breathing. Whether or not such neurologic findings are present, it is wise to obtain a lateral radiograph of the entire cervical spine in the emergency room as one of the first diagnostic studies on all patients with a significant head injury.

EVALUATION OF BRAIN FUNCTION

The neurologic examination is performed as thoroughly as feasible to establish the patient's baseline neurologic status. It is then repeated periodically to see if the patient is improving or worsening. In particular the examiner is looking for signs of increasing intracranial pressure from brain swelling or intracranial hematoma formation. Even with an uncooperative or unconscious patient, the examiner can obtain significant information about neurologic function in at least six categories:

1. Level of consciousness
2. Blood pressure and pulse
3. Pattern of respiration
4. Pupil function
5. Eye movement
6. Motor response to command or a painful stimulus

In 1974 Teasdale and Jennett of Glasgow introduced a clinical scale with which coma and impaired consciousness may be evaluated,[30] and in 1975 Jennett and Bond published a scale to assess outcome after severe brain damage.[12] These have come to be known as the Glasgow Coma Scale and the Glasgow Outcome Scale, respectively, and they are now used widely to evaluate patients with head injuries. Jennett and collaborators in Scotland, the Netherlands, and the Unit-

ed States have established a data bank in the three countries and recently analyzed in 1000 cases the relationship between clinical features of brain dysfunction in the first week after a severe head injury and outcome 6 months later.[13] They found that depth of coma, pupil reaction, eye movements, motor response pattern, and patient age are the most reliable predictors of outcome.

Pathophysiologic mechanism of craniocerebral trauma

The skull may be thought of as a rigid container with three main components: brain, blood, and CSF.[21] An increase in volume of any of the three components will increase the intracranial pressure unless it is compensated by a simultaneous reduction in volume of one or both of the other components. With head injury the bulk of the brain may increase by the development of cerebral edema, the blood component may increase by contusion or hematoma formation or by vascular engorgement secondary to loss of the normal vascular autoregulation, and the CSF may accumulate because of blockage by extravasated blood of the normal pathways of CSF reabsorption through the arachnoid granulations.[21,22] Any of these processes may be compensated initially by displacement of CSF into the spinal canal, and the intracranial pressure does not rise. However, additional units of intracranial volume have an increasingly significant effect on intracranial pressure (Fig. 7-1), and the patient's neurologic status may then deteriorate rapidly in the emergency room or during the hours after admission to the hospital.

To further complicate matters, focal increases in intracranial volume may cause cerebral herniation.[21,25,26] With a mass effect from pulped brain tissue or a hematoma affecting a portion of one cerebral hemisphere, three types of herniation may develop (Fig. 7-2). The cingulate gyrus may be herniated under the falx to the opposite side. More important, the uncus of the temporal lobe may be herniated

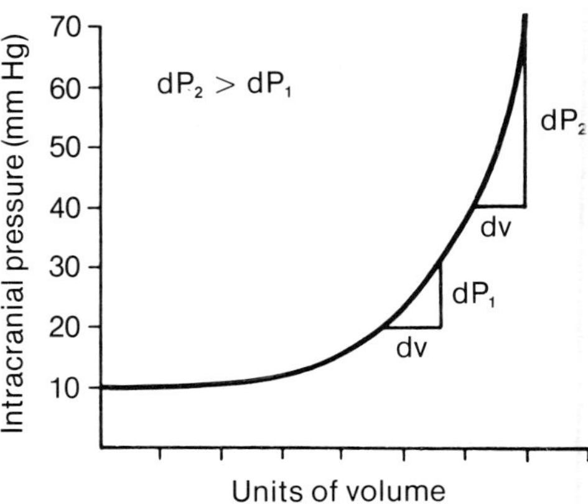

Fig. 7-1. Theoretical intracranial volume-pressure curve. As additional volume increases and intracranial pressure *(ICP)* rises, uniform increments of volume *(dv)* cause larger and larger rises of intracranial pressure *(dp)*. (From Miller, J.D.: Clin. Neurosurg. **22:**76, 1975.)

over the tentorial edge. The herniated tissue becomes wedged into the incisura like a cork in a bottle, and it exerts direct pressure against the side of the midbrain. The herniated uncus also frequently compresses the ipsilateral third cranial nerve, causing ipsilateral pupillary dilatation. Downward brainstem displacement, encountered with lesions involving one or both cerebral hemispheres, is also very important. Such brainstem displacement may cause angulation of the arteries supplying the midbrain and pons (Fig. 7-3), resulting in ischemia and then hemorrhagic infarction within these structures. Furthermore, the posterior cerebral artery on one or both sides may be drawn down against the tentorial edge, with arterial occlusion and occipital lobe infarction (Fig. 7-3). Finally, if a mass effect involves the posterior

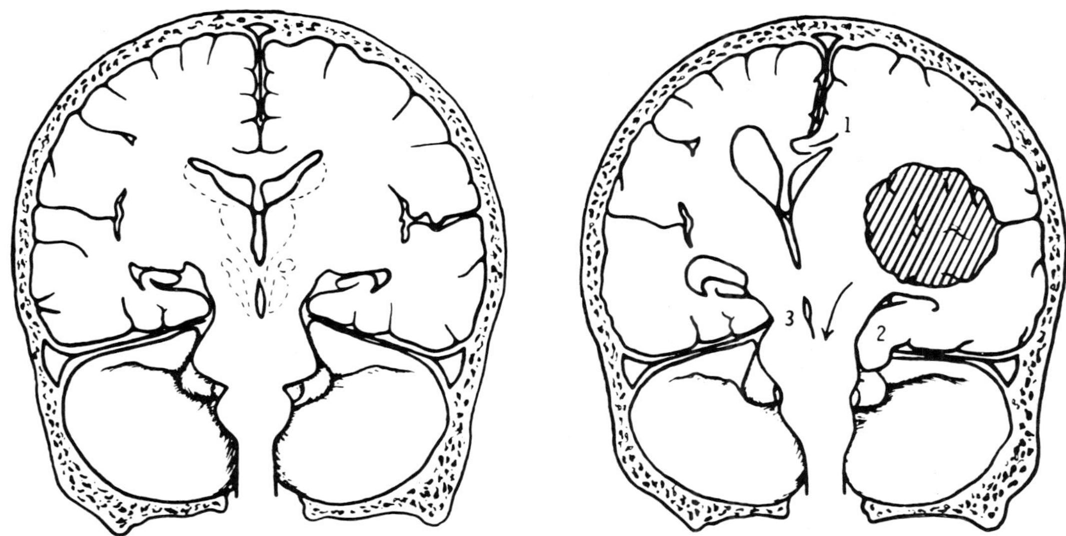

Fig. 7-2. Intracranial shifts with supratentorial lesions: *1*, herniation of the cingulate gyrus under the falx; *2*, herniation of the uncus of the temporal lobe into the tentorial incisura against the midbrain; *3*, downward displacement of the brainstem. (From Plum, F., and Posner, J.B.: The diagnosis of stupor and coma, Philadelphia, 1966, F.A. Davis Co.)

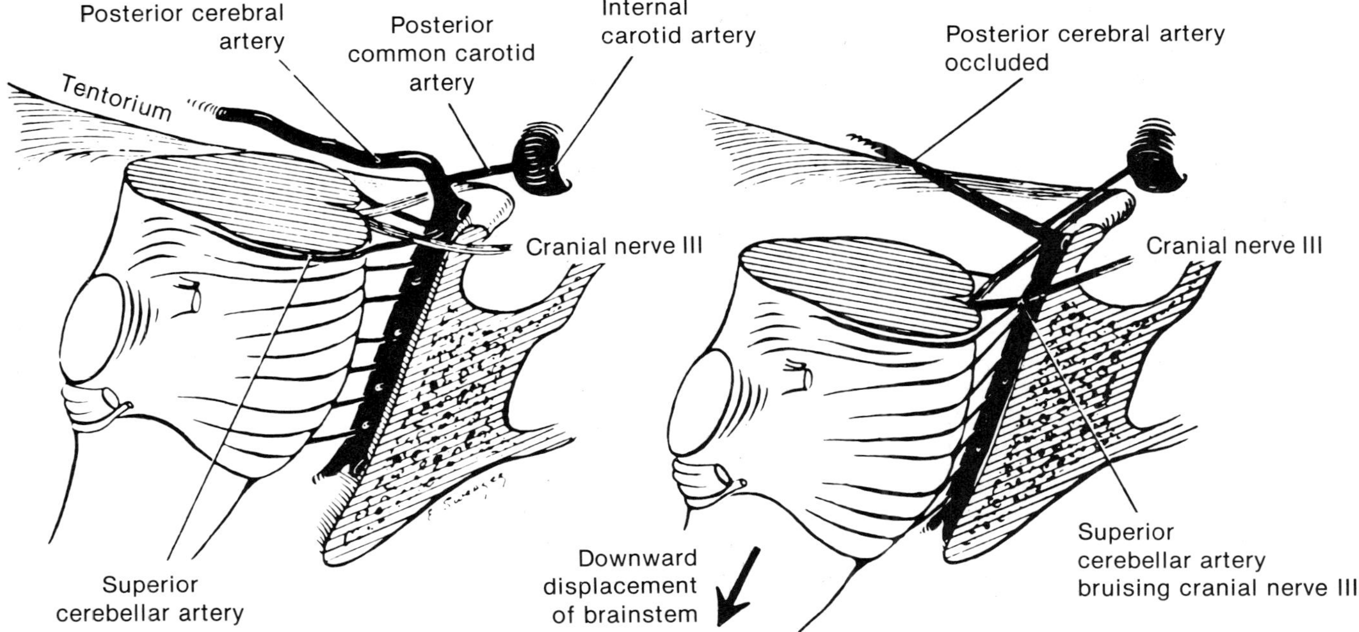

Fig. 7-3. Downward displacement of the brainstem, with stretching of the posterior cerebral arteries and branches of the basilar artery. (From Howell, D.A.: Brain **82:**524, 1959.)

cranial fossa, the cerebellar tonsil on one or both sides may herniate into the foramen magnum, becoming impacted against the medulla oblongata and compromising its vital functions.

The skull of a child is somewhat different from that of an adult. In the newborn the cranial bones are pliable, and they may indent like a Ping-Pong ball rather than actually fracturing in response to a localized blow. In addition, the cranial bones of a newborn have not yet fused together, and the unfused bones of the cranial vault may separate in the infant in response to an increase in intracranial volume. Under these circumstances there may be no major increase in intracranial pressure. For example, one of the main signs of a chronic subdural hematoma in a child is progressive head enlargement. The tension of the anterior fontanelle can be used as a rough index of intracranial pressure in a young infant; this fontanelle may remain open until 18 months of age. To monitor the intracranial pressure accurately in a patient of any age, however, the surgeon must insert an extradural, subdural, subarachnoid, or intraventricular pressure monitoring device.[22]

In regard to head injuries some other important empiric differences also exist. Compared with adults, children with head injuries have a higher incidence of diffuse cerebral swelling, a lower incidence of mass lesions (pulped brain, hematoma), and a lower mortality.[2,5] In one series of 53 children with severe head injuries, 34% developed diffuse cerebral swelling and 23% had mass lesions.[5] In three series composed of adults and children the mortality ranged from 49% to 52%.[5] In five pediatric series, in contrast, the mortality varied between 22% and 38%; in a sixth pediatric series the mortality was only 6%.[5] These data suggest that the pathophysiologic response of the child's brain to injury is different from that of the mature brain. However, the mechanisms and reasons for the differences are not yet well understood.

Clinical signs of craniocerebral trauma

When a head injury develops into a progressive generalized increase in intracranial pressure, the patient may experience a stepwise rostrocaudal loss of brain function.[25,26] If a focal lesion is also present, a focal deficit such as a hemiparesis or a dilated pupil (partial third cranial nerve palsy) may be superimposed on that basic pattern.

Of the various clinical parameters used to monitor a patient with a head injury, the most important is the patient's level of consciousness. As the intracranial pressure mounts and brain function deteriorates, the patient becomes restless and confused, lethargic, stuporous, and finally comatose. The level of consciousness is a sensitive indicator of cerebral function, and a reduction in consciousness usually implies immediate cerebral dysfunction from concussion or cerebral contusions or delayed dysfunction from brain swelling or intracranial hematoma formation. However, a decreasing level of consciousness also may be the result of other factors

that should not be overlooked. These include any process that impedes oxygenation of the blood (e.g., upper airway obstruction, pneumothorax, hemothorax), any process that interferes with cerebral perfusion (e.g., shock, traumatic carotid artery occlusion, fat emboli), and any process that interferes with cerebral metabolism (e.g., acidosis, traumatic diabetes insipidus).

Another sign of increasing intracranial pressure is the Cushing phenomenon, so named because it was studied in animals by Harvey Cushing at the turn of the century. This response consists of elevation of the systolic and diastolic blood pressures, widening of the pulse pressure, and bradycardia. When these changes begin, especially if they are accompanied by progressive lethargy, they should be viewed as early warnings of impending disaster and should prompt the responsible physician to take a more aggressive approach to diagnosis and therapy.

As rostrocaudal deterioration of neurologic function begins (early diencephalic stage), the Cheyne-Stokes respiratory pattern may appear, as may increased resistance to passive limb motion, bilateral Babinski's reflexes, and the doll's head–eye phenomenon. The doll's head–eye phenomenon is elicited as follows. The examiner holds the patient's eyelids open and rotates the head briskly from side to side or up and down. A positive response is transient conjugate eye deviation in the direction opposite that of the head movement. The doll's head–eye phenomenon is a brainstem reflex that is normally suppressed by cortical influences; it appears when cortical function is diminished but brainstem function has not yet been altered.

In the late diencephalic stage the patient also may develop decorticate posturing in response to painful stimulus. The upper limbs are flexed at the elbows and the trunk and lower limbs are extended.

At the midbrain–upper pons level of rostrocaudal neurologic deterioration, rapid regular breathing (central neurogenic hyperventilation) may replace Cheyne-Stokes respirations. The pupils become fixed to light and the doll's head–eye phenomenon is lost. The patient exhibits decerebrate posturing in response to a painful stimulus. The trunk and all four limbs are forcefully extended.

In the final stage of lower pontine–upper medullary function the patient is flaccid and unresponsive to stimuli, respirations are irregular, and the pupils often dilate widely.

When unilateral uncal herniation occurs from a focal lesion (e.g., an epidural hematoma in the temporal region), one of the first signs may be ipsilateral pupillary dilatation from direct compression of the third nerve by the herniating uncus. This is an alarming sign, because rapid neurologic deterioration frequently ensues.

The changes encountered in the early diencephalic stage are reversible with appropriate treatment. The early changes of uncal herniation also are reversible, but this usually requires surgical removal of the impacted uncus, in addition to removal of the initiating mass lesion (e.g., pulped temporal tip, epidural hematoma). Once the patient develops decorticate or decerebrate posturing or fixed pupils, recovery is doubtful, especially in an adult. These facts underscore the importance of repeated assessment of neurologic function in the head-injured patient and the *early* detection of deterioration, when something can still be done to correct it.

Because of the importance of the level of consciousness and pupillary responses in assessing patients with head injuries, such patients should not be given narcotic or hypnotic medications or mydriatic agents. The head-injured patient who is agitated and combative should be restrained; paraldehyde or chlordiazepoxide (Librium) may be given for mild sedation. Hypertension after a head injury is usually a response to increased intracranial pressure. The elevated blood pressure may be needed to maintain brain perfusion. Treatment should be directed toward lowering the intracranial pressure. If the systemic blood pressure is lowered before this is done, cerebral ischemia or infarction may result.

DIAGNOSTIC STUDIES

After the history has been obtained and the physical examination accomplished, certain diagnostic studies should be performed to allow as specific a diagnosis as possible. In part the performance of these studies depends on the patient's condition, which dictates the amount of time available for testing.

If the patient is in extremis in the emergency room, it may be worthwhile to rapidly drill a hole through the skull in the frontal area on each side with a twist drill or trephine to evacuate as much as possible of any extradural or subdural hematoma present and to deflate the lateral ventricles.[28] This maneuver may permit the diagnosis of any extradural or subdural hematoma. More important, twist-drill ventriculostomy, plus hyperventilation and the administration of a hyperosmotic agent such as mannitol or a diuretic such as furosemide, may result in enough clinical improvement to allow additional diagnostic steps (e.g., a CT brain scan) or definitive surgical treatment (e.g., a craniectomy or craniotomy in the operating room). The administration of adrenal steroids will probably not help in this situation. Although steroids are effective in reducing the cerebral edema that accompanies certain brain tumors, this type of medication, even in large doses, has no proven beneficial effect on traumatic brain swelling.

In a situation that is not so critical, plain radiographs of the skull and entire cervical spine of the head-injured patient should be obtained in the emergency room. These may reveal fractured or dislocated bones, intracranial air, or foreign bodies. However, plain radiographs of the skull do not provide the neurosurgeon with as much information as does the CT scan. This safe and noninvasive study shows blood, CSF, and brain tissue, in addition to the bones of the skull. It will reveal the position, size, and configuration of intracranial hematomas and the cerebral ventricles (Figs. 7-4 and 7-5). CT has replaced carotid arteriography as the most helpful test for acute assessment of head injuries. The latter test is now used only when a vascular lesion is suspected (e.g., traumatic carotid thrombosis, traumatic cerebral aneurysm).

In a recent study of 100 patients with an acute head injury, generalized cerebral swelling and subarachnoid hemorrhage

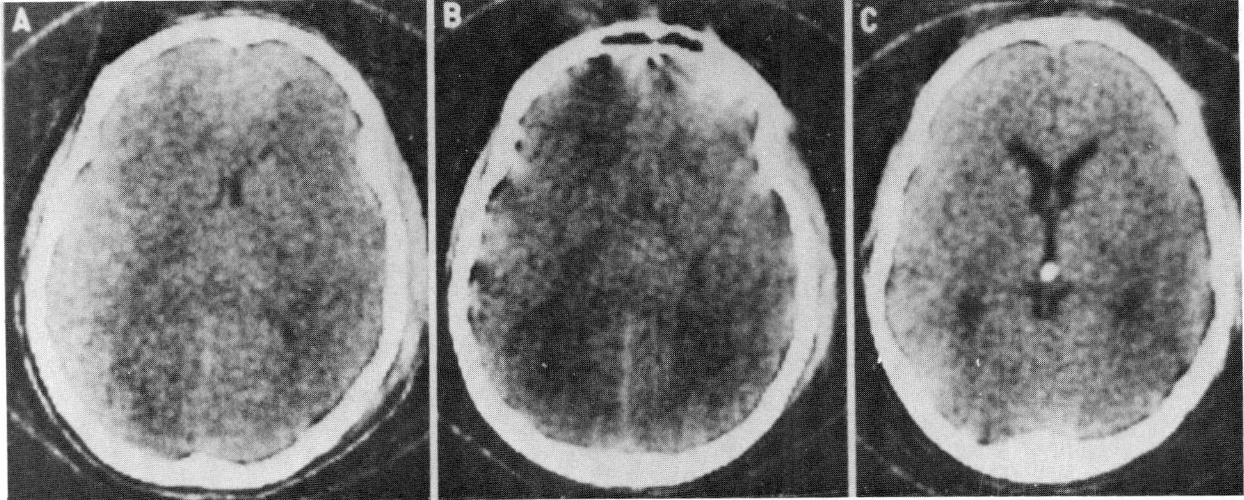

Fig. 7-4. Serial CT scans of an obtunded 17-year-old boy injured in an auto accident, showing hyperemic generalized swelling progressing to iatrogenic hyponatremic edema, with subsequent return to normal. *A,* On day 1 small ventricles, slightly increased brain density, and a scalp hematoma are present. *B,* On day 5 scan shows obliterated ventricles, decreased brain density, and a scalp hematoma. *C,* On day 24 scan shows normal ventricles, cisterns, and subarachnoid spaces. (From Zimmerman, R.A., Bilaniuk, L.T., Bruce, D., et al.: Radiology **126:**403, 1978.)

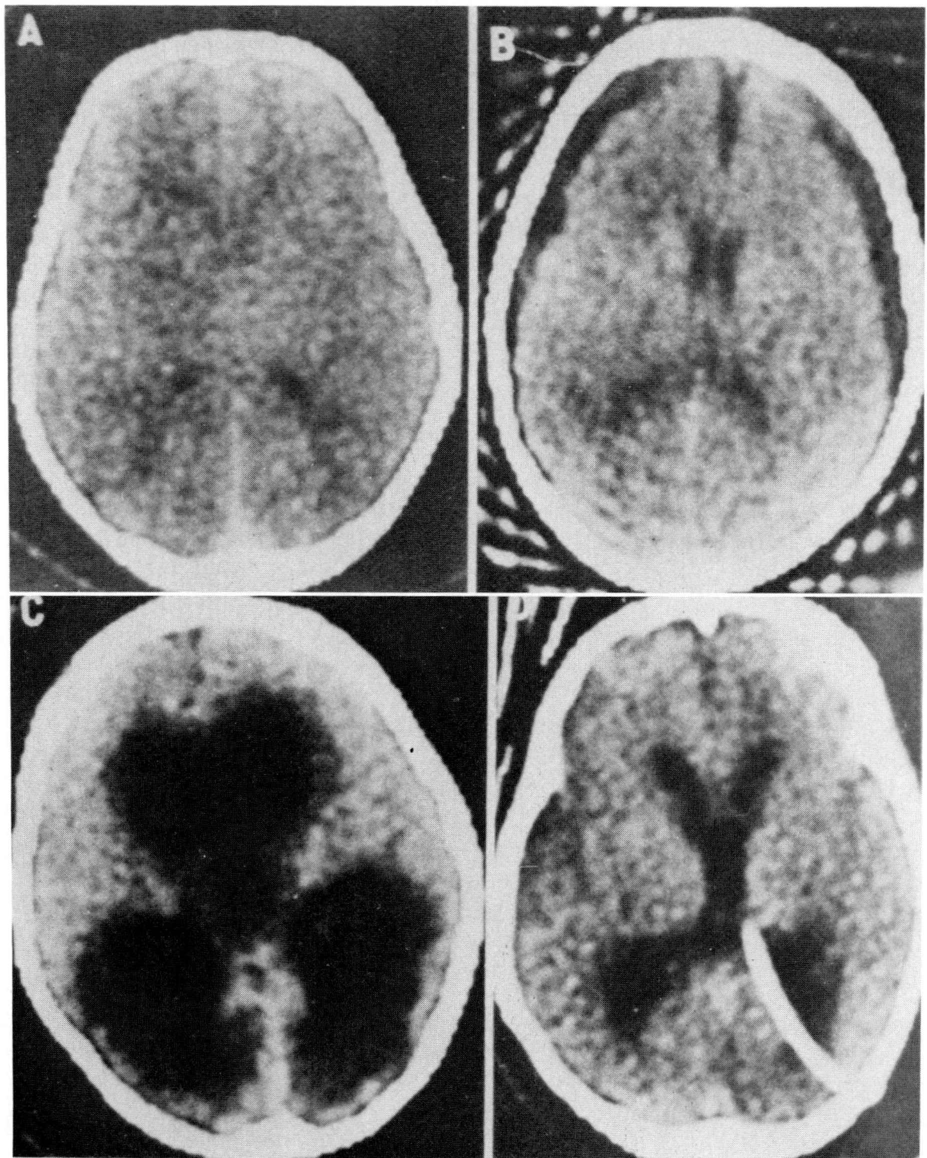

Fig. 7-5. Serical CT scans of a 3-year-old boy who was struck by a car and rendered unconscious, showing acute generalized cerebral swelling followed by subdural hygroma formation and then hydrocephalus. *A,* On day 2 scan shows obliteration of the ventricles and subarachnoid spaces and slightly increased brain density. *B,* On day 27 scan shows bilateral extracerebral collections of CSF density. *C,* On day 43 scan shows significant enlargement of the lateral ventricles. *D,* On day 219 the hydrocephalus has been treated with a shunt, and the ventricles are smaller, although not back to normal, suggesting some underlying brain damage. (From Zimmerman, R.A., Bilaniuk, L.T., Bruce, D., et al.: Radiology **126:**403, 1978.)

were the most common findings on CT.[33] The cerebral swelling was demonstrated on the CT scans as obliteration or compression of the lateral and third ventricles and the perimesencephalic cisterns (Figs. 7-4 and 7-5).

Radioisotope encephalography (radionuclide brain scan) or cisternography, electroencephalography (EEG), pneumoventriculography, and pneumoencephalography are of little value in evaluating craniocerebral injuries acutely, but one or more of these studies may be helpful in evaluating certain patients days to years after the injury.

During the acute stage after a head injury, lumbar puncture is of no help and may be dangerous if cerebral or cerebellar herniation is developing. Bloody CSF indicates that a significant injury has occurred, but it does not define the nature of the injury. Clear CSF provides no comfort because blood may still be present in the cranial subarachnoid space or within the brain. Normal CSF pressure may not reflect the actual intracranial pressure if uncal or tonsillar herniation has blocked free CSF communication through the incisura or foramen magnum. In fact, if such a herniation or downward brainstem displacement is present, it may be intensified by a lumbar puncture that reduces CSF pressure below the herniation (either by removal of fluid during the puncture or gradual leakage into the epidural space after the needle is removed).

Any child who is seen with a significant head injury may be the victim of child abuse.[3,11] Unless the cause of the injury is obvious, child abuse must be suspected. Under these circumstances there may be physical or radiologic evidence of fresh or old injuries to other parts of the body.

DEFINITIVE TREATMENT

Virtually any type of injury (e.g., abrasion, contusion, laceration) can occur at any level (e.g., scale, skull, dura, brain), but specific combinations occur preferentially. Some of the more common types of injury will be included in this discussion.

In general, the same basic guidelines of treating injuries elsewhere in the body also apply to the craniocerebral area. Yet there are a few important differences. Because of the convex configuration of the calvaria, it may be difficult to mobilize the scalp to directly close a traumatic defect having even a small amount of tissue loss; a rotation flap or some similar maneuver may be required. Wounds that breach the scalp, skull, and meninges must be closed to avoid meningitis and brain herniation. Finally, many antibiotics are irritating to the cerebral cortex and may cause seizures if they are applied directly to the brain (e.g., antibiotic irrigation of contaminated penetrating wounds). An antibiotic used commonly for irrigation of contaminated areas, without untoward effects, is bacitracin.

The patient with both craniocerebral trauma and injuries to the face or other parts of the body requires special consideration. If general anesthesia is used for repair of the extracranial injury, valuable parameters for monitoring brain function are lost, usually for a period of hours. Furthermore, the intracranial pressure may rise in response to the events surrounding the induction of anesthesia and the anesthetic agent used. Any remaining parameters, such as blood pressure and pulse, take on increased importance, and the physicians involved must keep in mind that the patient may be developing detrimental intracranial changes during the operation. If the craniocerebral injury also requires surgical treatment, this can be done before or simultaneously with the extracranial operation, using the same anesthetic.

Scalp injuries

Hematomas within or beneath (subgaleal) the scalp, or beneath the outer periosteum of one of the cranial bones (cephalohematoma) will reabsorb spontaneously. They do not usually require treatment. They should not be drained because of the risk of infection. A hematoma within the scalp may have a soft center and a firm edge; on palpation it may seem that a depressed skull fracture is present.

A scalp laceration should be dealt with after the scalp has been shaved around the laceration (the exception is the eyebrow, which is not shaved because of the resulting cosmetic defect). The laceration is inspected and palpated with a gloved finger to determine the extent of the injury and to detect any foreign bodies. It is cleansed and debrided, but with care taken to retain all viable tissue. It is then closed without buried sutures or a drain, both of which might promote wound infection.

If a portion of the scalp has been avulsed, the exposed skull should be covered, preferably with a full-thickness skin graft. This can be accomplished by various types of flaps, including a free flap of the avulsed scalp or a free flap from a donor site. Such a free flap is surgically attached by arterial and venous anastomoses involving one or more of the superficial temporal and occipital vessels.

Injuries to the skull and dura mater

Linear skull fractures develop and spring open at the moment of impact and then immediately snap shut. If the edges spring apart more than 2 or 3 mm, the dura mater adherent to the inner surface of the skull may be torn. In children this may permit gradual herniation of the arachnoid or brain, with or without cyst formation, between the bone edges. Such a process results in gradual enlargement of the fracture ("growing fracture of childhood").[31] If the scalp is lacerated at the same instant the skull is fractured, dirt, hair, and other debris may be trapped within the fracture as the bone edges snap shut. Linear skull fractures generally do not require surgical treatment. However, if it is suspected that contaminated material is trapped within the fracture line, this material should be removed via a narrow linear cranectomy along the fracture line. Similarly, if a linear fracture is demonstrated by inspection or by radiology to be more than 3 mm or so in width (implying that it was spread apart even farther at the moment of impact), it should be inspected surgically to repair any underlying dural laceration. With an open wound, dural closure will decrease the possibility of meningitis, and with either an open or closed wound it will prevent arachnoidal herniation and fracture enlargement.

If trauma results in a basilar skull fracture with laceration of the dura and arachnoid membrane, CSF rhinorrhea or otorrhea may result.[6] CSF rhinorrhea involves the escape of the CSF through the ethmoidal, sphenoidal, or frontal sinuses on one or both sides. A coexisting LeFort II or III facial fracture may be present. The nasal leakage causes the patient to frequently blow the nose, forcing air and bacteria into the cranial subarachnoid space. Air may even be forced into the brain substance (pneumocephalus) and ventricular system. CSF otorrhea implies leakage through the mastoid air cells, middle ear, or external auditory canal. The paranasal sinuses and mastoid air cells develop and enlarge during childhood; in infancy they have not yet begun to form or are still quite small. CSF rhinorrhea and otorrhea are rare in infants and unusual in children.

The management of CSF rhinorrhea or otorrhea begins with the demonstration of the nature and site of fluid leakage. If possible, the escaping fluid is collected and tested for its glucose content. Under normal circumstances the CSF glucose level is 45 to 70 mg/100 ml in adults and 70 to 90 mg/100 ml in children under 10 years of age. This amount of glucose establishes the fluid as CSF rather than tears, mucus, or saliva. The base of the skull in the appropriate area is studied by tomography to demonstrate the fracture, and the actual path of the leakage can sometimes be visualized by radioisotope cisternography or by the subarachnoid injection of a water-soluble contrast agent combined with CT scanning of the skull base. During radioisotope cisternography for CSF rhinorrhea, intranasal pledgets are usually placed near the openings of the paranasal sinuses on each side. Later they are removed and analyzed for radioactivity. In this way the site of the leak can usually be lateralized and roughly localized in an anteroposterior direction. Prophylactic antibiotics do not appear to prevent meningitis in patients with CSF rhinorrhea or otorrhea.[10,15] If the leakage does not stop spontaneously within a few days, the dural defect should be repaired surgically.

If the head injury results in a depressed skull fracture rather than a linear fracture, it ordinarily should be repaired surgically. The "Ping-Pong ball" indentations that occur before,[1] during, or shortly after birth will sometimes correct themselves spontaneously or can be elevated by suction, such as with a breast pump.[28] Otherwise depressed fractures should be treated surgically to remove pressure on the underlying cortex (and perhaps prevent subsequent gliosis) and to close any dural lacerations caused by the sharp edges of the fractured bone, not only for the reasons mentioned previously but also to prevent outward cerebral herniation through torn meninges, fractured bone, and lacerated scalp. A depressed fracture over one of the large dural venous sinuses should be elevated cautiously, with adequate exposure on all sides because the surgeon may have to quickly control vigorous bleeding from a previously tamponaded tear in the wall of the sinus. When a depressed fracture in any location is exposed surgically, the bone fragments are temporarily removed while the dura and brain are inspected, but they usually are cleansed and replaced in a more normal position, either at the same procedure or a later operation.[16] A less suitable alternative for closure of the skull defect in a child is an immediate or delayed cranioplasty with a plastic or metallic plate. The younger the child, the more likely is a bony defect to fill in with new bone formation from the dura mater, outer periosteum, and bone edges. Thus eventual bony restitution is to be expected in an infant and a cranioplasty is usually not necessary.

Extradural hematoma

Extradural hematomas are rare in infants and unusual in children.[8] Typically an extradural (epidural) hematoma occurs as a result of a tear in the middle meningeal artery that is sustained along with a linear fracture in the squamous portion of the temporal bone. This arterial blood collects outside the dura mater in the temporal area and may lead to ipsilateral uncal herniation, progressive neurologic decline, and death during the hours after the injury. However, more gradual arterial or venous bleeding may occur in association with fractures in the temporal region or elsewhere, and less acute extradural hematomas are occasionally encountered, especially in the frontal or suboccipital area. When a child sustains an extradural hematoma, it is more likely to be of this insidious type. The key to the management of an extradural hematoma is early diagnosis, before neurologic decline is far advanced. Treatment involves surgical evacuation of the hematoma through a craniotomy or craniectomy, with occlusion of the source or sources of bleeding. Any uncal herniation also must be treated, usually by surgical removal of the uncus from the tentorial incisura.

Subdural hematoma

In contrast to the extradural hematoma, the subdural hematoma is usually the result of venous bleeding. Typically the source of bleeding is one or more of the veins that bridge from the cerebral cortex to one of the major dural venous sinuses, especially the superior sagittal sinus. When the head is struck a blow from the front or back, the skull moves first and the brain follows. Similarly, at the end of the arch of movement the skull stops before the brain does. With such differential movement one or more veins may rupture on one or both sides of the sagittal midline (about 20% of patients with subdural hematomas have bilateral accumulations). The venous blood gradually accumulates in the subdural space, between the dura mater and the arachnoid membrane. After approximately 10 to 14 days membranes form over the outer and inner surfaces of the hematoma. The inner membrane is delicate and relatively avascular, but the outer membrane is thicker and contains numerous vessels that may be the source of additional bleeding, which leads to enlargement of the hematoma.

The acute subdural hematoma (<24 hours after injury) is usually discovered because a patient with a severe brain injury is being examined. The subdural hematoma may be adding little to the overall picture and its evacuation may not cause appreciable improvement. The high mortality (>50%) associated with acute subdural hematomas is mainly the result of the associated injuries to the brain.

The subacute subdural hematoma tends to have a consistency like currant jelly. Ordinarily a craniotomy or craniectomy is required to permit evacuation of the clotted blood.

A subdural hematoma is termed chronic after its investing membranes have become visible some 10 to 14 days after the injury. The central portion of a subdural hematoma is liquid, and the fluid can be removed by aspiration.[4,18] In an infant with open sutures such aspirations may be carried out on a daily basis through the coronal suture with a needle and syringe. If this does not result in a cure within 2 weeks, or if the patient is an older child without split sutures, some other procedure such as trephination, a craniectomy, or a craniotomy is required for evaluation of the hematoma. A temporary external drain or a permanent subdural-peritoneal shunt may also be required to permit gradual reexpansion of the brain. If such reexpansion is prohibited by the subdural membranes, these should be opened or removed. Occasionally a more radical revision of the calvaria is justified to correct the discrepancy between the size of the brain and the size of the skull, which became enlarged because of the underlying subdural hematoma(s).[27]

If the arachnoid membrane is breached at the time of injury, CSF may enter the subdural space, either alone (subdural hygroma) or in association with blood. Blood, either fresh or clotted, and CSF are easily demonstrated by the CT scan. However, if these are mixed, or if the blood is in the process of liquefying, the fluid may become isodense in relation to the brain and escape detection by CT scanning.

Traumatic subarachnoid hemorrhage

Subarachnoid hemorrhage is common in association with significant head injuries. The blood is ordinarily absorbed, and no active treatment is necessary. It is not unusual for the CSF absorptive pathways to be temporarily occluded by the subarachnoid blood, causing transient hydrocephalus. However, occasionally the hydrocephalus persists and requires a later CSF shunting operation.

Cerebral concussion

Cerebral concussion is a clinical diagnosis that refers to the transient loss of brain function (especially consciousness) after a head injury, with rapid and complete recovery except usually for some degree of amnesia. Cerebral concussion requires no treatment. However, cerebral concussion or cerebral contusions may be followed by a postconcussion or postcontusion syndrome that lasts up to several months and is characterized by irritability, dizziness, headaches, and other vague complaints. This ordinarily will resolve spontaneously, but the patient may require symptomatic therapy and reassurance.

Cerebral contusions

Cerebral contusions most frequently occur in the inferior portions of the frontal lobes and the tips of the temporal lobes. Contusions that occur immediately beneath the point of impact are referred to as *coup contusions,* and those on the opposite side of the brain are called *contrecoup contusions.* Physical disruption of the cerebral tissue and the

formation of cerebral edema frequently occur in the injured area, in addition to small hemorrhages.

If cerebral contusions are mild they will heal without treatment. However, if the involved portion of the brain is pulped to the degree that it causes an increase in intracranial pressure, various maneuvers may be necessary to reduce the pressure, such as the removal of ventricular CSF, institution of mechanical hyperventilation, or administration of a hyperosmotic agent, (e.g., mannitol, urea, glycerol), diuretic (e.g., furosemide), or barbiturate (e.g., thiopental, pentobarbital, secobarbital.)[2,3,5,22] If these techniques are not successful in controlling the pressure, and brain herniation is a threat, it may be beneficial to surgically excise the pulped portion of the brain (e.g., temporal tip).

Posttraumatic epilepsy

When the cerebrum is injured, with resulting physical disruption, hemorrhage, edema, or infarction, seizures may result. The occurrence of posttraumatic epilepsy is influenced by a number of factors, such as the type of injury, severity of injury, neurologic status, location of brain damage, and the occurrence of complications or early seizures. Those conditions believed to increase the possibility of posttraumatic epilepsy are a missile wound or dural penetration, loss of consciousness or posttraumatic amnesia of greater than 1 hour, skull fracture, persisting EEG abnormality, hemiparesis or aphasia, brain injury in the centroparietal area, intracranial hemorrhage or infection, and seizures during the first week after the injury.[7]

Prevention of posttraumatic epilepsy includes debridement of grossly damaged brain tissue and closure of dural defects. Prophylactic anticonvulsant drugs are seldom indicated except in high-risk patients.[32] However, if a seizure does occur after a head injury, appropriate anticonvulsant therapy should be given, and the other measures ordinarily used in the diagnosis and treatment of epilepsy should be employed as indicated.

Intracerebral hematoma

Traumatic intracerebral hematomas may be small or large, single or multiple, and immediate or delayed in onset. A patient with a large accessible hematoma may be helped occasionally by surgical evacuation of the hematoma, either by direct mechanical removal of the clot through a craniotomy or craniectomy or by stereotactic aspiration through a bur hole, using a suction device containing a rotating center similar to Archimedes' screw.

Secondary brainstem hemorrhages are commonly found at autopsy in patients dying of craniocerebral injuries. However, these are not a direct effect of trauma, but result from the brain herniations that develop in association with a unilateral or bilateral increase in supratentorial pressure. Although their exact pathophysiologic mechanism is debated, they correlate with the clinical signs of irreversible brainstem dysfunction discussed in the previous section concerning increased intracranial pressure and cerebral herniation.

Penetrating wounds of the brain

The skull of a child is not as thick or rigid as the skull of an adult, and it can be penetrated with less force; an object can easily penetrate the skull through the orbit. Penetration of the orbit by a wooden object such as a stick or pencil is especially dangerous.[20] If any of the wood is left behind when the object is removed, an intracranial abscess is likely to develop. Of 42 cases of periorbital traversing puncture wounds by sharp wooden objects reviewed by Miller et al.,[20] permanent neurologic sequelae occurred in 74%, many after an apparent trivial initial wounding. Furthermore, 25% of 28 patients treated in the antibiotic era died.

A penetrating object that is still in place when the child is brought to the emergency room should not be removed until appropriate diagnostic studies have been rapidly made. The preoperative preparations have been completed, the child has been anesthetized and is in the operating room, and the pertinent portion of the child's head has been shaved, cleansed, and draped. In this way, any resulting bleeding can be controlled and the wound can be treated definitively. With penetrating wounds of this type or with missile wounds, a craniotomy or craniectomy must be performed and the tract must be debrided down as far as the contamination to avoid subsequent meningitis or a brain abscess. The usual rule of thumb is to debride until all of the bone fragments have been removed. Low-velocity pellets also should be removed, if feasible, because they too may be contaminated. Then the dura and scalp are closed as barriers against infection from without and cerebral herniation from within.

SUMMARY AND CONCLUSIONS

Craniocerebral injuries are common among young people and are often accompanied by injuries to the face and other parts of the body. In an acute injury an airway must be established and the patient's circulation maintained. Examination of the head and neck may reveal direct and indirect evidence of cranial trauma.

Of more importance than external examination of the head is the evaluation of brain function through at least six parameters: level of consciousness, blood pressure and pulse, pattern of respiration, pupil function, eye movement, and motor response to command or pain. The examiner uses these parameters not only to assess immediate neurologic function, but also to determine whether the patient is improving, remaining the same, or worsening. Neurologic deterioration may occur as a stepwise rostrocaudal loss of brain function based on increasing intracranial pressure and one or more types of brain herniation. It is vital to the patient's outcome that such deterioration be detected early and that appropriate steps be taken to reverse the detrimental process if possible.

Compared with adults, children with head injuries have a higher incidence of diffuse cerebral swelling, a lower incidence of mass lesions, and a lower mortality. Since the cranial bones of the infant are not yet fused, the head may enlarge in response to brain swelling or to the development of an intracranial hematoma, thus minimizing the increase in intracranial pressure that otherwise would result. In infants a depressed skull fracture may occur as an indentation rather than being fragmented like the more rigid cranial bones of the older child or adult; it can sometimes be managed by nonsurgical measures. A wide linear skull fracture in a child may lead to herniation of the arachnoid membrane or brain between the bone edges, with or without cyst formation, leading to enlargement of the fracture. CSF rhinorrhea or otorrhea caused by basilar skull fractures are unusual in children because the paranasal sinuses and mastoid air cells have not yet developed fully.

Any child with a significant head injury may be a battered child. Unless the cause of the injury is obvious, child abuse must be a consideration.

Various diagnostic tests should be performed in the evaluation of the head-injured child. Of these, the CT brain scan is the single most helpful test. Treatment, of course, differs depending on the nature of the injury. The more common approaches to specific lesions have been discussed.

With present methods of management, the outlook for head-injured children is significantly better than it was just a decade ago. Children can recover from reduced levels of neurologic function that are deemed hopeless in the adult. The results obtained certainly justify an aggressive approach to the diagnosis and treatment of craniocerebral injuries in children.

REFERENCES

1. Alexander, E., Jr., and Davis, C.H., Jr.: Intrauterine fracture of the infant's skull, J. Neurosurg. **30**:446, 1969.
2. Becker, D.P., Miller, J.D., Ward, J.D., et al.: The outcome from severe head injury with early diagnosis and intensive management, J. Neurosurg. **47**:491, 1977.
3. Bell, W.E., and McCormick, W.F.: Increased intracranial pressure in children: diagnosis and treatment, ed. 2, Philadelphia, 1978, W.B. Saunders Co.
4. Blaauw, G.: Subdural effusions in infancy and childhood. In Vinken, P.J., Bruyn, G.W., and Braakman, R., editors: Handbook of clinical neurology, vol. 24, Injuries of the brain and skull, Amsterdam, 1975, North-Holland Publishing Co.
5. Bruce, D.A., Schutt, L., Bruno, L.A., et al.: Outcome following severe head injuries in children, J. Neurosurg. **48**:679, 1978.
6. Caldicott, W.J.H., North, J.B., and Simpson, D.A.: Traumatic cerebrospinal fluid fistulas in children, J. Neurosurg. **38**:1, 1973.
7. Feeney, D.M., and Walker, A.E.: A prediction of posttraumatic epilepsy: a mathematical approach, Arch. Neurol. **36**:8, 1979.
8. Hawkes, C.D., and Ogle, W.S.: Atypical features of epidural hematoma in infants, children, and adolescents, J. Neurosurg. **19**:971, 1962.
9. Hendrick, E.B., Harwood-Nash, D.C.F., and Hudson, A.R.: Head injuries in children: a survey of 4465 consecutive cases at the Hospital for Sick Children, Toronto, Canada, Clin. Neurosurg. **11**:46, 1964.
10. Ignelzi, R.J., and VanderArk, G.D.: Analysis of the treatment of basilar skull fractures with and without antibiotics, J. Neurosurg. **43**:721, 1975.
11. James, H.E., and Schut, L.: The neurosurgeon and the battered child, Surg. Neurol. **2**:415, 1974.

12. Jennett, B., and Bond, M.: Assessment of outcome after severe brain damage: a practical scale, Lancet **1**:480, 1975.
13. Jennett, B., Teasdale, G., Braakman, R., et al.: Prognosis of patients with severe head injury, Neurosurgery **4**:283, 1979.
14. Kihlberg, J.K.: Head injury in automobile accidents. In Caveness, W.F., and Walker, A.E., editors: Heat injury: conference proceedings, Philadelphia, 1966, J.B. Lippincott Co.
15. Klastersky, J., Sadeghi, M., and Brihaye, J.: Antimicrobial prophylaxis in patients with rhinorrhea or otorrhea: a double-blind study, Surg. Neurol. **6**:111, 1976.
16. Kriss, F.C., Taren, J.A., and Kahn, E.A.: Primary repair of compound skull fractures by replacement of bone fragments, J. Neurosurg. **30**:698, 1969.
17. Matson, D.D.: Neurosurgery on infancy and childhood, Springfield, Ill., 1969, Charles C Thomas, Publisher.
18. McLaurin, R.L., Issacs, E., and Lewis, H.P.: Results of nonoperative treatment in 15 cases of infantile subdural hematoma, J. Neurosurg. **34**:753, 1971.
19. Mealey, J., Jr.: Pediatric head injuries, Springfield, Ill., 1968, Charles C Thomas, Publisher.
20. Miller, C.F., II, Brodkey, J.S., and Colombi, B.J.: The danger of intracranial wood, Surg. Neurol. **7**:95, 1977.
21. Miller, J.D.: Volume and pressure in the craniospinal axis, Clin. Neurosurg. **22**:76, 1975.
22. Miller, J.D., Becker, D.P., Ward, J.D., et al.: Significance of intracranial hypertension in severe head injury, J. Neurosurg. **47**:503, 1977.
23. National Center for Health Statistics, Public Health Service, U.S. Department of Health, Education, and Welfare: Advance report, final mortality statistics, 1977, Monthly Vital Stat. Rep. Suppl. **28**(1):21, 1979.
24. National Center for Health Statistics, Public Health Service, U.S. Department of Health, Education and Welfare: Vital statistics of the United States: 1975, vol. 2, Mortality, Washington, D.C., 1979, U.S. Government Printing Office.
25. Plum, F., and Posner, J.B.: The diagnosis of stupor and coma, ed. 1, Philadelphia, 1966, F.A. Davis Co.
26. Plum, F., and Posner, J.B.: The diagnosis of stupor and coma, ed. 2, Philadelphia, 1972, F.A. Davis Co.
27. Porta, M., Rougerie, J., George, B., and Anquez, L.: Surgical treatment of chronic subdural hematomas in infants, Surg. Neurol. **11**:107, 1979.
28. Rand, B.O., Ward, A.A., Jr., and White, L.E., Jr.: The use of the twise drill to evaluate head trauma, J. Neurosurg. **25**:410, 1966.
29. Saunders, B.S., Lazoritz, S., McArtor, R.D., et al.: Depressed skull fracture in the neonate: report of the cases, J. Neurosurg. **50**:512, 1979.
30. Teasdale, G., and Jennett, B.: Assessment of coma and impaired consciousness: a practical scale, Lancet **2**:81, 1974.
31. Thompson, J.B., Mason, T.H., Haines, G.L., and Cassidy, R.J.: Surgical management of diastatic linear skull fractures in infants, J. Neurosurg. **39**:493, 1973.
32. Wohns, R.N.W., and Wyler, A.R.: Prophylactic phenytoin in severe head injuries, J. Neurosurg. **51**:507, 1979.
33. Zimmerman, R.A., Bilaniuk, L.T., Bruce, D., et al.: Computed tomography of pediatric head trauma: acute general cerebral swelling, Radiology **126**:403, 1978.

CHAPTER 8

Resuscitation and early management of the acutely burned child

JOSEPH A. MOYLAN

Major thermal injury is one of the significant challenges that faces the surgeon dealing with traumatized children. Of the 2½ million patients who require treatment for burn injuries in this country annually, more than half are pediatric patients. Hospital and medical costs for the treatment of this dreaded accident exceed a billion dollars annually. Surface burns are the third leading cause of accidental death and one of the primary causes of death in young patients in the United States. Recent advancements in burn care have significantly reduced the mortality but have imposed obligations for effective and long-term reconstructive programs for these unfortunate individuals. Properly and effectively treated after a thermal injury, these individuals can return to fully productive lives.

PATHOPHYSIOLOGIC MECHANISMS

The basic mechanism of injury with thermal trauma is partial or complete destruction of the cell membrane by increased temperature. The depth of the injury is proportional to the intensity, as well as duration, of the heat. It has been estimated that contact with a heat source above 170° F (82° C) for as little as 1 second will produce a full-thickness skin injury. The extent of the burn size is proportional to the total surface area in contact with the heat source.[12]

The two parameters used to determine the magnitude of the burn injury are size and depth. The size of the burn injury is determined by measuring the percentage of body surface damaged. The rule of nines is a convenient way to calculate this parameter. However, it should be remembered that an infant's head and neck area represents 21% of the body surface (Fig. 8-1). This proportion of body surface gradually decreases until about 12 years of age when the head and neck areas are comparable to the adult, or 9%.

The leg area is proportionally less and increases in size in reverse relationship with the head and neck area. A convenient way to measure irregular burns is to remember that the palmar surface of the hand represents approximately 1% of the body surface. Use of a standard burn diagram in sketching out each injured area of the body is the most accurate way to determine the extent of the burn.

Historically, the terms first, second, and third degree have been used to describe the depth of the burn. The first-degree burn involves just the epidermis and is initially seen as an erythematous, nonblistered insult to the surface of the skin, such as a sunburn. A second-degree burn extends down but not through the dermis. Initially it is erythematous, blistered, acutely swollen, and extremely painful, since both the capillaries and the nerve endings are preserved in the depth of the dermis (Fig. 8-2). A third-degree burn is an injury through the dermis into the subcutaneous tissue and is initially pale, dry, charred, and also anesthetic because the capillaries and nerve endings are completely destroyed at the time of the initial insult. More recently these historic terms have been abandoned and the terms *partial thickness* for second-degree burns and *full thickness* for a third-degree injury are clinically used.

Although the cause of the thermal injury may be helpful in determining the depth of the burn (e.g., spill scalds cause partial-thickness injury and immersion scalds cause full-thickness injury), these criteria have been consistently unreliable, particularly in small children because of the relative thinness of their skin.[7]

DISPOSITION AND TRIAGE OF THE BURN PATIENT

Decisions regarding the initial disposition and transfer to a major burn center, if indicated, are based on the serious-

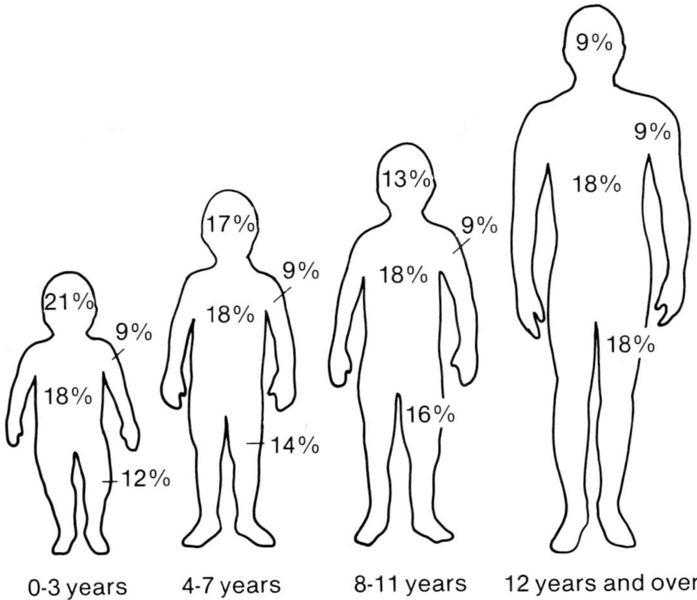

Fig. 8-1. ''Rule of nines'' for calculating the magnitude of the burn injury. Note that the infant's head and neck area represents 21% of the body surface. This area decreases proportionately until age 12 and older when the head and neck area account for 9% of the total body surface area.

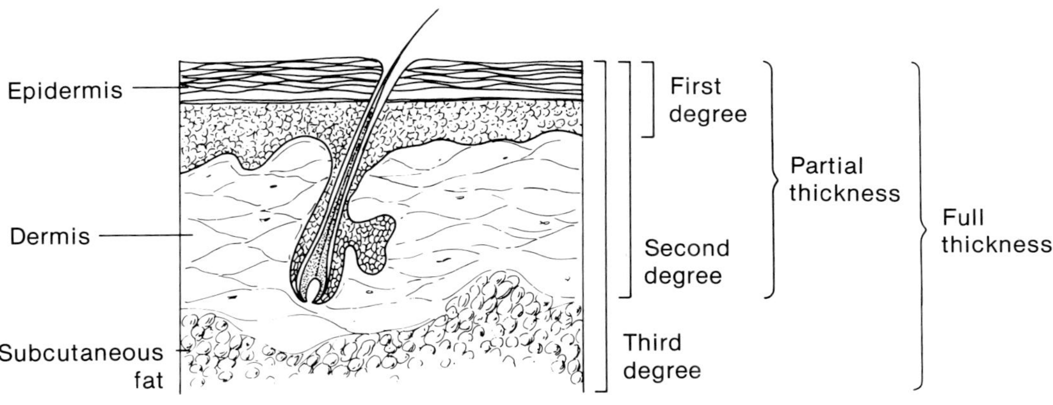

Fig. 8-2. Sagittal section of skin. Note that the relative depth of the burn injury determines whether or not regeneration is possible from residual epidermal elements.

ness of the burn injury. Burns have been classified as major, moderate, and minor based primarily on the size and depth of the injury in addition to the presence of any other injuries (Table 8-1). Minor burns in children include second-degree burns less than 10% of the total body surface and a full-thickness burn of less than 2%. These burns usually can be treated without hospitalization, and care can be instituted in the office or outpatient facility. Caution should be maintained with minor burns in children of less than 2 years of age, since a gastrointestinal ileus may develop, requiring short-term hospitalization. Moderate burns that require hospitalization include second-degree burns between 10% and 25% of the total body surface and third-degree burns measuring less than 10%. Burns of this magnitude usually can be treated effectively in the community hospital, provided that interested and experienced health professionals, including a surgeon, are available. Major burns include partial-thickness injuries involving more than 25% of the total body surface, third-degree burns involving more than 10%, and full- and partial-thickness injuries involving the face, hands, or genitalia where significant morbidity may arise if adequate treatment is not provided. In addition, burns complicated by respiratory tract injury, fractures, or extensive soft tissue injuries also are categorized as major burns. Burn patients in this category should be either treated initially or when stabilized at an institute with a designated burn service.

Table 8-1. Triage of burn injuries

Type	Depth	Percentage of total body surface (%)	Location of treatment
Minor	Partial thickness	<10	Outpatient
	Full thickness	<2	
Moderate	Partial thickness	10 to 25	Community hospital
	Full thickness	<10	
Major	Partial thickness	>25	Burn center
	Full thickness	>10	

EMERGENT THERAPY

The initial care of the burn patient is directed toward calculating the magnitude of the injury, providing initial stabilization, and diagnosing any early complications that resulted from the thermal accident itself. This initial treatment directly influences survival and functional recovery. A rapid, organized examination to determine the severity of injury includes assessment of the airway, location of associated injuries, and initial estimate of the extent and depth of the burn.

Small burns that are generally treated on an outpatient basis comprise about 95% of all burns seen in the United States. Generally these are superficial, first or second degree, and rarely exceed more than 10% of the total body surface. Initial treatment is directed toward relieving pain, cleansing the wound, debriding all loosely adherent tissue, administering a tetanus vaccine, and dressing the wound.

Pain and anxiety can be initially treated with an intramuscularly injected narcotic based on the age and weight of the pediatric patient. In children orally induced analgesia is often not effective because the initial treatment is somewhat painful, especially washing and debriding. Frequently, a cold towel to the burn parts will provide some pain relief. After the wound has been gently washed with a bland soap and rinsed, loose necrotic epithelium is carefully debrided. Soap containing alcohol (such as Hibiclens) should be avoided, since it may significantly not only increase the pain but also damage the injured tissue area. For very small burns, such as those less than 8 cm in diameter, it may be beneficial to leave the blister, since it provides some additional cover for the underlying epithelium and partial-thickness injury. For larger wounds, the blister should be broken and the protein-rich fluid evacuated since it provides an excellent medium for bacterial growth. Once the wound has been washed and debrided, placement of a greased gauze and a sterile bulky dressing will not only protect the wound but provide some additional pain relief. It is frequently necessary to use a large bulky dressing because small burn injuries may drain large volumes of serum, and small dressings may act as a wick for infection.

Tetanus prophylaxis is important to a patient with burn injuries. The tetanus toxoid booster should be given to any patient who has not had a booster in the last 5 years. Those persons not previously immunized should be given 250 units of tetanus immune globulin-human (Hyper-Tet) and the first dose of an active immunization series.

Once the initial treatment has been provided on an outpatient basis, an intermediate-strength oral analgesic should be prescribed for the first 2 or 3 days, although once the burn wound is covered with an occlusive dressing, the patient usually remains fairly comfortable. Early follow-up is important, particularly with burns from 8% to 10% of the total body surface. These children should be seen approximately 3 days after initial treatment at which time the bulky dressing should be removed down to the level of the greased gauze. If there is no evidence of infected discharge, a bulky dressing can be replaced and the patient evaluated again 5 days after the burn. Usually by this time the greased gauze dressing can be removed and the wound exposed to the air. Topical antibiotics are rarely indicated in the outpatient treatment of burns. Only those patients with a depressed immune response to infection such as patients with diabetes, leukemia, and those receiving cancer chemotherapy benefit from a topical treatment. Since the risk of infection is minimal in all other groups of patients, neither systemic nor topical antibiotics should be used because they predispose opportunistic infections from bacteria, yeast, or fungus.

MODERATE AND MAJOR BURNS
Replacement therapy

Burns covering more than 15% of the total body surface in children require initial fluid replacement by the intravenous route. The mortality in the first 48 hours has been vastly improved with the advent of effective shock replacement formulas. Many methods can be safely used in resuscitation provided that close attention is paid to the individual clinical response to these fluid administration programs.

Pathophysiology mechanism of burn shock

Immediate response to exposure to a thermal injury includes a significant increase in capillary permeability.[3] This permeability occurs not only in the damaged area itself but throughout the body and appears to be biphasic in that there is an initial rapid loss of plasma lasting minutes, then a slower prolonged capillary leak lasting in many instances more than 24 hours.[4]

Since there is selective loss primarily of plasma, the hematocrit level rises rapidly during this time due to red cell concentration. Since few red cells are lost initially, blood transfusions are rarely required during the first few days after injury. Because of the continued loss of fluid from the intravascular to the extravascular spaces, resuscitation is directed at replacing both the initial and continued losses until capillary permeability reverses to normal. Circulatory recovery usually occurs some time at 24 hours, but may be delayed as long as 36 hours. Even with reversal of the capillary leak, intravascular volume does not return to nor-

Table 8-2. Fluid resuscitation

Type of solution	Sodium concentration (mEq)	Volume/24 hours
Hypotonic	130 or less	4 ml times percentage of total body surface times kilogram
Isotonic	150 or less	3 ml times percentage of total body surface times kilogram
Hypertonic	300 or less	Maintain adequate urine output

mal until 72 hours in many instances, despite a hyperdynamic cardiovascular state as evidenced in increased cardiac output, an elevated metabolic rate, and mild hypertension.

Alterations in potassium balance also may occur during the initial resuscitation.[1] Careful monitoring of the serum potassium level is important because both mild hyperkalemia and hypokalemia can occur. Potassium losses are significantly exaggerated with the diuresis that begins at approximately 48 hours. It is frequently necessary to replace up to 200 mEq of potassium each day in children during this time.

Replacement formulas

A variety of approaches to fluid replacement have been effective as long as careful attention is paid to the individual patient response. These formulas provide an initial plan for estimating the amount of fluid that will be necessary for resuscitation. However, underresponse or overresponse to the fluid administration necessitates alteration in any formula. Failure to reverse hypotension or maintain an adequate urine output indicates the need for more fluid than the formula would estimate. Rapid return of vital signs with excessive urine outputs above 2 ml/kg/hr in a child indicates excessive fluid administration and requires some decrease in the volume of fluid administered.

Both clinical and experimental work has shown that colloid solutions such as plasma, plasmanate, and plasma expanders are frequently not necessary for effective resuscitation. Most current formulas, with the exception of the Brook formula, use primarily electrolyte solutions as either hypotonic, isotonic, or hypertonic sodium replacement (Table 8-2).

The Parkland formula

The Parkland formula is an outgrowth of initial work by Dr. Carl Moyer, suggesting that the sodium ion is the important element in burn resuscitation. Modification of this formula at the Parkland Hospital in Dallas standardized the approach.[2] The Parkland formula provides 4 ml of Ringer's lactate per kilogram for each percentage of the burn and uses no colloid- or electrolyte-free water during the first 24 hours. Usually 50% of the total calculated amount is administered in the first 8 hours after the injury and the remaining 50% in the subsequent 16 hours. In the second 24

hours, as capillary integrity is restored, no saline solution is used, and the functional volume is maintained with saline-free water, as well as colloid replacement, especially in children. Ordinarily in the second 24 hours, at least 1 unit of plasmanate or its equivalent in saline-poor albumin is administered. In burns that cover over 50% of the total body surface more colloid may be indicated.

Hypertonic lactated saline resuscitation

This formula uses a concentrated sodium chloride and sodium lactate solution providing a 300 mEq sodium solution.[6] The solution is administered at a constant rate, enough to maintain an hourly urine output at 0.5 to 0.75 ml/kg/hr. Advocates of the resuscitative technique state that this formula is valuable in preventing excessive edema formation peripherally, as well as pulmonary edema, and it is an important adjunct in treating children who have limited cardiopulmonary reserve. However, the margin of safety using this formula appears somewhat limited, especially with those physicians who have not had extensive experience. Significant hypernatremia may develop. If the serum sodium exceeds 160 mEq, serious seizure complications may develop in children.

Isotonic resuscitation

An isotonic solution providing 150 mEq/L of sodium is used at our institution.[11] This solution is formulated by adding half an ampule of sodium bicarbonate to each liter of Ringer's lactate. The solution is administered at a rate of 3 ml/kg for each percent of body surface burn. This formula has many significant benefits, including minimal edema formation, both in the burn and nonburn areas, a low incidence of pulmonary edema, a minimal ileus, an early diuresis, and a smaller net positive sodium balance. The only limitation of the formula is that infants with a burn less than 25% of total body surface usually require more fluid than the formula estimates.

Monitoring the resuscitation

Careful monitoring, both clinically and by laboratory parameters, is essential no matter what resuscitative formula is employed. Clinical signs include a clear mentation, normal blood pressure for age, and a pulse of good quality. Tachycardia is a normal response of burn injury even with adequate resuscitation; however, if this is coupled with a weak thready pulse, alteration in the fluid resuscitation is indicated. An indwelling Foley catheter is essential for monitoring significant burn injuries that require intravenous fluid administration. Urine output should be maintained at 0.5 to 0.75 ml/kg/hr. Ineffective urinary output is usually secondary to inadequate fluid replacement. With a low urine output, the volume of administered fluids each hour should be increased until an effective response can be obtained. Diuretics should be used only as a last resort, since they invalidate the urine output as a prime method of monitoring.

Usually changes in intravenous fluid replacement are not instituted until there has been a significant alteration in urine volume output for at least a period of 2 hours. Under these circumstances, the rate of fluid administration may be increased or decreased according to an inverse relationship with urine production.

Measurement of the arterial pH level and oxygen concentration is another important monitor for resuscitation. A low pH level is usually due to inadequate or delayed resuscitation resulting in metabolic acidosis. This change of pH level usually responds to augmentation in the volume replacement. A low PaO_2 may result from either inadequate resuscitation or pulmonary injury.

Central venous pressure monitoring is usually unnecessary during the initial resuscitation and may be hazardous if its limitation is not realized. With adequate resuscitation central venous pressure measurements during the initial 24-hour period are low, usually 0 to $+2$, since with increased capillary permeability the catheter is actually measuring more than the intravascular space. However, if an effective resuscitation cannot be obtained after a significant fluid replacement, central venous pressure measurements may be valuable, especially when high, in diagnosing excessive volume replacement and cardiac failure. With cardiac failure due to excessive fluid administration, the use of a diuretic or digitalis may be indicated. Again it should be emphasized that both of these agents are indicated only rarely in pediatric patients and that most resuscitation problems are related to inadequate fluid replacement and not myocardial failure.

With all resuscitation programs, further saline administration is not usually necessary after a 24-hour period. Most now encourage the use of plasma or plasmanate in children after 24 hours to maintain an adequate osmotic pressure. It should be pointed out that use of albumin, particularly in the first 12 postburn hours, has been associated with some complications, such as acute renal failure, probably due to protein deposition in the basement membrane of the kidney. However, after 24 hours there appears to be little risk of this complication. Salt-free fluids are usually administered to meet both the daily metabolic requirements and the evaporative water loss. A variety of formulas for daily metabolic needs of children have been suggested and are outlined in Chapter 5. Daily evaporative water losses vary from 0.5 to 1.5 ml/kg/day for each percent of burn. Monitoring serum electrolytes and daily weights provides an additional gauge to evaluate evaporative water losses and their replacement. Once ileus abets after the burn injury, most intravenous lines can be discontinued and all fluids replaced either orally or by enteral feeding.

EARLY POSTBURN COMPLICATIONS
Inhalation injury

An inhalation injury is a severe chemical tracheobronchitis produced by the inhaling of incomplete products of combustion. It is frequently incurred by patients who were trapped in fires in a closed space, in a blast accident, or exposed to noxious gases produced by burning plastics. The classic clinical signs of inhalation injury include wheezing, production of carbonaceous sputum, hoarseness, bronchorrhea, and shortness of breath. However, these clinical signs are frequently delayed 24 to 48 hours after the injury. Recent improvement in the diagnosis of inhalation injury has been associated with reduction in mortality and morbidity. With the use of fiberoptic bronchoscopy as part of the initial evaluation process, those patients with inhalation injuries can be identified before clinical complications develop.[8] Bronchoscopic criteria of inhalation injury include mucosal edema, erythema, and ulceration within the airway.

The levels of inhalation injury are upper airway injury involving the larynx, major airway injury involving the tracheobronchial tree, and parenchymal injuries involving the alveolar membrane. The two levels of inhalation injury, upper and major airway injury, can be diagnosed by fiberoptic bronchoscopy. Parenchymal injuries, which are extremely rare, are associated with immediate respiratory distress, hypoxia, and a pulmonary infiltrate on radiologic examination. Patients with major and upper airway injuries often have normal blood gases initially and normal chest radiographs on admission.

Complications from inhalation injury include upper airway obstruction, pneumonia, and progressive respiratory failure. Upper airway obstruction is associated with airway burns primarily of the larynx. As edema develops from the mucosal damage to the larynx, progressive occlusion of the airway occurs. The peak incidence time for airway occlusion is approximately 18 to 24 hours after the injury. When the diagnosis of an upper airway injury and impending obstruction is made, placement of a nasotracheal tube to splint the airway in the open position is indicated. Major airway injury results in damage to the cilia and mucosa of the trachea and bronchi, which reduces both mechanical clearing and the surface barrier to the development of bacterial infection. In addition, with progressive swelling of the inner lining of the airway, mucous plugs develop, producing distal obstruction. The result of this pathophysiologic process is the development of pneumonia and bacterial tracheobronchitis. Treatment includes frequent intermittent positive pressure breathing (IPPB), encouragement of coughing, and postural drainage. Daily culture of the airway is valuable so that if infection develops, it can be treated specifically with an appropriate antibiotic rather than broad-spectrum antibiotic therapy. Bronchial spasm frequently requires the use of a bronchodilator such as aminophylline. Damage to the alveolar membrane often is associated with gas-exchange problems, including hypoxia and hypercapnia. These patients require endotracheal intubation and ventilatory support. All efforts should be made to maintain a PaO_2 above 70 in these metabolically hyperdynamic patients.

In the past, steroids have been reported as valuable in the treatment of inhalation injury. Most recent experience shows that steroids are not only not beneficial in reducing edema and inflammatory response to an inhalation injury but are associated with increased infectious complications. The mortality associated with steroid therapy after inhalation injury is significantly higher.[9]

Limb ischemia

After the institution of intravenous fluid resuscitation and cardiovascular stabilization, immediate attention should be directed toward the adequacy of circulation of the distal limbs, particularly those with circumferential full-thickness burns. Edema formation beneath the circumferential eschar produces an increase in interstitial pressure that may result in obstruction to venous return. If venous return is completely stopped, arterial inflow will cease, resulting in limb ischemia and the loss of otherwise uninjured tissue. The presence of cyanosis, impaired capillary refilling, and progressive neurologic change have been clinical indications for surgical decompression of a circumferential burned limb (escharotomy). However, many of these signs are unreliable and appear late.

The ultrasonic Doppler flowmeter provides an objective assessment of peripheral flow even at the digital level and can be used effectively to monitor significantly swollen limbs.[10] If blood flow can be documented at the level of the palmar arch in the hand and the posterior tibial artery of the foot using the flowmeter, there is sufficient blood flow to maintain limb viability. Initial prophylactic treatment to minimize edema includes limb elevation and active exercise each hour during the first 24 to 36 hours after the injury. If, despite this vigorous prophylactic program, blood flow decreases or stops, an escharotomy should be performed along the medial and lateral aspects of the limb. Care should be taken not to incise the flexor or extensor surface of a limb where the tendons lie close to the skin. Fasciotomies are rarely indicated with thermal burns. Careful hemostasis is an important part of an escharotomy, since with return of skin blood flow, bleeding may occur.

In children, circumferential burns of the chest may produce a constricting effect, causing a decrease in ventilatory exchange with shallow respirations. The patient may become tachypneic, confused, anxious, and cyanotic. Palpation of the chest wall will reveal a tense, tight eschar that, unless decompressed, can further impair respiration. Ordinarily an incision in a shieldlike pattern over the anterior chest, along the anterior axillary line, and across the costochondral margin is used to decompress the eschar. Escharotomy of the limbs and chest should only be performed with full-thickness injuries and do not require general anesthesia. since third-degree burns are anesthetic.

NUTRITION

Progressive severe weight loss, hypermetabolism, and protein depletion are frequent features of extensive burns, more so than other types of injuries. In the absence of an aggressive nutritional program, major weight loss can be expected. This severe catabolic state may last until the wound is healed and is proportionate to the size of the injry. Once initial resuscitation has been completed and gastrointestinal motility returns, every effort should be directed toward providing a definite nutritional support plan.

Any child with a burn greater than 20% of total body surface has a distinctly increased nutrition requirement for protein and calories and also for growth. Unless adequate replacement is provided, infectious complications and growth suppression may occur. Weight losses of more than 10% of the preburn state are associated with increased mortality and morbidity. It is not unusual for a child with large burns to require 3500 to 4000 calories a day and 120 to 150 g of protein.[5]

To prevent the complications of an inadequate intake, a definite nutritional support plan should be implemented as soon as possible. The services of the hospital dietitian are valuable in formulating an initial plan, surveying patients' requirements, and recording daily protein and calorie intakes. Caloric requirements can be determined using an empirical formula of Curreri, which suggests that caloric needs are : (25 × preburn weight) + (40 × percent of total body surface burn).[2] The usual ratio is approximately 150 calories/g of nitrogen for proper utilization. Frequently in children, because of chronic depression and pain, oral intake may be inadequate even with the use of high-calorie supplements. If daily calorie requirements fall short of the estimated amount by 200 calories on 2 consecutive days, an enteral feeding tube should be installed and the patient fed continuously.

Most commercial solutions provide calories per milliliter, contain the proper ratio of calories to nitrogen, and can be administered through a feeding tube. Every effort should be directed at using an enteral rather than an intravenous feeding program. Although hyperalimentation provides an effective way for nutritional replacement, the mortality from septic complications with this technique runs as high as 50% in many series. Mechanical complications of catheter placement are also higher in pediatric patients.

Minor complications of an enteral feeding program include diarrhea, which usually can be controlled with antimotility agents such as paregoric. If the diarrhea is significant and prolonged, decreasing the volume of feeding temporarily may be effective in controlling this complication.

SUMMARY AND CONCLUSIONS

Surface burns are the third leading cause of accidental death and one of the primary causes of death in young patients in the United States. The rule of nines is a convenient way to determine the percentage of body surface damaged. In the infant the head and neck area represents 21% of the body surface area, whereas in the adult the head and neck occupies only 9% of the total body surface area. Children who have received second-degree burns on less than 10% of the total body surface area or full-thickness burns of less than 2% usually can be treated without hospitalization. Moderate burns that require hospitalization include second-degree burns between 10% and 25% of total body surface and third-degree burns measuring less than 10%. Major burns include partial-thickness injuries involving more than 25% of total body surface, third-degree burns involving more than 10%, and full-thickness injuries involving the face, hands, or genitalia. Burn patients in this category are at an extremely high risk. This is particularly true if the burns are complicated by injuries to the respiratory tract or other major trauma. These individuals should be transferred when stable to a designated burn service.

Several replacement formulas are available to govern fluid management in the acutely burned patient. Each method has its advocates. The most important factor ensuring success is familiarity with any of the methods selected. The isotonic resuscitation method is used at our institution. This solution is prepared by adding half an ampule of sodium bicarbonate to each liter of Ringer's lactate solution. An isotonic solution with 150 mEq/L of sodium is constituted. This solution is administered at a rate of 3 ml/kg for each percent of body surface burn.

During resuscitation the patient is carefully monitored. A urine output of approximately 0.5 to 0.75 ml/kg/hr should be maintained whenever possible. Measurement of the arterial pH level and oxygen concentration is another important monitor during resuscitation. Central venous pressure monitoring is usually unnecessary.

Patients trapped in fires in a closed, contained space may receive inhalation injuries. Clinical signs consisting of wheezing, hoarseness, shortness of breath, bronchorrhea, and carbonaceous sputum usually are not seen until 24 to 48 hours after the injury. Fiberoptic bronchoscopy is an integral part in the initial evaluation of these patients with inhalation injuries. Treatment includes IPPB, encouragement of coughing, and postural drainage. Steroids have not proven to be valuable adjuncts in management and are no longer used.

Extremities and digits must be carefully monitored in the early postburn state. Edema formation beneath the circumferential eschar may obstruct venous return. If venous return is completely obstructed, arterial insufficiency may develop with resulting limb ischemia and necrosis. The ultrasonic Doppler flowmeter is a useful adjunct to clinical observation in monitoring significantly swollen limbs. An escharotomy should be performed along the medial and lateral aspects of the limb if ischemia is suspected.

A thermal injury results in a hypermetabolic state with excessive protein depletion and caloric loss. It is not unusual for a child with large burns to require 3500 to 4000 calories a day and 120 to 150 g of protein. Commercial feeding solutions are available that provide sufficient calories and nitrogen to the burned patient and can be administered through a small feeding tube. Intravenous hyperalimentation in burn patients carries a high mortality, approximately 50% in many series. Its use should be avoided in enteral alimentation is possible.

REFERENCES

1. Baxter, C.R., and Shires, G.T.: Physiological response to crystalloid resuscitation of severe burns, Ann. N.Y. Acad. Sci. **150:**874, 1968.
2. Curreri, P.W., Richmond, D., Marvin, J., and Baxter, C.R.: Dietary requirements of patients with major burns, J. Am. Diet. Assoc. **65:**415, 1974.
3. Hayashi, H., Yoshinaga, M., Koono, M., et al.: Endogenous permeability factors and their inhibitions affecting vascular permeability in cutaneous arthus reactions and thermal injury, Br. J. Exper. Pathol. **45:**419, 1964.
4. Larkin, J.M., and Moylan, J.A.: Complete enteral support of thermally injured patients, Am. J. Surg. **131:**722, 1976.
5. Monafo, W.W.: The treatment of burn shock by the intravenous and oral administration of hypertonic lactated saline solution, J. Trauma **10:**575, 1970.
6. Moncrief, J.A.: The body's response to heat. In Artz, C.P., Moncrief, J.A., and Pruitt, B.A., editors: Burns: a team approach, Philadelphia, 1979, W.B. Saunders Co.
7. Moylan, J.A., Birnbaum, M., and Adib, K.: Fiberoptic bronchoscopy following thermal injury, Surg. Gynecol. Obstet. **140:**541, 1975.
8. Moylan, J.A., and Chan, C.K.: Inhalation injury—an increasing problem, Ann. Surg. **188:**34, 1978.
9. Moylan, J.A., Jr., Inge, W.W., and Pruitt, B.A., Jr.: Circulatory changes following circumferential extremity burns evaluated by the ultrasonic flowmeter: an analysis of 60 thermally injured limbs, J. Trauma **11:**763, 1971.
10. Moylan, J.A., Peters, C.R., and Filston, H.C.: Burn therapy updated, N.C. Med. J. **38:**594, 1977.
11. Shires, G.T., Carrico, C.J., Baxter, C.R., et al.: Principles in treatment of severely injured patients. V. Early resuscitation of patients with burns, Adv. Surg. **4:**308, 1970.
12. Zawacki, B.E.: Reversal of capillary stasis and prevention of necrosis in burns, Ann. Surg. **180:**98, 1974.

CHAPTER 9

Hemostasis: disorders and management of the pediatric patient

WALLACE H.J. CHANG

Under normal circumstances the body maintains a fine balance between coagulants and anticoagulants so as to maintain the fluidity of the blood and at the same time provide a ready mechanism to respond to vascular injuries with a series of reactions that leads to thrombus formation. Hemostasis is achieved by a complex interaction of tissue components, blood vessels, platelets, and the coagulation mechanism.

MECHANISMS OF COAGULATION

The usual textbook presentation separating the intrinsic and extrinsic pathways of thrombus formation has the great appeal of simplicity. In reality, however, the mechanisms of thrombus formation are anything but simple or yet totally understood.

Ratnoff[13,14] and Macfarlane[6] developed concomitantly a theory for clotting and coined the "cascade" or "waterfall" hypothesis based on the concept of sequential enzymatic activation of clotting factors. It is now apparent that not all clotting factors (Table 9-1) are involved in simple enzyme-substrate reactions.

Some of the factors act as co-catalysts; they accelerate a reaction without actually taking part in it. Thus the cascade concept is being replaced by the *complex-formation theory.* Clotting is activated by the formation of complexes between two or more clotting factors, which in turn work on the next substrate. The current concept (Fig. 9-1) makes little separation between the extrinsic and intrinsic pathways of clotting. Indeed, new evidence[4] suggests a link between the two pathways with kallikrein as the common catalyst for the activation of both factors IX and VII:

Factor XII to XIIa
Prekallikrein to Kallikrein
Factor VII to VIIa

Plasma kallikreins are enzymes that can increase vascular permeability, contract smooth muscles, decrease blood pressure, reduce pain, and provoke sticking of leukocytes to small blood vessels and migration of these cells into the extravascular space.[12] These responses are basically mediated through liberation of peptide kinins, notably bradykinin and kallidin (lysyl-bradykinin), which appear to act directly on the affected tissues. The kallidins exist in plasma as inert precursors but are readily activated by factor XIIa. Recent evidence has shown that the plasma kallidin not only participates in the liberation of kinins but in the clotting process itself.

Extrinsic pathways

Thrombin formation by this theoretical pathway begins when blood comes into contact with injured tissue. The

Table 9-1. Clotting factors

International nomenclature*		Common synonyms
Factor	I	Fibrinogen
Factor	II	Prothrombin
Factor	V	Proaccelerin
Factor	VII	Proconvertin
Factor	VIII	Antihemophilic factor (AHF)
Factor	IX	Christmas factor; plasma thromboplastin component (PTC)
Factor	X	Stuart factor
Factor	XI	Plasmathromboplastin antecedent (PTA)
Factor	XII	Hageman factor
Factor	XIII	Fibrin-stabilizing factor

*Factors III, IV, and VI are tissue thromboplastin, calcium ions, and activated factor V, respectively. They are no longer considered separate factors.

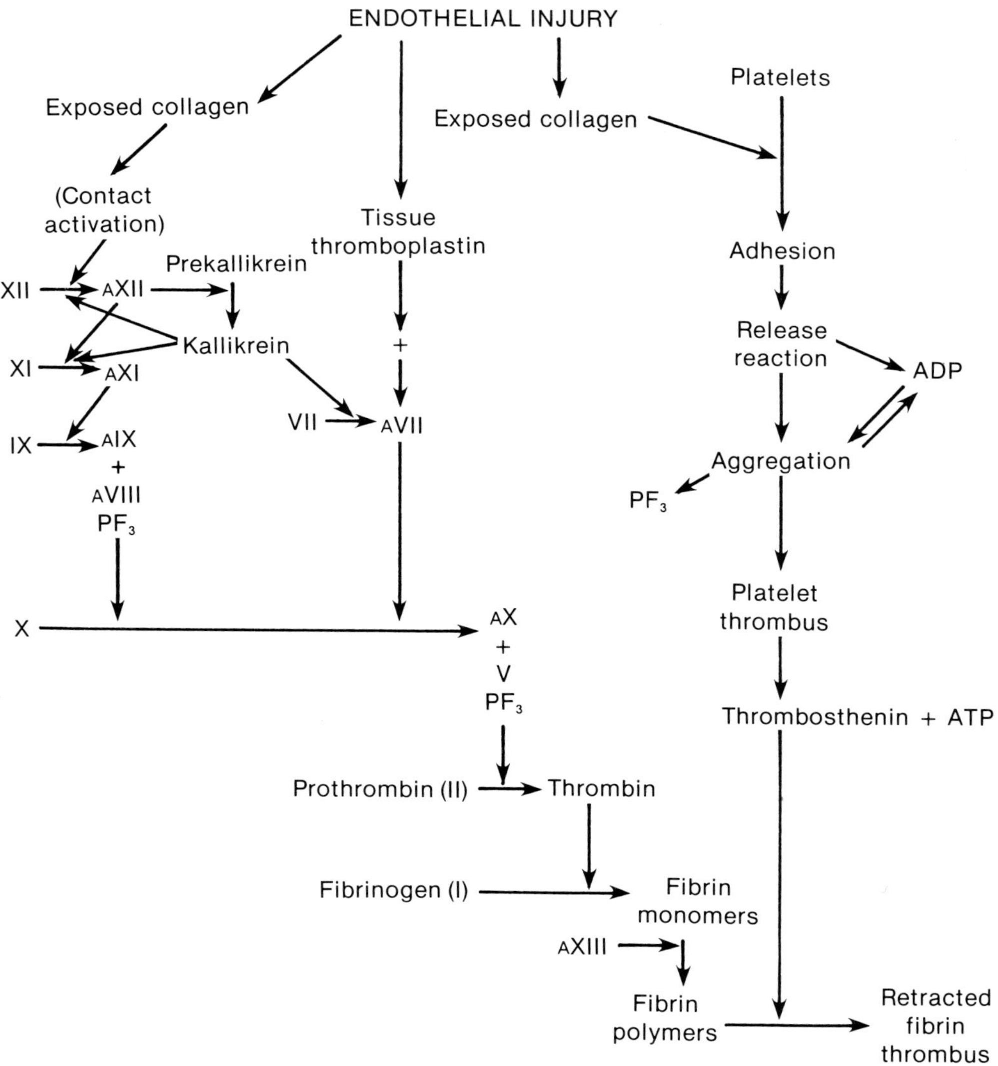

Fig. 9-1. Theoretical pathways of the coagulation mechanism. *A,* Activated.

active agent responsible for thrombin formation, tissue thromboplastin, has been localized subcellularly to the microsomes of various cells and to the cell membranes of fibroblasts and vascular endothelium.[19,20] Thromboplastin combines with the plasma protein, factor VII, to form an agent that "activates" factor X. This reaction depends on the presence of calcium ions and the phospholipid portion of thromboplastin. The phospholipid necessary for this reaction is present in the plasma itself, or it can be furnished by the platelets.[21]

Intrinsic pathways

A blood sample that comes in contact with the wall of a glass causes activation of factor XII, which then converts factor XI to an activated form by an enzymatic process. This agent in turn activates factor IX; the activated factor IX appears to form a complex with factor VIII. The complex

that forms as the result of these reactions changes factor X to its clot-promoting form. How the intrinsic pathway becomes active in vivo is unclear; however, collagen, certain mucopolysaccharides such as chondroitin sulfate, serum, and platelets have all been implicated as activators of factor XII.[8-10,15]

Activated factor X then converts prothrombin to thrombin through an enzymatic process involving the action of factor V, phospholipids, and calcium ions. Once thrombin has been elaborated, it cleaves two pairs of peptides, fibrinopeptides A and B, from each molecule of fibrinogen. The residual fibrin monomers then polymerize to form the visible clot,[1] a process that is accelerated by calcium ions. At this time the fibrin monomers are also bonded chemically through the action of factor XIII, a plasma transaminase. Although there seems to be a great disparity between the two theories of coagulation, it is anticipated that they will be combined into one that will satisfy both the chemical and clinical observations. Indeed, current evidence points to the steps of the intrinsic and extrinsic pathways merging at this point.

Platelets

The presence of platelets in thrombi was recognized as early as 1888. Eberth and Schimmelbusch[2] described masses of platelets on the edges of a wound induced in the wall of an artery. Although platelets have been known to exist in thrombi for nearly a century, evidence that they play a significant role in the formation of the thrombus has become more apparent during the past 10 years. The discovery that aspirin inhibits the capacity of platelets to undergo release of adenosine diphosphate (ADP) and aggregate after exposure to collagen places platelets in a central position in the scheme of the coagulation mechanism.[3,11,17,18]

Platelets originate in megakaryocytes, which are large cells about 35×160 m in diameter. During development the megakaryocytic cytoplasm develops granules and then an extensive network of tubules, which eventually subdivide the cytoplasm into platelet units. Regulation of platelet production is unclear but is believed to be mediated by a relative number of platelets in the circulating blood volume. In the peripheral blood the normal number of platelets is between 150,000 and 400,000/mm³. They survive an average of 8 to 10 days, becoming hemostatically less effective after 2 days of circulation. There is no nucleus in the platelets. The structure of the platelets generally consists of a peripheral zone that is involved in aggregation and coagulation, a sol-gel zone providing cellular support and contraction, and the organelle zone, which plays a role in storage and secretion. Under the exterior coat of the peripheral zone is a trilaminar membrane that is rich in lipoprotein and is considered to be of critical importance in the physiology of hemostasis, since it appears to be the source of platelet factor 3 (PF3), which is released from platelets during aggregation. In addition, the platelet granules located in the interior have similar lipoproteins that provide additional coagulating activity. At least three systems of fibers are present in the sol-gel zone: submembrane filaments, microtubules, and microfilaments. The most prominent of the three systems is the circumferential band of microtubules, which initiates the wave of contraction that takes place during the second wave of aggregation. The platelet contractile material is called *thrombosthenin* and consists of a myosin moiety and actinlike filaments. It is responsible for contraction of fibrin fibers and the clinical observation of clot retraction.

On an unfixed preparation platelets emit pseudopods, indicating ameboid movements; they reflect their ability to adhere by migrating to collagen or damaged endothelium. The three basic mechanisms that account for the functional activity of platelets in hemostasis are adhesion, contraction, and secretion-aggregation. Adhesion is necessary for platelets to form a hemostatic plug in areas of vascular injury. Aggregation gives rise to an increased mass of platelets

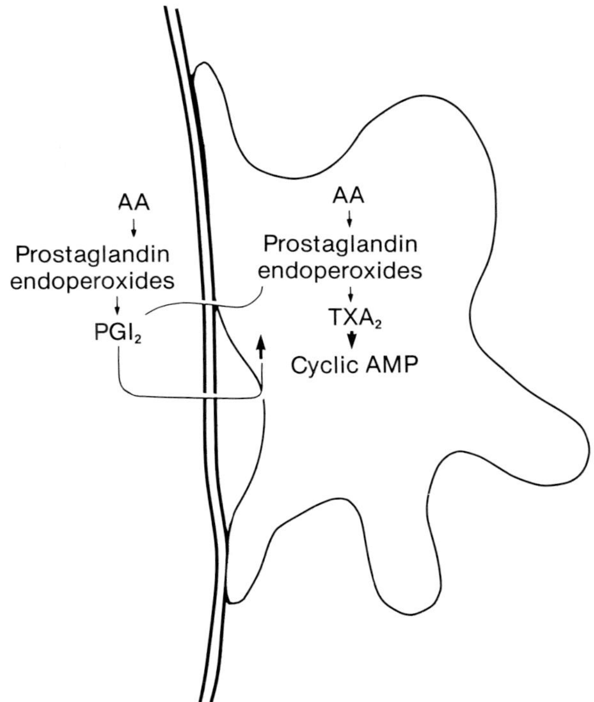

Fig. 9-2. Interaction of prostaglandins with the vessel wall and platelets. Stimulation of the platelets to aggregate releases prostaglandin endoperoxidase, which can either be converted to thromboxane A_2 (TXA$_a$) or escape and be used by prostacyclin (PGI$_2$) synthetase. PGI$_2$ also can be synthesized by the vessel wall from arachidonic acid. PIG$_2$ has a potent stimulatory effect on the adenylate cyclase of the platelets and will increase cyclic AMP levels and inhibit platelet aggregation.

formed in this plug. The contractile mechanism seals the loose mass of aggregated platelets into a hemostatic plug and retracts the platelet-fibrin meshwork. The precise mechanism of these processes is not completely understood.

When platelets are exposed to collagen they first adhere, then aggregate, to the area of the raw collagen. Collagen-induced platelet aggregation is believed to be mediated by the release of ADP from the platelet storage pool.[16] Since the ADP molecule is unable to cross the platelet membrane, its effect is believed to occur at the cell surface. In addition, external ADP can also induce platelet aggregation. Prostaglandins E_2 and F_2, as well as thromboxanes, are formed and released by platelets in response to thrombin or during aggregation by collagen, epinephrine, or ADP. It has been known that aspirin inhibits release reaction induced by ADP or collagen on platelets in vitro.[11,12] Smith and Willis[15] showed that aspirin inhibited prostaglandin production in platelets and implied that the inhibition of prostaglandin biosynthesis could account for the inhibitory effect of aspirin on platelet aggregation.

The prostaglandin endoperoxidases can be transformed enzymatically into two unstable products with potent biologic activity that are called *thromboxane A₂* and *prostacyclin (PGI₂)*. The former exerts a potent aggregating effect on platelets, whereas the latter is a powerful inhibitor of platelet aggregation. As further research elucidates this area of interaction between the platelets and the vessel wall, the known mechanisms of coagulation will have to be modified to include the opposing biologic effects of the proaggregatory thromboxane A_2 formed by the platelets and the antiaggregatory PGI_2 formed by the vessel walls (Fig. 9-2).

PROBLEMS PECULIAR TO THE PEDIATRIC PATIENT

Several coagulation factors such as factor I, vitamin K–dependent factors II, VII, IX, and X, and factor VIII are elevated during pregnancy. The newborn, however, has lower levels of some of these factors. Prothrombin times are prolonged in newborns and premature infants.[5] The administration of vitamin K to healthy term infants prevents a decrease in prothrombin activity and a prolongation of the prothrombin time that is normally observed during the first few days of life. Because of the routine administration of 1 mg of vitamin K_1 to all newborn infants, vitamin K deficiency as the cause of bleeding disorders is unlikely in a healthy newborn. Vitamin K deficiency, however, is likely to develop in an infant who is ill, eats poorly, and is receiving intravenous fluid or antibiotics. Levels of factors V and VIII are usually normal at birth, suggesting synthesis by the infants.

The administration of vitamin K antagonists to the mother may result in anticoagulation of the fetus as well, and, unless corrected several weeks before delivery, the fetal mortality may be quite high.

Other situations that predispose to hemorrhage in newborns are trauma, liver disease, disseminated intravascular coagulation (DIC), inherited bleeding disorders, thrombocytopenia, and platelet dysfunction. A reduction in the level of antithrombin III has been documented in normal newborns, with an even greater reduction in premature infants and those with idiopathic respiratory distress syndrome.[7]

Hereditary disorders of coagulation

The following tests can be used for detecting disorders of coagulation and hemostasis*:

Inherited disorders
    Complete blood cell (CBC) and platelet count
    Ivy bleeding time (if platelet count is 50,000/cu mm)
    Activated partial thromboplastin time (PTT)
    Quick prothrombin time
    Thrombin time (or screening test for factor I)
    Factor XIII screening test

---

*These procedures can be expected to detect virtually all significant disorders of coagulation and hemostasis. More specific assays of individual coagulation factors and tests of platelet function may be necessary to define the exact nature of the disorder.

Acquired disorders
    CBC and platelet count
    Ivy bleeding time (if platelet count is 50,000/cu mm)
    Activated PTT
    Quick prothrombin time
    Thrombin time
    Screening test for factor I
    Fibrinolytic profile
    Serum fibrin degradation products

Hemophilia A and B

Deficiencies in factors VIII and IX are indistinguishable clinically. Both diseases are inherited as X-linked recessive traits. The presence of the disease may be suggested by history. Manifestations of bleeding are infrequent during the first year of life. Spontaneous bleeding in soft tissues, bleeding caused by lacerations, acute hemarthrosis, bleeding after dental extractions, hematuria, and hemorrhage in the gastrointestinal tract are some of the clinical symptoms that strongly suggest coagulation defects.

Management of factor VIII deficiency

All patients should be prepared with factor VIII concentrate before undergoing surgical procedures, with replacement continued after surgery. Factor VIII levels should be maintained above 30% to 40% after major surgery. Minor bleeding or trauma may be handled by smaller doses (10 to 20 units/kg) for shorter periods of time.

The actual level of factor VIII achieved in patients and the factor's half-life depend on several variables: the rapidity of intravenous administration, the time and method of handling after the factor has been reconstituted or thawed, variability in the amount of factor VIII in different batches of cryoprecipitate, the stability of the particular factor preparation, loss of factor VII with blood loss, and extravascular distribution. It is therefore important to assay factor VIII levels for several days before and immediately after a dose of concentrate to assure the adequacy of the replacement therapy and the frequency of administration.

Factor IX deficiencies

Factor IX deficiencies are treated in a similar fashion. The concentrates used for replacement therapy contain all the vitamin K–dependent factors (II, VII, IX, and X), and, depending on which commercial product is used, variable amounts of other activated coagulation factors. The latter can result in thrombotic episodes or even in DIC in patients with liver disease. Therefore it has been recommended that before infusion, preparations with activated factors be mixed with 1 unit of heparin for every 10 units of factor IX. One unit of factor IX for each kilogram of body weight produces approximately a 1% to 1.5% rise in factor IX activity in the patient. The minimal level necessary for hemostasis after major surgery is probably about 30% to 40%. The actual frequency of administration is usually every 20 to 30 hours, based on the factor IX assay after transfusion of the concentrate.

von Willebrand's disease

Epistaxis, gingival or gastrointestinal bleeding, a tendency to bruise easily, bleeding after surgery, or excessive menstrual bleeding are some of the clinical symptoms in patients with von Willebrand's disease. The classic form of this disorder is inherited as an autosomal dominant trait and is expressed in a prolonged bleeding time and reduced levels of the factor VIII.

Management

There is controversy regarding the most appropriate parameters for predicting postoperative bleeding with von Willebrand's disease. If there is a concomitant abnormality in factor VIII, factor VIII levels should be maintained above 30% to 40% after major surgery. One of the current methods of management is to use 1 unit of cryoprecipitate for every 10 kg of body weight, repeated every 24 hours.

Factor XI deficiency

Factor XI deficiency has been documented mainly in Jewish patients. It is believed to be inherited as an autosomal recessive trait. An important aspect of the bleeding history is the variability in postsurgical bleeding. Operative bleeding after some surgical procedures may be normal, but severe bleeding can occur after others. Bleeding in such patients may start several hours to several days after surgery, as also occurs in hemophiliacs with factor VIII or IX deficiencies.

Management of deficiencies of factors V and XI

Patients with factor XI or V deficiency undergoing major surgery should have the levels maintained at about 20% to 25% with fresh, frozen plasma. The rise in factor XI activity with 1 unit of factor XI for each kilogram of body weight is approximately 2%. The rise in factor V is approximately 1.5%. In all factor deficiencies serial specific assays should be part of the routine follow-up after surgery or trauma to ensure an appropriate level of the clotting factors.

Factor XII deficiency

Factor XII deficiency is an autosomal recessive trait usually detected because of a prolonged PTT in asymptomatic patients. Such patients usually do not bleed extensively after surgical procedures.

Congenital afibrinogenemia and dysfibrinogenemia

Congenital afibrinogenemia reflects failure of the liver to synthesize fibrinogen. The mode of inheritance is autosomal recessive, and a history of consanguineity in the parents may be obtained. The low levels of fibrinogen in the plasma may not produce bleeding spontaneously and may bring about hemostasis in minor trauma. Severe and even fatal hemorrhage, however, may occur after surgery or other major trauma. Most patients with dysfibrinogenemia are asymptomatic, although a coagulation defect can be demonstrated by in vitro tests.

Management of afibrinogenemia

Afibrinogenemic patients can receive plasma, cryoprecipitate, or a commercial concentrate. Transfusion of 1 ml of plasma for each kilogram of body weight raises the fibrinogen level by 1% to 1.5 mg/100 ml. The minimal level for adequate hemostasis is perhaps 90 mg/100 ml.

Factor XIII deficiency

Congenital deficiency of this fibrin-stabilizing factor is often reflected in hemorrhage from the umbilical cord within days or weeks after birth. Such bleeding may occur in approximately 80% of the patients afflicted.

Diagnosis

A careful history is probably the most important single diagnostic aid available to the surgeon confronted with a patient suspected of having a bleeding disorder. A minimal effective combination of screening tests should include (1) a platelet count or visualization of platelets on a standard blood smear, (2) a bleeding time, (3) a prothrombin time, and (4) an activated PTT. The screening tests in Table 9-2 for detection of a hemorrhagic disorder will roughly distinguish between various types of coagulation factor deficiencies and a bleeding disorder based on platelet dysfunction.

An abnormal prothrombin time and normal PTT usually suggest a factor VII deficiency. A prolonged prothrombin time and PTT suggest a deficiency of one or more of the following: factors I, II, V, and X. A normal prothrombin time associated with an abnormal PTT suggests deficiencies of factors VIII, IX, XI, and XII. Factor XIII can be detected through a screening test that observes the stability of the fibrin clot in 5 M urea or 1% monochloroacetic acid. A deficiency of factor XIII usually is not a common clinical

Table 9-2. Screening tests for hemorrhagic disorders*

Disorder	Platelet count	Bleeding time	Prothrombin time	PTT
Vascular disorders	N	N/A	N	N
Platelet disorders				
Thrombocytopenia	A	A	N	N
Thrombasthenias	N	A	N	N
von Willebrand's disease	N	N/A	N	N/A
Coagulation factor deficiencies				
Fibrinogen	N	N/A	N/A	N/A
Prothrombin	N	N/A	A	A
Factor V	N	N/A	A	A
Factor VII	N	N/A	A	N
Factor X	N	N	A	A
Factor VIII	N	N	N	A
Factor IX	N	N	N	A
Factor XI	N	N	N	A
Factor XII	N	N	N	A
Factor XIII	N	N	N	N

*N, Normal values; A, abnormal values.

problem. Although the screening tests are useful in picking up gross patterns of coagulation disorders, a specific diagnostic workup and therapy are best done in consultation with a hematologist.

ACQUIRED BLEEDING DISORDERS
Disseminated intravascular coagulation

DIC is a syndrome that usually results from activation of coagulation mechanisms through contact activation of factors XII and XI (intrinsic system) or through activation of factor VII by tissue thromboplastin (extrinsic system), with the result that thrombin is generated in excess of the physiologic capacity to neutralize it. Numerous factors may precipitate or predispose a pediatric patient to DIC, including the following:

Sepsis
Shock
Acidosis
Hypoxia
Purpura fulminans
Hypotonic water (drowning) (release of ADP from red
   blood cells)
Mismatched transfusions
Extensive surgery
Brain injury
Pancreatitis
Liver disease
   Necrosis
   Hepatectomy
Widespread malignancy

In shock and other causes of hypotension, it is conceivable that factor XII is activated, which may result in generation of bradykinin through the kallikrein system. Immune complexes are also capable of inducing platelet aggregation and activate the coagulation mechanisms. The liver plays a vital role regulating the hypercoagulable state. In patients with liver disease DIC may follow stimuli such as shock, sepsis, or other antigen-antibody interactions. DIC is most often present in a low-grade or chronic form. The patient generally does not manifest an overt bleeding diathesis but shows abnormalities in the coagulation studies. Temporary correction of the syndrome with anticoagulants (heparin) is mandatory before further deterioration of the coagulation mechanism develops.

The patient with acute or severe decompensation intravascular coagulation syndrome has severe bleeding from several sites associated with conditions such as sepsis and shock. Large vessel thrombosis is rare. The characteristic coagulation findings are severe reduction in the levels of factors I, V, VIII, XIII, plasminogen, and platelets. As expected fibrin degradation products are usually elevated during the active phase. The levels of vitamin K–dependent factors that are affected, especially if there is liver dysfunction, are variable.

Management

The therapy must be directed at the cause of the DIC. If the precipitating cause is corrected, DIC is a self-limiting and self-correcting disorder. If the precipitating factor is not immediately apparent or amenable to therapy, the temporary use of heparin to neutralize the effect of thrombin, as well as other proteases of the coagulation cascade, allows the patient time to recover. Response to therapy is evidenced by rising factor I levels and decreasing amounts of large molecular fibrin degradation products (staphylococcal clumping test). The platelet count takes several days to recover and therefore is not a reliable parameter on which to base therapy.

Congenital heart disease

Patients with cyanotic heart disease frequently have thrombocytopenia and decreased levels of factors II, V, VII, IX, and X. These factors are synthesized in the liver and are more frequently abnormal in children with hematocrit levels above 60%. Thrombocytopenia with normal marrow megakaryocytes, shortened platelet life span, and large numbers of thrombocytes in children with cyanotic heart disease all attest to a rapid turnover of platelets.

Management

Wedemeyer and Lewis[17] have shown improvements in factors II, V, VII, IX, and X and platelets after a phlebotomy of 100 ml/sq m of body surface area. Maurer et al.[8] reported correction of platelet aggregation in response to ADP, collagen, and epinephrine after removal of 10 to 15 ml of blood for each kilogram of body weight with simultaneous administration of equal volumes of aged plasma.

Multiple transfusions with stored whole blood

The labile factors V and VIII are severely reduced during the 3 weeks of storage of whole blood. Platelet viability is also severely reduced. Factor I and the vitamin K–dependent factors, however, are not changed. Patients who require large numbers of stored, whole blood transfusions are likely to develop thrombocytopenia and coagulation defects.

Management

Patients requiring multiple transfusions should receive one unit of fresh whole blood for every two units of stored whole blood. As an alternative, one unit of fresh frozen plasma can be substituted with red cells after every two units of stored blood.

Liver disease

Reduced levels of vitamin K–dependent factors in normal newborns, even after vitamin K_1 is administered parenterally and the normalization of those levels between 2 and 4 months after birth is compatible with mild liver dysfunction. The development of slowly progressive hepatic damage after

12 months of age is also associated with a mild reduction of the vitamin K–dependent factors that is unresponsive to parenteral administration of vitamin K. Factor V is affected with further advancement in liver disease. With severe advanced liver disease, factor I levels also drop.

Hemangioma-thrombocytopenia syndrome (Kasabach-Merritt syndrome)

In certain patients with large mixed capillary-cavernous hemangiomas, thrombosis within the lesion consumes a large number of the circulating platelets. Thrombocytopenia becomes a potential hazard.

SUMMARY AND CONCLUSIONS

Current concepts of the coagulation sequence make little separation between the extrinsic and intrinsic pathways of clotting. New evidence suggests that kallikrein may be the common catalyst in both pathways.

Thromboxane A_2, synthesized from arachidonic acid, is released from platelets during aggregation by collagen or in response to an existing thrombus. It has a potent aggregating effect on platelets.

PGI_2 is synthesized in the endothelium from arachidonic acid. It has a potent stimulatory effect on adenyl cyclase of the platelets. Thus cyclic AMP levels are increased and platelet aggregation is inhibited. These opposing biologic effects (proaggregation versus antiaggregation) exist in delicate balance in the steady state. Disease, trauma, or medication may alter the coagulation sequence by affecting this balance.

A minimal effective combination of screening tests should include (1) a platelet count or visualization of platelets on a standard blood smear, (2) a bleeding time, (3) a prothrombin time, and (4) an activated PTT. These four modalities will distinguish between the various types of coagulation factor deficiencies and bleeding disorders from platelet dysfunction. An abnormal prothrombin time and normal thromboplastin time usually suggests factor III deficiency. A prolonged prothrombin time *and* PTT suggests a deficiency of one or more of factors I, II, V, and X. A normal prothrombin time associated with an abnormal PTT suggests deficiency of factors VIII, IX, XI, and XII.

REFERENCES

1. Blombäck, B., and Blombäck, M.: The molecular structure of fibrinogen, Ann. N.Y. Acad. Sci. **202:**77, 1972.
2. Eberth, C.J.: Die Thrombose nach Versuchen and Leichenbefunden, geschildert von C.J. Eberth and C. Schimmelbusch, Stuttgart, Germany, 1888, Ferdinand Enke.
3. Evans, G., Packham, M.A., Nishizawa, E.E., et al.: The effect of acetyl-salicylic acid on platelet function, J. Exp. Med. **128:**877, 1968.
4. Gjonnoess, H.: Cold promoted activation of factor VII. IV. Relation to the coagulation system, Thromb. Diath. Haemorrh. **28:**194, 1972.
5. Gross, S.J., and Stuart, M.J.: Hemostasis in the premature infant, Clin. Perinatol. **4:**259, 1977.
6. Macfarlane, R.G.: Hemostasis. In Biggs, R., editor: Human blood coagulation, hemostasis and thrombosis, Oxford, England, 1972, Blackwell Scientific Publications.
7. Mahasandana, C., and Hathaway, W.E.: Circulating anticoagulants in the newborn: relation to hypercoagulability and the idiopathic respiratory distress syndrome, Pediatr. Res. **7:**670, 1973.
8. Maurer, H.M., McCue, C.M., Robertson, L.W., and Haggins, J.C.: Correction of platelet dysfunction and bleeding in cyanotic congenital heart disease by simple red cell volume reduction, Am. J. Cardiol. **35:**831, 1975.
9. Moskowitz, R.W., Schwartz, H.J., Michel, B., et al.: Generation of kinin-like agents by chrondroitin sulfate, heparin, chitin sulfate and human articular cartilage: possible pathophysiologic implications, J. Lab. Clin. Med. **76:**790, 1970.
10. Niewiarowski, S., Bankowski, E., and Rogowicka, I.: Studies on the adsorption and activation of the Hageman factor (factor XII) by collagen and elastin, Thromb. Diath. Haemorrh. **14:**387, 1965.
11. Nossel, H.L.: Activation of factors XII (Hageman) and XI (PTA) by skin contact, Proc. Soc. Exp. Biol. Med. **122:**16, 1966.
12. O'Brien, J.R.: Effects of salicylates on human platelets, Lancet **1:**779, 1968.
13. Ratnoff, O.D.: Some relationships among hemostasis, fibrinolytic phenomena, immunity, and the inflammatory response. Adv. Immunol. **10:**145, 1969.
14. Ratnoff, O.D.: Some recent advances in the study of hemostasis, Circ. Res. **35:**1, 1974.
15. Smith, J.B., and Willis, L.: Nature **231:**235, 1971.
16. Walsh, P.N.: The role of platelets in the contact phase of blood coagulation, Br. J. Haematol. **22:**237, 1972.
17. Wedemeyer, A.L., and Lewis, J.H.: Improvement in hemostasis following phlebotomy in cyanotic patients with heart disease, J. Pediatr. **83:**46, 1973.
18. Weiss, H.J., and Aledort, L.M.: Impaired platelet/connective-tissue reaction in man after aspirin ingestion, Lancet **2:**495, 1967.
19. Weiss, H.J., Aledort, L.M., and Kochwa, S.: The effect of salicylates on the hemostatic properties of platelets in man, J. Clin. Invest. **47:**2169, 1968.
20. Zacharski, L.R., and McIntyre, O.R.: Membrane-mediated synthesis of tissue factor (thromboplastin) in cultured fibroblasts, Blood **41:**679, 1973.
21. Zeldis, S.M., Nemerson, Y., Pitlick, F.A., and Lentz, T.L.: Tissue factor (thromboplastin): localization to plasma membranes by perioxidase-conjugated antibodies, Science **175:**766, 1972.

CHAPTER 10

Surgery of scars

ERLE E. PEACOCK, Jr.

Unsightly scarring is a major complication of injury and repair in children and young adults; the problem unquestionably is multifactorial. Like almost all biologic phenomena, scar formation has cyclic characteristics. Between the ages of 2 and 20 years scars may not only be very important but unfortunately are more prominent than during other periods. Scars in young people tend to have hyperemia longer and more prominently than in infants and adults, and the amount of scar tissue is relatively greater than usually found in later life. The worst hypertrophic scars and keloids seem to occur in patients under 30 years of age; it is rare to find a new keloid developing after the age of 40. Although there is not much that can be done to reduce prominence or red tones in juvenile scars, the knowledge that youngsters develop prominent scars more readily than adults should be considered when planning elective reconstructive procedures, particularly in the head, neck, and upper chest regions. Scars in lower extremities of young people have a tendency to stretch and become wider more often than scars in the head and neck. Mercifully, such scars are not as likely to become hypertrophic of form a keloid as scars around the anterior chest, shoulders, face, and ears. Although little is known about the basic biologic differences between youngsters and mature adults that could account for such clinical observations, experience is helpful to the extent that it is seldom worthwhile trying to reduce surgically the width of a scar around the knee or the amount or redness of scar over the shoulders or face of a young patient. Plastic surgery techniques can change the position or characteristics of a scar, prevent or remove suture marks, and occasionally relieve the prominence by leveling edges or getting rid of shadows. The major problems caused by redness and too much scar tissue in the superior half of the body and the stretching or widening of scars in the lower extremities usually are not helped by present plastic surgery techniques. Some scars actually may be made significantly worse by

surgical revision. Humility, therefore, is an important aspect of plastic surgery experience when considering reconstructive surgery for a child or teenage patient. A severe hypertrophic scar or a frank keloid require relief, however, and most of this chapter will be directed to control of those lesions. A hypertrophic scar and keloid probably are expressions of the same basic abnormality but for clinical purposes have been separated arbitrarily by structure. Excessively large scars that still retain the shape of the original defect usually are called *hypertrophic scars*. Excessive collections of scar tissue that have no resemblance to the shape of the original wound and even spill over or become pedunculated or polypoid are called *keloids*.

THEORETICAL CONSIDERATIONS

It seems most likely at this time that both hypertrophic scars and keloids are the result of an imbalance between net collagen synthesis and deposition and collagenolysis. Such a conclusion is based primarily on failure to find any significant qualitative differences between collagen subunits in scars of different proportions. Deductions based on lack of data are subject to sudden refutation when data become available, but the concept of a quantitative rather than a qualitative abnormality has been strengthened over the years as new data concerning collagen synthesis and collagen destruction accumulate. Both collagen synthesis and collagenolysis by tissue collagenase acting at a neutral pH level are measurable in human scar tissue. The old concept that dense connective tissue is a static, adynamic, excelsior of the body therefore is not correct. Scar tissue has been shown to have an accelerated rate of collagen synthesis over unwounded tissue for at least 20 years after injury.[7] Collagenolysis can be measured in human scar tissue for a similar period of time.[15] Although quantitative measurements of tissue collagenase at a neutral pH level are not as accurate as other measurements of collagen metabolism, it is safe to assume that collagenolysis must be more active in scar tissue than in normal tissue (where it is often not measurable at all) and that collagenolytic activity is in equilibrium with accelerated collagen deposition in patients with stable scars. Such reasoning leads to the inescapable conclusion that hypertrophic scars and keloids are the result of abnormalities in the equilibrium between synthesis and lysis and that the imbalance favors collagen deposition. Whether such an imbalance is the result of abnormally accelerated synthesis or decreased lysis cannot be stated at this time. A major question, of course, is the ultimate control of an unbalanced metabolic equation that causes dense connective tissue to accumulate and finally become stable. A reasonable possibility is that, at some time, the mass of scar tissue outgrows its blood supply, and relative anoxia and shortage of nutrients control the deposition of additional collagen subunits. Although subject to all of the limitations of deductive reasoning, the theory of a metabolic imbalance between synthesis and lysis featuring abnormal deposition of dense connective tissue that ultimately becomes stable as it outgrows the blood supply provides a theoretical basis for future research and a sound biologic model for prevention and treatment of scar tissue in human beings.

BIOLOGIC CONSIDERATIONS IN THE CONTROL OF HYPERTROPHIC SCARS AND KELOIDS

Fundamental steps in synthesis, maturation, and removal of dense connective tissue involve intracellular synthesis of the collagen molecule, extracellular formation of intramolecular and intermolecular covalent cross-links, physical weaving of individual subunits, and removal of nonpurposefully oriented fibrils and fibers (remodeling of immature scar tissue). Each step offers the plastic surgeon at least one theoretical approach to control of unwanted scar tissue. For instance, agents are available that block translation and transcription so that formation of α- and β-chains on ribosomal aggregates is impossible. Some agents block storage and transport by the Golgi apparatus of the finished molecule across cell membranes. Other agents block specific reactions such as hydroxylation of proline to produce hydroxyproline near the end of the assembly process. Extracellular cross-linking can be prevented by administering specific monoamine oxidase inhibitors, and a number of agents have been identified that stimulate and inhibit tissue collagenase.[11] To be clinically useful such agents must be generally nontoxic, restricted in action to collagen metabolism, and readily reversible. It should never be forgotten that uncontrolled tampering with the kinetics of general collagen synthesis and destruction throughout the body has far-reaching implications on human health. An unsightly scar is a serious problem in some individuals, but the physical properties and amount of collagen composing the adventitia of the aorta, serosa of the colon, or leaflets of the heart valves (the function of which depends on the presence and stability of dense

connective tissue) are considerations of a far more serious nature than an ugly surface scar. The precise cause of such connective tissue abnormalities as scleroderma, cirrhosis of the liver, and stenosing cicatrix of tubular organs (esophagus, urethra, biliary tract, etc.) at one end of the scale, or a dissecting aneurysm of the aorta, diverticula of the colon, or abdominal wall hernia at the other end of the scale are all manifestations of, if not directly caused by, abnormal collagen metabolism.

The healing wound, featuring actively remodeling scar tissue during the first 2 to 3 weeks after repair, is selectively sensitive to the generally acting agents previously described because the kinetics of collagen synthesis and deposition are accelerated over normal, unwounded tissue.[13] Most pharmacologic agents that affect collagen synthesis are nonspecific and affect synthesis of many proteins in addition to collagen. Thus the major opportunity now to control collagen synthesis selectively in surface scar lies in taking advantage of the relatively rapid metabolism of scar tissue. Even nonspecifically acting drugs have a greater effect on rapidly remodeling scar tissue than slowly remodeling normal tissue. Many agents that presently are being investigated for clinical usefulness in controlling surface scar tissue in human beings are generally acting agents that affect collagen metabolism throughout the body. To produce a selective effect on scar tissue after repair of a skin wound without producing a significant effect on unwounded tissue, an agent must be administered during a carefully controlled time when the kinetics of collagen turnover in the wound are three or four times more rapid than in unwounded tissue. Failure to comprehend this basic pharmacodynamic principle could result in attenuation or disappearance of connective tissue in strategic areas throughout the body. For example, it has been common practice to administer oral penicillin in prophylactic doses to children with unusual or dangerous sensitivity to group A β-hemolytic streptococci. Streptococcal sensitivity diseases such as nephritis and rheumatic fever have been reduced by the use of prophylactic penicillin, but the late effects of long-term therapy on connective tissue in the rest of the body have not been assessed. Approximately 5% of orally administered penicillin is converted by gastric acid to penicillamine. Penicillamine, in addition to being a powerful copper chelator, also is a lathyrogenic agent that prevents cross-linking of newly synthesized collagen. Short-term administration of penicillamine does not affect mature collagen that already is firmly cross-linked. Long-term administration of penicillamine, however, may cause the collagen in the adventitia of the aorta, serosa of the colon, or transversalis fascia in the groin area to become lathyritic (under–cross-linked) and could result in a higher incidence of aneurysm, diverticula, or groin hernia during later life.

Considerations other than pharmacologic treatment are important in the management of unwanted scar tissue in human beings. The effect of tension on scar formation and the origin in the dermis of the signal to overcome entropy and accelerate collagen synthesis are two examples. The effect of tension on synthesis and deposition of collagen in a healing wound has been brought up repeatedly because of clinical observations that wounds under tension heal with excessive amounts of scar tissue. Data supporting the concept that tension across a healing wound increases collagen deposition are hard to obtain. Numerous experimental models have been designed but the problem is that it is very difficult to subject a wound or scar tissue to continuous tension without introducing significant artifacts.[16] Until scar tissue is synthesized and actually connects approximated skin edges and the sutures have been removed, the wound is not under tension; it is the sutures and the connection of the sutures to the skin that are tense. Despite the fact that basic data are not available, clinical experience, including empirical observations that relief of tension seems to help reduce scar formation, suggests that tension is a factor in deposition of excessive scar tissue and that the effects of tension must be considered by the plastic surgeon during treatment planning.

Although the actual stimulus to overcome entropy in wounded tissue and to start the healing process after a wound has occurred is unknown, the site or origin of the stimulus has been determined in the deepest layer of the dermis.[5] Interruption of physical integrity of the epidermis or even the superficial layers of the dermis does not result in significant measurable acceleration of collagen metabolism and is not followed by formation of a permanent scar after healing is complete. Interruption of physical integrity of the deepest layer of the dermis, however, is followed by accelerated connective tissue metabolism and always results in a permanent fibrous scar. The signal to overcome entropy seems to be limited to a radius of about 5 mm.[9,10] The biologcially oriented surgeon can use such data to control rate of collagen synthesis during excision and revision of excessively large scars.

Finally, anything that affects the inflammatory response, such as selection and placement of sutures, necrosis of tissue, and infection, has a sound theoretical basis in the clinical control of unwanted scar tissue. Inflammation up to the point of tissue necrosis increases and prolongs acceleration of net collagen synthesis and deposition. This general observation should not be extended, however, to mean that antiinflammatory agents such as steroids and antihistamines have any useful role in the clinical control of scar tissue. Antiinflammatory agents, particularly steroids, have no effect on the total collagen content of a scar; they only *delay* the rate of gain of tensile strength and the ultimate equilibrium between collagen synthesis and degradation.

MANAGEMENT OF PATIENTS WITH UNSIGHTLY SCARS

There are no safe and predictable methods of removing scar tissue in human beings other than surgical. External pressure will squeeze out water temporarily and internal pressure can cause central necrosis, but in my judgment neither technique is applicable to the problem of unwanted scar tissue in children, despite abundant claims to the contrary. Theoretically removal of collagen by enzymatic digestion from any area in a human being is likely to be too dangerous to be clinically practical, even if the process could be restricted to a fairly small area. There are only two enzymes that can digest collagen under physiologic conditions. Both tissue collagenase and bacterial clostridial collagenase are capable of digesting scar tissue, but difficulties in obtaining one and in controlling the other make digestion at a neutral pH level impractical at this time. The use of other enzymes such as papain or some of the acid hydrolases theoretically might be controllable in human scar tissue but presently are outside of the limits of acceptable clinical practice. Two methods of reducing surface scars that are widely believed to be clinically effective are being used so frequently that they deserve special consideration. They are external pressure by elastic garments and injection of steroids.

Although there is no question that reduction of the water content of scars and keloids can be accomplished by sustained external pressure from elastic coverings, no data support the popular notion that removal of water makes any permanent difference in the size of a scar. Sustained pressure on the dermis of a paralyzed patient does appear to stimulate collagenolysis, and digestion of dermis produces a typical trophic ulceration. There are no data, however, to support a similar stimulation of tissue collagenase by applying an elastic covering to an intact surface scar. The length of time, measured in months in most patients, required for continuous elastic pressure to reduce the size of a surface scar strongly suggests that the normal maturation process continues beneath the elastic covering and is responsible for most of the change. Children have suffered untold psychologic and physical discomfort from being made to wear gloves or elastic masks for months because of the notion that elastic compression reduces the collagen content of unsightly scars more than normal maturation. In some instances needed reconstructive surgery actually has been delayed while months of compression treatment elapsed. A side consideration, of course, is that lack of objectivity of surgeons prescribing elastic garments has resulted in a profitable business for the manufacturer that is not justified by clinical results in patients.

Although there was never a realistic biochemical of biophysical basis for the injection of steroids in excessive scar tissue, the practice has been popular because of early claims that massive scar tissue could be reduced. Such claims were probably based on factors other than the pharmacologic mechanism of steroids. An essential part of steroid injection is pressure. Dense connective tissue, as the name implies, is compact, and unless great pressure is used during injection it is usually impossible to introduce a significant amount of a viscous material into the scar tissue. It seems most likely now that previous beneficial reports of injecting triamcinolone (Kenalog) solution into excessive surface scar is more the effect of a central pressure necrosis similar to excision leaving a rim of keloid practiced some years ago than to any pharmacologic effect of steroids. In some respects central injection may have been a sort of medical debridement. Actually, there is a stronger theoretical basis for injecting substances such as urea than injecting Kenalog's solution. Urea has been shown to have an uncoupling effect on collagen, and I used it to try to reduce surface scar 30 years ago.[19] The fact that results were similar to saline controls and later triamcinolone solution points to the physical aspects of the process rather than the pharmacologic reactions that proponents of injection assigned to steroids.

Because there are no pharmacologic or biologic approaches (rather than time) to the problem of mature unsightly surface scars, treatment must start by removing the scar and then be directed toward controlling the amount of new scar that forms. The decision to embark on such a course is a complex one.

Revision of scars that are no unsightly because of the amount of scar present is relatively straightforward. Just because a wound was closed by someone other than a plastic surgeon, of course, is not an indication for a plastic surgeon to revise the scar. A scar with uneven edges that casts a shadow should be revised to produce a surface which does not become distorted when light is projected from one side. Shadows cause a hard look reminiscent of Rouge's Gallery photographs. Getting rid of shadows by producing an even surface softens the expression significantly. Prominent suture marks are another indication for revision of a scar; if suture marks are not too wide they often can be ellipsed out of the area. A wide scar sometimes can be improved, particularly if it is the result of secondary healing because of infection of dehiscence. It has been taught for many years that the width of a scar can be controlled by the use of permanent subcuticular sutures in the dermis; some recent studies have cast doubt on the accuracy of that principle, whereas others support it.[14,18] Width appears now to be more a function of remodeling, sometimes secondary to tension. Reduction in width of a scar is probably more often accomplished by changing the direction of the scar than by reopening it to insert permanent subcuticular sutures. In summary, scars should be surgically excised to make the coapted edges level, remove suture marks, change direction, and sometimes reduce width. The full thickness of skin must be excised for these conditions; repair is straightforward with permanent subcuticular sutures in the dermis and tiny sutures or tape coapting epithelium.

Timing, indications, technique, repair, and postoperative care are vastly more complicated when scar tissue is removed, because there is an excessive amount of collagen present. There are two main goals in such patients—to get rid of existing scar tissue and to rebalance the metabolic equation between collagen deposition and collagenolysis in favor of collagenolysis. Although complex and multifactorial, such goals can be achieved in many patients. Empirically, timing of the excision of excessive scar tissue seems important. Scientifically, we do not know for certain whether timing is important and, if it is, how timing affects surgical revision and within what limits. There is no question that the tendency to deposit excess scar tissue is temporal, just as the tendency to lyse normal dermis is cyclic in paralyzed patients. In addition to cyclic phenomena that may be present, there is also empirical recognition that the tendency to deposit excess quantities of scar tissue in healing wounds diminishes with life span and actually disappears completely after midlife in many patients. The three following principles based on consideration of time seem to be useful:

1. Scars that are still enlarging should not be excised as long as growth is measurable.
2. At least 18 months and often longer should elapse before considering revision of a scar because of the quantity of collagen present. Maturation or remodeling of an unsightly scar can be delayed for a year and still develop naturally.
3. Scars with obvious hyperemia, infection, and edema should not be revised when gross inflammation is present.

Complete excision of a hypertrophic scar or keloid after uncomplicated healing seldom results in improvement unless something different is done during or after closure. Something different during surgery usually means addition of skin in the form of a free graft. A local pedicle flap will change the direction of a scar and may improve part of it, but sometimes it only results in a longer scar of equally bad proportions. Excision and closure by suturing wound edges, no matter how carefully performed, usually makes a hypertrophic scar or keloid worse, presumably because there is more tension on the wound than during the initial healing process. Rarely excision and closure will not result in recurrence or an even worse collection of scar; such results are best explained by the temporal or unpredictable nature of collagen metabolism and not the ability of the surgeon to affect or even predict changes in collagen metabolism. For all practical purposes, excision of an unsightly scar must be followed by a reconstructive procedure that changes the conditions under which the next period of healing will occur. A free skin graft is the most reliable such procedure at this time.

Using free skin grafts in a patient already showing propensity for depositing more collagen than necessary introduces a number of important considerations, not the least of which is the fate of the donor site. A number of theoretical and practical considerations argue for thin split-thickness skin grafts rather than thick- or full-thickness grafts. One such consideration, of course, is the level where the stimulus to overcome entropy and accelerate collagen metabolism seems to be located. Because the signal appears to originate in activated macrophages and platelets as a result of interrupting physical integrity of the deepest layer of the dermis, it appears prudent at this time to avoid deep layers of dermis during excision of the lesion and harvesting the graft.[2,6] Because of this principle, a sort of tangential excision of the lesion and taking a thin skin graft from an area of very thick skin seems wise. Perhaps more important than the actual depth of keloid or scar excision is the principle that definitive excision should not include normal or unwounded dermis around the lesion.

Empirical observations that keloids can be controlled by performing a central excision of the scar and leaving a "picture frame" of remaining scar of keloid probably are the result of not overcoming entropy by entering unwounded dermis rather than leaving a rim of scar tissue to isolate the graft from peripheral tension. It is not necessary, however, to leave a grossly discernible rim of scar as was previously practiced. During scar excision, the biologically oriented surgeon concentrates on removing all of the scar that can be removed without penetrating unwounded dermis (Fig. 10-1). A tiny (often less than 1 mm) rim of scar tissue may be left when such a dissection is complete. Such a rim probably is of secondary importance, however, and may not contribute anything to the final result. The depth of scar excision in the center of the lesion is not determined by any basic data presently available. A few practical points may be worthwhile, however. Most of the keloid above the deepest layer is composed of swirls of collagen bundles with a high mucopolysaccharide content. The amount of highly

viscous discharge from such a surface is not ideal for grafting. If all of the thickness of a keloid is removed, fat will be exposed, which again does not produce an ideal surface for grafting. Moreover, the possibility that the deepest layer of scar or keloid contains macrophages that will be activated by physical stimulation is a theoretical possibility. It seems now, therefore, that excision in the center of the lesion should be at least at skin level to provide suitable contour and deep enough to be below the grossly discernible swirls with high mucous content. Dissection should not penetrate deep enough to expose fat. Dissection often resembles deep tangential excision of burned skin; the resulting defect is surrounded by a tiny rim of scar that isolates unwounded surrounding dermis and has a fibrous tissue base approximately level with surrounding skin.

Hemostasis, which is necessary for uncomplicated 100% take of a graft and healing completely by first intention, raises several questions. In keeping with the principle that secondary or prolonged healing would be avoided and that injury to macrophages in the deepest layers of unwounded dermis and scars should be avoided, cautery and ligation probably should not be used. Fortunately there are only capillaries to be dealth with in the type of dissection described; pressure and time suffice for most patients. Unfortunately, however, the capillary network in hypertrophic scar and in some keloids is extremely rich, even more than in normal skin; hemorrhage may be profuse even though only capillaries are involved. In these patients, particularly if the lesion is large (over 6 sq cm), a compression dressing should be applied and grafting delayed for 24 to 48 hours.

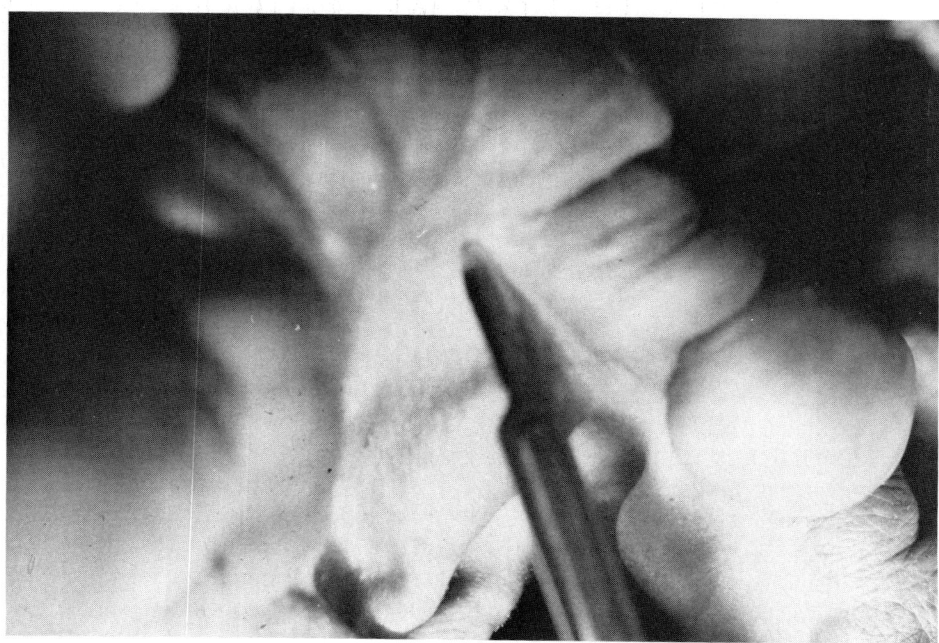

Fig. 10-1. Theoretical plane of excision deep to the keloid and superficial to the deepest layer of dermis where activation of collagen synthesis occurs.

Topical thrombin and epinephrine on the surface may help. Hemostasis must be so near perfect that the graft is not lost anywhere because of hematoma; even loss of a small spot in the center of a graft will introduce prolonged healing by secondary intention and will mitigate against balancing the metabolic equation.

Probably the best graft is taken from the surface of the keloid (Figs. 10-2 to 10-5). The surface of a hypertrophic scar is not adequate for a graft and by definition will be too small to resurfce the defect after dissection. Large areas of a keloid may contribute skin that can be dissected from the collagenous substrate and used as a free graft. This technique is particularly useful in grafting small areas of an earlobe that often contains large pedunculated smooth keloids. The obvious advantage of using skin from the surface of a keloid is protection from developing a keloid in a donor site; however, often the surface of a keloid is verrucous with infected crypts and sinuses and cannot be used. It is not possible, for example, to use the surface of verrucous or infected lesions to resurface a denuded area. An autogenous graft is needed. Wounds of the buttocks can produce atrocious hypertrophic scars, but they almost never form a true keloid. It may be that the thickness of skin over the buttocks assures that deep layers of the dermis will not be stimulated. Because other areas of thick skin such as the back and shoulders form terrible keloids, even with superficial injury, it seems possible that the skin of the buttocks may be relatively immune to keloid formation for other reasons. Regardless of the reason, however, the safest graft from the standpoint of donor site healing, is a thin split-thickness graft removed from the buttocks.

Postoperative care of the donor site is equally important as for the recipient area. Infection and delayed healing can lead to hypertrophic scar in the donor site that usually is not necessary. Exposure is the safest regimen. Ideally a dressing should not be applied, but patients should be positioned on the abdomen until a scab forms. Once the scab forms it should be protected until epithelialization beneath is complete.

Consistency in following the basic principle that unwounded dermis should not be exposed or penetrated requires a perfect fit of the graft and nothing more than tape

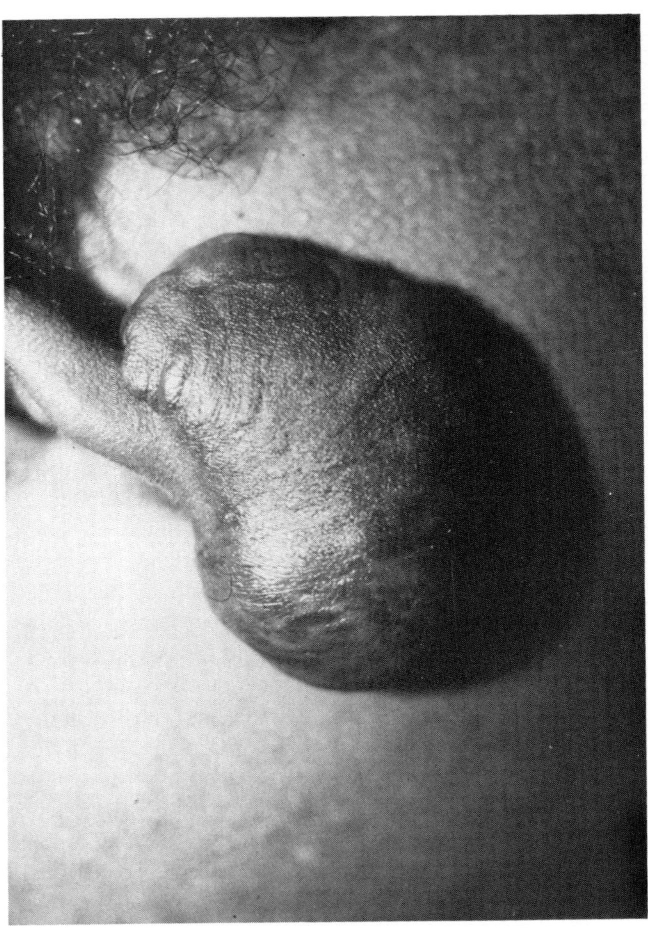

Fig. 10-2. Typical keloid deforming lobule of the ear after puncture wound.

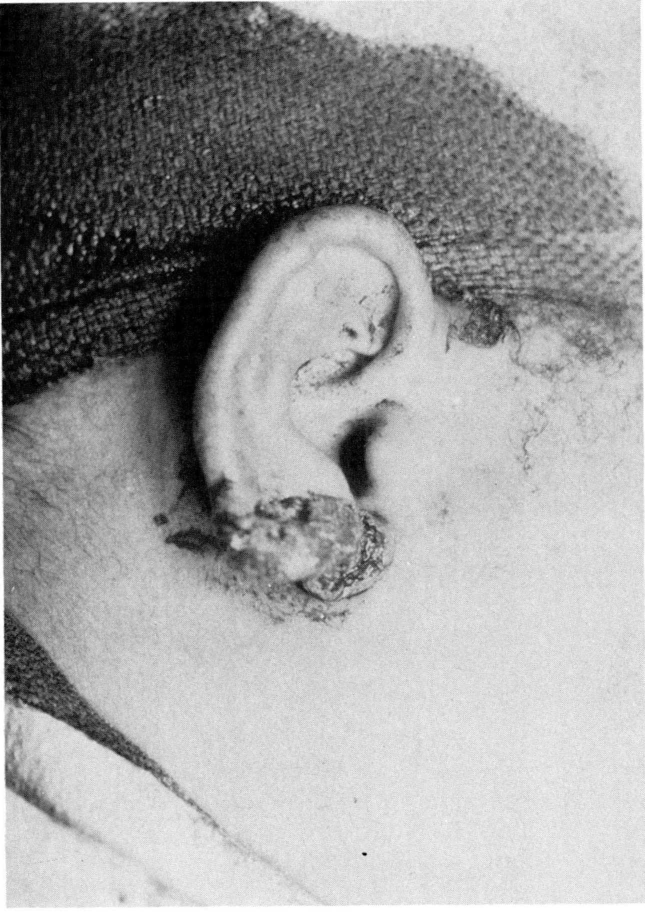

Fig. 10-3. Dissection of keloid to remove excess collagen without penetrating deep layer of normal dermis.

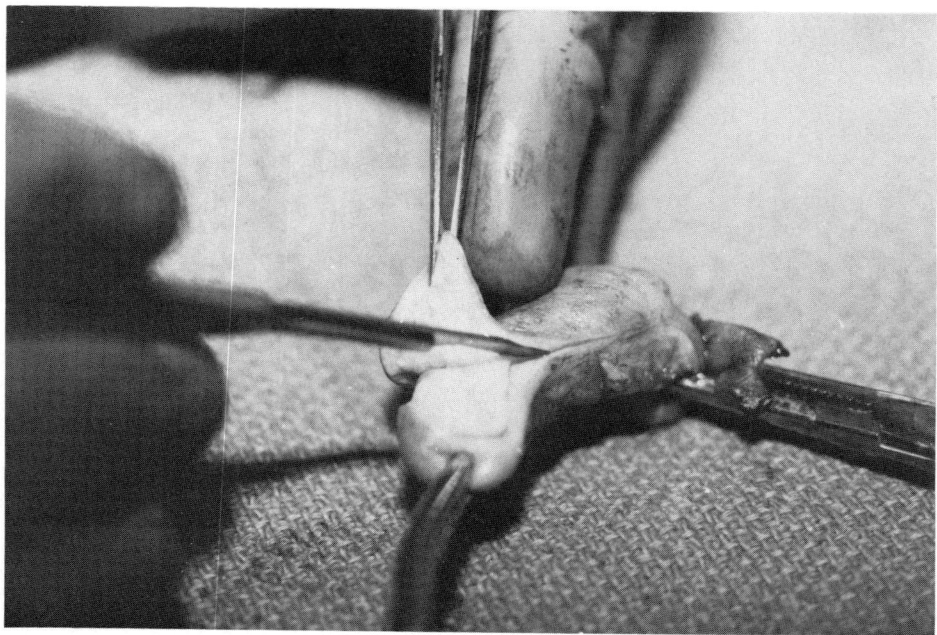

Fig. 10-4. Dissection of thick split-thickness skin graft from keloid to avoid a new donor site.

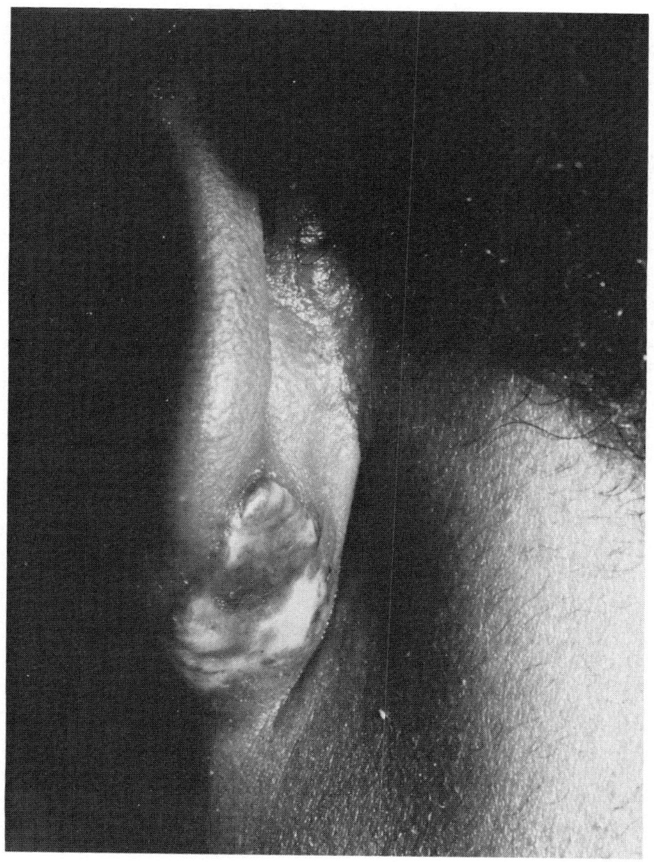

Fig. 10-5. Appearance of patient in Fig. 10-2 after grafting lobule with skin from keloid and administration of colchicine.

fixation. Certainly the graft should be cut to fit the defect perfectly so that no overlap of edges occurs. As far as epithelialization is concerned, contact inhibition is the best friend the surgeon has in controlling healing of the surface. The epithelium of the graft should touch epithelium of the recipient rim so accurately that cells will have little distance to span and no formidable obstacles to contact inhibition. It is not known whether such agents as chalones and other epithelium-stimulating factors are involved in keloid formation, but it does not seem wise to set up intentionally a secondary epithelializing wound by careless approximation or intentional overlap of epithelial edges.

Sutures can be used to secure the coapted edges of the graft and recipient rim but they should be epithelial sutures of fine material. Sutures should not pass through deep layers of the dermis if treatment is based on the premise that deep dermal stimulation is necessary to accelerate collagen metabolism. Large sutures that penetrate the dermis produce suture marks which can become classic keloids or bad hypertrophic scars some distance from the original injury. In addition to providing the most reliable and most accurate fixation, sutures also provide mild compression when tied over a bolus of cotton or Dacron. Delayed grafting can be performed using tape instead of sutures and exposure instead of a stent; primary grafts need the mild but important compression of a properly applied stent to diminish capillary oozing. Sutures should be removed early and, if a hematoma is found, immediate replacement of any graft that has been lost should be performed to prevent granulation tissue in secondary healing.

Postoperative management involves primarily drug therapy designed to increase tissue collagenase kinetics and alter newly synthesized collagen so that it will be more susceptible to enzymatic degradation than normal collagen. Although there are a number of theoretical and some practical methods to reduce collagen synthesis, none have been approved for human use at this time except radiation therapy. Postoperative radiation has been used to try to prevent excess collagen deposition for many years. Undoubtedly there is a dose of radiation that in some patients will destroy just the right number of fibroblasts to balance the metabolic equation between synthesis and lysis. How such a dose could be estimated, much less calculated, defies imagination. Although some uncontrolled beneficial results have been reported through the years, one can only surmise at this time that the correct dose was a matter of luck or that other factors, including surgical technique and timing, also were responsible. Many complications, including malignancy, are associated wth radiation. In my opinion there is no place for the use of radiation therapy in the control of scar tissue in young people at this time.

Present pharmacologic control of excess scar tissue in healing wounds is based on two studies. The first study revealed that abnormally or poorly cross-linked collagen is more susceptible to lytic degradation than normally cross-linked collagen.[3] The second study showed that colchicine accelerated tissue collagenase kinetics in rheumatoid arthritis synovial tissue in tissue culture.[4] From these two studies it has been hypothesized that if newly synthesized collagen in a healing wound can be made simultaneously deficient in intramolecular and intermolecular covalent cross-links and if normal tissue collagenase kinetics can be accelerated, the ultimate amount of collagen incorporated into permanent scar should be reduced. Approximately 50 human patients with severe keloids have been treated according to this deduction; the results to date are encouraging.[12]

Reduction in the number of intramolecular and intermolecular cross-links in newly synthesized collagen is the basic pathophysiologic mechanism in an ancient disease known as *lathyrism*. Lathyrism was first observed during the great famines when people ate ground peas of the genus *Lathyrus odoratus*. The disease can be induced artificially by ingesting sweet pea seeds or by taking a purified product called β-*aminopropionitrile*. There are other powerful lathyrogenic agents such as penicillamine, which is also a copper chelator currently used in treatment of Wilson's disease. All lathyrogenic agents do not work exactly the same way, which opens the possibility for multiple drug therapy in the future.

Administration of β-aminopropionitrile fumarate (BAPN) presently is under control of the Federal Drug Administration (FDA) and requires an investigational drug permit. In pure form the drug is safe; there have been no untoward reactions since the first study in which impurities apparently caused a hypersensitivity reaction in six patients. No hypersensitivity or any other untoward reactions have occurred since the drug has been purified and prepared for human use by a leading pharmaceutical firm. Penicillamine has been approved by the FDA and can be obtained and prescribed without special permission. It should be remembered, however, that administration of penicillamine to control surface scar is not considered routine use of the drug. Informed consent should be obtained from the patient and clearance by local human rights committees obtained before the drug is administered for control of surface scars.

The time of administration and the dosage of lathyrogenic agents may be vital to successful use. Neither has been determined accurately at this time. FDA regulations limit the use of BAPN to 4 weeks at an oral dosage of 1 g/day in 250 mg doses every 6 hours. It may be possible to administer smaller doses of BAPN for longer periods without damaging normal connective tissue throughout the body, but because carefully controlled studies reveal that 1 month at the level of 1 g/day had an almost selective action on wound healing without signifcant measurable effect on normal tissue, present regulations limit use of the drug to that extent. BAPN cannot be administered to children at this time. The course of administration of lathyrogenic agents has been set to coincide with data from studies which show that the maximal rate of net collagen synthesis and deposition in a healing wound is between 8 and 28 days after wounding.

The dose of penicillamine is variable. People have different tolerances to the drug and about 30 days often is required to build up tolerance. Since neurologists have the most experience in administering penicillamine, it is advantageous to consult one when administering penicillamine to children. There have been no untoward reactions in patients with keloids treated with penicillamine. An arbitrary period of 3 months of drug administration has been carried out in studies to date.

The colchicine dosage for optimal stimulation of tissue collagenase activity is, of course, unknown. The only available data have been derived from phase I, or tissue culture, experiments. Phase II (animal) experiments in rats reveal that colchicine does stimulate tissue collagenase at physiologic doses, but no human studies have been conducted to determine the optimal dose and course of colchicine to stimulate tissue collagenase in a healing wound.[1] Because the drug is relatively safe and has been administered to human beings over long periods without serious side effects, it has been given for 6 months to patients with keloids. The dosage in previous sutdies was one tablet three times daily. Of course colchicine should not be started until epithelialization of the donor site is complete. Colchicine interferes with spindle formation in dividing epithelial cells and would be a serious deterrent to healing of the donor site.

Data from recent studies in which surgical removal of a

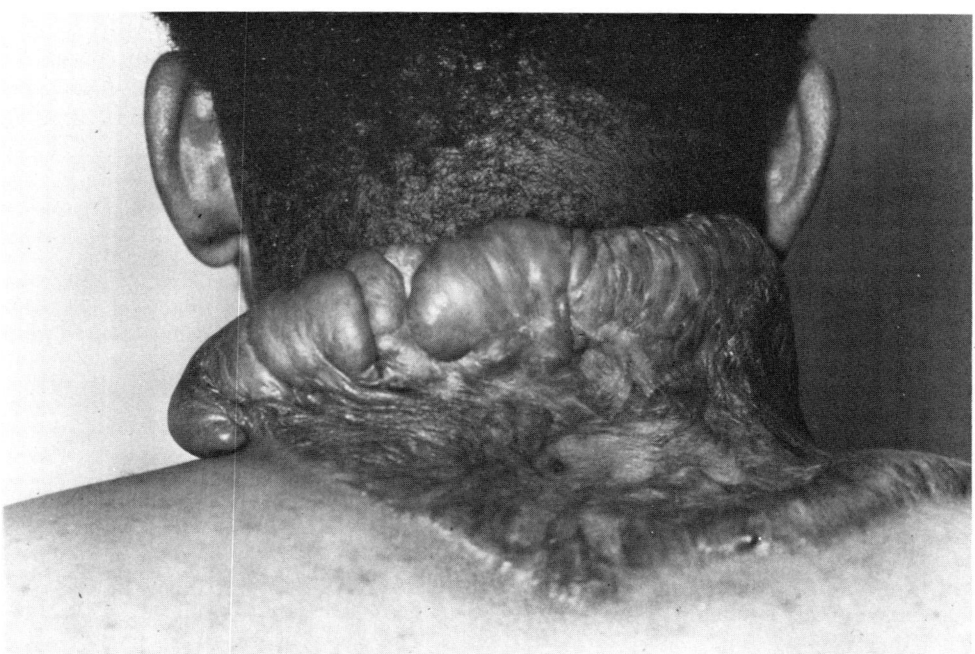

Fig. 10-6. Massive keloid in superior half of wound secondary to acne and sweat gland inflammation.

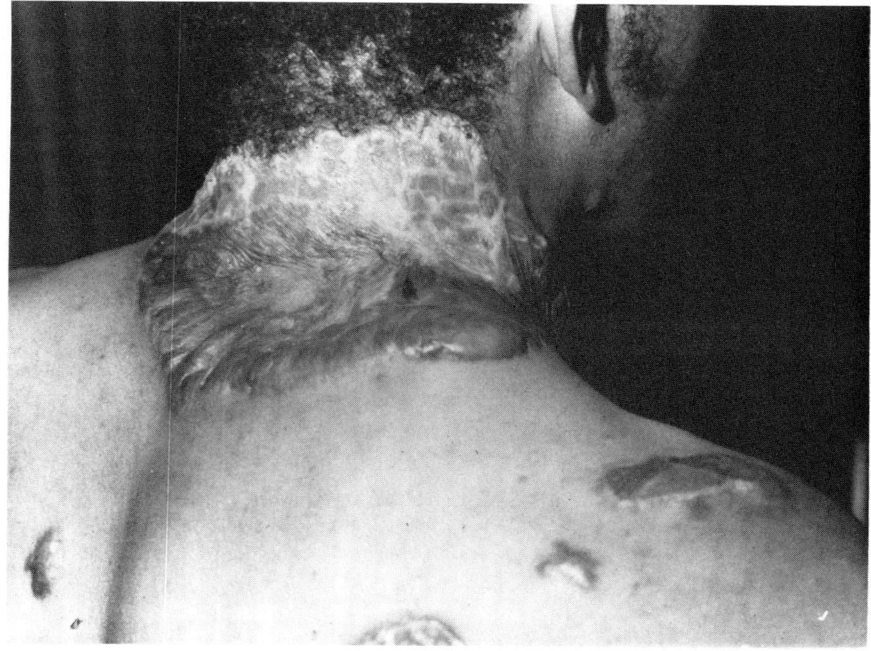

Fig. 10-7. Same patient as Fig. 10-6 2 years after postoperative treatment with BAPN and colchicine.

keloid followed by BAPN therapy beginning on the ninth postoperative day and continuing through the thirtieth postoperative day (or administering penicillamine starting on the tenth postoperative day and continuing for 3 months) and using colchicine for 6 months have been reported.[12] These studies can be summarized by stating that all patients improved—at least to the extent that a disabling verrucous keloid was converted into a moderately severe hypertrophic scar which did not cause physical disability (Figs. 10-6 and 10-7). No toxicity or untoward complications occurred from drug therapy, and there were no abnormal scars in donor sites (Fig. 10-8). It therefore seems that modern therapy

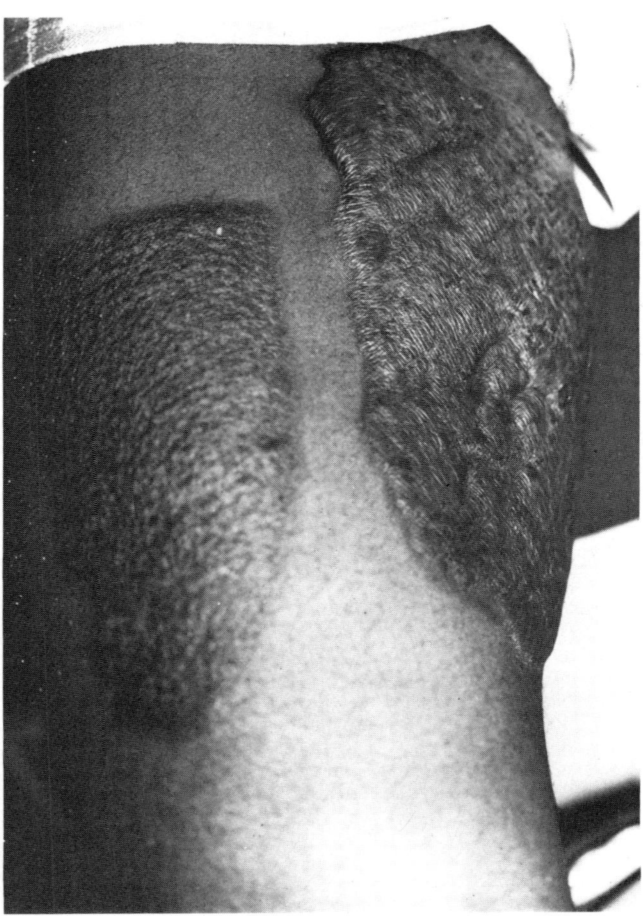

Fig. 10-8. Donor site with hypertrophic scar on right resulted from normal healing. Donor site on left healed under influence of BAPN and colchicine.

for keloids in children includes surgical removal of the lesion, resurfacing the area with a thin skin graft taken from the keloid or the buttocks, followed by a 3-month course of induced lathyrism with penicillamine and a 6-month course of colchicine to accelerate tissue collagenase kinetics. Studies have not been performed using similar treatment for hypertrophic scars. If a hypertrophic scar is significantly disabling, similar treatment might be justified, but for pure cosmetic reasons the results of pharmacologic adjuvant therapy do not seem adequate to justify taking two powerful drugs to control the appearance of a hypertrophic scar. Surgical revision and resurfacing according to the techniques described are probably the best that can be done for hypertrophic scars in children.

FUTURE CONSIDERATIONS AND CONCLUSIONS

The future holds much promise for the control of wound healing. It does not seem likely that acceleration of soft tissue healing will be possible even though the idea has been a favorite of many investigators for over 50 years. Actually, compared to the need to accelerate healing of osseous tissue, there is little need to accelerate soft tissue healing by formation of fibrous scar. Such processes as epithelialization, neovascularization, and aggregation of globular protein convey at least 100 g/linear cm of tensile strength to an experimental wound before any substantial amount or purposefully oriented collagen appears. Most patients have already left the hospital and usually have had sutures removed by the time scar deposition is a prominent feature of wound healing. Therefore from a practical standpoint there really is not much to be gained by increasing the tensile strength or accelerating the rate of gain of tensile strength 40% or 50% over normal values. Of course a 100% gain of tensile strength in a few hours or less (the spot-weld concept) would be of some value, and such a goal is not completely science fiction. As far as what cells can do in the way of multiplying, moving into proper position, cranking up protein synthesis machinery (rough endocytoplasmic reticulum), and discharging building blocks such as collagen and mucopolysaccharides, there is little likelihood of accelerating normal kinetics. The physiologic millieu for cellular function seems about ideal for maximal efficiency.[8] The concept of a spot weld therefore rests almost entirely on extracellular aggregation of already present building blocks rather than synthesis of new materials. Mature collagen, such as found in abundant quantity in dermal and fascial wound edges can be uncoupled and recoupled in laboratory preparations. Although present methods are too harsh to use in living patients, the concept that fascial or dermal integrity can be reestablished by depolymerizing or denaturing chemical cross-links in collagen followed by reaggregation to produce physical integrity with little or no seam remains theoretically possible.

The possibility that regeneration of compound tissue may be transiently regained, particularly in young patients, also is not science fiction. The knowledge that the architectural blueprint for organogenesis is present in the nucleus of all cells means that regeneration will not be impossible because the plans are not available. Undoubtedly totipotent germ cells are still present somewhere in the body, and the possibility that organ or area regeneration can be stimulated in mature human tissue by providing the proper cytoplasmic substrate remains viable even though there seems little probability now. Such discoveries as nerve growth factor, epithelial growth-stimulating factors, and electrical field stimulation are important early probes into the field of retaining or regaining some degree of regenerative capacity. The stimulation of bone healing and bone regeneration have been the most encouraging such studies.

It seems to me that the greatest rewards will come first in the ability to control physical properties of scar tissue and soon thereafter in the ability to control the amount of scar tissue. In all probability, similar to immunosuppression and cancer chemotherapy, success will come first from using multiple agents directed simultaneously at different stages in collagen metabolism. Antimetabolite drugs in low-toxicity doses have been used in animals to reduce some collagen synthesis and deposition.[17] Lathyrogenic agents such as penicillamine and BAPN are being used in phase III studies to block cross-linking simultaneously at multiple sites. Colchicine is being used to stimulate collagenolysis and anti–vitamin C agents and may be available for experimental use in the not too distant future. All such agents are toxic in large doses and probably will have to be used in conjunction with a number of other agents in small doses. The basic phase I and phase II experiments are now being moved into phase III (human) testing. The concept expressed so forcefully by Paré over a century ago, "I dressed the wound, God healed it," already can be modified significantly. Complete control over healing seems far from blasphemous in the decades ahead.

REFERENCES

1. Chvapil, M., Peacock, E.E., Jr., Carlson, E.C., et al.: Colchicine and wound healing, J. Surg. Res. **28:**49, 1980.
2. Diegelmann, R.F., Cohen, I.K., and Kaplan, A.M.: The role of macrophages in wound repair: a review, Plast. Reconstr. Surg. **68:**107, 1981.
3. Harris, E.D., and Farrell, M.E.: Resistance to collagenase: a characteristic of collagen fibrils cross-linked by formaldehyde, Biochim. Biophys. Acta **278:**133, 1972.
4. Harris, E.D., and Krane, S.M.: Effects of colchicine on collagenase in cultures of rheumatoid synovium, Arthritis Rheum. **14:**669, 1971.
5. Kassens, W.D., Jr., Tobin, G., and Peacock, E.E., Jr.: Preoperative induction of healing in skin wounds of rats, Surg. Forum **20:**60, 1969.
6. Knighton, D.R., Hunt, T.K., Thakral, K.K., and Goodson, W.H.: Role of platelets and fibrin in the healing sequence: an in vivo study of angiogenesis and collagen synthesis, Ann. Surg. **196:**379, 1982.
7. Madden, J.W., and Peacock, E.E., Jr.: Studies on the biology of collagen during wound healing. I. Rate of collagen synthesis and deposition in cutaneous wounds of the rat, Surgery **64:**288, 1968.
8. Peacock, E.E., Jr.: Production and polymerization of collagen in healing wounds of rats: some rate-regulating factors, Ann. Surg. **155:**251, 1962.
9. Peacock, E.E., Jr.: Some aspects of fibrogenesis during the healing of primary and secondary wounds, Surg. Gynecol. Obstet. **115:**408, 1962.
10. Peacock, E.E., Jr.: Variations in the amount of saline extractable collagen in skin distant to a healing wound, J. Surg. Res. **3:**250, 1963.
11. Peacock, E.E., Jr.: Control of wound healing and scar formation in surgical patients, Arch. Surg. **116:**1325, 1981.
12. Peacock, E.E., Jr.: Pharmacologic control of surface scarring in human beings, Ann. Surg. **193:**592, 1981.
13. Peacock, E.E., Jr., and Madden, J.W.: Some studies on the effects of beta-aminopropionitrile in patients with injured flexor tendons, Surgery **66:**215, 1969.
14. Raju, D.R., and Shaw, T.E.: Results of simple scar excision and layered repair with elevation of facial scars, Surg. Gynecol. Obstet. **148:**699, 1979.
15. Riley, W.B., and Peacock, E.E., Jr.: Identification, distribution, and significance of a collagenolytic enzyme in human tissues, Proc. Soc. Exp. Biol. Med. **124:**207, 1967.
16. Stopak, D., and Harris, A.K.: Connective tissue morphogenesis by fibroblast traction. I. Tissue culture observations, Dev. Biol. **90:**383, 1982.
17. Whitson, T.C., and Peacock, E.E., Jr.: Effect of alpha alpha dipyridyl on collagen synthesis in healing wounds, Surg. Gynecol. Obstet. **128:**1061, 1969.
18. Winn, H.R., Jane, J.A., Rodeheaver, G., et al.: Influence of subcuticular sutures on scar formation, Am. J. Surg. **133:**257, 1977.
19. Verzar, F.: The ageing of connective tissue, Gerontologia **1:**363, 1957.

CHAPTER 11

Cutaneous vascular lesions of children

JOHN B. MULLIKEN

Much of the confusion in diagnosis and management of pediatric cutaneous vascular lesions can be traced to a bewildering nomenclature. The word *hemangioma* has been applied to lesions that involute, never involute, and exhibit "malignant" behavior. The histologic term *cavernous* has been used clinically to describe lesions that predictably regress[39] and never regress.[1] Vascular lesions of lymphatic origin have been incorrectly called "lymphangioma" and "cystic hygroma," implying that they have the potential to grow and invade normal tissue. Hybrid and hyphenated terms, such as *lymphangiohemangioma* and *capillary-cavernous hemangioma,* further compound the confusion in the medical literature.

Studies of the endothelial features of cutaneous vascular birthmarks permit separation of two major categories. *Hemangiomas* are vascular tumors with increased endothelial turnover during the proliferative phase. *Malformations* are vascular anomalies with a normal endothelial cell cycle.[30]

A classification is justifiable only if it has diagnostic applicability, helps in planning therapy, and guides future studies of pathogenesis. Using this cell-based classification, the apparent myriad of vascular lesions becomes more understandable. Incorrect appellation of the word hemangioma can result in misinformation to parents about the potential for progression and, in some instances, to inappropriate management. Correct use of the terms hemangioma and malformation helps the clinician predict the natural history of lesions and choose proper therapy. Finally, this nosologic system is a guide to clinical and laboratory investigation of the pathogenesis of these lesions. Mast cells are associated with tumor angiogenesis and capillary migration.[3,34] These cells also are increased in proliferative phase hemangiomas and then fall to normal levels with involution. Mast cells are not elevated in vascular malformation tissue.[17] There are also in vitro differences between hemangiomas and vascular malformations. Endothelium derived from young heman-

giomas grows easily in tissue culture and forms capillary tubules, whereas endothelium from malformation tissue cannot be easily cultured and does not form tubules.[32] Recently, Sasaki and Pang reported elevated serum estradiol and increased tissue estrogen receptors in infants with hemangiomas. No evidence for hormonal markers was found in vascular malformations.[38]

HEMANGIOMAS
Diagnosis

Hemangiomas are the most common and most rapidly growing tumors of infancy. They are usually noted as a small red mark in 2.6% of newborns[22]; occasionally a large hemangioma is present at birth. The majority of hemangiomas first appear during the second to fourth week of life. By age 1 year, approximately 12% of children have a hemangioma with an equal frequency in premature and full-term infants.[20] Hemangiomas seem to predominate in white female infants and are uncommon in black children.

The hallmark of a hemangioma is an initial phase of proliferation followed by a slow, often protracted phase of involution (Fig. 11-1). The first sign can be an erythematous patch, pale spot, or localized telangiectasia surrounded by a pale halo.[19,36] Single, multiple, or extensive lesions can occur in any area of the body, but the head and neck region is the most common location. Hemangiomas that proliferate in the superficial dermis are bright red with a bosselated surface and are often raised from the surrounding skin. Hemangiomas also may grow in the lower dermis and subcutaneous tissue without involvement of the overlying skin. These lesions have a bluish hue or an entirely normal skin color. Hemangiomas may simultaneously proliferate in several areas of the body, for example, the gastrointestinal tract, liver, or central nervous system and lungs; this is called *hemangiomatosis.*[9] The histologic picture of a hemangioma in its growing phase is one of endothelial proliferation,

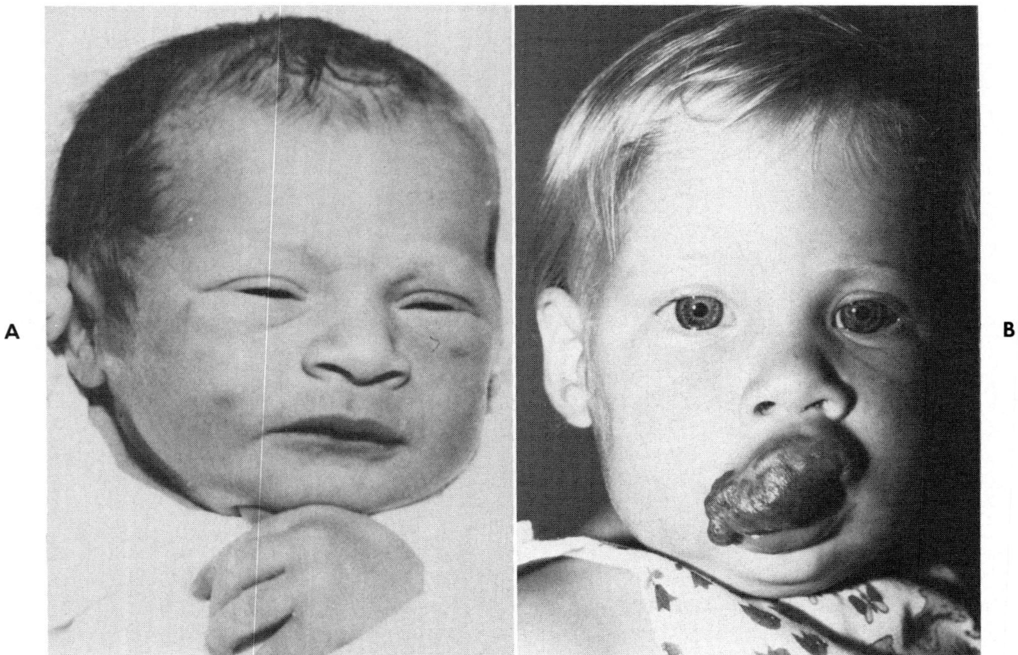

Fig. 11-1. Infant at 3 days (**A**) and 10 months (**B**) with a hemangioma of the upper lip. (From Mulliken, J.B., and Murray, J.E.: Natural history of vascular birthmarks. In Williams, H.B.: Symposium on vascular malformations and melanotic lesions, vol. 22, St. Louis, 1982, The C.V. Mosby Co.)

forming strands and syncytial masses with and without lumens.

Clinical course

Hemangiomas grow rapidly during the first year of life. Occasionally a lesion will proliferate to an alarming size and engulf the face (wildfire hemangioma). As the hemangioma grows beneath the epidermal basement membrane, minor trauma may cause repeated and annoying bleeding episodes. Spontaneous ulceration of the central portion of a rapidly growing hemangioma frequently occurs, particularly where the tumor is located just beneath the dermal-epidermal junction. DIC in association with extensive hemangioma was first reported by Kasabach and Merritt[23]; this is a rare but well-recognized entity.[40] There also are unusual instances of hemangiomatosis, widespread cutaneous and visceral lesions associated with high-output congestive heart failure. The mortality is reported to be 80% in untreated cases of this type.[6]

Hemangiomas usually enter an involution phase before the first 8 to 10 months of life. Several clinical studies confirm that complete resolution of hemangiomas occurs in over 50% of patients by age 5 years and in over 90% by age 7 years with continued improvement thereafter.[7,26,28,37] Conversely, a few hemangiomas show little clinical evidence of regression by this age. The earliest sign of involution is a fading of the original bright red color as the lesion takes on a deeper cherry red hue. Next the surface becomes covered with a grayish mantle and white flecks can be seen on close examination. The lesion becomes less tense and the involved skin becomes slightly wrinkled. These visible changes of involution seem to begin centrally with gradual centrifugal extension to the periphery of the lesion. On a cellular level involution is characterized by decreasing numbers of endothelial cells and diminishing cell turnover. Increased mast cells are still present during the early involution, but return to normal levels as involution is completed. Histologically involution is also marked by progressive and scattered fibrofatty infiltration of the parenchyma, with thin-walled vascular channels remaining in the areas previously occupied by proliferating endothelium. There is no histologic evidence for thrombosis or necrosis during involution.[30]

Some authors suggest that large hemangiomas are less likely to involute than small ones. However, experienced observers believe that the rapidity and completeness of regression are unrelated to the size of the lesion. It also is stated that deep subcutaneous hemangiomas involute more slowly than superficial lesions. This observation probably reflects our inability to monitor regression in these deep-seated lesions (Fig. 11-2).

Treatment

Fortunately, the natural process of involution is so predictable that the vast majority of hemangiomas should be allowed to regress spontaneously (Fig. 11-3). If ulceration

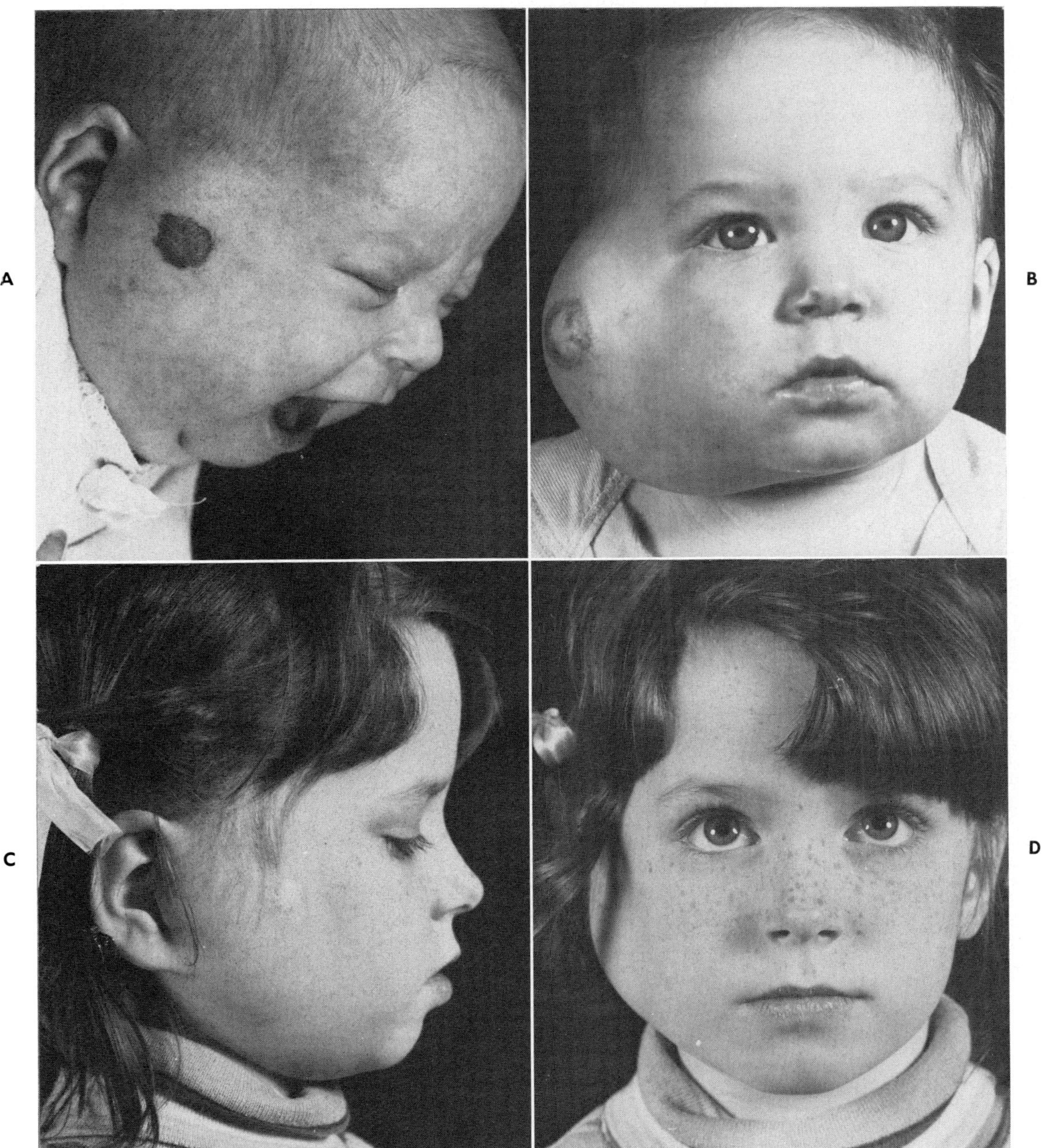

Fig. 11-2. A, Deep hemangioma of the right cheek with central superficial extension first noted at 1 month. **B,** Disproportionate growth occurs until age 1 year; signs of regression first seen in central area. **C** and **D,** Involution continues. Patient is 6 years old. (From Mulliken, J.B., and Murray, J.E.: Natural history of vascular birthmarks. In Williams, H.B.: Symposium on vascular malformations and melanotic lesions, vol. 22, St. Louis, 1982, The C.V. Mosby Co.)

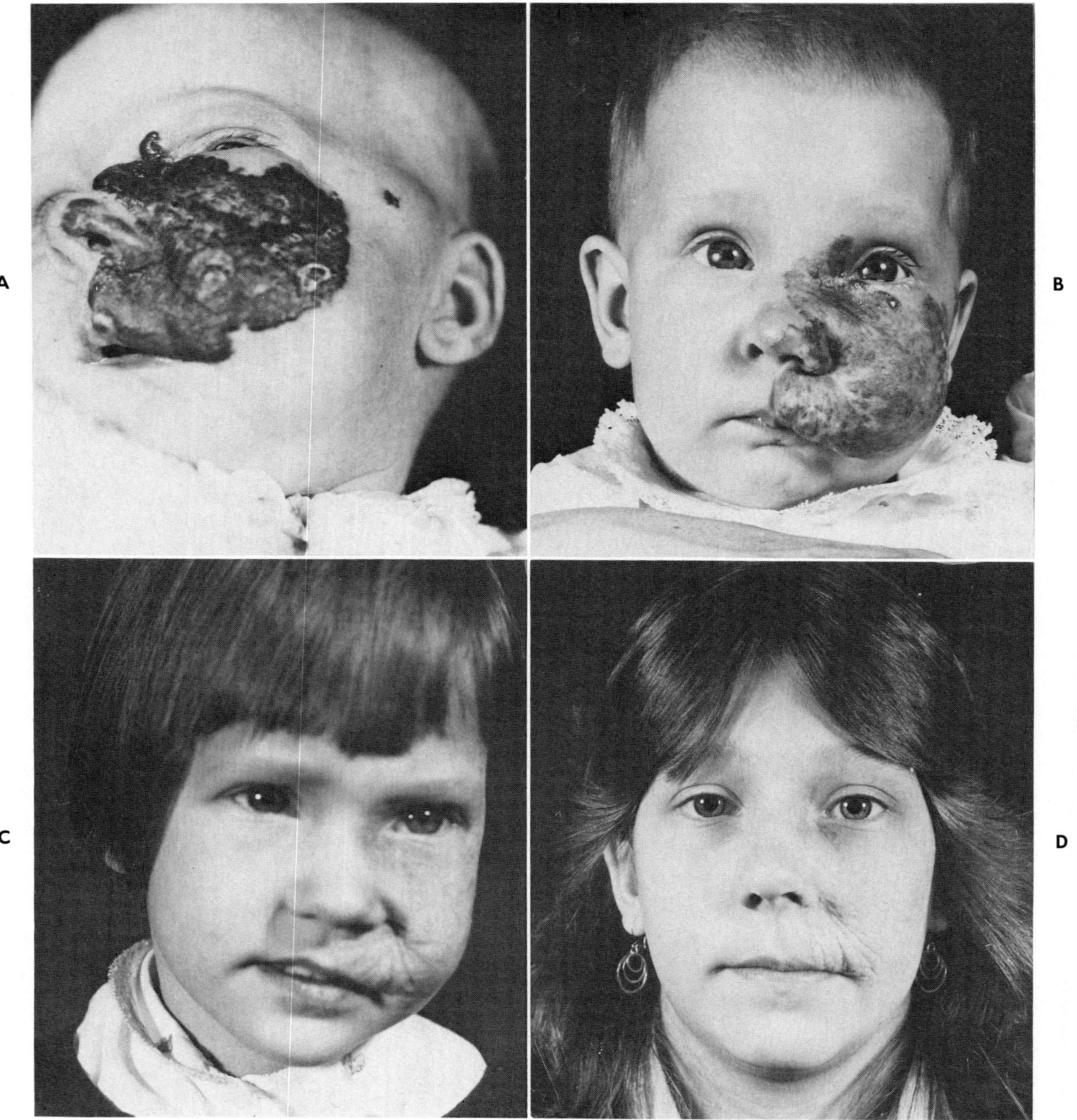

Fig. 11-3. This child appeared normal at birth. By age 2 months a hemangioma appeared on left side of face **(A).** No therapy was given. Same child at 1 year **(B),** 5 years **(C),** and 14 years **(D).** (From Mulliken, J.B., and Murray, J.E.: Natural history of vascular birthmarks. In Williams, H.B.: Symposium on vascular malformations and melanotic lesions, vol. 22, St. Louis, 1982, The C.V. Mosby Co.)

does occur, frequent cleansing and topical antibiotic application will ensure slow but predictable healing (Fig. 11-4). In rare instances bleeding and ulceration may be troublesome enough to necessitate steroid therapy.

Shrinkage of a large facial hemangioma coincident with systemic steroids was first reported by Zarem and Edgerton.[47] Subsequent investigators confirm that prednisone may accelerate the onset of involution in rapidly growing hemangiomas.[8,11] The response rate varies between 50% to 90% in published and unpublished reports. Systemic steroid therapy should be used only in selected patients: for example, a massive hemangioma distorting facial features, a lesion causing significant bleeding or ulceration, an upper eyelid lesion causing amblyopia, hemangiomatous obstruction of the trachea or external ear canals, or widespread hemangiomatosis causing high-output congestive failure.

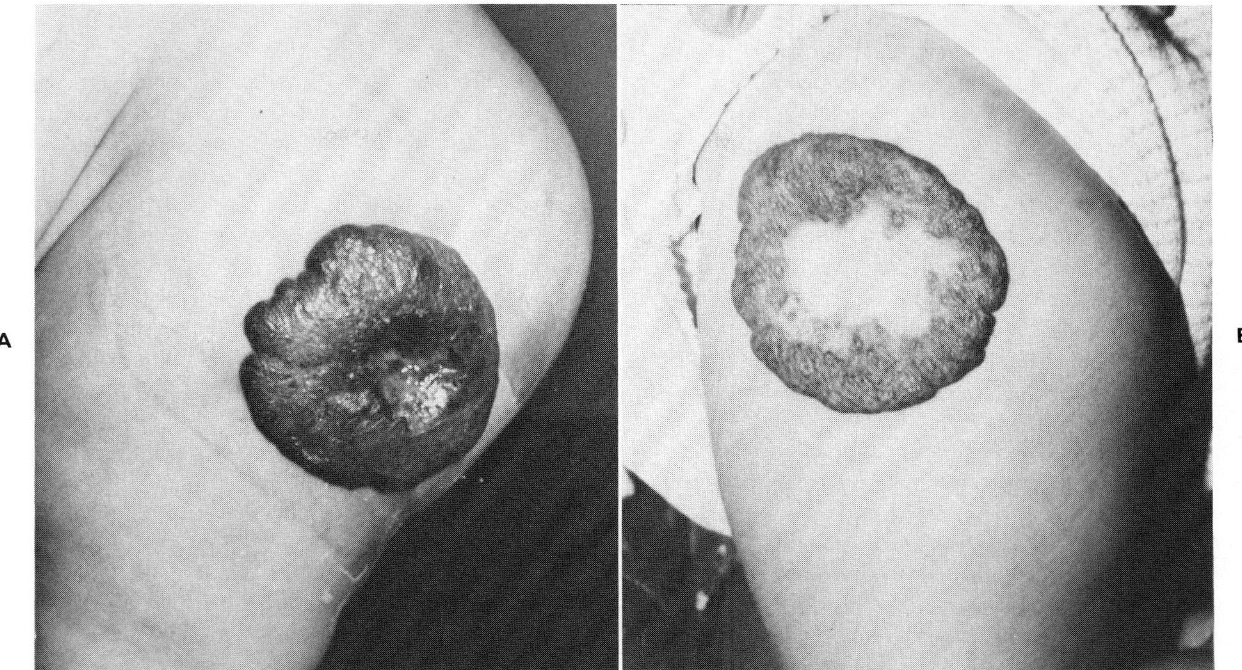

Fig. 11-4. A, Ulcerated hemangioma of the thigh in a 5-month-old child. **B,** At 1 year the central scarred area is still visible and involution is underway. (From Mulliken, J.B., and Murray, J.E.: Natural history of vascular birthmarks. In Williams, H.B.: Symposium on vascular malformations and melanotic lesions, vol. 22, St. Louis, 1982, The C.V. Mosby Co.)

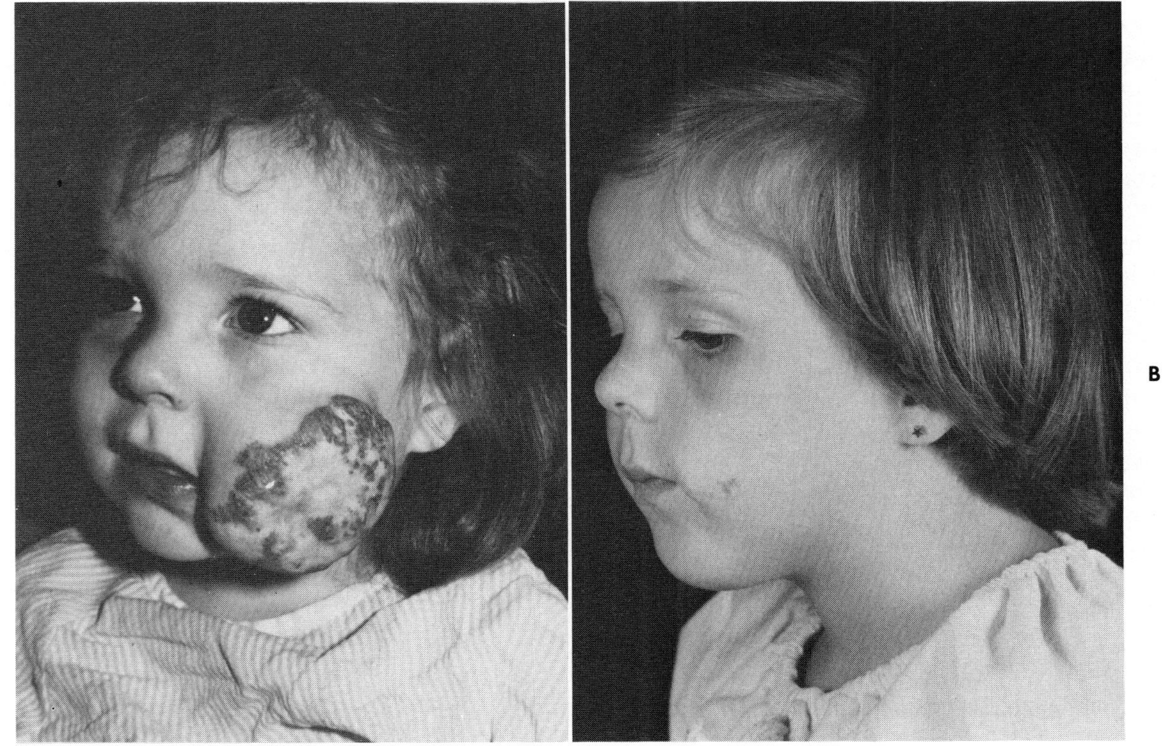

Fig. 11-5. This hemangioma began as a macular lesion of the cheek when child was 2 weeks old. Systemic prednisone was given for 6 months. **A,** At age 3 the hemangioma was excised because of psychologic problems. **B,** Result 1 year postoperatively.

Edgerton[15] emphasizes that treatment must begin when the child is less than 6 months of age; older hemangiomas are less responsive to steroids. The recommended dosage is 2 to 3 mg/kg/day given orally, for 2 to 3 weeks. If the lesion is sensitive, a response is usually noted within this time period and the dosage can be lowered to 1 mg/kg/day. Alternate-day regimens have been suggested to minimize possible systemic steroid side effects. The steroid dose should be tapered as soon as possible, depending on the response and maturity of the lesion. Rebound growth can occur at reduced steroid levels, and additional high-dosage therapy may have to be reinstituted. Complications, such as hypertension, salt and water retention, or permanent growth retardation, have not been clearly documented with this high-dose, short-course steroid regimen. Topical and intralesional steroid therapy for hemangiomas has been useful in some patients.[44]

In most cases, operative therapy of hemangiomas should be a contour excision of the fibrofatty residual tissue that remains after involution. In selected patients, however, early subtotal excision of a hemangioma may be necessary. For example, a localized lesion of the upper eyelid that causes amblyopia can be excised. Hemangiomas of the nasal tip notoriously cause psychologic problems.[43] Although lesions in this location do regress, albeit slowly, subtotal contour excision is occasionally indicated in the preschool years. Large pendant hemangiomas should be at least partially removed before a child goes to school. The excision should be kept within the lesion, and, if possible, with its axis along relaxed skin tension lines, care being taken not to excise too much tissue (Fig. 11-5).

Notwithstanding the excellent results after natural involution, prompt treatment of nascent hemangiomas would prevent potential anatomic and psychologic problems. There is no question that proliferative hemangiomas are exquisitely radiosensitive. However, radiation is not reasonable treatment for these benign tumors because of possible long-term sequelae, such as skin atrophy, hypoplasia of adjacent tissues, and the possibility of late tumor induction. There are scattered reports of the successful use of argon laser therapy for hemangiomas. The limited depth of penetration of the currently available laser beam and the potential for scarring in a child presently limit its usefulness for hemangiomas.

The common childhood hemangioma appears to be a problem of endothelial growth control. Only when the pathogenesis of this curious cycle of proliferation and involution is understood at a cellular level will truly biologic therapy be possible.

VASCULAR MALFORMATIONS

Vascular malformations are structural abnormalities that result from faulty morphogenesis of the embryonic vascular plexuses. By definition a vascular malformation is always present at birth, although the anomaly may not become obvious until early in the neonatal period. The growth of these lesions parallels the child's physical growth. There is no evidence that they proliferate by cellular hyperplasia or invade adjacent tissue.[30] Instead, hemodynamic and lymphodynamic characteristics determine the natural history of these lesions. Fortunately most vascular malformations are low flow capillary, venous, and lymphatic lesions. One type of abnormal vascular channel may predominate in a vascular malformation; however, frequently there are combined arterial, venous, and lymphatic components. The most worrisome lesions, arteriovenous malformations, contain fistulae and demonstrate high-flow characteristics such as pulsations, bruits, thrills, and increased skin temperature. These hemodynamically active lesions can expand with alterations in pressure or flow and with collateral formation secondary to trauma or attempts at operative therapy. Some malformations may enlarge by hormonal modulation during puberty or pregnancy or with estrogen therapy.

Port stains
Diagnosis

A port, or claret, stain is usually obvious at birth. They often occur in the distribution of the trigeminal nerve, or they may be diffusely scattered in geographic patterns over

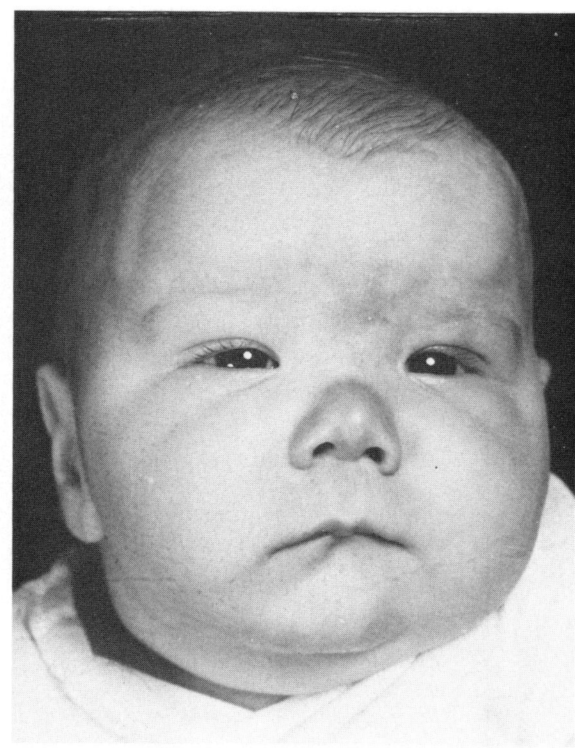

Fig. 11-6. A 2-month-old child with nevus flammeus of the glabella and left upper eyelid. These lesions predictably fade within 1 year. (From Mulliken, J.B., and Murray, J.E.: Natural history of vascular birthmarks. In Williams, H.B.: Symposium on vascular malformations and melanotic lesions, vol. 22, St. Louis, 1982, The C.V. Mosby Co.)

the trunk or extremities. Port stains are sharply demarcated and flat, but a pebbly or slightly raised surface can occur. On histologic examination numerous dilated capillary or venule-sized vessels are found in the superficial dermis with no evidence of endothelial proliferation.[30] Their characteristic pink color, seen in infancy, may lighten somewhat as the overlying skin thickens. The stain persists and deepens to a darker red hue with crying, fever, or increased environmental temperature. Port stains may be seen in combination with underlying venous or arteriovenous malformations. In rare instances a port stain may be a clue to a developmental vascular syndrome such as Sturge-Weber, Klippel-Trenaunay, or Beckwith-Wiedemann. There are localized port stain–like lesions with a verrucous surface that histologically exhibit hyperkeratosis; these are called *angiokeratomas.*

A very common vascular birthmark, *nevus flammeus,* may be confused with a port stain. This lesion, which occurs in one third of newborn infants, is also known as ''erythema nuchae,'' ''salmon patch,'' or ''stork bite.'' It consists of a macular, irregularly outlined area of pink intradermal staining, which despite its Latin name, is usually seen over the nasal bridge, glabella, eyelids, and nape of the neck (Fig. 11-6). These lesions tend to fade and disappear within the first year of life, leaving no residual evidence.[41] The nuchal patches fade somewhat more slowly than the anterior patches, and they can persist in adult life, only to become

obvious with blood pressure elevation, emotional episodes, or physical exertion. Nevus flammeus may be more of a physiologic phenomenon than a true dermatopathologic lesion.

Cutis marmorata is a rare type of vascular birthmark that also can be mistaken for port staining. Affected infants have prominent dermal veins and capillaries, giving their skin a mottled appearance. This cutaneous marbling effect is more pronounced when the infant is exposed to a low environmental temperature. It occurs in either localized or generalized distribution, the trunk and extremities being more commonly involved than the face and scalp. Almost all patients show steady improvement during the first year of life; however, the mottling may persist into adulthood. There are isolated reports of this disorder in association with defective growth of long bones and soft tissues and mental retardation.[42]

Clinical course

Port stains are permanent developmental defects. With time, the color usually darkens from pink to red to purple, and in adult years the lesion often becomes raised and nodular (Fig. 11-7).

Treatment

There is a long litany of attempts to erase port stains, including electrodesiccation, cryotherapy, thorium paste,

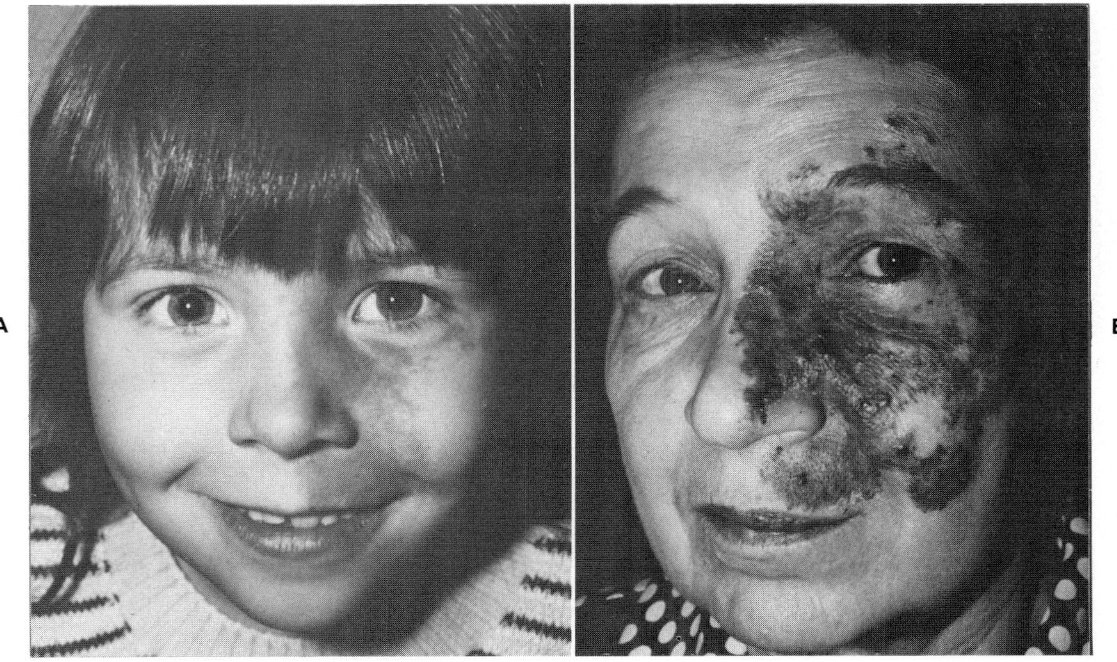

Fig. 11-7. A, Port stain located in the left trigeminal nerve distribution. **B,** In an adult a similar stain is a deeper color, raised, and nodular. (From Mulliken, J.B., and Murray, J.E.: Natural history of vascular birthmarks. In Williams, H.B.: Symposium on vascular malformations and melanotic lesions, vol. 22, St. Louis, 1982, The C.V. Mosby Co.)

and tattooing. Makeup can be used to hide the lesion but is objectionable to children, particularly little boys. In an older age group, excision and thick-splitness or full-thickness skin graft replacement can give satisfactory results, especially if the stain is deeply colored and nodular.[12]

Argon laser therapy for port stains is currently under investigation in several centers.[2,14,34,35] Noe et al.[34] believe that the color of the lesion, size of the anomalous channels, and patient's age are important determinants in predicting a successful result. He believes that the currently available argon laser should probably not be used to treat children, because they have pink staining, biopsy evidence of small channels, and a known tendency toward scarring, particularly in the central face (secondary to the thermal damage caused by the laser beam). Selected pediatric patients might benefit by laser therapy, but a biopsy and test patch should be done first.

Lymphatic malformations
Diagnosis

This type of vascular anomaly is often called *lymphangioma* or *cystic hygroma.* Cellular kinetic studies of these lesions demonstrate an exceedingly low rate of endothelial turnover; the suffix *-oma* is inappropriate. Since the lymphatics develop coevally with venous channels, combined venous and lymphatic vascular anomalies are common. These combined lesions are mistakenly labeled "lymphangiohemangiomas."

Lymphatic malformations present a wide spectrum of clinical findings from tiny, superficial mucosal or cutaneous blebs (lymphangioma circumscriptum) or solitary anomalies of the skin (lymphangioma simplex) to diffuse, cystic channels of the dermis, subcutaneous tissue, and muscle (lymphangioma cavernosum). Lymphatic malformations are commonly located in the head, neck, axilla, and groin; they may also occur in the mediastinum, mesentery, viscera, and bones. Extensive lymphatic malformations are often associated with hypertrophy of soft tissue, fat, and the adjacent skeleton.

Clinical course

Lymphatic malformations are typically low-flow vascular anomalies. They grow commensurately with the child. Superficial, dome-shaped, circumscribed vesicular lesions can bleed and may become infected, particularly when located in the oral mucosa, axillary folds, or perineum. Red blood cells frequently extravasate into these bleblike lesions. Cellulitis in a lymphatic malformation occurs frequently. Sepsis within a diffuse lesion of an infant oropharynx can cause airway obstruction (Fig. 11-8).

There are scattered cases reported of "regression" of lymphatic malformations.[18,45] Diminution of these lesions

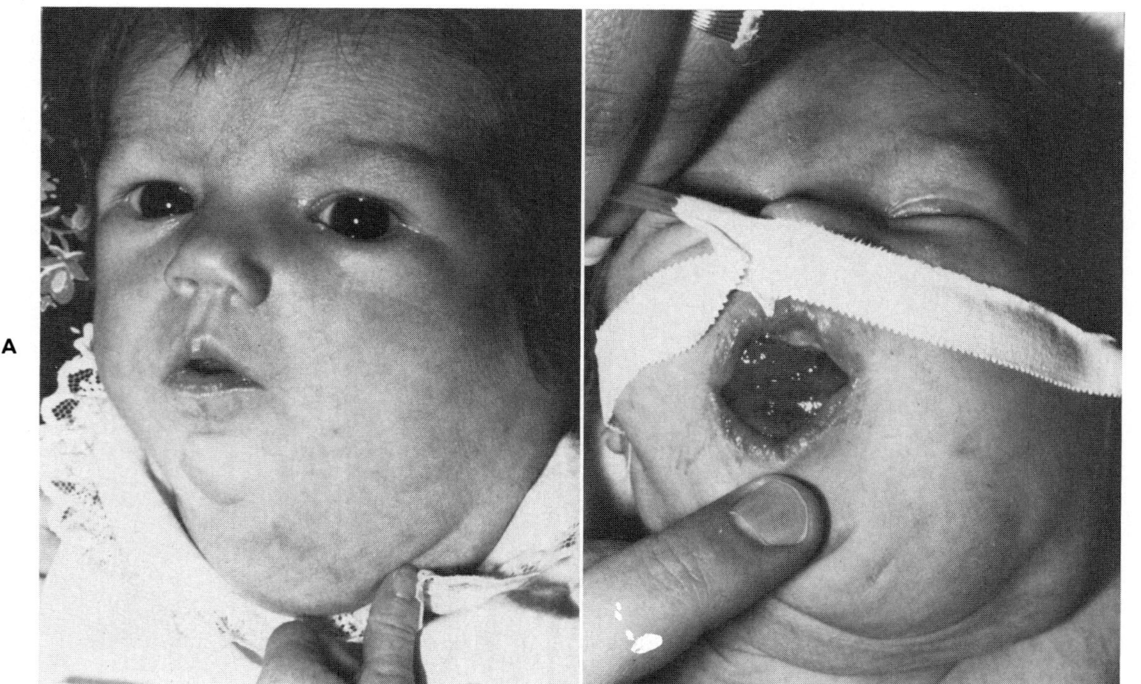

Fig. 11-8. A, Diffuse lymphatic malformation involving the left cheek, neck, and floor of the mouth in a 2-week-old infant. **B,** At 3 weeks the infant was admitted with cellulitis in the lesion and upper airway obstruction that necessitated intubation. (From Mulliken, J.B., and Murray, J.E.: Natural history of vascular birthmarks. In Williams, H.B.: Symposium on vascular malformations and melanotic lesions, vol. 22, St. Louis, 1982, The C.V. Mosby Co.)

may result from changes in flow via lymphaticovenous connections or possibly secondary to repeated bouts of inflammation.

Treatment

Cellulitis associated with lymphatic malformations usually responds to rest, elevation, warmth, and penicillin. Acute swelling of a lesion within the floor of the mouth may necessitate intubation. It is a good idea to keep a supply of penicillin in the home for prompt treatment of a lymphatic malformation that repeatedly becomes infected.

Well-localized lymphatic lesions can be totally excised (Fig. 11-9). However, all too often, these lesions are more extensive than they first appear, and excision is inadequate. The only therapeutic approach is staged excision with each procedure directed toward a defined anatomic area. Persistent serous drainage and hematoma formation are common complications after subtotal excision of a lymphatic malformation.

Venous malformations
Diagnosis

Cutaneous venous anomalies have a variable appearance from localized telangiectatic or large channel lesions to diffuse and extensive spongelike lesions. Venous malformations may be combined with capillary (port) stains or lymphatic or arterial anomalies. Pure venous anomalies, without arterial connections, grow commensurately with the child, with only a slight tendency to expand with age. In the head and neck region, venous malformations expand with the Valsalva maneuver. Venous malformations have a typical deep blue color, are easily compressed, and fill rapidly once pressure is released.

Clinical course

As long as arteriovenous connections are not open, venous malformations usually do not lead to life-threatening complications. These lesions may, however, expand with trauma, puberty, hormonal modulation, or attempted subtotal excision. Sluggish flow and turbulence within anomalous venous channels predisposes to thrombosis. Phleboliths can often be palpated or seen by radiographic study. Periodic localized pain and tenderness frequently occur in venous malformations of the extremities. These episodes may be the result of localized phlebothrombosis; classic thrombophlebitis also can occur in extremity venous lesions. There is some evidence that subtle coagulation defects occur in patients with diffuse venous malformations. In fact, the

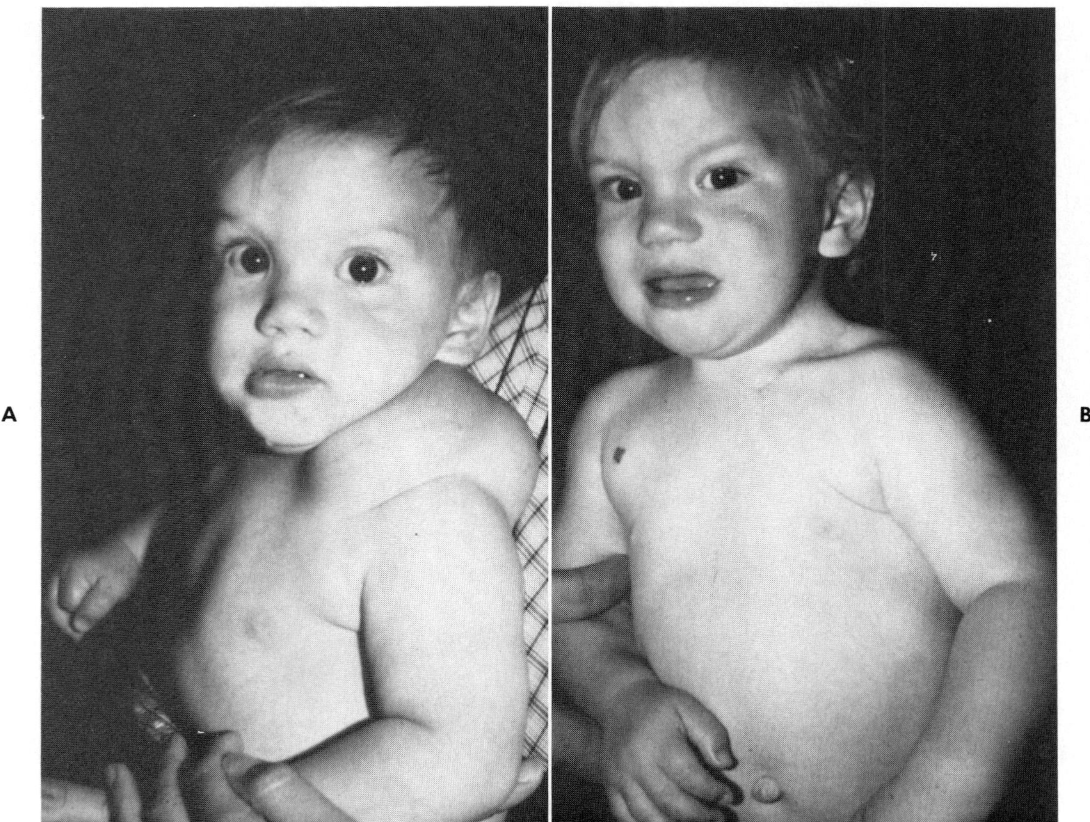

Fig. 11-9. A, One-year-old child with localized lymphatic anomaly of the left supraclavicular region. **B,** After excision incidental hemangioma of the chest was noted.

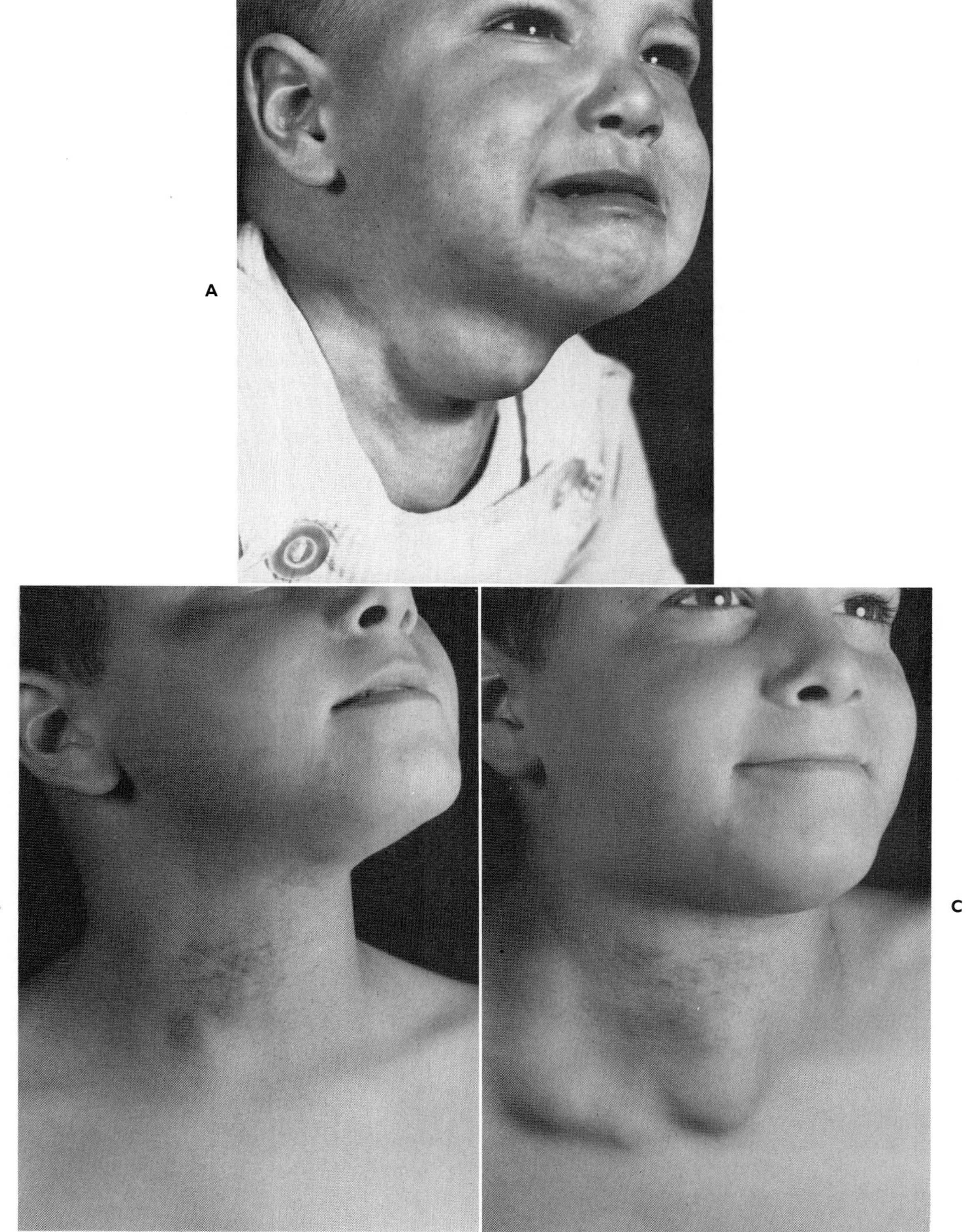

Fig. 11-10. A, Two-year-old boy with cervical venous malformation. **B,** At age 10, 5 years after excision, a superficial venous pattern is seen. **C,** Remaining lesions expands with Valsalva maneuver.

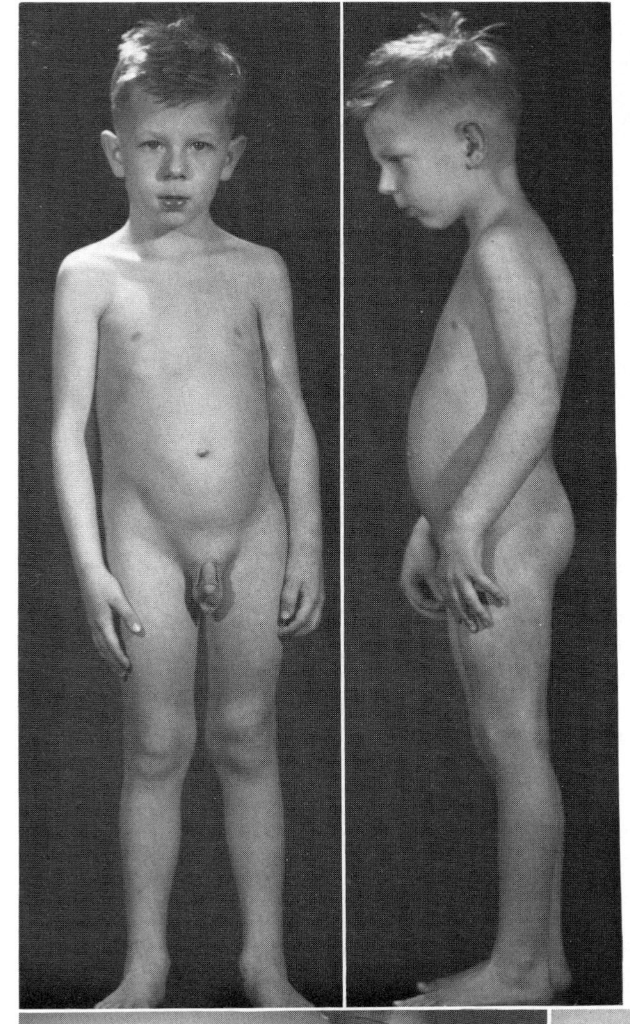

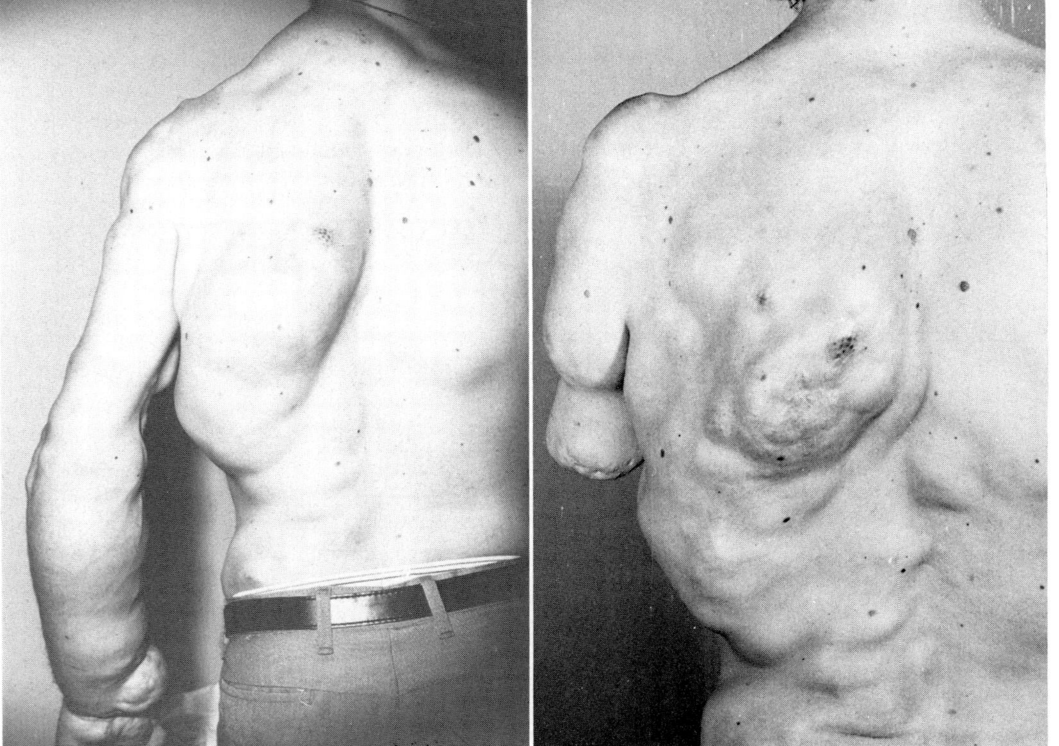

Fig. 11-11. A, Diffuse cutaneous vascular staining of the left side of the body. B, At age 15 the extensive arteriovenous malformation is obvious with associated DIC. C, Appearance after unsuccessful excision and heparin therapy. (From Mulliken, J.B., and Murray, J.E.: Natural history of vascular birthmarks. In Williams, H.B.: Symposium on vascular malformations and melanotic lesions, vol. 22, St. Louis, 1982, The C.V. Mosby Co.)

majority of reported cases of the Kasabach-Merritt syndrome are in patients with venous and arteriovenous malformations and not hemangiomas.

Treatment

Many localized and typically low-flow venous malformations are amenable to total or subtotal surgical excision (Fig. 11-10). The possibility of expansion of anomalous venous channels outside the operative field is always a potential problem with subtotal excision. Often these lesions are extensive and involve important anatomic structures in such a way that operative resection is impossible. Superselective angiography and arterial embolization are ill-advised for pure venous malformations. What is needed is a direct injection of a potent thrombosing agent that could somehow be confined within the lesion.

Arterial malformations

Diagnosis

Anomalies that demonstrate pulsations, increased skin temperature, and a bruit or thrill are arterial or arteriovenous lesions. These clinical signs of a high-flow state are usually unequivocal. Angiography is used to study the lesion's hemodynamics, particularly the pattern of artriovenous shunting. Angiography and CT scanning are both useful in delineating the anatomic extent of an arteriovenous malformation. Whereas venous malformations of the extremities are associated wtih hypoplastic lymphatics, extremities with arteriovenous fistulae demonstrate hyperplastic lymphatics.[25] In addition, low-flow lesions are associated with skeletal hypertrophy, and high-flow lesions are more likely to cause destruction of adjacent skeletal structures.

Clinical course

Arterial malformations are clinically labeled "unstable" because of their tendency to cause acute, often emergent problems. Expansion of such a lesion may be a precipitous event, for example, after trauma to the area, infection, or an attempted operative resection. Expansion may occur gradually and may be accelerated by hormonal changes, such as puberty, pregnancy, or estrogen therapy. In some patients increased cardiac output may progress to a state of high-output congestive failure. Arteriovenous anomalies of the extremities often result in ischemic necrosis of the distal limb. In lesions of the facial region frightening hemorrhage can occur after minor trauma or routine dental extraction. The treacherous natural course of these lesions is often only briefly interrupted by courageous attempts at resection, resulting in further tissue loss and "malignant" hemodynamic enlargement of persistent anomalous channels and collateral vessels.

Treatment

Therapy of an arteriovenous malformation is challenging, frustrating, and potentially as life threatening as the lesion itself (Fig. 11-11). Certain therapeutic principles have been learned from past mistakes. Whenever possible the entire lesion must be excised (Fig. 11-12). Residual anomalous vascular tissue at the margin of excision only invites further expansion. Numerous surgical disasters have taught us never to ligate "feeding" vessels proximal to an arteriovenous malformation. An underlying coagulation defect secondary to thrombotic consumption or destruction of clotting factors must be treated preoperatively.

Superselective angiography and embolization can be useful, particularly in experienced hands, such as the group led by Merland.[29] For some patients embolization alone can be therapeutic. For many patients, however, embolization can be considered only as a preliminary step to excision. Other maneuvers to minimize intraoperative bleeding include profound hypotensive anesthesia[33] and cardiopulmonary bypass with deep hypothermic circulatory arrest.[31] Hurwitz and Kerber[21] recommend that the defect after excision of an arteriovenous malformation should be reconstructed, whenever possible, with an axial or arterialized flap.

PYOGENIC GRANULOMA

Pyogenic granuloma is an acquired vascular lesion of childhood. It is a bright red polypoid growth that tends to crust and bleed easily with trauma. The lesions develop slowly, with occasional periods of rapid growth, until they reach several millimeters in diameter (Fig. 11-13). Histologically this lesion is similar to a proliferating phase hemangioma with newly formed capillaries in an edematous matrix. An infectious cause is implied by its name, but scientific basis for its pathogenesis is lacking. The lesion often occurs in sites of injury. The most common locations are the face and extremities.

Some lesions spontaneously undergo necrosis and regression. A pyogenic granuloma often has repeated episodes of ulceration, bleeding, and a history of unsuccessful topical therapy. It can be successfully removed by surgical excision. Electrodesiccation and argon laser therapy are also reported to be successful.

VASCULAR MALFORMATION SYNDROMES
Sturge-Weber syndrome

The Sturge-Weber syndrome consists of a port stain within the trigeminal nerve distribution and an ipsilateral vascular malformation of the leptomeninges either with or without calcifications, usually overlying the posterior parietal and occipital lobes. Port staining may also be present on the scalp, neck, trunk, and extremities, as well as intraorally.

Probably every child with a port stain in the trigeminal area should have an ophthalmic examination and skull radiographs, although only a small percentage will prove to have this syndrome. There is no strong evidence for genetic transmission of this condition.

Convulsions frequently occur in children with Sturge-Weber syndrome, and focal motor seizures are the most

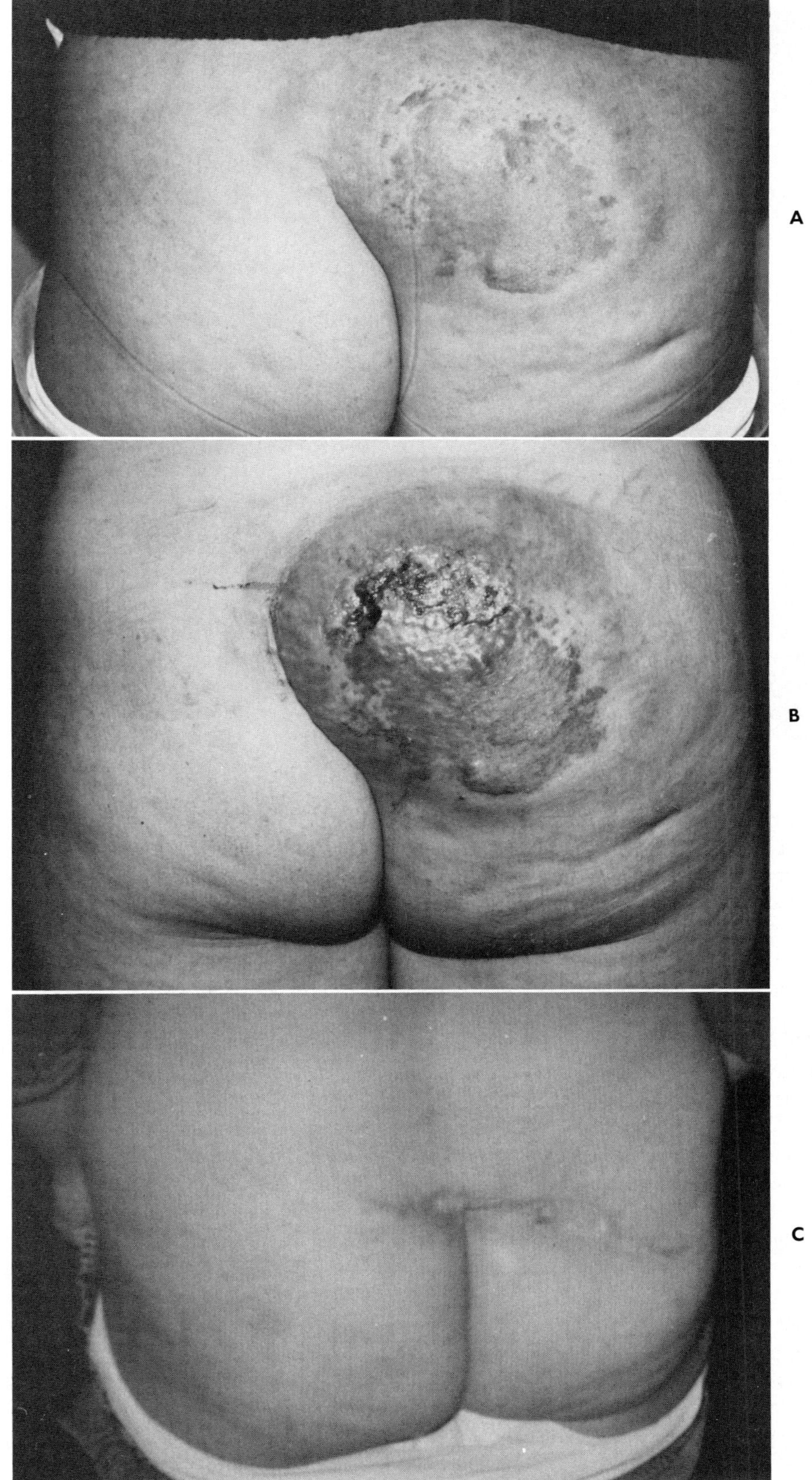

Fig. 11-12. A, Arteriovenous malformation of the buttock began to expand at puberty; at age 15 the lesion was warm and pulsatile. **B,** Months later there is ischemic ulceration of skin overlying the vascular anomaly. **C,** Appearance after wide excision, skin graft closure, and excision of the grafted area.

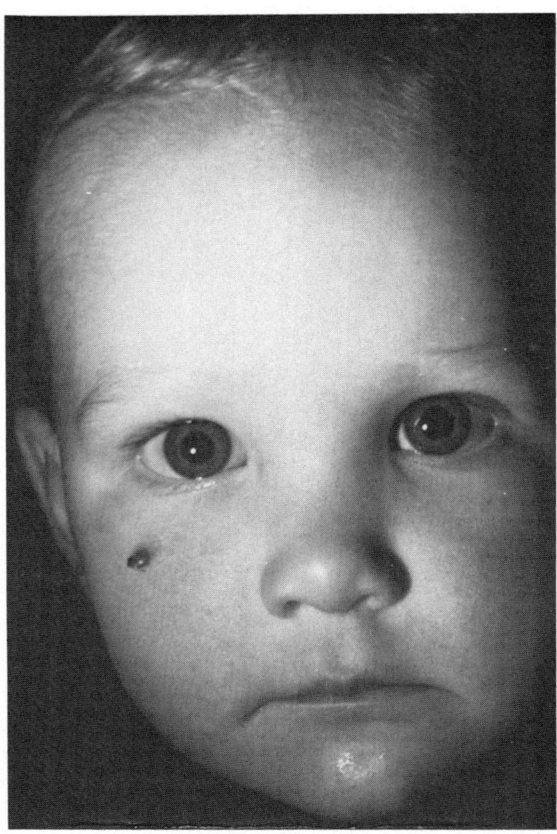

Fig. 11-13. Pyogenic granuloma of the cheek in a 1-year-old child; this lesion grew rapidly with repeated bleeding episodes.

common type. Hemiparesis and hemiatrophy, contralateral to the facial lesion, are less frequent findings. Ocular manifestations are common and include buphthalmos, glaucoma, choroidal vascular malformations, hemianoptic defects, and optic atrophy.[10] Anticonvulsant therapy and neurosurgical procedures can be of value. The prognosis depends on the extent of the intracranial lesion.

Klippel-Trenaunay syndrome

Involvement of an extremity with a patchy port stain and underlying combined venous and lymphatic malformations with associated skeletal hypertrophy constitute this syndrome. Arteriovenous fistulae are not present. Most often, it is seen in a single extremity, usually the lower leg; in some cases, both the ipsilateral lower and upper extremities may show typical anomalies. Bony overgrowth of the involved extremity is seen in over one half of the patients. However, in some patients, the involved limb may grow more slowly than the contralateral extremity.[46]

The superficial lymphatic blebs on the skin become infected easily, but will heal with topical therapy. Cellulitis may occur in the limb, presumably because of the deep lymphatic malformation component. Thrombophelbitis within the superficial and deep anomalous venous channels also can be a problem. Pulmonary embolism has been re-

ported in a patient with this vascular syndrome.[13] Custom-made elastic stockings provide symptomatic relief to these children, and elastic support may minimize dilatation of the anomalous vessels. The extremities must be observed closely for growth discrepancies, and appropriate epiphyseal stapling performed when necessary (Fig. 11-14).

Blue rubber bleb nevus syndrome

The blue rubber bleb nevus syndrome is a rare morphogenetic disorder, consisting of malformed vascular channels within the skin and bowel. The cutaneous lesions are sometimes present at birth, although they tend to appear throughout adolescence. The raised lesions are blue to purple in color, rubbery, and easily compressible. When blood is expressed from the bleblike lesions, the skin becomes a wrinkled sac. Still other lesions lie deep in the skin (Fig. 11-15). These malformed channels are also found in the gastrointestinal tract and may cause bleeding. These same lesions are also found in the liver, spleen, and central nervous system.[5]

Bowel lesions can be diagnosed with angiography; in some cases palliative resection of the involved intestinal segment may be necessary. The skin lesions can be painful or tender. Local subtotal excision can give symptomatic relief.

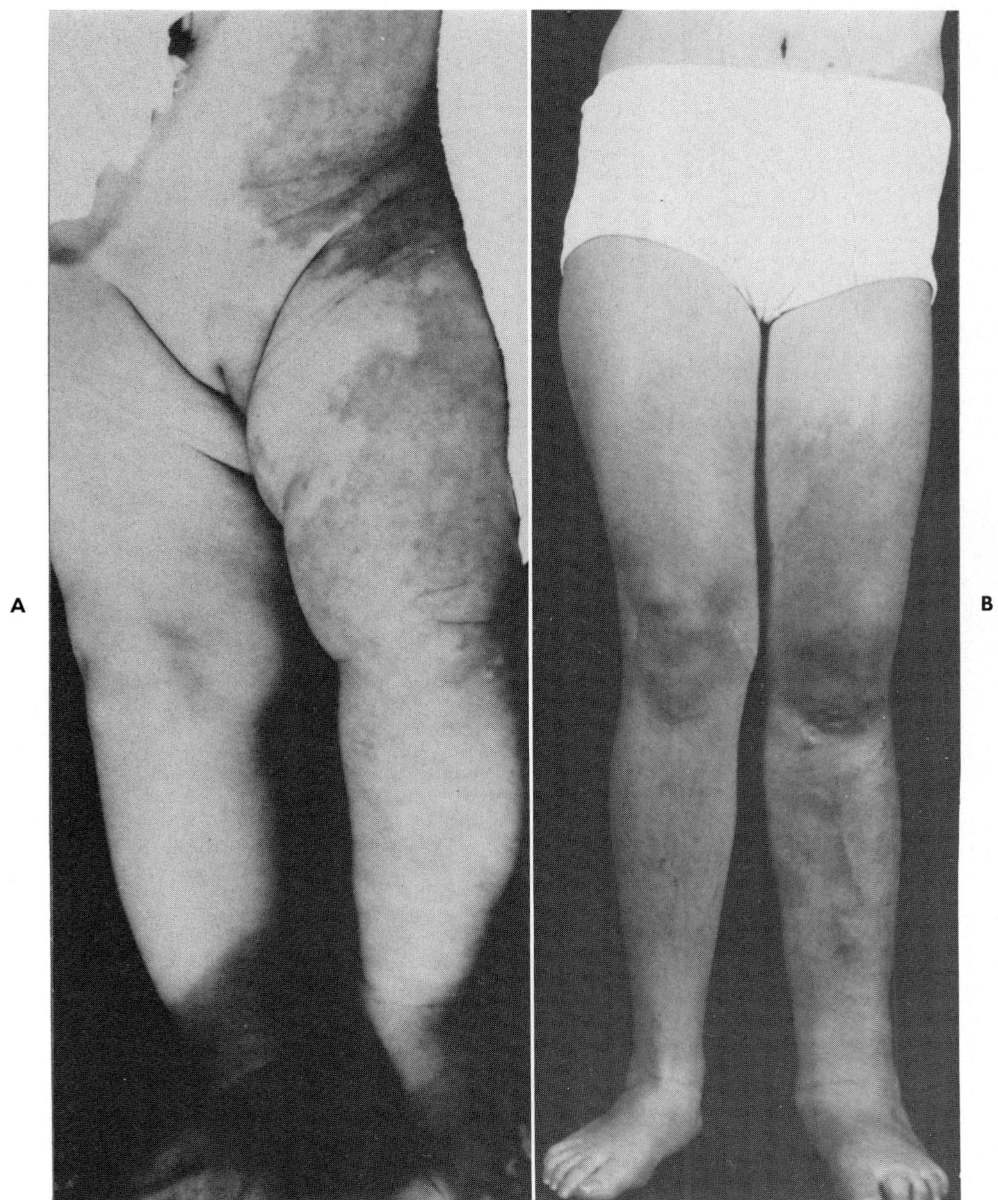

Fig. 11-14. A, Infant with dermal staining of the left lower extremity and flank with soft tissue enlargement, a combined venous-lymphatic malformation (Klippel-Trenaunay syndrome). **B,** At age 11, 2 years after contralateral distal femoral epiphysiodesis. (From Mulliken, J.B., and Murray, J.E.: Natural history of vascular birthmarks. In Willaims, H.B.: Symposium on vascular malformations and melanotic lesions, vol. 22, St. Louis, 1982, The C.V. Mosby Co.)

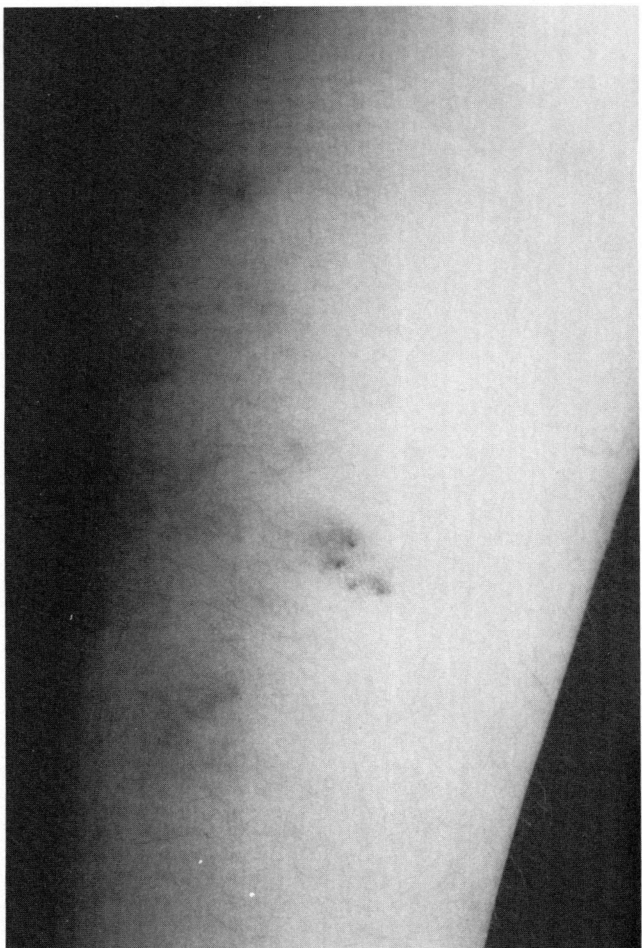

Fig. 11-15. Blue rubber bleb nevus syndrome in 8-year-old child. Child has painful vascular lesions of the forearm.

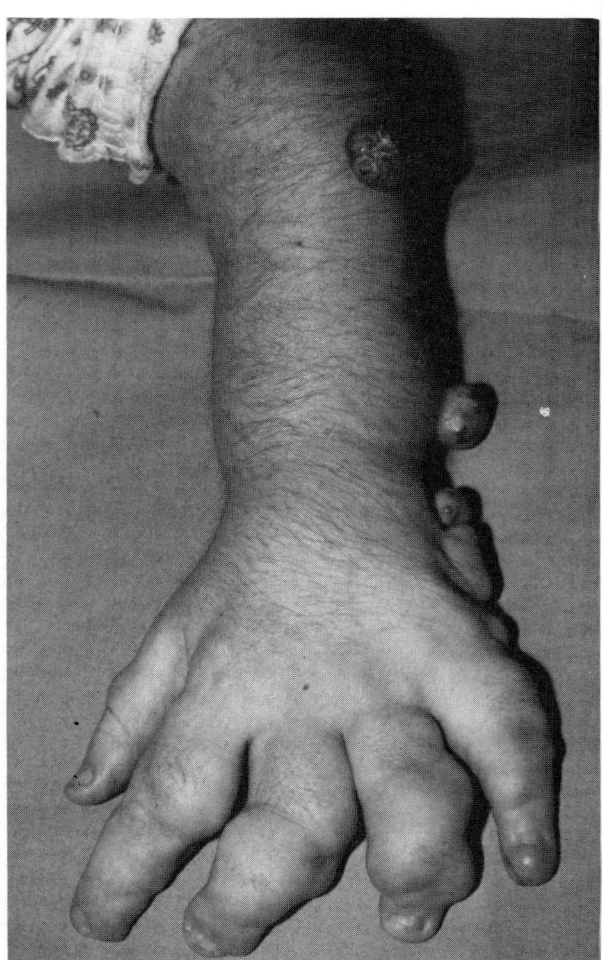

Fig. 11-16. Upper extremity with venous malformations and enchondromatoses (Maffucci's syndrome).

Rendu-Osler-Weber syndrome

The Rendu-Osler-Weber syndrome (hereditary hemorrhagic telangiectasia) is inherited in an autosomal dominant pattern. It is characterized by malformed ectatic vessels in the skin, mucous membranes, and viscera. The telangiectatic lesions often appear after puberty and increase in number with advancing age. Hemorrhage from lesions may appear as epistaxis, hematemesis, hematuria, or melena. Bleeding from telangiectasia in the brain or spinal cord can give neurologic symptoms.

Maffucci's syndrome

Malformed vascular channels in the presence of enchondromatosis constitute Maffucci's syndrome. The involved bones are usually shortened and deformed, with exostoses appearing on the fingers and toes, as well as on the proximal extremities. The vascular anomalies appear as localized papular or pedunculated lesions (Fig. 11-16). The distribution of the vascular lesions does not correspond to that of the skeletal lesions. Visceral vascular lesions also can occur.

Malignant tumors may develop in patients with this syndrome; chondrosarcoma has been reported in 20% of cases, and various intracranial tumors have been described.[27]

SUMMARY AND CONCLUSIONS

Studies of the endothelial features of cutaneous vascular birthmarks permit separation into two major categories: (1) hemangiomas are vascular tumors with increased endothelial cell turnover during the proliferative phase, (2) malformations are vascular anomalies with normal endothelial cell cycles. Mast cells are associated with tumor angiogenesis and capillary migration. These cells are also increased in the proliferative phase of hemangiomas and then fall to normal levels with involution. Mast cells are not elevated in tissue of vascular malformations. There are also in vitro differences between hemangiomas and vascular malformations. Endothelium derived from young hemangiomas grows easily in tissue culture and forms capillary tubules, whereas endothelium from malformations cannot be easily cultured and does not form tubules. Recently Sasaki and

Pang[38] reported elevated serum estradiol and increased tissue estrogen receptors in infants with hemangiomas. No evidence for hormonal markers was found in vascular malformations.

Hemangiomas are the most common and most rapidly growing tumors of infancy. They seem to predominate in white female infants and are uncommon in black children. The hallmark is an initial phase of proliferation followed by a slow often protracted phase of involution. Fortunately the natural process of involution is so predictable that the vast majority of hemangiomas should be allowed to regress spontaneously. If bleeding and ulceration occur, steroid treatment should be a consideration. Operative therapy for hemangiomas should be a contour excision of the fibrofatty residual tissue that remains after involution or early subtotal excision of a localized lesion, such as a lesion of the upper eyelid or nasal tip.

Vascular malformations are structural abnormalities that result from faulty morphogenesis of the embryonic vascular plexuses. By definition a vascular malformation is always present at birth. These lesions grow commensurately with the child. There is no evidence that they proliferate by cellular hyperplasia or invade adjacent tissue. Hemodynamic and lymphodynamic characteristics determine the natural history of these lesions. Fortunately most vascular malformations are low flow. High-flow malformations can be extremely destructive and often pose a treatment dilemma for the reconstructive surgeon.

Throughout the course of this chapter specific vascular malformations are discussed, as well as those malformations seen in recognized syndromes. Treatment is detailed and individualized.

Using the present system of classification an apparent myriad of vascular lesions becomes more understandable. This system is useful because it has diagnostic applicability, helps in planning therapy, and guides future studies of pathogenesis.

REFERENCES

1. Andrews, G.C., Domokos, A.N., Torres-Rodrigues, V.M., and Bembenista. J.K.: Hemangiomas—treated and untreated, J.A.M.A. **165**:1114, 1957.
2. Apfelberg, D.B., Maser, M.R., and Lash, H.: Argon laser treatment of cutaneous vascular abnormalities: progress report, Ann. Plast. Surg. **1**:14, 1978.
3. Azizkhan, R.G., Azizkhan, J.C., Zetter, B.R., and Folkman, J.: Mast cell heparin stimulates migration of capillary endothelial cells in vitro, J. Exp. Med. **152**:931, 1980.
4. Azzolini, A., Bertani, A., and Riberti, C.: Superselective embolization and immediate surgical treatment: our present approach to treatment of large vascular hemangiomas of the face, Ann. Plast. Surg. **9**:42, 1982.
5. Belsheim, M.R., and Sullivan, S.N.: Blue rubber bleb nevus syndrome, Can. J. Surg. **23**:274, 1980.
6. Berman, B., and Lim, H.W.P.: Concurrent cutaneous and hepatic hemangiomata in infancy: report of a case and a review of the literature, J. Dermatol. Surg. Oncol. **4**:869, 1978.
7. Bowers, R.E., Graham, E.A., and Tomlinson, K.M.: The natural history of the strawberry nevus, Arch. Dermatol. **82**:667, 1960.
8. Brown, S.H., Neerhaut, R.C., and Fonkalsrud, E.W.: Prednisone therapy in management of large hemangiomas in infants and children, Surgery **71**:168, 1972.
9. Burke, E.C., Winkleman, R.K., and Strickland, M.K.: Disseminated hemangiomatosis, Am. J. Dis. Child. **108**:418, 1964.
10. Chao, D.H.C.: Congenital neurocutaneous syndromes of childhood. III. Sturge-Weber disease, J. Pediatr. **56**:635, 1959.
11. Clemmensen, O.: A case of multiple neonatal hemangiomatoses successfully treated by systemic corticosteroids, Dermatologica **159**:495, 1979.
12. Clodius, L.: Excision and grafting of extensive facial hemangiomas, Br. J. Plast. Surg. **30**:185, 1977.
13. Cole, D.J., Sood, S.C., and Broomhead, I.W.: Pulmonary embolism associated with hemolymphangioma of lower extremity, Plast. Reconstr. Surg. **63**:265, 1979.
14. Cosman, B.: Experience in the argon laser therapy of port-wine stains, Plast. Reconstr. Surg. **65**:119, 1980.
15. Edgerton, M.T.: The treatment of hemangiomas, with special reference to the role of steroid therapy, Ann. surg. **183**:517, 1976.
16. Fost, N.C., and Easterly, N.B.: Successful treatment of juvenile hemangiomas with prednisone, J. Pediatr. **72**:351, 1968.
17. Glowacki, J., and Mulliken, J.B.: Mast cells in hemangiomas and vascular malformations, Pediatrics **70**:48, 1982.
18. Grabb, W.C., Dingman, R.O., O'Neal, R.M., and Dempsey, P.D.: Facial hamartomas in children: neurofibroma, lymphangioma, and hemangioma, Plast. Reconstr. Surg. **66**:509, 1980.
19. Hidano, A., and Nakajima, S.: Earliest features of the strawberry mark in the newborn, Br. J. Dermatol. **87**:138, 1972.
20. Holmdahl, K.: Cutaneous hemangiomas in premature and mature infants, Acta Paediatr. **44**:370, 1955.
21. Hurwitz, D.J., and Kerber, C.W.: Hemodynamic considerations in the treatment of arteriovenous malformations of the face and scalp, Plast. Reconstr. Surg. **67**:421, 1981.
22. Jacobs, A.J.: The incidence of birthmarks in the neonate, Pediatrics **58**:218, 1976.
23. Kasabach, H.H., and Merritt, K.K.: Capillary hemangioma with extensive purpura: report of a case, Am. J. Dis. Child. **59**:1063, 1940.
24. Kessler, D.A., Langer, R.S., Pless, N.A., and Folkman, J.: Mast cells and tumor angiogenesis, Int. J. Cancer **18**:703, 1976.
25. Kinmonth, J.B., Young, A.E., Edwards, J.M., et al.: Mixed vascular deformities of the lower limbs, with particular reference to lymphography and surgical management, Br. J. Surg. **63**:899, 1976.
26. Lister, W.A.: The natural history of strawberry nevi, Lancet **1**:1429, 1938.
27. Loewinger, R.J., Lichtenstein, J.R., Dodson, W.E., and Eisen, A.Z.: Maffucci's syndrome: a mesenchymal dysplasia and multiple tumor syndrome, Br. J. Dermatol. **96**:317, 1977.
28. Margileth, A.M., and Museles, M.: Cutaneous hemangiomas in children, J.A.M.A. **194**:523, 1965.
29. Merland, J.J., Tricot, J.F., Hadjean, E., et al.: Cervicocephalic vascular malformations: current protocol. Report of 230 cases, Phlebologie **33**:95, 1980.
30. Mulliken, J.B., and Glowacki, J.: Hemangiomas and vascular malformations in infants and children: a classification based on endothelial characteristics, Plast. Reconstr. Surg. **69**:412, 1982.
31. Mulliken, J.B., Murray, J.E., Castaneda, A.R., and Kaban, L.B.: Management of a vascular malformation of the face using total circulatory arrest, Surg. Gynecol. Obstet. **146**:168, 1978.
32. Mulliken, J.B., Zetter, B.R., and Folkman, J.: In vitro characteristics of endothelium from hemangiomas and vascular malformations, Surgery **92**:348, 1982.
33. Munro, I.R., and Martin, R.D.: The management of gigantic benign craniofacial tumors: the reverse facial osteotomy, Plast. Reconstr. Surg. **65**:777, 1980.
34. Noe, J.M., Barsky, S.H., Geer, D.E., and Rosen, S.: Port-wine stains and the response to argon laser therapy: successful treatment and the predictive role of color, age, and biopsy, Plast. Reconstr. Surg. **65**:130, 1980.
35. Ohmori, S., and Huang, C.K.: Recent progress in the treatment of portwine staining by argon laser: some observations on the prognostic value of relative spectroreflectance (RSR) and histologic classification of the lesions, Br. J. Plast. Surg. **34**:249, 1981.

36. Payne, M.M., Moyer, F., Marcks, K.M., and Trevaskis, A.E.: The precursor to the hamangioma, Plast. Reconstr. Surg. **38:**64, 1966.
37. Pratt, A.G.: Birthmarks in infants, Arch. Dermatol. **67:**302, 1967.
38. Sasaki, G.H., and Pang, C.Y.: Role of hormone in the pathogenesis of infant skin strawberry hemangiomas. Presented at the twenty-seventh annual meeting of the Plastic Surgery Research Council, March 16, 1982, San Diego.
39. Simpson, J.R.: The natural history of cavernous haemangiomas, Lancet **2:**1057, 1959.
40. Shim, W.K.T.: Hemangiomas of infancy complicated by thrombocytopenia, Am. J. Surg. **116:**896, 1968.
41. Smith, M.A., and Manfield, P.A.: The natural history of salmon patches in the first year, Br. J. Dermatol. **74:**31, 1962.
42. South, D.A., and Jacobs, A.H.: Cutis marmorata telangiectatica (congenital generalized phlebectasia), J. Pediatr. **93:**944, 1978.
43. Thomson, H.G., and Lanigan, H.: The Cyrano nose: a clinical review or hemangiomas of the nasal tip, Plast. Reconstr. Surg. **63:**155, 1979.
44. Weber, G.: The treatment of cavernous hemangioma with topical betamethasone 17-valerate, Br. J. Dermatol. **89:**648, 1973.
45. Williams, H.B.: Facial bone changes with vascular tumors in children, Plast. Reconstr. Surg. **63:**309, 1979.
46. Young, A.E.: Congenital mixed vascular deformities of the limbs and their associated lesions, Birth Defects **14:**289,1978.
47. Zarem, H.A., and Edgerton, M.T.: Induced resolution of cavernous hemangiomas following prednisolone therapy, Plast. Reconstr. Surg. **39:**76, 1967.

CHAPTER 12

Microsurgical composite tissue transplantation in children

DONALD SERAFIN and WILLIAM J. BARWICK

In this chapter we will attempt to define and explore those factors which are unique to the microsurgical transplantation of composite tissue in children. Are the vascular anatomy and histology in children similar to those found in adults? Is there a specific tolerance to hypoxia and anoxia peculiar to infants and children? Are patency rates after microvascular anastomoses lower in infants and children because of technical difficulties related to size or are other factors involved? After transplantation how are growth and function affected in transplanted tissue? What is the current status of allogeneic transplantation of composite tissue and organs in children and what does the future hold? Although answers are not always apparent, we will define the problems of tissue transplantation with the hope that future investigators will be able to provide much needed solutions.

BLOOD VESSELS
Arteries

Morphologic and histologic differences exist between arteries of varying sizes at any age. Arteries may be classified as small (arterioles); medium, and large.[14] Medium-sized arteries are the radial, brachial, anterior tibial, peroneal, posterior tibial arteries, and dorsal artery of the foot. Large arteries include the aorta, carotid, subclavian, and iliac arteries. In general the histologic appearance of an artery reflects its function. As blood is ejected from the heart in systole, much of the kinetic energy in the large arteries is transformed into potential energy by the elastic tissue of the vessel wall. This permits continued perfusion of distal parts with less pulsatile flow during diastole. Peripheral arteries in the limbs, in contrast, have a greater role in distributing arterial blood flow to various muscle and skin compartments.[14] This is reflected in the presence of a significant muscular layer. The arterial tree is a continuum with a gradation of the various histologic types present along its extent.

The *intima* of medium-sized arteries consists of three layers: (1) endothelium, (2) intermediate layer, and (3) internal elastic lamina.[14] The long axes of endothelial cells usually are arranged longitudinally along the vessel. The intermediate layer consists of delicate collagenous fibers and a few connective tissue fibers embedded in the connective tissue matrix. Isolated longitudinal muscle fibers are located in this layer, especially where branching occurs. The internal elastic lamina consists of closely interwoven elastic fibers.

The *media* of medium-sized arteries consists primarily of smooth muscle cells that are arranged in a circular fashion. Large arteries such as the aorta have a preponderance of elastic fibers arranged in a spiral fashion.[14] The walls of these vessels are thin compared to their diameter. This is a result of an increase in elastic tissue and a decrease in smooth muscle cells.

The *adventitia* in medium-sized arteries may be as thick as the media. It consists of collagenous and elastic fibers arranged longitudinally. There is a concentration of elastic fibers at the junction between the media and adventitia called the *external elastic lamina*. The vasa vasorum is located in the adventitia. A limited number of studies are available indicating changes noted in medium- or large-sized arteries with respect to age.

In newborns the intima and media of medium-sized arteries are quite thin (28 to 56 μm). At 3 to 4 years of age these layers become thicker (69 to 127 μm), primarily by development of longitudinal muscle fibers in the intima and circular muscle fibers in the media.[57]

The intima in newborns is quite thin (6 to 8 μm) but increases with age.[57] In 3- to 4-year-olds it is not fully developed, and its average thickness does not exceed 20 μm. Both the media and intima increase in size until adult thicknesses are reached by age 19. With increasing age the arterial wall becomes thicker, primarily in the intimal layer. In persons from 81 to 88 years, the intima is usually thicker than the media.

Early reports indicated that the vasa vasorum was confined to the adventitia in medium-sized limb arteries.[32] Vancov,[56,57] however, has demonstrated that the depth of penetration of these intramural capillaries depends on the thickness of the arterial wall (especially the intima) rather than the location of the medium-sized artery. No vascularization of the media was demonstrated in individuals under 20 years of age with vessels of normal thickness. Vascular penetration into the outer third of the media was noted in older patients with a notably thickened intima. The cause is still obscure. One could postulate that intimal changes, manifested histologically by thickening, act as a diffusion barrier from the vessel lumen. The media, particularly its outer third, is most affected by hypoxia. Neovascular mediating substances (prostaglandins) may act as the stimulus for ingrowth of capillaries from the vasa vasorum of the adventitia.[4]

Elastin fragmentation, fibrosis, and medionecrosis are changes seen in the media of the aorta with advancing age.[46] These changes are believed to represent the morphologic expression of injury and repair secondary to hemodynamic impact. Children under 20 years of age demonstrate minimal changes. In fact, the elastic layers within the media of the aorta are not completely differentiated until 25 years of age.[14]

The determination of vessel length and size in vivo and especially in vitro is most difficult. Not only is there a deficiency of such morphologic information available in the adult but especially in the child. In general, attempts to quantitate luminal diameter in an intact vessel are obscured by gross conjecture of vessel wall thickness and the continuous dilemma of vessel spasm. Angiography can provide useful information with regard to the presence of absence of donor or recipient arteries, the status of proximal or distal collateral circulation, and the appearance of the recipient artery at the site of transplantation. Only a gross estimation of luminal size, however, can be obtained with this technique. Furuyama[23] circumvented the effect of arterial contraction by measuring the length of the internal elastic lamina. This technique was modified by Pesonen, Martimo, and Rapola,[41,51] using a complicated mathematical model (error rate of 5%). Another study[50] demonstrated linear correlation between the size or large arterial ostia and body length in children from 25 weeks of gestational age to 9 years postpartum.

From the foregoing discussion it would seem that the optimal time to perform elective microsurgical procedures on the child would be after ages 3 to 4 years postpartum. The histologic appearance of the arterial wall at this age is becoming more mature, and the intima is becoming thicker. This is also a period of time associated with an increase in linear growth. Both donor and recipient arteries would be of a size and thickness suitable for anastomosis.

Veins

Smooth muscle in the media of superficial veins makes its appearance in the fifth month of gestation as it differentiates from mesenchyme. At birth the amount of smooth muscle cells in the media of superficial veins increases rapidly. The media of superficial veins is also two or three times thicker than the media of deep veins.[50]

In newborns only a circular layer of muscle is present. With advancing age the muscle layer increases twofold to fivefold.[50] At 4 months of age longitudinally oriented muscle cells appear in the intima of superficial veins. At 3 years of age longitudinal cells are clearly discernible in the intima and adventitia of superficial veins. Longitudinal muscle cells also appear in the intima of deep veins at this time. In general, the longitudinal muscle layer in deep veins appears later and is poorly developed. After the age of 40 the amount of longitudinal musculature in the adventitia of superficial veins greatly increases. An additional muscle layer also appears in a subendothelial location in veins with an intima greater than 50 μm thick.

The vasa vasorum in veins is well developed and appears to have a nutrient function. It is more pervasive and better developed in veins than in arteries. This network consists of a nutrient capillary plexus in the muscular layer and a vascular plexus for distribution and transportation in the adventitia.[34] In contrast to arteries, this vascular network occupies the entire thickness of the muscle layer, often extending to within 10 μm from the lumen.[50] Vascularization makes its appearance in superficial veins in the 32 cm fetus somewhat later than the appearance of smooth muscle cells, which can be identified in the 20 cm fetus. With advancing age (38 cm fetus) vascularization is detected in the deep veins. As the smooth muscle layer becomes thicker, vascularization of the media decreases. In the adult a vascular pattern, seen in arteries, is approached. An inner, subintimal avascular zone in the media can be identified and is seven or eight times greater than that seen in younger subjects.

As indicated previously, the smooth muscle content of superficial veins is considerably greater than that noted in deep veins. The difference is especially apparent in newborns and children below the age of 3 to 4 years.

In contrast to the distribution of smooth muscle cells, elastic fibers are present in greater concentration at birth in deep veins.[50] In general, elastic fibers are present in greater concentration in larger veins that have more of a reservoir function. It should be emphasized that the walls of veins are much thinner than arteries because of the reduction of both muscular and elastic[14] elements. The collagenous connective tissue component constitutes the bulk of the wall.

Based on the preceding discussion, certain observations on the timing of microvascular procedures in children can be made. In neonates and children below 3 or 4 years of age, arteries and veins will have thinner walls, primarily because of an incompletely developed muscular layer. Deep veins, particularly, will have thin, friable walls, making anastomosis more difficult. After the age of 3 or 4, the intima in arteries increases in thickness. This increase, which is partially related to an increase in collagen deposition, contributes further to the stability and strength of the arterial wall.

EFFECTS OF HYPOXIA AND THROMBOSIS

One characteristic of vascularized transplantation is that the composite tissue to be transferred always sustains a variable period of ischemia and anoxia. Success or failure depends on restoring the delivery of oxygen to the cells in the tissue before irreversible enzymatic changes occur and the cells die. Many factors influence the successful resumption of oxygen delivery to the cells besides such technical considerations as design of the flap or performance of the vascular anastomoses. The ability to withstand hypoxia varies with different tissue. In addition, factors within the microcirculation may result in alterations of blood flow and perfusion.

A brief discussion of intermediary metabolism is necessary before discussing the effects of ischemia and hypoxia. All work done within (or by) a cell requires energy. Intermediary metabolism refers to a series of chemical reactions that result in biologically usable energy. This energy is mostly in the form of adenosine triphosphate (ATP), created by the phosphorylation of adenosine disphophate (ADP). As ATP is consumed (i.e., reconverted to ADP), energy is released. Therefore a continuing production of ATP is necessary for cellular function.

Normally ATP is produced in the cytoplasm by glycolysis and in the mitochondria by oxidative phosphorylation and the Krebs cycle. When oxygen is abundant, 6 moles of ATP are produced for every mole of oxygen consumed by oxidative phosphorylation, and 36 moles of ATP are produced for each mole of glucose consumed by aerobic glycolysis.

Under anoxic conditions, the only available means of ATP production is anaerobic glycolysis, which converts glucose to pyruvate and lactate. This is a much less efficient method of energy production, only generating 2 moles of ATP for each mole of glucose consumed. The buildup of lactate results in lactic acidosis, which further inhibits cellular function. All mammalian cells must eventually return to aerobic conditions or cell death ensues.

Different tissues, however, are remarkably diverse in their capacity to function under and recover from anaerobic conditions. The brain, for example, has no capacity for anaerobic glycolysis and can withstand only minutes of anoxia. Skeletal muscles, on the other hand, can use stored glycogen for anaerobic glycolysis and can survive several hours of hypoxia. Peripheral nerve tissue, although similar to central nervous system cells in its sensitivity to anoxia, appears better able to recover with eventual return of function.[31]

Another type of tissue that appears very sensitive to anoxia is vascular endothelium. Vascular endothelium has a limited ability to convert to anaerobic glycolysis and depends on a continuing supply of oxygen for viability. After only several minutes of anoxia, endothelial cells demonstrate irreversible changes by electron microscopy.[38] Continued anoxia produces loss of cell membrane integrity and disruption of intercellular junctions. This results not only in an increase in capillary permeability, but also exposure of the subendothelium to the vascular space, with subsequent thrombosis. Even though endothelium regenerates readily, the damage from interstitial edema and thrombosis may be long lasting. This may well be one factor responsible for the "no-reflow phenomenon" seen in cerebral ischemia.[59]

Possible mechanisms by which loss of endothelial cell integrity results in thrombosis have come to light recently. The most important of these is the action of vascular mediators, principally prostacyclin and thromboxane. Since 1975 a considerable amount of investigation has been conducted into the function of prostaglandins as vascular mediators. Prostaglandins are formed from membrane-bound, long-chain fatty acids. Both prostacyclin and thromboxane are metabolites of arachidonic acid (bisenoic pathway). Two other pathways have been recognized but appear to be of lesser importance than the bisenoic pathway (the monoenoic pathway, derived from dihomolinolenic acid, and the trienoic pathway, derived from eicosapentenoic acid).

Arachidonic acid is present as a membrane phospholipid in both platelets and vascular endothelium. It is released by the action of an enzyme, phospholipase A2 to free arachidonic acid. This is then converted by the action of cyclooxygenase to an endoperoxide. Endoperoxides are then converted either into thromboxane A_2 (txA_2) or prostacyclin (PGI_2).

The enzyme necessary for the formation of TxA_2 is present mainly in platelets, and the enzyme necessary for the formation of PGI_2 is present mainly in vascular endothelial cells. Prostacyclin is a potent vasodilator and inhibitor of platelet aggregation. Thromboxane, on the other hand, is a potent vasoconstrictor and promotor of platelet aggregation. It appears that a balance between these two compounds is necessary to prevent intravascular thrombosis. One characteristic of vascular mediators that is shared by both prostacyclin and thromboxane is their extremely short half-life. Thromboxane has a half-life of approximately 30 seconds[26] and that of prostacyclin is approximately 3 minutes.[13] They are then converted to inactive metabolites.

A theoretical sequence of events can be formulated from the foregoing discussion. When ischemia or hypoxia is present, platelets are stimulated to release TxA_2-containing granules. If the surrounding vascular endothelium is also damaged by hypoxia or trauma, the balancing effect of the PGI_2 is lost and the TxA_2 comes into contact with the subendothelium, producing severe vasoconstriction and further platelet aggregation. Depending on the size of the vessel and the extent of endothelial damage, occlusion of the vessel by thrombus formation will result. Even though blood vessels are proportionately smaller in children, the enzymes necessary for the production of these vascular mediators are fully operational at birth. Thus, it would appear that any differences in thrombosis between adults and children are related to vessel size rather than biochemical mechanisms. Current literature, however, is deficient in this area; more research is required.

GROWTH OF TRANSPLANTED TISSUE
Kidney

A thorough literature review on the growth of autogeneic and allogeneic tissue after transplantation was generally disappointing. This in part was related to a limited number of cases with many variables, making interpretation of results difficult.

At birth the kidney weighs 50 g. It continues to grow until reaching its maximal size between the ages of 30 to 40, approximately 270 g. It then gradually decreases in size and weight until at age 90 years it weighs 185 g.[19] Dunnill and Halley[18] have demonstrated that both the increase in volume during early decades and the decrease in volume in later decades closely parallels changes in the absolute volume of the renal cortex. With approaching senescence two major changes in the arteriolar-glomerular units are demonstrable: (1) hyalinization and collapse of the glomerular tuft and obliteration of the lumen of the preglomerular arteriole and (2) the development of anatomic continuity between afferent and efferent arterioles during glomerular sclerosis in the juxtamedullary area.[52] The result of both of these changes is loss of glomeruli.

Physiologic maturity of the kidney is reached by the third decade. Functional parameters such as glomerular filtration rate, renal sodium handling, and renal concentrating ability increase with approaching maturity and decrease with advancing age.[19]

Most of the kidney transplants performed in children or from children are allogeneic. Such longitudinal studies suffer from variables introduced by long-term immunosuppression or by factors affecting local donor tissue rejection. Several studies directed specifically at growth of the donor kidney are available, however. Silber[47] found that four anephric adults who received kidneys from two children ages 4 to 5 years old demonstrated an increase in length of approximately 3 cm in a 5- to 9-month period. Renal volume was calculated to be 177% of the preoperative volume. The increase in length and volume was attributed to renal hypertrophy. In other studes Silber and Malvin[48] and Rist, Lee, and Gittes[44] demonstrated that functional hypertrophy is reversible. Obligatory growth is not reversible. In another study by Ingelfinger,[29] an increase in renal size and function was monitored for 2 months. The cadaveric transplant from a 16-month-old child increased in length from 7 to 11.5 cm during the 8 weeks of observation. Size determinations were made with ultrasound and renal scintiphotography. Unfortunately, in all these studies obligatory growth could not be differentiated from compensatory functional hypertrophy. The problem of using size or volume as criteria to assess growth may be confusing because any increase in size can represent acute rejection or acute tubular necrosis.

The accurate assessment of renal growth after transplantation in children is further complicated by a generalized growth arrest that occurs in patients with stable but moderately advanced renal insufficiency.[27] After transplantation compensatory growth will not occur. Even with alternate-day steroid therapy growth retardation can still occur.[12]

From the data and experience presented in the previous discussion, the following conclusions can be postulated:

1. Both compensatory and obligatory growth of a renal transplant in children does occur.
2. Growth of both the individual and the transplant is most likely to occur if transplantation can be performed at an early age before maturation arrest.
3. More information is needed to assess the extent and relative contribution to an increased renal size by compensatory or obligatory renal growth, both probably have varying degrees of retardation when matched with same-age, disease-free normal peers.
4. The closer and more sophisticated the tissue typing, the lower the incidence of rejection. As a corollary, long-term and high-dose immunosuppression with growth retardation could be minimized.
5. The transplantation of other organs and parts would have similar difficulties and probably similar alterations in growth.

Bone, joints, cartilage, and epiphyses

Success after the transplantation of bone is assessed by the achievement of structural strength, osteogenic capability, and growth.[8] After transplantation with nonvascularized bone, trabeculae or the graft must be replaced and new bone deposited by creeping substitution.[42] Progenitor mesenchymal cells come from a variety of sources in both the graft, recipient bone marrow cells, and surrounding soft tissues. In general, the osteogenic capability of the transplant is influenced greatly by the rapidity of ease of vascularization. Thus autogenous cancellous bone has become the standard by which all other types of grafts are judged.[8]

The strength of the transplant depends first on the osteogenic capability with resulting callus formation. Compressive forces and high oxygen tension encourage osteoblast formation.[2] Responding to these compressive forces, new trabeculae replace old, and the graft becomes incorporated in the recipient bone.

Growth occurs by apposition of new bone on an existing framework. Without contributions from an epiphysis, an increase in bone length is seriously limited.

Attempts to transplant nonvascularized epiphysis have generally given variable and usually unsatisfactory results. Germinal cells in the epiphyseal growth plate are sensitive to ischemia and do not survive well by diffusion alone.[8]

In contrast to bone and epiphyseal structures, cartilage is nourished and survives transplantation by diffusion. The matrix of cartilage acts as a mechanical barrier, preventing the ingrowth of vascular tissue.[28] Chondroblast formation appears to be stimulated by compressive forces and low oxygen tension.[2] growth of cartilage takes place by apposition from perichondrial cells and expansion of the interstitium by division of chondrocytes.[14] In a long-term follow-up of reconstructed auricles in children, Tanzer[54] demonstrated that the average increase in height of the reconstructed ear was 3.6 mm, compared to 4.4 mm for the normal ear. Although growth does occur, it is retarded.

Serial radiographs to assess bone and epiphyseal growth are useful but may be unreliable. The epiphysis may be open radiographically, but still be nonfunctional.[49] It may also be difficult to assess the contribution of growth to the epiphysis in question.

The microsurgical transplantation of bone, joints, cartilage, and epiphyses has contributed a great deal of information on the survival and growth of these composite tissues. Unfortunately, only a limited number of isolated longitudinal studies are available.

Successful replantation of upper limbs in children has demonstrated retarded longitudinal growth in long-term follow-up.[33,45,60] This can be explained by several reasons: (1) complete interruption and slow regeneration of all neural pathways has resulted in a delayed functional restoration of activity and (2) variable periods of ischemia, some prolonged, with incomplete tissue necrosis and ischemia to epiphyseal structures.[22] Experience with replantation of digits, thumbs, and hands in children also reveals diminution of longitudinal growth. Urbaniak, reporting on a series of 25 replanted digits in children, describes the average incurred growth to be 81% of the contralateral digit (range 21% to 118%). (See Chapter 65.) If epiphysial viability is preserved, growth may even be accelerated at times. In a single case report of a microvascular joint transplantation in a 4-year-old child, growth was "normal" in the 2½-year follow-up.[35] Isolated clinical reports of successful toe-to-thumb transplantations in children show evidence of continued growth of the transplant. (See Chapter 66.)

In an experimental study by Furnas[22] on replanted forelimbs in puppies, the limited clinical observations mentioned previously are supported. Longitudinal growth in most replanted limbs was normal. Two control animals in whom only the axillary plexus was transected (and repaired) demonstrated growth to be 98% of the contralateral normal limb. Of interest in this study was that a few of the replanted long bones actually became longer than control long bones. Other studies on vascularized epiphysial transplantation in puppies demonstrated growth that was two thirds of normal.[16,17]

Several conclusions can be postulated from these studies: (1) microsurgical transplantation of osseous, epiphyseal, or cartilaginous structures ensures complete survival and growth of all structures provided that blood flow is not interrupted for prolonged periods[55]; (2) longitudinal growth of proximally amputated limbs after successful replantation may be retarded by factors delaying the return of function and influenced by varying periods of ischemia; (3) after successful replantation of distal parts, longitudinal growth is also retarded but occasionally greater than normal; (4) after successful vascularized transplantation of cartilaginous or osseous structures containing viable epiphyses, normal growth can occur (alterations in normal growth often can be attributed to prolonged ischemia or failure to preserve the integrity of the epiphyseal blood supply during transplantation); (5) if functional requirements of the transplanted tissue at the recipient site exceed those at the donor site, an

increase in growth may occur; (6) if blood flow to the transplanted tissue at the recipient site is actually increased (e.g., dorsal artery of the foot to isolated second toe) then an increase in longitudinal growth might occur; and (7) a viable epiphysis is essential for longitudinal growth. Appositional and endosteal growth, however, are influenced by the integrity of the medullary or cortical circulation. In a recent experimental study, Berggren, Weiland, and Dorfman[5] have demonstrated that the preservation of both medullary and cortical circulation in transplanted posterior ribs results in a significant enlargement of cortical vascular canals and cortical resorption. Bone resorption was explained by a relative hyperemia and hyperoxia. Hyperemia was also believed to be a factor in cancellous bone formation in cortical bone. An improved growth potential was implied in this study because of a greater number of survival osteocytes and osteoblasts demonstrated in the transplanted osseous segment.

TRANSPLANTATION IMMUNOLOGY

The concept that organs or parts destroyed by disease or trauma can be replaced by healthy tissues from either living or deceased individuals is a very old one. References in Greek mythology to a chimera are common. Mythical accounts of transplantation also occur in ancient history. In 1907 Carrel described the first autogenic vascularized transplantation of intestine to replace a canine cervical esophagus. "Unfortunately a phlegmon of the neck developed the following day, and it was necessary to extirpate the loop of intestine.[11]

Carrel also described " . . . the homoplastic transplantation en masse . . . " of both kidneys, proximal ureters, adrenal glands, and corresponding segments of the aorta and vena cava.[11] The patient with this allogeneic transplant survived for 10 days. There were no long-term autogenic or allogenic transplant survivors, but survival from 1 week to 10 days was possible. Infection was common. Thus Carrel believed that if circulation to the transplanted part or organ could be reestablished and patency maintained through innovative vascular surgical techniques, the transplanted organ or part would survive indefinitely. Experiments with xogeneic transplantation were uniformly unsuccessful. Even initial viability eluded Carrel. An early understanding of an immunologic basis for transplant failure was expressed. "The transplanted organ must be prepared to support the serum of the animal on which it is to be grafted. *We do not yet know if such immunization is possible.*"[11] Modern transplantation immunology has its origin in the work of Medawar and Woodruff,[37] who during the 1940s and 1950s described and quantified first- and second-set skin homograft rejection. They demonstrated that such a transplant rejection was mediated by lymphoid cells. In the early 1950s dismal results with kidney transplants stimulated investigators to explore methods that would ameliorate graft rejection.

Allogeneic renal transplantation has been more successful tran transplantation with other composite tissues. In the early 1970s one could anticipate a 74% transplant survival rate at 2 years if the donor kidney came from a sibling. If the parent donated the kidney, a 68% transplant survival could be anticipated. Cadaveric transplants had less than a 50% 2-year survival rate.[54] Until recently transplant survival statistics were similar to these early experiences. In preliminary studies,[1,10] cyclosporin A improved the success of allogeneic renal transplantation. More recently Ferguson et al.[20] reported their experience in a prospective randomized trial of 100 mismatched, living related donor and cadaveric renal transplants. Cyclosporin A combined with prednisone was compared with standard immunosuppressive therapy using antilymphoblast globulin, prednisone, and azathioprine. The actuarial graft survival at 1 year was 93% in the cyclosporin A–prednisone group and 81% for patients treated with conventional immunosuppression.

In 1976 over 240 liver transplantations had been performed with only 29 patients surviving at the time of the report.[6] The longest survivor lived 6 years. A similar experience was found in cardiac transplantation. Over 280 heart transplants were performed, with 50 survivors present at the time of writing in 1976.[6] The longest a patient with a cardiac transplant lived was 7 years. Attempts to transplant the lung, larynx, pancreas, and adrenal glands laso have been reported, all with very poor results. More recently an awakening interest in allogeneic bone marrow transplantation has occurred, but has met with limited success. So far the greatest success has been obtained in patients with congenital immunologic deficiency where there is an associated defect in the rejection of allogeneic tissues.[6] Transplantation in patients with an intact immune mechanism still presents a formidable obstacle. The identification of graft-versus-host disease has complicated such transplantation efforts. Efforts to improve transplant survival statistics have been directed at histocompatibility antigens of both the donor and the recipient and a continued search for safer methods to regulate the immune response.

Histocompatibility antigens

The influence of ABO and other red blood cell groups in transplantation is well documented. In addition to being present on red blood cells, the antigens are also present on fixed tissue. Donor-recipient incompatibility results in the immediate hyperacute rejection of the transplanted tissue. In 1954 the HLA major histocompatibility system was serologically defined on leukocytes.[15] These antigens were also identified on fixed tissue.

During a recent international workshop a standardized battery of high-quality HLA typing reagents was shared among its members.[40] Typing for HLA-A, HLA-B, and HLA-C loci, as well as the new HLA-DR (B cell) locus was performed. Although the results are problematic, improved typing techniques may provide a stronger future correlation. The workshop concluded the following[40]:

1. The overall effect of HLA-A and HLA-B matching in cadaver transplantation is weak.
2. Apparently, transfusions have an improvement effect on graft survival that outweighs the influence of HLA incompatibility.
3. In nontransfused recipients matching appears to be valuable.
4. HLA-DR has a significant although not very strong effect on graft survival.
5. The results of this study demonstrate that HLA matching can be valuable in clinical transplantation.

Currently, investigation continues to define minor determinants of histocompatibility not coded for by the major histocompatibility system.

Immunosuppression-Immunoregulation

Other avenues being explored to enhance allogeneic transplant survival are improved methods of immunosuppression and immunoregulation. Until recently conventional methods of immunosuppression were nonspecific in their action. The entire host defense system was altered with an increased susceptibility to bacterial and viral infection and the potentiation of a malignancy. The introduction of cyclosporin A has permitted the select elimination of clones of lymphocytes that respond to stimulation by the antigens of the allograft, and at the same time spares other clones of lymphocytes that can respond to infectious agents.[1] Its action appears to be directed at interference with helper T lymphocytes early in the induction of the immune response, which is at the proliferative stage.[7] Nephrotoxicity associated with the administration of high-dose cyclosporin A is reversible. The addition of corticosteroids to the treatment regimen has permitted a decreased dose of cyclosporin A to be used without an increase in infectious complications. The potential for developing a lymphoma, particularly of the B lymphocyte type still exists as in other immunosuppressive regimens. The incidence appears to be lower, however.[7]

The advent of hybridoma technology has permitted the production of monoclonal antibodies.[25] Thus an antibody of a single class and specificity can be produced in culture in unlimited amounts. Its physical, chemical, and immunologic properties are constant and can be directed to one antigenic determinant of a complex antigen. Hybridoma antibodies are currently being developed to (1) recognize determinants for rapid and precise tissue typing for transplantation, (2) monitor quantitative and qualitative changes in immunoregulatory cells, thus predicting disease remission and exacerbations,[30,43] (3) serve as a source of blocking antibodies directed at specific HLA determinants (enhancement), (4) specifically react against T lymphocyte subpopulations involved in allograft rejection; and (5) facilitate marrow transplantation (without producing graft-versus-host disease) by selectively destroying past thymic cells.[25] Thus cells responsible for allogeneic graft rejection would be eliminated and replaced by stem cells (tolerance).

At the present time many investigators are searching for a technique that will permit the production of monoclonal antibodies in human cells. Initial enthusiasm for such a method to produce these antibodies from human hybridomas has been proven to be premature.[25,39] Unless human monoclonal antibodies can be produced, problems related to the antigenicity of allogeneic sera still exist and limit usefulness.

It is anticipated that within the next decade or two, immunosuppression will be replaced by immunoregulation. Then the transplant microsurgeon will be able to safely replace lost organs and parts, fulfilling the future predictions of Carrel. "It is not unreasonable to believe that some transplantations, as, for instance, the transplantaion of the arm a little below the elbow, may be successfully performed if an adequate technique is used."[11]

PRESENT SERIES

From 1977 to the present,* twenty-one patients underwent reconstruction with composite donor tissue of a variety of histologic types. Twenty-two separate microsurgical procedures were performed in these patients. The ages varied from 4 to 19 years with an average age of 10.6 years. Eight patients (38.1%) were 9 years old or less. Thirteen patients (61.9%) were between 10 and 19 years of age (Table 12-1). Problems requiring reconstruction were grouped according to regional anatomy. Five microsurgical procedures were performed in the head and neck region, three on the upper extremity, two on the genitalia, and twelve on the lower extremity.

The cause of the recipient defect was related to either trauma or congenital anomalies (Table 12-2). Fourteen problems related to trauma were noted in the older age group (ages 10 to 20). Only three problems related to trauma were noted in the 0 to 9 age group. All of the congenital anomalies

---

*Personal series of authors. This does not represent the total Duke University Medical Center experience.

Table 12-1. Relationship of age to location of recipient defect

Location	0 to 9 years	10 to 19 years
Head and neck	0	5
Upper extremity	3	0
Genitalia	2	0
Lower extremity	3	9
TOTAL	8/21 (38.1%)	13/21 (61.9%)

Table 12-2. Relationship of age to cause of defect

Cause	0 to 9 years	10 to 19 years
Trauma		
Avulsive	2	8
Burn	1	2
Chronic ulcer	0	2
Gunshot wound	0	2
SUBTOTAL	3/21 (14.3%)	14/21 (61.9%)
Congenital defects		
SUBTOTAL	5/21 (23.8%)	0/21 (0%)
TOTAL	8/21 (38.1%)	14/21 (61.9%)

in the present series were treated early in the 0 to 9 age group.

A variety of donor tissues were used in reconstruction (Table 12-3). A vascularized groin flap was employed in seven patients. The selection of this flap was related to our early evolving experience. With the advent of more reliable tissue the groin flap was decreasingly used. All of the vascularized groin flaps were transplanted before 1980. From 1979 to the present five vascularized latissimus dorsi musculocutaneous flaps and five vascularized scapular flaps were employed to provide flap coverage.

There was only one failure in the present series (4.5%), a vascularized groin flap in a 15-year-old girl. All of the other transplanted tissue survived completely.

Head and neck

In the head and neck region four patients were treated with five vascularized flaps, three vascularized groin flaps, and two vascularized scapular flaps. Three patients had previously sustained burns involving the head and neck region. All three patients were treated initially with split- or full-thickness skin grafts. As a result of growth of the patient and contraction of the graft, a neck contracture developed in all three patients. In two patients with the most extensive burns the deficiency of skin in the anterior neck region accentuated a lower lip ectropion deformity. The primary goal of reconstruction was to improve the mobility of the chin and neck, improve lip contour and function, and replace an unsightly contracting skin graft with a healthy well-vascularized skin cover. All three patients with the neck contracture underwent reconstruction with a vascularized groin flap (Fig. 12-1). The average size of the flap was approximately 10 × 22 cm. Vascular anastomoses in all cases were accomplished with an end-to-end arterial anastomosis of the donor superficial circumflex scapular artery to the recipient external facial artery. Venous anastomoses of the drainage vein of the flaps were also accomplished in an end-to-end fashion to an associated external facial vein or branch of the external jugular vein. In one patient a duplicated superficial circumflex iliac artery was identified. Both vessels were smaller in external diameter than if the artery were not duplicated (approximately 0.75 mm). To circumvent this

Table 12-3. Relationship of location of recipient defect to type of donor composite tissue

Recipient location	Donor tissue	Number of patients
Head and neck	Groin	3
	Scapula	2
Upper extremity	Second toe	3
Genitalia	Testicle	1
	Tensor fascia lata (innervated)	1
Lower extremity	Groin	4
	Latissimus dorsi	5
	Scapula	3

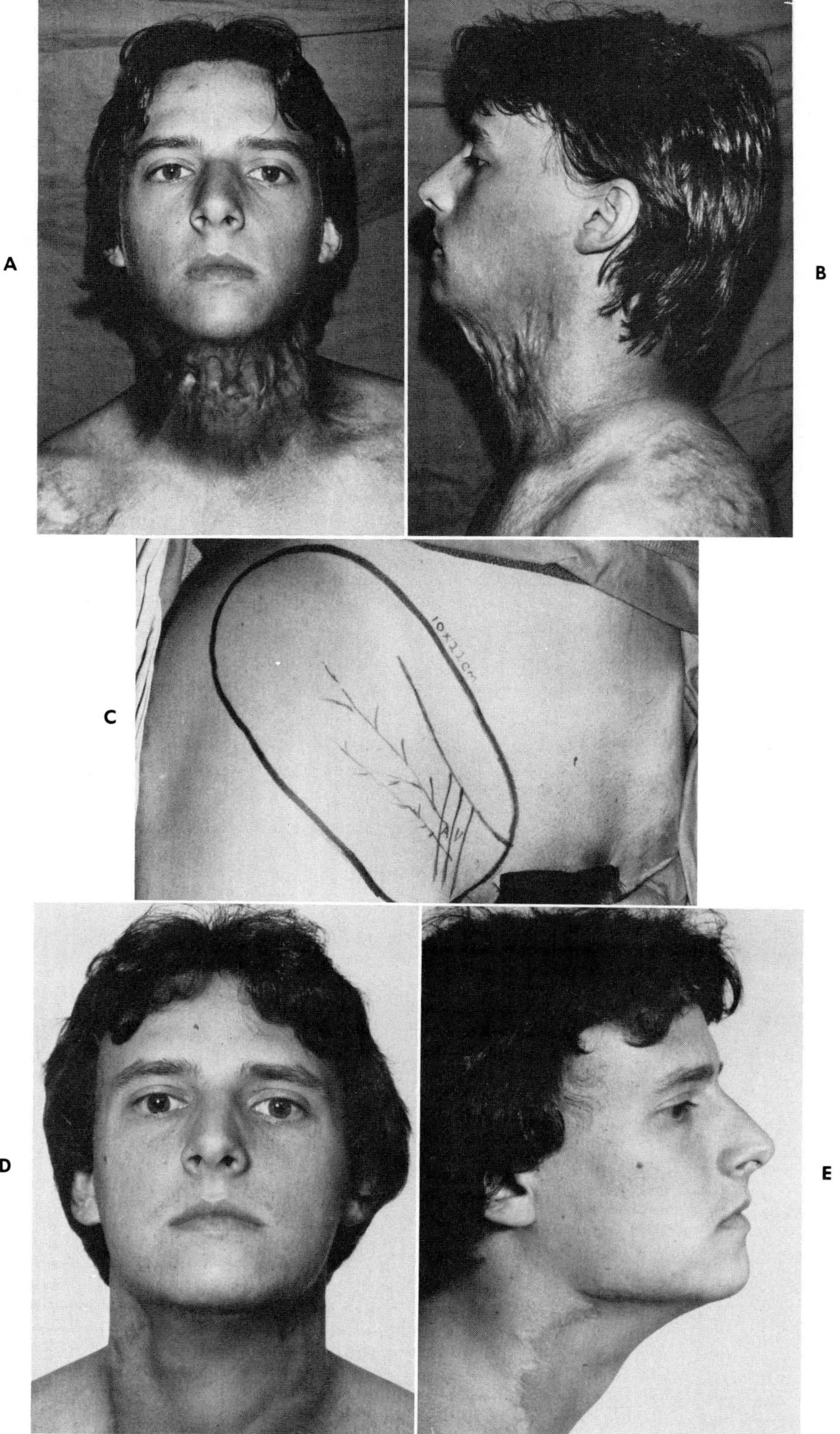

Fig. 12-1. A and **B,** Extensive scarring of the neck secondary to a third-degree thermal burn. **C,** Vascularized groin flap before transplantation. **D** and **E,** Successful vascularized groin flap transplantation.

problem, a Y-shaped segment of the external facial artery and a side branch was selected. An anastomosis was performed between each branch of the recipient artery and the corresponding branch of the superficial circumflex iliac artery. This finding of anomalous vascular arterial supply to the groin flap is consistent with our experience in adult patients. We believe that the relatively high frequency of anomalous vascular patterns in the groin flap contributes to a higher failure rate. The most distal portion of the vascularized groin flap with the duplicated superficial circumflex iliac artery did show signs of ischemia; however, the flap survived almost in its entirety. No secondary procedures were required for wound closure.

All three patients have been observed for approximately 4 years. After successful vascularized transplantation, the neck contracture did not recur. The growth of the transplanted tissues appeared to keep pace with the overall growth of the chin and neck. The lip ectropion responded to release of the neck contracture and did not require further grafting. No retardation of mandibular growth was noted.

One patient in this series sustained extensive head, neck, thoracic, and upper extremity burns (Fig. 12-2). No local or direct distant flaps were available for reconstruction. As outlined earlier, this patient underwent a vascularized groin flap to replace extensively scarred tissue of the chin and neck region. After the burn injury, the patient's entire forehead was grafted with a split-thickness skin graft. Several years later this patient was involved in an automobile accident in which the grafted forehead skin was avulsed and the exposed frontal bone denuded of periosteum. Healing was protracted and incomplete. The patient subsequently underwent reconstruction of the entire forehead with a vascularized scapular flap. Anastomoses were performed in an end-to-end fashion to the superficial temporal artery and vein. In patients with extensive third-degree burns, the vasculature in the subcutaneous tissue was relatively spared from extensive fibrosis. All of these patients were in their teens. Both arteries and veins were similar in size to that found in adults. The arteries retracted quite well when cut, suggesting an intact elastic lamina muscularis and minimal adventitial fibrosis. The intima was healthy and not friable. No problems were encountered during or after the anastomosis. One patient had an avulsive injury to the entire right side of the face. Bone was exposed. This patient also underwent reconstruction with a vascularized scapular flap. End-to-end anastomoses were performed between the donor vessels of the flap and the recipient external facial vessels. The donor sites in all four patients and in five flaps were closed primarily without the necessity of grafting.

Upper extremity

Three patients underwent thumb reconstruction by vascularized second toe transplantation. One patient had in utero amputation of the thumb just distal to the metacarpophalangeal joint (Fig. 12-3). Adjacent fingers and toes were also affected but to a lesser degree. A dowel-shaped peg was fashioned from the remaining proximal phalanx and placed in a drill hole within the central portion of the proximal phalanx of the transplanted toe. Follow-up on this patient was continued for 4 years. The transplanted toe has increased in size and subjectively appears to be larger than adjacent toes but smaller than the unaffected left thumb. Unfortunately, the contralateral second toe was not available for comparison because it had been previously amputated in utero. Skeletal radiographs at varying time intervals were examined and measurements made. Epiphyses of proximal, middle, and distal phalanges of the foot in both sexes close at approximately 18 years of age.[51] The metatarsal epiphyses close between 14 and 21 years of age. In the hand the epiphyses of the proximal, middle, and distal phalanges also close between 14 and 21 years of age.[51] This is true for the epiphyses of the first metacarpal bone. The present patient is now 12 years old. The second toe–to–right thumb transplantation was performed at age 8. Evaluation of the radiographs reveals open epiphyses but all appear to be closing. As indicated earlier, the recipient site contained a small portion of the proximal phalanx from which was fashioned a peg. This contained an epiphysis at the time of surgery. The epiphysis from the proximal phalanx of the transplanted second toe was removed. A drill hole was made in the proximal phalanx. The peg was then placed in the hole and both phalanges were maintained in fixation by an interosseous wire. The length of the transplanted second toe *exclusive* of the epiphysis of the proximal phalanx was 3.3 cm during the patient's most recent evaluation. The corresponding length of the third toe, *including* a viable epiphysis of the proximal phalanx, was also 3.3 cm (Table 12-4). A review of the data in Table 12-4 permits the following observations to be made:

1. The transplanted second toe has demonstrated slightly increased longitudinal growth when compared to the third toe. Unfortunately, the contralateral second toe was not available for comparison because it had been amputated in utero.
2. Growth of the transplanted second toe is considerably less than the contralateral left thumb.

On physical examination the length of the reconstructed right thumb was only 1 cm less than the normal left thumb. Careful inspection of the radiographs, however, revealed that the majority of the longitudinal growth was a result of an increase in length of a small segment of proximal phalanx with its intact epiphysis. Two-point discrimination of the patient's right index finger was approximately 0.5 cm. Two-point discrimination on the pulp space on the radial aspect of the transplanted toe was 0.6 to 0.7 cm. The joint measurements of the right thumb were as follows:

Metacarpophalangeal, 0 to 45 degrees

Proximal interphalangeal, +15 to 15 degrees

Distal interphalangeal, +15 to 35 degrees

These joint measurements reflect limited flexion and extension of the transplanted toe. This is consistent with Gilbert's observations.[24] Because the metatarsophalangeal joint

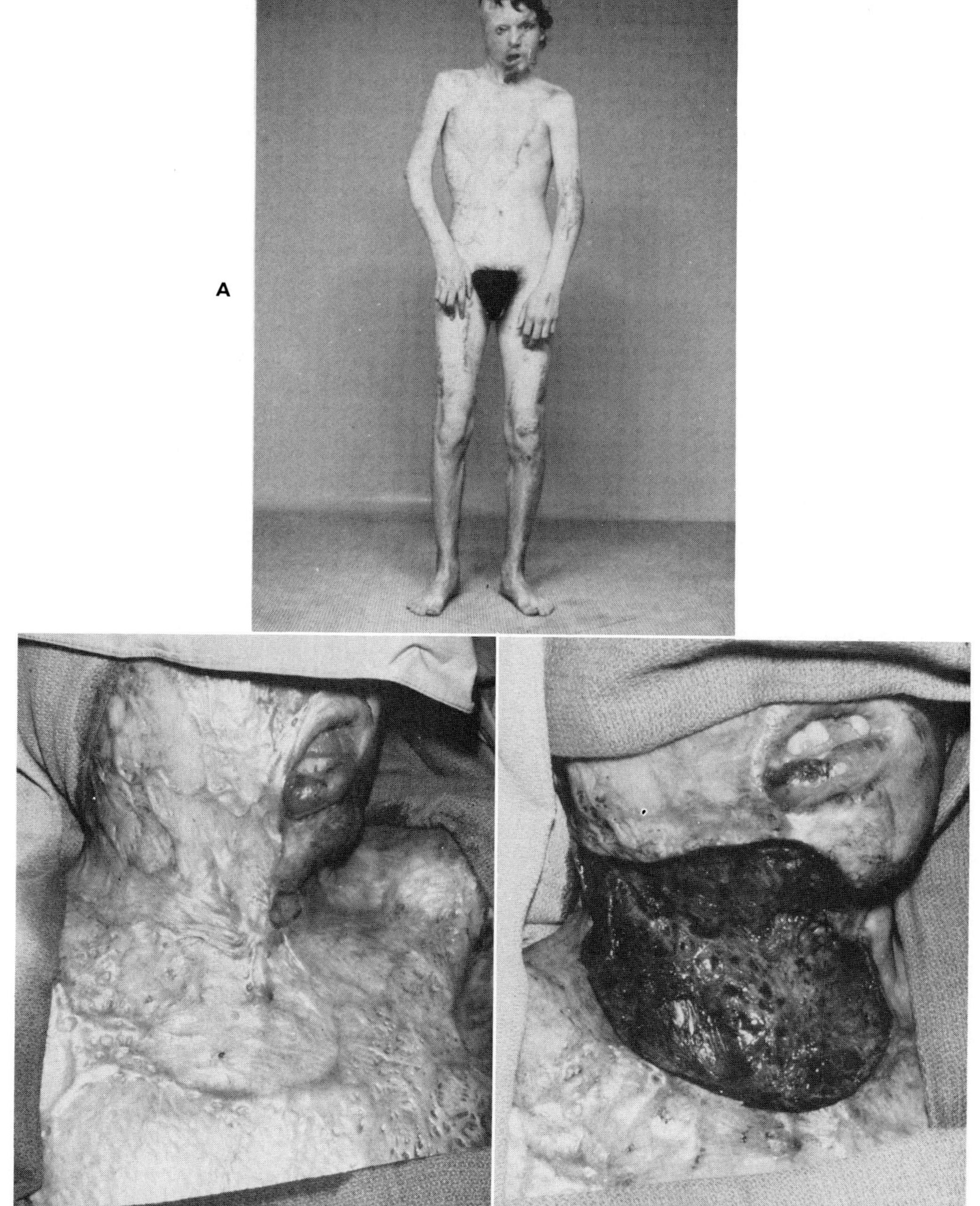

Fig. 12-2. A, Extensive thermal burns to upper thorax, arms, face, and neck. Donor sites for conventional flap transfer cannot be employed in reconstruction. **B,** Extensive scarring of anterior neck and chin with a lip ectropion. **C,** Incision and release of neck contracture. A minimal amount of scar tissue has been excised. Extensive cutaneous deficiency exists after release of neck contracture.

of the transplanted toe was eliminated, no hyperextension deformity ensued.

In a second patient an arrest of development of the patient's right hand was noted (Fig. 12-4). There was a total congenital absence of a thumb. In addition, a "mitten-type" syndactyly of all digits was apparant with poor distal differentiation of parts. In earlier stages of reconstruction the patient underwent separation of the radial from the ulnar ray. Motion was achieved primarily at the carpometacarpal joint level. A second toe transplantation to the thumb position was successfully accomplished during a subsequent procedure. Because additional length was needed for op-

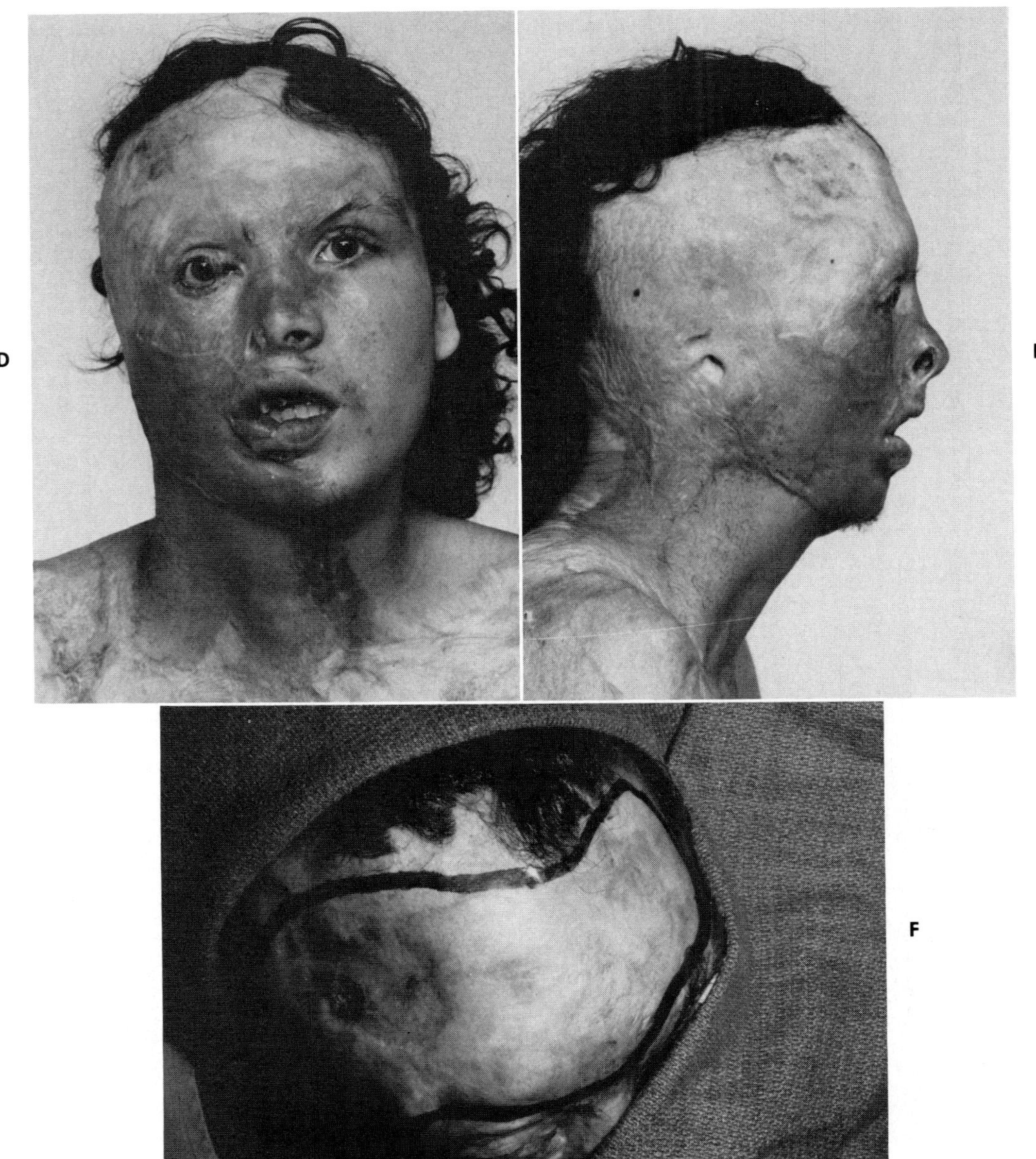

Fig. 12-2, cont'd. D and **E,** Successful vascularized groin transplantation to anterior neck. Note depression in the right frontal region secondary to extensive full-thickness loss of all tissue except a skin graft on the periosteum. **F,** Close-up of the right frontal region and forehead after an automobile accident in which the previously grafted area of the right frontal region was avulsed, exposing the frontal bone denuded of periosteum. *Continued.*

position, the distal metatarsal bone of the second toe was placed within a drill hole in one of the carpal bones at approximately a 60-degree angle with respect to the longitudinal axis of the hand. Despite what appeared to be a satisfactory position, a hyperextension deformity of the metatarsophalangeal joint ensued. This necessitated an osteotomy of the metatarsal bone approximately 1 year later to permit the transplanted toe and radial ray to be placed in better pulp-to-pulp opposition.

In a third patient both the thumb and index finger were deleted after an extensive burn to the right hand at approximately 2 years of age. In a previous operative procedure a pedicle groin flap was transferred to the dorsum of the hand after extensor tenolysis. A severe contracture with the wrist and the metacarpophalangeal joints in extension was corrected. During a subsequent procedure a second toe was transplanted to the thumb position. The thumb metacarpal bone had previously been completely destroyed except for the small portion of the metacarpal head. The metatarsal head of the transplanted toe was removed and the proximal phalanx was attached to the head of the first metacarpal bone. The volar plate and collateral ligaments of the metacarpophalangeal joint of the toe were also reconstructed.

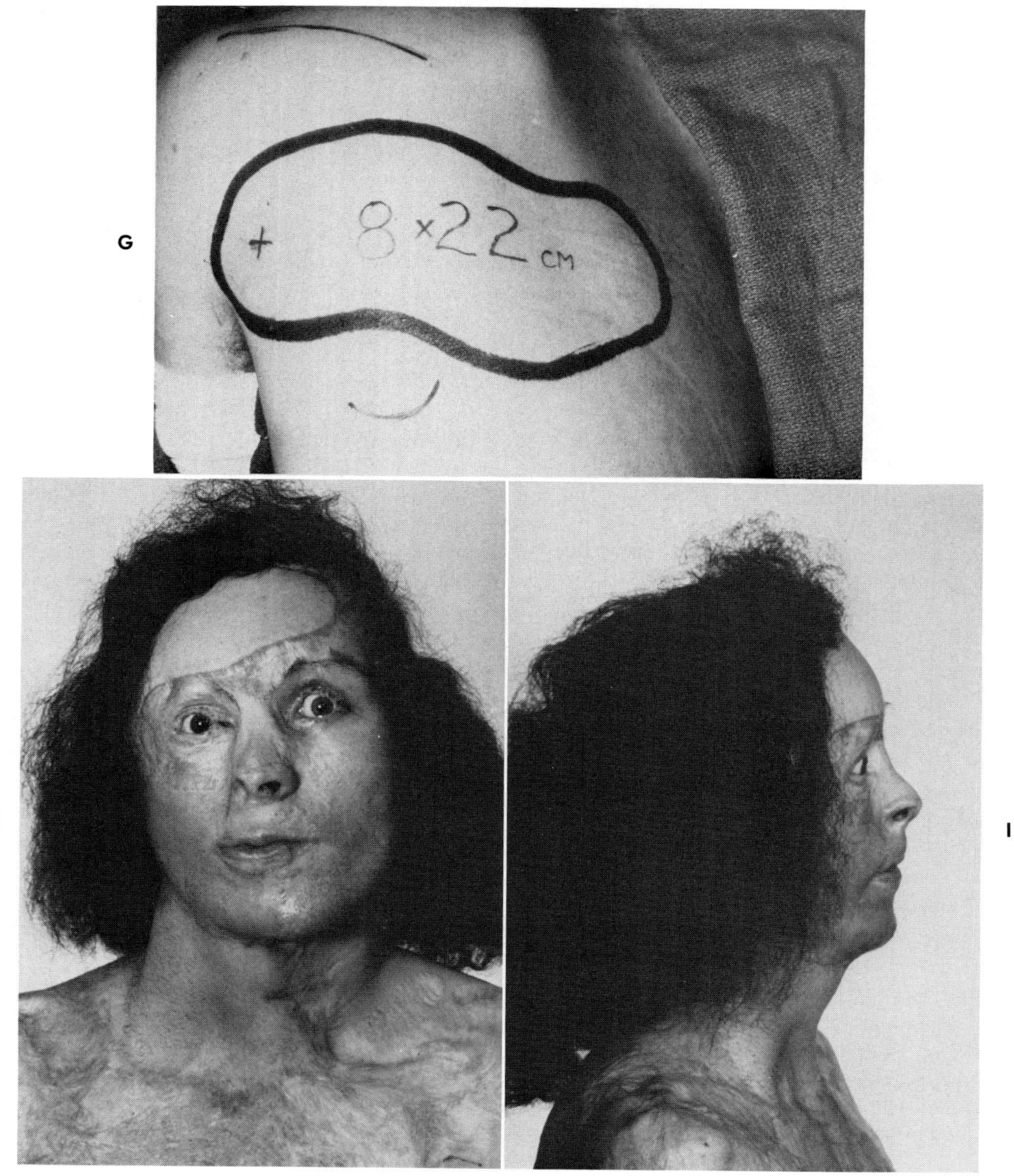

Fig. 12-2, cont'd. G, Vascularized scapular flap before transplantation. **H** and **I,** Successful vascularized scapular transplantation to forehead.

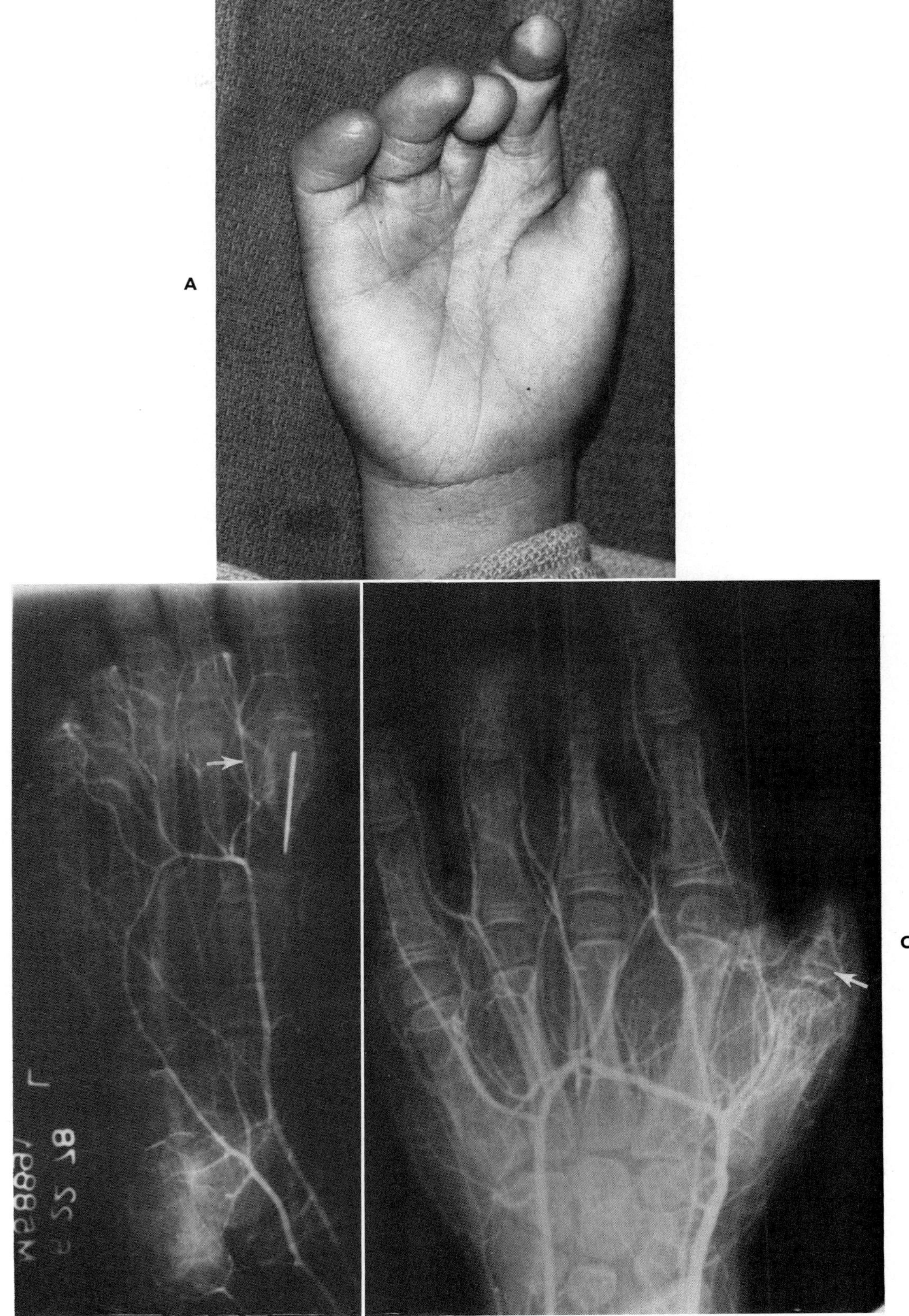

Fig. 12-3. A, Congenital amputation of thumb secondary to amnionic bands in utero. Adjacent fingers are similarly involved. **B,** Preoperative arteriogram of donor left foot. Note the patency of the dorsal metatarsal artery *(arrow)*. **C,** Preoperative arteriogram. The amputation occurred just distal to the proximal portion of the proximal phalanx. Arrow indicates open epiphyseal plate.

Continued.

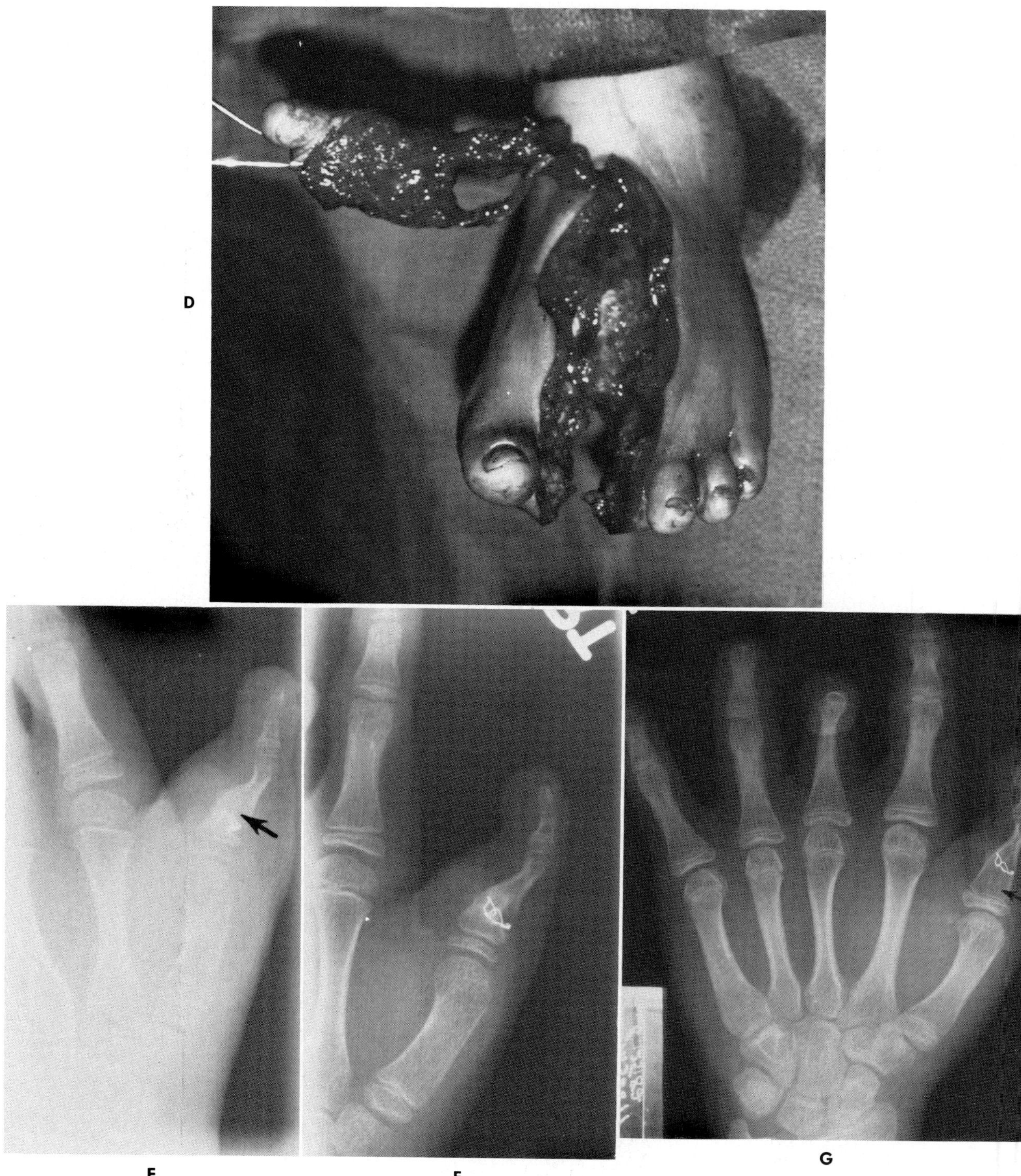

Fig. 12-3, cont'd. D, Isolated second toe on neurovascular pedicle just before transplantation. **E,** Radiograph 2 months postoperative. Note absence of the epiphysis of the proximal phalanx of the toe *(arrow).* **F,** Radiograph 9 months after surgery demonstrating continual longitudinal growth. **G,** Longitudinal growth continues 4 years after surgery. Growth occurs primarily from the retained portion of the proximal phalanx of the thumb *(arrow).* The epiphyseal plate remains open.

In one patient, with a 4-year follow-up longitudinal growth of the transplanted toe has continued. The epiphyses have remained opened. Although smaller in size than the unaffected contralateral thumb, it appears to be larger than an adjacent toe. In two patients growth cannot be assessed because there has been insufficient time after transplantation.

In second toe transplantation considerable planning must be directed toward achieving adequate skin cover adjacent to the transplanted toe, particularly in those patients who have an extensive loss either from trauma or as a result of a congenital birth defect. If a previous flap procedure is indicated, as in the patient with the extensively burned hand, provision should be made so that the bulk of the flap is in an area where the second toe is to be transplanted. This will facilitate wound closure and avoid the application of a split-thickness skin graft.

If all or the majority of the thumb metacarpal bone is absent, then attention must be directed to prevention of an extension deformity that frequently occurs at the metatarsophalangeal joint level. As indicated in previous publications, toes normally are positioned in slight extension.[11] This is related to the anatomy of the metatarsophalangeal joint. This posture may be accentuated after transplantation. One can prevent this by excising a portion of the volar metatarsophalangeal joint ligament or by placing the metacarpal head in a hyperextended position as described by Buck-Gramcko in pollicization procedures[9] (Chapter 54). The reconstruction is made more difficult if the additional length of the transplanted metatarsal bone is required to permit good pulp-to-pulp opposition of the transplanted toe to the index ray. As indicated before, in one patient a secondary osteotomy had to be performed because of a hyperextension deformity. When there is a severe deficiency of skin and total absence of the metacarpal bone, consideration should be given to a flap either transferred or transplanted with a

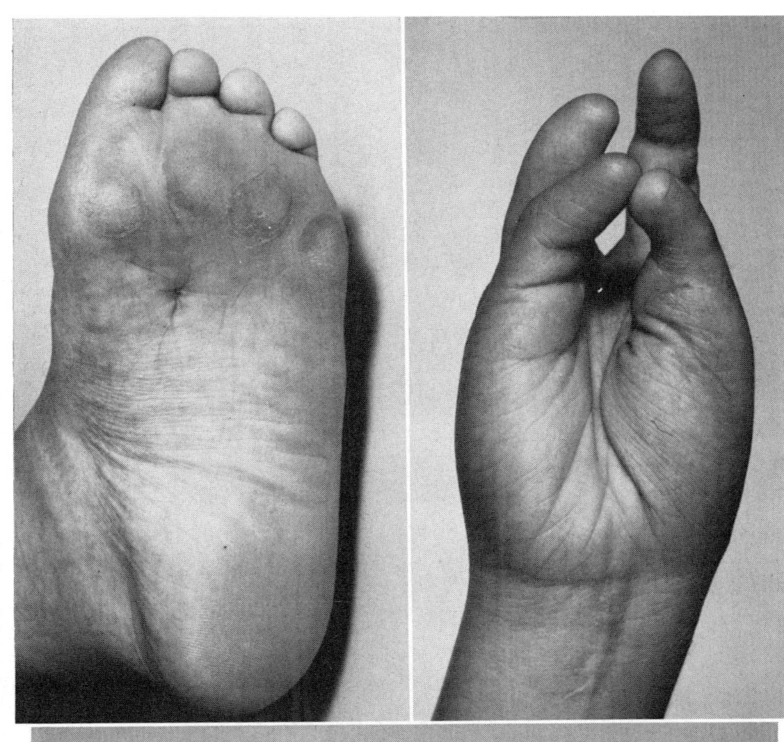

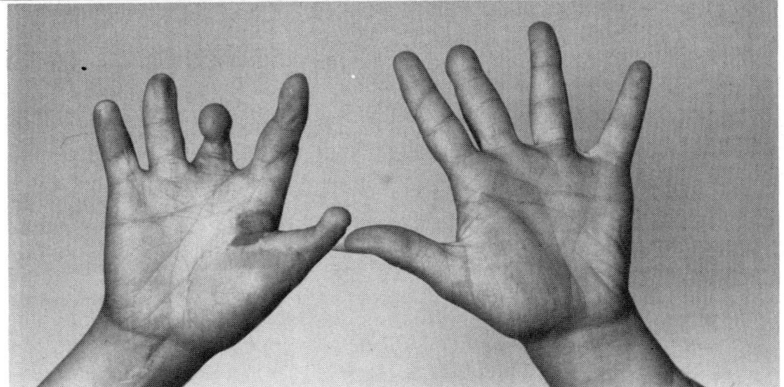

Fig. 12-3 cont'd. H, Minimal deformity of the donor foot. **I** and **J,** Final result.

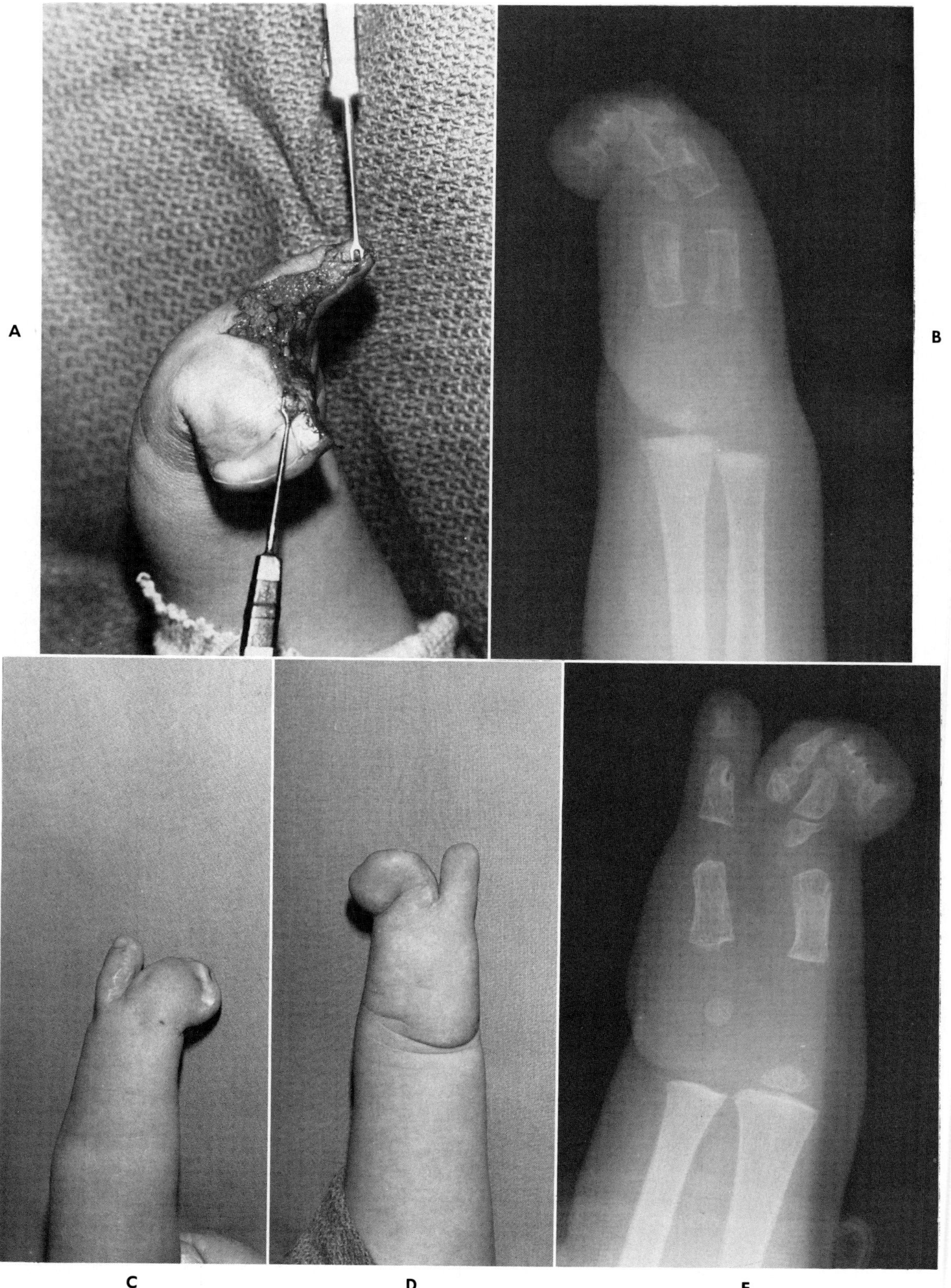

Fig. 12-4. A, Poor distal differentiation of parts with "mitten-like" deformity of right hand. Note separation of the index ray from hand. **B,** Preoperative radiograph demonstrating both a radial and ulnar metacarpal joint. Note absence of the metacarpal joint in the central ray. **C** and **D,** Result after separation of the index ray. **E,** Postoperative radiograph.

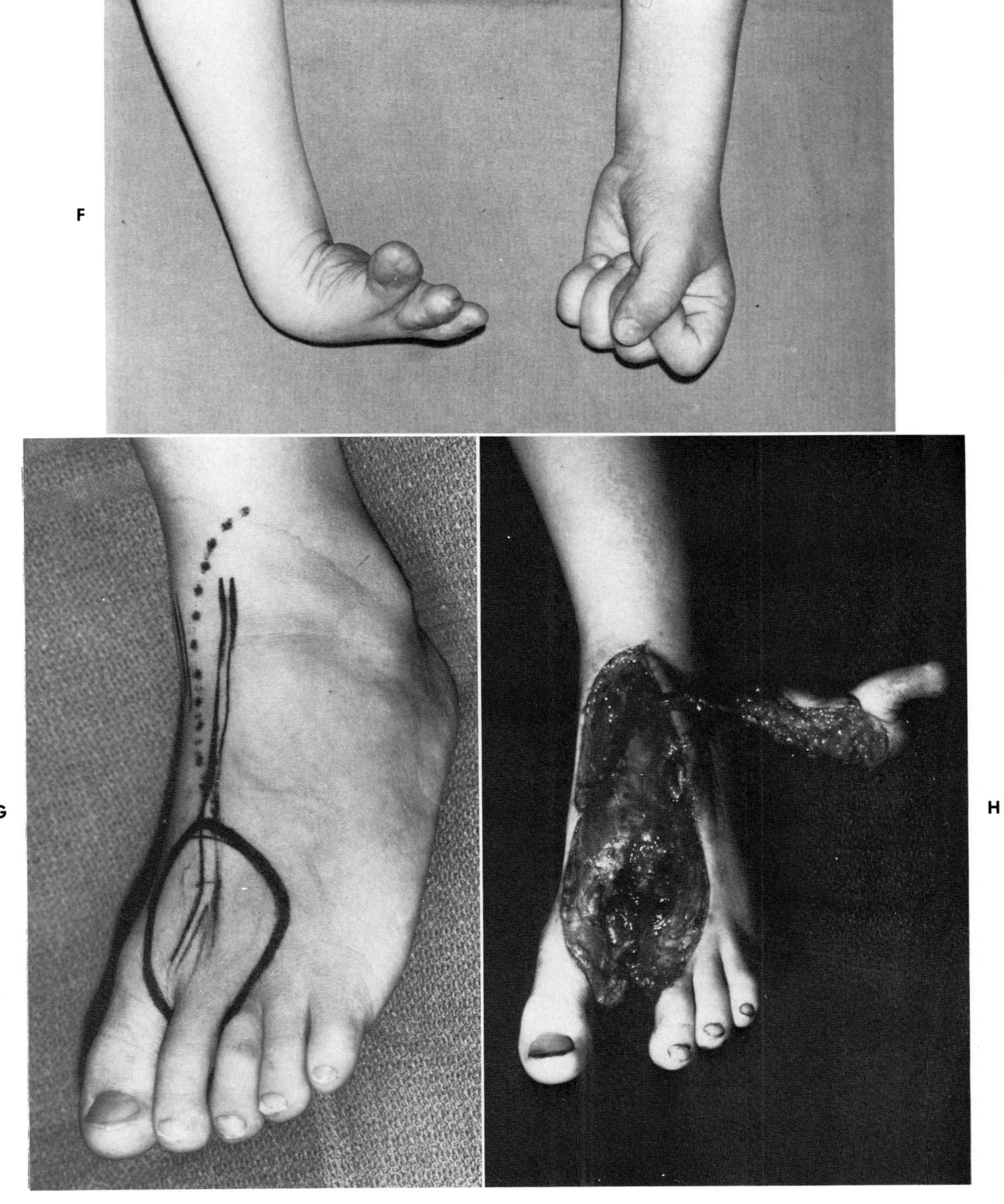

Fig. 12-4, cont'd. F, Result after separation of the index, central, and ulnar rray. There is good flexion and extension at the level of carpis with limited flexion of the radial and ulnar rays. **G,** Incisions required to isolate second toe before transplantation. **H,** Second toe isolated on neurovascular pedicle before transplantation.   *Continued.*

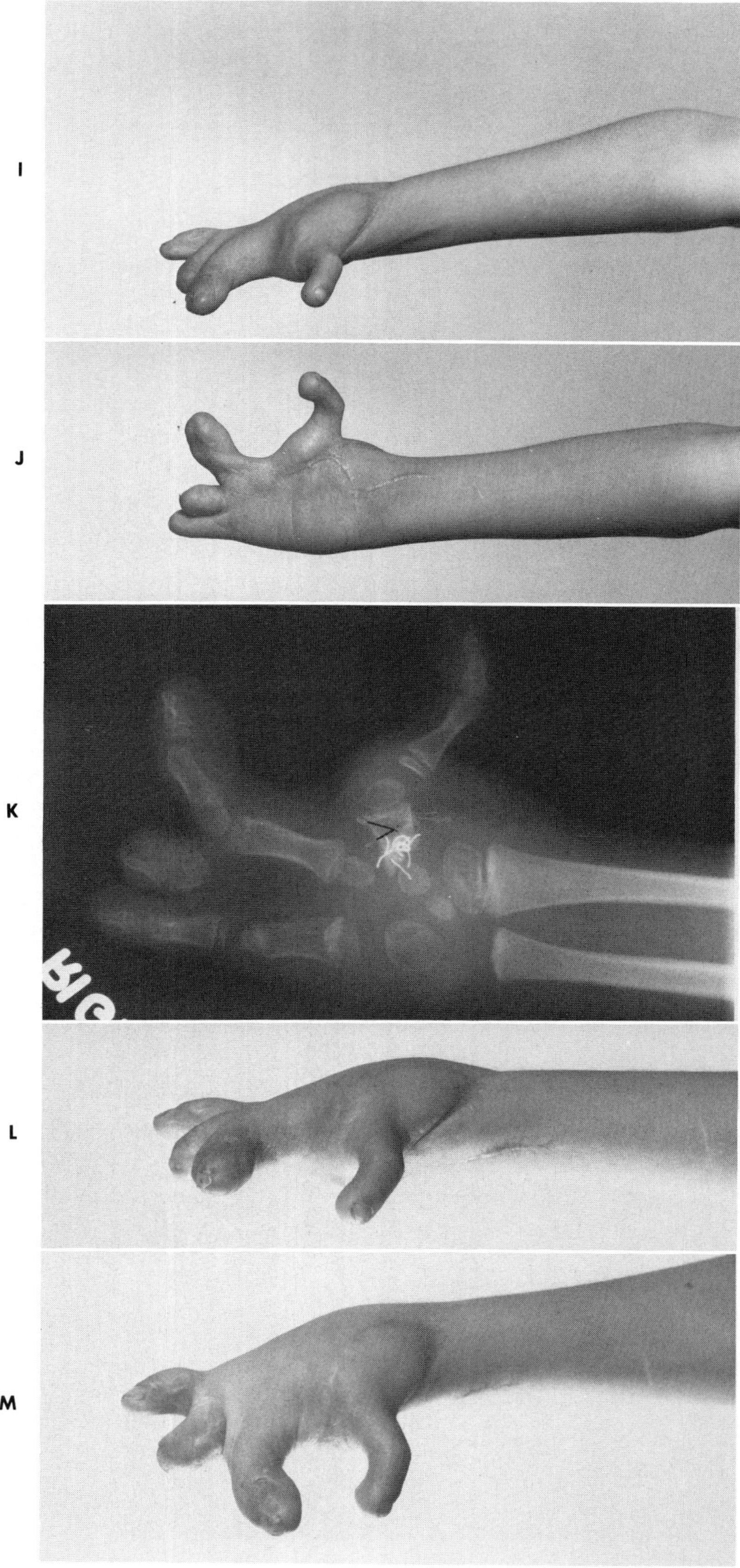

Fig. 12-4, cont'd. I and **J,** Result after successful transplantation. Note the hyperextension deformity at the level of the metatarsophalangeal joint. **K,** Radiograph after successful transplantation. Note the hyperextension deformity at the level of metatarsophalangeal joint. The metatarsal bone was placed at a 60-degree angle with reference to the radial longitudinal ray. Markings indicate the site of the wedge osteotomy. **L** and **M,** Postoperative result after wedge osteotomy.

Table 12-4. Growth characteristics of a transplanted second toe

	2 months		9 months		4 years	
	Length (cm)	Diaphyseal width (cm)	Length (cm)	Diaphyseal width (cm)	Length (cm)	Diaphyseal width (cm)
First metacarpal	3.3	0.8	3.5	0.9	4.4	0.9
First proximal phalanx (thumb)*	0.6	—	0.9	—	1.4	—
Second proximal phalanx (toe)*	1.5	—	1.5	—	1.7	—
Proximal phalanx (thumb and toe)	2.1	0.8	2.4	0.9	3.1	1.0
Second middle phalanx (toe)	0.8	0.3	0.8	0.3	1.0	0.4
Second distal phalanx (toe)	0.6	0.2	0.6	0.2	0.6	0.3
Second toe†	2.9	—	2.9	—	3.3	—
Reconstructed thumb‡	3.5	—	3.8	—	4.7	—
Third toe						
Proximal phalanx					1.7	
Middle phalanx					1.0	
Distal phalanx					0.6	
TOTAL LENGTH					3.3	

*No epiphyseal width.
†Second proximal phalanx plus second middle phalanx plus second distal phalanx.
‡First proximal phalanx plus second proximal phalanx, second middle phalanx, and second distal phalanx.

portion of the bulk of the flap in the first metacarpal area. During a later stage the second toe could then be transplanted with a long segment of the metatarsal bone. The metatarsal bone can then be placed within a hole drilled in bone and the volar plate excised and approximated with the joint in a slightly flexed position. The provision of an adequate skin envelope will permit adequate skin cover over the metatarsal bone and limit contracture, which contributes to a late extension deformity.[36]

In a recent publication, Gilbert[24] concluded that active motion of the transplanted toe is limited. This is especially true for patients with significant degrees of aplasia. In our limited experience, function is better when amputations occur distal to the metacarpophalangeal joint, preserving the thenar musculature. Limited goals should exist, however, in those patients with a missing metacarpal bone. Pulp-to-pulp pinch can be achieved with difficulty, but opposition is rarely achieved. In one case in which the metatarsophalangeal joint was preserved, Gilbert fixed the metatarsal head in extension. In this same study, growth of the transplanted toe was approximately the same as the index finger and slightly more than the nontransplanted toe.[24] As indicated previously, this may be related to an improvement in blood flow of the transplanted second toe isolated on and perfused by the dorsal artery of the foot.

Genitalia

Two patients underwent reconstruction for congenital defects of the genitalia. One patient was born with exstrophy of the bladder and a rudimentary penis (Fig. 12-5). Unfortunately, this child was reared as a male. A previous permanent ileal loop conduit was performed for urinary diversion. The dorsal sensory nerve to the penis was not present. This patient underwent successful transplantation of a tensor fascia lata flap. A neural coaptation was performed between the lateral cutaneous nerve of the flap and the recipient ileoinguinal nerve. Sensory recovery in the transplanted flap has yet to be determined. The dimensions of the tensor fascia lata flap were 8 cm wide and 18 cm long. Despite these large dimensions, flap closure was compromised more proximally and deferred. After muscle atrophy, future plans include completion of the tube and lining with a split-thickness graft. This will facilitate prosthesis placement and permit erection of the transplanted tissue.

A second patient was born with bilateral cryptorchism (Fig. 12-6). During exploration both testicles were in a juxtarenal position. The left testical was previously transferred into the scrotum using the conventional technique of Fowler and Stephens whereby the internal spermatic artery and veins are transected.[21]

Viability of the transferred testicle depends on circulation from the vas deferens. In 27% of patients testicular atrophy results.[21] Because of this significant failure rate after conventional transfer of a testicle, it was elected to transplant the right intraabdominal testicle into the scrotum using microsurgical techniques. At a second procedure the right juxtarenal testicle was transplanted into the scrotum. The internal spermatic artery and vein were anastomosed in an end-to-end fashion to the deep inferior epigastric artery and vein. Transplantation has been successful.

Testosterone levels in response to gonadotropin-stimulating hormone (GSH) ar elevated. Unfortunately, from these levels one cannot discriminate which testicle or both is responsible for this elevation.

Both testicles are now easily palpable, allowing early recognition of any testicular tumor that might develop. Castration would necessitate life-long hormonal replacement and obligatory sterility. A testicular biopsy is planned for a future date. The patient has now been observed for approximately 2 years. The transplanted testicle is significantly larger than the testicle transferred by more conventional means.

In performing testicular transplantation one must be aware that the internal spermatic vein is in reality a plexus of multiple small branching veins communicating with each other at different levels.[3] This internal spermatic plexus should be traced more proximally to its origin from the vena cava. On the left the internal spermatic plexus drains into the renal vein. At this high level the internal spermatic plexus forms a single vein, facilitating venous anastomosis after transplantation to the inguinal region. Adequate exposure often necessitates an intraabdominal exploration and isolation of the donor vasculature.

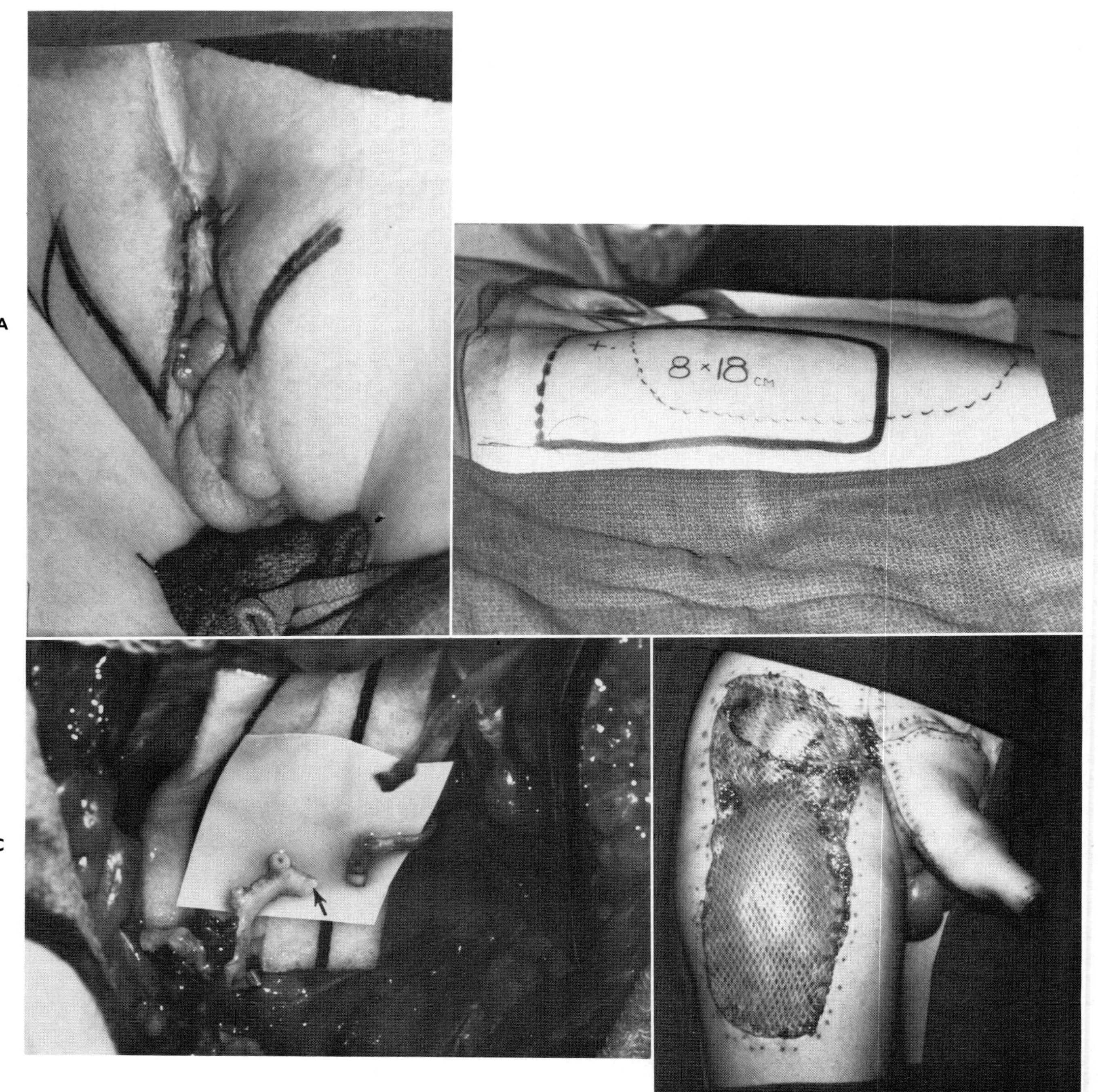

Fig. 12-5. A, Congenital exstrophy of the bladder with total absence of a penis. W-shaped flap markings are outlined to be used with tensor fascia lata musculocutaneous flap transplantation. The ectopic glans penis will be placed ventral to the reconstructed phallus. B, Outline of tensor fascia lata musculocutaneous flap. C, Donor artery *(arrow)* and recipient artery and vein. D, Successful transplantation of flap. Note the grafted donor site.

Lower extremity

In the our series 12 patients underwent lower extremity reconstruction with vascularized composite tissue. Four vascularized groin flaps, five latissimus dorsi musculocutaneous flaps, and three scapular flaps were employed in reconstruction. Nine of the twelve patients had extensive soft tissue defects involving the distal third of the extremity or foot. In 11 patients the cause was directly the result of trauma.

All arterial vascular anastomoses were performed in an end-to-side fashion, as well as most of the venous anastomoses. In three patients a significant size discrepancy existed between both the donor and recipient vein. In these

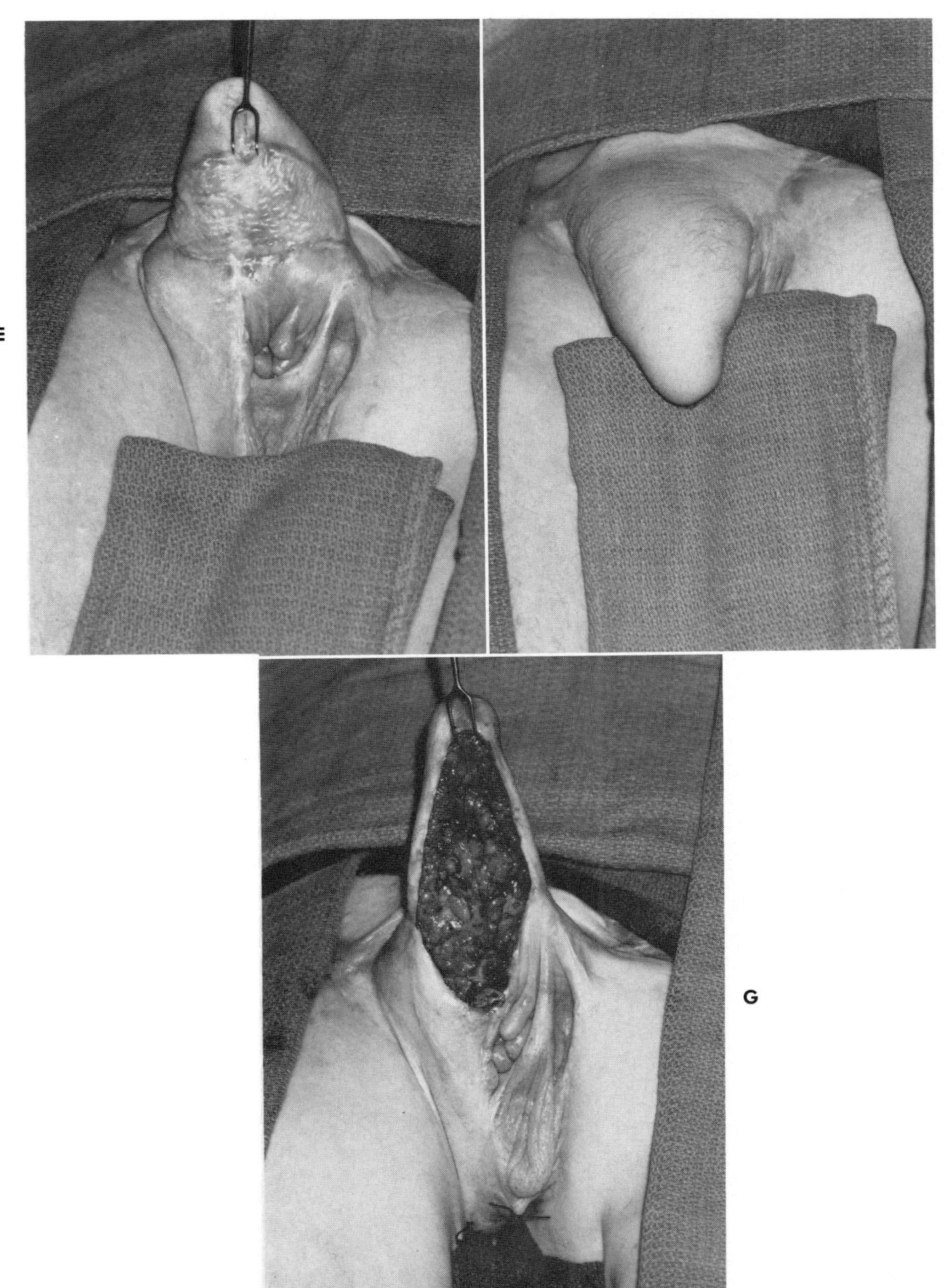

Fig. 12-5, cont'd. E, Graft on the ventral surface of the penis to facilitate wound closure and avoid tension. This graft will be excised at a later stage. **F,** Ventral aspect of the reconstructed penis after excision of a previously placed split-thickness graft. **G,** Graft excised.

Continued.

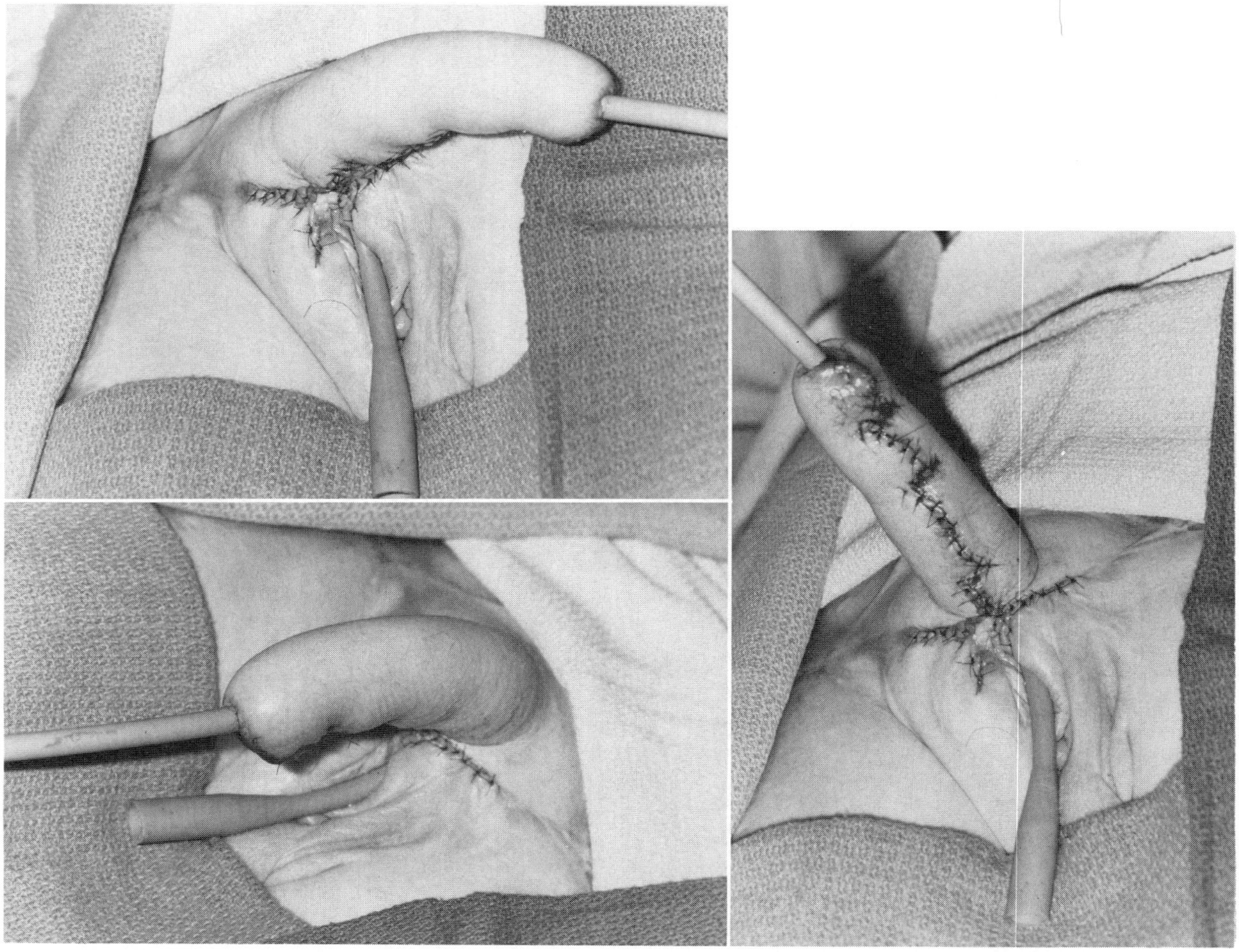

Fig. 12-5, cont'd. H to **J,** Postoperative result of graft excision and primary closure using multiple z-plasties on the ventral aspect of the penis to avoid scar contracture.

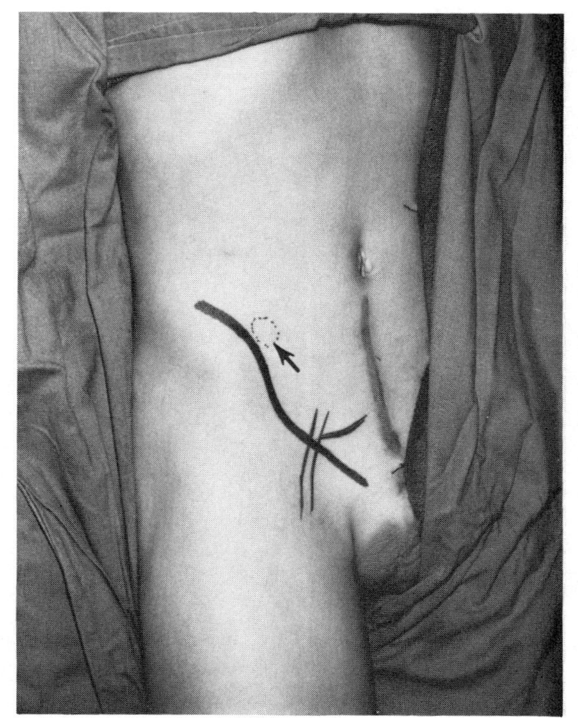

Fig. 12-6. A, Patient with bilateral cryptorchism through a previous intraabdominal incision. The left testicle was brought into the scrotum by the conventional technique of severing the internal spermatic venous plexus and artery. The right testicle is still in a retroperitoneal location *(arrow).*

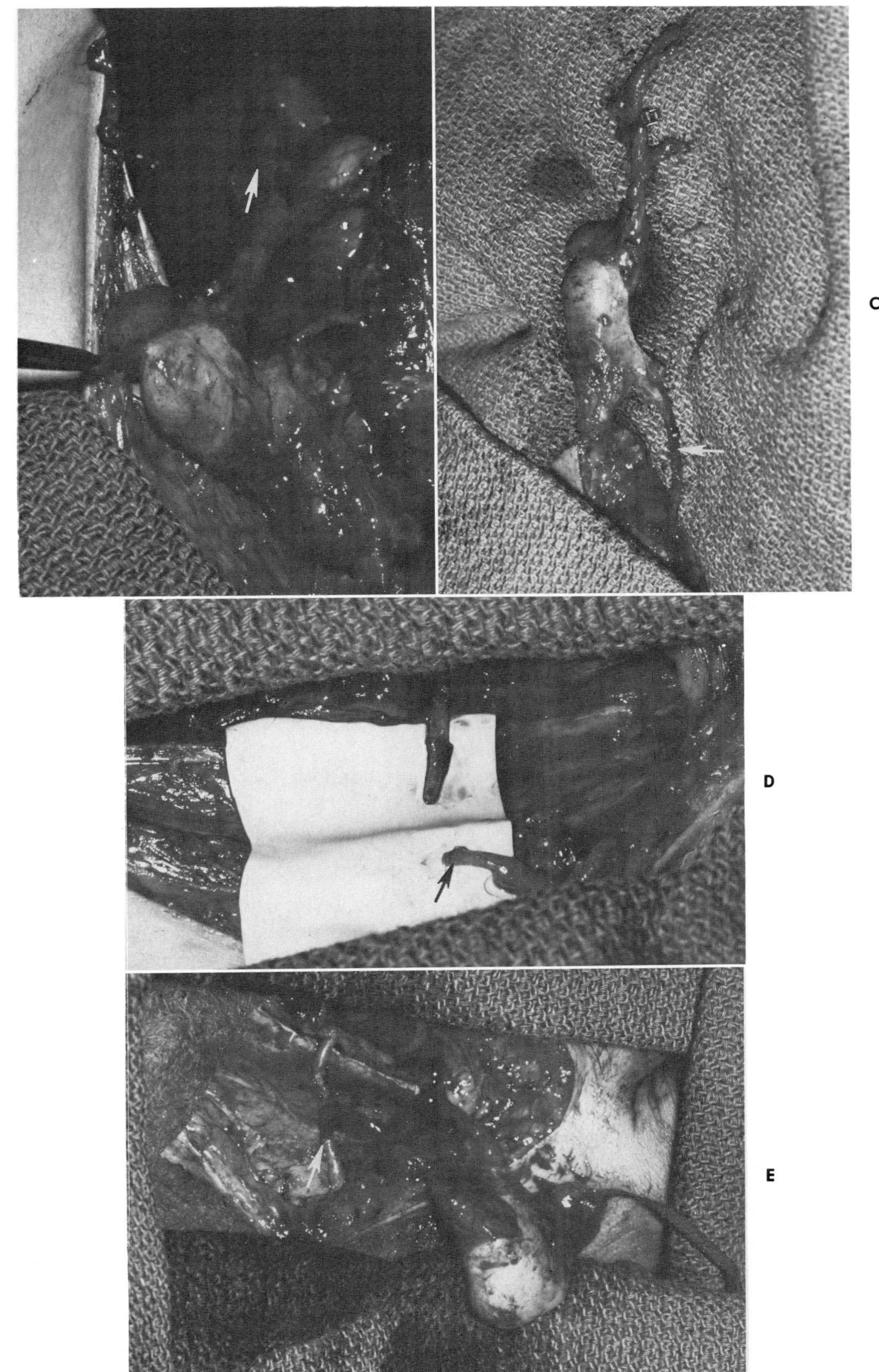

Fig. 12-6, cont'd. B, Internal spermatic venous plexus and internal spermatic artery *(arrow).* **C,** Vas deferens *(arrow).* Note donor vasculature superiorly. **D,** Donor *(arrow)* and recipient arteries. **E,** Testicle after revascularization. Arrow depicts venous anastomosis. Note arterial anastomosis more superiorly.

Continued.

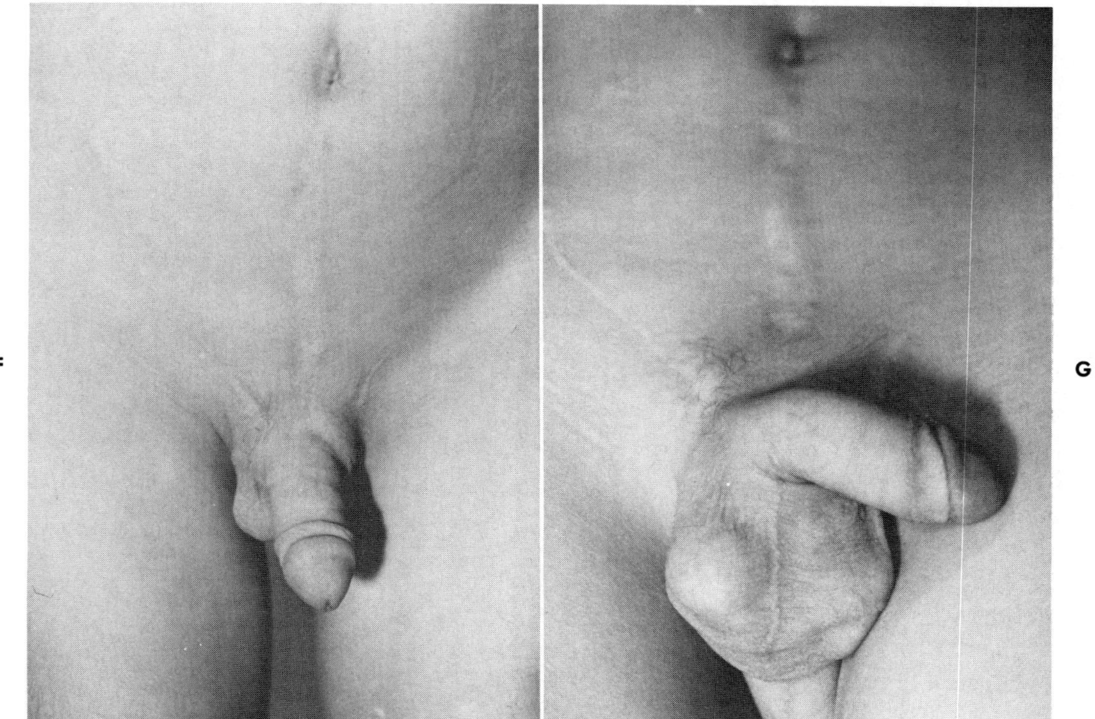

Fig. 12-6, cont'd. F and **G,** Viability of the transplanted testicle.

patients an end-to-side venous anastomosis was performed. The scapular and groin flaps were selected as donor tissue in seven patients. A deficiency in soft tissue cover existed in all patients. In patients with more extensive wounds, often associated with underlying comminuted fractures, a latissimus dorsi musculocutaneous flap was used (Fig. 12-7). It is believed that a muscle flap with its improved blood supply is more suitable donor tissue for a contaminated recipient bed.

One patient had a severe compound comminuted fracture of the tibia with extensive loss of soft tissue and approximately a 15 cm segmental loss of the tibia and fibula. This patient was first treated with a vascularized latissimus dorsi musculocutaneous flap, and primary wound healing was achieved. At a second procedure the Orthopaedic Service transplanted a vascularized fibula from the contralateral unaffected leg to achieve bony union and stabilization. The missing segment was so extensive that the fibula, rather than the iliac crest, was selected as donor osseous tissue.

With the exception of a vascularized groin flap that failed secondary to an anomalous arterial blood supply, all of the vascularized cutaneous flaps were completely successful and healed without infection, wound separation, or necrosis.

The vascularized scapular flap has replaced the groin flap as the donor tissue of choice when cutaneous cover only is needed in reconstruction. The flap is a relatively thin one of uniform thickness. The vascular pedicle is of adequate external diameter and approximately 10 cm in length. The vascular basis of the flap is the circumflex scapular artery. This artery can be traced proximally to its origin from the

subscapular artery if increased length or external diameter is desirable. Commonly there are two veins to the flap, frequently of disparate size. The largest of the two veins is approximately 4 to 5 mm in external diameter, the smaller vein is 1 to 3 mm in external diameter. A flap measuring 9 × 22 cm can be safely dissected with primary closure of the donor site. The resulting scar is a horizontal one, superior in location to that normally seen after a latissimus dorsi musculocutaneous flap. The scar is usually not an objectional one; however, it is not as well concealed as the scar from a vascularized groin flap. The dermis of the flap is quite thick and appears to be durable when transplanted to a recipient site in the distal lower extremity. The flap cannot be employed as a neurosensory flap. As indicated in Chapter 70, however, the vascularized scapular flap has been used successfully in weight-bearing areas. Peripheral neurotization from the surrounding skin is effective in providing protective sensation to the flap.

SUMMARY AND CONCLUSIONS

It would appear that the optimal time to perform elective microsurgical procedures in children would be after 3 to 4 years of age. At this age the histologic appearance of wall arteries and veins is similar to that seen in adult blood vessels. Both donor and recipient arteries and veins would also be of a size and thickness suitable for anastomosis. Microsurgical procedures can technically be performed in younger infants should this be necessary. Thus transplantation of epiphyseal growth centers in upper extremity reconstruction or reconstruction after trauma may require intervention at an earlier age.

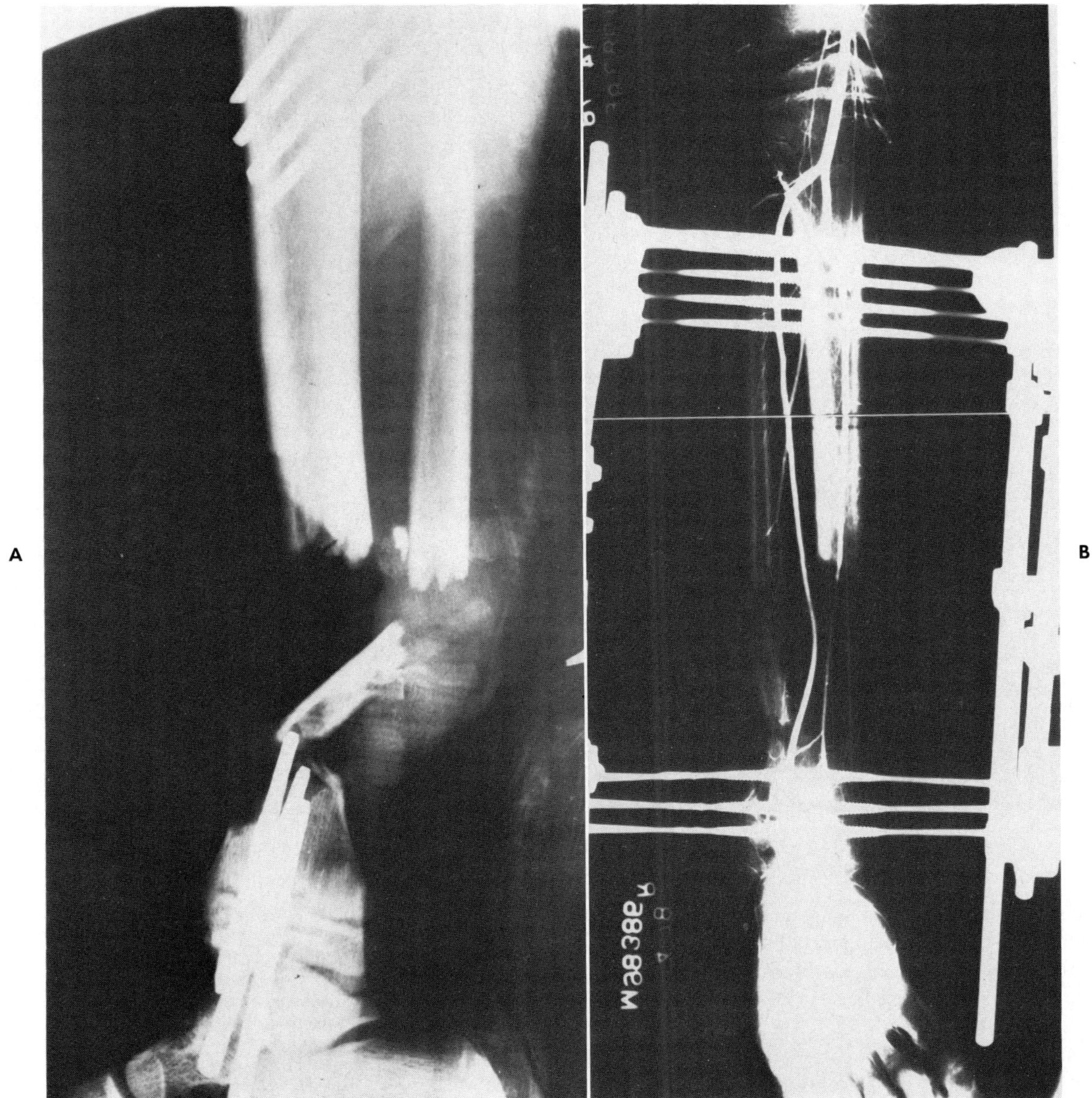

Fig. 12-7. A, Compound comminuted fracture. Note extensive loss (15 cm) of the tibia and fibula. **B,** Preoperative arteriogram demonstrating patency of only a single vessel to the distal lower extremity.

Continued.

After allogeneic renal transplantation both compensatory and obligatory growth of the renal transplant in children appears to occur. Growth of the individual and the transplanted organ is most likely to occur if transplantation can be performed at an early age before maturation arrest. Improved methods of tissue typing and the introduction of cyclosporin A have improved tissue survival statistics and reduced the deleterious effects of long-term immuno-suppression.

Microsurgical transplantation of osseous, epiphyseal, or cartilaginous structures ensures complete survival and growth of all structures, provided that blood flow is not interrupted for prolonged periods. Both the blood supply and function appear to influence growth of transplanted tissues.

Efforts are continuing to improve the success of immunoregulation. Recent research has been directed toward the production of monoclonal antibodies in human cells. Their production would provide a more improved and specific method for tissue typing and at the same time eliminate cells responsible for allogeneic graft rejection. It is anticipated that within the next decade or two the transplantation microsurgeon will be able to safely replace lost organs and parts, thus fulfilling the future predictions of Carrel.

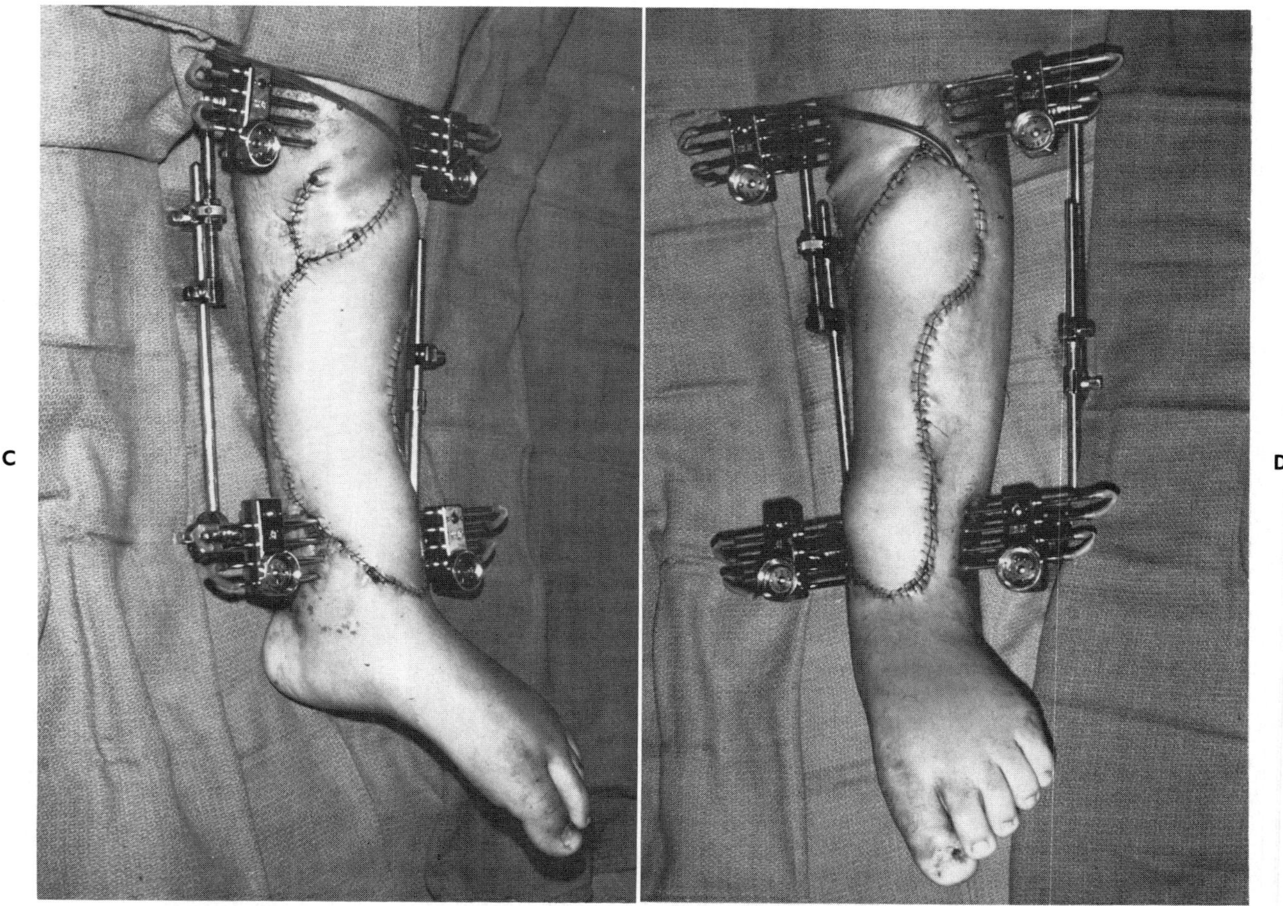

Fig. 12-7, cont'd. C and **D,** Early postoperative result of successful vascularized latissimus dorsi musculocutaneous flap transplantation to defect.

It is theorized that prolonged hypoxia results in the release of thromboxane from platelets promoting thrombosis. This is accentuated by a damaged vascular endothelium that is unable to produce sufficient PGI_2 to counteract this effect. It would appear that all enzyme systems resulting in clot formation and dissolution are present at birth. Problems increasing the frequency of thrombosis in children probably are related to vessel size rather than to their immaturity. This is especially true in children 3 to 4 years old.

Twenty-one patients underwent reconstruction with composite donor tissue of a variety of histologic types. Twenty-two separate microsurgical procedures were performed. Problems in reconstruction specifically related to children in various anatomic regions were examined and discussed in detail. Despite problems related to vessel size, only one failure occurred in the present series (4.5%).

It is hoped that unanswered questions throughout this chapter will serve as a stimulus to other investigators. The future role of microsurgical composite tissue transplantation both in children and in adults may be directed toward the replacement of parts from allogeneic sources.

REFERENCES

1. Allison, A.C., Garcia, R.C., Green, C., et al.: Effects of cyclosporin on a lymphoblast and the induction of tolerance to allografts. In Touraine, J.L., et al., editor: Transplantation and clinical immunology. XI, Amsterdam, 1979, Excerpta Medica.
2. Bassett, C.A.L.: Current concepts of bone formation, J. Bone Joint Surg. **44A:**1217, 1962.
3. Belker, A.M.: Urologic microsurgery: current perspectives. II. Orchiopexy and testicular homotransplantation, Urology **15:**103, 1980.
4. Ben Ezra, D.: Neovasculogenesis: triggering factors and possible mechanisms, Surv. Ophthalmol. **24:**167, 1979.
5. Berggren, A., Weiland, A.J., and Dorfman, H.: Medullary and/or periosteal circulation for survival of bone cells and "fracture" healing in composite bone grafts revascularized by microvascular anastomoses. (Manuscript in preparation.)
6. Bramis, J.P., and Taub, R.N.: Allograft reaction. In Castro, J.E., editor: Immunology for surgeons, Baltimore, 1976, University Park Press.
7. Brent, L.: Cyclosporin A: a discussion of its clinical and biologic attributes: summary of a workshop, Transplant. Proc. **12:**234, 1980.
8. Brown, K.L.B., and Cruess, R.L.: Bone and cartilage transplantation in orthopaedic surgery, J. Bone Joint Surg. **64A:**270, 1982.
9. Buck-Gramcko, D.: Pollicization of the index finger, J. Bone Joint Surg. **53A:**1605, 1971.
10. Calne, R.Y., White, D.J.G., Thiru, S., et al.: Cyclosporin A in clinical kidney grafting from cadaver donors. In Touraine, et al., editors: Transplantation and clinical immunology. XI, Amsterdam, 1979, Excerpta Medica.
11. Carrel, A.: The surgery of blood vessels, Johns Hopkins Hosp. Bull. **18:**25, 1907.
12. Chesney, R.W., et al.: Relationship of prednisone therapy to linear growth and bone mineral content in childhood glomerular disease, Am. J. Dis. Child. **132:**768, 1978.
13. Cho, M.J., and Allen, M.A.: Chemical stability of prostacyclin (PGI_2) in aqueous solutions, Prostaglandins **15:**943, 1978.

14. Copenhaver, W.M., Kelly, D.E., and Wood, R.L.: Bailey's textbook of histology, ed. 17, Baltimore, 1978, Williams & Wilkins.
15. Dausset, J.: Leuko-agglutinins IV, leuko-agglutinins and blood transfusion, Vox Sang. **4:**190, 1954.
16. Donski, P.K., Carwell, G.R., and Sharzer, L.A.: Growth in revascularized bone grafts in young puppies, Plast. Reconstr. Surg. **64:**239, 1979.
17. Donski, P.K., and O'Brien, B.M.: Free microvascular epiphyseal transplantation: an experimental study in dogs, Br. J. Plast. Surg. **33:**169, 1980.
18. Dunnill, M.S., and Halley, W.: Some observations on the quantitative anatomy of the kidney, J. Pathol. **110:**113, 1973.
19. Epstein, M.: Effects of aging on the kidney, Fed. Proc. **38:**168, 1979.
20. Ferguson, R.M., Rynasiewicz, J.J., Sutherland, D.E.R., et al.: Cyclosporin A in renal transplantation: a prospective randomized trial, Surgery **92:**175, 1982.
21. Fowler, R., and Stephens, F.D.: The role of testicular vascular anatomy in the salvage of the high undescended testis, Aust. N.Z. J. Surg. **29:**92, 1959.
22. Furnas, D.W.: Growth and development in replanted forelimbs, Plast. Reconstr. Surg. **46:**445, 1970.
23. Furuyama, M.: Histometrical investigations of arteries in reference to arterial hypertension, Tohoku J. Exp. Med. **76:**388, 962.
24. Gilbert, P.: Toe transfers for congenital hand defects, J. Hand. Surg. **7:**118, 1982.
25. Good, R.A.: Immunology, J.A.M.A. **245:**2197, 1981.
26. Hamberg, M., Suensson, J., and Samuelsson, B.: Thromboxanes: a new group of biologically active compounds derived from prostaglandin endoperoxides, Proc. Natl. Acad. Sci. U.S.A. **72:**2994, 1975.
27. Herrin, J.T.: Pediatric renal transplantation, Kidney Int. **18:**519, 1980.
28. Heyner, S.: The antigenicity of cartilage grafts, Surg. Gynecol. Obstet. **136:**298, 1973.
29. Ingelfinger, J.R., Teele, R., Traves, S., and Levey, R.H.: Renal growth after transplantation: infant kidney received by adolescent, Clin. Nephrol. **15:**28, 1981.
30. Kazmar, R.E., and Fathman, C.G.: Monoclonal antibodies: tools of the future, Mayo Clin. Proc. **55:**517, 1980.
31. Korthals, J.K., and Wisniewski, H.M.: Peripheral nerve ischemia. I. Experimental model, J. Neurol. Sci. **24:**65, 1975.
32. Lang, J.: Über die Vascularisation der Wand und des Einbaugewebes mittelgrosser Gefässe des Unterschenkels, Z. Anat. Entwicklungsgesch. **122:**482, 1961.
33. Malt, R.A., and McKhann, C.F.: Replantation of severed arms, J.A.M.A. **189:**716, 1964.
34. Marinov, G.: Some differences between the long and short saphenous veins as regards the structure and vascularization of the wall and location of the valves, Folia Morphol. **24:**221, 1976.
35. Mathes, S.J., Buchannan, R., and Weeks, P.M.: Microvascular joint transplantation with epiphyseal growth, J. Hand. Surg. **5:**586, 1980.
36. May, J.W., Smith, R.J., and Peimer, C.A.: Toe-to-hand free-tissue transfer for thumb reconstruction with multiple digit aplasia, Plast. Reconstr. Surg. **67:**207, 1981.
37. Medawar, P.B., and Woodruff, M.F.A.: The induction of tolerance by skin homografts in newborn rats, Immunology **1:**27, 1958.
38. Morrison, A.D., Berwick, L., Orci, L., and Winegard, A.I.: Morphology and metabolism of an aortic intima-media preparation in which an intact endothelium is preserved, J. Clin. Invest. **57:**650, 1967.
39. Olsson, L., and Kaplan, H.S.: Human-human hybridomas producing monoclonal antibodies of predefined antigenic specificity, Proc. Natl. Acad. Sci. U.S.A. **77:**5429, 1980.
40. Opelz, G., and Terasaki, P.I.: International workshop on HLA matching in cadaver kidney transplantation. In Touraine, J.L., et al., editors: Transplantation and clinical immunology. XII, Amsterdam, 1980, Excerpta Medica.
41. Pesonen, E., Martimo, P., and Rapola, J.: Histometry of the arterial wall: a new technique with the aid of automatic data processing, Lab. Invest. **30:**550, 1974.
42. Phemister, D.B.: The fate of transplanted bone and regenerative power of its various constituents, Surg. Gynecol. Obstet. **19:**303, 1914.
43. Reinherz, E.L., Kung, P.C., Goldstein, G., and Schlossman, S.F.: Separation of functional subsets of human T-cells by a monoclonal antibody, Proc. Natl. Acad. Sci. U.S.A. **76:**4061, 1979.
44. Rist, M., Lee, S., and Gittes, R.F.: Glomerular filtration rate and effective renal plasma flow in 4 kidney rats, Surg. Forum **26:**579, 1975.
45. Rosenkrantz, J.G., Sullivan, R.C., Welch, K., et al.: Replantation of an infant's arm, N. Engl. J. Med. **276:**609, 1967.
46. Schlatmann, T.J.M., and Becker, A.E.: Histologic changes in the normal aging aorta: implications for dissecting aortic aneurysm, Am. J. Cardiol. **39:**13, 1977.
47. Silber, S.J.: Renal transplantation between adults and children, J.A.M.A. **228:**1143, 1974.
48. Silber, S., and Malvin, R.L.: Compensatory and obligatory renal growth in rats, Am. J. Physiol. **226:**114, 1974.
49. Spira, E., and Farin, I.: Epiphyseal transplantation: a case report, J. Bone Joint Surg. **46A:**1278, 1964.
50. Stoinov, N.: Ontogenetic development of the structure and vascularization of the veins of the upper limbs, Folia Morphol. **25:**256, 1977.
51. Tachojian, M.O.: Pediatric orthopaedics, Philadelphia, 1972, W.B. Saunders Co.
52. Takazakura, E., Sawaby, K., Handa, A., et al.: Intrarenal vascular changes with age and disease, Kidney Int. **2:**224, 1972.
53. Tanzer, R.C.: Microtia—a long-term follow-up of 44 reconstructed auricles, Plast. Reconstr. Surg. **61:**161, 1978.
54. The Twelfth Report of the Human Renal Transplant Registry. Prepared by the Advisory Committee to the Renal Transplant Registry, J.A.M.A. **233:**787, 1975.
55. Van Beek, A.L., Wavak, P.W., and Zook, E.G.: Microvascular surgery in young children, Plast. Reconstr. Surg. **63:**457, 1979.
56. Vancov, V., and Marinov, G.: On the vascularization of lower limb arteries, Folia Morphol. **21:**188, 1973.
57. Vancov, V., and Marinov, G.: Growth characteristics of vascularization of the arterial wall in the lower limbs, with special reference to thickened parts of the arterial wall, Folia Morphol. **25:**379, 1977.
58. Van Meurs-Van Woezik, H., Klein, H.W., and Krediet, P.: Normal internal calibres of ostia of great arteries and of aortic isthmus in infants and children, Br. Heart J. **39:**860, 1977.
59. Waltz, A.G., and Sundt, T.M.: The microvasculature and microcirculation of the cerebral cortex after arterial occlusion, Brain **70:**681, 1967.
60. White, J.C.: Nerve regeneration after replantation of severed arms, Ann. Surg. **170:**715, 1969.

HEAD AND NECK

CHAPTER 13

Embryology of the head and neck

MALCOLM C. JOHNSTON and KATHLEEN K. SULIK

Recent technologic advances have greatly improved our understanding of normal and abnormal embryonic development of the head and neck. The complex sequences of developmental phenomena that are involved, such as extensive cell migrations and interactions, can be broken down in a progressive step-by-step manner. Once these sequences are put into perspective, they are much easier to understand.

This chapter first provides an overview of normal embryonic development of the head and neck and then details the normal development that is most pertinent to craniofacial malformations. Although alterations initiated during embryonic stages are emphasized, secondary alterations that manifest themselves in later development are briefly considered. Attention is also given to alterations initiated in the later (fetal) period of prenatal development. Even though some material has little apparent clinical relevance, it has been included primarily to provide a basis for a more complete understanding of normal and abnormal development. Wherever feasible, developmental alterations are related to counseling and clinical treatment.

OVERVIEW OF NORMAL DEVELOPMENT

This broad presentation of prenatal development provides a framework from which the reader may correlate normal and abnormal head and neck developmental alterations leading up to and away from "critical events" (e.g., lip formation). Developmental mechanisms peculiar to the embryonic period (e.g., massive cell migrations and interactions) are also introduced. Traditional morphologic treatment of human embryonic development may be found in a number of texts.[38,57,71]

Most information on embryonic developmental mechanisms comes from studies of subhuman vertebrates, especially those in which direct observation or experimental manipulation is possible. As more information accumulates, it is the similarity of mechanisms involved in head and neck

development of vertebrate embryos that is most striking. This evidence makes it possible to extrapolate the information to humans with a considerable amount of confidence; indeed, the gross morphology of higher vertebrate embryos is very similar (Fig. 13-1).

Advancing technology has greatly facilitated the comparison of both macroscopic and microscopic features of human and subhuman forms. One such technique—scanning electron microscopy—has been particularly useful because it permits three-dimensional observations at high magnifications; thus the cell structure characteristic of different aspects of developmental behavior (e.g., the bipolar morphologic appearance of migrating cells as shown in Fig. 13-12) can be observed.

The earliest stages of human development are illustrated schematically in Fig. 13-2, *A* to *C*. Only a small number of the "daughter" cells derived from the fertilized ovum are used to form the embryo (inner cell mass); the remainder (trophoblast) forms the placenta and other "support" tissues (Fig. 13-2, *D*). Little is known about the manner in which cells of the inner cell mass separate into two layers (epiblast and hypoblast) (Fig. 13-2, *E*). Migration of some of the cells from the upper layer (epiblast) into an underlying space, or potential space, between the layers (Fig. 13-2, *F*) forms the middle (mesodermal) layer of the three–germ layer embryo. Terms designating these three layers, *ectoderm, mesoderm,* and *endoderm* (Fig. 13-2, *F*), now replace the terms "epiblast" and "hypoblast." It appears that interference with mesoderm formation is related to the origin of some major craniofacial malformations.

Migration of cells to form the mesoderm is currently recognized as the first of numerous embryonic cell migrations. The significance of these migrations is that they bring different groups of cells into close proximity with one another, permitting them to "interact" and thereby alter their future development. The term *induction* refers strictly to an

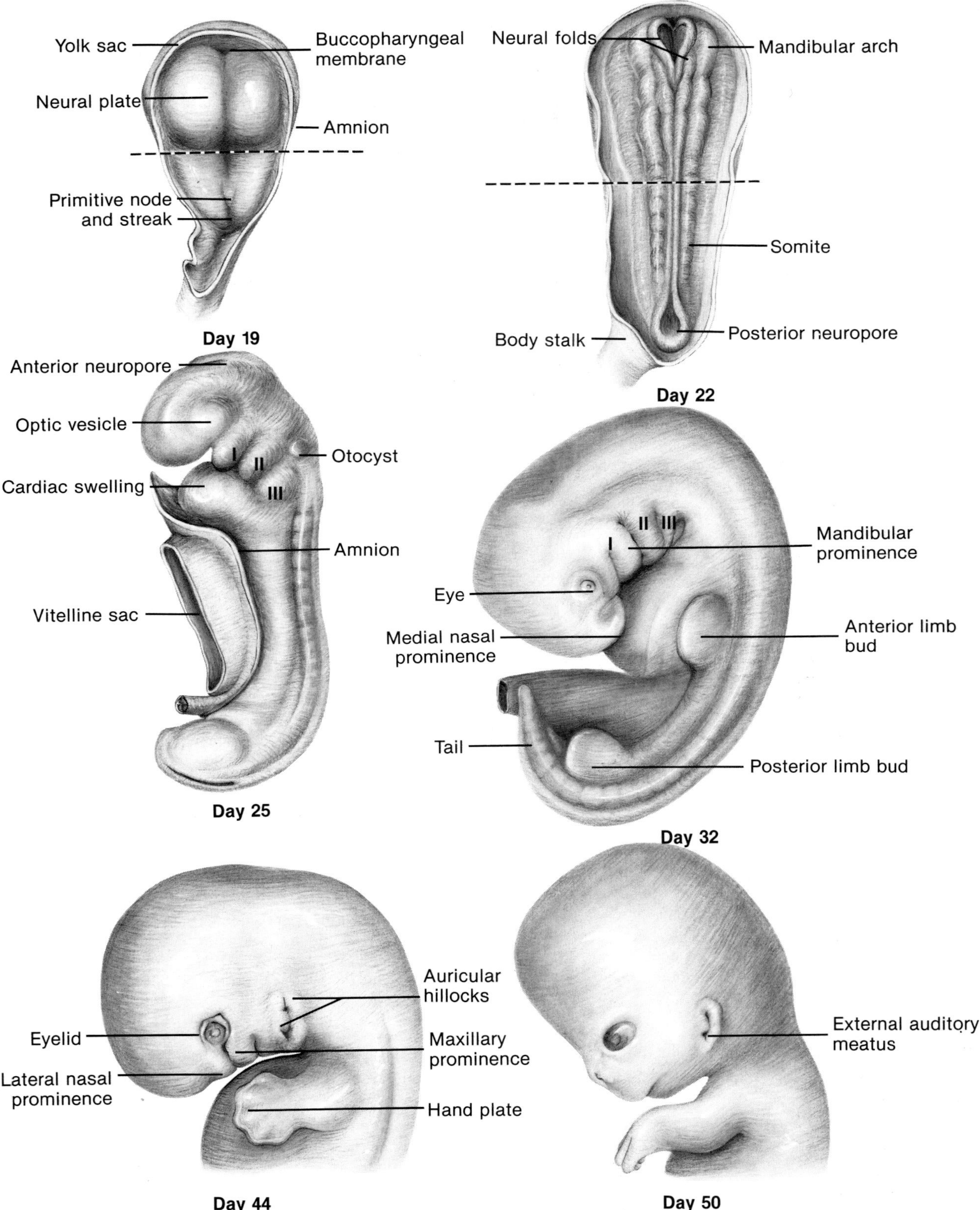

Fig. 13-1. Progressive development of the human embryo. Dorsal views are used for day 19 and day 22 embryos. Visceral arches are indicated by roman numerals. The external form of all higher vertebrate embryos is remarkably similar up to the stage of development seen in the day 32 embryo. Most malformations of the head and neck are easily identifiable by this stage of development. (See also Fig. 13-12.) (From Johnston, M.C., and Sulik, K.K.: Development of face and oral cavity. In Bhaskar, S.N., editor: Orban's oral histology and embryology, ed. 9, St. Louis, 1980, The C.V. Mosby Co.)

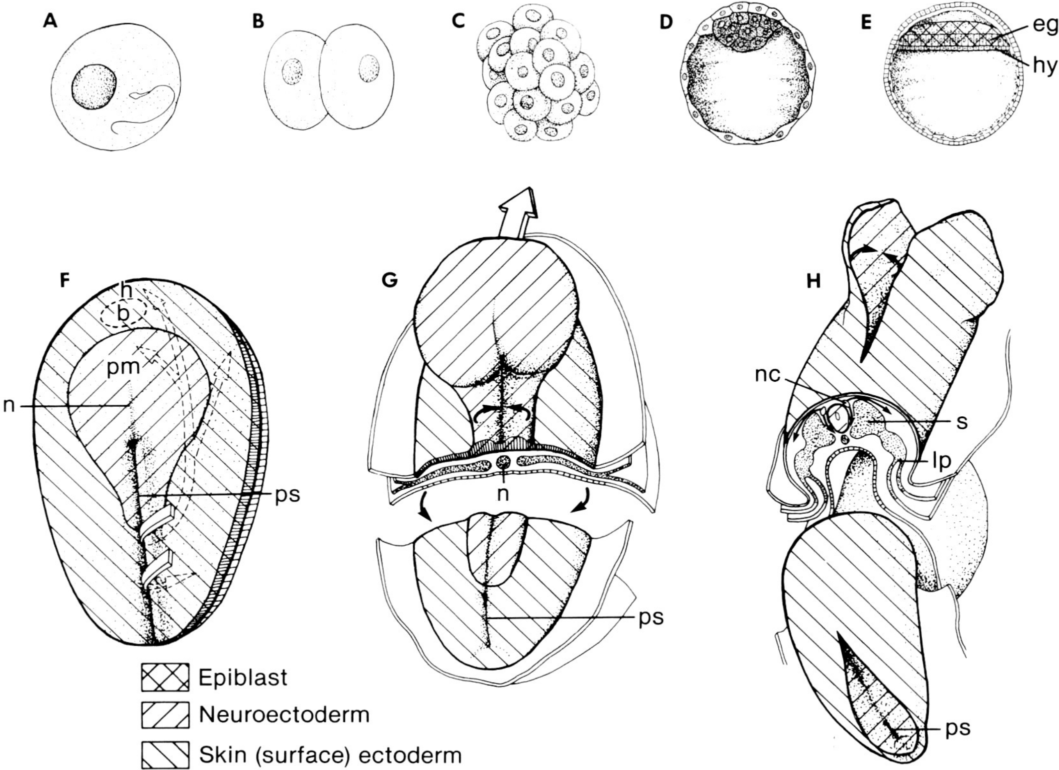

Fig. 13-2. Early stages of human embryonic development. **A** to **C,** Fertilization and earliest cell divisions. **D,** Sectioned blastocyst. A fluid-filled cavity has formed, and cells (darker area equals inner cell mass) that will form the embryo are distinct from other cells that will develop into support tissues (e.g., the placenta). **E,** Embryo-forming cells have now separated into two layers: the epiblast *(ep)* and hypoblast *(hy).* **F,** Dorsal view of an embryo slightly more advanced than the sectioned embryo illustrated in **E.** Gastrulation movements *(arrows)* bring cells from the upper layer through the primitive streak *(ps)* into the potential space between the two layers to form the middle germ layer. Mesodermal cells fail to penetrate between the ectoderm and endoderm at the oral plate (*b,* buccopharyngeal membrane), which later forms the embryonic partition between the oral and pharyngeal cavities. At this stage the heart primordium *(h)* lies anterior to the oral plate. The notochord *(n)* is formed from the anterior (cephalic) end of the primitive streak. The prechordal mesoderm *(pm)* is subjacent to the neural plate on the region between *n* and *b.* **G,** Early stages of neural tube folding and closure and folding of the lateral body walls *(solid arrows).* The anterior neural plate has begun to "overgrow" *(open arrow)* the heart primordium and future oral region, including the buccopharyngeal membrane. **H,** Embryo folding is nearing completion. Migration of cranial neural crest cells *(nc)* in the hindbrain region has been initiated. In contrast to the trunk crest cells, most of those forming in the head region migrate laterally under the surface ectoderm, but superficial to the somites *(s)* and lateral plate *(lp)* of the mesoderm.

embryonic phenomenon involving cellular interactions followed by "determination" of cell groups that can later develop without the continued presence of inducing cells. For example, a portion of the mesoderm induces the overlying ectoderm to form the neural plate (Fig. 13-2, *F*), which is then capable of proceeding on its own to form the brain, spinal cord, and portions of the eye.

Major form-shaping (morphogenetic) events involve folding of the neural plate to form a neural tube (Fig. 13-2, *G* and *H*), as well as folding of the lateral halves of the embryo to form the body wall and gut. Because of the latter, the endoderm becomes a tubelike structure (Fig. 13-2, *H*) that

eventually forms the epithelium lining most of the digestive tract and the epithelial components of its glandular derivatives.

A dominant feature of embryonic development of the head and neck is the role played by neural crest cells. These ectodermal cells form at the junction of the neural plate and adjacent surface ectoderm and usually migrate into underlying regions at about the time the neural folds are making contact to form the neural tube (Fig. 13-2, *H*). Unlike the trunk neural crest cells, which differentiate into pigment cells and cells of the peripheral nervous system, crest cells in the head region also form almost all of the skeletal and

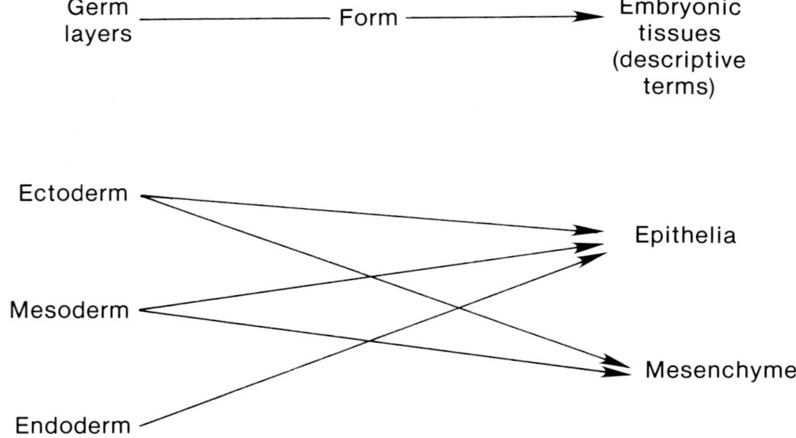

Fig. 13-3. Developmental biologists use the terms *epithelium* and *mesenchyme* to describe embryonic tissues according to histologic appearance (e.g., whether they have a small or large amount of extracellular matrix) without reference to the germ layer origin *(arrows)*.

connective tissues of the face (e.g., bone, cartilage, fibrous connective tissue, and most components of the teeth), a role reserved elsewhere for mesoderm. Head crest cells are induced to differentiate into the skeletal and connective tissues appropriate to their location by the pharyngeal endoderm, oral ectoderm, and other tissues with which they become closely associated (Fig. 13-13).

A source of continuing confusion, especially in clinically oriented publications, is use of the terms *mesenchyme* and *mesoderm*. Most developmental biologists use the terms *epithelium* and *mesenchyme* to describe embryonic tissues according to histologic appearance without reference to their germ layer origin (which sometimes is not known). Epithelial cells have extensive intercellular connections and little intercellular space, whereas mesenchyme has few (if any) intercellular connections and an abundance of intercellular space. Thus migrating neural crest cells are termed *mesenchymal cells* (Fig. 13-3).

At the completion of their major migrations, the crest cells form almost all of the mesenchyme in the upper facial region (above the oral cavity) and surround mesodermal cores in the visceral arches (Fig. 13-4, *A*). Initially cells of the mesodermal cores are involved in forming the endothelial cells of developing blood vessels. Later, other mesodermal cells that migrate from locations close to the neural tube are found in the cores of the arches. The "new" mesodermal cells eventually form myoblasts, which become the contractile cells of skeletal (voluntary) muscles, such as the masseter muscle and the muscles of facial expression. Recent studies indicate that virtually all other nonepithelial cells in the facial region are of crest cell origin.

Regional growth centers in the upper facial region give rise to surface elevations that are usually termed *facial processes*. We believe that the term *facial prominences* (as used by Slavkin[89]) is preferable, primarily because "processes"

is used for the description of cellular extensions as cell processes. The term *facial swellings,* as used by Streeter,[95] conveys the impression of fluid accumulation, which now appears to account for only a small amount of the regional growth.

There is little evidence that (crest) mesenchymal cells in the developing facial prominences undergo appreciable secondary migrations. This change in their migratory nature is consistent with the appearance of a very extensive mesenchymal "cell process meshwork" that is attached to the underlying epithelial surfaces (Fig. 13-4, *C*)[102] Differential growth rates may be explained by differences in "resident" cell proliferation rates. It is known that proliferation of facial prominence mesenchyme is maintained at much higher rates than in facial regions where little growth is occurring.[69,70]

The initial separation between the nasal pit and oral cavity is made much more extensive through growth, contact, and fusion of the medial nasal, lateral nasal, and maxillary prominences (Fig. 13-4, *C*). Details of this complex phenomenon, along with formation of the palatal shelves and their role in completing the separation of oral and nasal cavities, will be dealt with later. Both of these events involve *fusion,* a term designating epithelial contact and adhesion, followed by epithelial breakdown and mesenchymal consolidation across the contact area (Fig. 13-5, *A*). In contrast, simple filling in of grooves by coalescence of underlying mesenchymal growth centers (thereby pushing the bottom of the epithelial groove outward) is termed *merging* (Fig. 13-5, *B*).

Organogenesis, the period of organ formation during which almost all major malformations originate, is nearly completed by the end of the eighth week of human development. Long before organogenesis is completed, virtually all of the developing organs (e.g., the brain) are invaded by blood vessels. At the end of organogenesis, definitive

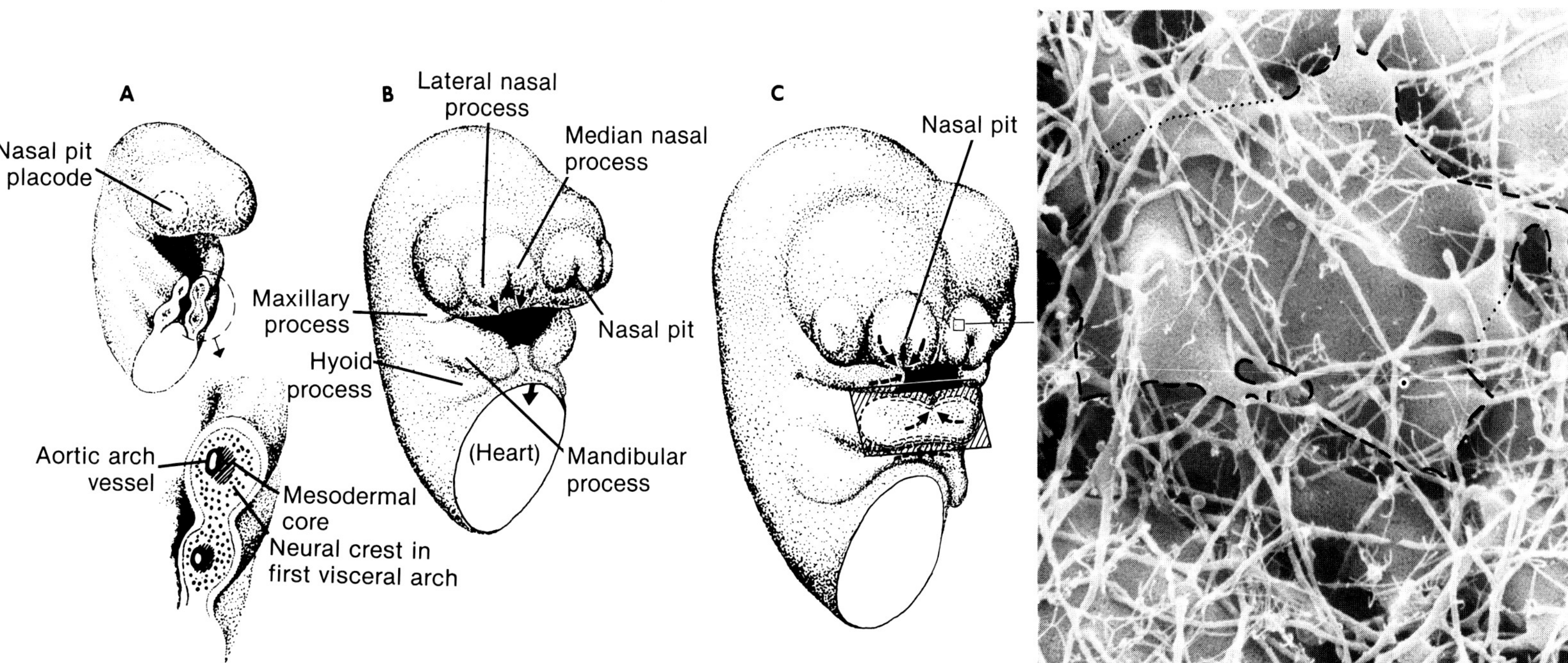

Fig. 13-4. A to **C,** Embryonic development from the completion of major crest cell migrations to fusion of facial prominences. The heart and contiguous portions of the visceral arches have been removed in **A.** The relations of the aortic arch blood vessels and the crest and mesodermal mesenchyme are indicated in the enlarged sketch of **A.** Arrows in **B** and **C** illustrate the growth directions of the facial prominences. **D,** The scanning electron micrograph illustrates the subepithelial mesenchymal cell process meshwork (after removal of the epithelial "patch") that may be involved in stabilizing epithelial-mesenchymal interrelations. (Modified from Johnston, M.C., and Sulik, K.K.: Development of face and oral cavity. In Bhaskar, S.N., editor: Orban's oral histology and embryology, ed. 9, St. Louis, 1980, The C.V. Mosby Co.)

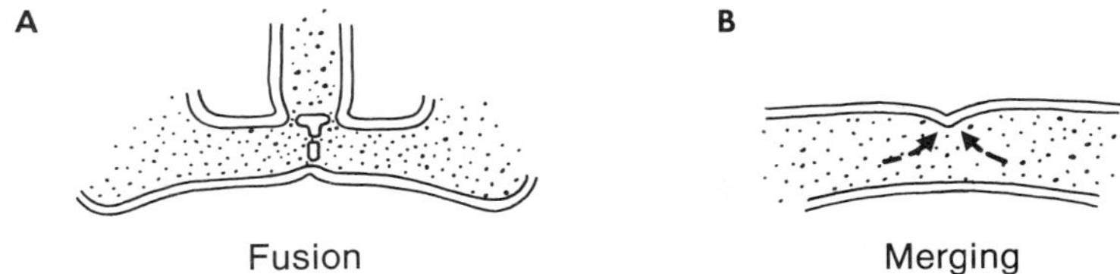

Fig. 13-5. A, Fusion of palatal shelves and nasal septum. **B,** Merging as in the developing mandibular arch. (See also Figs. 13-4, *C,* and 13-21, *B.*) Fusion involves contact of essentially "free-ended" structures, adhesion, epithelial breakdown, and mesenchymal consolidation as between the palatal shelves. Epithelial breakdown between the septum and palatal shelves has been initiated in **A.** Merging is the coalescence of growth centers whose already confluent mesenchyme appears to "push out" *(arrows)* and smooth intervening epithelial grooves **(B).**

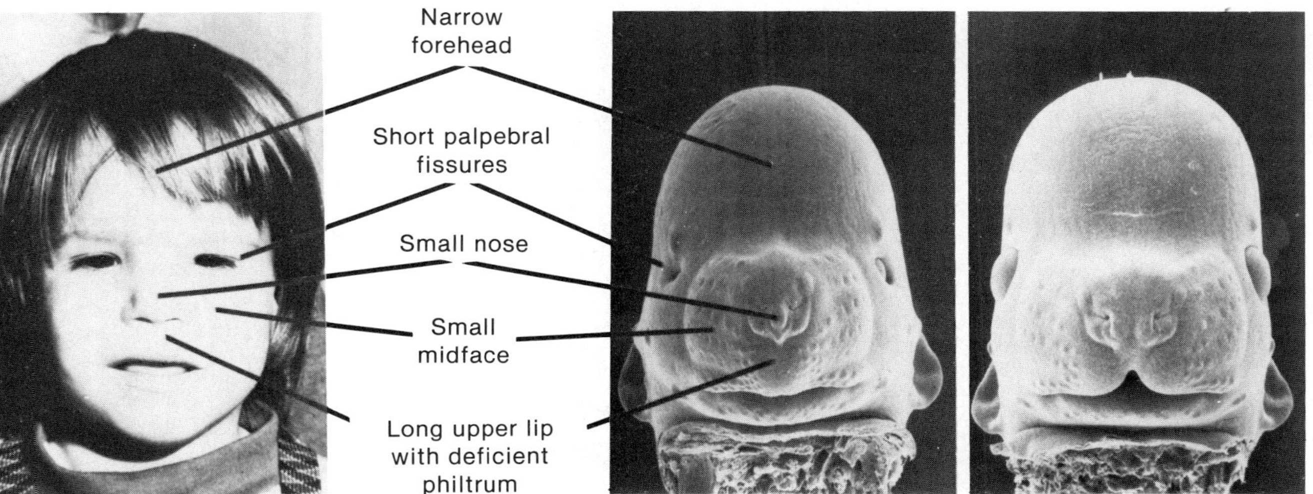

Fig. 13-6. A fetus *(center)* removed from a mouse to which alcohol (ethanol) had been administered early in pregnancy (gastrulation stage) shows numerous facial characteristics similar to those of a child with FAS. A control mouse fetus is shown on the right. (*Left* from Jones, K.L., and Smith, D.W.: The fetal alcohol syndrome, Teratology **12:**1, 1975.)

tissues such as bone and cartilage begin to make their appearance. These events mark the transition from embryonic to fetal life.

Human malformations usually occur at "critical points," when an essential phase of development fails to be completed. Failure at developmental critical points may depend on a number of prior developmental alterations resulting from genetic or environmental factors. An example of such a critical point is the attainment of sufficient contact for complete fusion of the embryonic facial prominences as illustrated in Fig. 13-4. If the prominences fail to make sufficient contact for the completion of fusion, the embryo is considered to be beyond the limit (threshold) for normal development, and cleft lip results. A number of prior developmental deviations, alone or in combination for each embryo, may lead to the contact failure. Further development of the face will be altered by the presence of the cleft. In the following discussions, the origins and progressive development of such malformations of the head and neck will receive detailed consideration.

GERM LAYER FORMATION AND ORGANIZATION OF ECTODERMAL AND MESODERMAL STRUCTURES

Evidence is accumulating that some malformations, such as those of the fetal alcohol syndrome (FAS) (Fig. 13-6), may result from interference with the formation of the mesodermal layer. Until recently abnormal development at these very early stages was believed to result either in prenatal death or a nonviable newborn having severe malformations, such as cyclopia.

Formation of the middle (mesodermal) germ layer is a complex phenomenon (Fig. 13-2, *F*). Large numbers of cells from the upper (epiblast) layer of the two-layer embryo migrate through the primitive streak to form mesodermal cells. As the anterior end of the primitive streak regresses, it appears to lay down the prospective notochordal cells from its anterior end (Hensen's node). The resulting notochord is an embryonic skeletal structure found beneath the midline of the neural plate except in the forebrain region. In this region, between the cephalic end of the notochord

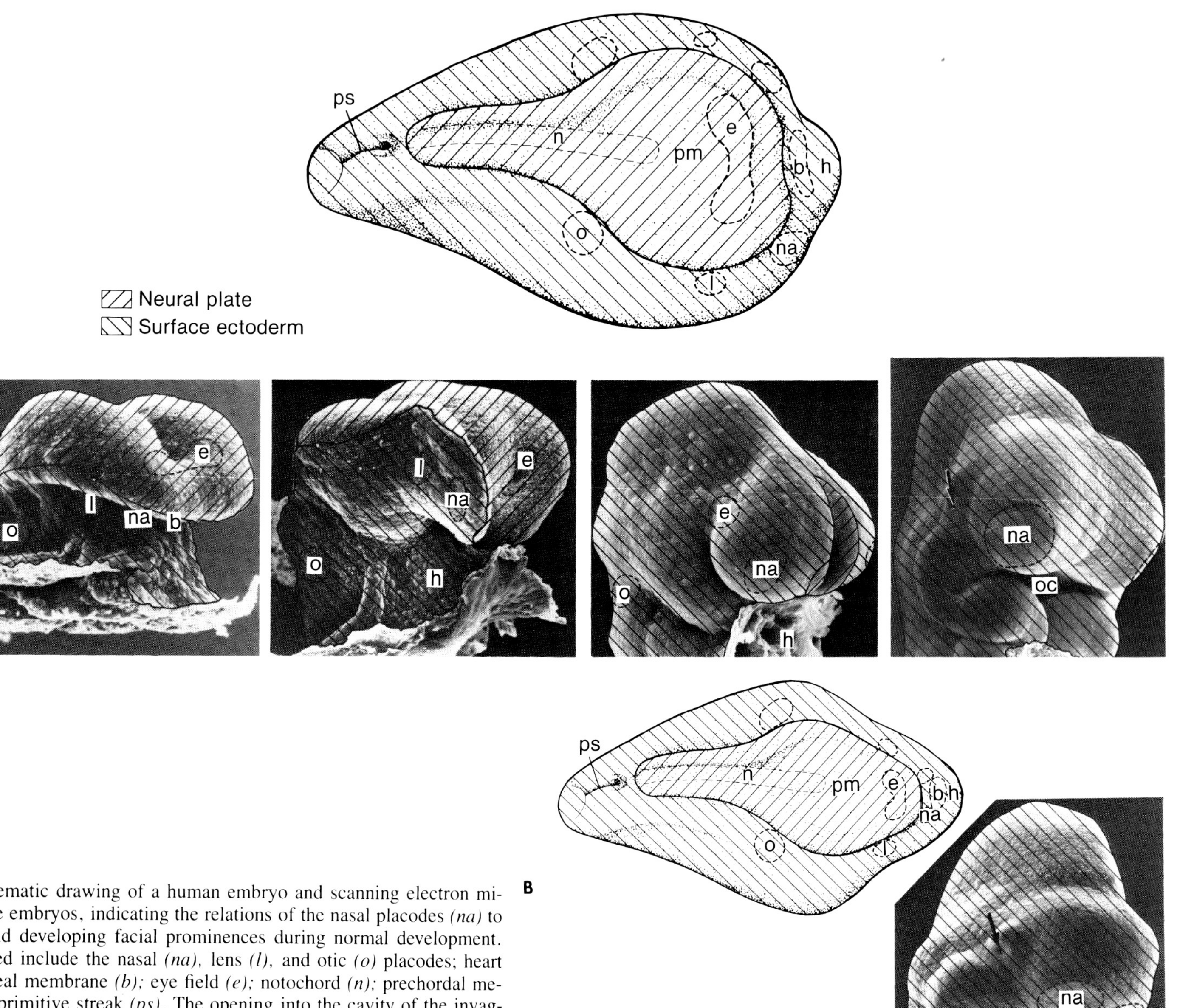

Fig. 13-7. A, Schematic drawing of a human embryo and scanning electron micrographs of mouse embryos, indicating the relations of the nasal placodes *(na)* to the neural plate and developing facial prominences during normal development. Structures illustrated include the nasal *(na)*, lens *(l)*, and otic *(o)* placodes; heart *(h)*; buccopharyngeal membrane *(b)*; eye field *(e)*; notochord *(n)*; prechordal mesoderm *(pm)*; and primitive streak *(ps)*. The opening into the cavity of the invaginating lens epithelium is indicated by the arrow on the scanning electron micrograph on the far right. The developing oral cavity *(oc)* is also shown. **B,** Altered development in embryos removed from ethanol-treated mothers. The nasal placodes are positioned much more closely to the midline in both the sketch and scanning electron micrograph.

and the oral plate, there is a special population of mesodermal cells termed the *prechordal mesoderm* (Fig. 13-2, *F*).

The development of a new FAS animal model[100,101,103] indicates that interference with gastrulation and associated deficiencies of the anterior neural plate may lead to a large variety of malformations of both the brain and face (Fig. 13-7). Such early developmental alterations may have little effect on embryonic viability. It is also possible that subtle developmental alterations of this type can lead to reduced mental capacity with little or no obvious morphologic change. Eye defects (e.g., microphthalmia) are common in the FAS animal model, just as in the human FAS. Since both the forebrain and most of the eye are derived from the anterior neural plate, underdevelopment of the eye is consistent with underdevelopment of the forebrain. Only a small lateral portion of the anterior neural plate gives rise to neural crest cells. These crest cells eventually form the mesenchyme of the frontonasal region, including the mesenchyme of the medial and lateral nasal prominences. Our studies provide no evidence that deficiencies of crest cells contribute to FAS.

Malformations in the holoprosencephaly series (Fig. 13-8) show considerable overlap with the FAS mouse model. The term *holoprosencephaly* indicates varying degrees of failure of the forebrain to divide into bilateral cerebral hemispheres. Human FAS might be considered to represent the mild end of the holoprosencephaly spectrum.[101] Although holoprosencephaly is seen in the severely affected offspring of ethanol-treated mice, cyclopia (the severe end of the holoprosencephaly spectrum) has been observed only rarely in our model[98] or in other similar models.[114] Phenotypic variability may be related to slight differences in timing of the insult, the specific tissue primarily involved,[1] and the degree to which anterior neural plate deficiency is confined to the midline region (Fig. 13-7). In our studies,[100,101] olfactory placode positioning (Fig. 13-7) is critical for the facial malformations observed. Olfactory placode induction (or positioning) depends both on the mesoderm and neuroectoderm (neural plate)[42], so that defects in both may be partly responsible for the olfactory placodes being too medially positioned with subsequent underdevelopment of the medial nasal prominences and their derivatives. Contact of the nasal placodes leads to severe or complete suppression of the formation of the medial nasal prominences and their derivatives.[49]

The FAS animal model indicates that abnormal cervical vertebrae may result from abnormal mesoderm formation. In the animal model mesodermally derived cervical somites (and the vertebrae that they form) are sometimes abnormal, as in human FAS.[98] We believe that defective mesoderm formation also may be responsible for defects seen in the Klippel-Feil syndrome, in which derivatives of both cervical and occipital somites may be defective (Fig. 13-9). Cleft palate is found in 5% to 20% of the patients with the Klippel-Feil syndrome[34] and is believed to result secondarily from inhibition of mandibular movement and palatal shelf elevation, although there is no experimental evidence for this hypothesis.

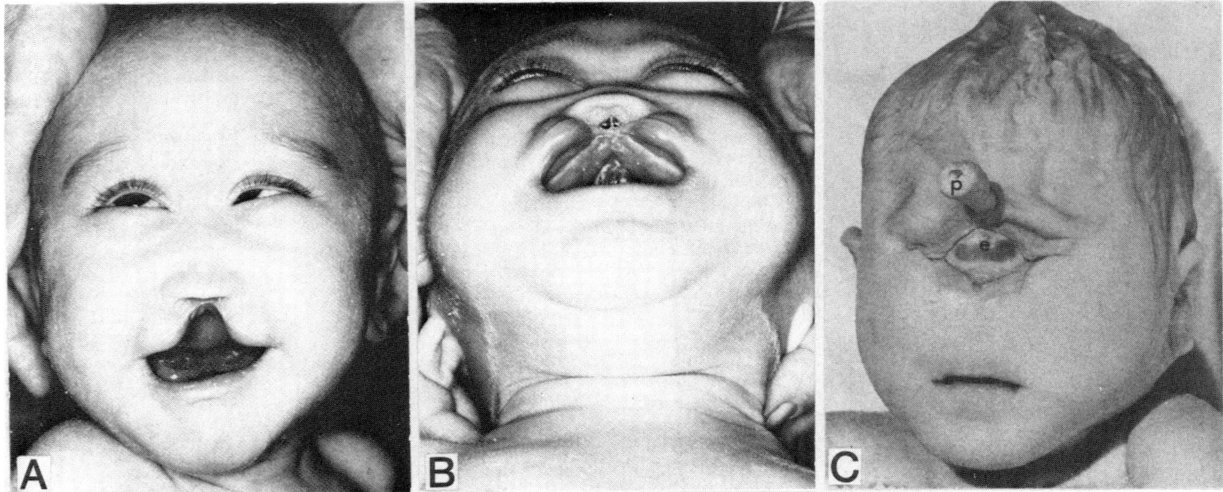

Fig. 13-8. A and **B,** Premaxillary agenesis (arhinencephaly) associated with trisomy 13, apparently results from midline contact of olfactory placodes and failure of medial nasal prominence formation. This malformation belongs to the holoprosencephaly series and represents an intermediate degree of severity, lying between the mild FAS malformations and more severe malformations, including cyclopia where the eye fields remain "fused." **C,** Cyclopia. A single proboscis *(p)* is located above the single midline eye *(e)*. The eyefields have failed to separate, and only one small olfactory placode has formed. (**A** and **B** from Ross, R.B., and Johnston, M.C.: Cleft lip and palate. © 1972, The Williams & Wilkins Co., Baltimore; **C** from Sedano, H.O., and Gorlin, R.J.: Oral Surg. **16:**823, 1963.)

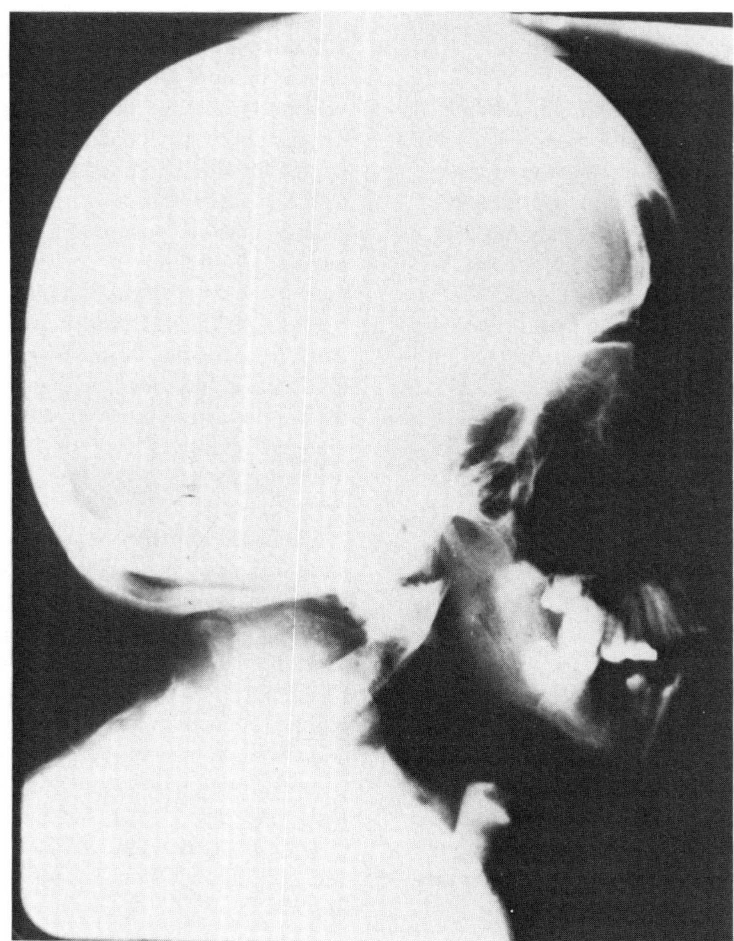

Fig. 13-9. Klippel-Feil syndrome. This patient had an anomalous cervical vertebrae, an enlarged foramen magnum, and cleft palate. (From Ross, R.B., and Johnston, M.C.: Cleft lip and palate. © 1972, The Williams & Wilkins Co., Baltimore.)

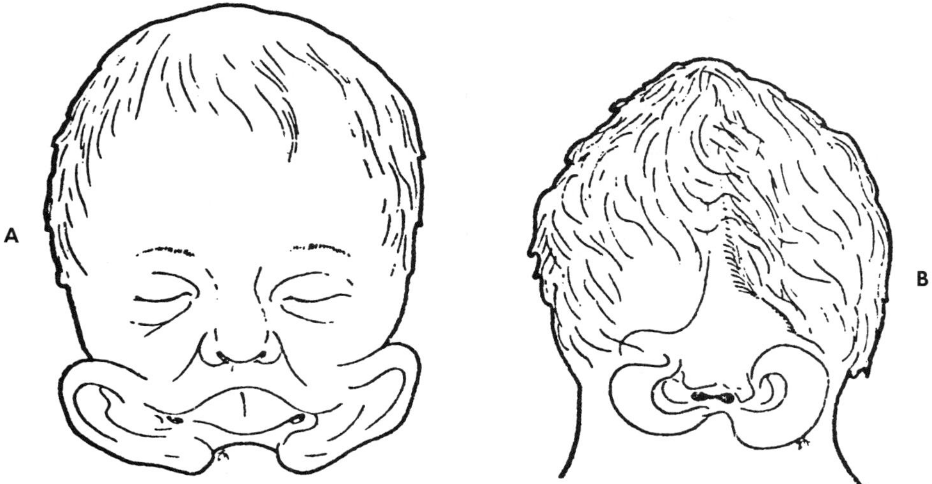

Fig. 13-10. Two gradations of otocephaly observed in humans. Study of an animal model indicates that such malformations result from early degeneration of head mesoderm. (From Duhamel, B.: Morphogenese pathologique, Paris, 1966, Masson et Cie.)

Otocephaly (Fig. 13-10) appears to be related to mesodermal degeneration as observed in a mouse model.[54,96] Although crest cells in the visceral arches of affected embryos appeared normal in the mouse model, they apparently were not able to maintain the integrity of the arches when the mesodermal cores underwent degeneration. The upper facial region consists almost entirely of crest mesenchyme and is much less likely to be affected than the mandibular arch, both in the animal model and humans (Fig. 13-10, *A*). In the most severely affected individuals, virtually no face is present (Fig. 13-10, *B*), suggesting early and more extensive mesodermal degeneration. In retrospect, this explanation appears much more reasonable than one of defective migration or other neural crest problems as postulated previously.[46,113]

EMBRYO FOLDING

Morphogenetic folding movements result in the formation of neural and gastrointestinal "tubes" (Fig. 13-2). The rapid growth of the developing brain relative to the heart is primarily responsible for "movement" of the heart from a position anterior to the oral plate (Fig. 13-2, *G*) to its final position in the thorax.

Neural tube closure is a complex phenomenon, apparently involving a concerted contraction of an actin-myosin complex close to the future luminal surface of the neural plate. Agents that interfere directly with actin-myosin function, such as cytochalasin D, can be used to experimentally induce exencephaly (failure of anterior neural tube closure).[61] Experimental interference with mesenchymal tissues adjacent to the closing neural tube also prevents its closure.

Of the folding movements, only problems of anterior neural plate closure are known to be involved to an appreciable extent in human craniofacial malformations. Failure of the anterior neural plate to close leads to neural tube defects (NTDs) such as exencephaly. Exencephaly eventually leads to degeneration of the developing cerebral and cerebellar hemispheres, and, although the resulting condition is termed *anencephaly* (literally meaning no brain), a partially functional brainstem is present, as are other structures of the head and neck that are not intimately related to the cerebral and cerebellar hemispheres (Fig. 13-11). Alterations (usually secondary) in the cranial base and facial structures are observed.[64] In most cases anencephaly is assumed to result from failure of anterior neural tube closure that is normally completed by or shortly after the twenty-sixth day of human gestation.[60] Although similar defects can be produced experimentally at later stages by causing degenerative changes and postclosure opening of the developing brain, their relevance for human anencephaly is not clear.

Anencephaly, as well as other common malformations such as cleft lip, may result from a host of causes or combinations thereof. The defect can be produced experimentally in guinea pigs by hyperthermia,[28] and there is some evidence in humans that a modest rise in maternal temperature of a few degrees Fahrenheit (such as that resulting from infectious diseases) is associated with anencephaly if the elevated temperature occurs at approximately the twenty-sixth day of gestation.[91] In both humans and the mouse FAS model, anencephaly is sometimes associated with features of the craniofacial malformations found in the holoprosen-

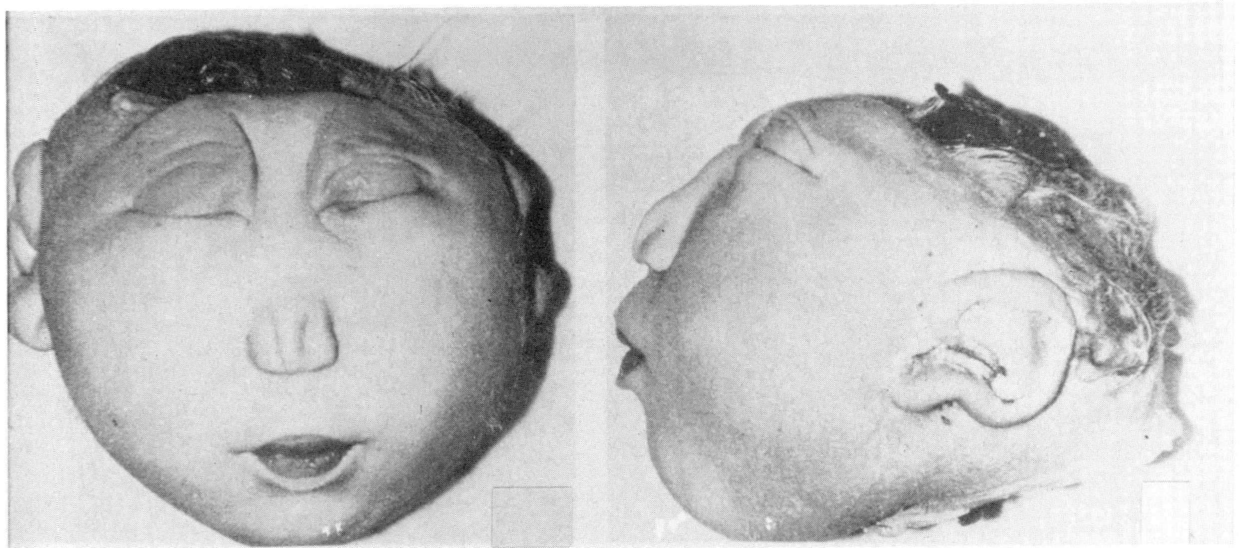

Fig. 13-11. In most patients with anencephaly the cerebral and cerebellar hemispheres are absent, and the ventral brainstem is at least partially functional. This patient has associated malformations of the face that are characteristic of holoprosencephalies. (From Lemire, R.J., Cohen, M., Jr., Beckwith, J., et al.: Teratology **23:**297, 1981.)

cephaly series, in which case the interference that causes the NTD would be considerably earlier (Fig. 13-11).

Recently some interesting studies conducted in England have indicated that anencephaly and other NTDs are frequently associated with nutritional deficiencies (particularly folic acid).[92-94] There is evidence from these studies that prenatal nutritional supplements in mothers who have previously borne a child with an NTD may drastically lower the recurrence rates for such defects. These findings potentially represent a major breakthrough in the prevention of a common malformation.

Since the possible prevention of other craniofacial malformations through dietary vitamin supplementation will be considered later in the chapter, some general comments regarding these procedures are in order. Most of the studies have used supplements, including many vitamins and large doses of folic acid and vitamin B_6. Studies using supplements of individual vitamins are proposed or underway, both for experimental animals[118] and humans. Such experiments are of considerable importance because, in addition to obvious advantages of shedding light on the relative importance and interactions of individual vitamins or groups of vitamins, large amounts of some (e.g., vitamin A) are teratogenic. More is not necessarily better!

Sometimes the membranes associated with the brain and spinal cord are fully formed, even though relatively small underlying neural tube closure defects remain. Pressure of CSF, which is then in direct contact with the membranes, usually distends the membranes, leading to meningoceles.

Encephaloceles (cephaloceles, meningomyeloceles) include both membranes and brain tissue, which evaginate or herniate into surrounding mesenchyme (part of which will form calvarial bones). The developmental relations between encephaloceles and meningoceles are not clear, nor is the causal relationship to some median facial clefts, where the NTD is found between two widely separated frontal bones (Fig. 13-20).[16,17,19,105] As will be seen in the discussion on the upper midface, the facial halves in this region initially develop somewhat independently, so that the presence of any abnormal midline structure could interfere with approximation (merging).

THE NEURAL CREST

As discussed previously, cell marking procedures have shown that neural crest cells make massive contributions to developing head and neck structures. After leaving the neural folds, crest cells are morphologically similar to most migrating embryonic cells; this has provided evidence for

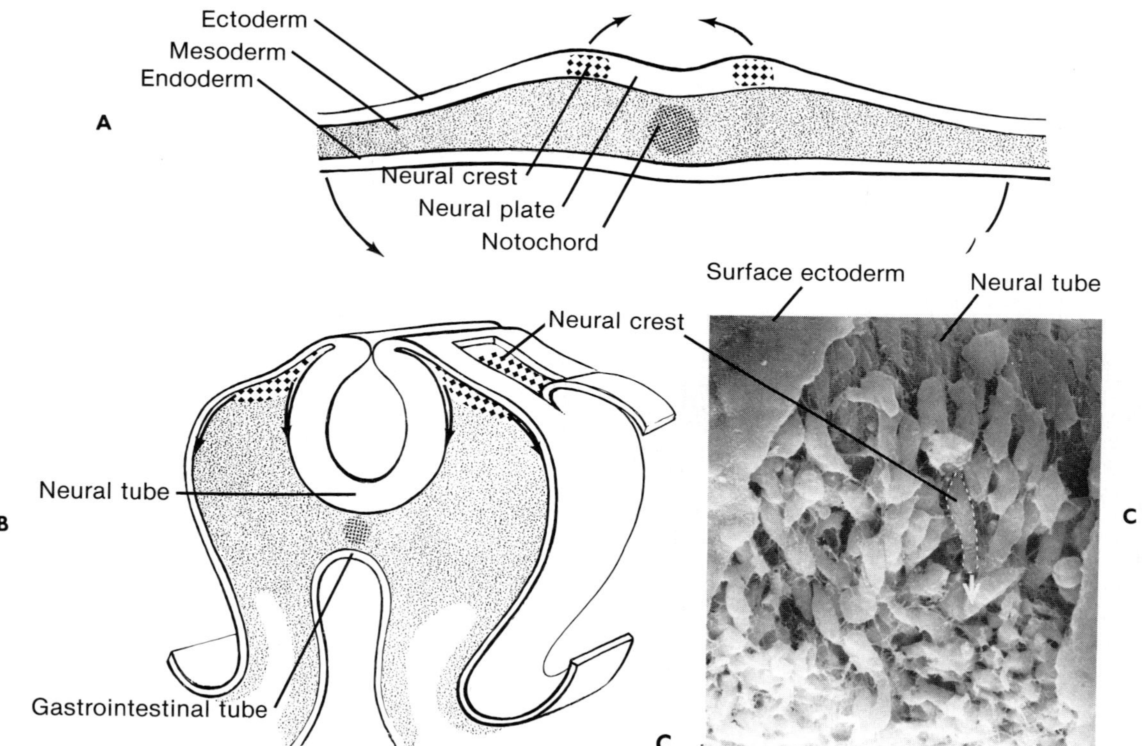

Fig. 13-12. Cross sections (see Fig. 13-1 for planes of sections) through embryos before (**A**) and after (**B**) the onset of crest cell *(diamond pattern)* migration. The ectoderm (**C**) has been peeled back (as in **B**), permitting direct visualization with scanning electron microscopy of underlying mouse embryo neural crest cells that, like crest cells in other species, are frequently bipolar and oriented *(arrow)* in the direction of migration. (From Johnston, M.C., and Sulik, K.K.: Development of face and oral cavity. In Bhaskar, S.N.: Orban's oral histology and embryology, ed. 9, St. Louis, 1980, The C.V. Mosby Co.)

the role of neural crest cells in embryos where no cell marking procedures have been used (Fig. 13-12, *C*).[44,58,59,77,78] Their eventual differentiation appears to depend on complex interactions both during and at the end of their migration (Fig. 13-13). The plasticity of crest cells may have phylogenetic importance, since they may provide the ability to add, with a minimum of developmental errors, increasingly massive amounts of mesenchyme and a wide variety of differentiated cell types to the head and neck in higher vertebrates.[31]

Although it is possible to produce many facial malformations through experimental interference with the number of crest cells formed[3,43,50] or with their migrations into the facial region, there is little evidence that a reduced number of crest cells plays a primary major role in the embryogenesis of many human facial malformations.[49,50] This is probably due to the extraordinary ability of crest cells to differentiate according to their environment and to compensate for the initial production of slightly or moderately deficient numbers.[43] The ability to compensate for abnormal numbers is also evident in experiments in which the addition of crest cells from donor embryos to normally developing hosts did not result in abnormally large facial structures.[18]

However, there is considerable experimental evidence that interference with crest cell migration contributes to at least some aspects of Treacher Collins' syndrome (Fig. 13-

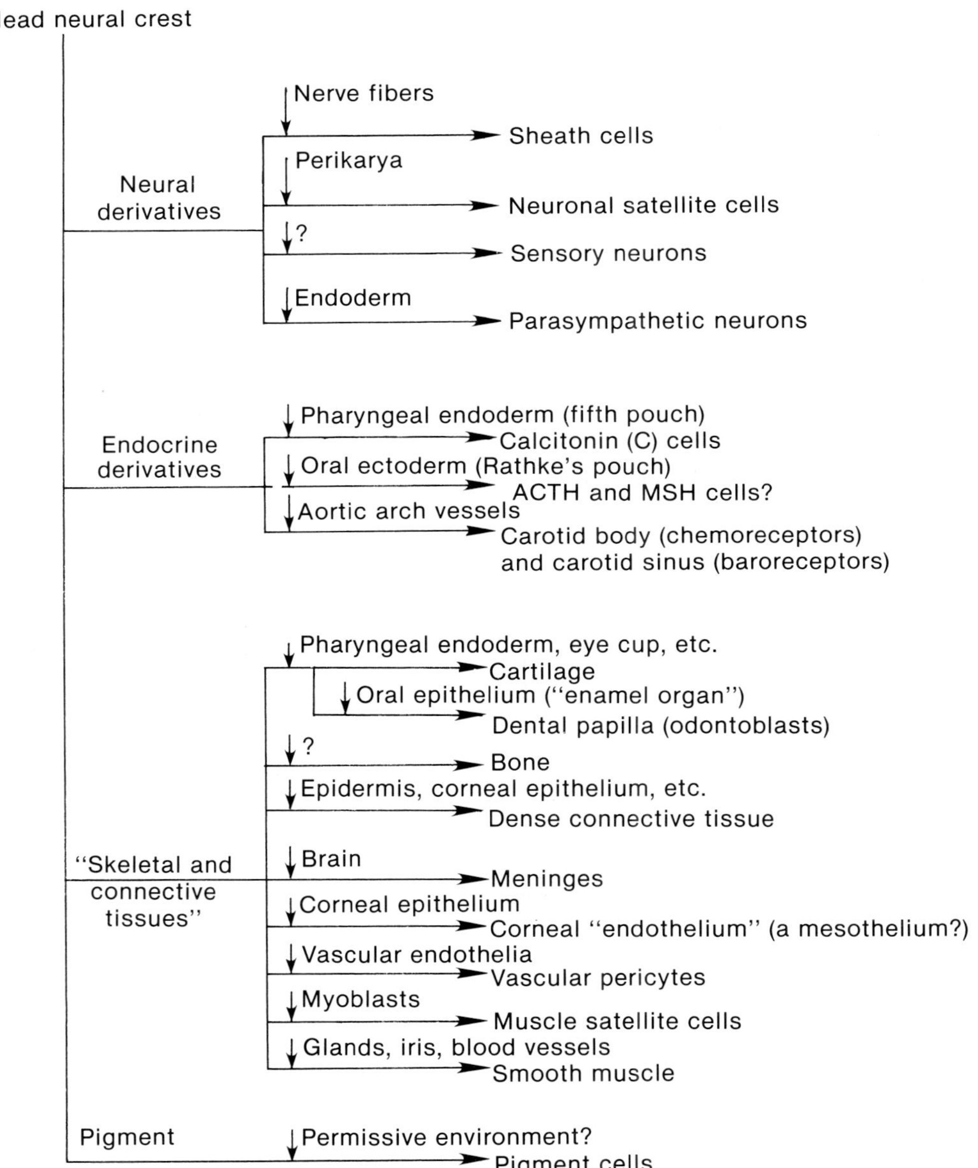

Fig. 13-13. Inductive interactions *(arrows)* and derivatives of head neural crest cells. Although numerous points need to be clarified, the development of new cell marking procedures has greatly expanded the number of known crest cell derivatives.

30).[9,37,39,72,84] Alterations involved in the development of this syndrome will be considered in more detail on p. 211.

Abnormalities of neural crest development are apparently responsible for Waardenburg's syndrome and for neoplasias that are sometimes referred to as *neurocristopathies*.[5,6] Both problems may involve abnormalities of crest cell responses to their environment. In Waardenburg's syndrome, developmental abnormalities include pigmentation deficiencies of the iris, hair, or skin; an elevated incidence of cleft lip (seen in about 5% of the patients); and a high incidence of deafness. Animal models, such as dancer[25,108] and twirler[62] mice, have major genes for cleft lip that also are associated with pigmentation deficiencies and inner ear defects related to vestibular function. Although pigmented cells in the inner ear are presumably of crest origin and are deficient in these animal models[24], their functions are unknown.

Neoplasias involving only crest cell derivatives are poorly understood and only of peripheral interest for this chapter; they provide another interesting problem[51] related to crest cell "differentiation." In individual patients, neoplasias may involve only one crest cell derivative (e.g., Schwann cells in neurofibromatosis) or a number of derivatives (e.g., medullary carcinoma of the thyroid[33]).

DEVELOPMENT OF THE FOREBRAIN, EYE, AND PITUITARY GLAND

The earliest stages of cephalic neural plate development were described in the discussion of germ layer formation and embryo folding. Considered here will be further development of one of the cephalic neural plate derivatives, the forebrain, and two structures, the eye and pituitary gland, which are partially derived from the anterior neural plate.

Well before the completion of neural tube closure in the forebrain region, the first indication of eye formation becomes evident (Fig. 13-7, *A*). Evagination of a portion of the anterior neural plate results in a vesicle that infolds to form a two-layered optic cup (Fig. 13-14). These two layers eventually become the neural and pigmented retinas, as well as most of the iris. The lens is derived from the overlying ectoderm after an inductive interaction with the underlying optic vesicles.[42] The epithelial layer of the cornea is also derived from overlying ectoderm (Fig. 13-14, *D*), whereas the remainder of the cornea and most of the remaining ocular tissues are derived from neural crest cells.[48]

Defects in eye formation can arise at virtually any stage of eye development.[21,63] Deficiencies of the anterior neural plate, occurring before any morphologic evidence of eye formation is apparent, have already been discussed.[100,103] Defects in the lens, iris (e.g., defective pigmentation in the Waardenburg syndrome), and other ocular structures are genetically determined or result from a variety of insults.[63] The developmental origins of some abnormalities (e.g., epibulbar dermoids in Goldenhar's syndrome) are unknown. At least some eyelid abnormalities are related to incomplete facial prominence formation or merging.

The initiation of pituitary gland development involves an interaction between the ventral forebrain and the ectoderm of the roof of the oral cavity (Fig. 13-15). The initial primordium of the anterior pituitary gland (that portion which gives rise to the anterior lobe, pars intermedia, and pars tuberalis) develops from the oral ectoderm and is later invaded by neural crest cells. The crest cells then form the connective tissue stroma and possibly adrenocorticotropic and melanocyte-stimulating hormones (Fig. 13-13). The forebrain-derived portion of the gland forms the posterior pituitary (neurohypophysis), and it is in this structure that most physiologic (neuroendocrine) interactions between the hypothalamus and pituitary occur. The pituitary gland is variably affected in the holoprosencephalies, including those of a mouse model for the FAS.[114]

UPPER MIDFACIAL DEVELOPMENT

Included in the upper midfacial region are structures above the oral cavity and between and under the eyes. Development of the embryonic primordia of these structures occurs in two phases: growth, contact, and fusion of the medial nasal, lateral nasal, and maxillary prominences, followed at a later time by growth, elevation, and fusion of the palatal shelves. There is some confusion, even in standard texts, concerning the appropriate terminology to describe embryonic structures in this region. During the first phase of upper midfacial development, the initial separation between the olfactory (nasal) pit and buccal (oral) cavity is further developed by fusion of the medial nasal, lateral nasal, and maxillary prominences (occurring, approximately during gestational days 30 to 37) (Fig. 13-16). The derived structure that intervenes between the oral and nasal cavities is sometimes referred to as the *primary palate,* even though only a small portion of it will be incorporated into the definitive hard palate, with the major portions forming parts of the dentoalveolus (teeth and supporting structures) and lip. Moore[71] uses the term *intermaxillary segment* to describe that portion of the upper midface between the two maxillary prominences (essentially the medial nasal prominences). The primary palate and intermaxillary segment are not quite coextensive as illustrated in Fig. 13-17. Since the term primary palate is confusing and the intermaxillary segment gives rise to a very limited portion of the upper midface, both terms will be avoided. During a later phase of upper midfacial development (approximately occurring during gestational days 50 to 60) (Fig. 13-21), growth, elevation, and fusion of the palatal shelves gives rise to the "secondary palate" (from which develops the remainder of the hard and all of the soft palate).

Growth, contact, and fusion of the medial nasal, lateral nasal, and maxillary prominences (including formation of the primary palate)

Although all three facial prominences are involved in upper midfacial development, the underlying mechanisms are not well understood. A primary event is the formation

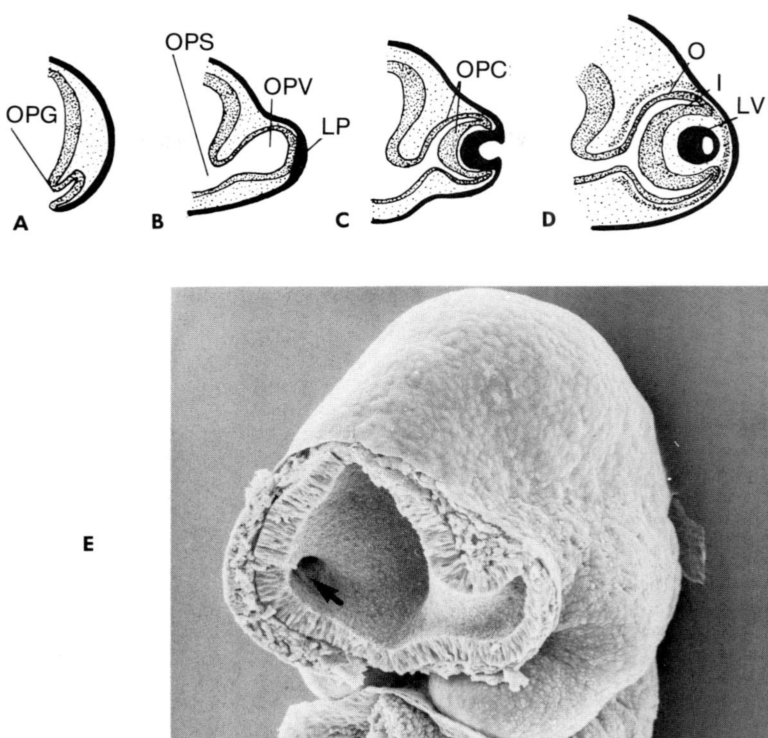

Fig. 13-14. Frontal sections of the developing eye. **A,** The evagination indicated by the optic groove *(OPG)* leads to close contact of the optic vesicle *(OPV)* with the overlying ectoderm. **B,** With later thickening this overlying ectoderm forms the lens placode *(LP)*. *OPS,* Optic stalk. **C,** Invagination of the placode leads to formation of the lens vesicle *(LV)*. The *OPV* has also invaginated to form the optic cup *(OPC)*. **D,** The outer *(O)* and inner *(I)* layers of the optic vesicle will differentiate into pigmented and neural retinas, respectively. **E,** The section of this specimen is similar to that of the sketches. On the embryo's right side, the section is anterior to the section through the embryo's left side. It is slightly less advanced than the specimen illustrated in **B.** The arrow points into the cavity of the optic stalk. The first and second visceral arches are evident because the heart has been removed. (**A** to **D** from Waterman, R.E., and Meller, S.M.: Prenatal development of the oral cavity and paraoral structures in man. In Shaw, J.H., Sweeney, E.A., Cappuccino, C.C., and Meller, S.M., editors: Textbook of oral biology, Philadelphia, 1978, W.B. Saunders Co.)

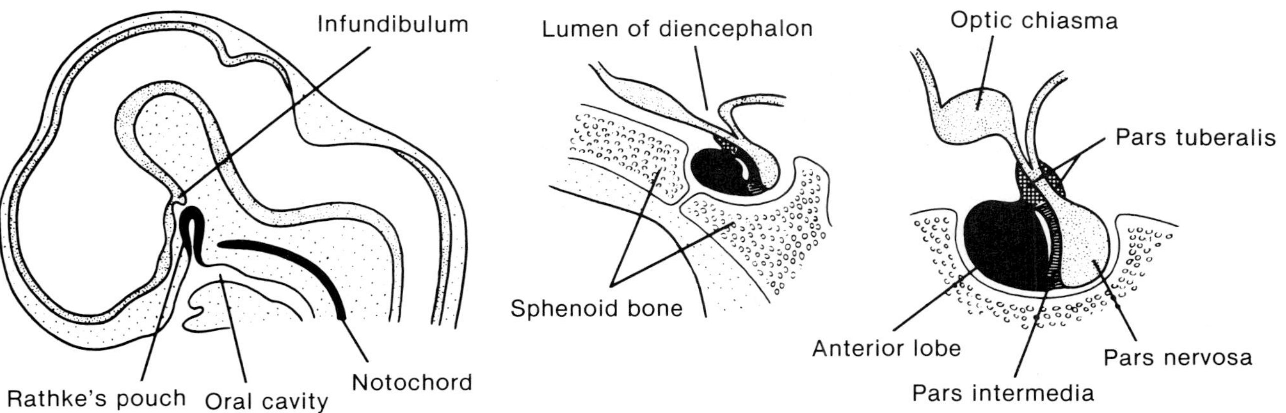

Fig. 13-15. Sagittal sections illustrating development of the pituitary gland. The initial primordium of the pars nervosa (posterior pituitary) develops from ventral forebrain *(light stipple)*, whereas the initial primordia of the anterior lobe and pars intermedia *(black* and *horizontal hatching)* arise from oral ectoderm. (From Langman, J.: Medical embryology, ed. 4. © 1981, The Williams & Wilkins Co., Baltimore.)

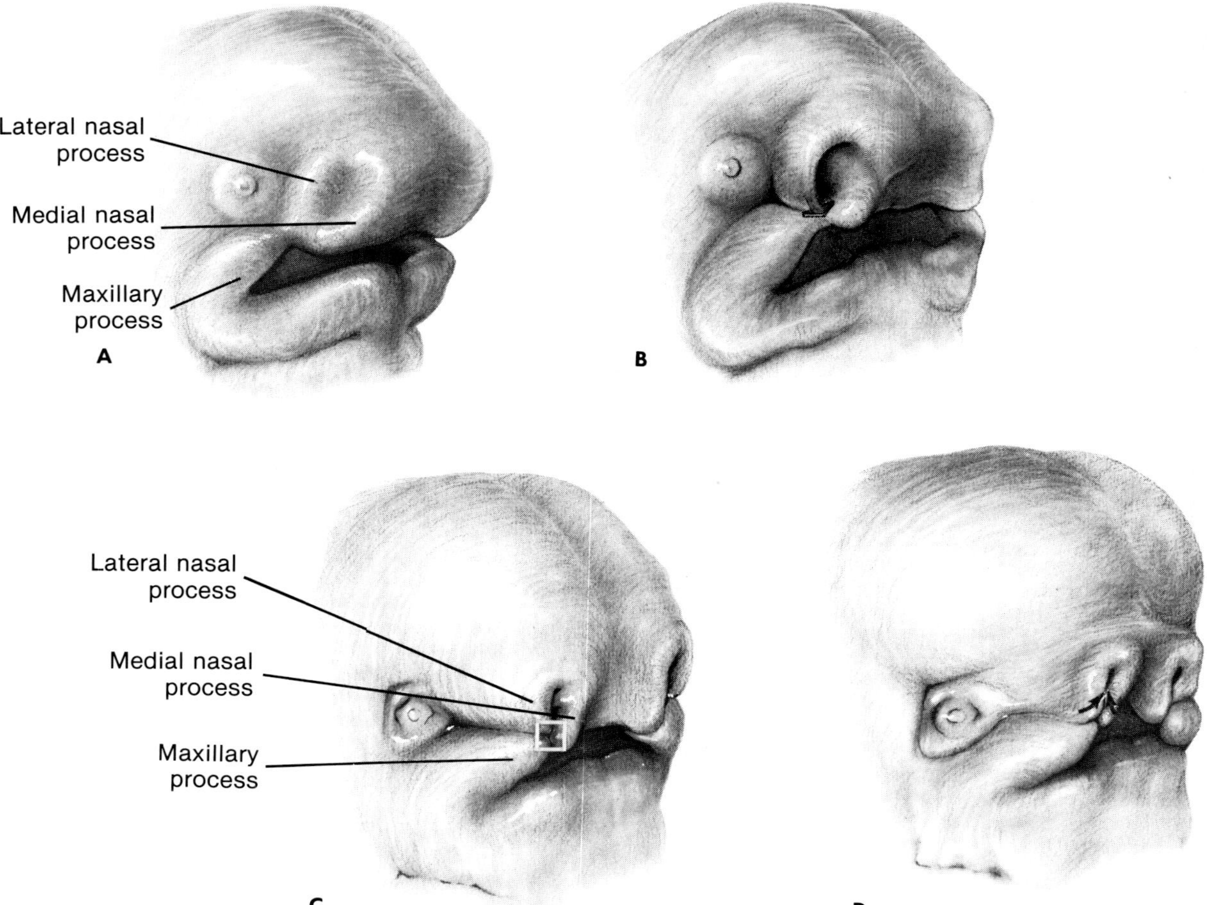

Fig. 13-16. Fusion and merging of the medial nasal, lateral nasal, and maxillary prominences (primary palate development) further separates the oral and nasal cavities. **A,** Early stage of development (approximately gestational day 30). The medial and lateral nasal prominences are starting to form on either side of the invaginating nasal (olfactory) placode, and the maxillary prominence is enlarging anteriorly under the eye. **B,** All three prominences have made contact, and the lateral nasal prominence is rapidly growing forward *(arrow)*. **C,** An epithelial seam is formed between contacting prominences, which breaks down only in that portion deep to the area indicated by the square. Mesenchymal cells of the three prominences consolidate the "fusion" by becoming confluent in the area of epithelial breakdown. The epithelium behind the area of breakdown "hollows out" to establish a connection between the base of the nasal pit and the roof of the primitive oral cavity. (See also Fig. 13-17, *D*.) **D,** The fusion is further consolidated by a merging phenomenon with the epithelia "zipping up" *(arrows),* accompanied by elevation of the base of the epithelial groove. (From Johnston, M.C., and Sulik, K.K.: Development of face and oral cavity. In Bhaskar, S.N.: Orban's oral histology and embryology, ed. 9, St. Louis, 1980, The C.V. Mosby Co.)

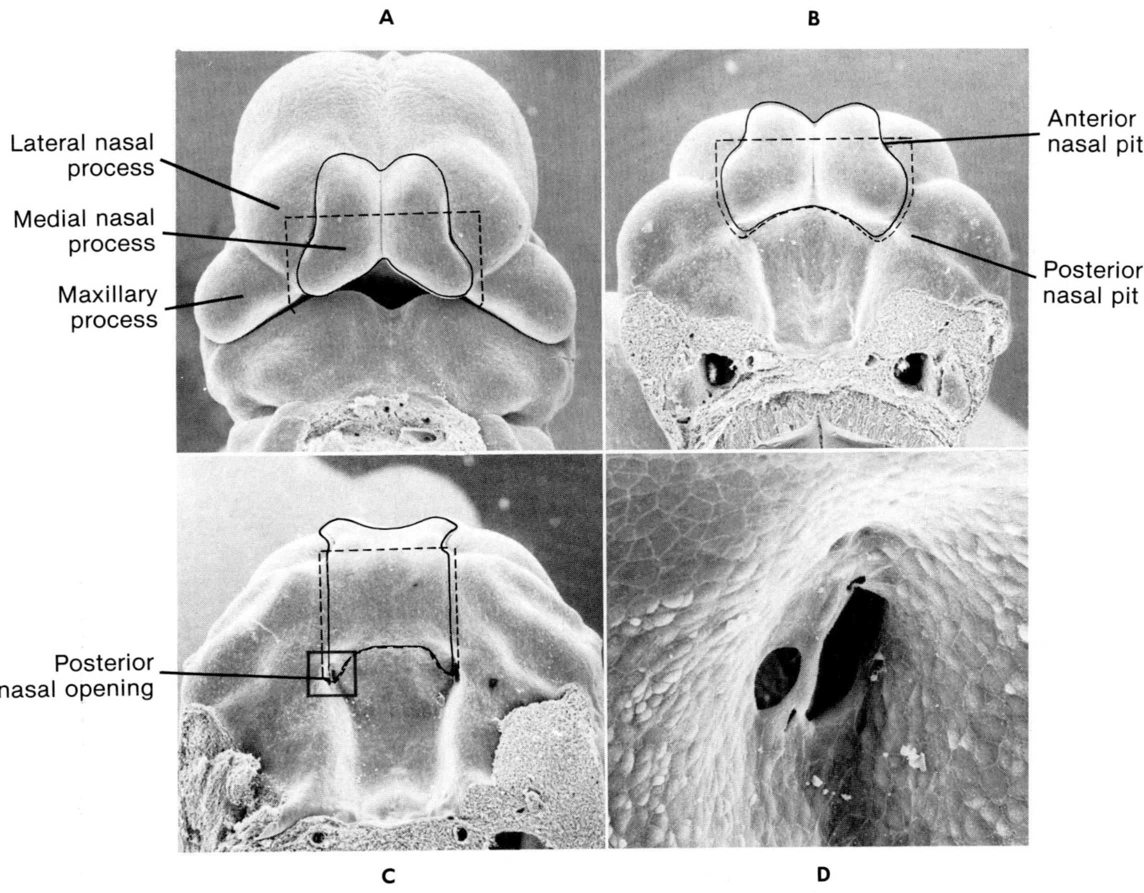

Fig. 13-17. Upper midfacial development of mouse embryos. **A** to **C**, The intermaxillary segment is outlined by solid lines and the primary palate by broken lines. **B** and **C**, Palatal shelves are beginning to grow from the medial aspect of the maxillary prominences. **C** and **D**, The "hollowing out" or stretching and disruption of the epithelial connection between the base of the nasal pit and the roof of the primitive oral cavity has reached an advanced stage in the older specimen. (Modified from Johnston, M.C., and Sulik, K.K.: Development of face and oral cavity. In Bhaskar, S.N.: Orban's oral histology and embryology, ed. 9, St. Louis, 1980, The C.V. Mosby Co.)

and invagination of the olfactory placodes (Fig. 13-16, *A*). Proliferation of mesenchymal cells in the surrounding medial and lateral nasal prominences and in the maxillary prominence is maintained at a relatively high rate, whereas proliferation of mesenchymal cells in areas that are not growing rapidly, such as in the roof of the primitive oral cavity, falls off rapidly after the stage of olfactory placode formation.[69,70] Incomplete separation of the eye primordia, as occurs in synophthalmia and cyclopia (Fig. 13-8, *C*), physically separates the olfactory placodes and surrounding tissues from the maxillary prominences. In these cases the placodes are usually also in contact ("fused"), and a symmetrical outgrowth around them gives rise to a single proboscis. In milder cases, where there is separation of the eyes and only partial contact of the placodes, premaxillary agenesis (Fig. 13-8, *A* and *B*) may occur.[49,101] If there are unfused but medially positioned placodes, the result is un-

derdevelopment of the medial nasal prominences, as is frequently observed in trisomy 13.

Alterations of epithelial cells in the zone of fusion of the medial nasal, lateral nasal, and maxillary prominences, as observed in mouse embryos, indicate that these cells may be involved in bringing facial prominences together or promoting their adhesion (Fig. 13-18).[65,66] Epithelial activity in this zone is very much reduced in CL/Fr mouse embryos (as compared to A/J and C57B1/6J embryos) and may increase the embryo's problems in achieving contact and fusion between the medial nasal and lateral nasal prominences.[65] This difference may be responsible for the discrepancy between the higher reported spontaneous incidences of cleft lip of 18% to 36% for the CL/Fr strain and 0% to 15% for the A/J strain.

Little is known about the mechanisms that regulate growth, both in terms of rate and direction, in the facial

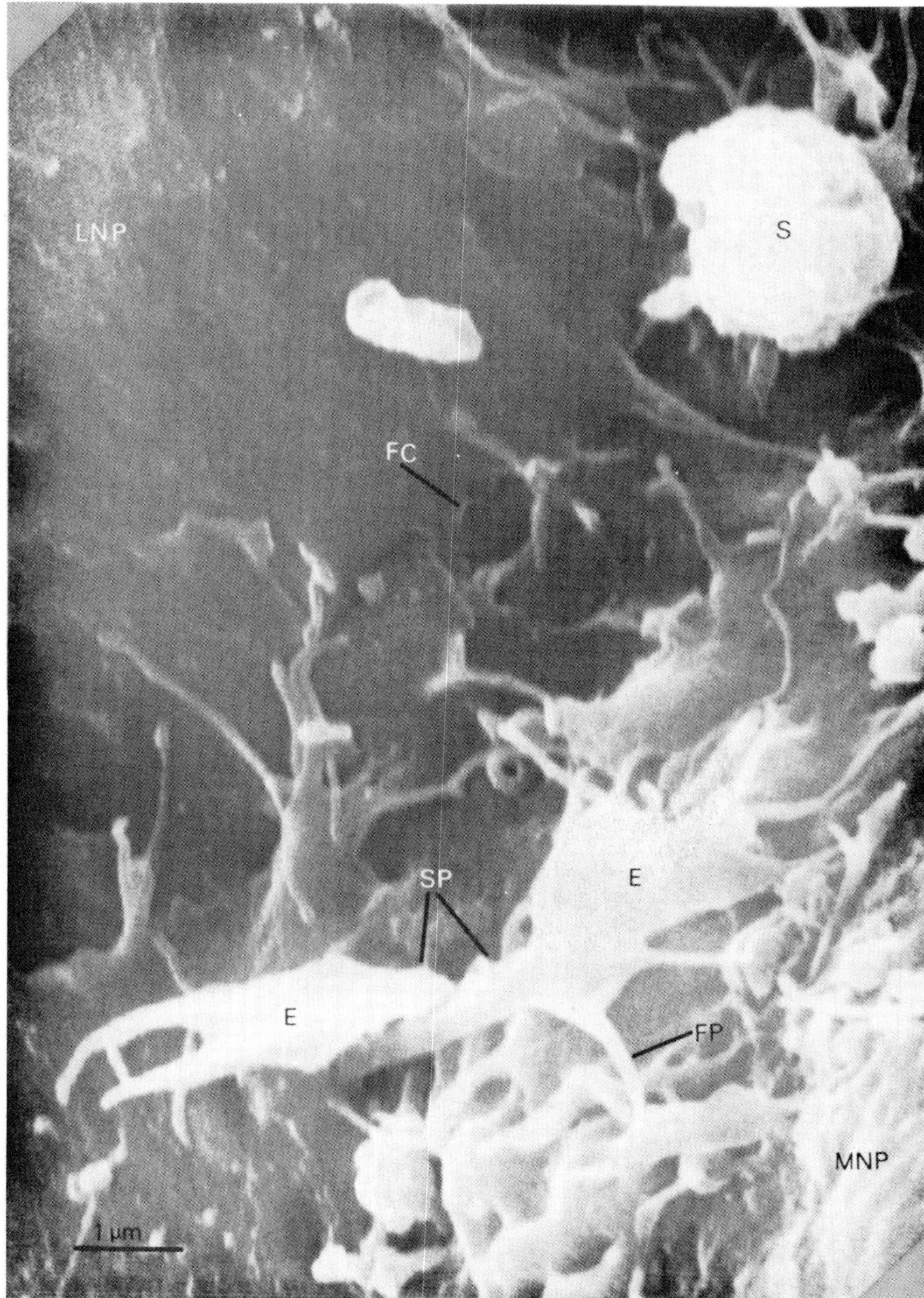

Fig. 13-18. Normal epithelial ''activity'' in the fusion line between the lateral nasal *(LNP)* and medial nasal *(MNP)* prominences of a mouse embryo. The structure of active epithelial cells varies from flattened cells *(FC)* to secondary projections *(SP)* with enlargements *(E)* to filipodial processes *(FP)*. This activity, which is believed to promote approximation of the prominences, is much reduced in CL/Fr and phenytoin-treated A/J mice embryos, both of which are predisposed to cleft lip. The spheroidal particles *(S)* are believed to be cell debris. (From Millicovsky, G., and Johnston, M.C.: J. Embryol. Exp. Morphol. **63:**53, 1981.)

C57B1/6J   CL/Fr

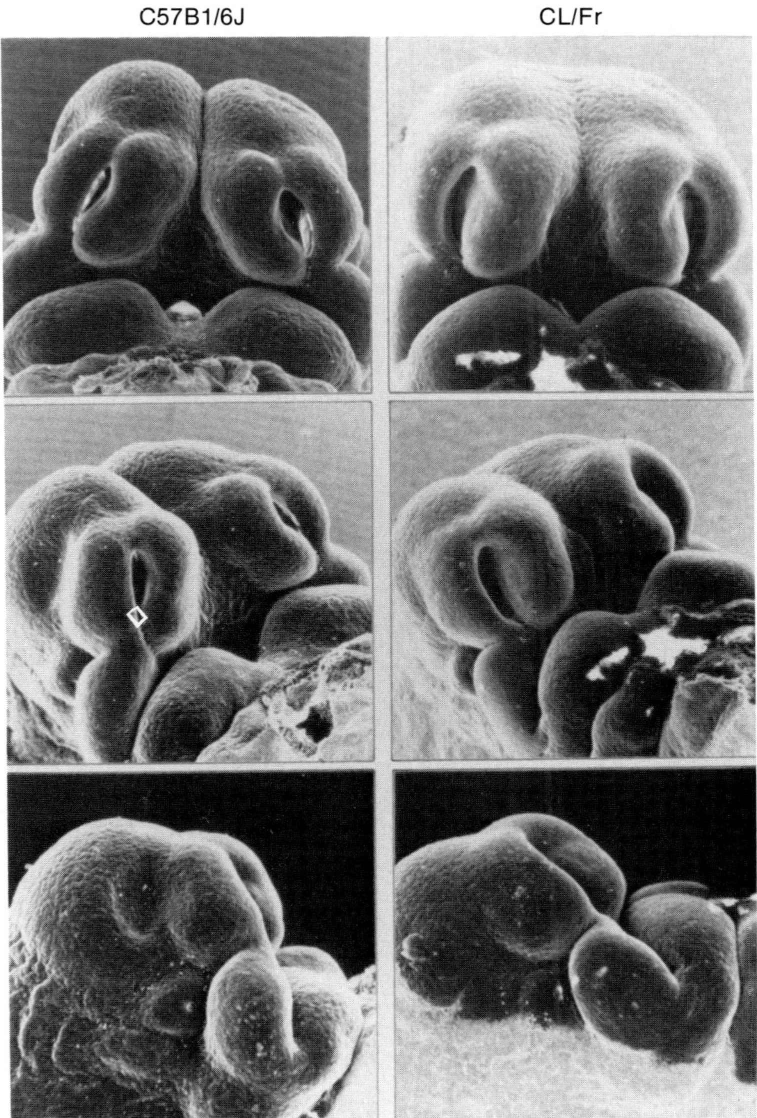

Eight tail somites

Fig. 13-19. Frontal, quarter, and lateral views comparing development of the medial nasal, lateral nasal, and maxillary prominences just before contact and fusion in C57B1/6J (little or no spontaneous cleft lip) and CL/Fr (approximately 36% incidence of spontaneous cleft lip in our colony) mouse embryos. The growth direction of the medial nasal prominences of CL/Fr (and A/J) mouse embryos is more medially directed and consequently less convergent on the lateral prominences than in C57B1/6J embryos. This difference, coupled with decreased epithelial activity in the fusion line, may predispose CL/Fr embryos to cleft lip. The rectangle on the quarter view of the C57B1/6J specimen approximates the position of Fig. 13-18. (From Millicovsky, G., Ambrose, L.J.H., and Johnston, M.C.: Am. J. Anat. **164**:29, 1982.)

prominences.[69,70,79] The growth direction of the medial nasal prominences in A/J[108] and CL/Fr[65] mouse embryos is more medial than that of a strain (C57B1/6J) which is genetically resistant to cleft lip (Fig. 13-19); this factor may be at least partly responsible for a genetic predisposition to cleft lip and the development of spontaneous cleft lip in these closely related strains. As shown in Fig. 13-19, growth of the medial nasal prominence in a more medial direction (i.e., more parallel to the midline) is less convergent with the growth direction of the lateral nasal prominence and would be expected to put the embryos at a greater than normal risk for contact failure and clefting.

Clefts of the lip (with or without cleft palate)* in CL/Fr and phenytoin-treated A/J[102] animal models seem comparable to clefts of the lip observed in most humans. The narrow nasal cavities of unaffected twins of monozygomatic pairs discordant for these clefts would be consistent with medial positioning of nasal placodes or a medial direction of growth of the medial nasal prominences.[47] The fact that parents of children with such clefts have some reduction in their overall midfacial size[30] is consistent with decreased formation or growth of facial mesenchyme. A moderate reduction in the size of facial prominences, which is particularly severe for the lateral nasal prominences in the phennytoin-treated A/J mouse model,[102] is consistent with these observations. It is possible that both problems (i.e., abnormal facial prominence size and positioning) are involved in at least some cases.

Clefts of the lip (and alveolus) are usually associated with clefts of the hard palate and all of the soft palate. The association is usually assumed to result from a wedging action by the tongue in the existing (lip) cleft that separates the midfacial segments, so that the now widely separated palatal shelves are not able to make midline contact after elevation. Although Smiley, Vanek, and Dixon[90] have shown that such increases in maxillary width are associated with cleft lip in A/J mouse embryos, the eventual failure of palatal shelves to elevate at all in affected specimens complicates interpretation of their findings. A reduction in the size of developing maxillary prominences (that tissue from which the palatal shelves are derived) could account for the cleft lip/cleft palate association.

It is possible to experimentally reduce the incidence of both phenytoin-induced cleft lip in A/J mice and spontaneous cleft lip in CL/Fr mice through maternal respiratory hyperoxia.[67,68] Preliminary scanning electron microscopy studies indicate that the decreased incidence is accomplished through stimulation of facial prominence growth. Although the reverse (maternal respiratory *hypoxia*) has been shown to increase the incidence of cleft lip in CL/Fr mice,[68] associated alterations in embryonic development have not been studied. These and other observations demonstrating that it is possible, through environmental manipulation, to experimentally move embryos back and forth across the threshold for cleft lip raises the possibility for cleft lip prevention, at least in some human pregnancies.

Recent studies concerning NTDs (anencephaly and spina bifida) in humans and the above observations (see also pp.

193-194) provide a theoretic basis for considering the possible prevention of cleft lip. The studies demonstrated apparent reduction, to about 10% of the expected in one study,[93] in the recurrence rate for NTDs brought about by dietary supplements in pregnancies subsequent to the birth of an affected child. Both NTDs and cleft lip (like the other three of the five most common major malformations observed in humans) are believed to result from the action of multiple genetic and environmental factors operating in each case. There is, however, much less evidence for environmental factors contributing to the cause of cleft lip and other common human malformations in comparison to NTDs.[12,13] Despite this, separation of families with cleft lip from those with isolated cleft palate, in a similar vitamin-supplement study conducted by Briggs[8] demonstrated a reduction in cleft lip incidence to one third of the controls in his relatively small sample. Recently larger reductions in cleft lip incidence have been reported for a similar study by Tolarova.[106] Both the NTD and cleft lip studies emphasized folic acid dietary supplementation. An experimental dietary deficiency of folic acid has long been known to be capable of inducing cleft lip.[2] It should be pointed out that the diets also contained antifolates. There is some evidence that depression of embryonic folate levels may be a factor in experimental phenytoin teratogenicity as well.[74] However, the studies of Neidyl and co-workers[73] have failed to demonstrate a correlation between cleft lip and reduced maternal folate levels. Kenney et al.[55] have been unable to reduce the incidence of phenytoin-induced cleft lip in A/J mice with tetrahydrofolate, the active form of folic acid. More recent studies conducted by Smithells and co-workers[92] indicate that dietary folate requirements for individual pregnant mothers may be highly variable, suggesting that dietary folate supplementation might be effective in birth defect prevention only for selected pregnancies.

Failure of facial prominences to merge apparently gives rise to a number of different kinds of rare facial clefts. Reference has already been made to median facial clefts (Fig. 13-20), including the possible involvement of defects in anterior neural tube closure. There is obvious heterogeneity in the median cleft face syndrome, with some investigators finding large amounts of abnormal tissue (which may not be of neural origin) in the interorbital region. These latter observations suggest that abnormal tissues between the facial halves may prevent their approximation. It seems more likely, however, that most medial facial clefts result from a failure of midline merging of the median nasal prominences (Figs. 13-4, *B*, and 13-5).

Although there is only a minor notch of the lip in the patient illustrated in Fig. 13-20, median cleft lip may be the dominant feature of midfacial clefts, with little or no clefting of the nose or higher structures. Such median clefts of the lip occur fairly often according to a study on blacks in Nigeria.[41] Similar lip clefts have been produced experi-

---

*Clefts of the lip usually lead to, or are otherwise associated with, clefts of the palate, both in humans and in experimental animals. The term *cleft palate* is often used to include all types of cleft lip or palate, even though cleft palate (without cleft lip) is almost invariably an etiologically different problem. Because of the confusion, the term *cleft lip* will be used to describe cleft lip with or without associated cleft palate, and cleft palate will be used to describe cleft palate without cleft lip.

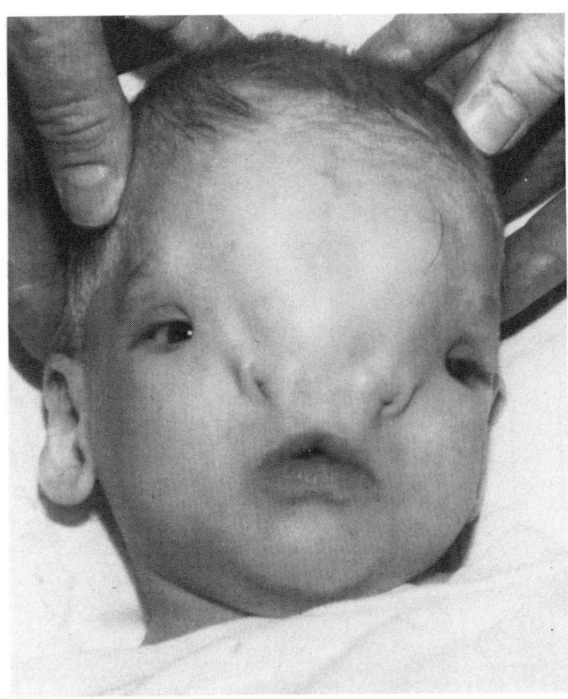

Fig. 13-20. Failure of upper facial structures to coalesce in the midline results in a median facial cleft. (From Sedano, H.O., Cohen, M.C., Jirasek, J., and Gorlin, R.J.: J. Pediatr. **76:**906, 1970.)

mentally in mice with agents that interfere with development of the medial nasal prominences.[11,108]

We are unaware of any relationship between these clefts and midline clefts of the mandible and associated structures, although this would also appear to be a problem of merging. "Cleft mandible" may be associated with defects of the hand,[34] suggesting that similar developmental mechanisms or critical time periods may be involved in both mandibular arch and limb development. Similar associations exist between lateral ("common") cleft lip and limb defects in the genetically determined ectrodactyly ectodermal dysplasia clefting syndrome.[4]

Oblique facial clefts are usually assumed to result from failure of merging between the maxillary and lateral nasal prominences. Early studies[95] and more recent scanning electron microscopy studies of human embryos[98] suggest that multiple growth centers in each facial prominence are involved in head and neck development (Fig. 13-27, *A* and *B*). Failure of merging between the centers could lead to some of the rare facial clefts, such as macrostomia (Fig. 13-27, *C* and *D*).

Other rare facial clefts will be discussed later. Such clefts are of interest in that they indicate some of the basic mechanisms involved in embryonic development of the head and neck. A small number of facial clefts apparently result from physical pressure exerted by folds of amniotic membranes (amniotic bands).[52]

Palatal shelf growth, elevation, and fusion (secondary palate development)

The palatal shelves develop as outgrowths from the medial surfaces of the maxillary prominences, extending downward in mammals, lateral to the tongue (Fig. 13-21). Coleman[20] first provided evidence that shelf elevation in the hard palate region is different from shelf elevation occurring in the region from which the soft palate forms. The more anterior portion swings upward in "barn door" fashion, whereas closure in the posterior area is attained more by "remodeling" (Fig. 13-21, *C* and *D*). An intrinsic shelf force of the palate is indicated by the observation that experimental removal of the tongue just before the normal time of elevation leads to at least partial shelf elevation.[113]

In normal palatal development a number of factors seem to be involved in moving the tongue from between the shelves. A major role is apparently played by a mandibular growth spurt, which appears to depend largely on the growth of Meckel's cartilage.[26] Also it has long been postulated that mandibular movements promote tongue removal from between the shelves,[111] and such movements have been observed[97] in cinefilms of human embryos and fetuses made in England by Marlow using fiberoptics.

A considerable amount of study has concentrated on the epithelial changes in shelf edges that are related to contact adhesion, epithelial breakdown, and mesenchymal condensation.[36] The programing of epithelial changes apparently

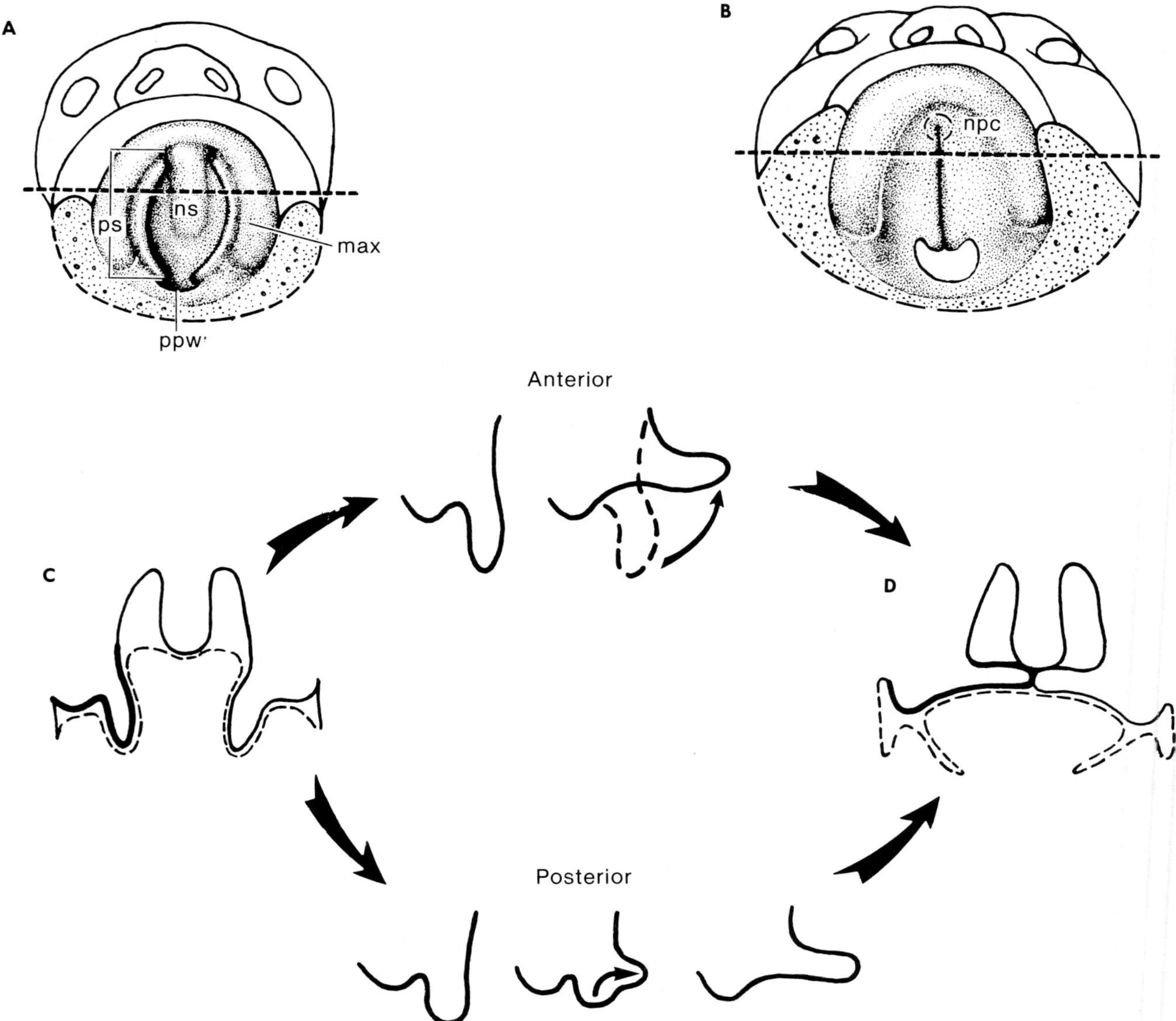

Fig. 13-21. Elevation and fusion of the palatal shelves (secondary palate development). Roof of the embryonic oral cavity (mandible and tongue removed) before (**A**) and at the completion of (**B**) shelf elevation. The anteroposterior length of the right palatal shelf *(ps)* is indicated in **A** as are the nasal septum *(ns)*, basal maxilla *(max)*, and posterior pharyngeal wall *(ppw)*. The region of the nasopalatine canal *(NPC)* is outlined by the circle in **B**. Coronal sections of palatal shelves before (**C**) and at the completion of (**D**) shelf elevation. Although the result is much the same, shelf movement *(heavy outlines)* in the anterior (hard palate) region appears to take place in "barndoor" fashion, whereas that in the posterior (soft palate) region involves "remodeling." (From Johnston, M.C., Hassell, J.R., and Brown, K.S.: Clin. Plast. Surg. **2:**195, 1975.)

begins at or before the initiation of shelf formation[109] and later involves complex signaling at the biochemical level (e.g., increased cyclic AMP and decreased epidermal growth factor related to cessation of proliferation).[86] Although interference with this programing in laboratory animals results from exposure to the environmental pollutant dioxin,[85] there is little evidence that it does so in humans.

However, it is possible that a primary problem of fusion is involved in the mixture of lip and palate clefts associated with the van der Woude syndrome.

A preliminary study of unaffected monozygotic twins of pairs where the affected twin has cleft palate[76] indicates that an excessively large tongue may provide at least part of the genetic predisposition for cleft palate in humans. Although

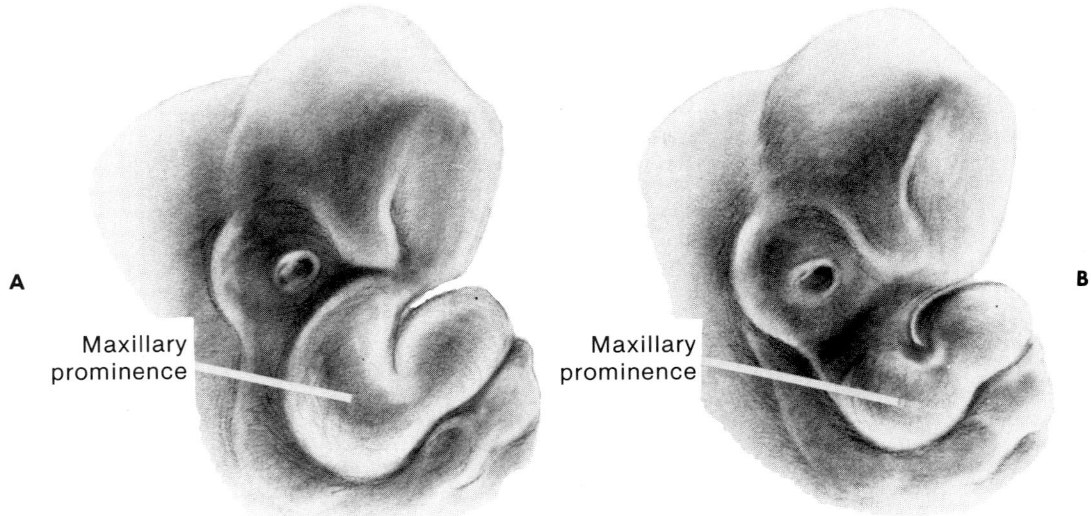

Fig. 13-22. Delay in the initiation of maxillary prominence formation by hypervitaminosis A. **A,** Control. **B,** Treated mother. Subsequent delay in palate shelf development results in small palatal shelves and cleft palate.

a large tongue could interfere with shelf elevation (Figs. 13-21, *C* and *D*), no such genetically susceptible animal model is available. The lack of cleft palate associated with the macroglossia seen in the Beckwith-Wiedemann syndrome suggests that interpretation of the twin study may be more complex than indicated.

In experimental animal studies interference with adequate shelf contact appears to be the most common manner by which cleft palate can be induced experimentally. Inadequate shelf contact can result from a decrease in the size of palatal shelves, inhibition of their elevation, or a combination of both. One of the cleanest pieces of evidence concerning inhibition of shelf elevation is experimental withdrawal of amniotic fluid,[82] which physically inhibits mandibular opening movements and mandibular growth. The malformation complex that results (mandibular underdevelopment associated with cleft palate) is similar to that seen in the Pierre Robin syndrome. Although there is obviously heterogeneity of symptoms with this syndrome, the major features are micrognathia (mandibular underdevelopment), glossoptosis (normally sized tongue forced back into the airway), and in about 30% of the cases a wide (''horseshoe'') cleft palate.

Interference with shelf growth may be achieved experimentally at many different stages. An example of early interference is that caused by hypervitaminosis A, when the vitamin is administered as the maxillary prominence is just beginning to form. Growth of this prominence is delayed (Fig. 13-22), and growth of the palatal shelves is severely retarded, the latter eventually leading to contact failure.[99] Palatal shelf underdevelopment occurs in animal models with defects closely resembling defects of Treacher Collins'

syndrome, in which the incidence of cleft palate is approximately 17%.[34]

A combination of growth retardation and delayed shelf elevation seems to be involved in corticosteroid-induced cleft palate. Natural and synthetic corticosteroids have been the most popular experimental cleft palate–inducing teratogens since they were first introduced by Fraser and Fainstat.[29] However, these agents are commonly administered later in gestation than is vitamin A. Shelf elevation is delayed by corticosteroids, and when the shelves become elevated, little or no contact occurs.[27] There is a good correlation between strain sensitivity and the numbers of steroid receptors in palatal shelves.[88,117] Recent experimental interest in strain sensitivity and the H_2 haplotype (the mouse H_2 locus is comparable to the HLA locus in humans) is somewhat controversial.[7,110]

One of the most difficult problems in assessing human relevance in terms of experimental animal studies on palate closure results from the fact that the secondary palate develops very late, at a time when few structures other than the secondary palate and brain remain sensitive to the usual teratogens. Because of this, very high doses can be (and usually are) administered at late embryonic stages to give a high incidence of cleft palate, usually without a major reduction in the viability of the embryos. Of possibly greater human relevance are studies conducted by Yoneda and Pratt,[118] in which supplementary vitamin B_6 decreased the incidence of cortisone-induced cleft palate.

THE VISCERAL ARCHES, TONGUE, AND EAR

Some aspects of maxillary prominence (a derivative of the first arch) development and its relation to the secondary

Table 13-1. Visceral arch–derived craniofacial structures

Branchial arch	Cranial nerve	Muscles	Skeletal structures
First	V (Mandibular branch)	Muscles of mastication (temporal, masseter, medial and lateral pterygoid), mylohyoid and anterior belly of digastric; tensor muscle of tympanic membrane and palatine curtain	Meckel's cartilage, malleus and incus, mandible, sphenomandibular ligament, Reichert's cartilage
Second	VII	Muscles of facial expression (cheek, occipitofrontal, auricular, occipitofrontal, platysma, orbicular), stapedius, stylohyoid, posterior belly of digastric	Stapes, styloid process, lesser cornu of hyoid, upper part of body of hyoid bone, Stylohyoid ligament
Third	IX	Stylopharyngeal and upper pharyngeal	Greater cornu of hyoid, lower part of body of hyoid bone
Fourth, fifth, and sixth	X (superior laryngeal and recurrent laryngeal branch)	Pharyngeal and laryngeal	Thyroid, arytenoid, corniculate, and cuneiform cartilages

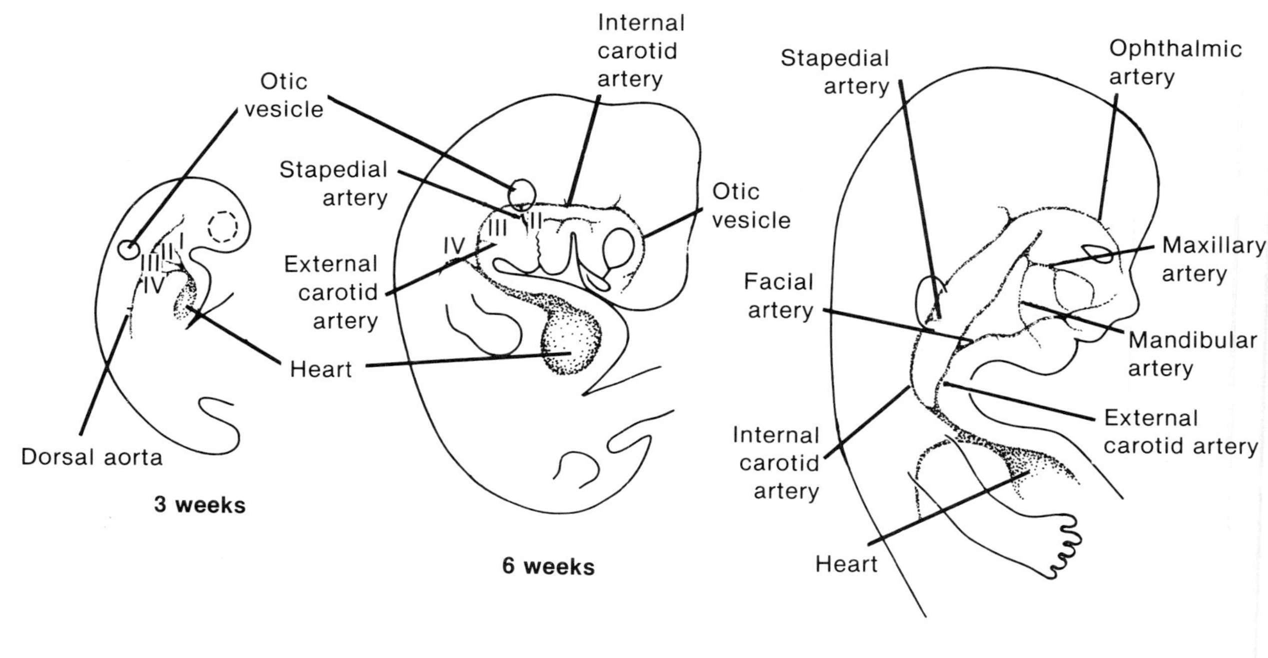

Fig. 13-23. Development of the arterial system serving the facial region with emphasis on its relation to the visceral arches. In the 3-week human embryo the visceral arches are little more than conduits for blood traveling through aortic arch vessels (indicated by Roman numerals according to the visceral arch containing them) from the heart to the dorsal aorta. Other structures indicated are the eye *(broken circle)* and otic vesicle. In the 6-week embryo the first two aortic arch vessels have regressed almost entirely, and the distal portions of the arches have separated from the heart. The portion of the third aortic arch vessel adjacent to the dorsal aorta persists and eventually forms the stem of the external carotid artery by fusing with the stapedial artery. The stapedial artery, which develops from the second aortic arch vessel, temporarily (in humans) provides the arterial supply for the embryonic face. After fusion with the external carotid artery, the proximal portion of the stapedial artery regresses. The aortic arch vessel of the fourth visceral arch persists as the arch of the aorta. By 9 weeks the primordium of the definitive vascular system of the face has been laid down. (From Ross, R.B., and Johnston, M.C.: Cleft lip and palate. © 1972, The Williams & Wilkins Co., Baltimore.)

palate have been discussed. A number of other malformations involving visceral arch derivatives also involve the maxillary prominence.

The term "branchial," instead of "visceral" or "pharyngeal," is sometimes used when describing the arches. The use of branchial to describe the mandibular and hyoid arches is technically incorrect, since the term is derived from descriptions of arches with gill "branches" found only caudal to the mandibular and hyoid arches in fish and larval amphibia.

As with all vertebrates, visceral arch development in humans constitutes a prominent aspect of their embryology. Each of the visceral arches has a set of sets of structures (Fig. 13-4 and Table 13-1) that change progressively during development.

The mesodermal cores and surrounding sheaths of neural crest cells were described earlier. Also noted were the aortic arch arteries whose endothelial lining develops from the mesodermal cores. The visceral arch arterial pattern and further development of the facial arterial system are illustrated in Fig. 13-23. The potential significance of this complex pattern of vascular development for at least some cases of hemifacial microsomia will be considered at the end of this discussion.

Later in development, mesodermal cells in the arches differentiate into the contractile cells of skeletal (voluntary) muscles (Fig. 13-24). Since the definitive locations of these muscles are often at some distance from the original arch position, they must undergo fairly extensive migrations. Each migrating group of myoblasts takes with it a branch of the appropriate nerve for that particular arch, for example, branches of the facial nerve for the second arch.[32] The ex-

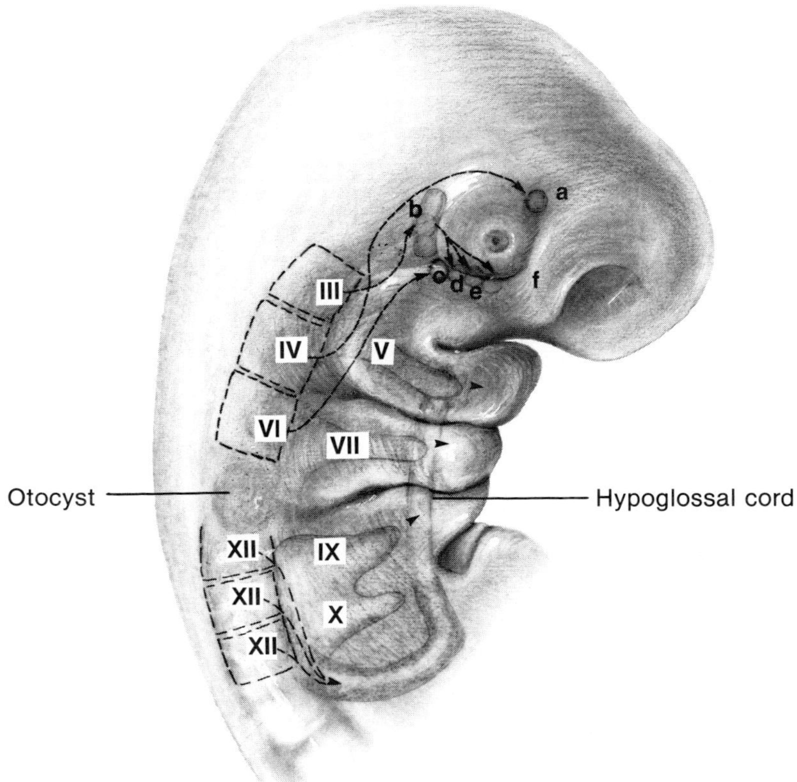

Fig. 13-24. The visceral arches also play a major role in the development of facial skeletal (voluntary) musculature. After development of the vascular system, the original mesoderm forming the cores of the visceral arches is replaced by presumptive myoblasts migrating *(arrowheads)* from proximally located mesoderm, which may be homologous with the myotomes of postotic somites. The myotomes of the first three postotic somites give rise to the hypoglossal cord, which supplies the myoblasts of the tongue and other muscles supplied by the twelfth cranial nerve. The myoblasts of extrinsic ocular muscle are derived from poorly defined myomeres[104] supplied by the third, fourth, and fifth cranial nerves. The extrinsic ocular muscles are as follows: *a,* superior oblique; *b,* superior rectus; *c* to *e,* lateral, medial, and inferior rectus; and *f,* inferior oblique. (From Johnston, M.C., and Sulik, K.K.: Development of face and oral cavity. In Bhaskar, S.N.: Orban's oral histology and embryology, ed. 9, St. Louis, 1980, The C.V. Mosby Co.)

trinsic ocular muscles originate from preotic "myomeres,"[104] and they also undergo long and complex migrations (Fig. 13-24). The most complex migrations involve the lateral rectus muscle, a factor which may contribute to the frequency of developmental abnormalities of this muscle and the high incidence of internal strabismus.

Besides motor nerve fibers, the nerve for each arch also has at least some sensory fibers. Apart from proprioceptive neurons (which monitor "muscle stretch," positional sense, etc.), whose cell bodies remain in the central nervous system, sensory fibers of the cranial nerves originate from neurons in cranial sensory ganglia. Although some of these neurons originate from neural crest cells and others from ectodermal placodes, neither the functional nor evolutionary significance of the dual origins is known.[23,45] All of the autonomic nervous system neurons and all of the supporting (e.g., Schwann) cells are of crest origin.

Skeletal structures derived from each of the visceral arches are illustrated in Fig. 13-25. They will be given further consideration in relation to middle ear development. Finally, a number of endocrine glands (e.g., thyroid and parathyroid) develop from the endoderm that lines the internal surface of the arches (Table 13-2).

The structure of the developing arches and tongue is illustrated in Fig. 13-26. In the sectioned visceral arches (Fig. 13-26, *B* and *D*) mesodermal core cells cannot be distinguished morphologically from surrounding sheaths of crest cells (Fig. 13-4, *A*).

Development of the tongue is complex (Fig. 13-26, *E* to *G*). The bilateral lingual swellings presumably result from

the accumulation of hypoglossal cord myoblasts (Fig. 13-24), which are derived from the myomeres of the occipital somites.

"Growth centers" forming the external ear (pinna) are illustrated in Fig. 13-27. The external and middle ear develop after the otic (inner ear) epithelium has invaginated into the underlying mesoderm as an otocyst (Fig. 13-28). Later the otocyst is much closer to the location of the external ear (Fig. 13-27, *B*). Early separation of the otocyst from other ear primordia may partially explain the infrequency of association between inner ear abnormalities and other ear abnormalities.

Failure of the growth centers of the external ear (auricular hillocks) and adjacent growth centers (Fig. 13-27) to develop or merge gives rise to abnormalities of the external ear and face. Such abnormalities may be in the form of rare facial clefts, ear tags, and an abnormal pinna or external auditory meatus, as in macrostomia (Fig. 13-27, *C* and *D*).

Table 13-2. Derivatives of the pharyngeal pouch endoderm

Pouch	Derivatives
First	Middle ear and eustachian tube epithelia, mastoid air cells
Second	Palatine tonsil
Third	Inferior parathyroid and thymus glands
Fourth	Superior parathyroid gland
Fifth	Ultimobranchial body

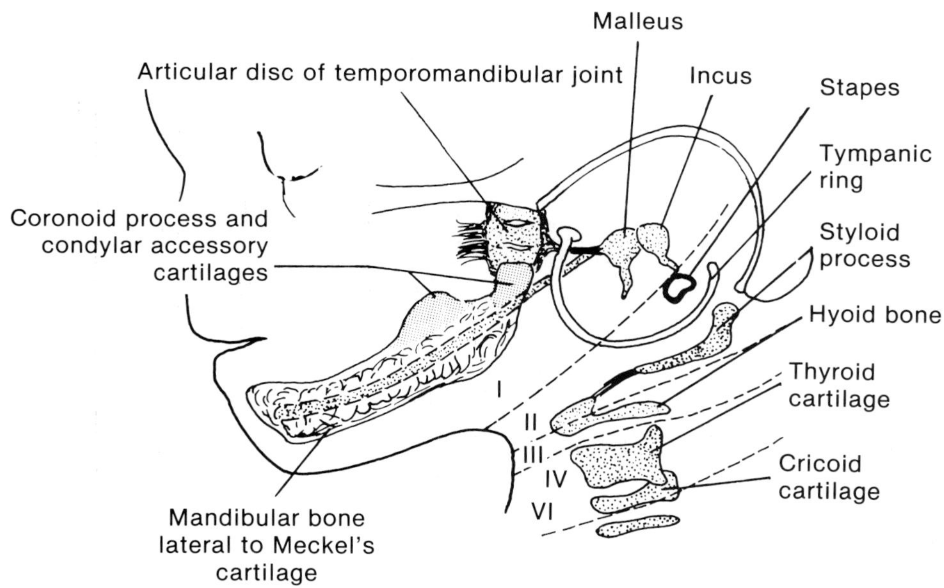

Fig. 13-25. Fetal skeletal components of the visceral arches (Roman numerals) and their relation to the developing temporomandibular joint. (From Waterman, R.E., and Meller, S.M.: Normal facial development in the human embryo. In Shaw, J.H., Sweeny, E.A., Cappuccino, C.C., and Meller, S.M., editors: Textbook of oral biology, Philadelphia, 1978, W.B. Saunders Co.)

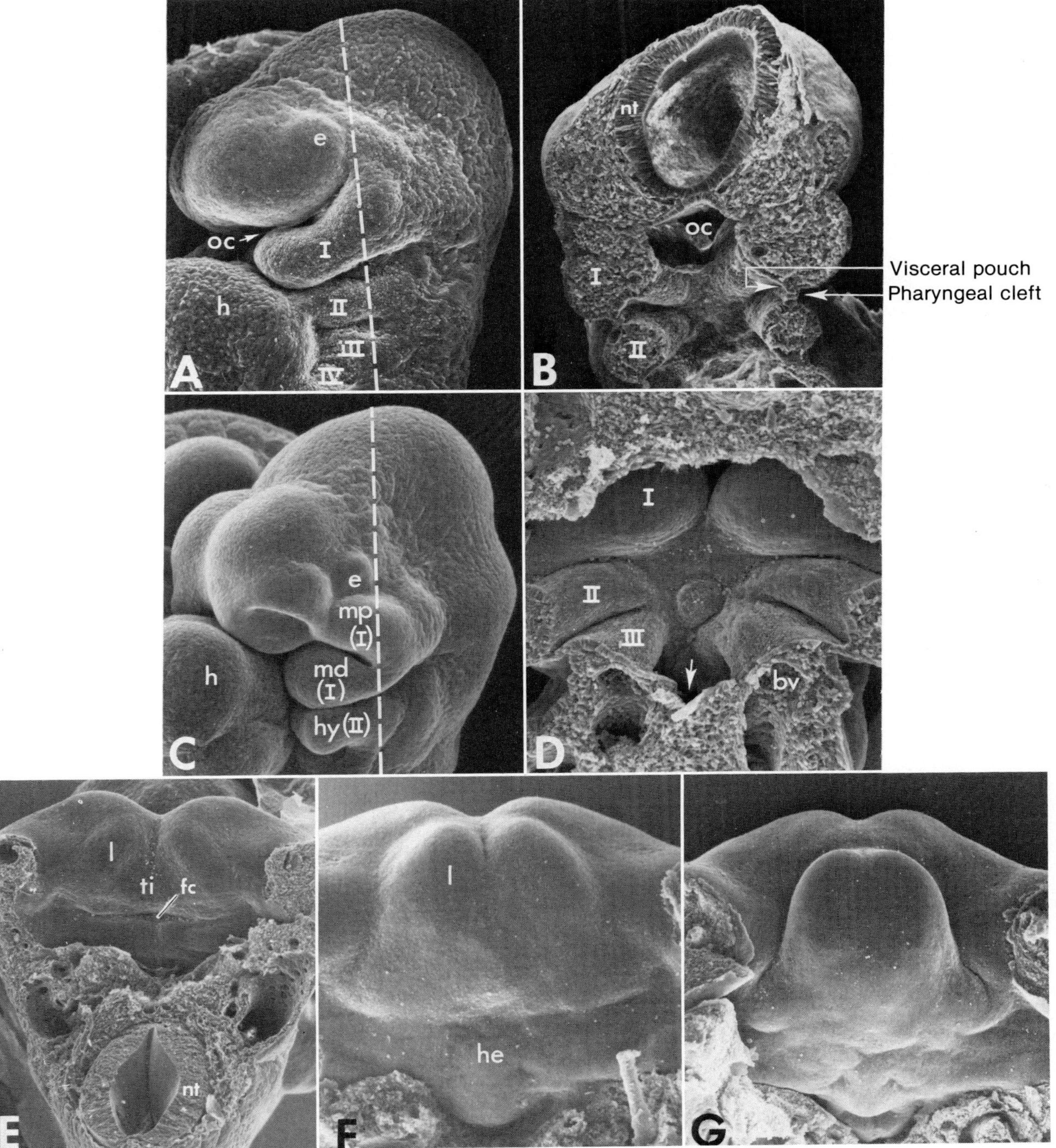

Fig. 13-26. Scanning electron micrographs of the developing visceral arches and tongue of mouse embryos. The planes of section illustrated in **B** and **D** (dorsal views of floor of pharynx) are shown in **A** and **C**. **A** and **B**, Embryos whose developmental age is approximately equivalent to that of human 30-day-old embryos. (See Fig. 13-1.) Development of the medial and lateral nasal prominences has yet to be initiated. The visceral arches are indicated by Roman numerals. The first (mandibular) arch is almost separated from the heart *(h)*. Other structures indicated are the eye *(e)*, oral cavity *(oc)*, and neural tube *(nt)*. **C** and **D**, These are comparable to 35-day-old human embryos. The mandibular arch now has two distinct prominences, the maxillary prominence *(mp)* and the mandibular prominence *(md)*. The second arch is called the hyoid arch *(hy)*. In **D** the blood vessel exiting from the third arch is labeled *bv*. The arrow indicates entry into the lower pharynx. **E** to **G**, Older specimens, prepared in a manner similar to **B** and **D**, illustrate development of the tongue. The lingual swellings *(l)* presumably represent accumulations of myoblasts derived from the hypoglossal cord. The tuberculum impar *(ti)* also contributes to the anterior two-thirds of the tongue. The foramen cecum *(fc)* is the site of endodermal invagination that gives rise to epithelial components of the thyroid gland. It lies at the junction between the anterior two thirds and posterior one third of the tongue. The hypobranchial eminence *(he)* is the primordium of the epiglottis.

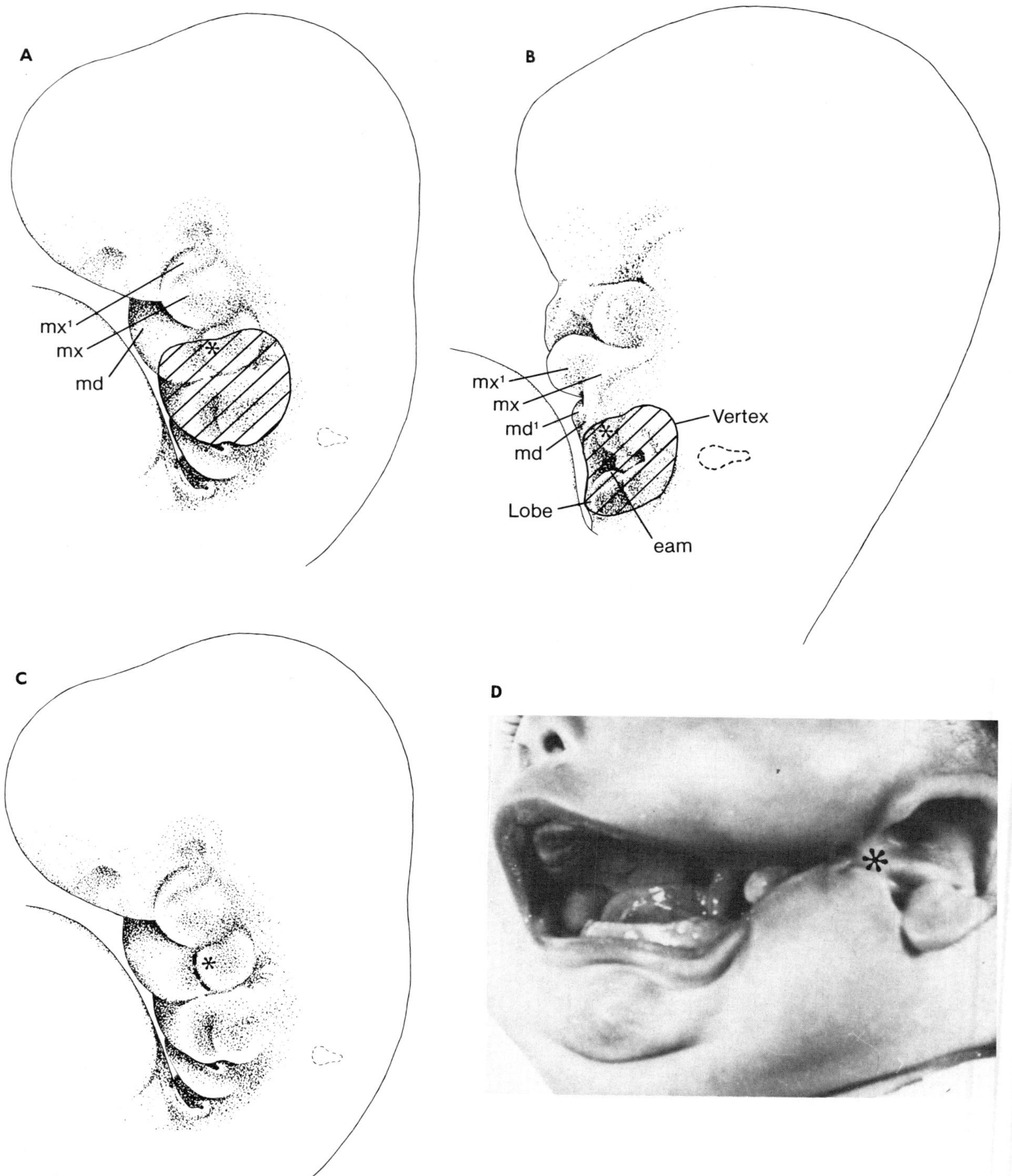

Fig. 13-27. Growth centers related to development of the external ear (pinna and external auditory meatus) and contiguous facial structures. **A** and **B,** Two stages of development. The position of the tragus and its embryonic primordium is indicated by asterisks. The developmental primordia (auricular hillocks) of the external ear are indicated by oblique hatching. These primordia are still close to the ventral (anterior) midline of the neck in **B** and have not achieved their final orientation (*vertex* and *lobe*). The inner ear epithelium or otocyst *(broken line)* is relatively much closer to the external ear in the older embryo. The orientation, position, size, and structure of the external ear are altered in a large number of malformations. **C** and **D,** Failure of merging of these growth centers may result in rare facial clefts such as lateral facial clefts (macrostomia). (**C** and **D** from Gorlin, R.J., Pindborg, J.J., and Cohen, M.M.: Syndromes of the head and neck, New York, 1976, McGraw-Hill, Inc.)

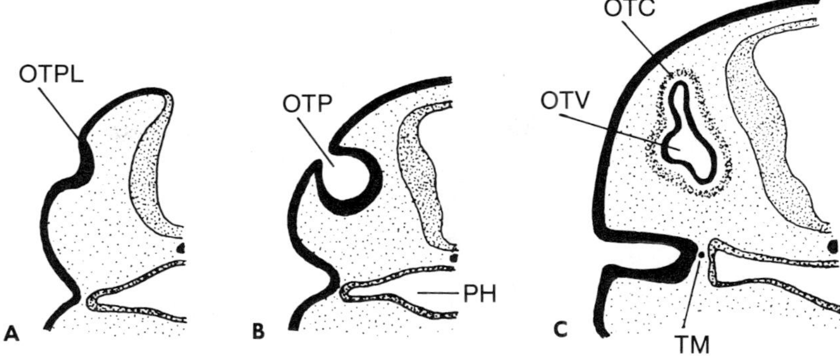

Fig. 13-28. Development of the inner ear. **A,** The otic placode *(OTPL)* invaginates into the underlying mesoderm to form the otic pit *(OTP)* as illustrated in **B. C,** Eventually the inner ear epithelium becomes separated from the surface and forms the otic vesicle *(OTV),* which becomes surrounded by the cartilaginous otic capsule *(OTC).* The tympanic membrane *(TM)* and location of the pharynx *(PH)* are also shown. (Modified from Waterman, R.E., and Meller, S.M.: Normal facial development in the human embryo. In Shaw, J.H., Sweeny, E.A., Cappuccino, C.C., and Meller, S.M., editors: Textbook of oral biology, Philadelphia, 1978, W.B. Saunders Co.)

These structures are also affected in Treacher Collins' syndrome and hemifacial microsomia. Accurate descriptions of human embryos presented in the early part of this century,[95] recent human scanning electron microscopy studies,[98] and detailed descriptions of clinical cases[105] should provide considerable insight into these problems.

The middle ear and temporomandibular joint have interesting interrelations, both in evolution and embryonic development. The evolutionary history of reptiles and primitive mammals indicates strongly[22] that the primitive reptilian jaw joint, which is located posterior to the ''modern'' temporomandibular joint is replaced by the latter in more advanced reptiles. This ''frees up'' skeletal mandibular arch components of the earlier jaw joint, and they become incorporated into the middle ear as the incus and malleus. The (new) temporomandibular joint (Fig. 13-25) is much more versatile than the primitive reptilian jaw joint, permitting complex movements in speech and mastication. The condylar cartilage represents a ''secondary'' (''accessory'') cartilage that is histologically and physiologically different from ''primary'' cartilages found in other joints and synchondroses.[80] Its peculiar origin may be relevant to the condylar regeneration sometimes seen after fracture and resorption of the original condyles in children.

The embryonic origins of the visceral arch skeletal components are illustrated in Fig. 13-25 and Table 13-1. The anterior portion of Meckel's cartilage becomes incorporated into the developing mandible, whereas only the perichondrium of the posterior portion persists in the form of the sphenomandibular segment (Fig. 13-25). Similarly, the perichondrium of Reichert's cartilage gives rise to the stylohyoid ligament, styloid process, and stapes.

The possible developmental origins of so-called first arch malformations will now be considered. The two most common, hemifacial microsomia and mandibulofacial dysostosis (Treacher Collins' syndrome), will be emphasized.

There is experimental evidence[83] that hemorrhage at the point of fusion between the external carotid and stapedial arteries (Fig. 13-23) may be responsible for at least some cases of hemifacial microsomia (Fig. 13-29). Such hemorrhages can be induced in a mouse model,[83] and they appear to interfere with development of structures in the region. As in the human malformation (Fig. 13-29), these structures include the temporomandibular joint, middle and external ear, muscles of mastication, and parotid gland. Poswillo[83] also provided some evidence that thalidomide might produce similar malformations in primates, including humans.

The developmental origins of Treacher Collins' syndrome (Fig. 13-30) are apparently complex. As indicated in the earlier discussion of neural crest development, many of the manifestations of the syndrome can be induced with hypervitaminosis A. Evidence was presented that the major early developmental change resulted from interference with crest cell migration.[39,72,84] Many of the upper facial changes can be induced by administering vitamin A at the initiation of maxillary prominence development.[99] Since a period of several days or more is apparently required for elimination of vitamin A,[56] it is possible that the early administration of vitamin A (before crest cell migration) might still have some effect at the initiation of maxillary prominence development.

DIFFERENTIATION AND MORPHOGENESIS OF SKELETAL TISSUES

At the end of the embryonic period, terminal differentiation into mature tissues has been initiated in most regions of the body. Although growth and morphogenesis continues, most tissues are resistant to common teratogens.

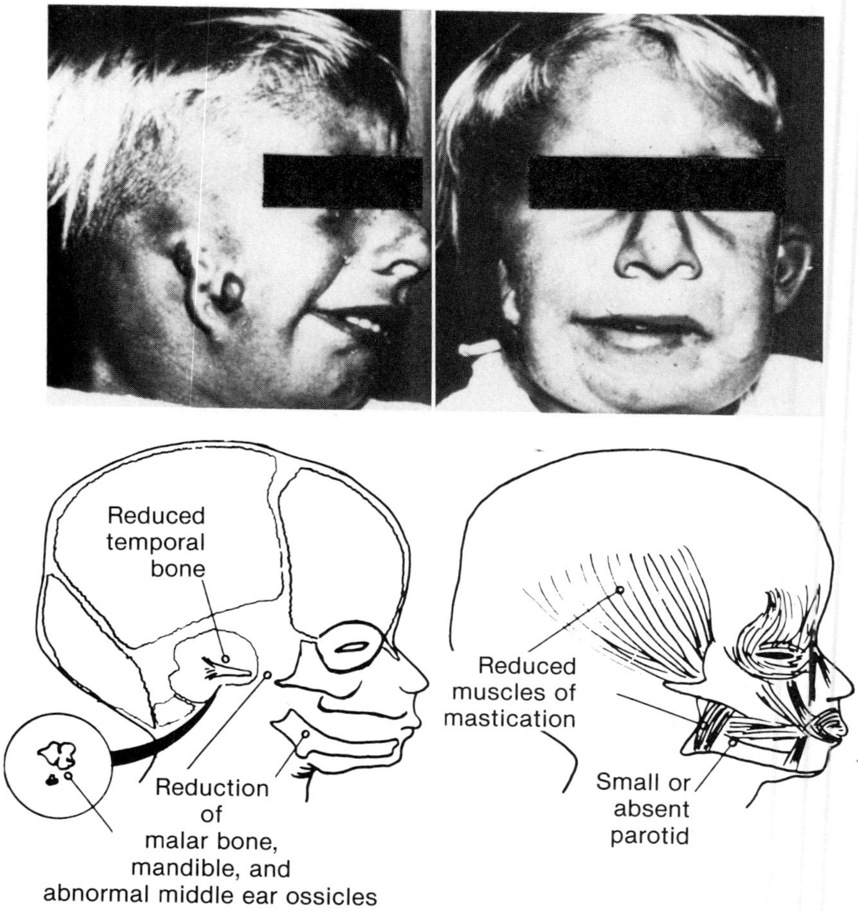

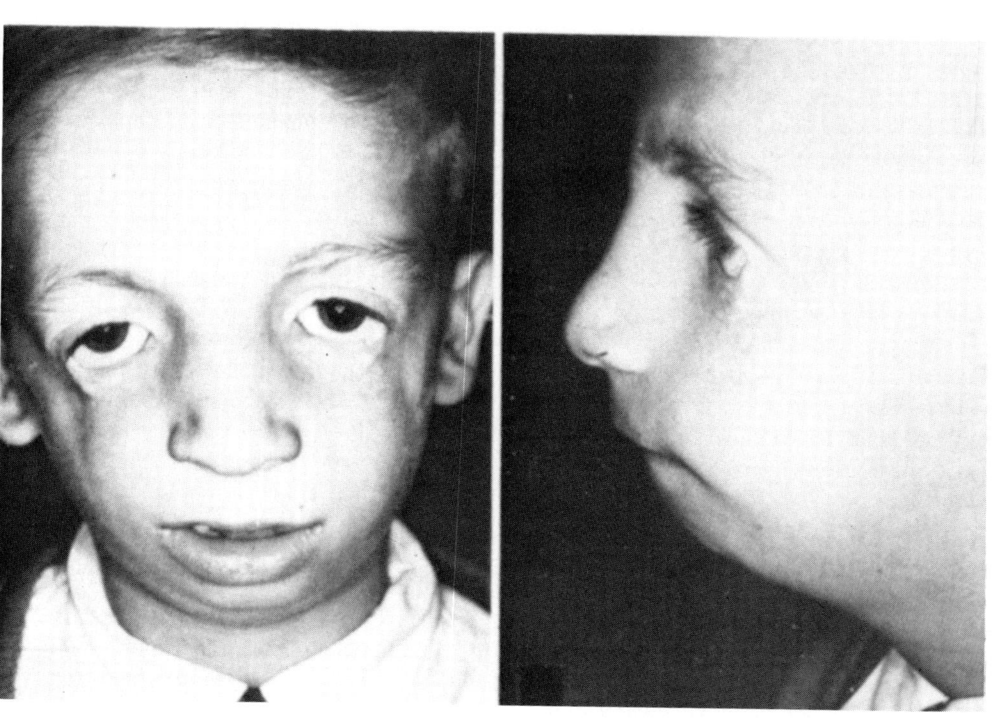

Fig. 13-29. Major features of hemifacial microsomia. In addition to a small deformed pinna, this patient has regional reductions and deficiencies of all underlying tissues, including those in and around the temporomandibular joint, middle ear ossicles, muscles of mastication, and parotid gland. (Modified from Poswillo, D.: Oral Surg. **35**:302, 1973.)

Fig. 13-30. Patient with Treacher Collins' syndrome. Deficiency in the zygomatic region, lateral lower lid gap (coloboma), and micrognathia are present. The patient also has a cleft palate. (From Ross, R.B., and Johnston, M.C.: Cleft lip and palate. © 1972, The Williams & Wilkins Co., Baltimore.)

Growth of cartilage may be deficient in genetically determined conditions such as achondroplasia. Such defects result in characteristic craniofacial malformations.

Intramembranous (i.e., nonendochrondral) bones are common in the head. Their development is initiated as an ossification center. Usually there is one ossification center for each bone, and bone formation stops before contact and fusion of the centers, with sutures remaining between the bones. Bone growth occurs by apposition at the sutures and is apparently secondary to expansive growth forces exerted by soft tissues. If premature closure of sutures (synostosis) occurs, growth may be inhibited. Premature closure may be genetically determined, such as Crouzon's disease (craniofacial dysostosis), or may result from premature contact and fusion of (cranial vault) bones because of excessive intrauterine pressure secondary to oligohydramnios.[35] Excessive intrauterine pressure may also result in deformations.[37]

In Crouzon's disease both cranial and facial sutures are affected. Involvement of cranial vault sutures may be somewhat variable both in time of onset (first through fifth year) and location.[34] Exophthalmos readily distinguishes Crouzon's disease from achondroplasia. It is primarily related to deficient growth of the periocular bones but may be partially due to downward pressure from the developing brain, leading to remodeling of the orbital roof. Increased intracranial pressure in unoperated cases may be associated with mental retardation. Although the basic nature of the developmental defect is unknown, it is inherited as an autosomal dominant trait.

Although most of the craniofacial manifestations seen in Apert's syndrome are similar to those of Crouzon's disease, it appears that the two conditions are etiologically different. The developmental disturbances in Apert's syndrome are always present at birth, more widespread, and, in addition to premature suture closure, include syndactyly and clefts of the soft palate in about 30% of the cases.[34] Most of the patients are mentally retarded. Although few patients reproduce successfully, it appears that most cases result from abnormal autosomal dominant genes.

The initial primordia of the teeth (the dental laminae and associated mesenchyme) form at about the time of fusion of the medial nasal, lateral nasal, and maxillary prominences. Failure of fusion of these prominences leads to cleft lip and alters further development of teeth in the fusion area with a peculiarly wide spectrum of supernumerary and missing teeth and unusual structures of those teeth which are present.[87] Tooth abnormalities may be associated with a wide variety of craniofacial malformations,[34] or there may be abnormalities of structure, form, size, or numbers not associated with other malformations.[10] Since enamel and dentin do not undergo remodeling, as do other mineralized tissues, they may provide evidence of the timing of more generalized developmental disturbances, such as those occurring at birth.

CONCLUSION

Recent advances have greatly improved our understanding of both normal and abnormal embryonic development of the head and neck. Accurate descriptions of craniofacial malformations by plastic surgeons and other clinicians have been helpful, particularly in the assessment of the suitability of animal models for human malformations. For the first time it appears possible to prevent certain craniofacial malformations both in animals and humans through manipulation of the "environment." Rapid progress is expected.

REFERENCES

1. Adelmann, H.B.: The embryological basis of cyclopia, Am. J. Ophthalmol. **17:**890, 1934.
2. Asling, C.W.: Congenital defects of the face and palate following maternal deficiency of pteroylglutamic acid. In Pruzansky, S., editor: Congenital anomalies of the face and associated structures, Springfield, Ill., 1961, Charles C Thomas, Publisher.
3. Been, W., and Lieuw Kie Song, S.H.: Harelip and cleft palate conditions in chick embryos following local destruction of the cephalic neural crest: a preliminary note, Acta Morphol. Neerl. Scand. **16:**245, 1978.
4. Bixler, E., et al.: The ectrodactyly-ectodermal dysplasia-clefting (EEC) syndrome, Clin. Genet. **3:**43, 1971.
5. Bolande, R.P.: The neurocristopathies: a unifying concept of disease arising in neural crest maldevelopment, Hum. Pathol. **5:**409, 1974.
6. Bolande, R.P.: Neurofibromatosis—the quintessential neurocristopathy: pathogenetic concepts and relationships, Adv. Neurol. **29:**67, 1981.
7. Bonner, J.J., and Slavkin, H.C.: Cleft palate susceptibility linked to histocompatibility-2 (H-2) in the mouse, Immunogenetics **2:**213, 1975
8. Briggs, R.M.: Vitamin supplementation as a possible factor in the incidence of cleft lip/palate deformities in humans, Clin. Plast. Surg. **3:**647, 1976
9. Brown, K., and Harne, L.C.: The genetics of two traits: cleft palate and anencephalus in the oel strain of mice (abstract), Teratology **9:**14, 1974.
10. Brown, K.S.: Evolution and development of dentition, Birth Defects. (In press.)
11. Burks, D., and Saddler, T.W.: Morphogenesis of median facial clefts in mice treated with diazo-oxy-norleucine (DON), Teratology **27:**385, 1983.
12. Carter, C.O.: Genetics of common disorders, Br. Med. Bull. **25:**52, 1969.
13. Carter, C.O.: Principles of polygenic inheritance, Birth Defects **13(3A):**69, 1976.
14. Chatot, C.L., and Klein, N.W.: Teratogenic activity of serum from human epileptic subjects studied by rats embryo culture (abstract), Teratology **23(2):**30, 1981.
15. Chatot, C.L., Klein, N.W., Piatek, J., and Pierro, L.J.: Successful culture of rat embryos on human serum: use in the detection of teratogens, Science **207:**1471, 1980.
16. Chernoff, G.F.: Personal communication, 1982.
17. Chernoff, G.F., and Golden, J.A.: Strain differences in the dose response and morphology of heat induced neural tube defects in two strains of mice, Presented at the David W. Smith Conference on Malformations and Morphogenesis, 1982, Hickory Knob, S.C.
18. Chibon, P.: Personal communication, 1977.
19. Cohen, M.M., and Lemire, R.J.: Syndromes with cephaloceles, Teratology **25:**161, 1982.
20. Coleman, R.D.: Development of the rat palate, Anat. Rec. **151:**107, 1965.
21. Coulombre, A.J., and Coulombre, J.L.: Abnormal organogenesis in the eye. In Wilson, J.G., and Fraser, F.C., editors: Handbook of teratology, New York, 1977, Plenum Press.
22. Crompton, A.W., and Parker, P.: Evolution of the mammalian masticatory apparatus, Am. Sci. **66:**192, 1978.

23. D'Amico-Martel, A., and Noden, D.M.: Contributions of placodal and neural crest cells to avian sensory ganglia, Am. J. Anat. (In press.)

24. Deol, M.S.: The relationship between abnormalities of pigmentation and the inner ear, Proc. R. Soc. Lond. **175:**201, 1970.

25. Deol, M.S., and Lane, P.W.: A new gene affecting the morphogenesis of the vestibular part of the inner ear in the mouse, J. Embryol. Exp. Morphol. **16:**543, 1966.

26. Diewert, V.M.: Differential changes in cartilage cell proliferation and cell density in the rat craniofacial complex during secondary palate development, Anat. Rec. **198:**219, 1980.

27. Diewert, V.M., and Pratt, M.: Cortisone-induced cleft palate in A/J mice: failure of palatal shelf contact, Teratology **24:**149, 1981.

28. Edwards, M.J., Warner, R.A., and Mulley, R.C.: Exencephaly in fetal hamsters following exposure to hyperthermia, Teratology **14:**3203, 1976.

29. Fraser, F.C., and Fainstat, T.D.: Causes of congenital defects, Am. J. Dis. Child. **82:**593, 1951.

30. Fraser, F.C., and Pashayan, H.: Relation of face shape to congenital cleft lip, J. Med. Genet. **7:**112, 1970.

31. Gans, C., and Northcutt, R.G.: Neural crest and the origin of vertebrates: a new head, Science **220:**268, 1983.

32. Gasser, R.F.: The development of the facial muscles in man, Am. J. Anat. **120:**357, 1967.

33. Gorlin, R.J., and Mirkin, B.L.: Multiple mucosal neuromas, pheochromocytoma, medullary carcinoma of the thyroid and marfanoid body build with muscle wasting, Z. Kinderheilkund **113:**313, 1972.

34. Gorlin, R.J., Pindborg, J.J., and Cohen, M.M.: Syndromes of the head and neck, New York, 1976, McGraw-Hill, Inc.

35. Graham, J.M., deSaxe, M., and Smith, D.W.: Sagittal craniostenosis: fetal head constraint as one possible cause, J. Pediatr. **95:**747, 1979.

36. Greene, R.M., and Pratt, R.M.: Developmental aspects of secondary palate formation, J. Embryol. Exp. Morphol. **36:**225, 1976.

37. Greer-Walker, D.: Malformations of the face, Edinburgh, 1958, E.S. Livingstone.

38. Hamilton, W.J., and Mossman, H.: Human embryology, ed. 4, Cambridge, England, 1972, W. Heffer & Sons, Ltd.

39. Hassell, J.R., Greenberg, J.H., and Johnston, M.C.: Inhibition of cranial neural crest cell development by vitamin A in the cultured chick embryo, J. Embryol. Exp. Morphol. **39:**267, 1977.

40. Hassell, T.H., Johnston, M.C., and Dudley, K.H., editors: Phenytoin-induced teratology and gingival pathology, New York, 1980, Raven Press.

41. Iregbulem, L.M.: Midline clefts of the upper lip, Br. J. Plast. Surg. **31:**63, 1978.

42. Jacobson, A.G.: Inductive processes in embryonic development, Science **152:**25, 1966.

43. Johnston, M.C.: The neural crest in vertebrate cephalogenesis, doctoral dissertation, New York, 1965, University of Rochester.

44. Johnston, M.C.: A radioautographic study of the migration and fate of cranial neural crest cells in the chick embryo, Anat. Rec. **156:**143, 1966.

45. Johnston, M.C., and Hazelton, R.B.: Embryonic origins of facial structures related to oral sensory and motor function. In Bosma, J.F. editor: Oral sensory perception: the mouth of the infant, Springfield, Ill., 1972, Charles C Thomas, Publisher.

46. Johnston, M.C., Morris, C.M., Kushner, D., and Bingle, G.D.: Abnormal organogenesis of facial structures. In Wilson, J.G., and Fraser, F.C., editors: Handbook of teratology, vol. 2, New York, 1977, Plenum Press.

47. Johnston, M.C., and Niswander, J.D.: Unpublished data, 1983.

48. Johnston, M.C., Noden, D.M., Hazelton, R.D., et al.: Origins of avian ocular and periocular tissues, Exp. Eye Res. **29:**27, 1979.

49. Johnston, M.C., and Sulik, K.K.: Some abnormal patterns of development in the craniofacial region, Birth Defects **15**(8):23, 1979.

50. Johnston, M.C., and Sulik, K.K.: The neural crest. In Shields, E.D., Burzynsky, N.J., and Melnick, M., editors: Craniofacial dysmorphology: genetics, etiology, diagnosis and treatment, Littleton, Mass., 1983, John Wright/PSG, Inc.

51. Johnston, M.C., Vig, K., and Ambrose, L.: Neurocristopathy as a unifying concept: clinical correlations, Adv. Neurol. **29:**97, 1981.

52. Jones, K.L., Smith, D.W., Hall, B.D., et al.: A pattern of craniofacial and limb defects secondary to aberrant tissue bands, J. Pediatr. **84:**90, 1974.

53. Juriloff, D.M., and Fraser, F.C.: Genetic maternal effects on cleft lip frequency in A/J and CL/Fr mice, Teratology **21:**167, 1980.

54. Juriloff, D.M., Sulik, K.K., and Roderick, T.H.: Morphogenesis of spontaneously occurring otocephaly in a newly developed mouse mutant (abstract), Teratology **21:**47, 1980.

55. Kenny, J., et al.: Unpublished data, 1982.

56. Kochar, D.M.: Transplacental passage of label after administration of (^{3}H) retinoic acid (vitamin A acid) to pregnant mice, Teratology **14:**53, 1976.

57. Langman, J.: Medical embryology, ed. 4, Baltimore, 1981, Williams & Wilkins.

58. Le Douarin, N.: A biological cell labelling technique and its use in experimental embryology, Dev. Biol. **30:**217, 1973.

59. Le Lievre, C., and Le Douarin, N.M.: Mesenchymal derivatives of the neural crest: anlysis of chimeric quail and chick embryos, J. Embryol. Exp. Morphol. **34:**125, 1975.

60. Lemire, R.J., Cohen, M., Jr., Beckwith, J., et al.: The facial features of holoprosencephaly in anencephalic human specimens. I. Historical review and associated malformations, Teratology **23:**297, 1981.

61. Linville, G.P., and Shepard, T.H.: Neural tube closure defects caused by cytochalasin B. Nature **236:**246, 1982.

62. Lyon, M.F.: The developmental origin of hereditary absence of Otoliths in mice, J. Embryol. Exp. Morphol. **3:**23, 1955.

63. Mann, I.: Developmental abnormalities of the eye, London, 1937, Cambridge University Press.

64. Marin-Padilla, M.: Study of the skull in human cranioschisis, Acta Anat. **62:**1, 1965.

65. Millicovsky, G., Ambrose, L.J.H., and Johnston, M.C.: Developmental alterations associated with spontaneous cleft lip and palate in CL/Fr mice, Am. J. Anat. **164:**29, 1982.

66. Millicovsky, G., and Johnston, M.C.: Active role of embryonic facial epithelium: new evidence of cellular events in morphogenesis, J. Embryol. Exp. Morphol. **63:**53, 1981.

67. Millicovsky, G., and Johnston, M.C.: Hyperoxia and hypoxia in pregnancy: simple experimental manipulation alters the incidence of cleft lip and palate in CL/Fr mice, Proc. Natl. Acad. Sci. U.S.A **9:**4723, 1981.

68. Millicovsky, G., and Johnston, M.C.: Maternal hyperoxia greatly reduces the incidence of phenytoin-induced cleft lip and palate in A/J mice, Science **212:**671, 1981.

69. Minkoff, R., and Kuntz, A.J.: Cell proliferation during morphogenetic change: analysis of frontonasal morphogenesis in the chick embryo employing DNA labelling indices, J. Embryol. Exp. Morphol. **40:**101, 1977.

70. Minkoff, R., and Kuntz, A.J.: Cell proliferation and cell density of mesenchyme in the maxillary process and adjacent regions during facial development in the chick embryo, J. Embryol. Exp. Morphol. **46:**65, 1978.

71. Moore, K.L.: The developing human, ed. 2, Philadelphia, 1977, W.B. Saunders Co.

72. Morriss, G.: Abnormal cell migration as a possible factor in the genesis of vitamin A–induced craniofacial anomalies. In Neubert, D., editor: New approaches to the evaluation of abnormal mammalian embryonic development, Stuttgart, 1976, Georg Thieme.

73. Neidyl, S., et al.: Personnel communication, 1983.

74. Netzloff, M.L., Streiff, R.R., Frias, J.L., and Rennert, O.M.: Folate antagonists following teratogenic exposure to diphenylhydantoin, Teratology **19:**45, 1979.

75. New, D.A.T.: Whole embryo culture, Biol. Rev. **53:**81, 1978.

76. Niswander, J.D., and Johnston, M.C.: Unpublished data, 1983.

77. Noden, D.M.: Interactions directing the migration and cytodifferentiation of avian neural crest cells. In Garrod, D.R., editor: Specificity of embryological interactions, vol. 5, London, 1978, Chapman & Hall, Ltd.

78. Noden, D.M.: Patterns and organizations of craniofacial skeletogenic and myogenic mesenchymes. In Dixon, A., and Sarnat, B., editors: Factors and mechanisms influencing bone growth, New York, 1982, Alan R. Liss, Inc.

79. Patterson, S., Minkoff, M., and Johnston, M.C.: Autoradiographic

studies in cell migration during primary palate morphogenesis, J. Dent. Res. **58A:**113, 1979.

80. Petrovic, A.J., Stutzmann, J., and Oudet, C.: Control processes in the postnatal growth of the condylar cartilage of the mandible. In McNamara, J.A., Jr., editor: Determinants of mandibular form and growth, Monograph No. 4, Craniofacial Growth Series, Center for Human Growth and Development, Ann Arbor, 1975, The University of Michigan.

81. Petter, C., Bourbon, J., Maltier, J.P., and Jost, A.: Prevention des amputations congenitales hereditaries du lapin par une hyperoxie maternelle, C.R. Acad. Sci. **273:**2639, 1971.

82. Poswillo, D.: Observations of fetal posture and causal mechanisms of congenital deformity of the palate, mandible and limbs, J. Dent. Res. **45:**584, 1966.

83. Poswillo, D.: The pathogenesis of the first and second branchial arch syndrome, Oral Surg. **35:**302, 1973.

84. Poswillo, D.: The pathogenesis of the Treacher-Collins syndrome (mandibulofacial dysostosis), Br. J. Oral Surg. **13:**1,1975.

85. Pratt, R.M.: Personal communication, 1983.

86. Pratt, R.M., and Martin, G.R.: Epithelial cell death and cyclic AMP increase during palatal development, Proc. Natl. Acad. Sci. U.S.A. **72:**874, 1975.

87. Ross, R.B., and Johnston, M.C.: Cleft lip and palate, Baltimore, 1972, Williams & Wilkins.

88. Saxén, I.: Association between oral clefts and drugs taken during pregnancy, Int. J. Epidemiol. **4:**37, 1975.

89. Slavkin, H.C.: Developmental craniofacial biology, Philadelphia, 1979, Lea & Febiger.

90. Smiley, G.R., Vanek, R.J., and Dixon, A.D.: Width of the craniofacial complex during formation of the secondary palate, Cleft Palate J. **8:**371, 1971.

91. Smith, D.W.: Personal communication, 1979.

92. Smithells, R.W.: Personal communication, 1982.

93. Smithells, R.W., Sheppard, S., Schorah, C.J., et al.: Possible prevention of neural-tube defects by periconceptional vitamin supplementation, Lancet **1:**339, 1981.

94. Smithells, R.W., Sheppard, S., Schorah, C.J., et al.: Apparent prevention of neural tube defects by periconceptional vitamin supplementation, Arch. Dis. Child. **56:**911, 1981.

95. Streeter, G.L.: Developmental horizons in human embryos, description of age groups XV, XVI, XVII, and XVIII, Contrib. Embryol. **32:**133, 1948.

96. Sulik, K.K.: Unpublished data, 1980.

97. Sulik, K.K.: Unpublished data, 1981.

98. Sulik, K.K.: Unpublished data, 1983.

99. Sulik, K.K., and Johnston, M.C.: Cleft palate investigations in T1Wh mice, Anat. Rec. **190:**555, 1978.

100. Sulik, K.K., and Johnston, M.C.: Sequence of developmental changes following ethanol exposure in mice: craniofacial features of the fetal alcohol syndrome (FAS), Am. J. Anat. **166:**257, 1983.

101. Sulik, K.K., and Johnston, M.C.: Embryonic origin of holoprosencephaly: interrelationship of the developing brain and face, Scanning Electron Microscopy **1:**309, 1982.

102. Sulik, K.K., Johnston, M.C., Ambrose, L.J.H., and Dorgan, D.R.: Phenytoin (Dilantin)-induced cleft lip: a scanning and transmission electron microscopic study, Anat. Rec. **195:**243, 1979.

103. Sulik, K.K.., Johnston, M.C., and Webb, M.A.: Fetal alcohol syndrome: embryogenesis in a mouse model, Science **214:**936, 1981.

104. Tam, P.P.L., and Meier, S.: The establishment of a somitomeric pattern in the mesoderm of the gastrulating mouse embryo, J. Anat. **164:**209, 1982.

105. Tessier, R.: Anatomical classification of facial, cranio-facial and latero-facial clefts, J. Maxillofac. Surg. **4:**69, 1976.

106. Tolarova, M.: Periconceptional supplementation with vitamins and folic acid to prevent recurrence of cleft lip, Lancet **2:**217, 1982.

107. Trasler, D.C.: Pathogenesis of cleft lip and its relation to embryonic face shape in A/J and C57B1 mice, Teratology **1:**33, 1968.

108. Trasler, D.G., and Leong, S.: Mitotic index in mouse embryo with 6-aminonicotinamide-induced inherited cleft lip, Teratology **25:**259, 1982.

109. Tyler, M.S., and Koch, W.S.: Epithelial-mesenchymal interactions in the secondary palate of the mouse, J. Dent. Res. **53:**64, 1974.

110. Vekemans, M., and Fraser, F.C.: Stage of palate closure as one indication of liability to cleft palate, Am. J. Med. Genet. **4:**95, 1979.

111. Walker, B.E.: Correlation of embryonic movement with palate closure in mice, Teratology **2:**191, 1969.

112. Walker, B.E., and Patterson, A.: The mechanism of cortisone-induced cleft palate, J. Dent. Res. **53:**63, 1974.

113. Walker, B.E., and Quarles, J.: Palate closure in embryonic mice after excising the tongue, Teratology **7:**4, 1973.

114. Webster, W.S., Walsh, D.A., and Lipson, A.H.: Teratogenesis after acute alcohol exposure in inbred and outbred mice, Neurobehav. Toxicol. Teratol. **2:**227, 1980.

115. Weston, J.A.: The migration and differentiation of neural crest cells, Adv. Morphogen. **8:**41, 1970.

116. Wright, S., and Wagner, K.: Types of subnormal development of the head from inbred strains of guinea pigs and their bearing on the classification and interpretation of vertebrate monsters, Am. J. Anat. **54:**383, 1934.

117. Yoneda, T., and Pratt, R.M.: Glucocorticoid receptors in palatal mesenchymal cells from the human embryo: relevance to human cleft palate formation, J. Craniofacial Genetics Dev. Biol. **1:**411, 1981.

118. Yoneda, T., and, Pratt, R.M.: Vitamin B_6 reduces cortisone-induced cleft palate in the mouse, Teratology **26:**255, 1982.

CHAPTER 14

Growth and development of the craniofacial skeleton

RALPH A. LATHAM

The emergence of a rudimentary facial form in the fifth week of development (ovulation age) involves migration of cells from the neural crest to presumptive skeletal sites. Here mesectodermal cell masses develop and produce the surface features described as facial processes in the oronasal region. During the fifth week, only soft tissues are seen in the internal structure of the embryonic head.[4]

THE CHONDROCRANIUM

The first skeletal support for the embryo is provided by cartilaginous tissue. In the head region the first functional skull is formed of cartilage and is referred to as the *chondrocranium*. In the face it first develops at about 37 days when a condensation of prechondroblast cells in the midline heralds the formation of the nasal septum and the cranial base. Soon after, bilateral rods of cartilage (Meckel's car-

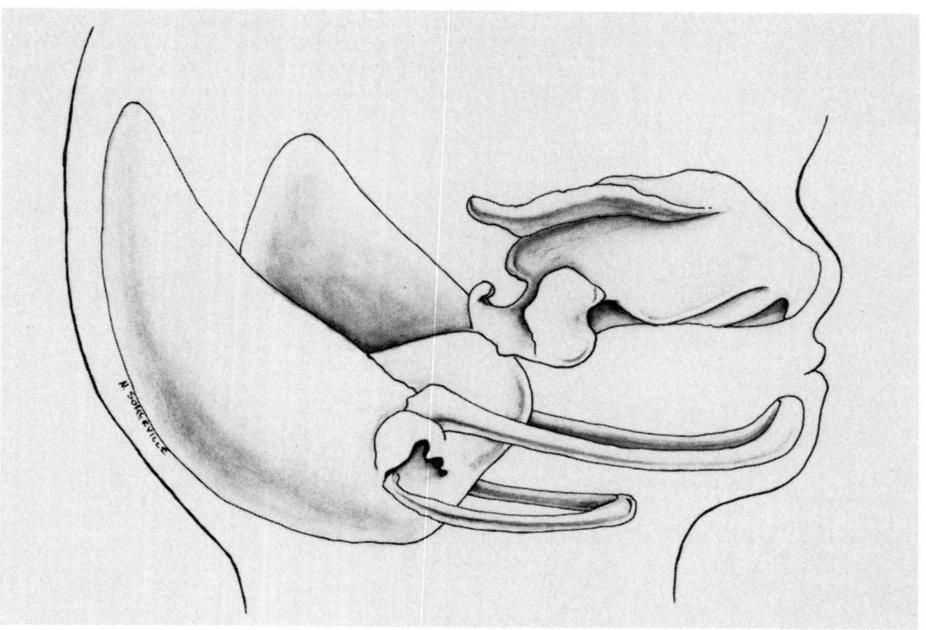

Fig. 14-1. Lateral view of chondrocranium of a 10-week human embryo. (Modified from Wynne, T.H.M.: Observations on the development of the human chondrocranium, doctoral thesis, Liverpool, England, 1966, University of Liverpool.)

tilage) develop in the mandibular arch as supportive precursors of the mandible. The chondrocranium has four basic components (Fig. 14-1):

1. Mandibular arch cartilage (Meckel's cartilage)
2. Nasal capsule (supported by the nasal septum)
3. Basal plate (also termed parachordal plate)
4. Otic capsules

The mandibular arch cartilage remains a free structure that articulates at the meckelian joint where its dorsal part later becomes the malleus of the middle ear. The other three parts of the chondrocranium join together into a continuous one-piece structure.[16]

Nasal capsule

The nasal capsule is a supporting cartilaginous structure that is closely related to the olfactory organ and supports

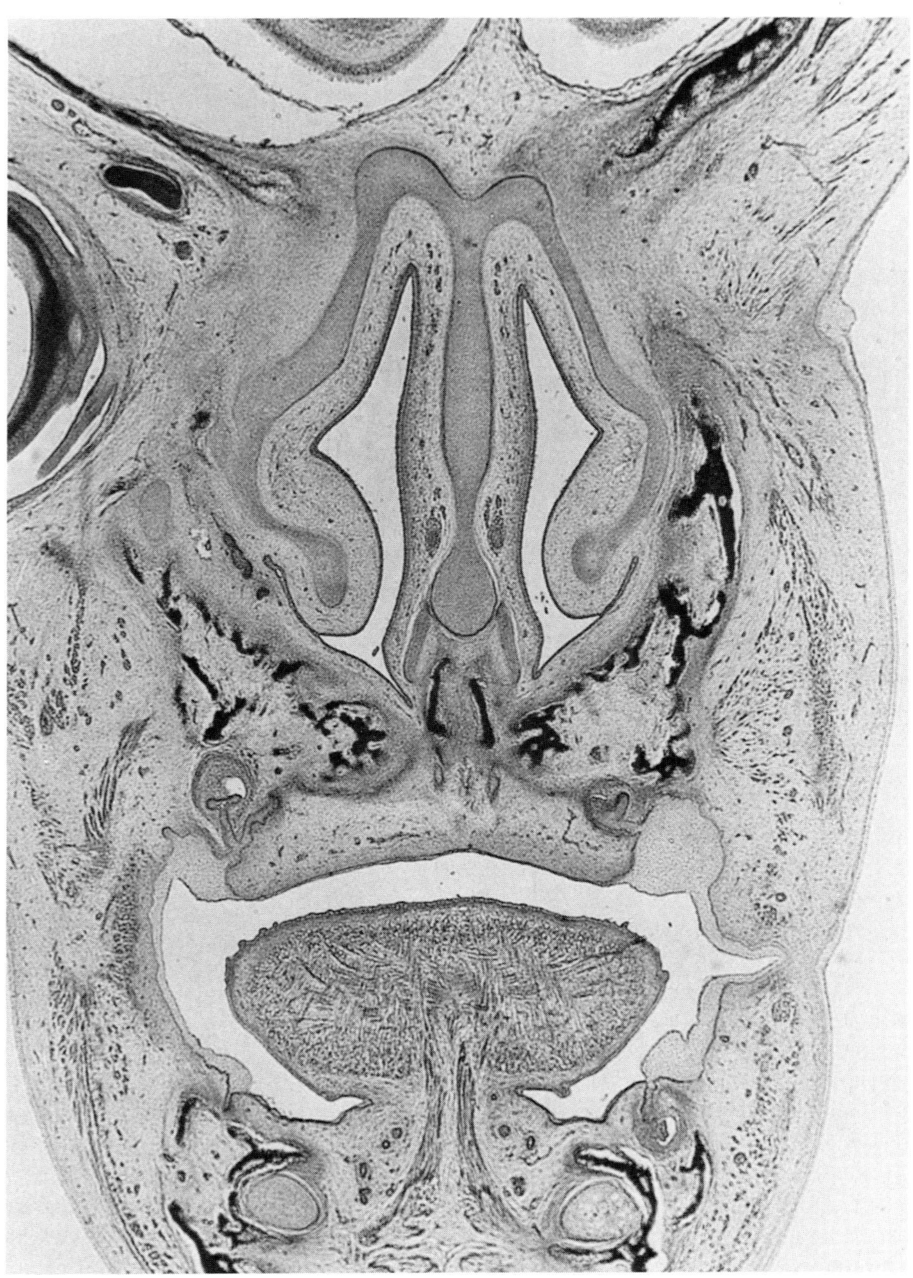

Fig. 14-2. Coronal section of an 11-week human fetus showing cartilagenous nasal capsule supporting the midface, nasal cavities, and inferior concha. Note thickened inferior part of the cartilaginous nasal septum that provides septal reinforcement anteroposteriorly. (From McNamara, J.A., editor: Factors affecting the growth of the midface, Ann Arbor, Mich., 1976, The University of Michigan Press.)

the olfactory and respiratory mucous membranes of the nose in the embryonic periods. The nasal septum is continuous superiorly over the nasal cavities with the lateral lamina of the nasal capsule (Fig. 14-2). The lower border of the lateral lamina turns medially and supports the inferior nasal concha; this part is replaced later by bone of the inferior nasal concha. Posteriorly the nasal septum merges with the basal plate that is later to become the basisphenoid and basioccipital parts of the cranial base. The nasal septum and nasal alar cartilages are the only structures of the nasal capsule remaining at birth.

Mandibular arch cartilage

The cartilage bar of the first branchial arch supports the embryonic lower jaw. The two halves of the arch cartilage are joined together at the midline by fibrous tissue. The mandibular arch cartilage appears to fulfill an important supporting role for the mandible for a period of about 8 weeks, from 6 to 14 weeks. It contributes to the beginning of the osseous mandible in its initial size and form. Hypoplasia, or agenesis, of Meckel's cartilage might have far-reaching effects in facial development and may be a factor in some cases of the Pierre Robin syndrome with mandibular hypoplasia and cleft palate. The arch cartilage may be a form-determining factor and growth pacemaker (for the mandible) during early development.

The chondrocranial role

Once established by the processes of organogenesis, the chondrocranium exhibits a number of characteristics that, in contrast to properties of bone, appear to suit it for an embryonic role. First, its structural tissue is relatively simple when compared to bone. In the less–well vascularized tissues of the embryo, it may be better adapted for development and function than bone. Second, its cartilage is ready to function as a supporting tissue immediately after differentiation; thus it provides the earliest form of skeletal support. Although the ossification centers for some of the membranous bones (mandible and maxillae) differentiate at about the same time as much of the cartilage, they cannot provide skeletal support until after a period of growth. Third, a capacity for rapid growth is evident. Cartilage can grow by an internal swelling or interstitial growth that results from internal cell mitosis and matrix formation, as well as by surface addition. Fourth, the chondrocranium appears to have a form-determining role. Basic features of the facial phenotype may be determined by this stage. Its parts may serve as growth pacemakers for adjacent structures whose growth may be guided and stimulated. Some evidence found in the unilateral cleft lip and palate condition points to a growth relationship between the nasal septum and the middle third of the face.[6,7]

The chondrocranium reaches maximal development at about 10 to 12 weeks; thereafter, signs of regression may be seen in the mandibular arch cartilage and in the cranial base as the osseous cranium progresses.

THE OSSEUS CRANIUM

Bones of the skull develop in two ways: (1) by intramembranous or periosteal ossification and (2) by replacing a cartilaginous structure that undergoes endochondral ossification.

Intramembranous ossification

At about the same time as cartilage differentiates, ossification centers appear for the mandible and maxillae. These membrane bones appear as small centers of ossification that require a longer period of time to develop functionally. The mandibular center of ossification appears at about 39 to 40 days, immediately after that for the clavicle, which develops first of all. The maxillary center of ossification appears at about 40 days and the premaxillary centers at about 41 days. The ossification center for the mandible arises in close relation to the mandibular arch cartilage whose anterior part is later incorporated.

In a 41-day embryo having an immature face in which cartilage is commencing to differentiate, the ossification center for the maxilla appears as a ribbon-like structure. In the premaxillary region there are small islets of ossification for the premaxillary bone. The human maxilla and premaxilla appear to develop separately, but they are enveloped within a common condensation of mesectoderm, and the bony centers unite rapidly to form one bone. The maxillary ossification center forms first in relation to the canine tooth lateral to the chondrocranial nasal capsule. It then extends superiorly, medially and laterally, and posteriorly. Ossification centers for other facial bones appear in mesectoderm of the facial region.

Ossification time sequence

There is a time-related pattern in the development of the initial ossification centers of the skull bones.[11] An interesting anteroposterior sequence of appearance of ossification centers may be seen in the following scheme:

Intramembranous ossification

Group I	39 days	Mandible
	40 days	Maxilla
	41 days	Premaxilla
Group II	56 days	Zygomatic, frontal, parietal bones
	57 days	Vomer, palatine, nasal bones

Endochondral ossification

Group III	65 days	Basioccipital parts of cranial base
	83 days	Basisphenoid parts of cranial base

Group I comprises the jaws, which appear about 15 days before the rest of the intramembranous facial bones of group II. Group III represents bones formed by endochondral ossification.

The first priority of the intramembranous cranial bones is to establish joints, or sutures, with adjacent bones before functioning as a skeletal system. After the establishment of joints, the individual bones are held together and become mutually supporting.

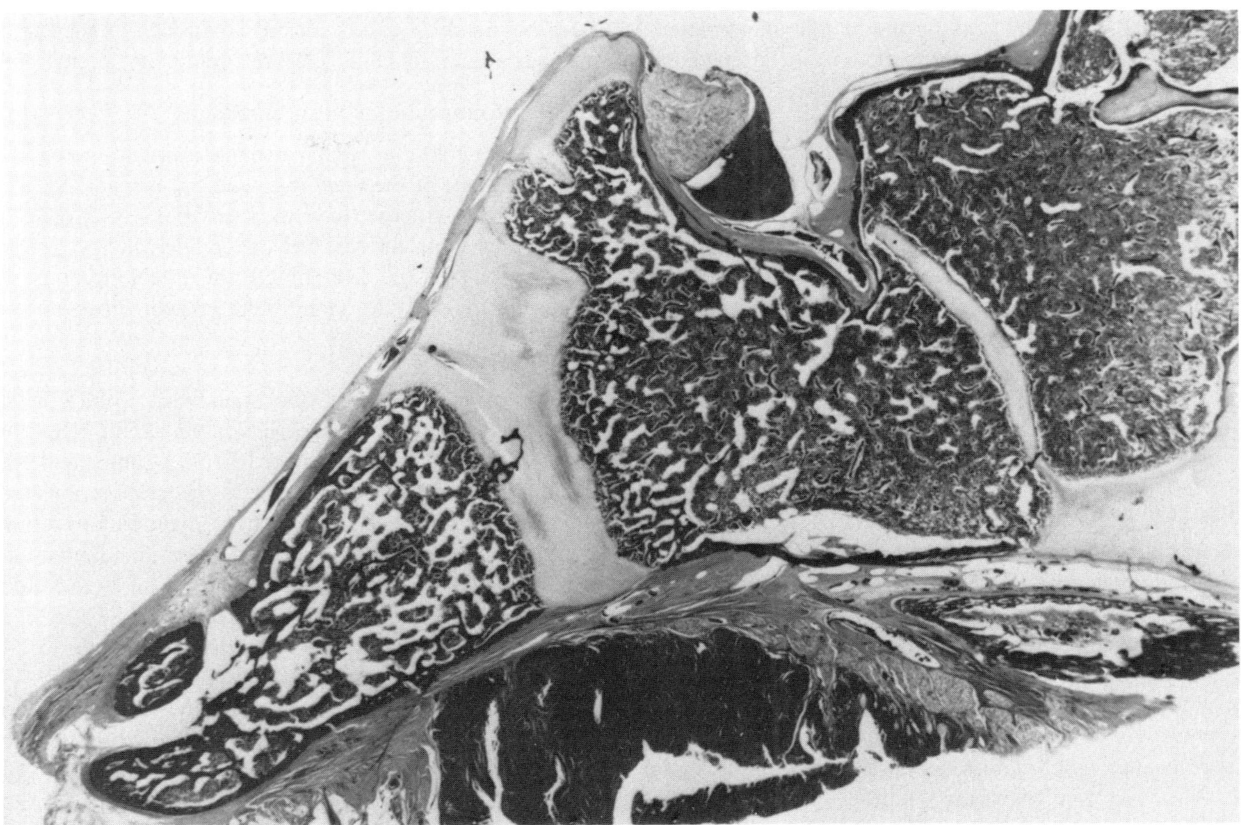

Fig. 14-3. Histologic sagittal section of a 6-month-old fetus through the cranial base to show the sellar-synchondrosal plate of cartilage between the basioccipital and basisphenoid bones.

Endochondral ossification

Vascular channels penetrate the cartilage of the chondrocranium as it is removed by chondroclasts. A framework of cartilage is left on which osteoblasts differentiate; having moved in with the blood vessels, these osteoblasts then deposit bone on the cartilaginous framework. At about 10 weeks the cranial base is still totally formed of cartilage; in a sagittal section through the midline, cartilage extends from the foramen magnum posteriorly to the nasal septum anteriorly. Ossification of the cartilage in the cranial base commences in the occipital and sphenoid regions at about 10 and 12 weeks, respectively.

In histologic sections endochondral bone is formed of a network of trabeculae that have areas of calcified cartilage in their central parts—a feature that is helpful in distinguishing the endochondral pattern of ossification. Ossification proceeds until all the cartilage is replaced. In the base of the skull a plate of cartilage persists between the basioccipital and basisphenoid bones (Fig. 14-3). A histologic picture of cartilage proliferation appears along the margin of each bone, and mensural evidence indicates that it is a growth site.[9] Bones originating within the cartilage of the chondrocranium are rapidly covered on their surfaces by periosteal bone. The perichondral capsule is transformed into a periosteal capsule with the capacity for surface bone

formation. Internally endochondral ossification may continue. With histologic study it is usually quite easy to recognize bone formed by endochondral ossification and that formed at a periosteal site.

THE MANDIBLE
Early ossification

The mandible first appears as a dense band of preosteoblasts on the lateral side of the inferior dental and incisive nerves. Ossification first occurs in the angle formed by the incisive and mental nerves. It spreads backward to form a trough for the inferior dental nerve and forward to enclose the incisive nerve in the incisive canal. In this way the body of the mandible is established from the midmandibular joint at the midline to the mandibular foramen posteriorly.

The ramus

The mandibular ramus is produced by a backward extension of bone of the body. The coronoid and condylar processes are to a large extent formed by the tenth week. In the developing mandibular condyle of the ramus secondary cartilage differentiates and subsequently makes a great contribution to the growth of the mandible. At 10 weeks it forms a cone-shaped mass of cartilage that contributes both the whole of the condylar process and extends downward and forward into the ramus as far the mandibular foramen. It undergoes endochondral ossification from before backward, so that at birth it is reduced to a layer of cartilage covering the condylar head.

Temporomandibular joint

As the mandibular condyle develops in close relation to the temporal bone an intervening strip of dense tissue to which the lateral pterygoid muscle is attached becomes the interarticular disc. Joint cavities develop above and below this strip to establish the articulating surfaces of the temporomandibular joint. The mandibular condyle is functional from the twelfth week in prenatal life. The articular eminence of the temporal bone develops after birth and attains its typical form after eruption of the primary teeth.

Midmandibular joint

The fibrous joint between the two parts of the mandibular arch cartilage becomes extensively enlarged by the growth of bone of the mandibular bodies. By 14 weeks the arch cartilage is embedded in bone in the upper third of the joint between the halves of the bony mandible. These medial ends of the cartilages at the joint persist until birth, continuing to grow with the rest of the bony joint surfaces. The entire joint undergoes synostosis during the 6 months after birth. After this time growth in width of the anterior region

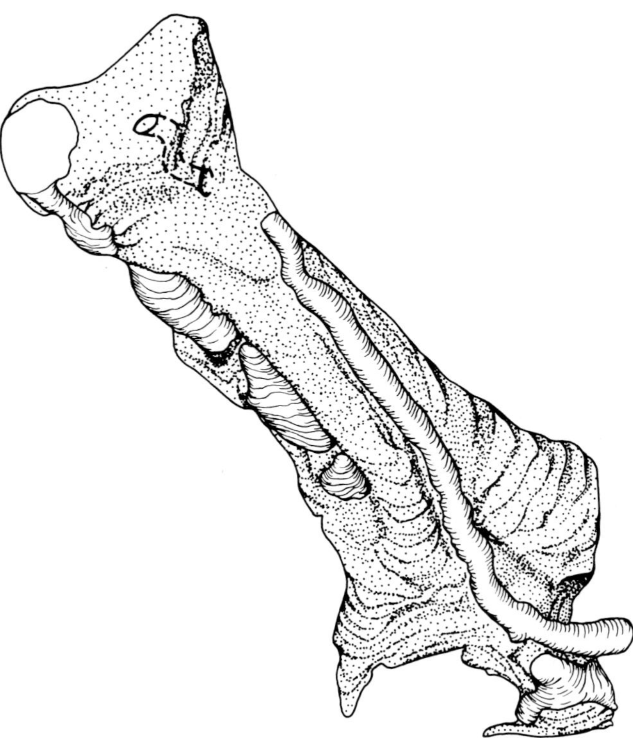

Fig. 14-4. Medial view of the mandible in a reconstruction of the skull of an 18-week human fetus. Note mandibular arch cartilage lying on the medial aspect and entering the mandible at about the level of the canine tooth.

of the mandible can occur only by bone remodeling, osteogenesis laterally, and bone resorption on lingual surfaces.

Fate of mandibular arch cartilage

The mandibular arch cartilage is incorporated into the anterior part of the mandible where it is resorbed (Fig. 14-4). Where it emerges from the mandibular body on its medial aspect at about the level of the canine tooth, it breaks free at the end of the fifth month. It is not involved in any significant way with mandibular growth subsequently.

Mandibular growth

Increased length of the mandibular body is mainly achieved by backward growth of the ramus. New bone is added along the posterior border of the ramus and compensatory resorption of bone occurs on the anterior border of the ramus. Vertical growth of the mandibular body occurs mainly on the alveolar process. The mandibular alveolar process continues to extend posteriorly on the medial aspect of the ramus. Developing molar teeth may lie buried in bone medial to the ramus, but will come to lie anterior to it by the time their eruption into the mouth commences.

Vertical growth of the mandibular ramus occurs mainly along its superior border by upward growth of the coronoid process and mandibular condyle. There may be compensatory bone resorption at the inferior border of the ramus, particularly in brachyfacial (short-faced) individuals.

Mandibular condylar cartilage

The mandibular condylar cartilage grows throughout the growing period. After birth it is reduced to a thin layer of cartilage that has a number of distinct structural layers. A knowledge of this structure is necessary for an understanding of the unique character of the condyle with regard to mechanisms controlling its growth activity (Fig. 14-5). The articular surface of the mandibular condyle is composed of a layer of fibrous tissue. Beneath this is a more cellular layer in which cell mitosis is active with the production of prechondroblasts. This important germinative layer is sensitive to stimuli that influence mandibular growth and is called the *prechondroblast proliferation zone*. Next a layer of cells with cartilage characteristics represents the transition from prechondroblast to chondroblast cells. The latter produce the cartilage matrix and become enlarged. A layer of mature chondrocytes is then seen. These have no particular arrangement and are not in columns. A major part of the growth effect is achieved in this zone by cell swelling or hypertrophy and further maturation of the chondrocytes. At a deeper level a zone of endochondral ossification forms an interface between the hypertrophic cartilage layer and bone. This zone is characterized by calcification of remaining cartilage, chondrocyte death, partial resorption of cartilage, and a progressive front of osteogenesis that results in bone deposition on the remaining cartilage. The spaces left by chondrocytes are penetrated by connective tissue and blood capillaries.

Recent research indicates that the mandibular condylar cartilage is not of the same type as that at the epiphyseal plate of long bones. As well as having developmental differences, the condylar cartilage originates from membranous connective tissues (periosteum) of the mandibular bone territory and the epiphyseal plate originates from the primary cartilage of the long bone, there are differences in histologic structure and growth control mechanisms.

Two views of condylar growth

The mandibular condyle is an important growth site and has held a traditional place of importance as a growth center. Accordingly condylar growth has been regarded as the primary event causing the entire mandible to be projected downward and forward. Bone formation occurring at the posterior and upper borders of the ramus was then seen as compensatory and secondary to stimulus from the condyle.

Evidence obtained from experimental studies indicates that condylar cartilage growth is probably secondary to tractional effects of soft tissues within and attached to the mandible, such as the tongue, muscles of mastication (particularly the lateral pterygoid muscle), and salivary glands. According to this view the condylar cartilage only grows to maintain contact with the glenoid fossa of the temporal bone. This concept was advocated by Moss,[12] Koski,[3] and Petrovic[14] and is based on research of the past 15 years.

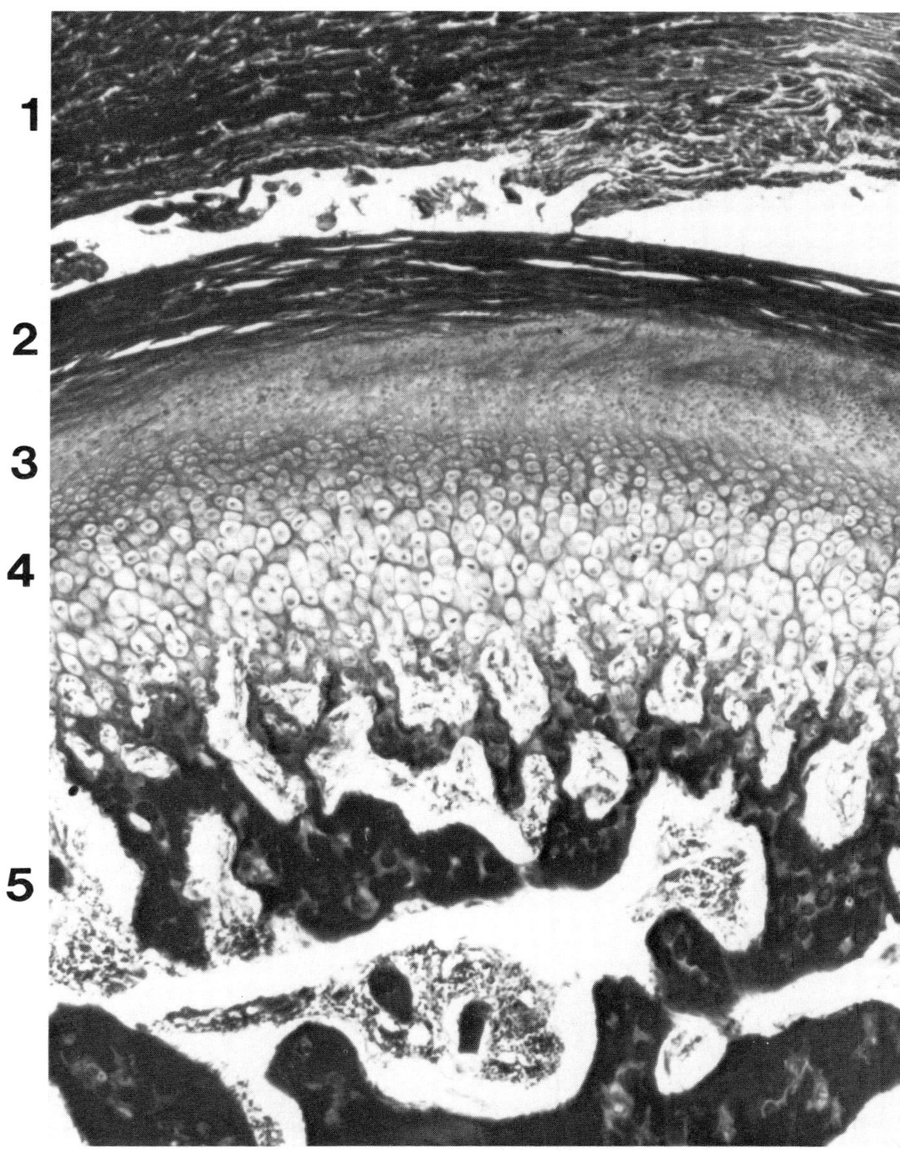

Fig. 14-5. Histologic sagittal section of the mandibular condyle from a young rhesus monkey. From top to bottom the following zones can be seen: *1*, fibrous articular surface; *2*, prechondroblast; *3*, chondroblast; *4*, chondrocyte maturation; *5*, endochondral ossification. ($\times 60$.)

The mandible appears to continue growing after growth of other skull bones is completed. Its growth period is believed to extend to near the end of the second decade of life. Both boys and girls show a slowdown of growth just before puberty, which is then followed by a pubertal growth spurt. There is a sex difference in the general time at which the growth spurt occurs; it is usually in the range of 11 to 13 years for girls and 13 to 15 years for boys.

THE MAXILLA
Establishing form

The maxillary ossification center appears at 40 days and lies lateral to the cartilage of the nasal capsule; it is located over the developing canine tooth and close to the infraorbital nerve. The next 2 weeks is a period of developing skeletal connections when slender bony processes extend toward other facial bone areas. The maxillary ossification center spreads anteriorly to fuse with the premaxillary center and overgrows it on the facial aspect. From both the maxillary and premaxillary centers a frontonasal process extends superiorly between the eye and the nose. These individual processes of the maxillae and premaxilla rapidly unite so that from this time no maxillopremaxillary suture appears between them on the facial aspect.

The interpremaxillary suture is the first sutural joint to form as a result of extension of the palatal processes of the maxillae toward the midline. It is present at about 45 days and long before any other facial sutures because of the later development of adjacent bones of the midface. The timing of the development of the interpremaxillary suture is of interest for two reasons. First, it establishes a skeletal bridge across the embryonic primary palate from the earliest possible time. Developing into this bridge at the same time is the septopremaxillary ligament from the anterior border of the cartilaginous nasal septum (Fig. 14-6). Growth tensions appear to be present in the face as it rapidly develops between the fifth and seventh weeks. The forward-growing nasal septum is believed to act as a primary force not only in the formation of the early facial profile, but also in the development of midfacial bones. Early development of the interpremaxillary suture supports the primary palatal region and ensures equal loading of each side of the face to the growing septum. Disruption of the primary palate, as when a developmental cleft occurs, is quickly followed by a widening of the cleft and facial asymmetry. Second, having noted that a midline suture is in place in the primary palate toward the end of the seventh week (45 days), it may be observed that the palatal shelves of the secondary palate still have to fuse in the eighth week and will not be fully supported by bone of the hard palate until about 12 weeks.[8] At 12 weeks the remainder of the midpalatal suture is established—the intermaxillary and interpalatine parts. Hence for a period of 5 weeks a midline union of the maxillary bones is present only in the premaxillary region. There is a considerable developmental time lag between the premaxillary and maxillary parts of the midpalatal suture. In the event of primary palatal clefting, the possibility of malformation is increased. This explains why facial deformity accompanying a unilateral cleft of the primary palate only is frequently as severe in appearance as when the cleft is

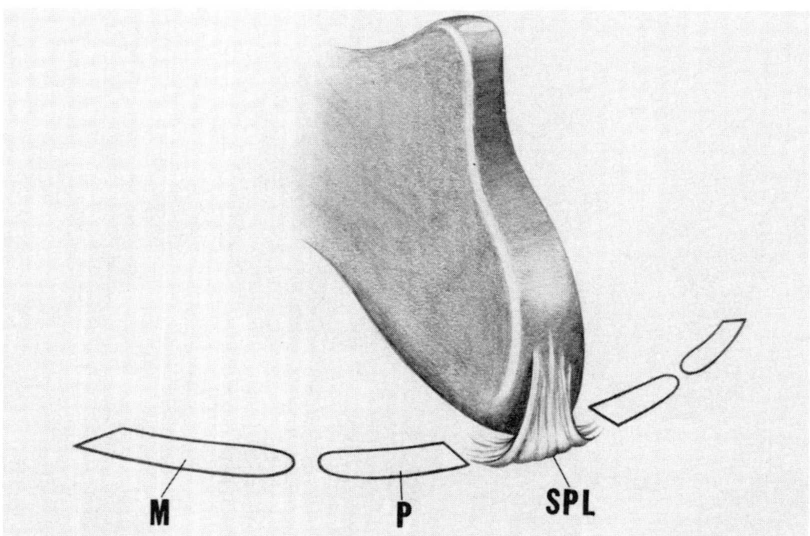

Fig. 14-6. Septopremaxillary structures seen in a 41-day human embryo. Maxillary *(M)* and premaxillary *(P)* ossification centers, very soon after their first appearance, are connected to the nasal septum by a septopremaxillary ligament *(SPL)*. (From Latham, R.A.: Maxillary development and growth: the septopremaxillary ligament, J. Anat. **107:**471, 1970.)

completely through both the primary and secondary palatal regions.

Ossification spreads posterolaterally below the orbit toward the zygomatic bone and posteromedially in relation to the palatine bone and pterygoid plates. A wide posterior surface thus develops between the palatine and zygomatic bones and becomes an important site of maxillary growth (Fig. 14-9).

The septopremaxillary growth mechanism

When the maxilla has established basic form, growth occurs mainly in a backward direction by osteogenesis on the retromaxillary surface. This surface forms a boundary for the pterygopalatine fossa and faces the infratemporal region. In initiating the pattern of osteogenesis on the posterior maxillary surface, it appears that the maxillary attachment to the nasal septum anteriorly by the septopremaxillary ligament is a factor. As the nasal septum grows forward it applies a pull on the maxillae at the insertion of the ligament on the anterior nasal spine. The maxillae then move forward, sliding between the zygomatic and palatine

bones (Fig. 14-7). Thus the early facial sutures perform a function of constant adjustment in the sutural collagen fibers to allow the bones to slide parallel to the sutures.

Cranial sutures: structure and function

The cranial sutures are primarily skeletal joints of the syndesmosis type. They are also sites of osteogenesis and skeletal adjustment. The latter is a function of collagen adjustment in fiber bundles of the connecting system. Structurally, the facial suture is composed of two periostea, one from each adjoining bone. Each periosteum is composed of an outer fibrous layer and an inner cambial layer; up until the neonatal stage a middle zone composed of loose connective tissue and blood vessels usually can be seen between the two fibrous layers (Fig. 14-8). This five-layer structure was originally described by Pritchard, Scott, and Girgis.[15] The sutures of the cranial vault may not show all five layers distinctly. As all sutures mature with age, the middle zone disappears; after growth has ceased, bundles of fibers may be traced directly from one bone to the other.

Maxillary sutures with the zygomatic and palatine bones

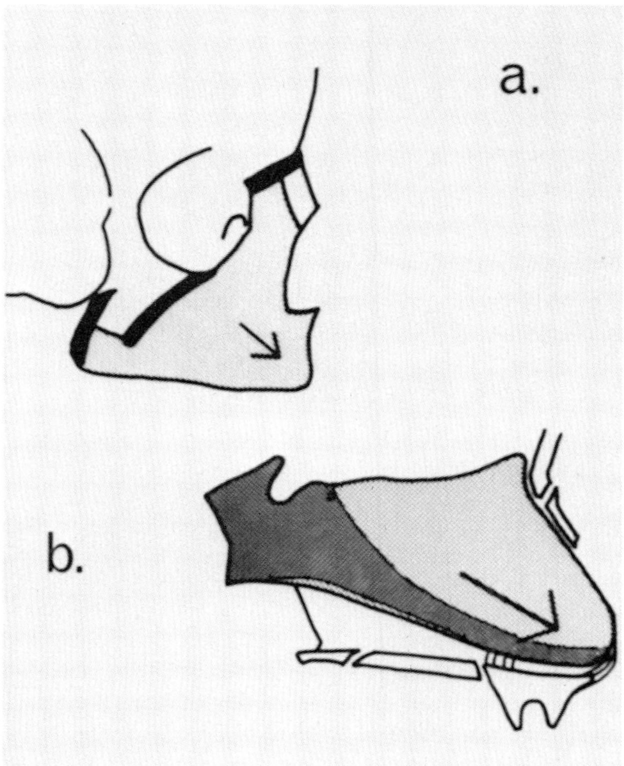

Fig. 14-7. Prenatal septal mechanisms for maxillary growth. **a,** Displacement downward and forward from adjoining skull bones. **b,** Sutural adjustment and maxillary growth are indicated by black lines. The nasal septum thickened along its inferior border applies traction in the region of the anterior nasal spine of maxillae with the septopremaxillary ligament.

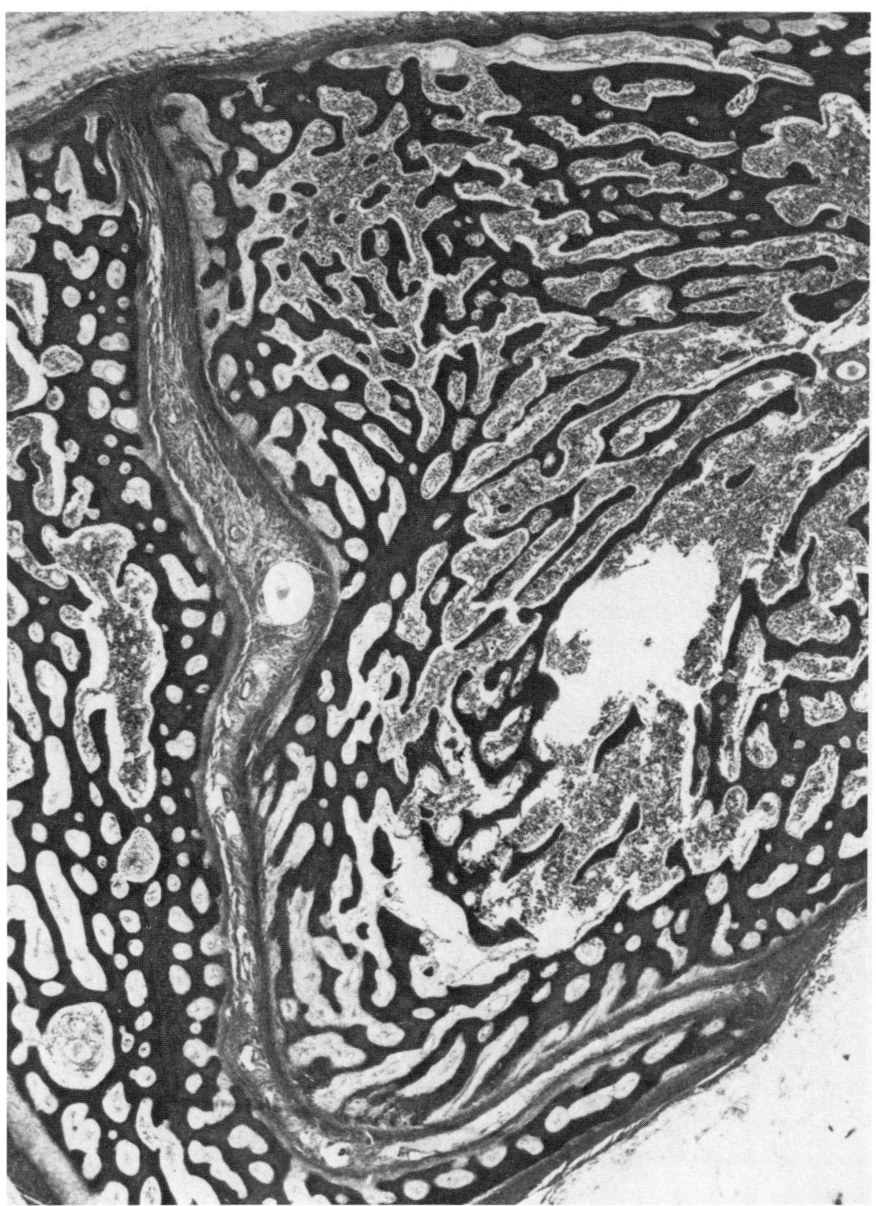

Fig. 14-8. Coronal section of the zygomaticomaxillary suture at birth. The suture shows five structural layers; it courses mainly in a vertical direction and inferiorly turns out around the zygomatic bone. (×9.5.)

consist at first of a simple overlapping of one bone on the other (Fig. 14-9). During prenatal life the overlap relationship provides a capacity for rapid movement of the bones in response to growth forces. Observations have shown that growth of the fetal and infant skull was characterized by a simple sliding of one bone in relation to its sutural fellow along the sutural plane. Furthermore, the sutural planes tended to be similar to the direction of growth. This sutural sliding is a function of the adjustment mechanism in the sutural soft tissues, particularly the collagen fiber bundles that perform the jointing role. The five-layered structure of the early sutures, in which the sutural fiber bundles are mainly parallel to the bone margins, appears to facilitate sutural sliding. This mechanism provides for rapid adaptive adjustment in intrauterine life and infancy and has generated interest and the clinically exciting possibility that rapid correction of facial bone positions may be possible in response to orthopedic forces in facially deformed infants.

Interlocking sutures

The interlocking, or serration, of skull sutures appears to develop where sutures are under some tension during growth of the bone edges (Fig. 14-10). The interlock structure can be analyzed as a response to the two main functions of the

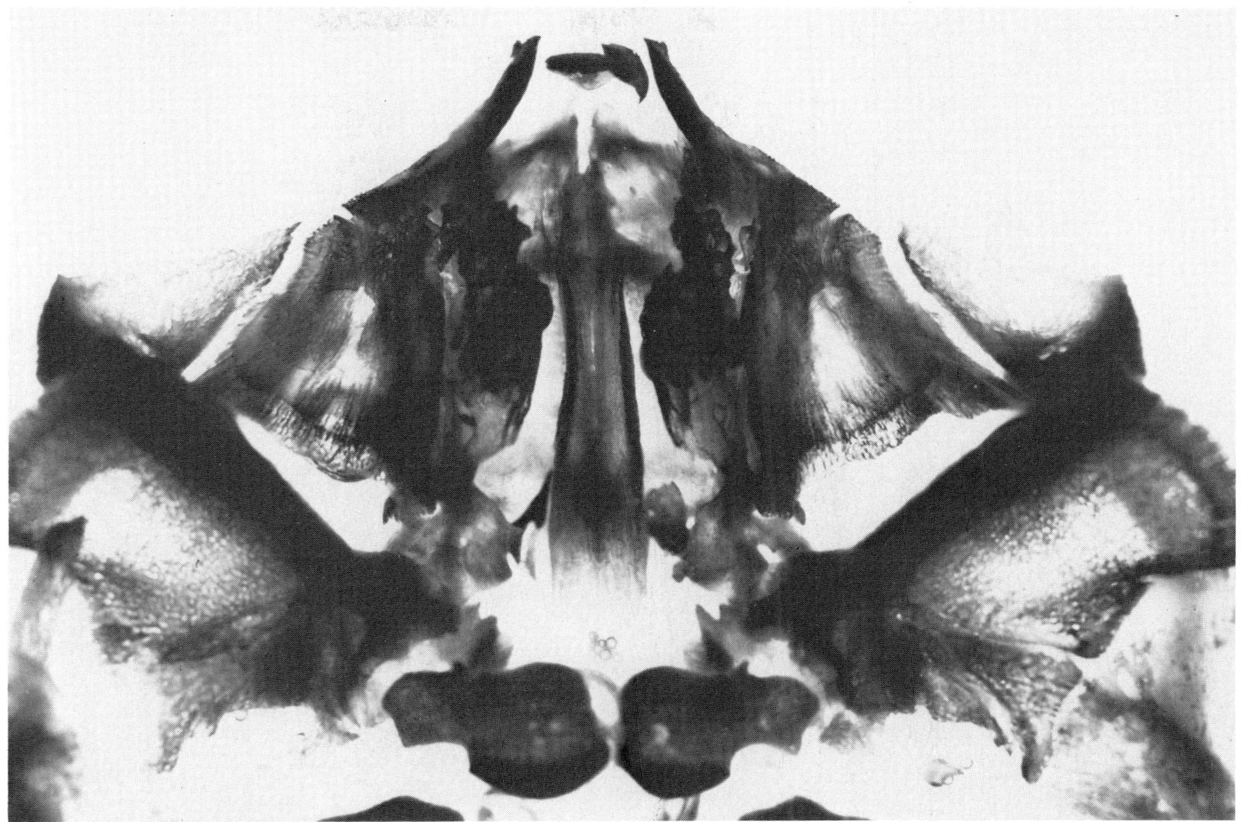

Fig. 14-9. Maxillae and adjacent bones of a 20-week fetus viewed from above. The orientation of zygomaticomaxillary sutures allows maxillae to slide forward as new bone is added mainly at the broad retromaxillary surface. Specimen cleared, and stained with alizarin and the frontal bones removed. (From Latham, R.A.: Trans. Eur. Orthod. Soc., 1968, p. 53.)

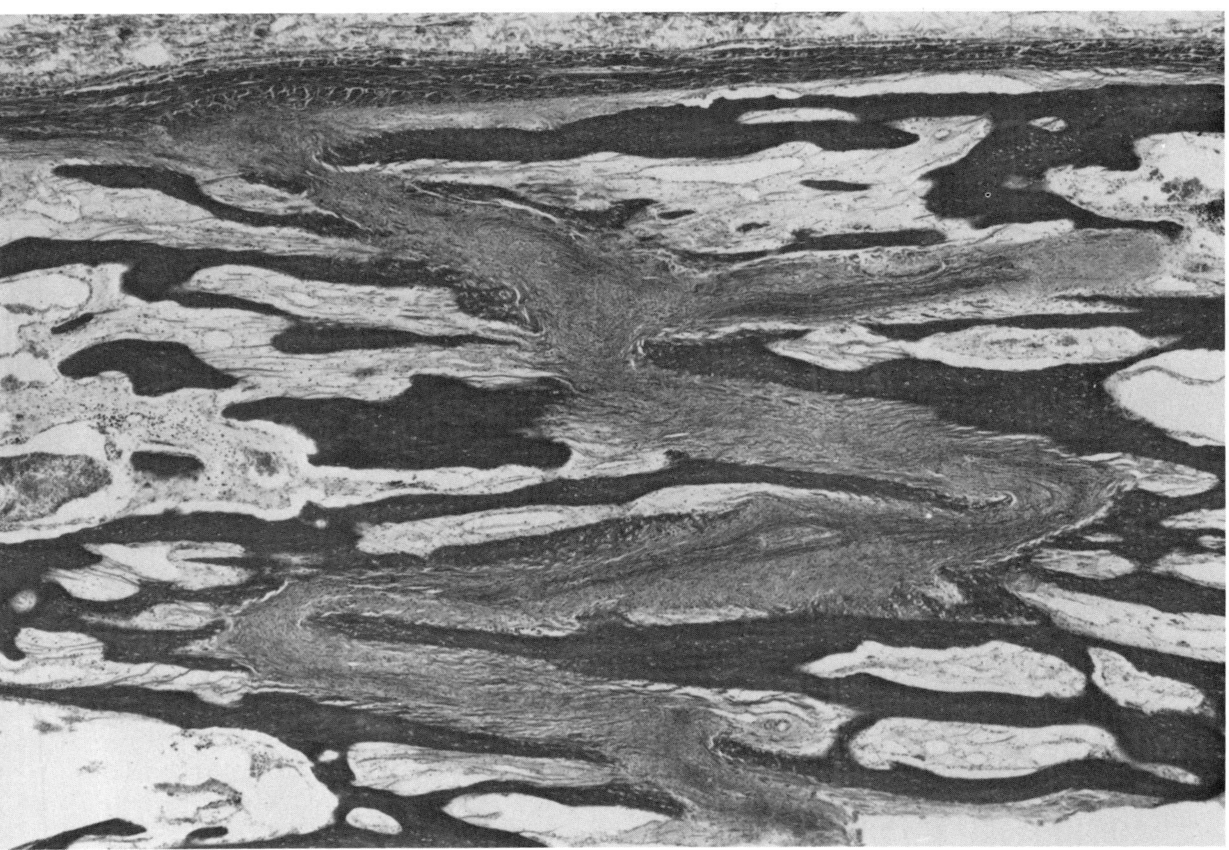

Fig. 14-10. Transverse section of a human coronal suture from a 6-month-old infant. Note the interlocking course of the suture and coarse jointing bundles of fibers in relation to the sides of the socket formations. Two peg-and-socket units are shown. ($\times 21$.)

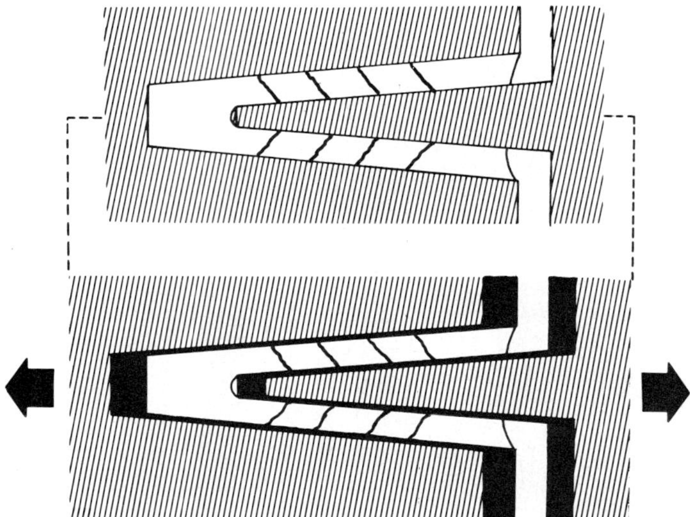

Fig. 14-11. Main sites of bone formation in a suture consisting of peg-and-socket units. As bones separate, new bone is formed at the bottom of the socket and point of the opposite peglike structure. The least amount of bone forms on the sides of the socket and peg where the jointing mechanism operates to advantage. Note that the sides of the sockets and pegs form a sliding growth mechanism.

suture: joint function and growth. By developing a peg-and-socket arrangement, the jointing mechanism operates mainly between the sides of the peg and the socket. The osteogenesis required as the bones separate occurs mainly at the bottom of the socket and at the point of the peg (Fig. 14-11). A localization of the functions of jointing and osteogenesis may be seen that provides each with a favorable environment. Again the principle of sutural sliding operates at the sides of the socket and peg where bone surfaces are aligned in the direction of growth, and movement parallel to the bone margins requires collagen bundle adjustments. The formation of interlocking in a suture may be seen as an adaptation that permits jointing and growth to occur simultaneously.

Maxillary growth

The maxilla establishes definitive form while under the influence of the nasal capsule of the chondroncranium. Growth of the nasal capsule provides the space and stimulus for maxillary growth. After about the third month in fetal life, the only important interaction is between the nasal septum and the maxillae by means of the septopremaxillary ligament. The nasal septum, in growing downward and forward, tends to exert a "pull" on the premaxillary bone. The septal cartilage has a firm base in the basisphenoid region of the cranial base and is reinforced along its inferior border to the site of the septopremaxillary ligament (Fig. 14-7, *B*). At this time in fetal life the maxillary sutures act primarily as sliding planes, not as sites of bone growth. The main sites of maxillary growth are the posterior and superior free surfaces, namely, the pterygopalatine and orbital surfaces (Fig. 14-9).

During the 1960s it became apparent that after birth the nasal septum was no longer a pacemaker for maxillary growth. It continued to have an important role in skeletal support of the nose and nasal bones. Reports concerning growth of the face in conditions of facial deformity, such as cyclopia, arrhinencephaly, and cleft lip and palate showed that the maxillae could continue to grow throughout infancy and childhood unaided by the nasal septum or even nasal cavities.[5,10,13] There are two hypotheses available to help the clinician understand maxillary growth in the child: the functional matrix concept[12] and the intrinsic maxillary growth concept.[5,10] The functional matrix concept ranks the growth of bone as secondary to a stimulus from soft tissue organs and capsules. Two examples will illustrate the relationship. The mandible encloses the muscular organ—the tongue—and various other muscles and glands. Systemic function and growth of these organs tends to reposition the mandible downward and forward; then growth of the mandibular ramus upward and backward takes place secondarily to maintain normal relationships with the base of the skull. Another example would be the orbital cavity that enlarges by growth in response to a prior increase in size of the eyeball and orbital contents. The useful aspect of the functional matrix concept is that surgical alteration of the soft tissues of the face may be expected to have an influence on growth and development of adjacent facial bones.

The intrinsic maxillary growth concept places bone at a higher level in the control of its growth behavior. It recognizes that the growth sites are specially adapted to increase the size of the bone and that plasma-borne stimuli may be primary factors stimulating bone cell mitosis and osteogenesis. In the case of the maxilla, which has been shown to

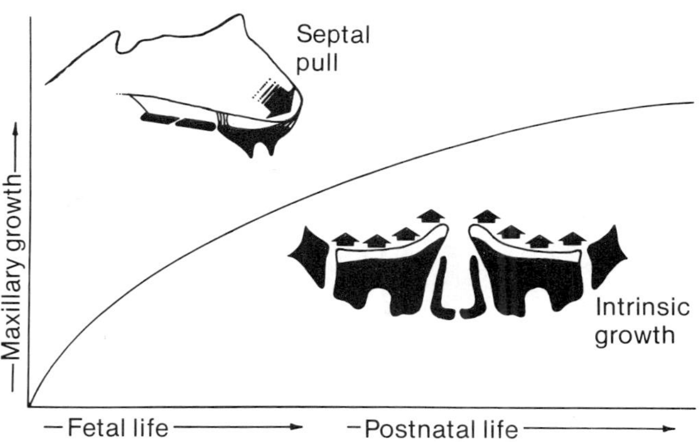

Fig. 14-12. Two different mechanisms postulated to influence maxillary growth at different times in development. First, the embryonic mechanism of septal pull occurs. Then in later fetal life and thereafter the intrinsic maxillary growth mechanism is in effect. Both contribute to normal maxillary growth and displacement downward and forward. (From Latham, R.A.: Cleft Palate J. **6**:404, 1969.)

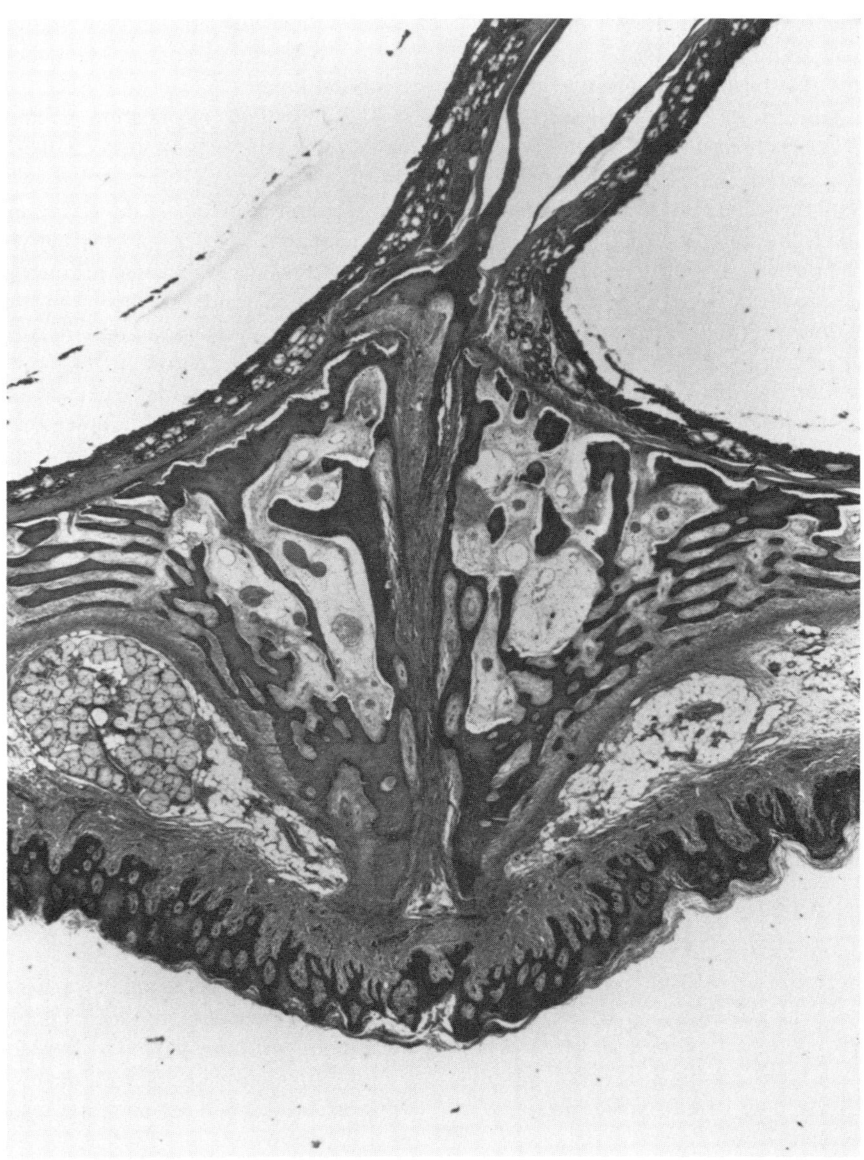

Fig. 14-13. Transverse section of the palate at the midpalatal suture to show the pattern of bone formation on the oral aspect (inferiorly) and resportion at the floors of the nasal cavities. This patient was 2 years and 2 months old, when sutural activity is much reduced. (× 16.)

grow in the absence of the nasal septum and nasal cavities, the posterosuperiorly oriented growth sites are postulated to have potential for intrinsic maxillary growth. In terms of developmental osteology it is proposed that once the maxillary growth sites are activated, then the cellular proliferation within the periosteum develops enough pressure against adjacent orbital and retromaxillary fat pads to displace the maxillae downward and forward. The effective periosteum has a large surface area whose cumulative growth pressure becomes a force that acts on the maxillary sutures. This force initiates displacement of the entire maxillae, and adjustment occurs in the sutures (Fig. 14-12). The advantage of this hypothesis is that it permits the surgeon to identify the maxillary growth sites and to preserve freedom for the maxilla to displace in the process of normal growth.

The anterior surfaces of the maxilla are not involved in new bone formation and, indeed, have been found to be sites of bone resorption[2] in association with growth posterosuperiorly. The midpalatal suture contributes to growth in width until about 6 months after birth. After this time growth may continue at a much slower rate.[1,8] The oral surface of the palate generally is a site of bone formation throughout the growing period in association with bone resorption on the floors of the nasal cavities (Fig. 14-13). The crest of the alveolar process in both the maxilla and mandible is a growth site throughout the growing period. With it the teeth are moved in an occlusal direction. Maxillary teeth have a pattern of forward drift during growth. This provides additional room at the back of the maxilla for newly erupting molar teeth, especially after the displacement method of maxillary growth has ceased between 5 and 7 years of age. The pattern of drift of the mandibular teeth is more variable and is affected by facial muscle tone, malocclusion, and facial growth (i.e., horizontal, normal, or vertical). Typically the mandibular teeth are carried in an occlusal direction by alveolar bone growth. Room for developing mandibular molar teeth is provided by the backward extension of the alveolar process medial to the mandibular ramus. The erupted teeth tend to stay in contact at interproximal surfaces because of the transeptal fibers that course from the neck of each tooth directly across the septum of alveolar bone to an insertion at the neck of the adjacent tooth. Spaces in the dental arch caused by extraction or developmental absence tend to close by drift of adjacent teeth, particularly of the later developing molar teeth.

SUMMARY AND CONCLUSIONS

The first skeletal support for the developing embryo is provided by cartilaginous tissue. In the head region the first functional skull is formed with cartilage and is referred to as chondrocranium. The chondrocranium has four basic components: (1) mandibular arch cartilage (Meckel's cartilage), (2) the nasal capsule (supported by the nasal septum), (3) the basal plate, and (4) otic capsules.

Bones of the skull develop by intramembranous or periosteal ossification or by replacing a cartilaginous structure that undergoes endochondral ossification. The mandibular center of ossification appears at about 39 or 40 days, whereas the maxillary center of ossification appears about 40 days. The premaxillary centers appear at about 41 days. Ossification progresses in an anteroposterior sequence. At about 10 weeks of gestation the cranial base is still totally formed of cartilage. Ossification occurs in the occipital region at approximately 10 weeks of gestation and in the sphenoid, at approximately 12 weeks.

Increased length of the mandibular body is mainly achieved by backward growth of the ramus. Vertical growth of the mandibular body occurs mainly on the alveolar processes. Evidence obtained from experimental studies indicates that the condylar cartilage growth is probably secondary to tractional effects of soft tissues within and attached to the mandible such as the tongue and muscles of mastication. According to this view the condylar cartilage only grows to maintain contact with the glenoid fossa of the temporal bone.

The maxillary ossification center appears at approximately 40 days of gestation. It then spreads anteriorly to fuse with the premaxillary center, which makes its appearance at approximately 41 days. The interpremaxillary suture is of interest for two reasons: (1) it establishes a skeletal bridge across the embryonic primary palate from the earliest possible time, and (2) developing into this bridge at the same time is the septopremaxillary ligament from the anterior border of the cartilaginous nasal septum. The forward-growing nasal septum is believed to act as a primary force on the septopremaxillary ligament in formation of the early facial profile and development of the midfacial bones.

After the maxilla has established basic form, growth occurs mainly in a backward direction by osteogenesis on the retromaxillary surface. As the nasal septum grows forward it applies a pull on the maxilla at the insertion of the septopremaxillary ligament.

Cranial sutures function as sites of osteogenesis and skeletal adjustment. The interlocking, or serration, of skull sutures appears to develop where sutures are under some tension. This structure may be seen as an adaptation that permits jointing and growth to occur simultaneously.

After birth the nasal septum no longer functions as a pacemaker for continued maxillary growth. Two hypotheses are available to help the clinician understand maxillary growth in the child: (1) the functional matrix concept ranks the growth of bone as secondary to a stimulus from soft tissue organs and capsules, and (2) the intrinsic maxillary growth concept places bone at a higher level in the control of its growth behavior. Once maxillary growth sites are activated, perhaps by plasma-borne stimuli, then cellular proliferation within the periosteum develops pressure against adjacent orbital and retromaxillary fat pads to displace the maxilla downward and forward.

REFERENCES

1. Bjork, A., and Skieller, V.: Growth in width of the maxilla studied by the implant method, Scand. J. Plast. Reconstr. Surg. **8:**26, 1974.
2. Enlow, D.H.: Handbook of facial growth, Philadelphia, 1975, W.B. Saunders Co.
3. Koski, K.: The mandibular complex, Trans. Eur. Orthod. Soc., 1974, p. 53.
4. Kraus, B.S., Kitamura, H., and Latham, R.A.: Atlas of developmental anatomy of the face, New York, 1966, Harper & Row, Publishers, Inc.
5. Latham, R.A.: A new concept of the early maxillary growth mechanism, Trans. Eur. Orthod. Soc., 1968, p. 53.
6. Latham, R.A.: The pathogenesis of the skeletal deformity associated with unilateral cleft lip and palate, Cleft Palate J. **6:**404, 1969.
7. Latham, R.A.: Maxillary development and growth: the septopremaxillary ligament, J. Anat. **107:**471, 1970.
8. Latham, R.A.: The development, structure and growth pattern of the human mid-palatal suture, J. Anat. **108:**31, 1971.
9. Latham, R.A.: The sella point and postnatal growth of the human cranial base, Am. J. Orthod. **61:**156, 1972.
10. Latham, R.A.: An appraisal of the early maxillary growth mechanism. In McNamara, J.A., Jr., editor: Factors affecting the growth of the midface, Ann Arbor, Mich., 1976, The University of Michigan Press.
11. Mall, F.P.: On ossification centers in human embryos less than one hundred days old, Am. J. Anat. **5:**433, 1906.
12. Moss, M.L.: The functional matrix. In Kraus, B.S., and Reidel, R.A., editors: Vistas in orthodontics, Philadelphia, 1962, Lea & Febiger.
13. Moss, M.S., Bromberg, B.E., Song, I.C., and Eisenman, G.: The passive role of nasal septal cartilage in mid-facial growth, Plast. Reconstr. Surg. **41:**536, 1968.
14. Petrovic, A.G., Stutzmann, J.J., and Oudet, C.L.: Control processes in the postnatal growth of the condylar cartilage of the mandible. In McNamara, J.A., Jr., editor: Determinants of mandibular form and growth, Ann Arbor, Mich., 1975, The University of Michigan Press.
15. Pritchard, J.J., Scott, J.H., and Girgis, F.G.: The structure and development of cranial and facial sutures, J. Anat. **90:**73, 1956.
16. Wynne, T.M.H.: Observations on the development of the human chondrocranium, doctoral thesis, Liverpool, England, 1966, University of Liverpool.

CHAPTER 15

Pediatric cephalometrics

PETER J. COCCARO

DEVELOPMENT OF CEPHALOMETRICS

The development of accurate techniques for cephalometric radiology of infants and children has made possible longitudinal studies of the growth and development of craniofacial structures.* Interest in the early detection, interception, and correction of craniofacial disorders in children creates the need for a radiographic technique that will effectively and satisfactorily document the character of the abnormalities over a period of time. Knowledge of normal growth standards permits the clinician to better understand deviant patterns of skeletal and soft tissue growth and development at various age levels.†

Important information can be obtained from analyzing cephalometric films of a variety of anatomic regions of the head and neck. In addition to the developing dentition, skeletal components making up the face, cranium, and cervical vertebrae can be studied along with the contiguous soft tissue structures.[3,9,16,27] Areas of investigation vital to diagnosis and treatment planning include the integumental profile, tongue, soft palate, epiglottis, tonsils, and adenoids. Dimensional changes vertically and horizontally of the nasopharynx intimately associated with the increased respiratory needs of the growing child can be assessed from longitudinal cephalometric radiographs.[10,16,23,27]

Since Broadbent[4] introduced and developed the method of radiographic cephalometry, much important work has been carried out in the investigative areas of craniofacial growth.[5-7,19] An advantage of cephalometry is that the same child can be studied at chosen intervals over a long period of time. The contribution of cephalometric radiology as a research tool for studying craniofacial growth is well established.‡ It has been widely used in the treatment of clinical problems by the orthodontist, speech pathologist, plastic surgeon, and prosthodontist, as well as many other specialties. Thus the advent of the Broadbent-Bolton radiographic cephalometer heralded the beginnings of clinical and research orthodontics.[4]

CLINICAL APPLICATIONS OF CEPHALOMETRICS

Cephalometrics has been adapted for routine use in clinical practice as an aid to diagnosis and treatment planning. Through it the description and identification of craniofacial abnormalities becomes more apparent.

The interrelationships of craniofacial skeletal and soft tissue structures may create a favorable or unfavorable facial appearance. A good example of this is found within the first and second branchial arch anomaly (hemifacial microsomia).[12,14] As a group they reflect a hypoplasia of the pterygomandibular complex. The absent or hypoplastic condyle has a negative effect on the development of the glenoid fossa. In addition, the anomaly has an adverse effect on the development of other contiguous anatomic structures, such as the zygomatic process of the temporal bone, pterygoid processes of the sphenoid bone, malar bone, and maxilla. The condylar abnormality with its affected altered muscular development and function indirectly affects other areas.

A differential diagnosis can be made through the use of cephalograms, particularly to determine the size and position of the anomalous craniofacial structures. Specific clinical entities such as ocular hypertelorism, craniofacial synostosis, hemifacial microsomia, cleft palate, and trauma can be measured with cephalometry. Within these groups growth and development and the impact of surgical or nonsurgical treatment procedures on craniofacial structures may be studied.*

---

*References 1, 2, 7, 9, 15, 17, 20, and 23.
†References 5-7, 18, 19, 24, and 25.
‡References 1, 2, 18, 20, 24, and 25.

---

*References 3, 8, 11, 13, 14, and 21.

RESEARCH

Long-term cephalometric studies have documented growth and development of the craniofacial structures in infants and children without any discernible defects.[5,7,18] Serial cephalometric studies also have been carried out on children with cleft lip and palate.[9-11] Increased interest in craniofacial synostosis has led investigators to use cephalometrics for diagnosis and treatment.[13]

Data on the unaffected population provide a basis for comparison when studying the syndrome population.[8] Cephalometrics also supplies needed information to help identify those factors responsible for anatomic structural imbalances that exist within patients with syndromes.

Furthermore, documentation of the favorable or unfavorable effect specific treatment procedures have on craniofacial structures is possible with cephalometric research. The cephalometer and x-ray source are positioned in a fixed relation to each other. The anode target of the x-ray tube is placed exactly 5 feet (1.5 m) from the center of the cephalometer with the central ray of the tube at right angles to

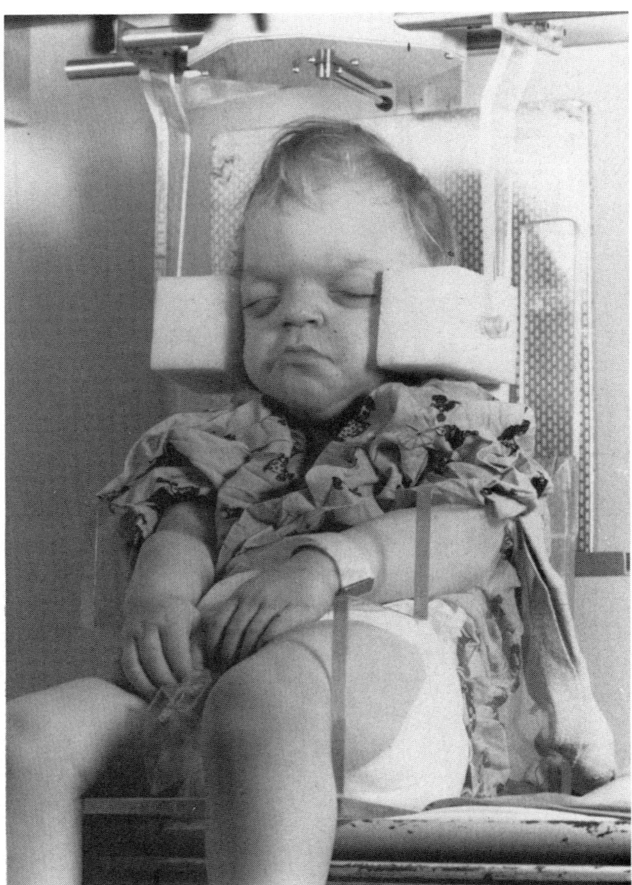

Fig. 15-1. Sedated 2-year-old patient with Crouzon's disease positioned in the cephalometer for obtaining lateral and posteroanterior cephalometric radiographs. Note "carlike" seat to assist in positioning the patient.

the film. The cephalometer and x-ray tube relationship is a critical constant, whereas the distance from the instrument center (object) to the film is a variable.

Motion is the main cause of a blurry image. Therefore suitable measures must be taken to immobilize the head. The ear rods of the cephalometer serve this purpose.

Sharpness is improved when the focus-film distance is increased, and magnification and distortion are reduced. In the final analysis the purpose of the cephalogram is to bring before the examiner the maximal amount of information about the anatomic regions under study.

A complete description of the instrument and its use is excellently reported by Broadbent, Broadbent, and Golden.[5] Since there may be problems in securing the desired cephalograms on infants and children, adequate management is an essential prerequisite. Sedation of the patient and modification in the armamentarium have been employed to obtain satisfactory radiographs in infants. Pruzansky and Lis[22] have reported on such methods. Coccaro and Curry have used a "carlike seat" (Fig. 15-1) and sedation to position the infant within the conventional headholder. A combination of drugs (meperidine, 2 mg/kg of body weight; promethazine and chlorpromazine, each 1 mg/kg of body weight) is administered by a pediatrician 1 hour before each record-taking procedure.

TRACING CEPHALOMETRIC RADIOGRAPHS

Matte acetate tracing paper (0.0003 inch) is placed over the cephalogram, and then both are placed over an illuminating view box. With a No. 2 pencil cephalometric landmarks are identified and registered on the tracing paper. Outlines of the anatomic structures as seen in the lateral and posteroanterior films are carried out so that relationships between them can be used in any analysis (Fig. 15-2). Fig. 15-3 shows cephalometric landmarks that are useful in a variety of analyses. A glossary for these landmarks is included at the end of the chapter. Once the landmarks are identified and traced, linear and angular measurements may be obtained to assist in the diagnosis and treatment plan. Areas of particular importance in the growing child are the cranial base, upper face, lower face, and nasopharyngeal region (Figs. 15-4 to 15-7).

LATERAL ANATOMIC STRUCTURES
Cranial base

The cranial base (Fig. 15-4) is a logical starting place for cephalometric analysis, since the facial skeleton receives support from and attaches onto the base of the cranium. The landmarks nasion (N) and basion (Ba) (which is the anterior projection of the foramen magnum) serve as division marks between the neurocranium and facial skeleton. A straight line drawn from Ba to N does not, however, provide much information as to this relationship. The addition of the sella turcica (S) into the cranial base landmarks provides an angular measurement of the neurocranial relationship to the

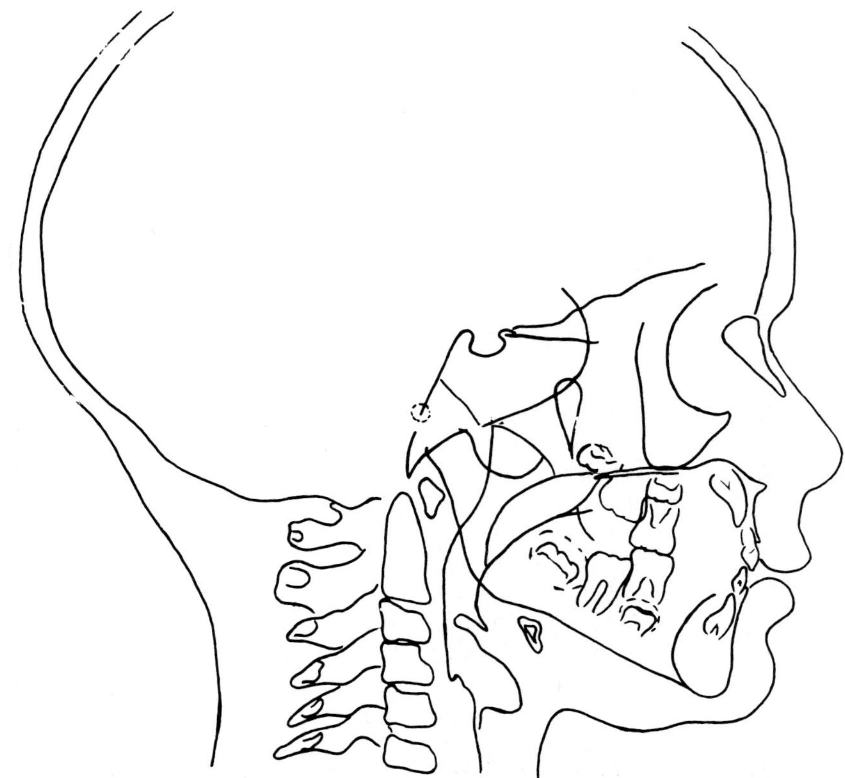

Fig. 15-2. Lateral cephalometric radiograph of a normal 5-year-old boy.

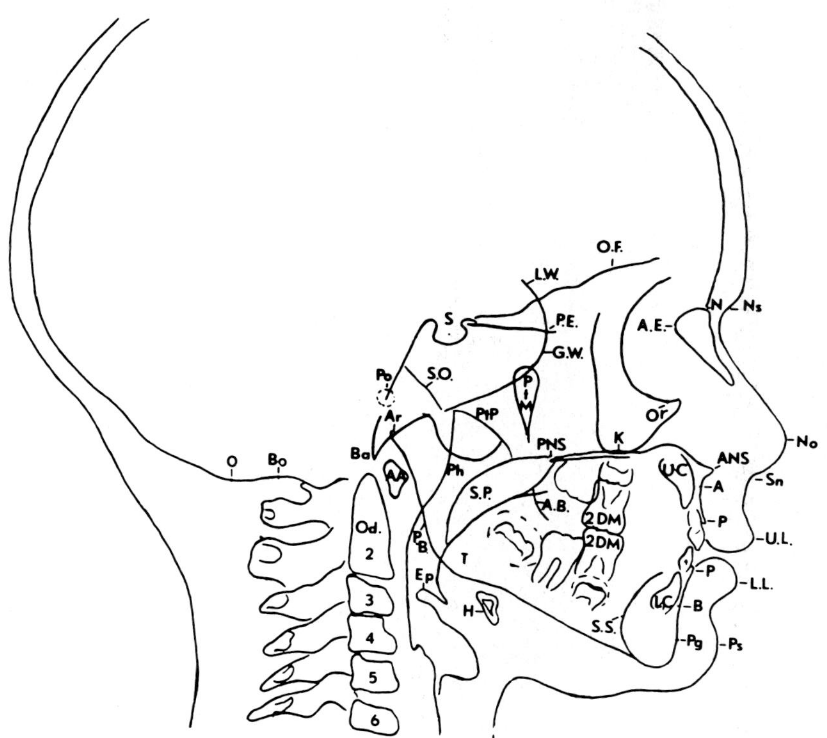

Fig. 15-3. Lateral cephalometric film tracing showing the location of many of the pediatric cephalometric landmarks. (See glossary at the end of the chapter.)

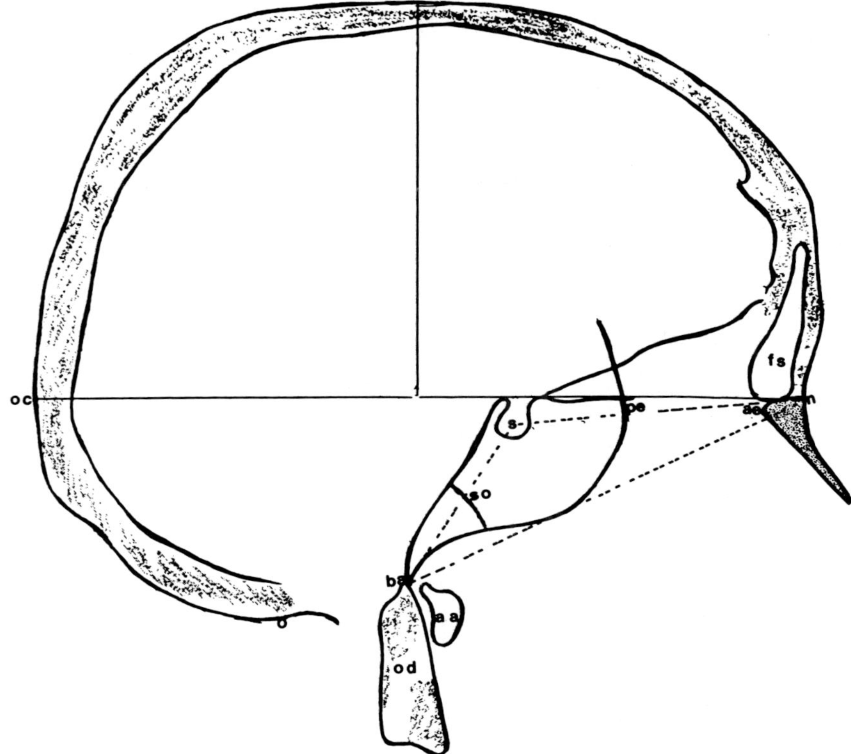

Fig. 15-4. Schematic tracing of the *cranial base* region outlining anatomic areas and the landmarks for linear and angular measurements of the cranial base. The skull height and depth in the midsagittal plane also may be measured.

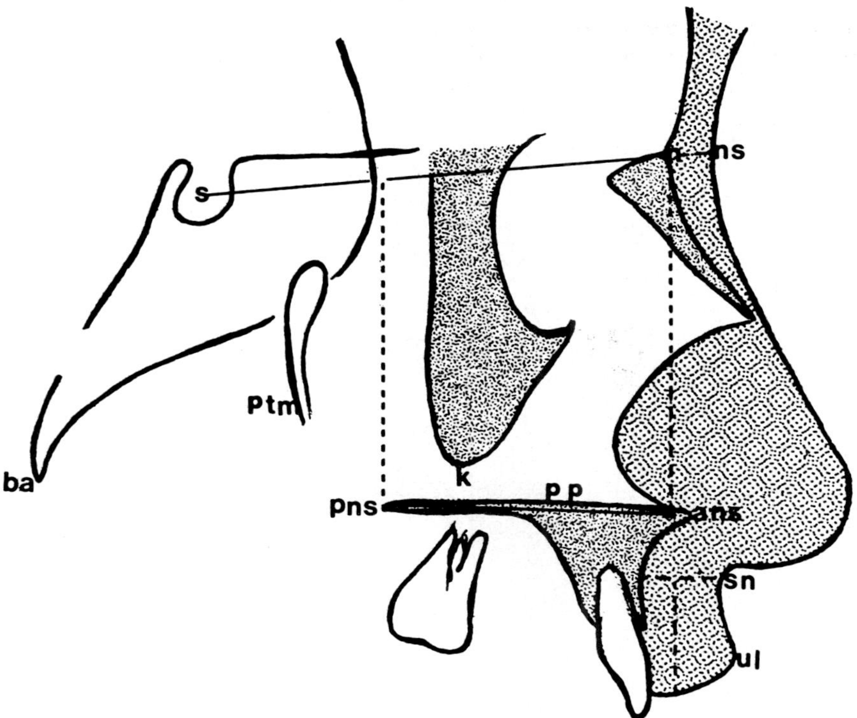

Fig. 15-5. Specific areas of importance in the analysis of nasomaxillary growth and development in an anteroposterior dimension are shown. Linear and angular measurements may be used in a variety of analyses to demonstrate changes in size and position of nasomaxillary structures in the affected and unaffected population relative to the cranial base and lower face.

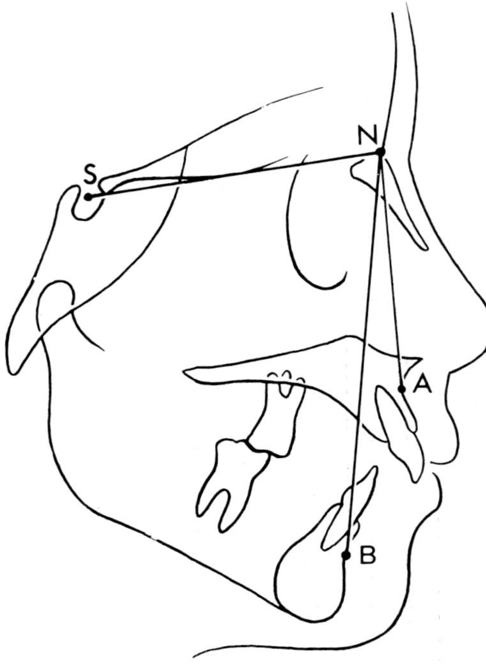

Fig. 15-6. Lateral radiograph showing the most frequently used angular measurements to express the horizontal position of the maxilla and mandible. Angle *SNA* compares the maxillary position to the base of the skull; *SNB* compares the mandibular position to the cranial base; and *ANB* compares the maxilla to the mandible. Normative data for these and other common cephalometric measures are provided in Table 15-1.

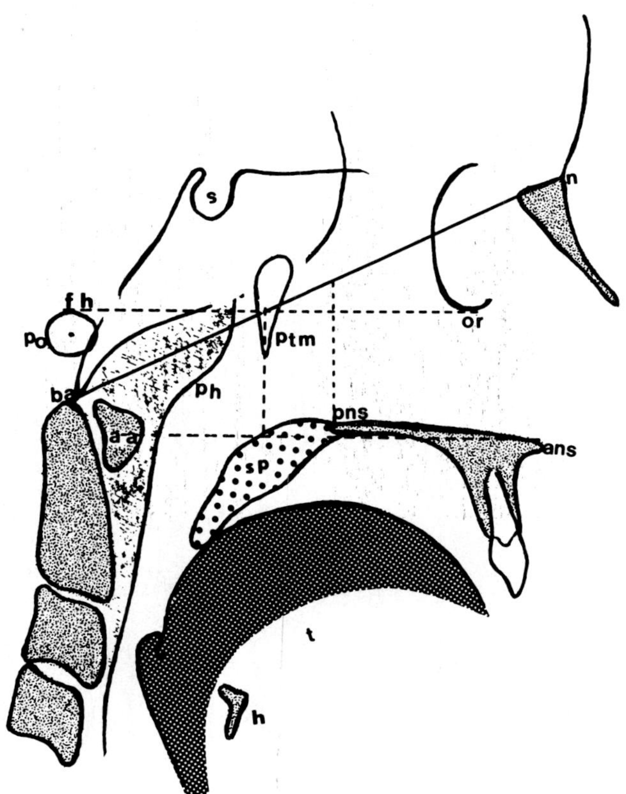

Fig. 15-7. Morphologic character of the nasopharyngeal area in the midsagittal plane is shown, as well as its relationship to the cranial base, upper face, tongue, hyoid bone, and cervical vertebrae. It permits assessment of the epipharynx, mesopharynx, and hypopharynx in normal and abnormal situations.

facial skeleton. The normal cranial base angle, as measured from N to S to Ba is 130 degrees $\pm$ 6 degrees. Consequently, a cranial base angle of 145 degrees would indicate an obtuse cranial base. In such a situation one would be expected to find the glenoid fossae positioned posteriorly along with the other cranial structures, and a downward growth pattern tendency of the face could be partially explained on this basis. An acute cranial base angle, such as 110 degrees, could possibly contribute to a reduced nasopharyngeal dimension and a forward growth tendency of the face. Although there are no absolutes in facial growth that relate to the cranial base, the angulation of the cranial base aids in the description of the basic framework from which the tissues of the facial skeleton arise and ultimately find attachment.

To establish dimensional changes within the anterior and posterior cranial base, distances between S, N, and Ba are measured. To obtain the overall inferior cranial base measurement, a line from Ba to N is used. An angular measurement to demonstrate the degree of flexion of the cranial base at the sphenooccipital (SO) junction is formed by S-Ba-N. In studying the anterior cranial base (S-N) it is essential to know the distance between the anterior limits of the cribriform plate of the ethmoid bone (AE) and the posterior limits of the cribriform plate of the ethmoid bone (PE). S-N has a great impact on the overall anterior cranial base measurement, particularly during the first 3 years of life. It is an area that reflects discernible differences for patients with craniofacial anomalies when compared to unaffected persons. Other linear measurements for depth and height of the skull also can be made by using N and opisthion (O).

Upper face

In the midsagittal plane the upper face may be defined as being bounded superiorly by the plane of the cribriform plate of the ethmoid bone and inferiorly by the nasal floor or palatal plane (Fig. 15-5). The anterior nasal spine (ANS) and the posterior nasal spine (PNS) make up the anterior and posterior limits of the maxilla. Upper facial height is an expression of the relocation of the maxilla away from the cranial base; when this does not occur as it should, variations in midface development result. To measure facial height anteriorly and posteriorly, parallel lines are projected upward from the ANS and PNS to a point of intersection with the plane formed by the cribriform plate of the ethmoid bone. Discernible changes in length of the maxilla may be noted by obtaining linear measurements from the ANS and PNS. Deviations in length could reflect a smaller than average maxilla, or it could indicate that the maxilla has migrated away from the cranial base but that it is hypoplastic and thus smaller, as seen in some patients with cleft palate. In patients with craniofacial dysostosis the maxilla is not only hypoplastic, it is also severely retruded, suggesting that it has failed to relocate adequately because of freedom at the sutural sites.

The most useful measurement of maxillary position to the plastic surgeon is the horizontal position of the maxilla in relationship to the neurocranium (Fig. 15-6). The angles SNA (from sella to nasion to point A) express this relationship well. A normal SNA is 82 degrees $\pm$ 4 degrees. This would imply that an SNA measure of 70 degrees would indicate midfacial retrusion, or that a measure of 90 degrees would indicate maxillary protrusion. Although this is usually so, the SNA is only one of several measures to be considered. One variable that can affect the SNA measurement is a low sella position. This may have to be corrected in selected patients for an accurate cephalometric portrayal of the facial characteristics.

Lower face

The mandible has a direct impact on the development of the lower face. Its development and position is intimately associated with the muscles and ligaments attached to it. Their functional activity can influence the morphologic makeup of the mandible, as well as dictate its position relative to the rest of the face. The interrelationship it has with the tongue, hyoid bone, and nasopharyngeal complex makes its position and development closely allied to the physiologic actions of respiration, mastication, deglutition, and speech.

The plastic surgeon will be especially interested in measuring the horizontal position of the mandible in relation to the maxilla and cranial base. The most used measurement for mandibular position is SNB (sella to nasion to point B). This measurement is a means of assessing the horizontal relationship of the mandible to the cranium (Fig. 15-6). The norm is 79 degrees $\pm$ 3 degrees. The SNB, in combination with the SNA measurement of the maxilla, provides a simple means of determining whether a given patient has a true prognathism or a pseudoprognathism.

Although SNA and SNB relate the maxilla and mandible to the cranial base, the measurement point A to nasion to point B (ANB) is a means of relating the maxilla to the mandible. An ANB of 0 to 5 degrees is considered to be within the normal range, with 3 degrees representing the norm (Table 15-1).

Nasopharyngeal region

In the newborn the palatal plane is in close proximity to the cranial base, thus creating a smaller height and depth to the nasopharynx (Fig. 15-7). With early and rapid growth of the nasomaxillary complex, incremantal gains are made in both dimensions by virtue of the maxilla moving down and forward away from the cranial base.[7,13,16] This is consistent with growth needed in this area to satisfy the increased respiratory needs of the infant. To demonstrate this cephalometrically one can superimpose on the S-N plane and graphically illustrate the direction of the maxilla and its influence on the changing pharyngeal dimensions. Height measurements may be taken from the PNS or pterygomax-

Table 15-1. Normal cranial base and maxillary-mandibular relationships

Relationship	Cephalometric value	
Cranial base relation- ships		
S-N-Ba (saddle length)	130 degrees ± 6	
S-N length	83 mm ± 4	77 mm ± 4
S-Ba length	50 mm ± 4	46 mm ± 4
Ba-N length	120 mm ± 4	112 mm ± 5
Maxilla to cranium		
Horizontal		
SNA	82 degrees ± 4	
S-N-ANS	87 degrees ± 4	
Vertical		
N-ANS	60 mm ± 4	56 mm ± 3
Eth-PNS	55 mm ± 4	50 mm ± 3
Mandible to cranium		
SNB	79 degrees ± 3	
S-N-Pg	79 degrees ± 3	
N-Pg-Fh (facial plane)	85 degrees ± 5	
Mandible to maxilla		
ANB	3 degrees ± 2	

illary fissure (Ptm). Lines parallel to the palatel plane are projected upward to a point where they meet the cranial base plane (Ba-N).[26] The migration away from the posterior wall of the pharynx may be recorded by virtue of measurements going from the PNS to the posterior wall of the pharynx at the level of the palatal plane or to a bony landmark such as the anterior border of the anterior arch of the atlas. In patients with anomalies these dimensions vertically and horizontally are greatly reduced when compared to those in an unaffected population.[13]

FRONTAL-ORBITAL-NASAL REGION

Frontal cephalometric radiographs are used for making width measurements in the frontal-orbital-nasal regions. To demonstrate changing dimensions between the bony orbits on a time basis or for assessment of abnormal divergence of the bony orbits, measurements are made from interorbital distance to interorbital distance (IOD-IOD). IOD measurements contribute information in patients with frontonasal dysplasia and in cases of true ocular hypertelorism. With normative data it helps establish information that can be used in assessing the degree of deviation of bony orbits seen in pathologic conditions (Fig. 15-8).[18,24]

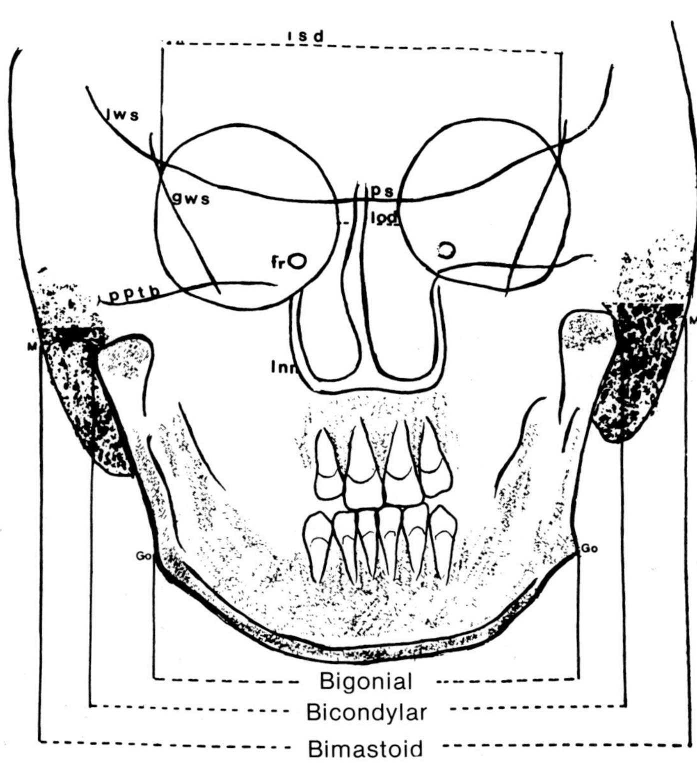

Fig. 15-8. Anteroposterior cephalometric radiograph demonstrates specific landmarks that are useful in the analysis of dimensions in width for the frontal-orbital-nasal regions. It also permits assessment of lateral growth in the areas of the condyle, mastoid, and gonion.

To determine the width at the cranial base level, measurements are taken from a point of intersection of the greater wing of the sphenoid bone with the superolateral rim of the bony orbit (GW-GW) and also with the lesser wing (LW-LW). Furthermore, to demonstrate the influence of the frontoorbital width on the width at a lower level (nasal floor), measurements are taken from the lateral nasal notch to the lateral nasal notch (LNN-LNN). Other measurements in width that may be closely identified with the developing regions of the mandible are the mastoid (M-M), bicondylar (Co-Co), and bigonial regions (Go-Go).

SELECTED SKELETAL DYSPLASIAS
Ocular hypertelorism

Posteroanterior cephalometric radiographs are used to demonstrate the outline and position of the bony orbits (Fig. 15-9) relative to each other and to contiguous cranial base structures. Landmarks such as the LW and GW permit an assessment of the relationships between the bony orbits and the cranial base. The radiopaque outlines of the bony orbits as seen on posteroanterior cephalometric films permit analysis of the interorbital and intraorbital dimensions. All of these measurements are useful in the diagnosis and treatment

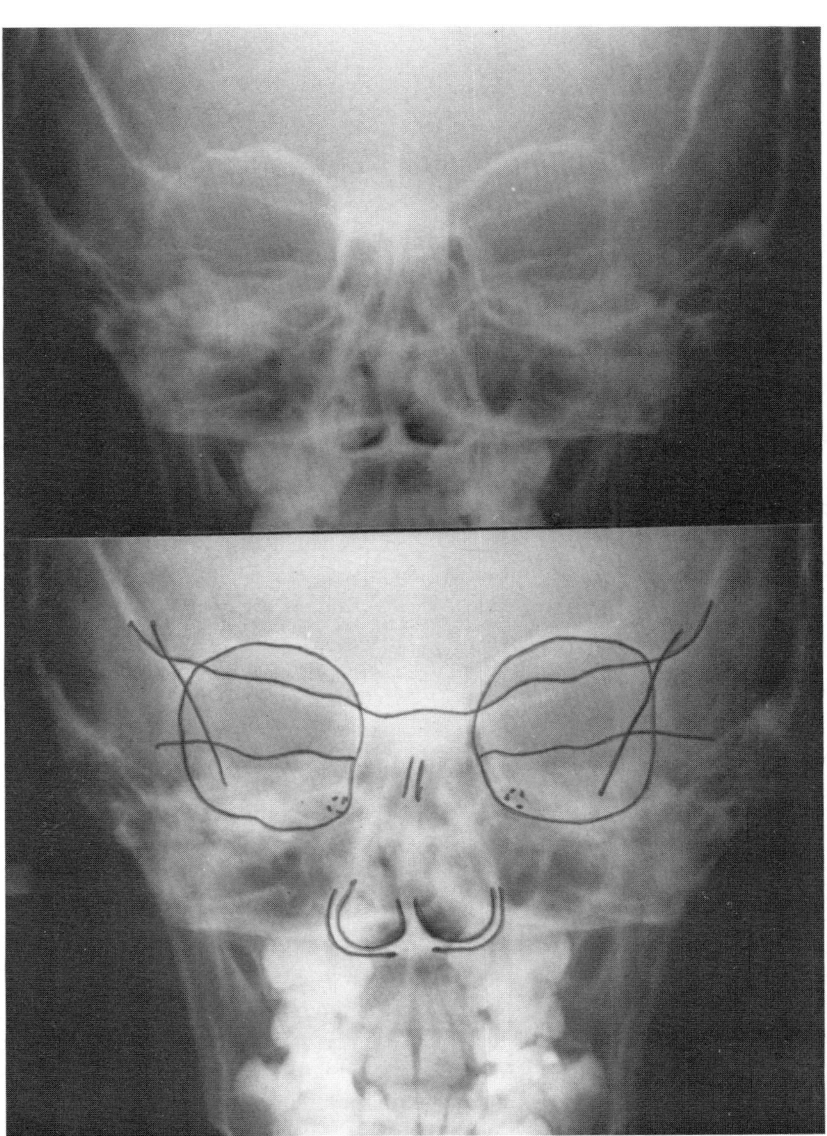

Fig. 15-9. Posteroanterior cephalometric radiograph shows landmarks used for studying orbital dimensions.

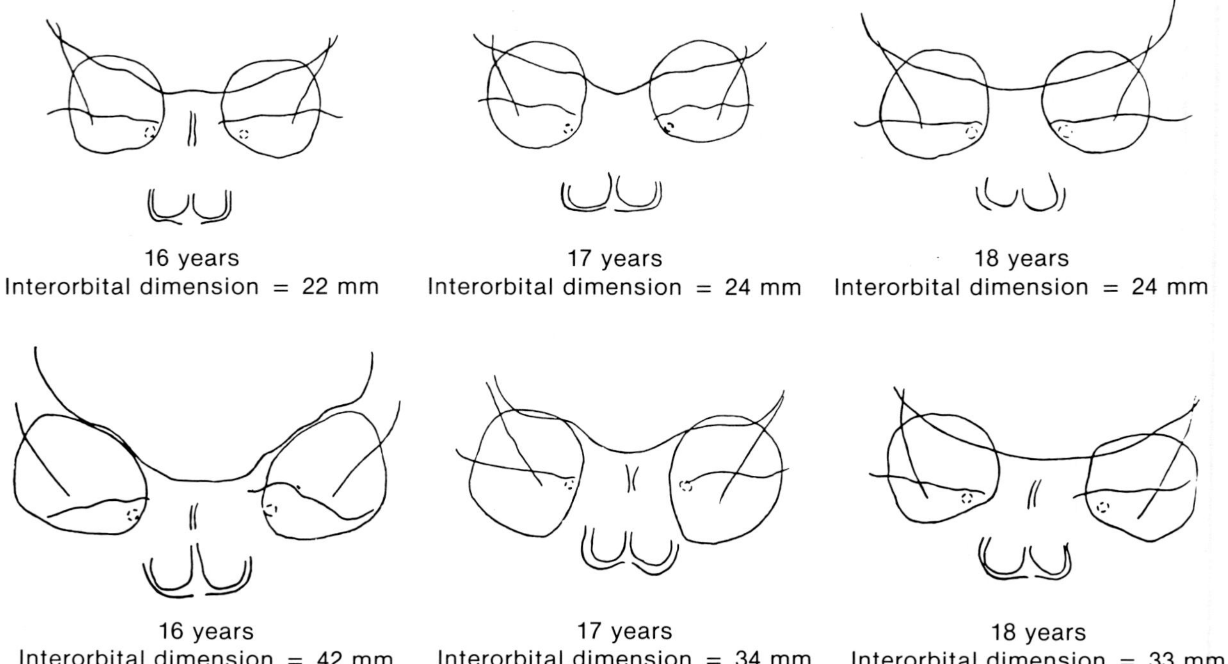

Fig. 15-10. Posteroanterior cephalometric radiograph of the orbital dimensions for three ages. *Top,* Dimensions in normal persons. *Bottom,* Persons with hypertelorism.

of ocular hypertelorism. A large number of patients with this condition have a frontonasal dysplasia contributing to the notable divergence of the bony orbits (Fig. 15-10).

Craniofacial synostosis

Clinical findings common to many of the patients with this syndrome are exophthalmos, midfacial underdevelopment, and facial prognathism. The exophthalmos is intimately related to the smaller anterior cranial base and the failure of the maxilla to relocate adequately in a vertical and horizontal direction. Thus the accompanying facial prognathism is more apparent than real. The hypoplasia of the maxilla is due to the lack of dimensional increase at the sutural sites associated with the premature closure of these sutures. One that appears to have particular significance to growth in length of the maxilla is the transverse palatine suture. Lack of growth at this site appears to occur very early in life.[13]

Lateral cephalometric radiographs depict the character of the deformity within the cranial, upper face, lower face, and nasopharyngeal regions. A notable difference exists between cleft palate and craniofacial synostosis, in which the maxilla fails to move away from the cranial base in a satisfactory manner (Fig. 15-11). As a result, the posterior border of the hard palate, to which the soft palate is attached, is buttressed up against the pharyngeal wall. The diminution in height and depth of the nasopharynx, at an age when growth and development within this area are essential to the increased needs for respiration, is intimately related to fail-

ure of the maxilla to migrate sufficiently in a downward and forward direction.[13]

Growth and development in a patient over a 6-year period from ages 5 to 11 are documented in Fig. 15-11. Tracings of serial cephalograms reflect that no discernible maxillary growth occurred in a vertical and horizontal direction. But in the absence of maxillary growth, demonstrable growth continued in the mandible and resulted in an exaggeration of the facial prognathism. The cephalometric records also document the changes within the epipharynx, mesopharynx, and hypopharynx before and after a LeFort III procedure. Thus the use of cephalometrics in the growing child with a congenital deformity contributes information on growth of facial structures, as well as needed data for the establishment of a treatment plan.

Hemifacial microsomia

Patients with a first and second branchial arch anomaly demonstrate varying degrees of abnormalities about the ear and mandible. There appears to be no correlation between the severity of the ear deformity and the accompanying mandibular abnormality. Facial asymmetry is a common finding within this group of patients and is associated with the degree of anatomic aberration in the temporomandibular complex. The external pterygoid muscle on the affected side is underdeveloped or missing and results in the failure of this muscle to contribute in the motions of protrusion and opening of the mandible.[12,14]

Using a conventional head holder for obtaining cephalo-

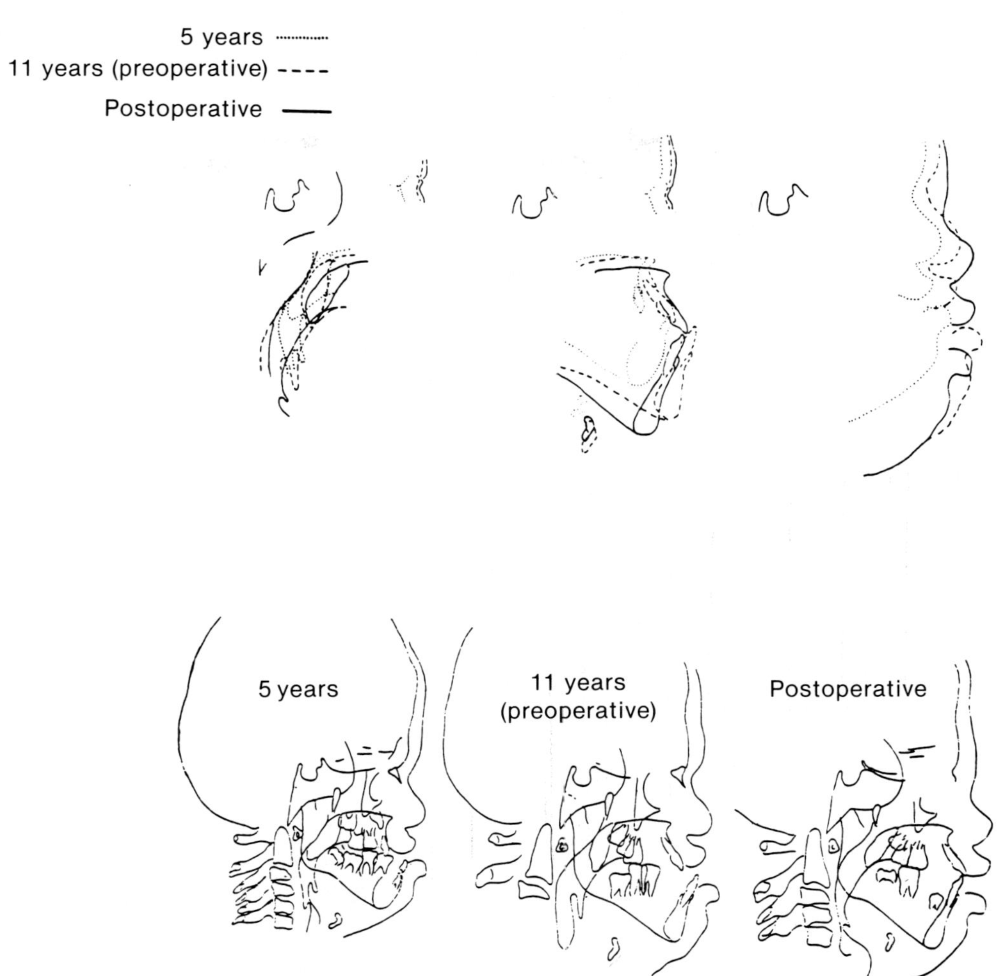

Fig. 15-11. Serial lateral cephalometric radiographs in a patient with Apert's syndrome depict the status of the craniofacial structures at three different age levels (5 to 8 and 11 years). Note the changes within the nasopharyngeal area. No discernible maxillary growth has occurred, whereas demonstrable growth is noted for the mandible during the 6-year period. Changes are also documented for the skeletal and soft tissue areas after a LeFort III surgical advancement procedure.

metric radiographs of patients with this syndrome poses a problem, since the ear on the affected side may be malpositioned, malformed, or completely missing. The patient's head is positioned with the unaffected ear within the ear rod, and the other ear rod is placed at a comparable level on the affected side. The Frankfort horizontal plane is used to obtain a satisfactory, standardized head position.

Fig. 15-12 demonstrates the character of the abnormality within the temporomandibular region. It exhibits the changes coincidental to growth on a time basis. The lateral cephalometric film (Fig. 15-12) illustrates changes that have occurred in the ramus height and body length on the affected side and the unaffected side. Note the relationship of the condyle to the Ptm area. The differences between the two sides at this site are in a superoinferior and anteroposterior

direction. It is somewhat suggestive that the syndrome has involved the maxilla, as well as the mandible. The posteroanterior films support the changes observed in the lateral films, showing the growth and associated diminution in facial asymmetry (Fig. 15-13). Schematic tracings of both sides of the mandible indicate demonstrable growth on the affected side over a 10-year period, with some disparity still evident (Fig. 15-14).

Cleft lip and palate

Cephalometry for cleft palates has resulted in many studies in growth and development of the craniofacial structures [9-11,21] (Fig. 15-15). Serial radiographs have been used for the study of developing dentition and malocclusions. Surgeons have used preoperative and postoperative films to

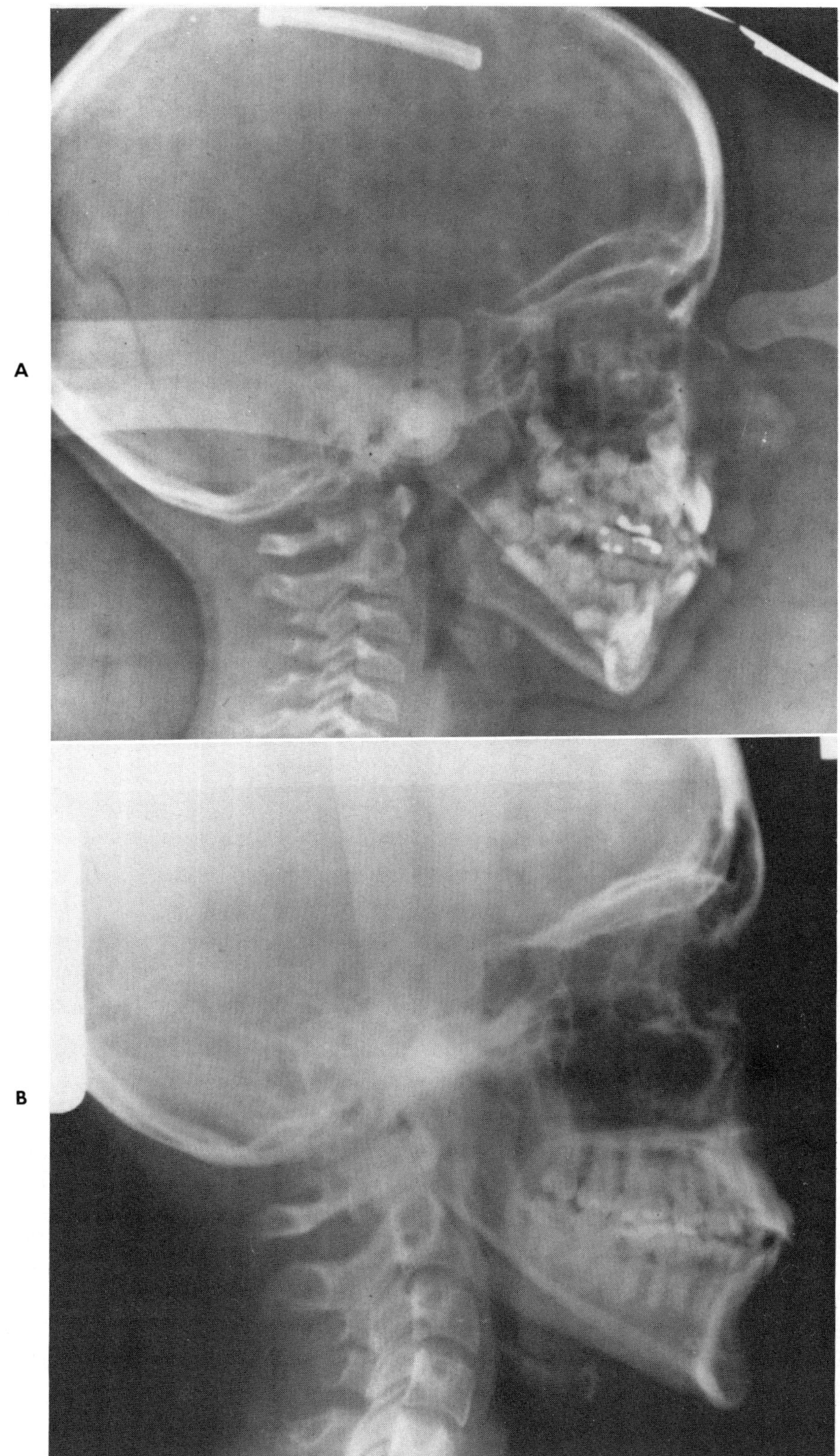

Fig. 15-12. Lateral cephalometric radiographs for a patient with hemifacial microsomia. **A,** Patient at 5 years of age. Note the differences in morphologic pattern of mandibular development between the affected and unaffected sides. On the affected side note the location of the angular process of the mandible relative to the odontoid process. **B,** At 21 years of age (16 years after the initial film) note the location of the angular process relative to the odontoid process. The cephalometric films document the changes on a time basis in a patient with a congenital deformity.

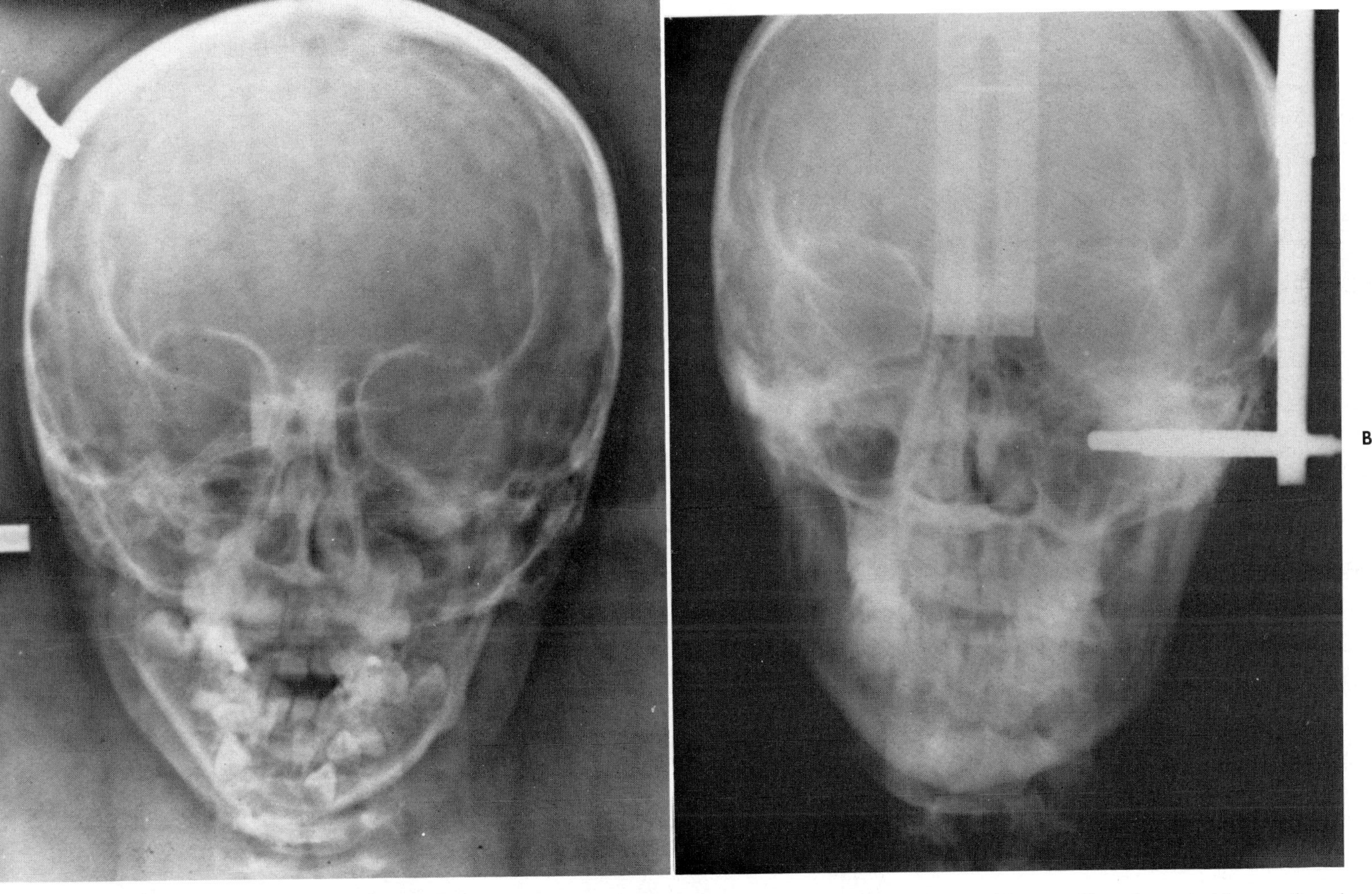

Fig. 15-13. Posteroanterior cephalometric radiographs for patient in Fig. 15-12. **A,** Patient at 5 years. **B,** Patient at 21 years. Note demonstrable growth and development on the affected side.

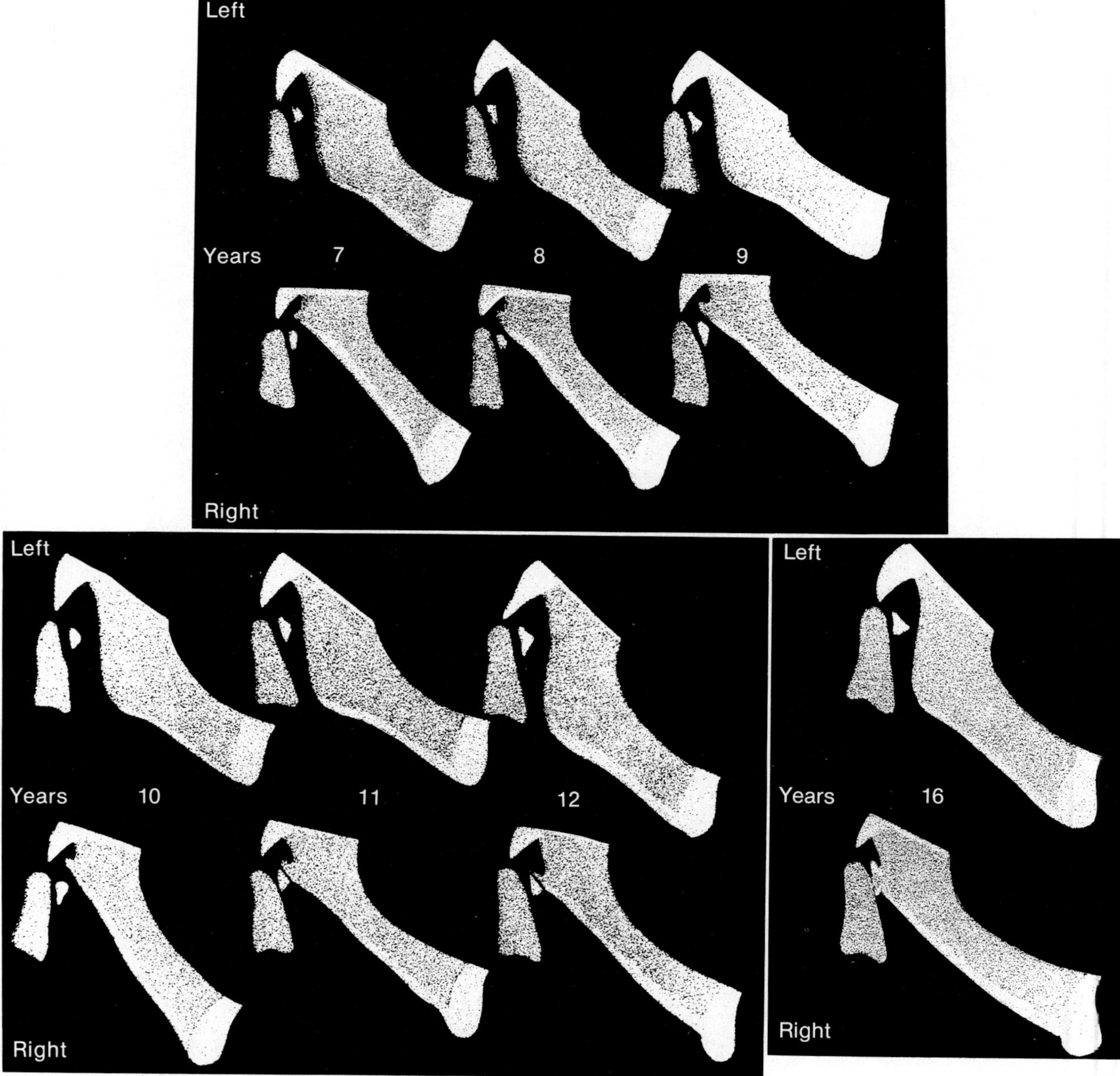

Fig. 15-14. Schematic tracings of the mandible relative to the odontoid process for patient in Figs. 15-12 and 15-13. From ages 7 to 16 observe the changes in the ramus and body of the mandible from the affected to the unaffected side.

demonstrate the impact of surgery on skeletal and soft tissue anatomic structures. Speech pathologists have used lateral films taken during sustained phonation to demonstrate the character of the pharynx and the quality of velopharyngeal movement in diagnosing hypernasality. Longitudinal studies on the growth of the skeletal and soft tissue structures have been carried out in conjunction with surgical and orthodontic treatment procedures. Altogether, the static cephalogram has been an effective tool in the diagnosis and treatment of these patients.

Patients with cleft lip and palate have a hypoplastic maxilla that, although deficient and distorted, tends to show a growth pattern similar to the unaffected population. They differ from patients with craniofacial synostosis in this regard. In craniofacial synostosis the maxilla does not express satisfactory directional growth, but it does with cleft palate. However, because of the potential for a deficient maxilla to move away from the cranial base with growth, speech problems may arise. This occurs because of the presence of the shortened soft palate and the changing position of the max-

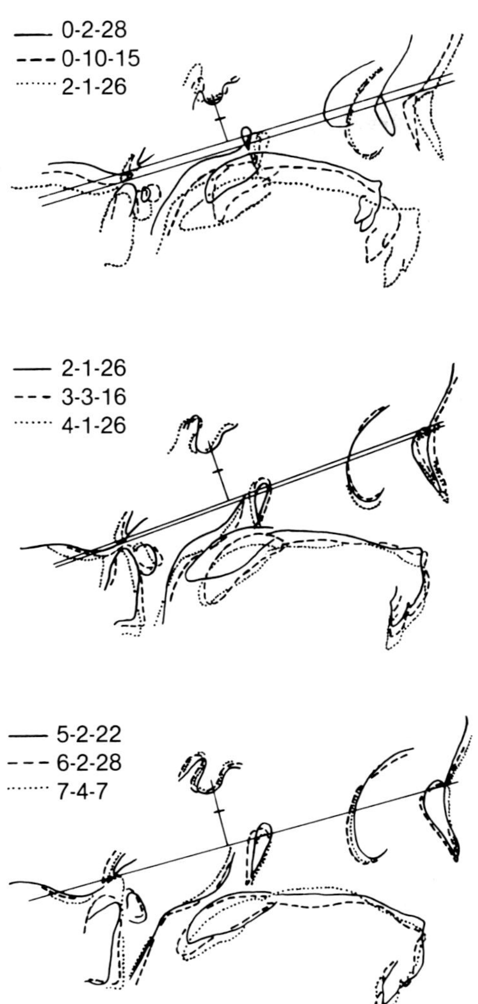

Fig. 15-15. Lateral cephalometric radiographs of a patient with a bilateral cleft lip and palate, superimposed for the period of 3 months to 7 years. Serial records permit the documentation of changes within the craniofacial areas. (From Coccaro, P.J., Subtelny, J.D., and Pruzansky, S.: Growth of soft palate in cleft palate children, Plast. Reconstr. Surg. **30:**43, 1962.)

illa. Thus the increased dimensional change in nasopharyngeal depth plus the shorter palate creates the potential for hypernasality. Facial abnormalities may persist because of the deficiency of the maxilla and continued growth of the mandible.[9-11]

SUMMARY AND CONCLUSIONS

The availability of cephalometric radiology provides the clinician with an extremely important diagnostic tool, as well as a mechanism to document the natural history of various malformations. A great variety of cephalometric measurements and normative data are available to assist the clinician and researcher in studying syndromes.

Characteristics of the normal and abnormal cranial base, upper face, lower face, and nasopharyngeal areas were discussed from the lateral cephalometric projection. The frontal film provides valuable information, including the transverse dimensions associated with the orbits and jaws.

Discussion focused on selected patients with skeletal dysplasias. These included ocular hypertelorism, craniofacial synostosis, hemifacial microsomia, and cleft lip and palate. Some key characteristics of each condition were presented.

Overall, the cephalometric radiograph provides one of the most accurate and useful parts of the data base in the examination sequence of the patient from infancy through adulthood.

GLOSSARY OF CEPHALOMETRIC RADIOGRAPHIC LANDMARKS

A   Point A. The most posterior point on the labial curve of the maxilla located between the anterior nasal spine and prosthion (supradentale).

AA   Anterior arch of the atlas.

AB   Anterior border of the ramus. The most posterior point on the concave outline of the anterior border of the mandible.

AE   Anterior limits of the cribriform plate of the ethmoid bone. May also be defined as posterior nasion. As viewed in the normal lateral plane, it may be seen as the most posterior point in the midline where the nasal bone articulates with the frontal and ethmoid bones inferior to the frontal sinus.

ANB   The angle formed by lines joining point A, nasion, and point B.

ANS   Anterior nasal spine. The most anterior point of the maxilla in the midsagittal plane. A sharp anterior bony projection of the maxilla at the level of the palatal plane.

Ar   Articulare. The point of intersection of the inferior cranial base surface and the posterior surface of the upper limits of the neck of the mandibular condyle.

B   Point B. The most posterior point on the anterior surface of the symphyseal contour of the mandible, located between the prosthion (infradentale) and pogonion.

Ba   Basion. Lowest and most posterior point on the anterior margin of the foramen magnum.

Bo   Bolton point. The point at the height of curvature of the junction of the occipital condyle with the lateral portion of the occipital bone. May be located between the basion and opisthion (center of the foramen magnum)

DM   Deciduous molar.

Ep   Epiglottis. Leaflike structure projecting upward behind the root of the tongue in the area of the third and fourth cervical vertebrae.

Fh   Frankfort horizontal plane. Plane established by connecting a point 4.5 mm above the geometric center of the ear rod and orbitale.

Fr   Foramen rotundum. May be seen on the frontal cephalogram. It is located within the shadow of the bony orbital outline at its medioinferior margin.

Fs   Frontal sinus. As seen on the normal lateral radiograph, it lies above the root of the nose bounded in front and behind by the tables of the skull.

Go   Gonion. Located by bisecting the posterior ramal plane and the mandibular plane angle.

Gn   Gnathion. The most anteroinferior point on the bony chin contour obtained by bisecting the angle formed by the mandibular plane and the facial plane (nasion to pogonion).

GW   Greater wing of the sphenoid bone. On the frontal cephalogram it appears as an oblique line through the lateral aspect of the bony orbit shadow.

H   Hyoid bone.

IOD   Interorbital distance. From the medial wall of the orbit at the point of greatest convexity in the region of the frontal process of the maxilla.

ISD   Intersphenoidal distance. Distance between the point of intersection between the lateral orbital rim and the greater wing of the sphenoid bone.

K   Key ridge. The lowermost point on the contour of the zygoma located at the anterior wall of the infratemporal fossa.

LC   Lower incisor.

LL   Lower lip. The most prominent spot of the lower lip.

LN   Lateral nasal notch of the maxilla. It constitutes the lateral margins of the piriform opening of the anterior nasal aperture.

LW   Lesser wing of the sphenoid bone.

M   Mastoid bone. Most lateral point of the contour of the mastoid process of the temporal bone.

MP   Mandibular plane. This plane is defined by the menton anteriorly and the lowermost border of the ramus posterior to the antegonical notch.

N   Nasion. The junction of the frontonasal suture as seen on the normal lateral radiograph.

No   Nose. The most anterior point on the soft tissue contour of the nose.

Ns   Soft tissue nasion. Located by extending the S-N line anteriorly to a point where it intersects the soft tissue overlying the nasion.

O   Opisthion. The most dorsal point of the bony margin of the foramen magnum.

OC   Opisthocranium. The most posterior point on the occipitocranium.

Od   Odontoid axis. The second cervical vertebrae.

OF   Orbital process of the frontal bone (roof of the orbit) in the midsagittal plane.

Or   Orbitale. The lowermost point on the infraorbital margin in the midsagittal plane.

P   Prosthion. The most anterior and inferior alveolar point (for the maxilla) and anterior and superior point (for the mandible) situated between the central incisors.

PB   Posterior border of the ramus. It may be defined as a point opposite the anterior border of the ramus located by a line drawn through the ramus from the anterior border at right angles to the ramal plane.

PE   Posterior limits of the cribriform plate of the ethmoid bone. Located at the intersection of the planum sphenoidale with the greater wing of the sphenoid bone.

Pg   Pogonion. The most anterior point on the bony chin contour in the midsagittal plane.

Ph   Pharyngeal wall. Radiopaque contour of the pharyngeal wall in a midsagittal plane demonstrating the epipharynx, mesopharynx, and hypopharynx.

PNS   Posterior nasal spine. The most posterior point on the bony palate in the sagittal plane.

Po   Porion (cephalometric). The highest point on the superior surface of the soft tissue of the external auditory meatus. The true, or anthropometric, porion is located on the superior bony surface of the external auditory meatus. It may be approximated by measuring 4 mm vertically from the center of the superimposed orientation rings.

PP   Palatal plane–nasal floor. A plane perpendicular to the midsagittal plane going through the anterior and posterior nasal spines.

Ps   Soft tissue pogonion. The most anterior point on the soft tissue chin contour.

PS   Planum sphenoidale.

Ptm   Pterygomaxillary fissure. A teardroplike outline formed by the maxillary tuberosity anteriorly and the anterior margin of the pterygoid plates posteriorly.

Ptp   Pterygoid plate. As seen behind the pterygomaxillary fissure.

S   Sella turcica. The center of the pituitary fossa of the sphenoid bone determined by inspection.

Sn   Subnasale. A soft tissue point situated on the lower edge of the nasal septum where the columella joins the upper lip.

S-N   Sella-nasion line. Line going from the center of the sella turcica to the nasion.

SO   Sphenooccipital synchondrosis.

Sp   Soft palate. The radiopaque mass seen anteriorly at the posterior nasal spine and pterygomaxillary fissure and positioned caudally above the tongue and below the inferior outline of the cranial base.

SS   Symphyseal shadow of the mandible.

T   Tongue.

UC   Upper incisor.

UI   Upper lip. A soft tissue point representing the most prominent spot of the upper lip.

REFERENCES

1. Baum, A.: A cephalometric evaluation of the normal skeletal and denture pattern of children with excellent occlusion, Angle Orthod. **21**:96, 1951.
2. Bjork, A.: Cephalometric x-ray investigations in dentistry, Int. Dent. J. **45**:718, 1954.
3. Brader, A.C.: A cephalometric x-ray appraisal of morphological variations in cranial base and associated pharyngeal structures: implications in cleft palate therapy, Angle Orthod. **27**:179, 1957.
4. Broadbent, B.H.: A new x-ray technique and its applications to orthodontia, Angle Orthod. **1**:35, 1931.
5. Broadbent, B.H.: The face of the normal child, Angle Orthod. **7**:209, 1937.
6. Broadbent, B.H., Sr., Broadbent, B.H., Jr., and Golden, W.H.: Bolton standards of dentofacial developmental growth, St. Louis, 1975, The C.V. Mosby Co.
7. Brodie, A.G.: On the growth pattern of the human head from the third month to the eighth year of life, Am. J. Anat. **68**:209, 1941.
8. Coccaro, P.J., D'Amico, R., and Chavoor, A.: Craniofacial morphology of parents with and without cleft lip and palate children, Cleft Palate J. **9**:28, 1972.
9. Coccaro, P.J., and Pruzansky, S.: Longitudinal study of skeletal and soft tissue profile in children with unilateral cleft lip and cleft palate, Cleft Palate J. **2**:1, 1965.
10. Coccaro, P.J., Pruzansky, S., and Subtelny, J.D.: Nasopharyngeal growth, Cleft Palate J. **4**:214, 1967.
11. Coccaro, P.J., Subtelny, J.D., and Pruzansky, S.: Growth of soft palate in cleft palate children: a serial cephalometric study, Plast. Reconstr. Surg. **30**:43, 1962.

12. Converse, J.M., Coccaro, P.J., Becker, M., and Wood-Smith, D.: On hemifacial microsomia: the first and second branchial arch syndrome, Plast. Reconstr. Surg. **51**:268, 1973.
13. Firmin, F., Coccaro, P.J., and Converse, J.M.: Cephalometric analysis in diagnosis and treatment planning of craniofacial dysostosis, Plast. Reconstr. Surg. **54**:300, 1974.
14. Grabb, W.C.: The first and second branchial arch syndrome, Plast. Reconstr. Surg. **36**:485, 1965.
15. Graber, T.M.: A critical review of clinical cephalometric radiography, Am. J. Orthod. **40**:1, 1954.
16. King, E.W.: A roentgenographic study of pharyngeal growth, Angle Orthod. **22**:23, 1952.
17. Krogman, W.M.: Validation of the roentgenographic cephalometric technique, Am. J. Orthod. **44**:933, 1958.
18. Krogman, W.M., and Sassouni, V.: A syllabus in roentgenographic cephalometry, Philadelphia, 1957, Philadelphia Center for Research in Child Growth.
19. Lande, M.J.: Growth behavior of the human bony facial profile as revealed by serial cephalometric roentgenography, Angle Orthod. **22**:78, 1952.
20. Margolis, H.I.: Standardized x-ray cephalometrics, Am. J. Orthod. **26**:725, 1940.
21. Moss, M.L.: Malformations of the skull base associated with cleft palate deformity, Plast. Reconstr. Surg. **17**:226, 1956.
22. Pruzansky, S., and Lis, E.: Cephalometric roentgenography of infants—sedation, instrumentation, and research, Am. J. Orthod. **44**:159, 1958.
23. Rosenberger, H.C.: Growth and development of the nasorespiratory area in childhood, Ann. Otol. Rhinol. Laryngol. **43**:495, 1934.
24. Salzmann, J.A., editor: Roentgenographic cephalometrics, Philadelphia, 1961, J.B. Lippincott Co.
25. Sassouni, V.: Diagnosis and treatment planning via roentgenographic cephalometry, Am. J. Orthod. **44**:433, 1958.
26. Subtelny, J.D.: A cephalometric study of the growth of the soft palate, Plast. Reconstr. Surg. **19**:49, 1957.
27. Subtelny, J.D.: A longitudinal study of soft tissue facial structures and their profile characteristics defined in relation to underlying skeletal structures, Am. J. Orthod. **45**:481, 1959.

CHAPTER 16

Speech patterns and disturbances associated with clefts and craniofacial anomalies

JOHN E. RISKI, LuVERN H. KUNZE, KAREN R. NAILLING, and JUDITH G. MANN

A cleft of the lip is caused by failure of the medial nasal and maxillary processes to fuse during the embryonic stage of development. A cleft palate is caused by failure of the palatal shelves to fuse. A cleft occurs in approximately 1 in every 700 live births. The child born with a palatal cleft faces a number of obstacles to the development of normal conversational speech. These obstacles include velopharyngeal incompetency, maxillary arch and dental malformations, and hearing loss. The most severe detriment is velopharyngeal incompetency (VPI). Primary palatal surgery is effective in producing a competent velopharyngeal mechanism in approximately 70% to 80% of the cases.[6,11] The remaining 20% to 30% will require some form of secondary palatal management.

A VPI predisposes an individual to speech disturbances of two types: disorders of articulation and disorders of oral-nasal resonance balance. Often the diagnosis of VPI and recommendations for management are made by the speech pathologist, and the management procedure (pharyngoplasty) is carried out by the plastic surgeon. Therefore effective evaluation and management of VPI depends on the cooperative efforts of a cleft palate or craniofacial team with active participation by and communication between the plastic surgeon and the speech pathologist. The purpose of this chapter is to illustrate the methodology for evaluating and managing VPI and the necessary communication between professionals.

TERMINOLOGY

The terms in this discussion encompass the primary concepts to be considered in the evaluation and treatment of speech disorders in patients with cleft palate and craniofacial anomalies.

Language is the use of symbols that are ordered by rules (grammar) to communicate thoughts or feelings. Language may be verbal (speech and audition), or it may be nonverbal (reading and writing). Speech is the use of vocal or oral symbols for communication. *Articulation* is the movement and placement of speech structures that serve to interrupt and modify the voiced or unvoiced airstream into meaningful sounds. Among the articulators are the lower jaw, lips, tongue, hard palate, and soft palate.

Oral-nasal resonance is a balance between oral resonance and nasal resonance. It is achieved when the velopharyngeal valve appropriately couples the oral and nasal cavities from the remainder of the vocal tract during speech. Three English sounds require the nasal cavity to be coupled with the vocal tract (i.e., /m/, /n/, /ng/). All other sounds require the velopharyngeal valve to close, thus isolating the nasal cavity from the vocal tract. *Nasality,* or *hypernasality,* is the quality perceived by the listener when inappropriate nasal coupling with the vocal tract occurs during speech. That is, excessive nasality appears during sounds which are typically characterized by oral resonance. As a counterpart to hypernasality, *nasal air emission* is defined as audible or measurable air escape through the nasal cavities and is also associated with inappropriate nasal coupling.

Denasality, or *hyponasality,* is at the opposite end of the spectrum from hypernasality. This quality is perceived as a partial or complete obstruction of the nasal tract during production of those sounds which are normally associated with nasal resonance. The obstruction may be posterior (e.g., hypertrophied adenoids) or anterior (e.g., hypertrophied turbinates). The speaker with a head cold is typically hyponasal.

Thus a normally functioning velopharyngeal valve permits *oral-nasal resonance balance*. Disturbance of this balance can be to either end of a continuum. That is, there can be an excess of nasal resonance (hypernasality) or lack of nasal resonance (hyponasality).

Oral-nasal resonance and nasal air emission are intimately related to *velopharyngeal competency*. Velopharyngeal competency represents that range of velopharyngeal function during speech that extends from complete closure of the portal to a small (probably less than 20 mm²) velopharyngeal opening. An opening greater than 20 mm² generally results in (**VPI**).[24]

ARTICULATION
The English sound system

The phonemes within the English sound system are classified as consonants and vowels. The consonant sound system of English is illustrated in Table 16-1. Consonants are described by their *place of articulation* (the location of articulators in the oral cavity) and by the *manner of articulation* (the way in which the sound is produced). *Plosives* are made by a brief interruption of the airstream. *Fricatives* are made by constricting the airstream. Some consonants require intraoral air pressure, whereas others do not. Intraoral air pressure is developed behind the active articulators and requires velopharyngeal competency for consonant production. Some sounds are voiced (that is the vocal cords within the larynx vibrate during the production), and other sounds are unvoiced.

Vowels in the English sound system are described by the position of the tongue within the oral cavity (Fig. 16-1). The horizontal position of the tongue is described as front, middle, or back, and the vertical position is described as high, middle, or low. A high tongue carriage offers more resistance to sound energy as it exits the oral cavity. Thus in the presence of a VPI, high vowels are more susceptible to hypernasal resonance than low vowels.

Compensatory articulation in the child with VPI

A child with an incompetent velopharyngeal mechanism during the articulation development years will find it difficult or impossible to produce sounds that require intraoral breath pressure. Frequently a child with VPI will resort to using the laryngeal valve to produce plosive sounds. This sound is called a *glottal stop*. It appears naturally in English only infrequently. An example of a naturally appearing glottal stop is in ''uh huh'' and ''uh uh.''

Table 16-1. Classification of American-English consonants

	Manner									
	Pressure						Nonpressure			
	Plosive		Fricative		Affricative		Nasal		Semivowel	
Place	UV*	V*	UV	V	UV	V	UV	V	UV	V
Bilabial	/p/ pie	/b/ boy						/m/ me		/w/ water
Labiodental			/f/ fan	/v/ van						
Interdental or lingual-dental			/θ/ thin	/ð/ this						
Lingual-alveolar	/t/ tie	/d/ do	/s/ sun	/z/ zoo				/n/ no		/l/ love
Palatal			/ʃ/ shoe	/ʒ/ vision	/tʃ/ chair	/dʒ/ jump				j yes
Velar	/k/ cat	/g/ go						/ŋ/ sing		/r/ run
Glottal		/ʔ/† uh huh	/h/ horse							
Pharyngeal			/ħ/‡							

*UV, Unvoiced; V, voiced.
†Glottal stop.
‡Pharyngeal fricative (no example in English).

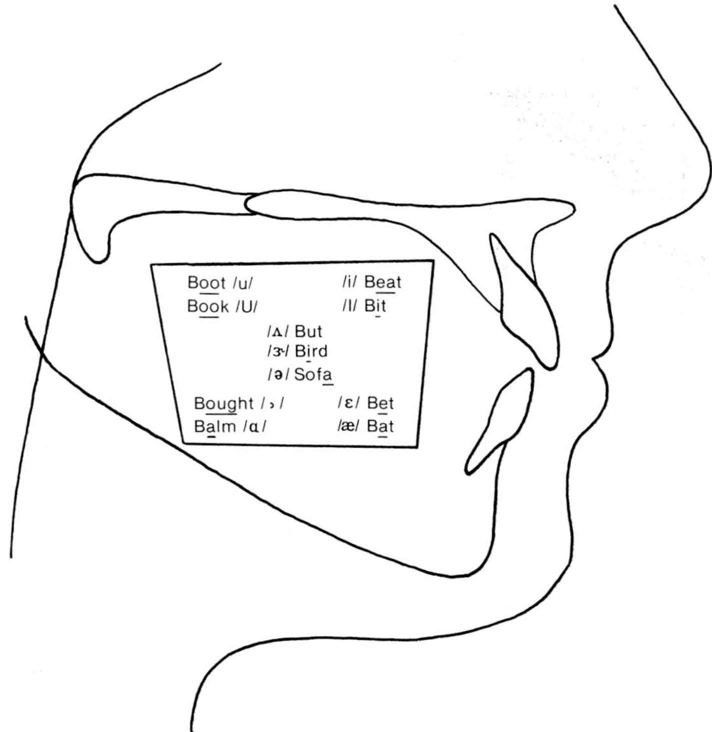

Fig. 16-1. Vowel quadrangle superimposed on the oral cavity.

A child with an incompetent velopharyngeal mechanism might also learn to use a pharyngeal fricative for the oral fricative sounds. In producing a pharyngeal fricative the airstream is constricted by approximating the tongue at some point along the posterior pharyngeal wall. The pharyngeal fricative does not appear naturally in the English sound system.

Normal speech development

Normal development of articulation serves as a gauge by which the articulation skills of children with clefts can be measured.* An in-depth discussion will not be conducted, rather some generalizations will be made from these studies.

The accuracy of articulation skills improves with age and generally reaches a mature state when the child is 8 years old. Studies completed more recently have demonstrated that children are acquiring articulation skills earlier, possibly because of the influence of television. Girls generally develop articulation skills faster than boys. The maturation of articulation skills generally proceeds from nasal sounds (e.g., /m/, /n/) to plosives (e.g., /p/, /t/) to fricatives (e.g., /s/, /f/) to consonant combinations (e.g., /bl/, /tr/) to semivowels (e.g., /l/, /r/).

---

*References 1, 9, 10, 18, 22, and 25.

Speech development in children with cleft palate

In 1959 Spriestersbach and Powers [20] concluded that the articulation skills of individuals with cleft palate vary as a function of their ability to impound oral air pressure. Van Demark[23] concluded that articulation deficiency is most closely related to factors of velopharyngeal competency and maturation. Van Demark added that the velopharyngeal competency factor contributes three times as much to the judged articulatory defectiveness as does the maturational factor.

Several studies of articulation development in children with cleft palate have been completed by Riski et al.[13,15-17] Most recently they have analyzed the longitudinal articulation development of 108 children from the Lancaster Cleft Palate Clinic in Lancaster, Pennsylvania. This series included 84 children who did not require pharyngeal flaps and 24 children who did require pharyngeal flaps for VPI.

The researchers concluded that the severity of the articulation deficit varies with the severity of the cleft type (Fig. 16-2). In general, children who require pharyngeal flaps demonstrate poorer articulation skills than those who do not require flaps. Children who require flaps do not make significant gains in articulation acquisition until after flap surgery.[11] Cleft type is a signfiicant factor in the nonflap group only between palatal and nonpalatal clefts. Age is a signif-

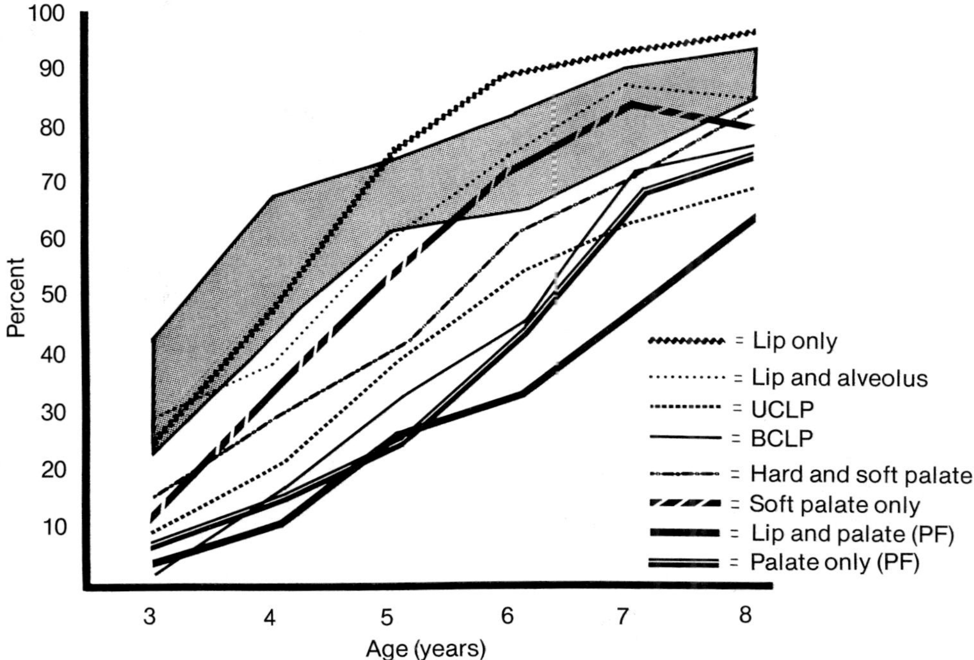

Fig. 16-2. The percentage of sounds produced correctly on the Templin-Darley 50-Item Screening Test. The scores of 84 children in six cleft types who did not require pharyngeal flaps and 24 children in two cleft types who required pharyngeal flaps are compared to Templin's norms *(gray area).*[22] The top of the gray area represents Templin's mean score, and the bottom approximates −1 standard deviation. The number of patients represented in each group is: lip only, 16; lip and alveolus, 12; unilateral cleft lip and palate *(UCLP)*, 26; bilateral cleft lip and palate *(BCLP)*, 7; hard and soft palate, 18; soft palate only, 5; lip and palate with pharyngeal flap *(PF)*, 8; palate only with pharyngeal flap *(PF)*, 16.

icant factor, but appears to be influenced by the severity of the defect. The articulation development period is prolonged in cleft palate children when compared to the noncleft peers. Sex is not a significant factor.

Speech development in children with craniofacial anomalies

Cleft palate occurs in over 154 of the recognized craniofacial anomalies.[3] For this reason, the efforts of many cleft palate teams are focused on individuals with craniofacial malformations. However, a cleft palate is only one of the hinderances to speech and language development. Another frequent cause for speech and language aberrancies in groups with craniofacial anomalies is mental retardation. Mental retardation may be consistently severe, as in orodigitofacial dysostosis, or it may be mild or absent, as in Crouzon's disease.

In some craniofacial disorders the articulation errors are due in part to dental and arch anomalies. Patients with Apert's syndrome typically have a V-shaped maxillary dental arch and irregular positioning of the dentition. A severe Class III malocclusion also is typically present. Maxillary hypoplasia contributes to the Class III malocclusion and

small nasopharyngeal dimensions. When coupled with a large velum, hyponasal resonance may be present. Other dental and arch anomalies include the congenital absence of teeth, malpositioned teeth, enamel hypoplasia, and lateral swelling of the palatal vault, leaving only a narrow median groove. This narrow median groove may be misdiagnosed as a palatal cleft.

Speech and language development may be disrupted to some degree by loss of hearing. In some groups of patients, such as those with Apert's syndrome and Crouzon's disease, hearing loss is precipitated by deficient eustachian tube function that results in chronic otitis media. In other groups of patients, such as those with mandibulofacial dysostosis, a hearing loss may be precipitated by unilateral or bilateral deformities (e.g., atresia of the external and middle ear).

Surgical advancement of the middle third of the face is becoming a more common treatment for the management of maxillary hypoplasia. Clinical experience with midfacial advancement suggests that a VPI rarely occurs after advancement procedures for Crouzon's disease and Apert's syndrome. This is probably due to the shallow nasopharynx that exists preoperatively. Moreover, resonance usually moves from a hyponasal quality in the preoperative state to

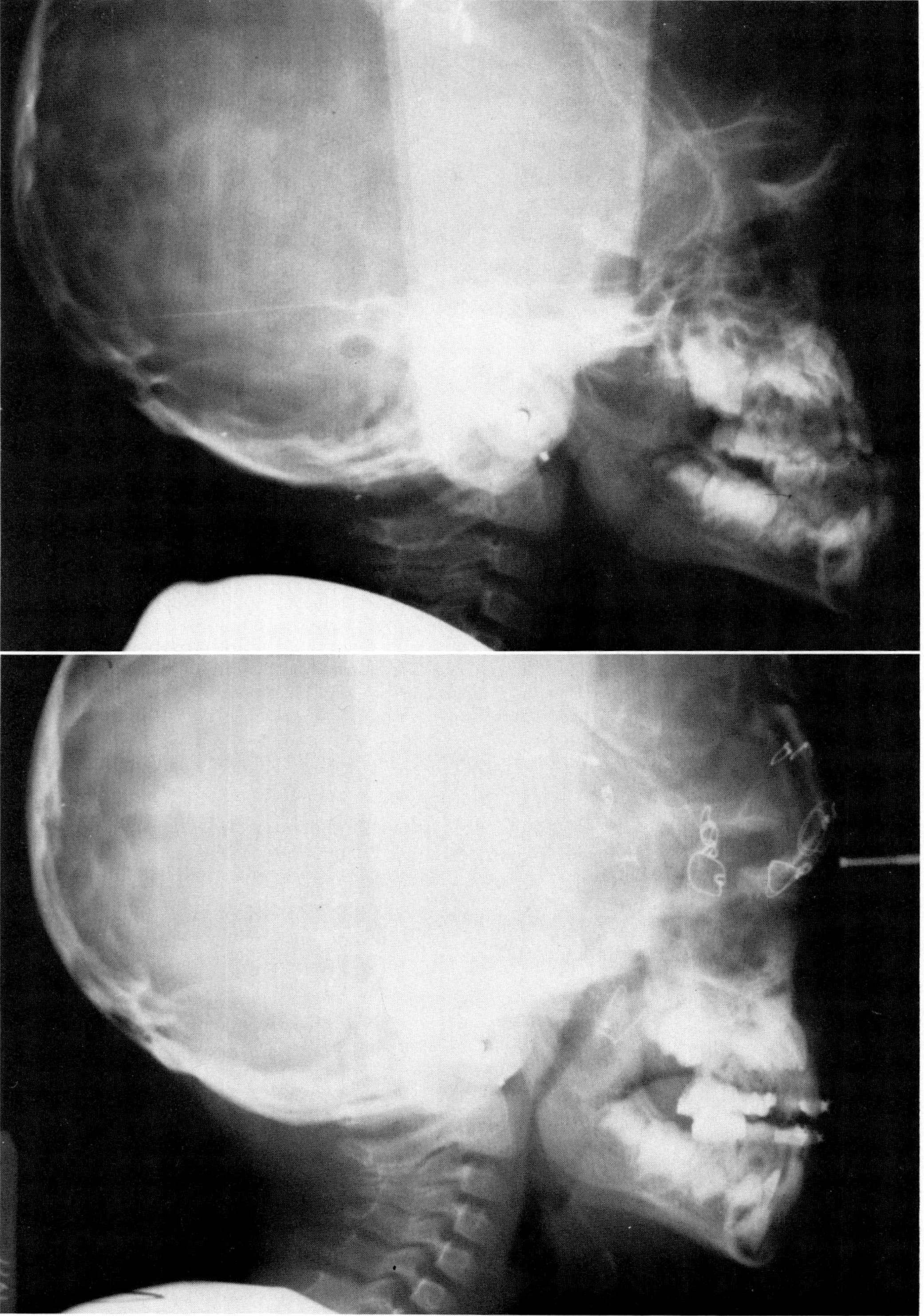

Fig. 16-3. Lateral radiographs before and after midfacial advancement demonstrating increased nasopharyngeal air space and improved dental arch relationships.

a more normal resonance in the postoperative state. Articulation skills are generally improved postoperatively. This improvement in the acoustic production of speech is due to the construction of a more normal dental arch relationship (Fig. 16-3).

VELOPHARYNGEAL COMPETENCY

Velopharyngeal competency is the primary goal of cleft palate management. A competent velopharyngeal mechanism enables the speaker to achieve two goals: (1) to consistently produce speech that is perceived to have normal oral-nasal resonance balance and (2) to develop oral pressure for articulation without audible nasal air emission. Achievement of these goals depends on the interaction of respiratory effort and velopharyngeal orifice size (Table 16-2).[24]

Completely acceptable resonance is achieved when the velopharyngeal orifice size is 10 mm^2 or less. An orifice size from 10 to 20 mm^2 generally produces mild hypernasality. Any opening greater than 20 mm^2 produces significant hypernasal resonance.

Differential oral-nasal air pressure is similarly affected by velopharyngeal orifice size. When copmlete closure of the portal occurs on the production of a word containing no nasal consonants (e.g., peat), the air pressure in the oral cavity will be 3 cm H$_2$O, or higher, depending on the respiratory effort. If an opening occurs in the portal, the oral pressure will vary with the size of the opening and the respiratory effort. The consequence of this pressure loss will be an auditory perception of air escape, hypernasality, and inadequate production of pressure phonemes.

PHYSIOLOGY OF VELOPHARYNGEAL CLOSURE

The work of Skolnick, McCall, and Barnes[19] illustrates that a VPI may appear in many shapes and sizes. Their work also shows that as a three-dimensional structure, the velopharyngeal portal should be observed in at least two planes of space in order to adequately evaluate the shape and size of the VPI. Fig. 16-4 illustrates several of the patterns of velopharyngeal closure documented by Skolnick, McCall,

Table 16-2. Relationships pertinent to velopharyngeal competence

Resonance rating	Velopharyngeal competency	Velopharyngeal orifice size	Differential oral-nasal air pressure
Normal resonance, infrequent hypernasality	Competent	Less than 10 mm^2	Greater than 3 cm H$_2$O
Normal resonance, infrequent hypernasality, or consistent slight hypernasality	Borderline competency	Between 10 and 20 mm^2	1 to 2.99 cm H$_2$O or may vary above and below 3 cm H$_2$O
Consistent hypernasality: slight, moderate or severe	Incompetent	Greater than 20 mm^2	Less than 1 cm H$_2$O

Based on data from Warren, D.: Cleft Palate J. **16**:279, 1979.

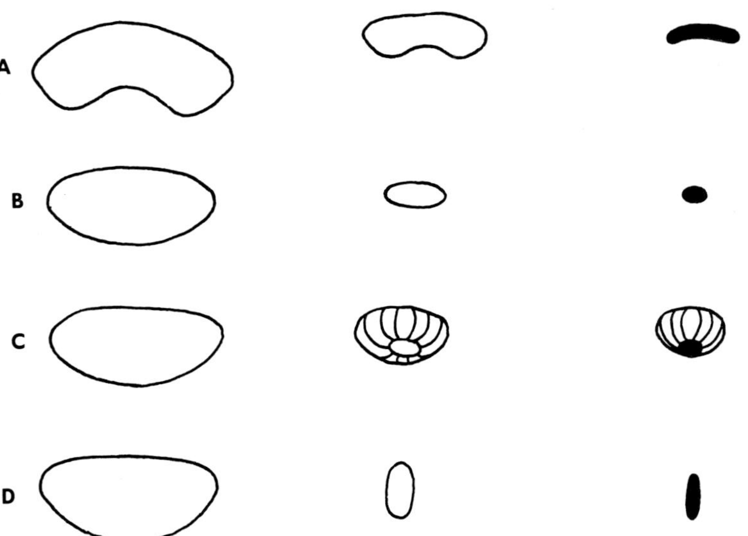

Fig. 16-4. Patterns of velopharyngeal closure as viewed from the nasopharynx. **A,** Coronal pattern. **B,** Circular pattern without Passavant's ridge. **C,** Circular pattern with Passavant's ridge. **D,** Sagittal pattern.

and Barnes.[19] Some individuals achieve velopharyngeal closure primarily by the posterior and superior elevation of the velum to make a broad contact against the posterior pharyngeal wall (Fig. 16-4, *A*). In other individuals mesial movement of the lateral pharyngeal walls combines with velar elevation to develop a sphincteric pattern (Fig. 16-4, *B* and *C*). Active development of a bulge or Passavant's ridge on the posterior pharyngeal wall may accompany either of these patterns (Fig. 16-4, *C*). Passavant's ridge has been found to contribute to velopharyngeal closure in a large percentage of individuals (37%) in whom the ridge is observed.[5] Often, however, Passavant's ridge appears below the point of velar elevation and does not contribute to velopharyngeal closure. One last pattern of velopharyngeal closure was described by Skolnick, McCall, and Barnes.[19] In this pattern there is little velar elevation but extremely active mesial movement of the lateral pharyngeal walls. It is the contact of one lateral wall to the other that achieves closure of the portal (Fig. 16-4, *D*).

EVALUATING VELOPHARYNGEAL FUNCTION

A three-step evaluation of velar function is the most expedient. The first step rates the qualities of oral-nasal resonance balance and intraoral air pressure. The second step involves a screening of velopharyngeal competency using indirect measures. A screening test identifies patients with a velopharyngeal opening and distinguishes them from those who make complete closure. Patients who fail the screening and are candidates for management of the VPI are then evaluated using objective measures. The results of this third stage are used for planning and documenting the results of management.

The purpose of the following discussion is to describe methods for rating and screening patients for velopharyngeal closure and then objectively measuring the parameters of VPI. Although the discussion will deal primarily with cleft palates, the procedures for diagnosing, quantifying, and managing VPI are applicable to VPI as a sequela to adenoidectomy, submucous cleft, neuromotor disorders, or hearing loss.

Rating scales of velopharyngeal function

The most important assessment of velopharyngeal competency, which is the least sensitive, is that made by rating certain characteristics of the individual's conversation speech. The ratings represent a listener's perception of speech qualities as they appear in a natural speaking situation. The decision to manage a VPI rests heavily on this rating.

A simple scale of oral-nasal resonance balance might include the following categories: (1) hyponasality, (2) acceptable resonance balance, (3) borderline hypernasality, and (4) obvious hypernasality. One word of caution, hypernasality and hyponasality may appear in one individual simultaneously. The most frequent cause is the presence of

a VPI and an anterior nasal obstruction (e.g., inflamed mucosa, enlarged turbinates, or a deviated septum).

Oral breath pressure behind the pressure consonants and nasal air emission also should be assessed. In most instances oral breath pressure is the inverse of nasal air emission. As one increases, the other is reduced. Thus they represent a continuum and may be represented on the same scale. Oral breath pressure is that pressure which develops behind the oral articulators. For example, the breath pressure that develops behind the closed lips differentiates the /b/ from the /m/ sound. During conversation listen to the force of the airstream behind the pressure consonants /p/, /b/, /t/, /d/, /k/, /g/, and the other pressure consonants. (See Table 16-1.) The presence of grimacing is typically a positive indicator of VPI. Grimacing is an attempt to occlude the nasal airway anteriorly. It is never successful.

Screening velopharyngeal closure

Screening procedures make use of any one of many indirect, clinical tests of velopharyngeal closure. The materials needed are inexpensive and readily available in most clinical settings. The procedures are easily performed, and noninvasive and are used to confirm the presence or absence of velopharyngeal closure.

The ability to detect closure varies with the sensitivity of the index used. A rating scale of oral-nasal resonance balance is possibly the least sensitive of the indices that we use. On the other hand, the listening tube is one of the more sensitive screening devices.

The ability to detect the various components of VPI (i.e., hypernasality or nasal air emission) also varies with the index used. One index might be more sensitive to detecting nasal airflow (e.g., an air paddle), whereas another index might be more sensitive to nasal resonance (e.g., cul-de-sac test).

Cul-de-sac test

The cul-de-sac, or nasal flutter, test is particularly sensitive to hypernasal resonance. The examiner asks the patient to repeat each word twice, holding the nose the second time. If the nasal cavity is coupled to the oral cavity during the repetition of these words, there will be a distinct difference in the resonance tone between the two repetitions. A difference in resonance tone is a positive indicator of VPI. Since the cul-de-sac test is especially sensitive to resonance, the words "beat," "bat," "boot," and "bought" are useful in a routine screening. These words incorporate simple, early learned, voiced consonant sounds to eliminate the influence of articulation deficiency, as well as an assortment of high and low vowels.

Nasal listening tube

One of the most sensitive assessments of nasal resonance can be made with the nasal listening tube.[2,12,26] The listening tube is an 18-inch (45 cm) length of rubber tubing with a nasal tip or olive attached to either end. The nasal listening tube, like the stethoscope, requires experience to use it successfully. One olive is placed in the patient's most free-breathing nostril and the other in the clinician's ear while the patient repeats the speech sample.

Since both hypernasal resonance and nasal air emission may be acoustic events, the nasal listening tube is particularly appropriate. With the appropriate speech sample, the nasal listening tube is equally able to assess the presence of hypernasal resonance or the presence of nasal air emission. The words "beat," "bat," "boot," "bought," "people," "paper," "puppy," and "sixty-six" are helpful when using the listening tube.

With some training the clinician is able to detect the presence of "pharyngeal flutter," which results from a borderline or touch contact of the velopharyngeal structures. This has diagnostic and planning implications as suggested below.

The clinician will find that some children who are judged with the unaided ear to exhibit normal resonance will exhibit nasal resonance or touch closure with the nasal listening tube and cul-de-sac tests. These children usually fall within the "borderline" closure category and are not typically candidates for physical management. However, this finding does yield important diagnostic information. If radiographic data demonstrate that the velum is elevating against a large adenoid pad, a VPI could be created if the adenoids were removed or if the adenoids involute. These children should be monitored closely.

In summary, there are many simple screening methods for VPI without the use of exotic, expensive, or invasive techniques or exposing the patient to radiation. We did not discuss airpaddles, scape scopes, or many other simple, available instruments. Those few discussed are some of the more useful techniques.

Quantifying velopharyngeal competency

Once the diagnosis of VPI has been made with the screening procedures, it is important to quantify the parameters of the VPI. This is important for two reasons. The test results allow us to compare the patient to a normative sample and to quantify the patient's preoperative and postoperative status. Thus they provide the means for quantifying the results of management procedures.

Pressure flow instrumentation

Warren[24] presents a technique and instrumentation for assessing velopharyngeal competency during speech by differentially measuring oral and nasal air pressures. The PERCI-II (Palatal Efficiency Rating Computed Instantaneously) simultaneously records the differential pressure between the oral and nasal cavities, measures airflow in the nasal cavity, provides an estimate of velopharyngeal orifice size, and measures airway conductance. Any one of the four parameters can be selected for digital display. Analog signals are available from output jacks. These outputs allow simultaneous recordings of these parameters when the PERCI-II is joined with an analog chart recorder (Fig. 16-5).

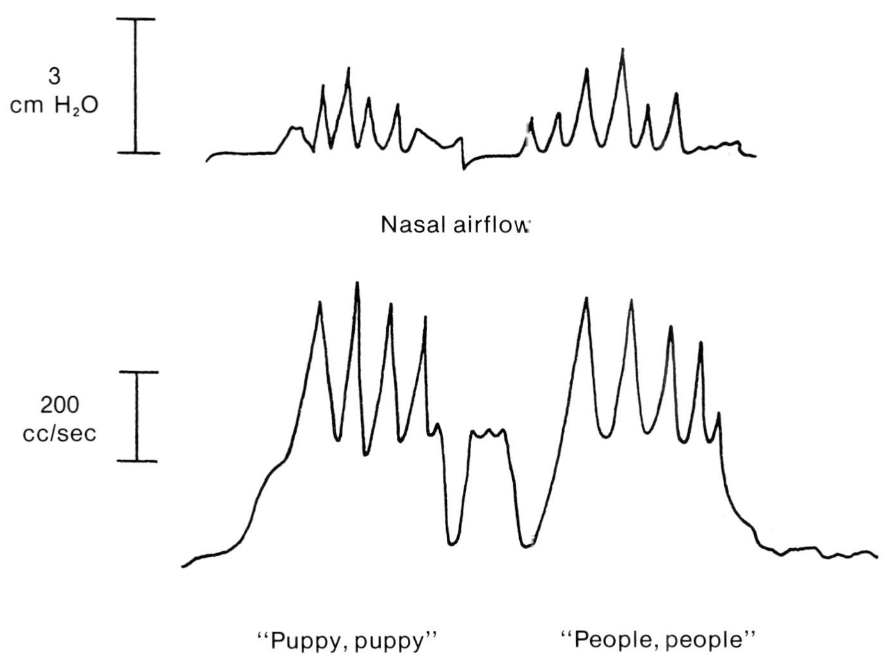

Fig. 16-5. Strip chart recording of differential oral-nasal air pressure *(top)* and rate of nasal airflow *(bottom)*. This patient falls within the range of borderline velopharyngeal competency.

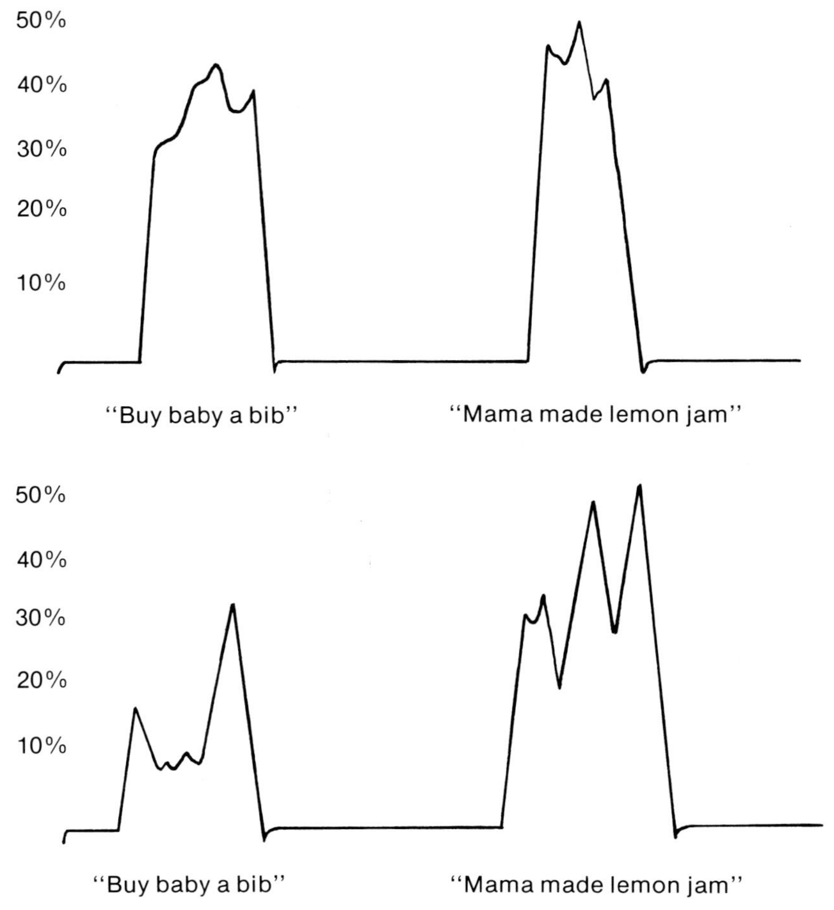

Fig. 16-6. X-Y plotter recording nasality ratios from TONAR-II.[4] An oral and a nasal speech sample are contrasted preoperatively *(top)* and postoperatively *(bottom)*.

Oral-nasal acoustic ratio

The objective measurement of nasality is one of the reported features of TONAR-II, or The Oral-Nasal Acoustic Ratio.[4] TONAR-II simultaneously measures the intensity of the auditory signals emerging from the oral and nasal cavities. It then provides electronically computed ratio readouts that are converted into a digital reading in the percentage of nasality. During an oral speech sample 0% to 20% nasality indicates normal oral-nasal resonance balance. Ratios above 20% indicate increasing degrees of VPI.[4] TONAR-II analog signals are available from output jacks, thus providing a hard copy when coupled with an analog recorder (Fig. 16-6).

Visualizing the velopharyngeal portal

Although the instruments just discussed provide quantitative measures of parameters associated with VPI, they do not provide any information about the amount or type of velopharyngeal movement, nor do they define structurel abnormalities. Such important information can be provided only from visualizing the velopharyngeal portal. Since the velopharyngeal mechanism demonstrates several movement patterns and is a three-dimensional structure, its analysis also requires observation of the mechanism at different angles in order to assemble a three-dimensional picture of velopharyngeal movement. Currently, it appears that this goal can be achieved best by a combination of lateral cinefluoroscopy and nasal endoscopy.

Cinefluoroscopy

Clinicians working in hospitals have access to fluoroscopic units. By adding a television or motion picture camera to the unit it is possible to achieve video or cinefluoroscopic studies of velopharyngeal function. The midsagittal view is the most frequent study employed. Frontal, basilar, or oblique views of the portal can be obtained, but similar information can be obtained using a nasal-endoscopic examination that does not expose the patient to additional radiation.

Cinefluoroscopy has certain advantages over still lateral radiographs. The most important advantage is that it allows observation of the velopharyngeal mechanism during speech

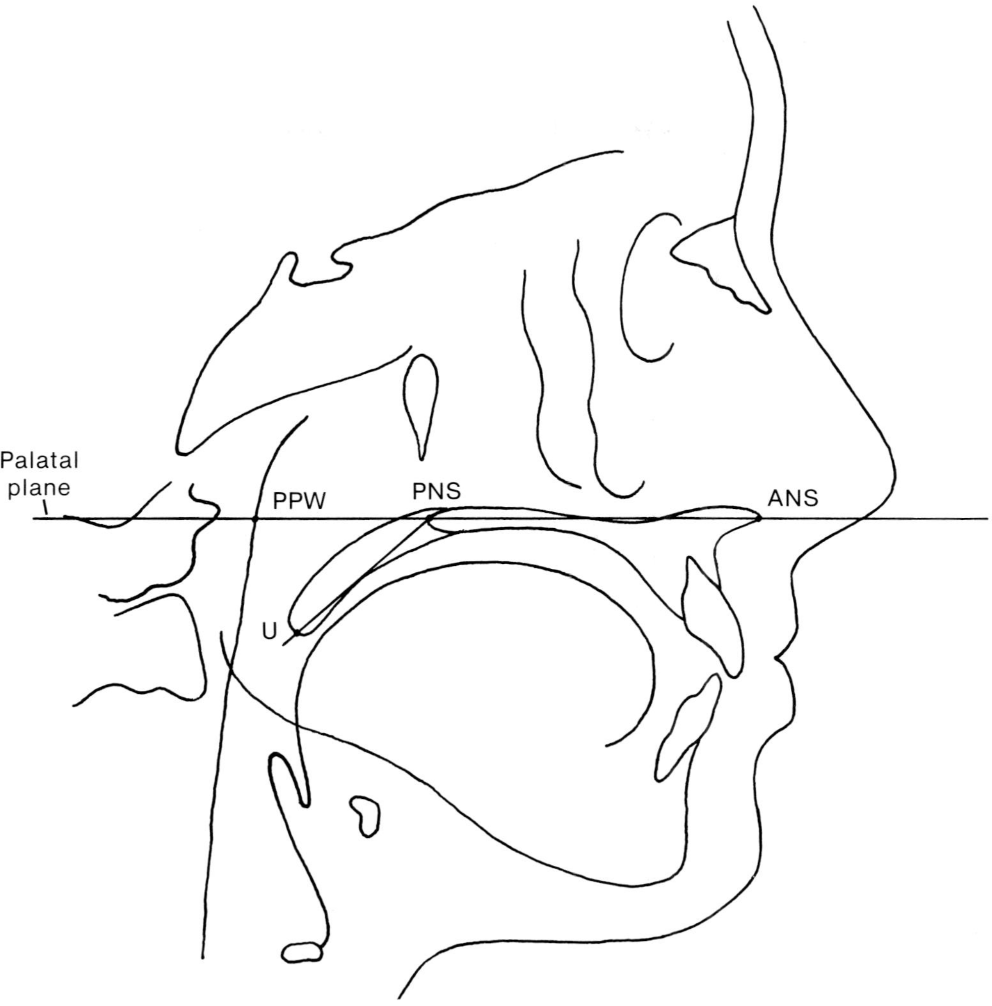

Fig. 16-7. Line drawing of a lateral radiograph demonstrating measurements of velar lengths *(PNS-U)* and nasopharyngeal depth *(PNS-PPW)*. These measurements can be compared to normal values compiled by Subtelny.[21] Analysis of the Subtelny data suggests that the normal length-to-depth ratio is 3:2. *ANS,* Anterior nasal spine; *PNS,* posterior nasal spine; *U,* distal tip of uvula; *PPN,* posterior pharyngeal wall.

function, not just during sustained phonation. Thus the appropriateness and timing of movement can be observed. This is important, since the movement of the velum during sustained phonation is not indicative of its movement during conversational speech.[27,28]

Measurements of velar length and depth of the nasopharynx also can be obtained from radiographs (Fig. 16-7). For the sake of analysis, these measures can be compared to the normative data assembled by Subtelny.[21]

A cinefluoroscopic study often provides valuable information that supplements the oral examination. An oral examination includes estimating the length of the soft palate and the depth of the nasal pharynx; however, such judgments are difficult and frequently misleading. For example, a 14-year-old girl who had a repaired cleft of the hard and soft palate was recently seen by the Cleft Palate Board. On oral examination she seemed to have an excessive distance between the inferior border of the soft palate and the posterior pharyngeal wall. However, listening to her conversational speech indicated oral-nasal resonance to be within normal limits, and adequate oral air pressure was present for consonant sound production. Moreover, a cinefluoroscopic study completed 2 years earlier demonstrated that the velum made appropriate and consistent contact against a large adenoid pad just above the first cervical vertebrae. Because of the height of the adenoids, they were not visible on oral examination. The velum was making contact with the posterior pharyngeal wall, which was displaced anteriorly by adenoid tissue that was not visible on oral examination (Fig. 16-8).

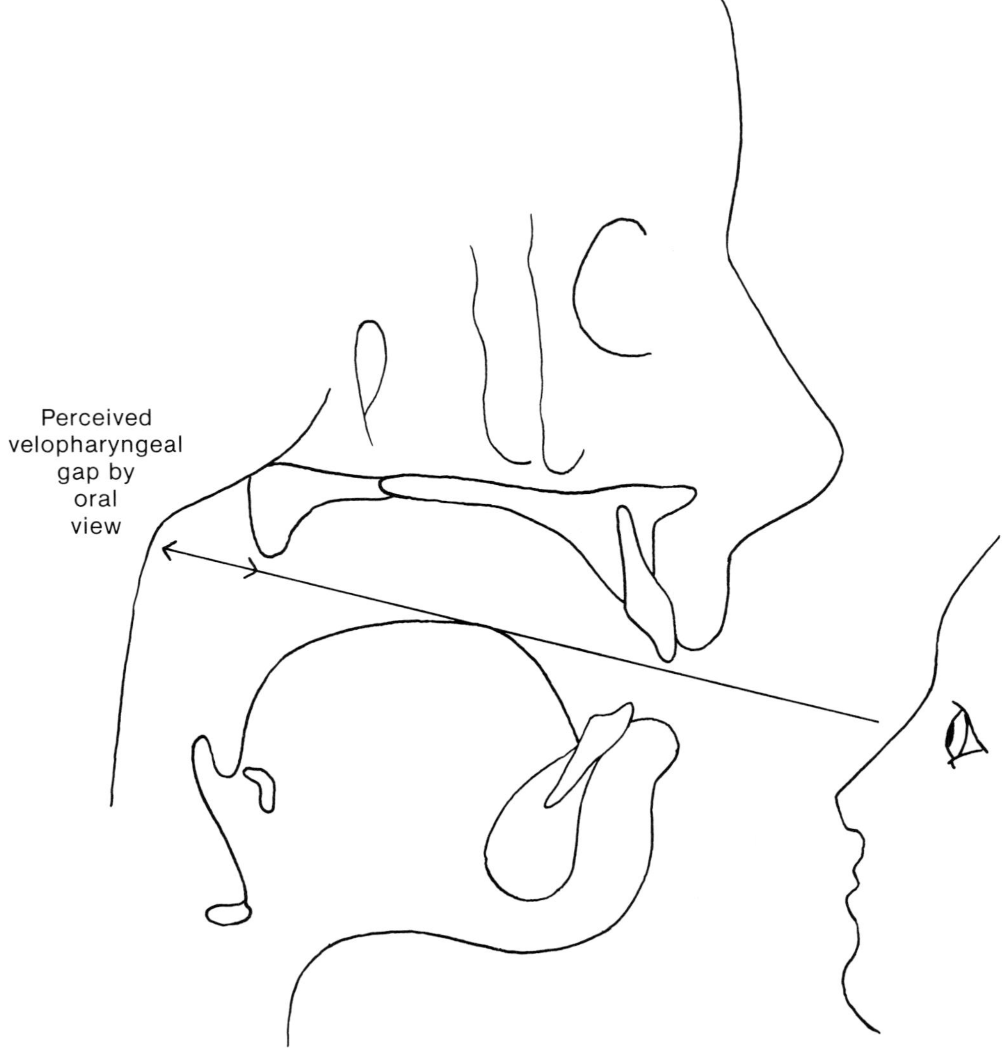

Fig. 16-8. Line drawing of a lateral radiograph demonstrating velopharyngeal closure against an anteriorly displaced adenoid pad. The line of sight *(arrow)* on oral examination would suggest a deep nasopharynx and a large velopharyngeal opening.

Nasal endoscopy

The development of the flexible fiberoptic nasal endoscope has added to the armamentarium of the clinician who wishes to visualize the velopharyngeal portal. The Machida ENT-US-25 endoscope is 3.9 mm in diameter, and the distal tip can be deflected downward by the examiner to view the portal. The scope can be attached to a video camera, 35 mm camera, or movie camera for the purpose of making records.

Like cinefluoroscopy, nasal endoscopy enables the clinician to view the portal during speech function. From the superior view the contributions of the lateral pharyngeal walls in narrowing the portal can be assessed. Observations can be made of the size and shape of the VPI. This view also provides an excellent vantage point for assessing the mass of the vulva on the nasal side of the velum, as well as any deformities of the torus tubarius.

Nasal endoscopy provides added information and supplements the oral examination. Recently a 13-year-old boy with a repaired cleft of the lip and palate and an inferiorly based pharyngeal flap appeared for treatment. On oral examination the flap was visible; it appeared to extend from the inferior third of the velum to the posterior pharyngeal wall approximately 1 cm below the resting soft palate. The flap was very narrow, approximately 5 to 6 mm wide. There was an anterior oral-nasal fistula that did not contribute to nasal airflow. Conversational speech was characterized by audible nasal emission of air on sibilant sounds and mild hypernasal resonance.

Because of the pharyngeal flap, a lateral cineradiographic

study was deferred, and a nasal endoscopic examination was completed to evaluate the effectiveness of the pharyngeal flap for obturating the nasopharynx. The pharyngeal flap was visualized. However, on phonation, the soft palate elevated and obscured the view of the pharyngeal flap. Further examination revealed that the velum elevated consistently for the speech sample studied. A very wide but shallow velopharyngeal gap remained even at the best attempts at closure. Mucus pooled along this line could be seen bubbling throughout the speech sample. There was no mesial movement of the lateral pharyngeal walls toward the low pharyngeal flap. Our assessment suggested that the pharyngeal flap was not at a sufficient height to assist in the pharyngeal closure.

MANAGING SPEECH ABERRANCIES: THE COOPERATION OF SPEECH PATHOLOGISTS AND PLASTIC SURGEONS

After the evaluation of the speech mechanism and its function, the role of the speech clinician is to provide management for aberrant speech behaviors. During the remediation process, interaction among the team members continues. Frequently treatment is staged so that as management by one professional is completed, management by another begins. Successful management therefore depends on successful communication among team members and continued assessment of the patient's needs. Surgical management of VPI is discussed in Chapter 21. The purpose of this discussion is to illustrate the role of the speech pathologist in the management of speech disorders associated with VPI and to demonstrate interaction among team members during a management regimen.

Functional VPI

As stated earlier, *functional* speech disorders exist because of faulty learning. They exist in the presence of an adequate speech mechanism. Although their initial cause might have been a structural defect, they continue to exist despite successful management of the structural defect.

Faulty use of the velopharyngeal valve has been described by Peterson-Falzone[7,8] and Riski and Paone.[14] Riski and Paone[14] described a "functional" VPI (or a "sound-specific" VPI) in patients who (1) had a transient, or previously managed VPI; (2) exhibited faulty learning of oral-nasal valving; and (3) exhibited a moderate hearing loss. A functional VPI was characterized as follows:

1. Normal oral-nasal resonance balance
2. Adequate oral breath pressure for some consonants, usually the plosives
3. Substitutions of nasal air emission or pharyngeal fricatives for specific phonemes, usually the silibants (e.g., /s/, /sh/) or affricates (e.g., /ch/, /dg/)

Treatment of these speech deficits falls within the realm of the speech/language pathologist.

Case 1. D.L. was a 23-year-old woman who had bilateral, moderately severe, precipitous, sensorineural hearing loss.

The hearing loss was diagnosed at 21 years of age. Conversational speech was characterized by both hyponasality and nasal emission of air, particularly for the /s/ sounds. This misarticulation was not the result of VPI. It was caused by inadequate auditory feedback. This speech disturbance, as noted earlier, qualifies as a functional VPI. The patient was subsequently fitted with a hearing aid and enrolled in an aural rehabilitation program in the community.

Speech therapy when surgery is contraindicated

In some instances other medical concerns must take precedence over palatal surgery so that a child is left with a longstanding VPI. When this happens therapy is often indicated to aid in language and articulation development. When the VPI is managed, the child has a competent auditory and kinesthetic feedback system for monitoring velopharyngeal valving.

Case 2. N.A. was born with multiple anomalies, including velar paresis, a ventricular septal defect, congenital agenesis of the auricles, stenosis of the external ear canals, a tracheoesophageal fistula, and right facial paresis. Her history included feeding problems such as nasal regurgitation, choking, and difficulty chewing. Initial speech evaluation at 3 years, 10 months of age revealed severely hypernasal speech secondary to a short, immobile palate. Spontaneous speech was generally unintelligible, with only vowels and the consonant /m/ employed. A 7- to 8-month receptive language delay was found. The plastic surgeon believed that palatal surgery could not be performed until the heart condition was improved. She underwent open heart surgery at 6 years, 6 months of age and pharyngeal flap surgery at 7 years, 4 months of age. During the 3½ years between the initial evaluation and palatal surgery, she received speech therapy with the goals of improving receptive language skills, developing syntactic structures, teachinig correct production of nonpressure phonemes within her present abilities (/l/, /n/, /ng/, /w/, /h/, /r/) to increase speech intelligibility, and teaching her air pressure and airflow sounds with the nares occluded by the clinician. In the last speech evaluation before palatal surgery, receptive language skills were within normal limits, with expressive language deficits occurring primarily in the use of selected rules of grammar. She was using all consonant phonemes that were not significantly affected by lack of intraoral air supply, and she was achieving recognizable approximations of (/d/, /t/, /f/, and /g/).

Trial therapy to assess potential for speech

In some cases, the presence of a severe VPI can be diagnosed, but the presence of other problems may suggest that it is inappropriate or unnecessary to manage the VPI.

Case 3. A 5-year-old boy (A.H.) had congenital cranial nerve involvement and a repaired cleft of the hard and soft palate. Cranial nerves VI, VII, X, and XII were involved. He had a masklike facies an found it difficult to approximate his lips. In addition, little or no tongue movement was visible. During chewing, A.H. moved a bolus of food from one side of the mouth to the other using his fingers. When necessary he would also push the bolus of food to the back of the mouth to be swallowed. Swallowing was completed by a very infantile pattern in which the mandible assisted tongue elevation. The velum was not observed to move during an oral examination. Subsequent cineradiographic study confirmed that there was no velar movement. Conversational speech was characterized by consistent use of the glottal stop and hypernasal distortion. Intelligibility was poor to a naive listener, even though the mother had little difficulty in understanding the patient. Because of the limited tongue and lip movement, it was questioned whether or not this patient had the potential to develop any oral communication. It was suggested that a period of trial speech therapy for 1 year be undertaken to assess this potential. The goal of the therapy program was to establish consistent lip closure for the consonants /m/, /p/, and /b/ and to assess the ability of the tongue to retract to produce a /k/ and /g/ sound. For the pressure sounds /p/, /b/, /k/, and /g/, a swimmer's nose clip was used during speech therapy to occlude the nasal airway and allow intraoral pressure to develop. The patient was reevaluated after 1 year of speech therapy. During the reevaluation it was demonstrated that with the swimmer's nose clip in place the patient could consistently produce the pressure phonemes /p/, /b/, /g/, and /f/ in single words and with adequate oral air pressure. Conversational speech without the use of the nose clip remained distorted by hypernasal resonance and marked by consistent use of the glottal stop. It should be noted that this type of therapy regimen does not offer much in the way of carry-over into conversational speech, since the patient is able to generate intraoral breath pressure only with the nose clip in place. After reevaluation it was recommended that a wide superiorly based pharyngeal flap be constructed to establish velopharyngeal competency. The pharyngoplasty has now been completed, and the child has normal oral-nasal resonance. In addition, adequate breath pressure and complete velopharyngeal closure is observed for sounds not affected by poor tongue mobility.

SUMMARY

In summary, the child born with a palatal cleft faces severe hazards to normal speech and language development. These hazards include VPI, dental arch malformations, and hearing loss. The most significant problem is usually VPI. The presence of a velopharyngeal opening may be evaluated using simple, noninvasive diagnostic tests. Furthermore, velopharyngeal function may be quantified using pressure flow instrumentation and visualized using radiography and nasal endoscopy. Management is often a two-step procedure: (1) management of the VPI and (2) management of the aberrant compensatory misarticulations. Therefore management of a VPI involves the cooperative efforts of a cleft palate team with special input from the plastic surgeon, dental specialist, and speech pathologist.

REFERENCES

1. Arlt, P.B., and Goodban, M.T.: A comparative study of articulation acquisition as based on a study of 240 normals, aged three to six, Lang. Speech Hear. Serv. School **7:**173, 1976.
2. Blakeley, R.W.: The practice of speech pathology: a clinical diary, Springfield, Ill., 1972, Charles C Thomas, Publisher.
3. Cohen, M.M.: Syndromes with cleft lip and palate, Cleft Palate J. **15:**306, 1978.
4. Fletcher, S.G.: Diagnosing speech disorders from cleft palate, New York, 1978, Grune & Stratton, Inc.
5. Glaser, E.R., Skolnick, M.L., McWilliams, B.J., and Shprintzen, R.J.: The dynamics of Passavant's ridge in subjects with and without velopharngeal insufficiency—a multi-view videofluoroscopic study, Cleft Palate J. **16:**24, 1979.
6. Morris, H.: Velopharyngeal competence and primary cleft palate surgery, 1960-1971: a critical review, Cleft Palate J. **10:**62, 1973.
7. Peterson-Falzone, S.J.: Nasal emission as a component of the misarticulation of sibilants and affricates, J. Speech Hear. Disord. **40:**106, 1975.
8. Peterson-Falzone, S.J.: Nasal distortions and compensatory articulations in velopharyngeal competent speakers, Presented at the Fourth International Congress on Cleft Palate and Related Craniofacial Anomalies, Acapulco, Mexico, May 1981.
9. Poole, I.: Genetic development of articulation of consonant sounds in speech, Elem. Eng. Rev. **11:**159, 1934.
10. Prather, E.M., Hedrick, D.L., and Kern, C.A.: Articulation development in children age two to four years, J. Speech Hear. Disord. **40:**179, 1975.
11. Riski, J.E.: The development of articulation skills and oral nasal resonance in children with cleft palate receiving pharyngeal flaps, Cleft Palate J. **16:**421, 1979.
12. Riski, J.E., and Millard, R.T.: Processes of speech: evaluation and treatment. In Cooper, H.K., et al., editors: Cleft palate and cleft lip, Philadelphia, 1979, W.B. Saunders Co.
13. Riski, J.E., Millard, R.T., Watt, C., et al.: Longitudinal analysis of speech development in children with clefts from three to eight years, San Francisco, 1976, American Cleft Palate Association.
14. Riski, J.E., and Paone, C.A.: Functional velopharyngeal incompetency: diagnosis and management, Detroit, 1980, American Speech and Hearing Association.
15. Riski, J.E., and Williams, W.N.: Articulation development in children with palatal clefts, Chicago, 1977, American Speech and Hearing Association.
16. Riski, J.E., and Williams, W.N.: The influence of age and cleft type on articulation development of children with cleft lip/palate, San Diego, 1979, American Cleft Palate Association.
17. Riski, J.E., Williams, W.N., and DeLong, E.: Longitudinal appraisal of the effects of age and cleft type on the articulation development of 108 children with cleft lip/palate, Proceedings of the International Association of Logopedics and Phoniatrics, Washington, D.C., Aug. 1980.
18. Sander, E.K.: When are speech sounds learned? J. Speech Hear. Disord. **37:**54, 1972.
19. Skolnick, M.L., McCall, G., and Barnes, M.: The sphincteric mechanism of velopharyngeal closure, Cleft Palate J. **10:**286, 1973.
20. Spriestersbach, D.C., and Powers, G.R.: Articulation skills, velopharyngeal closure and oral breath pressure of children with cleft palate, J. Speech Hear. Res. **2:**318, 1959.
21. Subtelny, J.D.: A cephalometric study of the growth of the soft palate, Plast. Reconstr. Surg. **19:**49, 1957.
22. Templin, M.C.: Certain language skills in children, Minneapolis, 1957, The University of Minnesota Press.
23. Van Demark, D.R.: Misarticulation and listener judgments of the speech of individuals with cleft palates, Cleft Palate J. **1:**232, 1964.
24. Warren, D.: Perci: a method for rating palatal efficiency, Cleft Palate J. **16:**279, 1979.
25. Wellman, B.L., Case, I.M., Mengert, I.G., and Bradbury, D.E.: Speech sounds of young children, University of Iowa Studies in Child Welfare, vol. 5, 1936.
26. Westlake, H., and Rutherford, D.: Cleft palate, Englewood Cliffs, N.J., 1966, Prentice-Hall, Inc.
27. Williams, W.N., and Eisenbach, C.R.: Assessing VP function: the lateral still technique vs. cinefluorography, Cleft Palate J. **18:**45, 1981.
28. Williams, W.N., Eisenbach, C.R., Bzoch, K.R., et al.: Clinical guidelines in selecting a speech sample for the radiographic assessment of velopharyngeal function, Gainesville, Fla., May 1976, Florida Cleft Palate Association.

CHAPTER 17

Psychologic considerations: patients with clefts and craniofacial malformations

EDWARD CLIFFORD

Birth defects and their sequelae are significant problems for our society. Although the nature of the defect is of crucial importance and has implications for treatment, its significance extends beyond the individual. A chain of reactions follows such births. The family and the primary health care professionals are immediately involved. Shortly thereafter, a number of other relevant professionals may be consulted. Later speech pathologists, audiologists, dentists, teachers, and others will become involved.

The defect itself is not static. It can be rightfully stressed that clefts of the lip and palate are repairable. After the primary repair individuals and professionals actually deal with the sequelae associated with the cleft rather than with the original cleft condition. Similarly, a growing number of the more severe craniofacial malformations are now amenable to surgical intervention, the later effects of which we will examine.

My purpose in this chapter will be to examine cleft lip, cleft palate, and other craniofacial anomalies from a psychologic perspective. More specifically I will examine several themes in the clinical and research literature about these patients. Within each theme I will examine underlying assumptions and stated or unstated hypotheses and examine them in the light of available supporting evidence. The following thematic areas will be presented:

1. The impact of the affected child on parents and the family
2. The effect of the defect on the developing personality
3. The status of patients at maturity
4. The effects of treatment on patients

THE IMPACT OF THE AFFECTED CHILD ON PARENTS AND THE FAMILY

From a developmental perspective it is taken for granted that early growth experiences universally influence the expression of later behaviors. For the parent of a child with a defect, as well as for the child, emerging psychologic processes may be additionally affected by a simple fact— the child was born with a defect. In the developmental sequence of events we turn to the birth because it is a commonly recognized beginning point; the parents and society see the child for the first time. When the child is born with a defect, it is often assumed that initial parental reactions will be indicative of their subsequent reactions to the child, ultimately affecting the emerging personality.

Parental first feelings

Giving birth to a baby with a defect initially evokes negative, rather than positive, feelings because the defect almost universally is perceived to be undesirable. These first reactions are usually intense, and a relatively broad range has been reported, including confusion, disappointment, disbelief, resentment and shock.[1,7,50,51] The initial intense parental reactions form part of the context in which affected babies must take their place, and they ultimately may be affected. It has been stressed that since strong emotions are expressed and intense emotions may be disorganizing, family disintegration follows because of the overwhelming nature of these feelings. There is evidence that in birth defects such as cerebral palsy[58] or in severe mental retardation,[20,21] family disintegration may be present in a significant number of cases.

Although no data are available about family disintegration and severe craniofacial malformations, a number of clinical and research investigations have examined parental reactions to the birth of a child with a cleft.* The evidence about families where a cleft palate is present tends to reject the hypothesis that family disintegration will follow. On the contrary, there is evidence that the birth of a baby with a cleft palate may have integrative effects. Couples reported positive changes in themselves after the birth of the affected baby. Independently spouses reported increases in marital satisfaction after the birth of the affected baby. Apparently husbands and wives gave each other mutual support in the face of the crisis, aiding each other to cope with the situation.[8,16,50,51]

There are some cases in which the initial aversive feelings persist, and one or both parents may be incapable of coping with the new set of circumstances. In such cases, family disruption can occur. Spriestersbach[51] reports that 7% of the fathers and 10% of the mothers in his sample believed that their marital relationship was adversely affected.

Some writers imply that these initial reactions continue unabated for relatively lengthy periods of time.[3,20,34] However, there is evidence that for most cases the initial shock-like reactions dissipate about the time the mother and baby leave the hospital.[8,50] Feelings of depression lasted only up to 4 days in a study of 13 sets of parents of babies with cleft lip and palate.[24] Once parents were able to overcome their initial reactions and master them, they were able to express love and compassion for the baby.[54] It has been suggested that there are several steps in the process of accommodating to the affected baby. The initial shock is succeeded by a feeling of unreality, followed by feelings of anxiety, anger, and sadness. A relatively lengthy period of adaptation follows, which evolves into a reorganization that leads to a more rewarding level of interaction with the affected infant.[19]

Continuing effects of the child on parents

Emerging psychologic processes and experiences are often affected by functional and structural limitations associated with a defect. Frequent concomitants of cleft palate are functional limitations of speech, hearing, and dentition. Visual and hearing impairments often are associated with other craniofacial anomalies. Although the health care professional is aware that such limitations are probably in the offing, parents are usually unaware of the true nature of the functional disorders until they emerge later in the course of development. Parents may have accommodated to the existence of the birth defect, but they still must make additional adjustments.

---

*The term *cleft palate* will be used to refer to all cleft conditions, unless a specific cleft type is mentioned. This generic use of the term is common practice if there are too few cases within a study to make meaningful differentiations, or if an author combines various cleft groupings because there are no statistically significant differences among them.

The mere existence of the defect induces a variety of adaptations, in part related to the nature of the defect and the presumed implications for the future. At the same time, parents and others are accommodating to the baby as a person. The baby born with a defect is an evolving, developing, dynamic individual who will be in constant interaction with others in the environment. During these interactions the baby will be affected by and influence all with whom he comes in contact.

Accommodations to appearance

Appearance begins to play a more central role for the parents as the child grows older. Infants are exposed to ever-increasing numbers of strangers who may further sensitize the parents to the child's appearance. Frequently a chance remark about the baby, a question about the child's condition, or frank staring takes place in circumstances over which parents have little or no control and for which they have to adopt defensive strategies.

Many parents have stated to me that the child with a craniofacial malformation becomes an object of staring during infancy and the preschool period. Various coping mechanisms are used, some of them oriented toward avoiding situations in which the likelihood of being stared at is high. Other coping mechanisms involve defensive strategies such as explaining what a cleft is to strangers or becoming hostile toward those who stare. Still other parents state that the curiosity is natural, despite the fact that it makes them uncomfortable.

A variety of parental feelings may be attached to the necessity of coping with staring or questioning about the child's appearance. A factor to be considered is whether the affected child represents a threat to the parents' competence, in which the appearance of the child is attributed to some fault in the parents.[57] It has been my clinical experience that parents express a degree of ambivalence about the situation. They express anger at the attitudes and behaviors of strangers, often accompanied by embarrassment, and at the same time, they express a willingness to explain the child's appearance. Some parents may feel that the anomaly has been imposed on them, whereas others believe they bear this burden as proof of their strength. It is possible that they are also ambivalent, loving the child, while feeling anger about the upset the child's condition has caused.

Accommodations to environment

Perhaps because of the staring problem and their heightened sensitivity, parents continue to be affected by the fact that the child has a cleft palate. A large number of activities are viewed by the parents as being problematic, and questions arise about performing routine tasks because of parental uncertainty about the amount of care and supervision the affected child will require.[57] From a purely clinical point of view, it is believed that children with cleft palates are raised in socially restrictive environments because the parents wish to avoid social contacts.[7] Research data, however, cast doubt on this speculation. In an extensive study, questionnaires were given to approximately 175 mothers and 175 fathers of normal children and a similar number of mothers and fathers of children with clefts.[51] Cleft palate had no demonstrable effects on the parents' social life, entertainment patterns, and recreational activities. No information is available about the environments provided for children with more severe craniofacial anomalies.

Either because of appearance factors or because the child's defects are viewed as handicapping conditions, the child can be seen as having special needs. These perceptions can be translated into providing a protective environment. It is believed that children with congenital anomalies are less likely to be taken out of the home and that they are provided with fewer opportunities to interact with friends and acquaintances. It also has been stated that these children are given no voice in family matters, are rarely given the opportunity to talk about their defect, are discouraged when they ask questions, and are rarely given appropriate responsibilities. In short the atmosphere in which they grow is seen as relatively restrictive, and their parents are perceived as being overly-solicitous or overprotective.[28,40,41,56] However, these speculations have not been substantiated.[12,52]

Early parent-child interactions

By the end of the preschool period, the child probably has had one or more surgical procedures, has been hospitalized and separated from parents and family, and has experienced a number of evaluations by various members of a cleft palate or craniofacial team. During infancy and the preschool period many parents begin to realize that their child's treatment involves more than surgery and that the diagnosis has other implications. There may be speech problems, hearing problems, orthodontic problems, or a combination of problems. The existence of these problems can tax family and personal resources, possibly affecting the nature of the parent-child relationship.

Early experiences related to the management of cleft palate can have effects on parental, as well as child, behaviors. A remarkable degree of passivity has been observed in these children in psychiatric interviews.[55] It was believed that the children were forced into this state because their mothers could not protect them. Mothers could only participate as passive onlookers when decisions about surgery and hospitalization were made. Mothers could not prevent the potential trauma of surgery and the enforced separation that hospitalization entails. These experiences might then induce feelings of helplessness and powerlessness in the parent and child. Unfortunately, almost no other data are available with which to corroborate or refute this position. This hypothesis was tested in samples of older children with cleft palate and their mothers and nonaffected peers and their mothers. The groups of mothers did not differ in their beliefs about the

extent to which their lives were controlled by external forces.[16]

The weight of the evidence cannot support the clinical speculations about the effect of cleft palate in particular on parents. It can be demonstrated that parents are upset at the birth of a baby with a defect. It can also be demonstrated that in general parents are able to cope with their feelings. Having a child with cleft palate may leave a mark on the parents, and they may become sensitized as a result, but the effects appear to be limited. These parents appear to cope with the problems presented rather than succumb to them.

THE EFFECT OF THE DEFECT ON THE DEVELOPING PERSONALITY

One of the major problems a person with a craniofacial defect must face, as do many with cleft palate, is the presence of a visible facial disfigurement. Patients with facial anomalies face discrimination and may suffer psychologic consequences.[29] Since the disfigurement deviates from the normal level of acceptability, the person's feelings about how others regard him and self-concepts can be negatively affected.

During infancy and the early years of development a child accumulates ever-increasing amounts of information about himself. Within the context of the family, parents and other family members act as social mirrors and provide feedback information. From these early experiences most children abstract a sense of being valued, of being accepted. In conjunction with developing competencies, the child's emerging concepts of the self are influenced.

Those responsible for management of the defect are also important sources of information about the child. Treatment efforts for the child with cleft palate, for example, take place during the crucial formative years, during which the child must make some accommodation to changes in appearance and functioning. The management of these patients usually involves repeated visits to hospitals and clinics for long-term treatment and evaluation. Children can and do abstract information about themselves during the course of treatment. In a sense professional efforts can lead the patient to feel defective of deficient in some way. In a similar manner, self-concepts and attitudes toward the body may be influenced by the therapeutic attempts devoted to correcting the defect.

The distillations of experiences, feelings, and attitudes toward the body—including its functioning and appearance—and self-judgments are integrated into the sense of self. Somewhere in the multiplicity of ongoing behaviors, the defect and its consequences are built into the self-system.

Craniofacial malformations and competency

Competency becomes an issue because the presence of any craniofacial malformation has implications beyond that of appearance. Brain function can be affected, resulting in intellectual deficits. Neurologic and sensory impairments are possible, leading to questions about integrity of visual-motor performance. Fluctuating hearing losses and pathologic speech can have an impact on the ability of the affected person to perform adequately. In sum, questions have been asked about the general competency of those with the defects.

Intelligence

Intellectual level is an important characteristic because it has implications for academic achievement and for the person's ultimate role as an adult. There may be associated mental retardation in some of the craniofacial anomalies, such as Apert's syndrome. In many craniofacial syndromes, as well as in cleft palate, however, retardation is not an invariant. Detailed information about the measured intelligence of children with specific craniofacial malformations is lacking. Of the children I see, however, many of them with more severe craniofacial malformations perform at an average level. Children with cleft palate are found to operate within the normal range of intelligence, although the intellectual level can be affected by the presence of other additional anomalies.[32] Although consistently lower scores have been obtained for children with cleft palate when compared to normal children,[23,26,45,59] these children are not remarkably different from their siblings when such factors as socioeconomic status, the parents' intellectual level, and the child's age, sex, and hearing status are systemically controlled.[46]

Visual-motor performance

On a clinical basis I have observed impaired performances in children with craniofacial malformations, such as Crouzon's disease, on tests of visual perception. No research data are available, however. Difficulties with perceptual motor tasks have been noted in children with cleft palate.[56] However, when these children are compared with their unaffected siblings, others find they perform similarly on tests of visual-motor integration.[25,45,46]

School achievement

School introduces the child to a formal learning process in which the what, when, how, and why of materials to be learned are in the hands of professional educators. It is expected that children will be ready developmentally for school. School readiness is age related and first-grade entrance usually occurs in the fall when the child is 6 years old, the age at which most children with cleft palate enter school as well.[51] A variety of academic tasks are set for the child, to which conformity is expected. These expectations are usually met. Children with craniofacial malformations who live at home do learn to read, write, spell, communicate, manipulate numbers, and solve a variety of problems with degrees of success differing among them as they do among other children.

How well children with cleft palate or other craniofacial

anomalies actually perform in school is still open to question. The academic achievement level of children with cleft palate is similar to their nonaffected siblings,[46] yet they perform more poorly than their nonaffected peers.[5,42] In part the performance level demonstrated may be related to the teachers' attitudes about appearance and about the effects of cleft palate. The teacher's impression of a child's intelligence quotient (IQ) has been found to be influenced by the presence of a visible defect. For example, teachers overestimate the ability of less bright children with cleft palate, whereas they underestimate the ability of brighter children with clefts.[43] In my experience teacher behavior is affected by the presence of more severe craniofacial malformations as well. Because of the defect the child is not expected to perform as well as classmates. Expectations of the child's performance in school are also influenced by appearance; the effects of unacceptable appearance on teachers' judgments have been amply demonstrated.[2]

Personality and adjustment

A possible stress point for the child and family occurs when the child is first introduced into the school system. Up to this point the parents have been able to exert some control over the child's environment, but their influence usually cannot be extended into the classroom. For example, the parents cannot prevent classmates or teachers from remarking on the child's appearance or speech. Children who are teased in school have to develop the means of coping with the teasing themselves. Thus one of the penalties a facial disfigurement exacts is being noticed, commented on, and teased. Although children develop a variety of ways of coping, a residue of ill feeling may remain. Teasing appears early in the school history of the child. In my interviews, however, many children report a precipitous drop in teasing by the end of second grade, and little or no teasing is reported at older age levels.

One means of coping with teasing about appearance or communication ineffectiveness is to adopt withdrawal behaviors, such as shyness and passivity. Parents of children with craniofacial anomalies characterize them as uncomfortable in the presence of strangers, quiet, and shy.[28] Compared to their normal peers children with cleft palate are described as more dependent, self-effacing, and compliant and less mature, confident, or socially outgoing.[31,51] Psychiatric evaluations reveal that children with cleft palate are noted for passivity and for exhibiting excessive dependency problems.[48] Teachers of children with cleft palate rate them as being more inhibited in the classroom than their parents do at home.[44] Clinically there appears to be consensual validation for a cluster of related behaviors found in those with cleft palate.

A more recent psychologic investigation about cleft palate emphasized two variables: locus of control and field articulation. Locus of control refers to the degree to which a person's life is believed to be under self-control or under the control of others. Children who see themselves as being controlled by fate, destiny, or outside forces have an external locus of control, whereas those who view their lives primarily as being self-determined have an internal locus of control. Field articulation refers to the relative influence of internal proprioceptive cues versus external visual cues on the person making perceptual judgments. When the influence of internal cues is high, the individual is field independent; when the influence of the visual context is high, the individual is field dependent. Adolescents with clefts are more external in their locus of control and are more field dependent than children without congenital defects.[5] Thus those with cleft palate appear to be more sensitive to environmental contexts.

Self-concepts and body image

The assumption that a defect has negative consequences on the person is central to the examination of self-concepts and body image. Experiences associated with the defect, including its sequelae, have a direct bearing on feelings of being accepted by one's parents, self-esteem, and attitudes toward one's body.

Feelings about parental acceptance

One approach to assessing feelings about parental acceptance is to ask the person with a congenital defect to imagine how his parents might have reacted to his birth. Since recall of the experience is not possible, it is assumed that these imagined responses are related to what the child was told about the birth, his own feelings about it, and his current feelings about his parents. The "when I was born" test was constructed for this purpose and used with various samples, including normal adolescents, adolescents with cleft palate, and adolescents with craniofacial anomalies.[9,14,15]

Affected adolescents with cleft palate or other craniofacial anomalies, in contrast to normal adolescents, perceive their parents as expressing more negative feelings about their birth, experiencing greater anxiety, exhibiting less pride in them at the time, and as having their infant-care practices more negatively affected. Clearly adolescents with these anomalies feel less accepted by their parents, presumably as a result of a birth defect.[5]

Self-concepts

It was already noted that affected children exhibit characteristics of shyness and passivity. This is coupled with characteristics of external locus of control and field-dependent perceptual organization. These characteristics, in combination with the birth defect, influence self-perceptions. The reported self-esteem of adolescents with cleft palate is high and positive.[9] When a number of self-concept measures are combined, self-esteem remains high and positive, even to the extent of being significantly more positive than that of normal peers.[4] Similarly, I find high and positive self-esteem in my patients with more severe craniofacial mal-

formations. This high level of self-regard can come about as a result of successful coping with the defect and its sequelae. In a sense self-esteem can be enhanced by the belief that the management of the defect has been successful.

Body image

With children who have visible body (facial) defects it is implied that the defect must induce a necessary and mandatory dissatisfaction as reflected in their body image. The term *body image* refers to a number of attitudes and reactions to the body and its functioning, as well as to a composite of a number of these. Many conflicting approaches have been used to measure body image, and this concept is still problematic.[53,60] It is rare, for example, that identical body image measures are used by differing investigators.

Paralleling the high self-esteem with which affected adolescents hold themselves, their degree of satisfaction with body parts and body functioning is equivalent to that of their normal age mates.[10,49] When a multiplicity of body image measures are used, adolescents with cleft palate cannot be differentiated from their normal peers. When they are compared to significantly obese adolescents, however, it can be demonstrated that the poorer body images of the latter are associated with obesity rather than with cleft palate.[4] It can also be demonstrated that the presence of cleft palate has subtle rather than gross effects on the body images of adolescents with this anomaly. Despite high overall satisfaction with their bodies, when degrees of satisfaction for each body part and each body function are examined, those with cleft palate are relatively and significantly less satisfied with voice, lips, nose, talking, speech, and teeth than are their normal peers.[49]

THE STATUS OF PATIENTS AT MATURITY

More information is available about the adult status of patients with clefts than about those with other craniofacial malformations. This is due in part to a long history of successful treatment of cleft palate and to the existence of the American Cleft Palate Association, which provides a forum for research about cleft palate. With the advent of newer intracranial surgical approaches, the growth of craniofacial treatment centers, and greater emphasis on and support for research about the more severe craniofacial defects, the paucity of information about these patients may well be corrected.

Status of patients with cleft palate

An examination of the roles patients with cleft palate occupy later in their lives can give us important information about the psychologic and social effects of being born with this defect.

Social relationships

The passivity noted in early life may be continued into adulthood. For example, adults with cleft palate clearly prefer passive to active leisure time activities. Passivity also may be reflected in their reporting that it is difficult for them to meet new people. They participate less frequently in voluntary social groups than do their unaffected peers. They have fewer friends but see them quite frequently.[38]

Marriage

A cleft has little influence on the dating behavior of adolescents with cleft palate.[17] Although dating may not be affected, fewer persons with cleft palate marry than do their siblings, and a larger proportion than their normal peers or siblings never marry. When they do marry, it occurs at a later age.[33,35] Although they report being satisfied with their marriages, childless marriages occur more frequently when one of the spouses was born with a cleft, and they tend to have fewer children.[17,35]

Educational status

The educational levels attained by those with cleft palate is similar to the rest of the population. Those with cleft palate do not demonstrate a higher dropout rate than the rest of the population, and the overwhelming majority finish high school (73% to 80%) or have further education.[17,18,27,33,36]

Vocational status

The vocational and economic status of adults born with cleft palate are within normal limits and cannot be differentiated from their siblings, fathers, or random controls.[17,33,37] Employment stability and job satisfaction seem not to be affected by having a cleft, although when those adults are unemployed, they are out of work longer than are unaffected individuals but not longer than their siblings.[37] A wide range of occupations is represented, many of which are associated with high socioeconomic status.[17]

Status of patients with craniofacial anomalies

In contrast to the child with cleft palate, surgical correction for the child with a craniofacial anomaly occurs much later in life. For many such patients surgical correction may not have been attempted until adulthood. Others have not experienced surgery. This obviously affects the adult status of these patients. In addition, there are relatively few patients, making controlled scientific study difficult. Most of our information about them therefore comes from clinical practice.

Social relationships

Craniofacial anomalies are often deterrents to the establishment of social relationships. Persons with visible defects are more readily accepted as casual acquaintances than as friends or in more intimate relationships.[30,47] Because such relationships are restricted, the facially disfigured, in my clinical experience, lead relatively restricted social lives. They are aware of the effects of their appearance on others and have, to the extent possible, accommodated to these social restraints. Many of them hope that corrective surgery will change their social lives.

Marriage

As well as experiencing general social restrictions in forming social relationships with others, the facially disfigured often fail to have opportunities to practice and experience appropriate sex-role behavior.[47] Those severely disfigured are less likely to be accepted as marriage partners.[30,47] They believe strongly that they do not have free choices when they try to establish heterosexual relationships and thus must content themselves with any available partner.[6] With rare exceptions adults with craniofacial malformations in my practice are single. Not only are they single, but they believe they have little chance for marriage.

Educational status

There is also little information available about the educational status of these patients. Many of the adult candidates for craniofacial surgery that I have interviewed finished high school. A few have gone to college. In an examination of 50 consecutive patients undergoing craniofacial surgery, half of the children under the age of 12 who were eligible for school were not in school, whereas adolescent or adult patients were either attending or had completed school.[39]

Occupational status

No hard data are available about the occupational status of adults with craniofacial malformations. Clinical case studies ascribe a marginal status to the facially disfigured adult and stress that as a result of being stigmatized the person is devalued or discounted.[22] Their stigmatization is reflected in the economic marketplace. Adults with these defects, even with an appropriate educational background, experience difficulty in obtaining jobs and are employed at levels below their actual capabilities.[30]

EFFECTS OF TREATMENT ON PATIENTS

The effects of treatment regimens are directly related to the general atmosphere of hope and encouragement that treatment offers. In contrast to those born with cleft palate, to whom positive assurances can be given because of the long history of successful management and successful outcomes, less confidence is possible with those suffering severe facial disfigurements. Families of both groups are aware of this information.

Management of clefts

When a child is born with a cleft that is not part of another syndrome, a support system is generated for the parents and child. Parents are given information about clefts in which the repairable nature of cleft palate is emphasized. Those facial disfigurements related to clefts of the lip are surgically managed within the first few months of the child's life. Each professional is able to make fairly definite statements about the probable status of the child. In effect, by their professional expertise, those who manage the treatment of cleft palate become part of the psychologic support system available to patient and family.

This support system and the repairability of the defect may account for the relatively benign psychologic reactions to cleft palate. Although there is an initial focus on appearance factors, within a relatively short time emphasis shifts toward functioning. In the attempt to improve function, the attitude can be conveyed that the child can improve his own function with the assistance of the professional. In receiving speech therapy, for example, the child is reinforced by the therapist for improving performance. This gives both feedback about the quality of speech and rewards active work toward meeting the goals of improvement.

Even when appearance remains an issue, the patient and parents are often led to understand that improved appearance will be possible at a later age. It is not unusual for an older child or adolescent to request surgery in an effort to gain further improvement in appearance. Despite the fact that hospitalization and surgery may be frequent, these experiences are interpreted by the patient as a chain of necessary events, all geared to the improvement of ultimate status rather than being viewed negatively.

During the course of cleft palate treatment the patient is provided with information that beomes integrated into self-concept. Possibly cleft palate treatment heightens sensitivity, thus contributing to the patterns of shyness and withdrawal frequently described in these patients. It is possible as well that the long-term treatment involved in the management of cleft palate affects decisions about marriage and having children. These effects cannot be attributed solely to the treatment of cleft palate, but the experiences of these patients with cleft palate team members probably influences the general pattern of life they ultimately adopt.

Management of craniofacial malformations

Psychologic motivations rather than physical or functional factors cause families and patients to seek surgical treatment for craniofacial malformations. It is clear that patients with these facial disfigurements endure a number of problems because of societal attitudes about persons who are physically unattractive.[11] Before the introduction of newer surgical techniques and their improvement, it was difficult to provide hope or optimism for this group of patients. In contrast to the situation of persons with cleft lip, in which intervention takes place very early, it is questionable at this time whether or not early intervention is the treatment of choice for a large number of craniofacial cases. Thus they experience the primary defects for longer periods of time than do those with cleft lip. In addition, craniofacial surgery carries a higher surgical risk factor than does cleft palate. This risk affects attitudes toward surgery and places patients and parents in conflict between the possible good effects of surgery for a non–life-threatening condition and placing oneself or one's child in jeopardy.

Once the decision is made, the surgical treatment of craniofacial deformities has positive effects on patients and families. Before treatment, expectations of craniofacial surgery are uniformly high. Parents and patients indicate they expect surgery to have significant positive effects on all aspects of life. Postsurgical evaluations demonstrate that they are satisfied with the results.[13,39] They report being pleased specifically with their faces and heads, as well as with their bodies in general.

In part, expressed satisfaction seems related to the actual change in apperaance or function experienced by the patient. It is also possible that the patient, having invested great energy and suffering in the decision to have surgery, has no choice but to be satisfied. As a result of the high involvement in the decision, the patient and family members must find the changes congruent with their expectations. Thus, as a result of very high investments in the craniofacial surgery, expressed satisfaction will be high to justify the decision made.

A distinction can be made between the specific results of surgery in improving appearance and expectations of the results of surgery in other areas of life. These patients, it will be remembered, expect changes in many aspects of their lives because of the surgery. There are psychologic problems, however, associated with craniofacial surgery. Appearance modification does not always have positive effects. Even the patient who is satisfied with the change in appearance will probably have difficulty in changing lifelong behaviors, which may include depending on the malformed appearance as a way of coping with the world. The sudden transformation in appearance after surgery may disrupt the person's ability to know what to expect and how to deal with others. It may not have the desired effects because changes in other behaviors and ways of thinking have not occurred simultaneously. The patient may be ill prepared for dealing with changed social situations in which apperaance does not have the effects it did previously. Once appearance becomes nonremarkable, the individual may be confronted with an inability to meet social expectancies. Social acceptance becomes dependent on the patient's psychologic and social resources. When these resources are inadequate, anxiety may be exacerbated. Depressive reactions may follow, and the person may be as socially reclusive as before surgery. Another area of possible disappointment for these patients lies in the expectation of change in occupational status after surgery. No evidence of occupational mobility exists for this group of postsurgical patients.[13]

With younger patients, parents report a high degree of satisfaction with the surgery. In general, they believe the surgery has been beneficial and see improvement in their children. Despite the reported improvement, however, some children become management problems.

Before surgery the craniofacial malformation affects the

child-rearing atmosphere so that demands for the child's conformity were either virtually nonexistent or moderated. With surgical correction, parents begin to react as if the deformity never existed. Parent attitudes and expectations introduce new factors into the parent-child relationship. As a result parents experience more difficulty and frustrations in child management, and the child begins to act out against new restrictions and the apparently inexplicable changes.

Many of the psychologic problems arising after craniofacial surgery come about because of insufficient psychologic assistance before and after the surgery. Since craniofacial surgery has significant psychologic implications, it is reasonable, if not imperative, to have psychologic treatment available to patients and their families. The postsurgical period in particular may require the patients to adapt to a new set of circumstances for which they are ill prepared unless they are offered assistance in modifying their behaviors.

SUMMARY AND CONCLUSIONS

Initially strong, negative parental feelings are elicited when a baby with a cleft or craniofacial malformation is born. These first parental reactions moderate and are followed by a lengthy period of parental adaptation to the affected baby. Adaptations include accommodation to the baby's appearance, when this is a factor, and possible adjustments to the child's functioning, particularly in the areas of feeding, speech development, and hearing. In general, parents cope effectively with the affected child in the family, although some may experience difficulties in the management of the infant.

Most children born with clefts function within the normal range of intelligence and are not significantly different from their siblings and nonaffected peers in visual-motor performance and school achievement. Insufficient evidence is available about the performance levels of children with more severe craniofacial malformations to draw sound conclusions.

Having a craniofacial or a cleft birth defect may be a point of stress for the child. There have been some clinical observations, for example, concluding that these children exhibit a greater degree of shyness, withdrawal, or passivity than do their nonaffected peers. Despite this, however, most of the affected children behaviorally function within normal limits.

The adulthood of persons born with clefts is also essentially nonremarkable. Pathologic behavior is noted by its absence, although the degree of passivity described persists; fewer persons with clefts marry, and those who do marry tend to do so at later ages than their peers or siblings. Most finish high school; their vocational status and occupational stability is similar to their nonaffected peers.

Again little research evidence is available about the adult status of those born with more severe craniofacial malformations. Inferring from knowledge of the effects of other facial disfigurements, the social relationships, marital status, and vocational status of these adults may be marginal.

There are major differences between the long-range effects of treatment for patients with clefts and those found for patients with other craniofacial anomalies. The team treatment of cleft palate is well established and has enjoyed a high degree of rehabilitative success. Team members emphasize that a cleft is a repairable defect and stress that educational, social, and behavioral outcomes fall within the normal range.

Team treatment of patients with other craniofacial defects is comparatively recent. Some remarkable advances have been made with significant improvements in appearance and functioning. Information is lacking, however, about the overall rehabilitative success. Short-term effects have been positive, and patients and parents are pleased with the results; the longer term outcome is not so clear. Despite significant improvements in appearance, some patients still fall below a level of social acceptability in physical attractiveness, which continues to adversely affect their behavior.

It is evident that the birth defects under consideration have both subtle and gross effects on children and their families. For the most part, they cope more or less effectively with the sequelae. The possibility of treatment and the existence of teams of caring professionals significantly affect their ability to meet day-to-day problems and influence their hopes for being able to achieve a semblance of a normal status.

REFERENCES

1. Barker, R.G.: The social psychology of physical disability, J. Soc. Iss. **4:**29, 1948.
2. Berscheid, E., and Walster, E.: Physical attractiveness. In Berkowitz, L., editor: Advances in experimental social psychology, New York, 1974, Academic Press, Inc.
3. Boles, G.: Personality factors in mothers of cerebral palsied children, Genet. Psychol. Monogr. **58:**159, 1959.
4. Brantley, H.T., and Clifford, E.: Congenitive, self-concept, and body image measures of normal, cleft palate, and obese adolescents, Cleft Palate J. **16:**177, 1979.
5. Brantley, H.T., and Clifford, E.: Maternal and child locus of control and field-dependence in cleft palate children, Cleft Palate J. **16:**183, 1979.
6. Bryt, A.: Psychiatric aspects. In MacGregor, F.C., Abel, T.M., Bryt, A., et al., editors: Facial deformities and plastic surgery, Springfield, Ill., 1953, Charles C Thomas, Publisher.
7. Castellanos, M.C., and Stewart, M.: Psychosocial implications in plastic surgery. In Converse, J.M., editor: Reconstructive plastic surgery, Philadelphia, 1964, W.B. Saunders Co.
8. Clifford, E.: Effects of giving birth to a cleft lip-palate baby, Paper presented to the Plastic Surgery Research Council, Durham, N.C., 1968.
9. Clifford, E.: The impact of symptom: a preliminary comparison of cleft lip-palate and asthmatic children, Cleft Palate J. **6:**221, 1969.
10. Clifford, E.: Body satisfaction in adolescence, Percept. Mot. Skills **33:**119, 1971.
11. Clifford, E.: Psychosocial aspects of orofacial anomalies: speculations in search of data. In Werz, R.T., editor: orofacial anomalies: clinical and research implications, report No. 8, Washington, D.C., 1973, American Speech and Hearing Association.
12. Clifford, E.: Psychological aspects of cleft palate. In Bzoch, K.R., editor: Communicative disorders related to cleft lip and palate, ed. 2, Boston, 1979, Little, Brown & Co.

13. Clifford, E.: Psychological aspects of the craniofacial experience. In Converse,J.M., McCarthy, J.G., and Wood-Smith, D., editors; Symposium on the diagnosis and treatment of craniofacial anomalies, St. Louis, 1979, The C.V. Mosby Co.

14. Clifford, E., and Bentz, E.: When I was born: a comparative study of normal and clinical samples, Presented to the American Cleft Palate Association, New Orleans, 1975.

15. Clifford, E., and Brantley, H.T.: When I was born: perceived parental reactions of adolescents, J. Pers. Assess. **44:**604, 1977.

16. Clifford, E., and Crocker, E.C.: Maternal responses: the birth of a normal child as compared to the birth of a child with a defect, Cleft Palate J. **8:**298, 1971.

17. Clifford, E., Crocker, E.C., and Pope, B.A.: Psychological findings in the adulthood of 98 cleft lip-palate children, Plast. Reconstr. Surg. **50:**234, 1972.

18. Demb, N., and Ruess, A.L.: High school dropout rate for cleft palate patients, Cleft Palate J. **4:**327, 1967.

19. Drotar, D., Baskiewics, A., Irvin, N., et al.: The adaptation of parents to the birth of an infant with a congenital malformation: a hypothetical model, Pediatrics **56:**710, 1975.

20. Farber, B.: Family organization and crisis: maintenance of integration in families with a severely mentally retarded child, Monogr. Soc. Res. Child Dev., vol. 25, 1960.

21. Farber, B., and Jenne, W.C.: Family organization and parent-child communication: parents and siblings of a retarded child, Monogr. Soc. Res. Child Dev., vol. 28, 1963.

22. Goffman, E.: Stigma, Englewood Cliffs, N.J., 1963, Prentice-Hall, Inc.

23. Goodstein, L.: Intellectual impairment in children with cleft palate, J. Speech Hear. Disord. **4:**287, 1961.

24. Koch-Schulte, R.: Family adjustment of the newborn with cleft lip and palate, Presented to the American Cleft Palate Association, Miami Beach, 1958.

25. Lamb, M.M., Wilson, F.B., and Leeper, H.A.: A comparison of selected cleft palate children and their siblings on the variables of intelligence, hearing loss, and visual-perceptual abilities, Cleft Palate J. **9:**218, 1972.

26. Lamb, M.M., Wilson, F.B., and Leeper, H.A.: The intellectual function of cleft palate children compared on the basis of cleft type and sex, Cleft Palate J. **10:**367, 1973.

27. Latti, A., Rintals, A., and Soivio, A.I.: Educational levels of patients with cleft lip and palate, Cleft Palate J. **11:**36, 1974.

28. Lauer, E.: The family. In MacGregor, F.C., Abel, T.M., Bryt, A., et al., editors: Facial deformities and plastic surgery, Springfield, Ill., 1953, Charles C Thomas, Publisher.

29. MacGregor, F.C.: Some psychological hazards of plastic surgery of the face, Plast. Reconstr. Surg. **12:**123, 1953.

30. MacGregor, F.C., Abel, T.M., Bryt, A., et al., editors: Facial deformities and plastic surgery: a psychosocial study, Springfield, Ill., 1953, Charles C Thomas, Publisher.

31. McWilliams, B.J.: Speech and language problems in children with cleft palate, J.Am. Med. Wom. Assoc. **21:**1005, 1966.

32. McWilliams, B.J., and Mathews, H.P.: A comparison of intelligence and social maturity in children with unilateral complete clefts and those with isolated cleft palates, Cleft Palate J. **16:**363, 1979.

33. McWilliams, B.J., and Paradise, L.P.: Educational, occupational and marital status of cleft palate adults, Cleft Palate J. **10:**223, 1973.

34. Norval, M., Larson, T., and Parshall, P.: The impact of the cleft lip and palate child on the family: a preliminary survey, mimeographed report, Minneapolis, 1964, Minnesota Crippled Children's Services.

35. Peter, J.P., and Chinsky, R.R.: Sociological aspects of cleft palate adults. I. Marriage, Cleft Palate J. **11:**295, 1974.

36. Peter, J.P., and Chinsky, R.R.: Sociological aspects of cleft palate adults. II. Education, Cleft Palate J. **11:**443, 1974.

37. Peter, J.P., Chinsky, R.R., and Fisher, M.J.: Sociological aspects of cleft palate adults. III. Vocational and economic aspects, Cleft Palate J. **12:**193, 1975.

38. Peter, J.P., Chinsky, R.R., and Fisher, M.J.: Sociological aspects of cleft palate adults. IV. Social integration, Cleft Palate J. **12:**304, 1975.

39. Phillips, J., and Whitaker, L.A.:The social effects of craniofacial deformity and its correction, Cleft Palate J. **16:**7, 1979.

40. Richardson, S.A.: The effects of physical disability on the socialization of the child. In Goslin, D.A., and Grass, D.C., editors: The handbook of socalization theory, New York, 1969, Rand McNally & Co.

41. Richardson, S.A., Hastorf, A.H., and Dornbusch, S.M.: Effects of physical disability on a child's description of himself, Child Dev. **35:**893, 1964.

42. Richman, L.C.: Behavior and achievement of cleft palate children, Cleft Palate J. **13:**4, 1976.

43. Richman, L.C.: The effects of facial disfigurement on a teacher's perception of ability in cleft palate children, Cleft Palate J. **15:**155, 1978.

44. Richman, L.C.: Parents and teachers: differing views of behavior of cleft palate children, Cleft Palate J. **15:**360, 1978.

45. Ruess, A.L.: A comparative study of cleft palate children and their siblings, J. Clin. Psychol. **21:**354, 1965.

46. Ruess, A.L., and Lis, E.F.: A multidimensional study of handicapped children, Final report to Maternal and Child Health Sevices, Grant No. Mc-R-170007-04-0, Washington, D.C., 1973, Health Services and Mental Health Administration, Department of Health, Education, and Welfare.

47. Sieka, F.L.: Facial disfigurement: impact of sex role evaluation and its relationship to acceptance of disability, doctoral dissertation, 1970, State University of New York at Buffalo.

48. Simonds, J.F., and Heimburger, R.E.: Psychiatric evaluation of youth with cleft lip-palate matched with a control group, Cleft Palate J. **15:**193, 1978.

49. Sinicrope, P.E., and Clifford, E.: Effects of cleft lip-palate on body satisfaction, Presented to the Cleft Palate Association, Oklahoma City, 1973.

50. Slutsky, H.: Maternal reaction and adjustment to birth and care of cleft palate child, Cleft Palate J. **6:**425, 1969.

51. Spriestersbach, D.C.: Psychological aspects of the "cleft palate problem," Iowa City, 1973, University of Iowa Press.

52. Spriestersbach, D.C., Dickson, D.C., Fraser, F.C., et al.: Clinical research in cleft lip and cleft palate: the state of art, Cleft Palate J. **10:**113, 1973.

53. Stricker, G., Clifford, E., Cohen, L.K., et al.: Psychosocial aspects of craniofacial disfigurement, Am. J. Orthod. **76:**410, 1979.

54. Tisza, V.B., and Gumpertz, E.: The parents' reaction to the birth and early care of children with cleft palate, Pediatrics **30:**86, 1962.

56. Tisza, V.B., Irwin, E., and Scheide, E.: Children with oral-facial clefts, J. Am. Acad. Child Psychiatry **12:**292, 1973.

56. Tisza, V.B., Silvertone, B., Rosenblum, D., and Hanlon, N.: Psychiatric observations of children with cleft palate, Am. J. Orthopsychiatry **28:**416, 1958.

57. Voysey, M.: Impression management by parents with disabled children, J. Health Soc. Behav. **13:**80, 1972.

58. Winick, M.: Comprehensive approach to a child with a birth defect, Bull. N.Y. Acad. Med. **43:**819, 1967.

59. Wirls, C.J.: Psycho-social aspects of cleft lip and palate. In Grabb, W.C., Rosenstein, S.W., and Bzoch, K.R., editors: Cleft lip and palate: surgical, dental, and speech aspects, Boston, 1971, Little, Brown & Co.

60. Wylie, R.C.: The self-concept, rev. ed., vol. 1, A review of methodological considerations and measuring instruments, Lincoln, Neb., 1974, University of Nebraska Press.

CHAPTER 18

The unilateral cleft lip

D. RALPH MILLARD, Jr.

When Dr. Georgiade invited me to write this chapter, I was less than enthusiastic, not having totally recovered from the 810 pages recently written on this subject.[10] He sympathized that I had probably used up all my cases in *Cleft Craft*[10] and offered to lend me a few of his. Since the overall value of a method is better estimated by the results of other surgeons than those of the originator, I accepted Dr. Georgiade's generous offer and therefore include four of his cases, three incomplete and one complete cleft (Figs. 18-1 to 18-4).

Unilateral cleft of the lip, apart from the actual clefting, has the perverse distortion of asymmetry. Actual closure of the cleft offers no great obstacle except the necessity of a scar. Correction of asymmetric distortion is the key to success, and in my opinion the principles of rotation-advancement with adept craftsmanship have been shown to accomplish this better than previous approaches. Although the normal side is the model by which the cleft side must be fashioned, it represents an almost unconquerable challenge.

In this chapter emphasis will be placed on the recurring mistakes seen in postoperative results, with details on how to avoid these minor problems. Within reason they are minor because secondary corrections along the rotation-advancement tract are relatively easy.

PLATFORM

The first concern in the management of a cleft is whether the alveolus and hard palate are cleft. If they are uncleft, then the platform on which the lip and nose rests is symmetric, and the problem is merely a soft tissue rearrangement. If the alveolus and hard palate are cleft, then there will be varying degrees of asymmetry of the platform as the noncleft premaxillary-maxillary element rotates laterally and forward, leaving the cleft-side maxillary element behind. This creates a distorted platform that resists both cleft closure and achievement of symmetry. In my opinion pre-

surgical orthopedics, as started by McNeil[8] and Burston,[2] used by Hotz[6] and Gnoinski,[5,6] simplified by Hagerty, Mylin, and Hess,[4] and modified by Georgiade and Latham,[3] is a method of atraumatic positioning of premaxillary and maxillary parts into a temporary relative symmetry to facilitate the primary surgery. Unfortunately, I do not have readily available this adjunct and thus am forced to use the adhesion principle to mold the premaxillary and maxillary elements without subjecting the final lip scars to the unnatural pull and pounding required for maxillary platform correction.

ADHESION

The principle of lip adhesion first employed by Simon,[13] Johanson and Ohlsson,[7] Millard,[9] and later Randall[11] achieves a quick, easy, and effective method of applying a constricting band across the cleft. This band not only reduces the width of the cleft, but molds the maxillae into better alignment while stalling for catch-up growth and pacifying the parents that something positive is being done for their child. The adhesion is carried out at about 3 to 5 weeks and left to work for about 6 months. Usually at this operation as much of the posterior soft palate as possible is united to achieve posterior molding and early coordination with the posterior pharyngeal musculature. With experience the adhesion has become more sophisticated, incorporating some nasal correction.

TECHNIQUE

The standard marking for a rotation-advancement procedure is made so that flaps *L* and *M* can be taken and the adhesion created without intrusion on natural landmarks (Fig. 18-5, *A*). Flaps *L* and *M*, which are merely an economical means of freshening the cleft edges, are fashioned well within the marks for safety. Flap *L* is used to fill the gap developed when the alar base and lateral nasal vestibule

Text continued on p. 274.

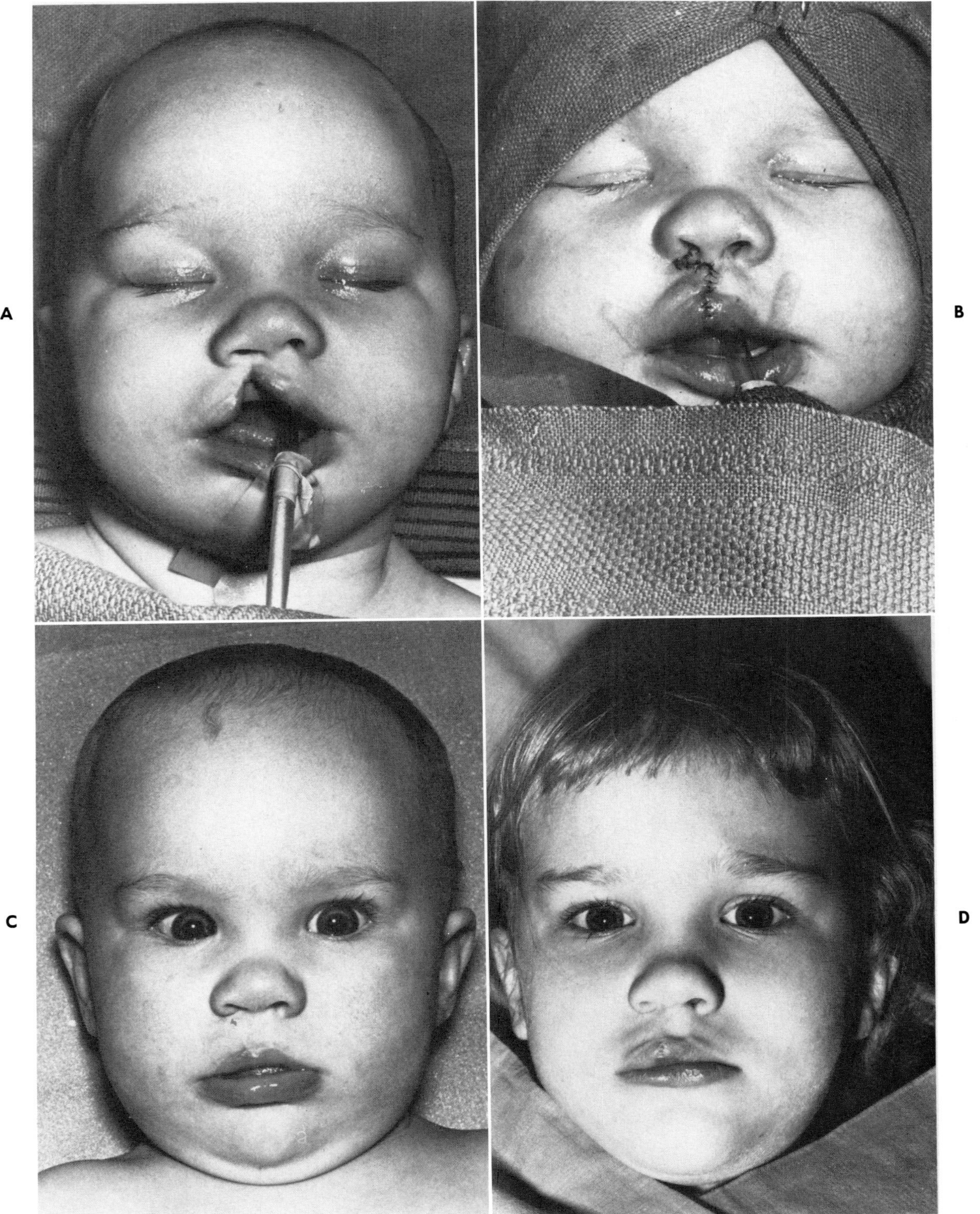

Fig. 18-1. A, Incomplete cleft of the lip. **B,** After rotation-advancement showing the old method of using flap *c* across into the lip as nostril sill, which does not aid lengthening of the unilateral columella shortness. **C,** Postoperative results just under 4 months. **D,** Results 4 years after surgery.

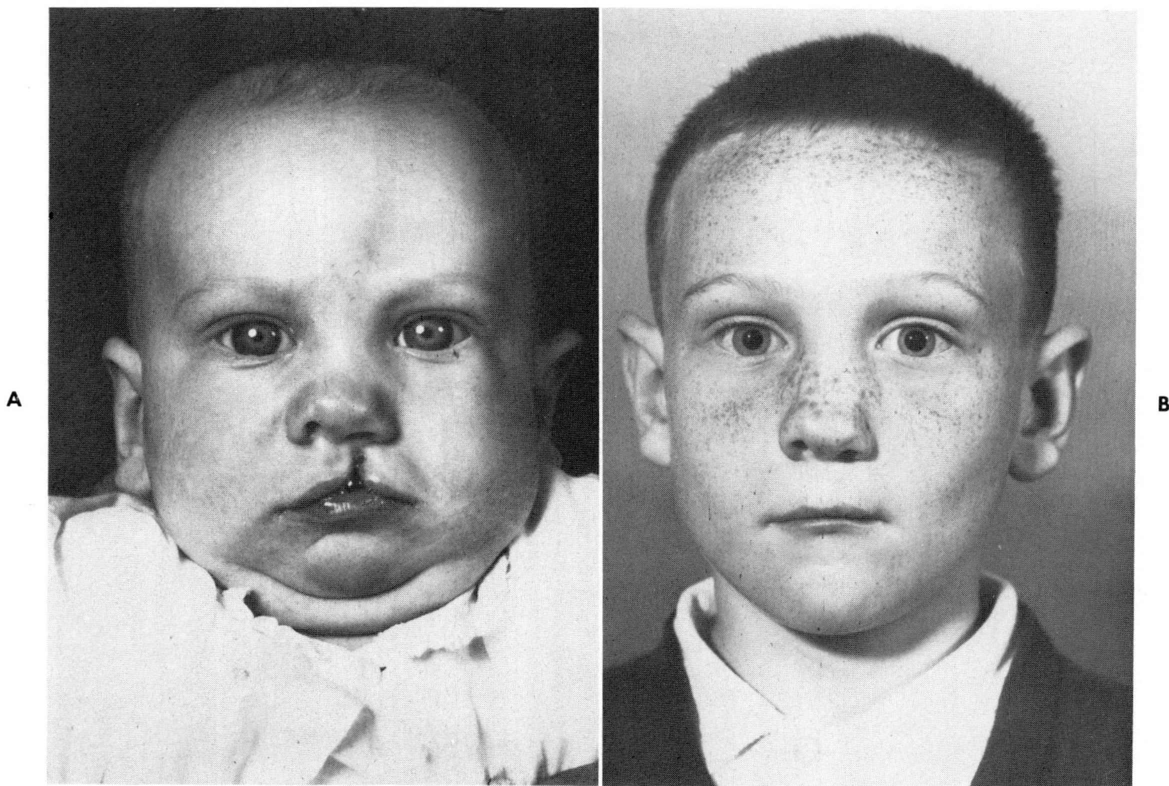

Fig. 18-2. A, Incomplete cleft of the lip. **B,** Result of rotation-advancement of the lip after 8 years.

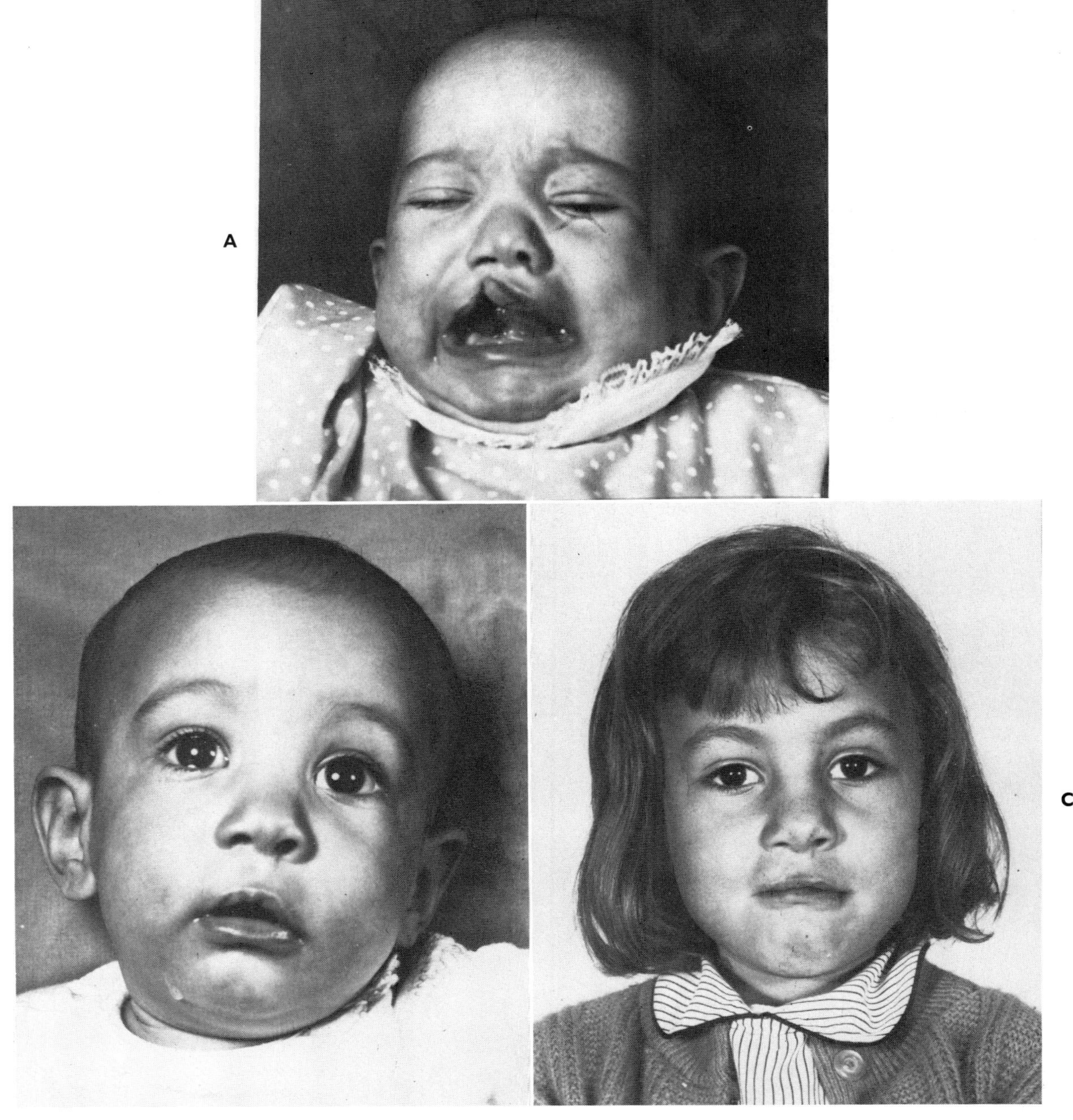

Fig. 18-3. A, A more severe incomplete cleft of the lip with alveolar clefting and distortion. **B,** Results at 4 months after rotation-advancement. **C,** Result after 5 years.

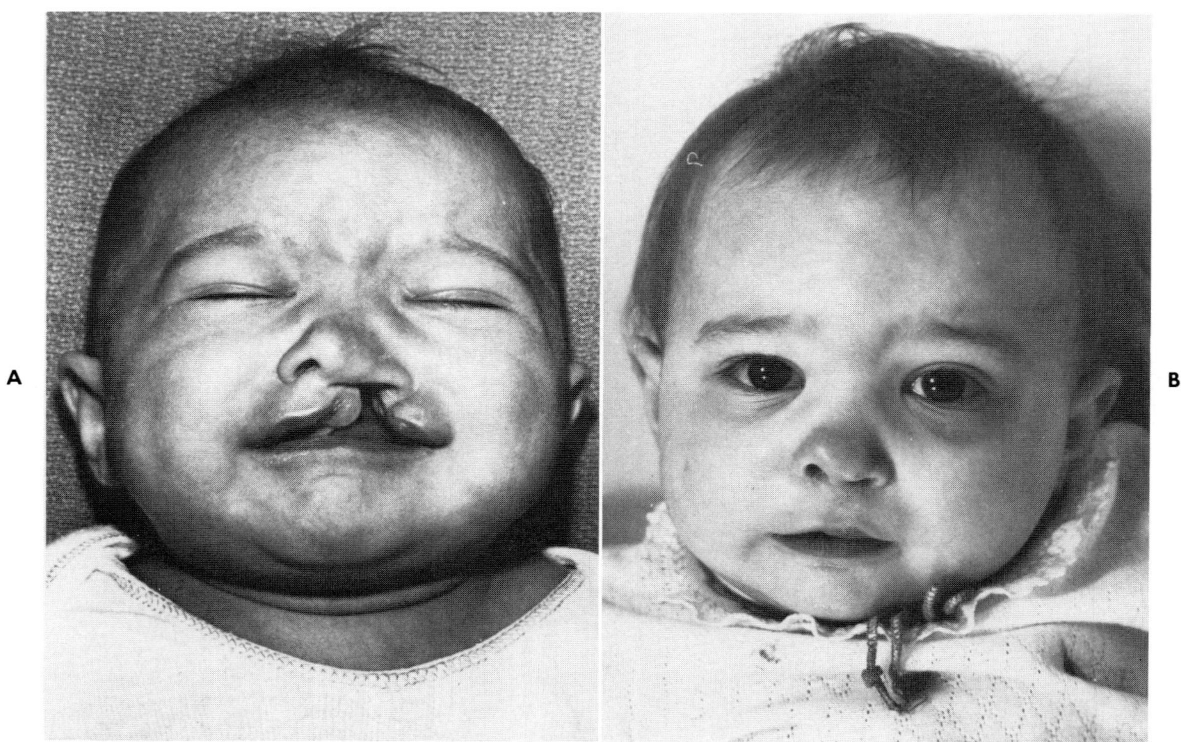

Fig. 18-4. A, A complete unilateral cleft of the lip with the usual severe nasal distortion. **B,** One year after rotation-advancement of the lip.

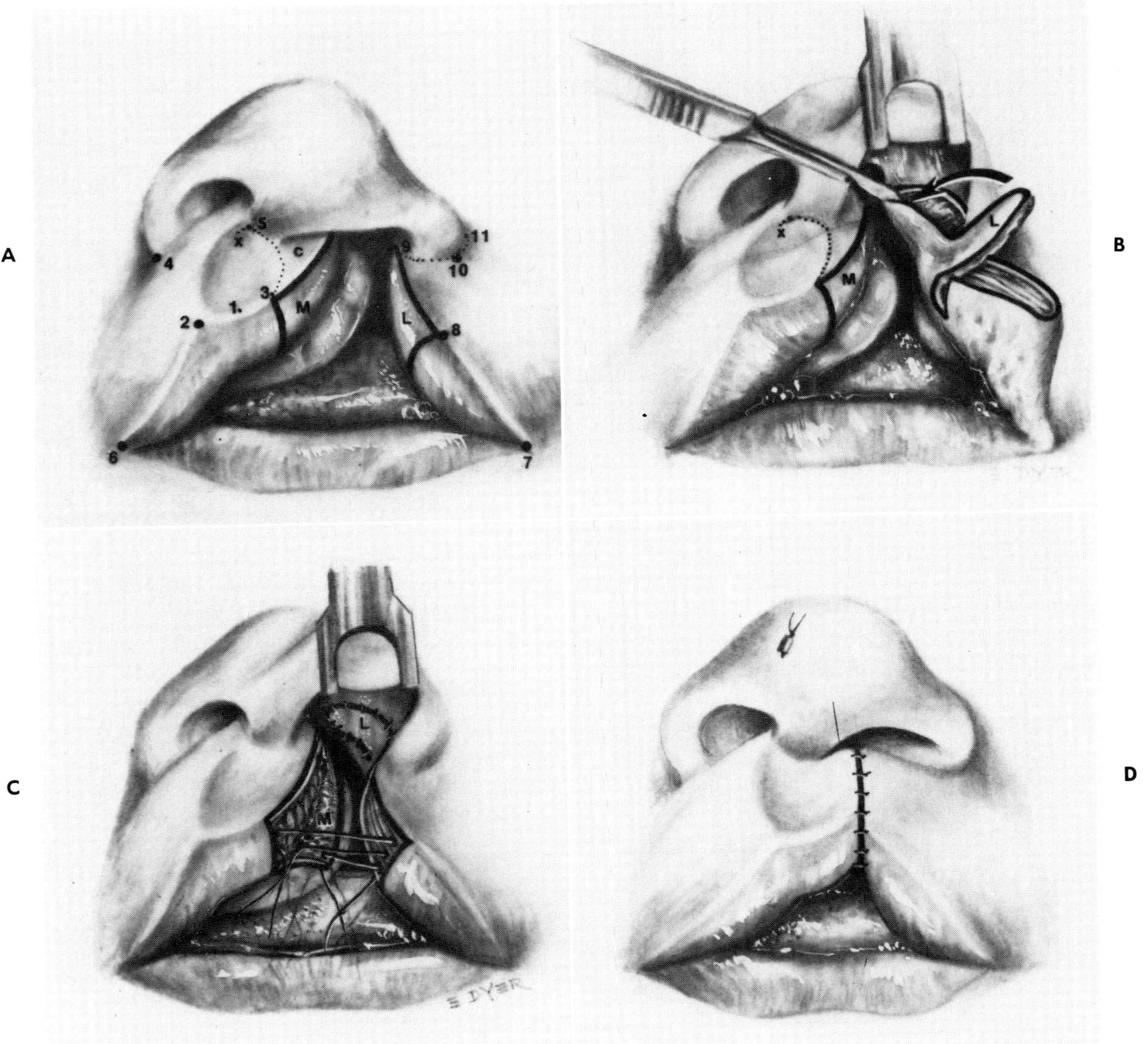

Fig. 18-5. A, Markings for an adhesion in a complete cleft lip. Medial *(M)* and lateral *(L)* flaps are marked on the cleft edge mucosa *(c)* to achieve freshening of the edges within natural landmarks. *1* to *2* = *1* to *3*, *3* to *5* to *x* = *8* to *9*, *2* to *6* = *7* to *8*, *2* to *4* = *8* to *10*. **B,** Flap *L* is based superiorly and is used to fill the defect created when the alar base is released from the retropositioned lateral maxillary element. **C,** Flap *L* is in its new position; Flap *M* is turned over and used in the posterior lip closure. Mattress sutures bring the muscles together. **D,** When the slumped alar cartilage is freed from the nasal skin, an external through-and-through mattress suture can help the lift temporarily. The skin is sutured with silk.

are released from their posterior retropositioned attachments to the underdeveloped cleft side maxilla (Fig. 18-5, *B*). Through this releasing incision, a curved scissor can free the nasal skin from the slumped alar cartilage on the cleft side to allow some sliding as the alar base moves medially. This rearrangement can be fixed with external through-and-through mattress sutures as described by Blair and Brown.[1] Transposition of the mucosal flap *L* is fixed with 5-0 chromic catgut. Flap *M* is merely turned over "leaf of book" fashion to make up for mucosa used in flap *L* and to aid in the posterior closure of the adhesion (Fig. 18-5, *C*). Several 4-0 chromic catgut sutures are placed in the muscles, 6-0 silk sutures are used to close the skin, and a Logan bow is applied (Fig. 18-5, *D*). A complete cleft has now been turned into an incomplete one.

DEFINITIVE LIP CLOSURE

The adhesion is turned into a rotation-advancement closure 3 to 6 months later. The adhesion tissue of scar and excess skin between the rotation and advancement incisions can be retained with a superior base and used to cover raw alveolus or in any other desired capacity.

Rotation

The medial element, carrying two thirds of a cupid's bow, one philtrum column, and the dimple, is to be rotated down into normal balanced position. The rotation incision mimics the philtrum column on the opposite side and is carried to the base of the columella, extending about two thirds of the way across the base before turning down in the back-cut to *x*. The distortion of the lip and twist of the nose often misleads the surgeon as to how far to extend the rotation. Often it is *not* extended far enough. It is vital that the incision

not cross the normal philtrum column but remain medial to it. The back-cut speeds up the pivot of the total rotation, and the terminal point x may differ slightly in each case (Fig. 18-6, *A*). The average back-cut is not more than 2 to 3 mm and rarely requires another millimeter. After the muscles have been divided deep into the chink of the back-cut, there will be a release of the entire medial lip element down into normal position. The short-cleft-side columella will rise, leaving a triangular gap at its base and side.

It is at this point that many surgeons still do not follow the modern design (Fig. 18-6, *B*). With the aid of a unilateral membranous septal incision, the short side of the columella is freed and advanced upward. The point of flap *c* swings around into the rotation gap to fill the upper half of the back-cut and wrap the lengthened columella with a triangle flap to complete the balance of the columella.[10] Flap *c*, taking up part of the rotation gap increase by the back-cut *x*, allows the tip of the lateral lip advancement flap to slice in below it and fill the lower half of the *gap* in a natural union of lip and nose. Note that the side and not the tip of flap *c* forms the columella base of the nostril sill. After adequate rotation of the medial lip element, the orbicular muscle fibers of the mouth are correctly aligned. The total rotation action is effective and can achieve a drop of as many millimeters as is necessary. The claim by Randall[12] that a difference of 3 to 4 mm between the height of the two peaks of the cupid's bow marks the limit of rotation is incorrect. As much as 8 to 9 mm have been corrected.

Alar base

The nostril sill–alar base component is cut as a flap and the excess end denuded of epithelium to be used as a buried tether to the septum, ducking under the side of flap *c* (Fig.

Fig. 18-6. A, The definitive rotation-advancement closure skirts the adhesion scar. The cupid's bow is marked from its midline *1* to noncleft peak *2*, a similar distance to the cleft side peak *3*. The rotation incision starting at *3* curves up toward the base of the columella, imitating the opposite normal philtrum column curve. The incision crosses under the columella base one half to two thirds its width to point *5*, and then well short of the normal philtrum column it turns down in a slant for another couple of millimeters to point *x*. This leaves a triangular skin flap *c* to lengthen the columella. To mark the advancement flap, the high horizontal incision snugly skirts the nostril sill and alar base, taking as much flap at *9* as there is good skin and extending around to *10* or *11*, depending on the amount of alar base flaring. A key measurement is the normal distance of commissure *6* to the cupid's bow peak on the noncleft side *2*. This identical distance is marked on the cleft side from *7* to *8* with the lateral lip element under gentle traction to offset its contraction. The white roll of the mucocutaneous junction flap can be used to interrupt the scar if desired. *1* to *2* = *1* to *3*, *3* to *5* to *x* = *8* to *9*, *2* to *6* = *7* to *8*, *2* to *4* = *8* to *10*. **B,** Unilateral membranous septal incision being made to advance flap *c*. The tip of flap *c* rotates around into the rotation back-cut. The alar base flap is cut free from the lip element and denuded of epithelium at the tip. **C,** The nostril sill–alar base flap, denuded of epithelium at its tip, is tucked under the side of flap *c* and sutured to the base of the septum to correct the alar flare. **D,** Moderate freeing of the orbicular muscles of the lateral lip element enable better positioning of the fibers. Small flaps of muscle can be used to cross the midline in the closure when indicated. **E,** The final closure achieves lengthening of the columella, creation of the nostril sill, positioning of the alar base, balancing of the lip scar and the normal philtrum on the noncleft side, correction of the cupid's bow position, and balance of the free-border vermilion.

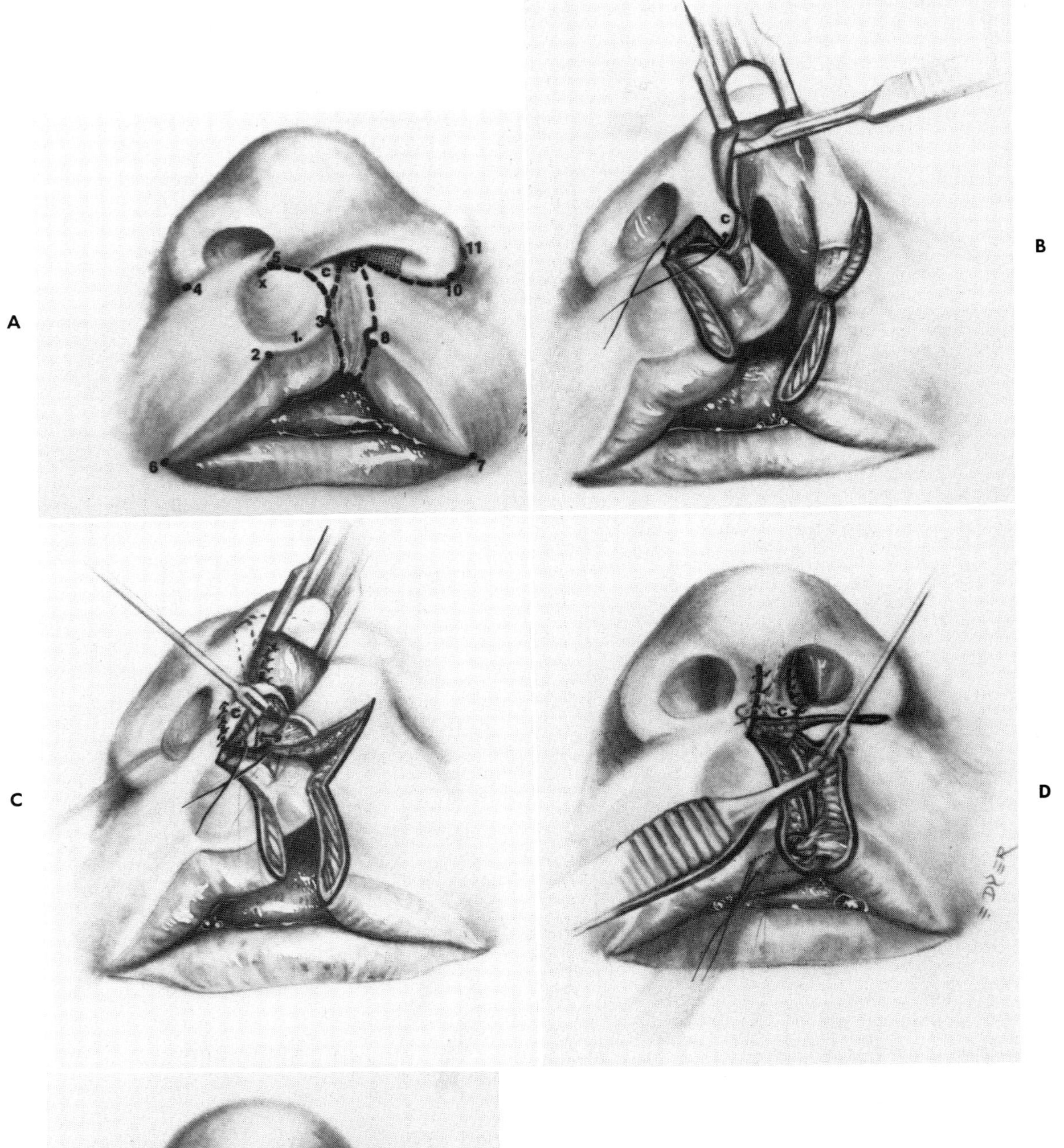

Fig. 18-6. For legend see opposite page.

18-6, *B* and *C*). This corrects the alar flare without the tendency toward lateral alar drift. The skin cuff of the alar base flap joins the side of flap *c* to construct the natural flow of the nostril sill into the columella base.

Advancement

The high horizontal incision of the advancement flap closely skirts the nostril sill and hooks around the alar base.

The vertical incision that freshens the cleft edge of the advancement flap starts as high in the vestibule at *9* as there is good skin (Fig. 18-6, *A*). This incision skirts the edge of the cleft, extending laterally just above the white roll of the mucocutaneous junction. The length of this incision must equal the length of the rotation incision from *3* to *5* to *x*. It is important to measure the distance from the commissure to the height of the bow (*6* to *2*) on the normal side. Re-

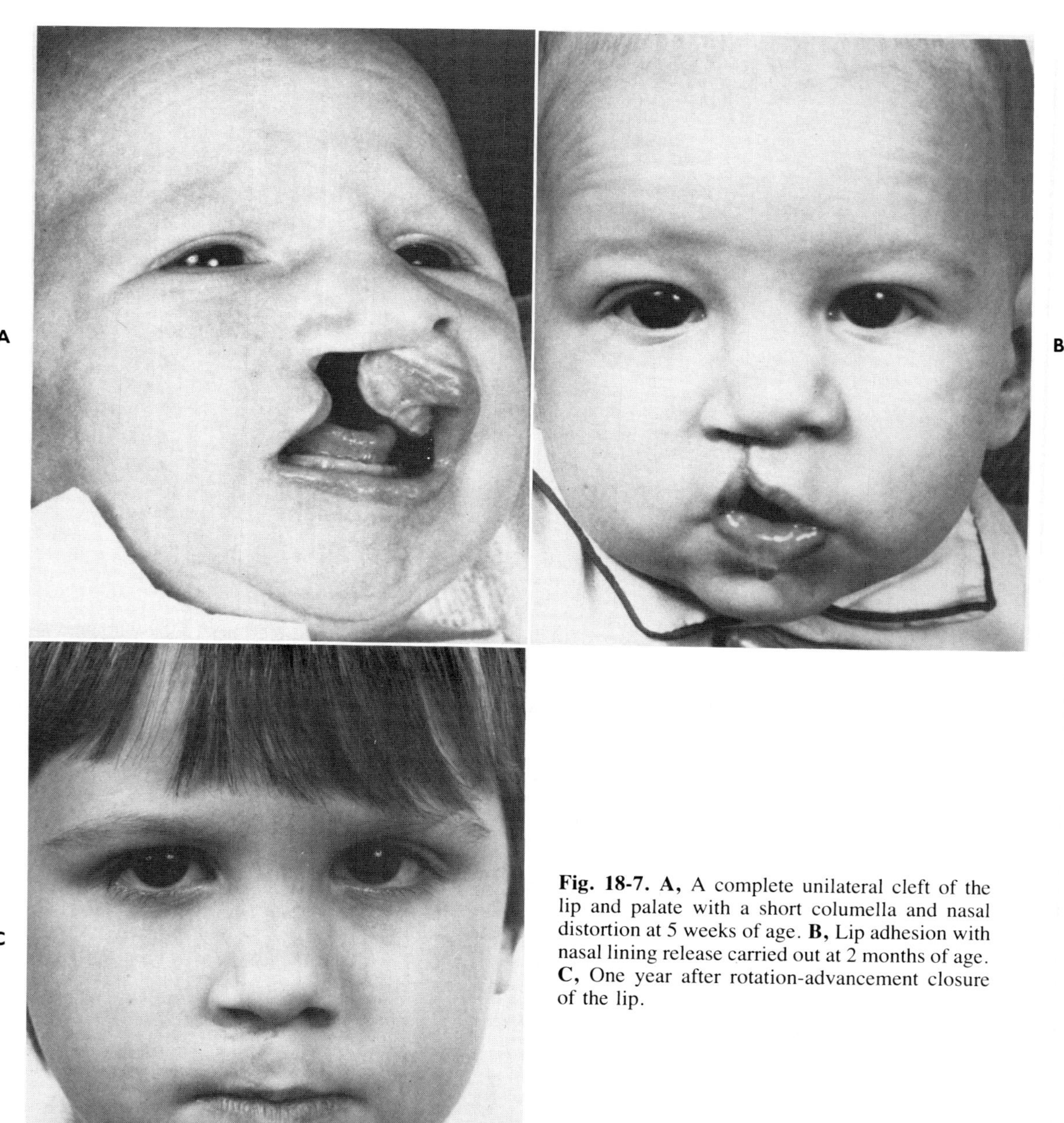

Fig. 18-7. A, A complete unilateral cleft of the lip and palate with a short columella and nasal distortion at 5 weeks of age. **B,** Lip adhesion with nasal lining release carried out at 2 months of age. **C,** One year after rotation-advancement closure of the lip.

membering that the cleft-side element is contracted, stretch it medially with a gentle pull using the finger and thumb or forceps and mark an equal normal distance from this commissure to a point medially along the mucocutaneous line of the lip. This point *(8)* marks the limits within 2 mm for lateral paring of the lateral lip element. Extend the lateral paring from *9* for a distance equal to *3* to *x*, but keeping within the bounds of mark *8*. The lateral lip advancement flap is cut free from the maxilla along the upper sulcus, dividing the tiny fistula formed by the base of flap *L* during the adhesion. The key suture advances the tip of the advancement flap into the rotation gap in the lower half of the back-cut *x*. Undermining of the lateral muscle elements with some rotation of the fibers improves their alignment for suturing with 4-0 chromic catgut (Fig. 18-6, *D*). The white roll flap can be used to cross the union scar at the muco-

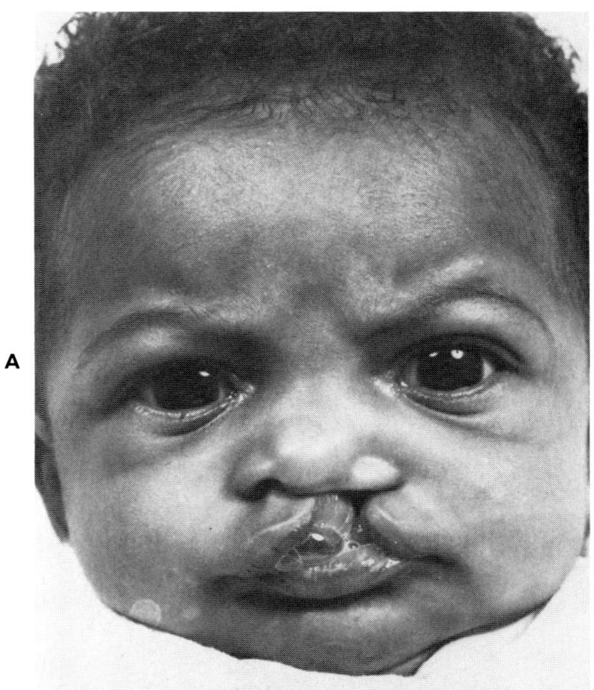

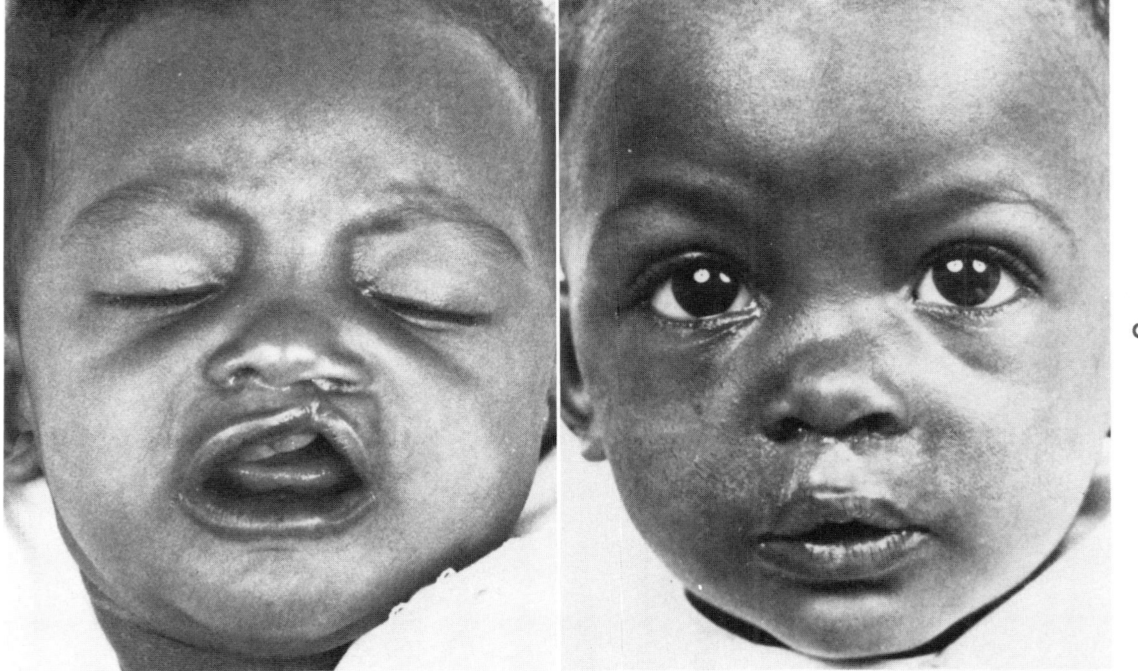

Fig. 18-8. A, Complete unilateral cleft of the lip and palate with nasal deformity at 1 month of age. **B,** Lip adhesion, nasal lining release, and soft palate closure at 3 months of age. **C,** Rotation-advancement closure of the lip at 8 months of age.

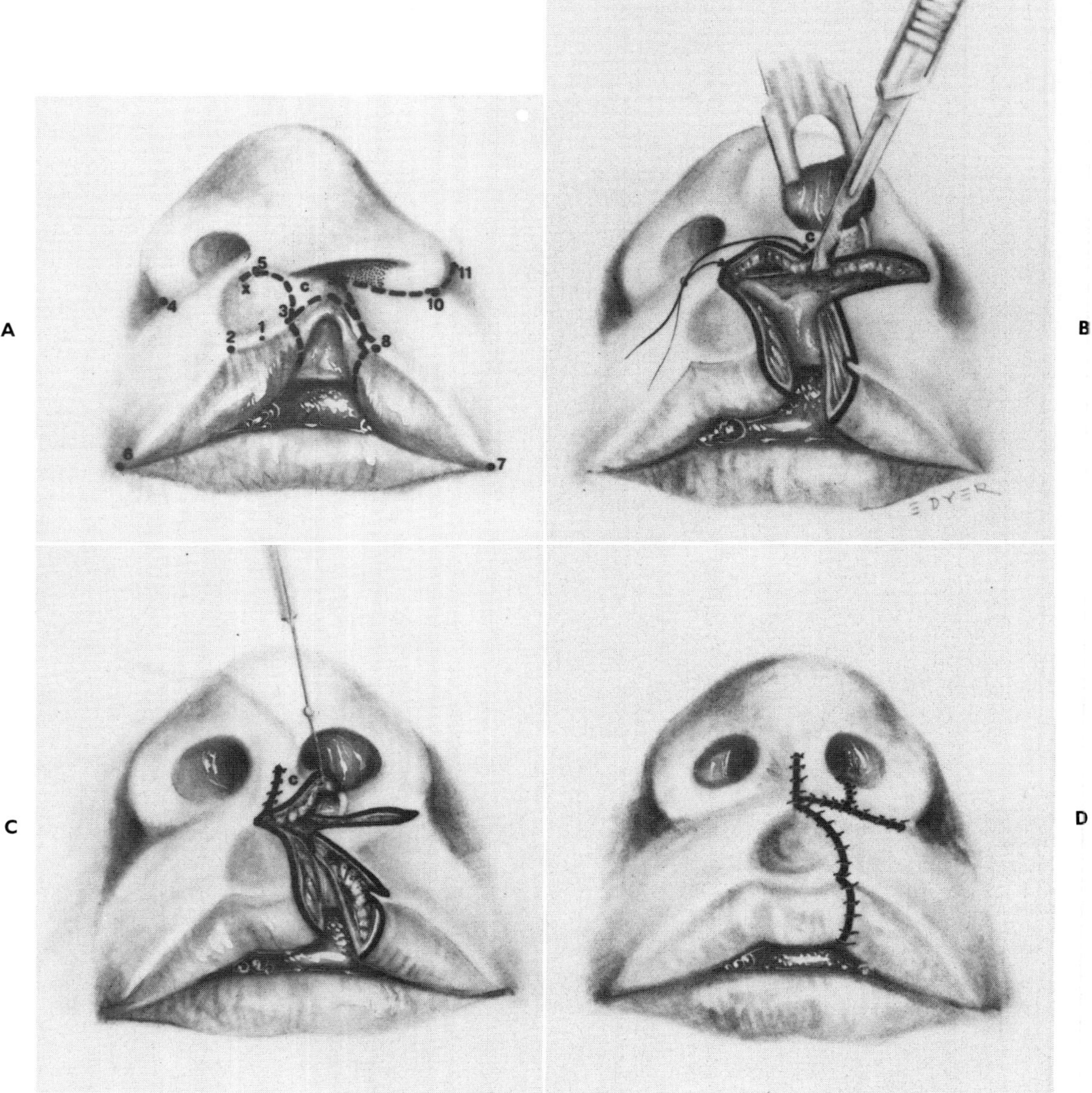

Fig. 18-9. A, In incomplete clefts the marking of the rotation incision *3* to *5* to *x* and advancement incision *8* to *9* to *10* to *11* is similar to that for the complete cleft. Simonart's band is used in the advancement flap, alar flap, or flap *c,* but the excess unusable skin and mucosa can be retained and based superiorly to cover any raw maxilla. *1* to *2* = *1* to *3, 3* to *5* to *x* = *8* to *9, 2* to *6* = *7* to *8, 2* to *4* = *8* to *10.* **B,** Flap *c* is used for unilateral columella lengthening. The denuded tip of the nostril sill–alar base flap is divided. **C,** The denuded portion of the nostril sill–alar base flap dips under the side skirt of flap *c* and is attached to the base of the septum. The lateral muscles are freed for better alignment. **D,** The lateral lip flap has been advanced into the rotation gap. Flap *c* has lengthened the columella and formed the medial portion of the nostril sill as it joins the alar base.

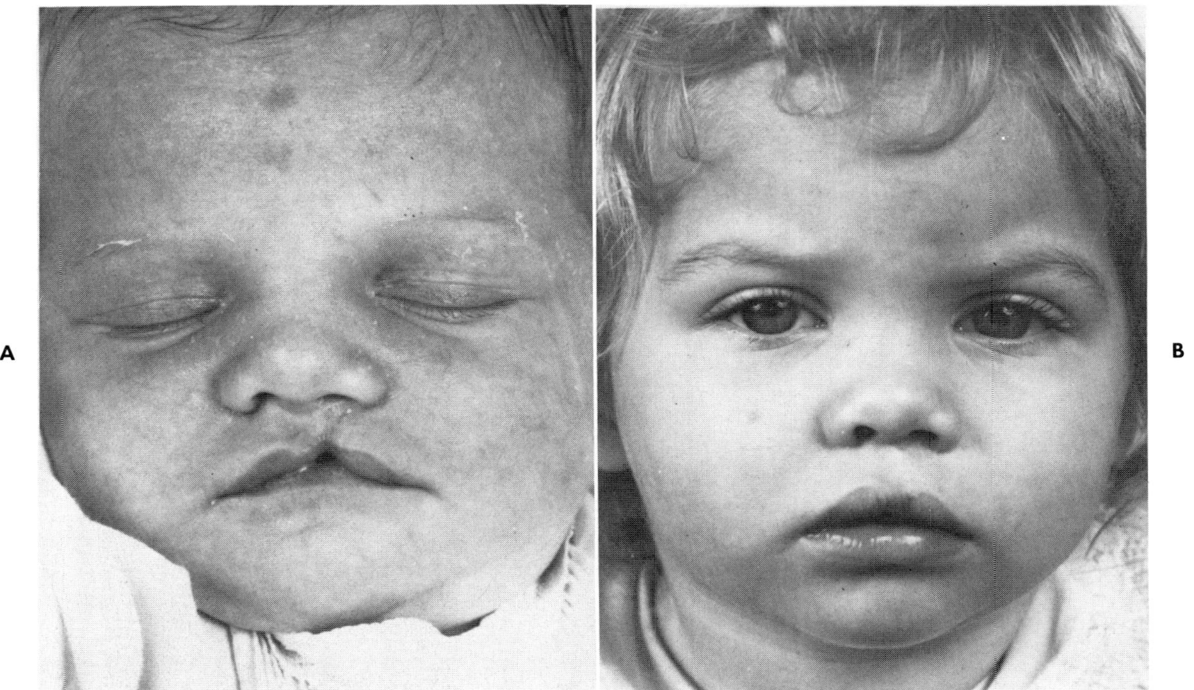

Fig. 18-10. A, Incomplete cleft of the lip at 1 month of age. **B,** Result at age 16 months after rotation-advancement closure of the lip at 7 months.

cutaneous line, and a small muscle flap can be used to cross the union wherever it is needed (Fig. 18-6, *D*). The anterior free border vermilion is closed in a straight line with a strong suture in the muscle at this inferior point. Closure of the posterior mucosa usually involves one mucosal flap in an interdigitation out of sight to discourage contraction of an otherwise relatively straight line, and the mucosa is closed with 4-0 chromic catgut; the skin is closed with 6-0 silk (Fig. 18-6, *E*).

A Logan bow is applied and an antibiotic ointment spread over the suture line to protect against nasal discharge. Arm restraints are placed. The sutures are removed in 4 days, the bow at 1 week, and the arm restraints at 2 weeks.

INCOMPLETE CLEFT

An incomplete cleft lip is similar to a complete cleft after an adhesion except that the premaxillary-maxillary platform probably has far better symmetry, and there is more inherent tissue present for use in the lip construction. Despite the variation in each deformity, the general plan and markings are about the same, and an incomplete cleft can be done any time after 3 months, but preferably at 4 to 6 months of age to allow increase in the size and strength of the tissues being manipulated and united (Figs. 18-9 and 18-10).

SUMMARY AND CONCLUSIONS

The unilateral cleft lip, apart from the actual clefting, suffers the perverse distortion of asymmetry. The first con-

cern in the management of a cleft is whether the alveolus and hard palate are also cleft. Before surgical correction of the cleft lip, the platform on which the lip and nose rest should be symmetric. Correction of a distorted platform can be corrected with either presurgical orthopedics or a lip adhesion technique. When the platform is symmetric, usually 3 to 6 months after a lip adhesion, rotation-advancement closure of the cleft is performed.

The surgical procedure for correcting the cleft lip deformity consists of a rotation-advancement closure. It is vital that the rotation incision does not cross the normal philtrum column but remains medial to it. After adequate rotation of the medial lip element the orbicular muscle fibers of the mouth are correctly aligned. The tendency of the alar base to flare is minimized when the nostril sill–alar base component is cut as a flap and the excess end denuded of epithelium is tethered to the septum under the side of flap *c*. The length of the advancement incision must equal the length of the rotation incision. The lateral lip advancement flap must be separated from the maxilla along the upper sulcus. The anterior border of the vermilion is closed in a straight line, whereas the posterior mucosa is closed with a mucosal flap in an interdigitation to minimize contracture if necessary.

REFERENCES

1. Blair, V.P., and Brown, J.B.: Mirault operation for single harelip, Surg. Gynecol. Obstet. **51:**81, 1930.
2. Burston, W.R.: The early orthodontic treatment of cleft palate condition, Dent. Practitioner **9:**41, 1958.

3. Georgiade, N.G., and Latham, R.A.: Maxillary arch alignment in the bilateral cleft lip and palate infant, using the pinned coaxial screw appliance, Plast. Reconstr. Surg. **56:**52, 1975.

4. Hagerty, R.F., Mylin, W.K., and Hess, D.A.: The prosthetic closure of cleft palate. In Sanvenero-Rosselli, G., and Boggio-Robutti, G.: Transactions of the Fourth International Congress of Plastic Surgery, Amsterdam, 1969, Excerpta Medica Foundation, International Congress Series No. 174.

5. Hotz, M., and Gnoinski, W.: Effects of early maxillary orthopaedics in coordination with delayed surgery for cleft lip and palate, J. Maxillofac. Surg. **7:**201, 1979.

6. Hotz, R.: The role of orthodontics in treatment management of cleft lip and palate, Cleft Palate J. **7:**371, 1970.

7. Johanson, B., and Ohlsson, A.: Bone grafting and dental orthopaedics in primary and secondary cases of cleft lip and palate, Acta Chir. Scand. **122:**112, 1961.

8. McNeil, C.K.: Oral and facial deformity, London, 1954, Pitman Publishing, Ltd.

9. Millard, D.R., Jr.: Refinements in rotation-advancement cleft lip technique, Plast. Reconstr. Surg. **33:**26, 1964.

10. Millard, D.R., Jr., editor: Cleft craft: the evolution of its surgery, 2 vols., Boston, 1976, Little, Brown & Co.

11. Randall, P.: A lip adhesion operation in cleft lip surgery, Plast. Reconstr. Surg. **35:**371, 1965.

12. Randall, P.: The unilateral cleft lip. In Georgiade, N.G., and Hagerty, R.F., editors: Symposium on management of cleft lip and palate and associated deformities, St. Louis, 1974, The C.V. Mosby Co.

13. Simon, G.: Ueber die Uranoplastik mit besonderer Berücksichtgung der mittel zur Wiederherstellung einer reinen (Nicht Naselnden) Sprache, Greifswalder Medicinishe Beitrage **2:**129, 1864.

CHAPTER 19

The bilateral cleft lip

GREGORY S. GEORGIADE, NICHOLAS G. GEORGIADE,
and RALPH A. LATHAM

The management and surgical repair of the newborn with a bilateral cleft lip can be a relatively simple surgical procedure, or it can be quite complex, depending on a number of factors.

The bilateral lip clefts may be incomplete on both sides, unilateral complete, opposite side incomplete, or bilateral complete. The premaxillary segment can be intact or partially cleft on one or both sides or completely detached from the maxillary segments with varying degrees of protrusion of the premaxillary segment.

The concept of management of the bilateral cleft lip patient, particularly those with complete clefts and the often associated protrusion of the premaxilla, has gradually changed at our institution over the past 20 years. An ongoing study of the possibility of suitably adjusting the maxillary segments and simultaneously repairing the bilateral cleft and carrying out a gingivoplasty has been our goal. Minimizing the number of surgical procedures, anesthetics, and hospitalizations and yet attaining a more satisfactory result were considered to be essential. The attainment of these goals had heretofore not been possible using the multiple-staged procedures involving lip adhesion techniques, unilateral repairs with resultant surgical premaxillary deformities.

EMBRYOLOGY

Formation of the lip originates with the formation of the primary plate in the embryo. The primary plate initially consists of enlargement of the ectoderm of the frontonasal processes which are termed *nasal placodes*. Further development in this area gives rise to the lateral and medial nasal processes. Fusion occurs gradually as the medial and lateral nasal processes join. Failure of this embryonic structure (the primary plate) to fuse by the fourth week in the embryo will lead to the formation of either a unilateral or bilateral cleft of the lip. The lack of sufficient numbers of mesen-

chymal cells being present at this time in the medial and lateral nasal processes appears to be critical for fusion of these processes.[4]

ANATOMY

The anatomy of the bilateral cleft lip will vary, depending on the completeness of the cleft of the lip. In the incomplete bilateral cleft lip, the orbicular muscle of the mouth penetrates from the lateral lip segments to the midportion of the lip (philtrum). In the complete cleft on one side of the lip and an incomplete cleft of the other side, the orbicular muscle fibers will advance only to the midportion of the prolabium and not extend to the portion of the prolabium on the cleft side. In the complete bilateral cleft the orbicular muscle fibers will turn and follow the lateral borders of the cleft, with the muscle fibers inserting laterally in a spiral fashion at the base of the nasal alae. The branches of the facial nerve and arterial supply also follow this pattern in the orbicular muscle. The prolabium therefore does not contain any muscle fiber initially but as has been described, obtains its muscle and motor innervation from the lateral lip segments in varying degrees, depending on the severity of the cleft deformity.[12]

OBJECTIVES

Repair of the bilateral cleft lip should also encompass suitable management of the premaxillary segment so that the maxillary segments can be aligned. A gingivoperiosteoplasty at the same time as the lip repair should also be carried out. Stabilization and subsequent growth of the maxillary segments in unison is the ultimate goal.

TECHNICAL FACTORS

Repair of the bilateral cleft is usually initiated when the birth weight has been regained and an increase of 0.5 kg has occurred. This is usually at 8 weeks of age. Feeding is managed quite successfully using a suitable formula or mother's milk given through a rubber-tipped Chetwood-type syringe.

Surgical repair of the bilateral cleft lip is basically the same, regardless of the configuration of the lip clefts. Planning and marking for the repair is as follows:

1. The length of the desired lip is determined by placing points *A* and *A'* at the desired new nostril floor. The *B* points will be marked at what will be the height of the new cupid's bow. *B'* will be marked on the lateral lip, equaling the length of *A* to *B*. This point must be placed at a point of full thickness of vermilion to prevent notching (Fig. 19-1, *A*).
2. The mucosa on the premaxillary segment is reflected to form the new labial mucosal lining and is attached to the superior portion of the mucosa between points *A'* to *B'*, which is also reflected labially (Fig. 19-1, *B*).
3. The lateral orbicular muscle fibers are dissected free in the incomplete bilateral cleft lip repair, incised along their insertion in the alar areas, and rotated medially and sutured to the op-

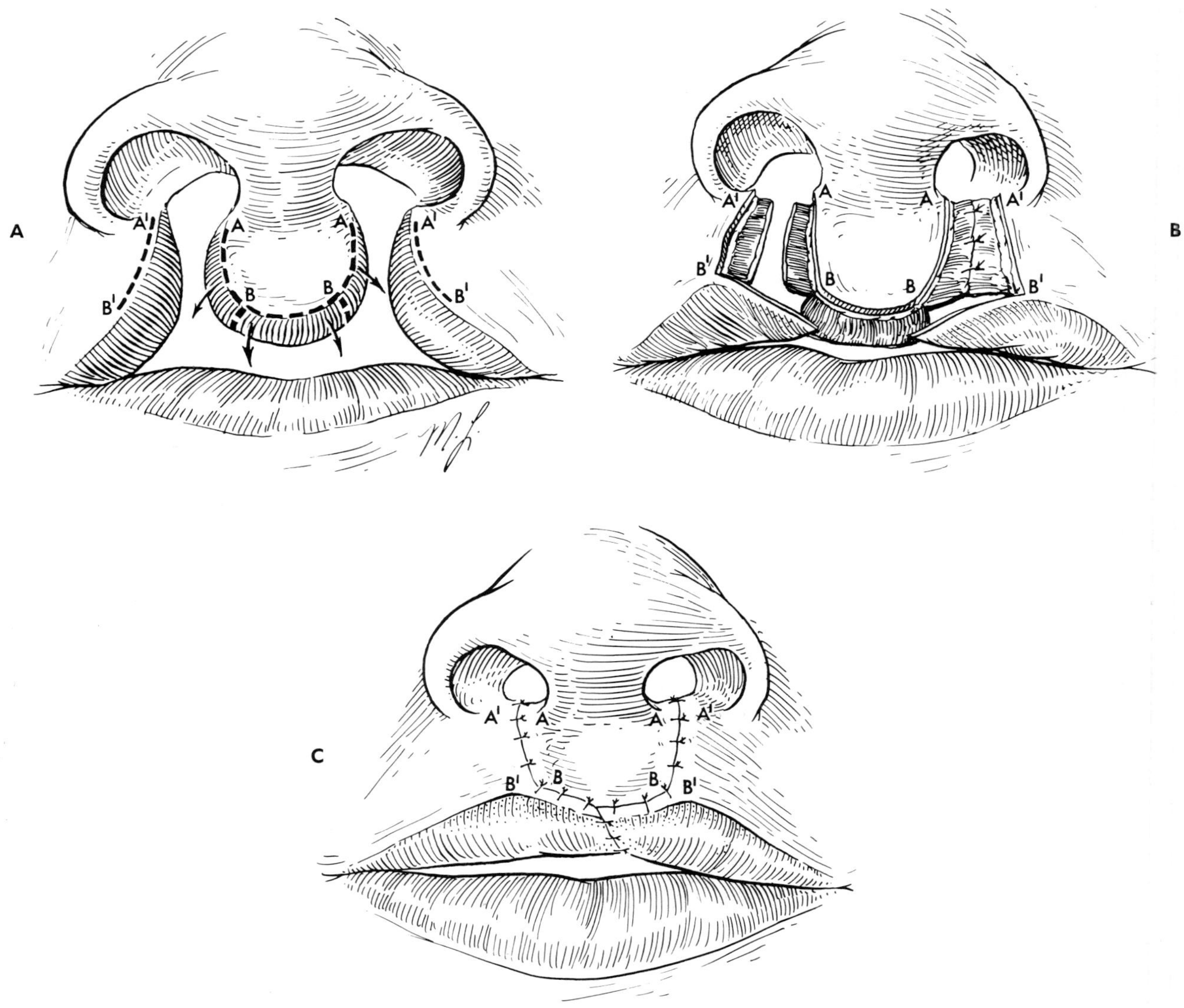

Fig. 19-1. A, Points *A* and *A'* are placed at the points for the new nostril floor. Point *B* on the philtrum is to be the height of the cupid's bow and is placed on the curve of the philtrum. Point *B'* is placed at the point where the lateral lip has full-thickness vermilion. **B,** The mucosa of the premaxillary segment is shown reflected and sutured to the lateral lip segments to form the new labial mucosa. The mucosa on the prolabium is reflected to give added length to the labial sulcus. The lateral vermilion segments are rotated to the midline to form the new upper lip. A small rim of additional skin above the vermilion is carried with the flaps. **C,** The lateral lip flaps are shown with creation of the new cupid's bow. Note the thin rim of normal skin above the vermilion.

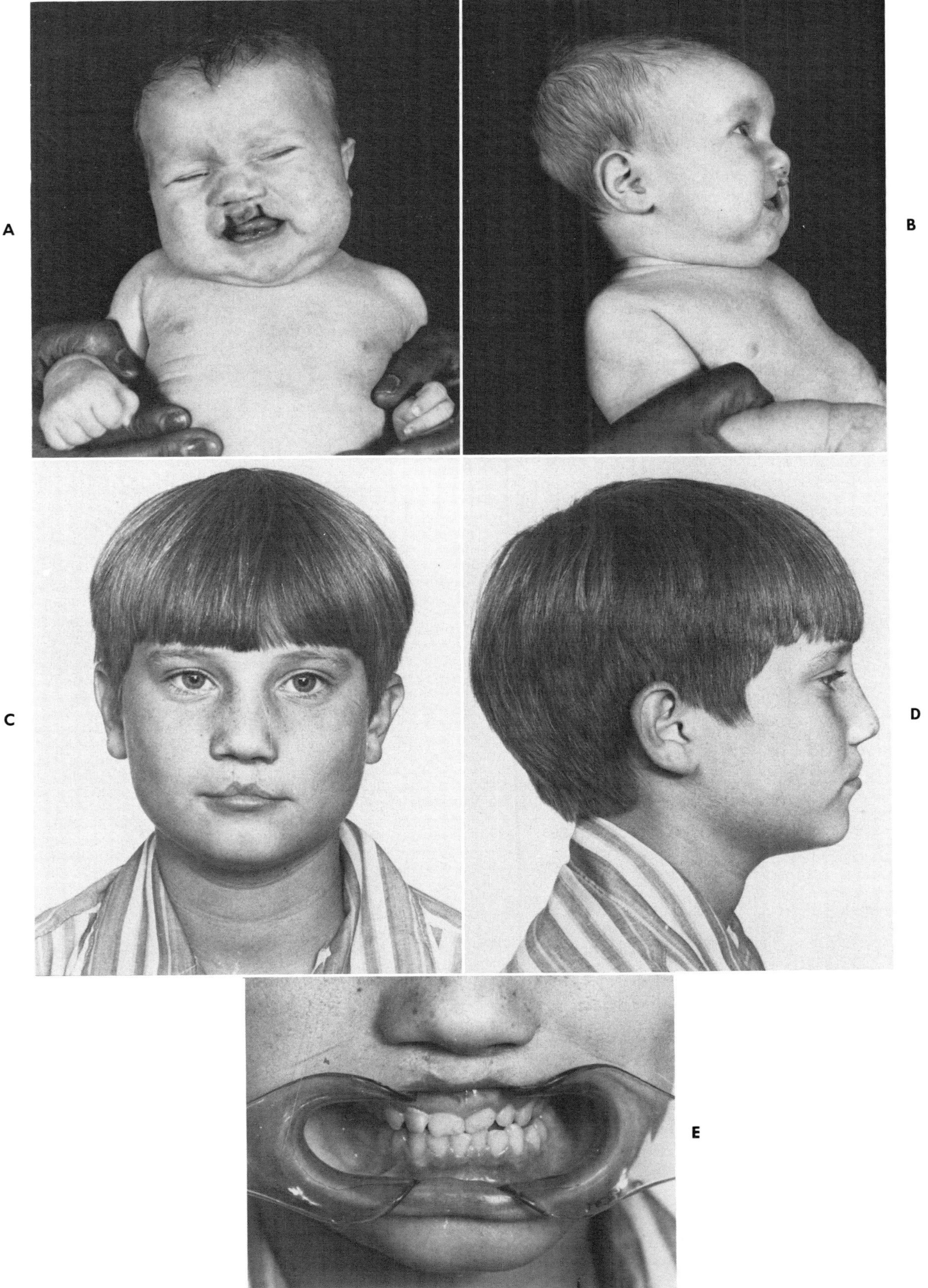

Fig. 19-2. A and **B,** Preoperative appearance of vermilion with a bilateral incomplete cleft of the lip. **C** to **E,** Postoperative appearance of the same infant 14 years later. No lengthening of the columella appears to be needed.

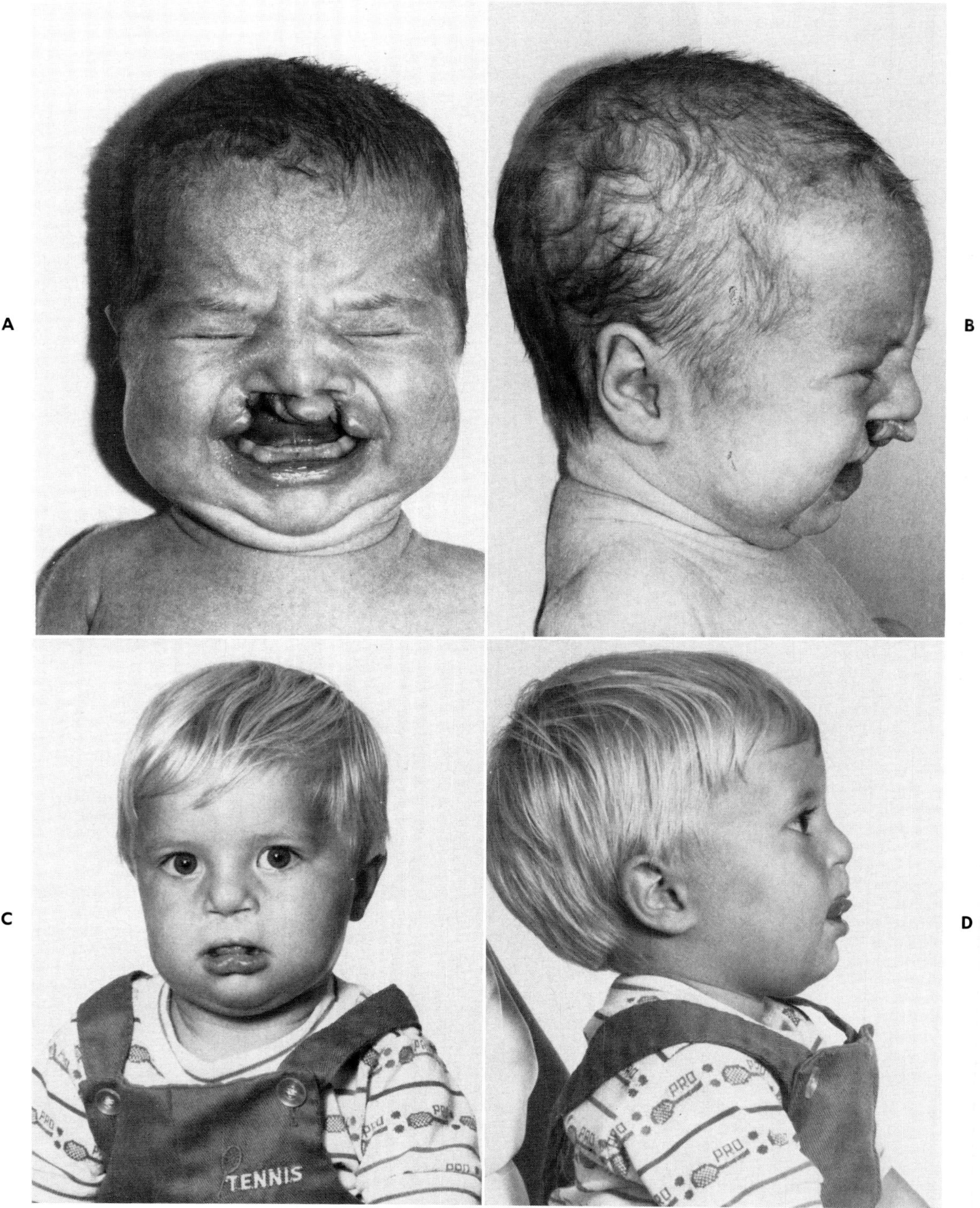

Fig. 19-3. A and **B,** Newborn with complete bilateral cleft of the lip and alveolus with some premaxillary protrusion. **C** and **D,** Appearance 2 years after bilateral cleft lip repair.

posite muscle fibers in the prolabial subcutaneous layer. All of the prolabial tissue is used (Fig. 19-1, *C*). Although this yields a wider than desired philtrum width, this tissue can be used at a later date for the fork flap in giving length to the columella. Adjustments are made in the cupid's bow at the same time. The prolabial mucosa was originally used by us to form part of the midportion of the vermilion; however, subsequent growth has shown that there is a disparity in the color and that it yields an undesirable esthetic length. This technique has been discarded, and only the lateral vermilion flaps are used to create the entire lip height (Figs. 19-2 and 19-3).

The infant with a bilateral cleft lip and associated protruding premaxillary segment is the most challenging of problems. In many instances a bilateral collapse of the maxillary arches is associated with the protrusion. To meet this anatomic challenge, a coaxial arch alignment appliance has been designed (Georgiade-Latham-Mark III).[3] The appliance consists of bilateral expandable arms with a prosthesis fitted to each maxillary segment and is stabilized by a staple pin fixation. (Fig. 19-4). The saddle component of the appliance is pinned into the premaxillae anterior to the premaxillary-vomerine suture and posterior to the tooth buds using a stainless steel pin 0.035 inch in diameter. The long arm of the appliance consists of two knurled thumbscrews on coaxial shafts. The larger, or anterior, thumbscrew (Fig. 19-4, *1*) when turned will cause a gradual posterior movement of the premaxillary segment toward a more normal anatomic relationship with the maxillary segments. One complete turn will move the appliance posteriorly 1 mm and will gradually allow retrusion of the premaxillary segments. Initially there will not be a noticeable change in the retropositioning of the premaxillary segment, but usually within 3 days this will become more evident. Caution must be observed against turning the screw more than necessary to compress the retraction safety spring, or the pin may pull out of the premaxillary bone.

Turning the smaller, more posterior, thumbscrew will cause expansion of the maxillary segments, so that the premaxillary segment can be brought into suitable relationship with the maxillary segments (Fig. 19-4, *2*). It takes approximately 10 days or more for the protruding premaxillary segment to be in a position to carry out a gingivoplasty (Fig. 19-5). At the time of bilateral lip repair, the coaxial palatal, premaxillary appliance is removed, and a gingivoplasty is first carried out bilaterally followed by the lip repair as described[8] (Fig. 19-6).

If a substantial union of the gingivoalveolar ridge is ac-

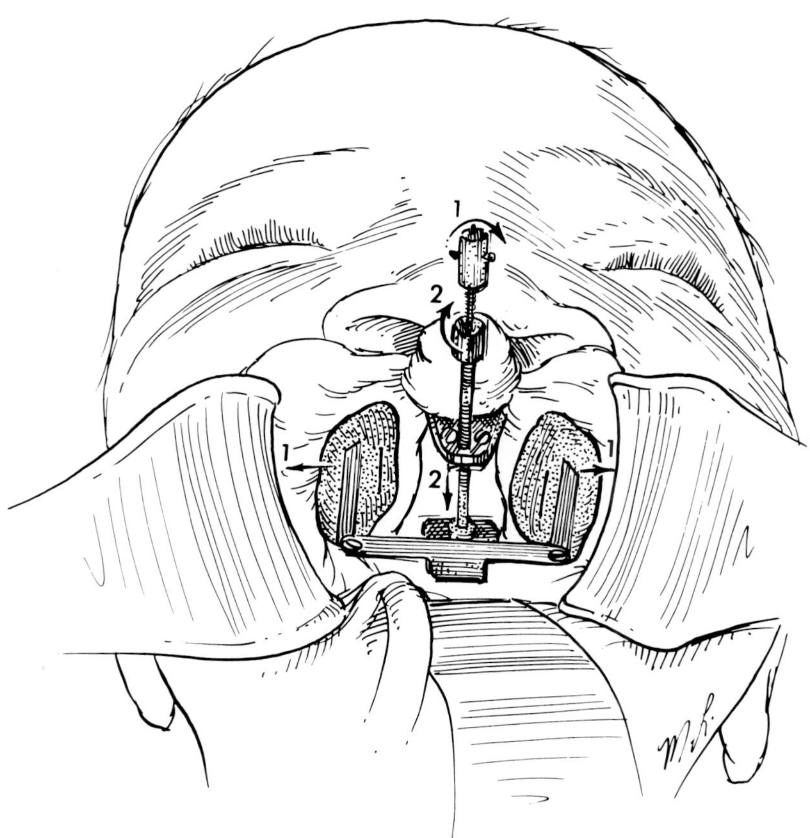

Fig. 19-4. Appearance of the maxillary-premaxillary appliance in place. Note that turning knob *1* will expand the maxillary segments. Turning knob *2* will cause the premaxilla to be pulled back closer to a satisfactory relationship with the maxillary segments.

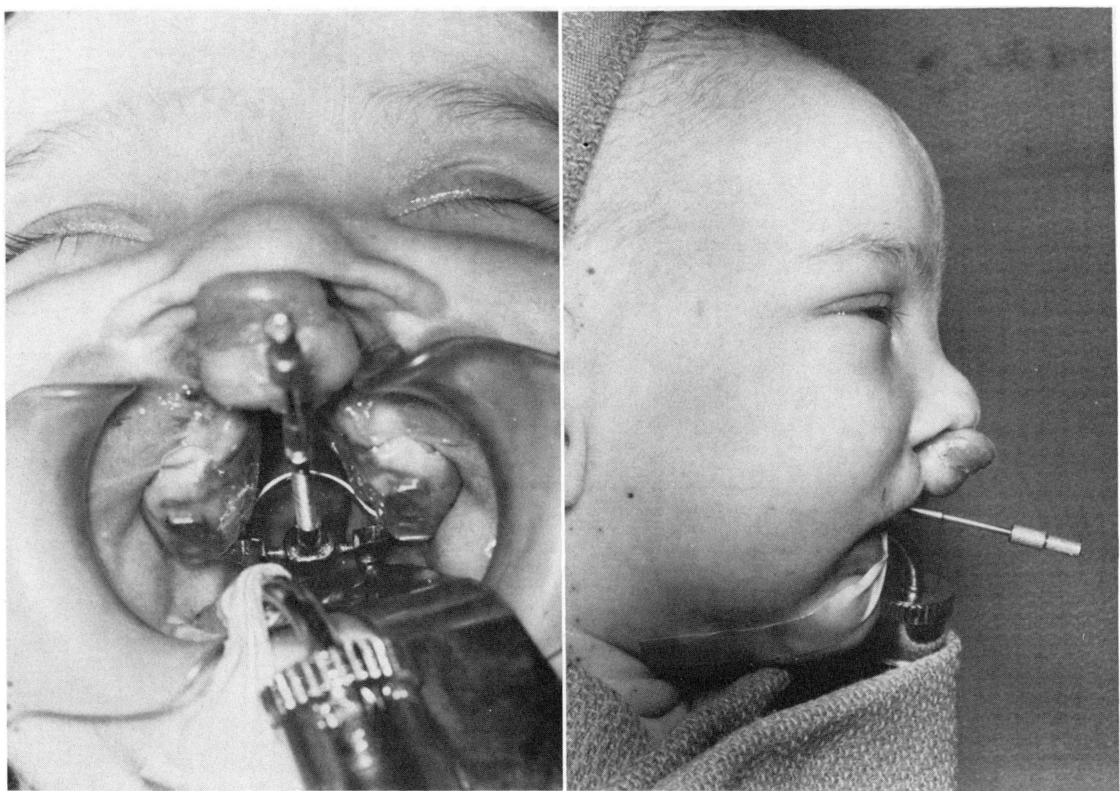

Fig. 19-5. The coaxial maxillary appliance is shown in position attached to the maxillary segments and premaxilla.

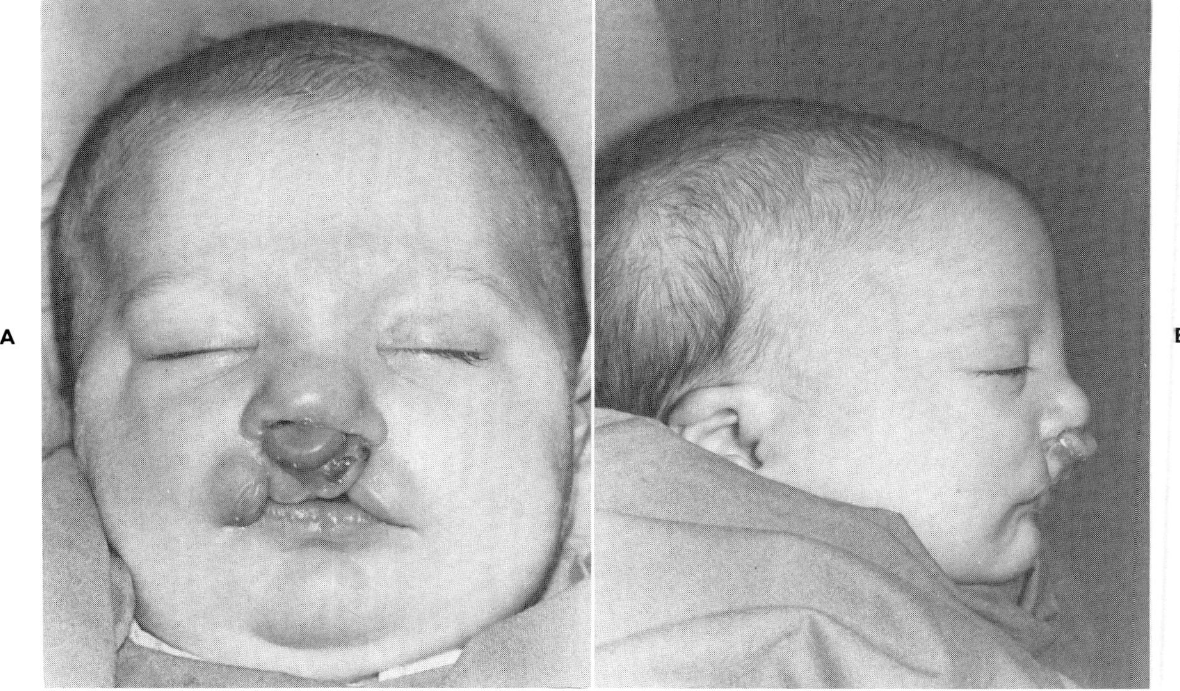

Fig. 19-6. A and **B,** Newborn with extensive protrusion of the premaxilla and accompanying bilateral lip clefts.

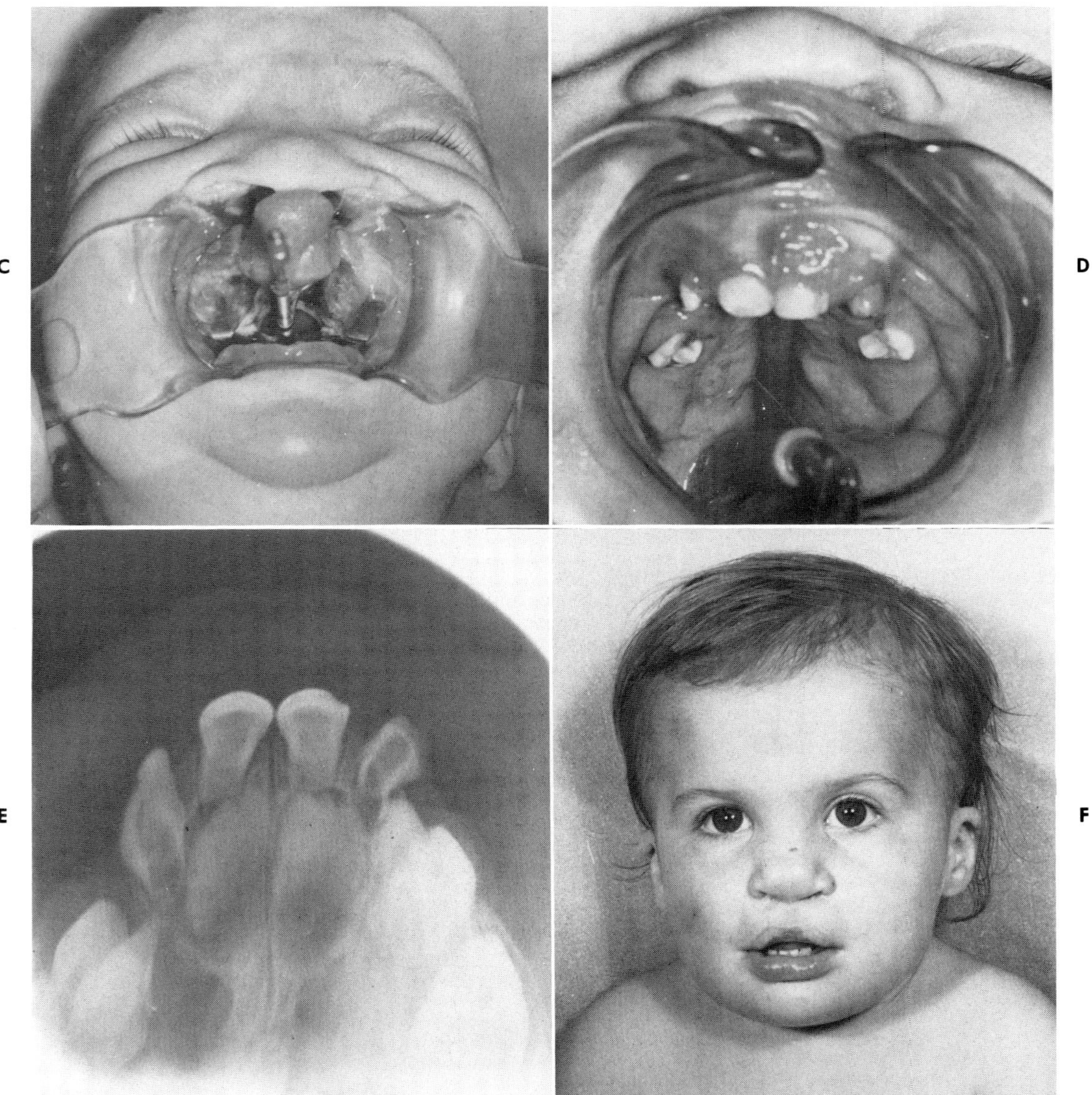

Fig. 19-6, cont'd. C, The coaxial appliance is shown in position and after positioning of the premaxilla in a more suitable alignment with the maxillary segments, just before bilateral gingivoperiosteoplasty. **D,** Appearance of maxillary alignment 13 months after gingivoplasty. **E,** Occlusal radiograph reveals bony union of maxillary segments. **F,** Appearance of same patient 13 months after one-stage alignment of maxillary segments and bilateral cleft lip repair.

complished, even if only on one side, the expansion appliance must be reinserted to splint the maxillary segments during healing. They should be held for about 3 months in an expanded, ideal arch form. Failure to do this in the past has been the pitfall of much previous work in this area. The goal is to obtain stable bony support for well-aligned palatal segments from periosteal ossification across the healed surgical sites.

POSTOPERATIVE CARE
Immediate care

A suitably sized Logan-type bow is invariably placed across the newly repaired lip. This appears to minimize the stress on the lip during the immediate postoperative phase and also to protect the lip repair when the infant turns or moves a hand over the lip area.

The intravenous fluid is maintained until the infant has

started taking sufficient fluids by mouth, and it is then removed. Feeding by mouth is initiated with water and clear liquids, followed by a predetermined formula. The fluids are administered via a rubber-tipped Chetwood syringe; after the first postoperative day, the mother is encouraged to feed the infant so that she can continue this when returning home.

Intermediate care

The 6-0 Prolene* sutures are removed on the fifth or sixth postoperative day under light anesthesia. The newly repaired area is then supported with sterile paper strips for an additional 5 days.

Maternal massage of the lip scar is initiated the second postoperative week twice a day. Rotary pressure is applied, using some light baby cream for ease of massage.

MANAGEMENT OF NASAL TIP DEFORMITY

There is no general agreement on the management of the columella in the repair of the bilateral cleft lip. The points of controversy mainly center around reduction of the prolabial to philtrum dimension and developing forked flaps at the original time of repair. Millard has reported the technique of banking the fork flaps between the upper lip and alar bases in the whisker position.[6,7] These flaps are to be used at a later date for columella lengthening. The other alternative is to maintain as much tissue as possible during the initial repair leaving a wide prolabium[1,5] that can be tailored at a later date using these tissues for flaps. This seemingly has the advantage of not subjecting the infant to a number of years of unsightly whisker fork flaps beneath the alar areas bilaterally. At the time of the construction of the forked flaps for columella lengthening and narrowing the philtrum to any appropriate width, the orbicular muscle from the lateral flaps is dissected free from the base of the nasal alae and transferred and joined under the philtrum (Fig. 19-7).

SUMMARY AND CONCLUSIONS

The basic concept in management of the patient with the bilateral cleft is that all available lip tissue should be conserved and used. A staged construction of the lip and nasal area should be taken into consideration. Radical attempts at creating a normal length in the columella, bringing the orbicular muscle together, and carrying out a satisfactory lip repair at the same time usually are not within the realm of possibility or practicality. A more conservative approach is to repair the lip and construct a satisfactory cupid's bow and vermilion lip line (Fig. 19-6). At a later date, usually in the early school years, creation of a continuous muscle layer with a suitable lengthening of the columella is carried out. Careful approximation of the lip tissues after a fork flap procedure should result in a scar equal to that which can be attained in the initial repair. Alignment of the maxillary and premaxillary segments, which are now carried out before the initial surgical repair, appears to be the procedure of choice.

REFERENCES
1. Broadbent, T.R., and Woolf, R.M.: Correction of cleft lip nasal deformity. In Georgiade, N.G., and Hagerty, R.F., editors: Symposium on management of cleft lip and palate and associated deformities, St. Louis, 1974, The C.V. Mosby Co.

---

*Prolene-Ethicon suture, Somerville, N.J.

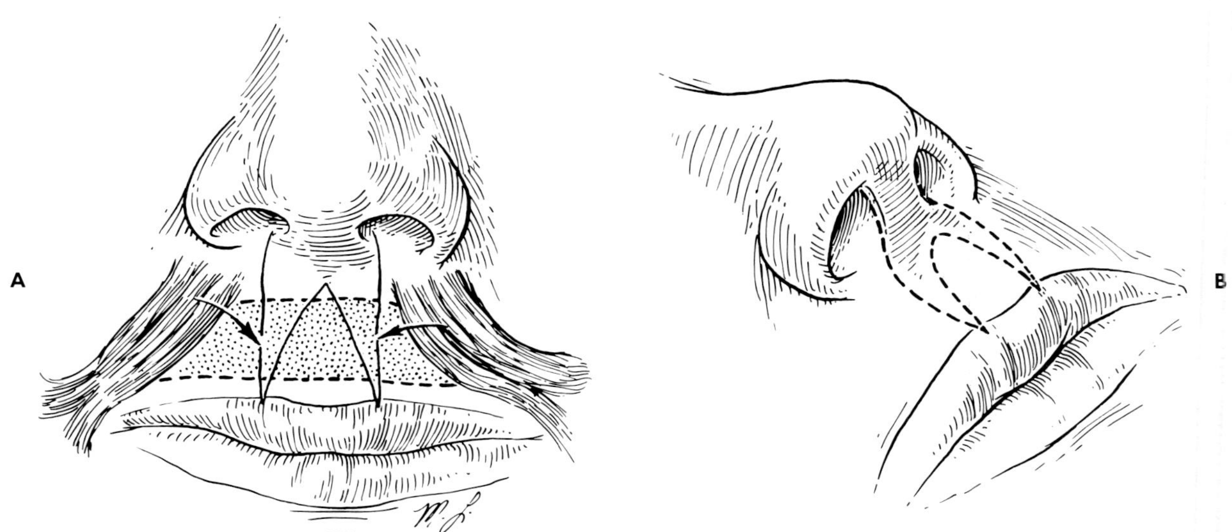

Fig. 19-7. A, Outline for developing fork flaps. **B,** Relationship of orbicular muscle fibers. Note their position in close proximity to the nasal alae. These fibers must be identified and rotated medially to meet the opposite muscle components at the time the fork flaps are created.

2. Fara, M.: The anatomy of cleft lip, Clin. Plast. Surg. **2:**204, 1975.
3. Georgiade, N.G., and Latham, R.A.: Maxillary arch alignment in the bilateral cleft lip and palate infant, utilizing the pinned coaxial screw appliance, Plast. Reconstr. Surg. **56:**52, 1975.
4. Johnston, M., Hassell, J., and Brown, K.: The embryology of cleft lip and palate, Clin. Plast. Surg. **2:**195, 1975.
5. Manchester, W.M.: A method of primary cleft lip repair. In Hueston, J.D., editor: Transactions of the fifth International Congress of Plastic and Reconstructive Surgery, Melbourne, 1971, Butterworths, Pty., Ltd.
6. Millard, D.R., Jr.: Closure of bilateral cleft lip and elongation of columella by two operations in infancy, Plast. Reconstr. Surg. **47:**324, 1971.
7. Millard, D.R., Jr.: Cleft craft: bilateral and rare deformities, vol. 2, Boston, 1977, Little, Brown & Co.
8. Skoog, T.: The use of periosteal flaps in the repair of clefts of the primary palate, Cleft Palate J. **2:**332, 1965.

CHAPTER 20

Cleft of the alveolus and palate

PETER RANDALL

Surgery of cleft palate remains a challenging and exacting field of plastic surgery. Challenging because we are achieving only 75% to 80% good speech results, and we should be doing better; exacting because the velopharyngeal mechanism has to work as quickly, easily, and effortlessly as a blink, or speech is likely to be severely affected.[14,57,78] Meaningful comparisons of techniques are almost completely lacking because objective comparisons are exceedingly difficult and take years to collect. In recent years the cooperative efforts by teams of specialists, including speech pathologists, plastic surgeons, dental specialists, pediatricians, otolaryngologists, and radiologists, and the American Cleft Palate Association have improved the overall care of these patients.

This chapter will cover chronologically embryology, timing of surgery, initial surgical repair, follow-up, and secondary palatal procedures. Brief mention will also be made of the problems with the alveolar segments and concomitant middle ear disease, although these areas are not strictly within the cleft palate area.

EMBRYOLOGY

Cleft palate appears to be a multifactorial anomaly, and indeed several different types of clefts are evident.* They vary in their anatomic configuration, as well as their extent (Fig. 20-1).

Clefts of just the soft and hard palate (i.e., the secondary palate extends from the incisive foramen posteriorly as opposed to the primary palatal clefts, or clefts of the prepalatal structures, which extend from the incisive foramen anteriorly) appear to be strictly midline defects, as are those clefts associated with bilateral prepalatal clefts. Clefts of the palate associated with unilateral prepalatal clefts have a

---

*References 15, 20, 30, 31, 46, 48, and 80.

lateralizing component in that the vomer is usually attached to the hard palate on the noncleft side.

Delay in the shift of the palatal shelves from a vertical position alongside the tonue up to a horizontal position and their eventual fusion can conceivably be responsible for clefts. This would account for a higher percentage occurring on the left side because the left palatal shelf usually reaches the horizontal position shortly after the one on the right, thus making it vulnerable to a teratogen for a longer period of time than the right palatal shelf.[15,79] On the other hand, the cleft usually seen with the Pierre Robin syndrome and perhaps caused by delay in straightening of the cephalic flexion of the embryo is almost always a cleft of the secondary palate only and might be due more directly to delay in the descent of the tongue from a position up between the palatal shelves.[64]

The most rudimentary type of cleft is a bifid uvula, which has a surprisingly high incidence of 2% in the American population.[45] Since most of these do not apparently have a functional deficiency, they are unrecognized and indeed need no treatment. The anteroposterior dimension in bifid uvula, however, can be short, and it is ill advised to remove the adenoid tissues in these patients unless adequate palatal length and velopharyngeal closure can be ascertained. Bifid uvula is often associated with a submucosal cleft palate, which can be recognized by a very thin membranous central portion of the soft palate, the zona pellucida and diagonal ridges lateral to this, indicative of the levator muscles being displaced from their normal transverse position to a more longitudinal position with insertion along the edges of the bony cleft. A notch in the posterior edge of the hard palate usually can be palpated. Rarely, the levator muscle can be in this abnormal position without a bifid uvula. Occasionally VPI can result from the following: a congenitally short palate without evidence of a submucosal cleft, or a neuromuscular

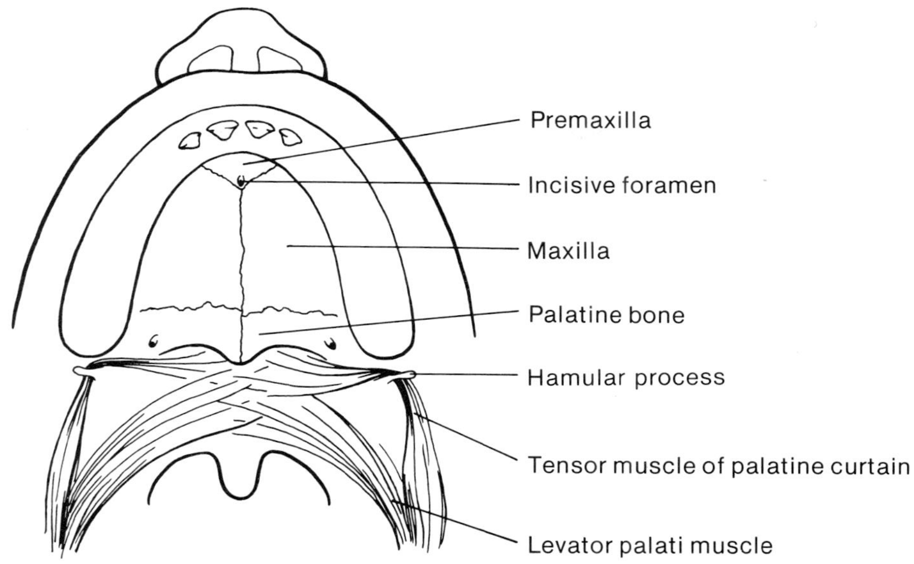

Fig. 20-1. Normal anatomy. Note the position of the incisive foramen separating the anterior structures, which are involved in the prepalatal (primary) palatal clefts, from the posterior structures, which are involved in the palatal (secondary) palatal clefts. Also note the transverse orientation of the levator muscles.

deficiency in the levator mechanism, or an unusually deep nasal pharynx which is often due to a cervical spine anomaly.[20,64]

Extension of the cleft through the alveolus is usually associated with a deficiency of the bony tissue on the side of the cleft. Although the lateral maxillary segment is usually too far lateral at birth, eventually it is more likely to be medially placed, producing a lateral crossbite. A difference of opinion exists as to whether it is better to treat this orthodontically (or "orthopedically") in the infant, before the primary dentition has erupted, or whether to wait until after the eruption of the permanent dentition so that manipulating these segments in the infant and at the time of the primary dentition might just as well be omitted and the problem cared for at the time of the permanent dentition.[6,17,18,32] Initial enthusiasm for early bone grafting of the alveolar cleft in infancy after orthodontic alignment of the alveolar segments, although once very popular, has now waned, except in a few clinics. Interference with maxillary growth was found, but a few teams are showing very nice results.*

A more difficult problem to handle is a deficiency of vertical growth at the margins of the cleft, causing the teeth adjacent to the cleft to be angled into the cleft, rather than in the usual vertical plane. In the bilateral cleft, the premaxillary structures are frequently displaced too far anteriorly, often with a considerable amount of labial angulation. Here again, a difference of opinion exists as to whether the

maxillary structures should be expanded and the premaxillary segment brought back into the maxillary arch at an early age, or whether the anterior position of the premaxilla should be maintained until the eruption of the permanent dentition. The greatest deficiency in growth, as seen in the adult patient, is an anteroposterior deficiency, and many of these patients will end up with a Class III malocclusion and an anterior crossbite rather than with the incisor teeth being too far forward.[17-19,50]

TIMING

In the United States most people prefer to close clefts of the palate at about 12 to 18 months of age. The belief is that by this time the patient is a good anesthetic risk, has already achieved an appreciable amount of facial growth, and the palate will be closed before it is needed for speech. Customarily in some European and Eastern European countries this time is postponed until 24 months of age or even later.[20,37] Two questions arise. The first concerns whether this is the best time for closure of the hard palate, and the second has to do with whether soft palate closure should best be done at a much earlier age.

Currently there is enthusiasm for closing the soft palate at the usual time, obturating the hard palate and alveolar cleft until full eruption of the primary dentition, and then closing the hard palatal cleft at 5 to 7 years of age when additional facial growth has occurred.[3,10,14,27] Having tried this approach for several years, I have lost my enthusiasm for this timing for a number of reasons. First, it is difficult to maintain obturation through the eruption of primary and

---

*References 1, 5, 6, 16, 17, 29, 33, 35, 42, 54, 61, 68-71, and 72.

secondary dentition. Second, even with good obturation, articulation of the anterior consonant sounds was often distorted. Finally, it was my impression (although no hard data exist) that these patients had just as many problems with lateral crossbite and anterior crossbite as those who had had the hard palate and alveolar cleft closed at the time of soft palate surgery or even at the time of the primary lip repair.

Early closure of the soft palate cleft is a different matter; however, few data exist to show a significant advantage.[37,38,65] Palatal function is a complex series of actions that require the exact synchronous control of a number of different muscles. This is needed not only for *speech,* but also for adequate maintenance of an *airway,* particularly while eating, and also for *swallowing* liquids and solid food. These three functions are not only extremely basic, but are called into play immediately after birth.[58,59] Furthermore, I have never seen a newborn with a cleft palate who did not already have a well-developed Passavant's ridge, which is believed to be a compensatory mechanism causing a forward projection of the posterior pharyngeal wall through an overaction of the superior pharyngeal constrictor or palatopharyngeal muscles. There is good evidence that swallowing is necessary in utero and that respiratory actions also occur. It should be obvious that the ''programming'' of the central nervous system for the control of these actions must be exceedingly complex, and, if they are not working properly, compensatory mechanisms would be called into play. Since these compensatory patterns are likely to become more and more firmly established in the early months of development, it would follow that for the proper normal control of these structures for speech, there would be a real advantage in closing the soft palate cleft at a much younger age, such as 3 to 6 months, rather than waiting until 12 to 14 months of age. Since 1964 I have been doing this in selected cases. These patients do seem to have overcome the problem of fluid collection in the middle ear space at an earlier age. Those with good speech appear to have particularly good speech with an easy, quick, and accurate production of critical articulatory sounds as opposed to a good, although perhaps more sluggish and stressed, way of speaking for those closed in the older age group. Some of these patients have required secondary pharyngoplasty, which is not surprising, but only about a quarter as many have needed secondary pharyngoplasties as in my patients whose soft palates were closed at 12 to 18 months of age.[65]

PRIMARY PALATAL PROCEDURES

At the time of surgery the child should be in good condition and free from respiratory tract infections. However, patients with unrepaired clefts usually have some mucopurulent nasal discharge. Virtually 100% of these children do not have good function of the eustachian tubes and will have serositis, which is probably best treated by myringotomies, evacuation of the fluid, and placement of ventilating tubes in the myringotomy incision.[67,82] Endotracheal anesthesia by a competent anesthetist and an intravenous line appear to be essential, although in developing countries, anesthesia by insufflation with a heavy stitch in the tongue to control the airway is probably better than endotracheal anesthesia attempted by an inexperienced person. I usually take the footpad from the operating table and put it halfway between the hinge on the headpiece and the head of the table so that the child's shoulders can rest on the footpad. With the head on the headpiece, a moderate amount of hyperextension can be achieved, and an extreme amount of hyperextension can be achieved by dropping the headpiece. Tape across the baby's thighs will help prevent slipping. A Dingman mouth gag provides good exposure, but the endotracheal tube is likely to be compressed unless small stainless steel lugs are added at the level of the alveolar ridge or a Ring tongue blade is used. The areas of incision are injected with 1% lidocaine (Xylocaine) with epinephrine 1:100,000 in small amounts and well distributed.[20] It is advisable to wait 7 minutes after injection before making an incision.

The important steps in closure (Fig. 20-2) appear to be wide freeing up of the palatal tissues so they can be approximated with little or no tension, repositioning and reconstruction of the levator palati muscle, possibly a V-Y lengthening of the palate with lengthening of the nasal mucosa either with a large Z-plasty or with flaps from the nasal floor, a vomer flap closure of the hard palatal cleft, a buccal sulcus flap for closure of the alveolar cleft, and possibly a superiorly based posterior pharyngeal flap to increase the efficiency of the soft palate closure.* NOTE: This primary posterior pharyngeal flap is not used when the palate is closed at 3 to 6 months of age or in children with possible airway obstruction, such as those with the Pierre Robin syndrome or the Treacher Collins' syndrome.[65] I usually prefer a primary posterior pharyngeal flap for a child without airway problems operated on after the ages of 12 to 18 months and certainly when the primary operation is done after 3 years of age.[81] The edges of the cleft are incised, and the edges of the uvula are excised. A relaxing incision is made from just anterior to the anterior tonsillar pillar, around the posterior maxillary tubercle, and then forward to about the level of the premolar teeth. Mucoperiosteal flaps are elevated from the hard palate, isolating the major palatine vessels, and stretching them out of their canals. Dissection is then carried *medial* from the pterygoid hamulus along the posterior edge of the hard palate. The hamulus can be fractured medially if need be without fear of interfering with eustachian tube function.

The edge of the cleft is then picked up with a skin hook and the dissection carried posteriorly from the bony surface at the posterior edge of the hard palate between oral mucosa and the levator muscle. This will show the longitudinal position of the levator palati muscle, and its abnormal in-

---

*References 11, 20, 26, 40, 80, and 81.

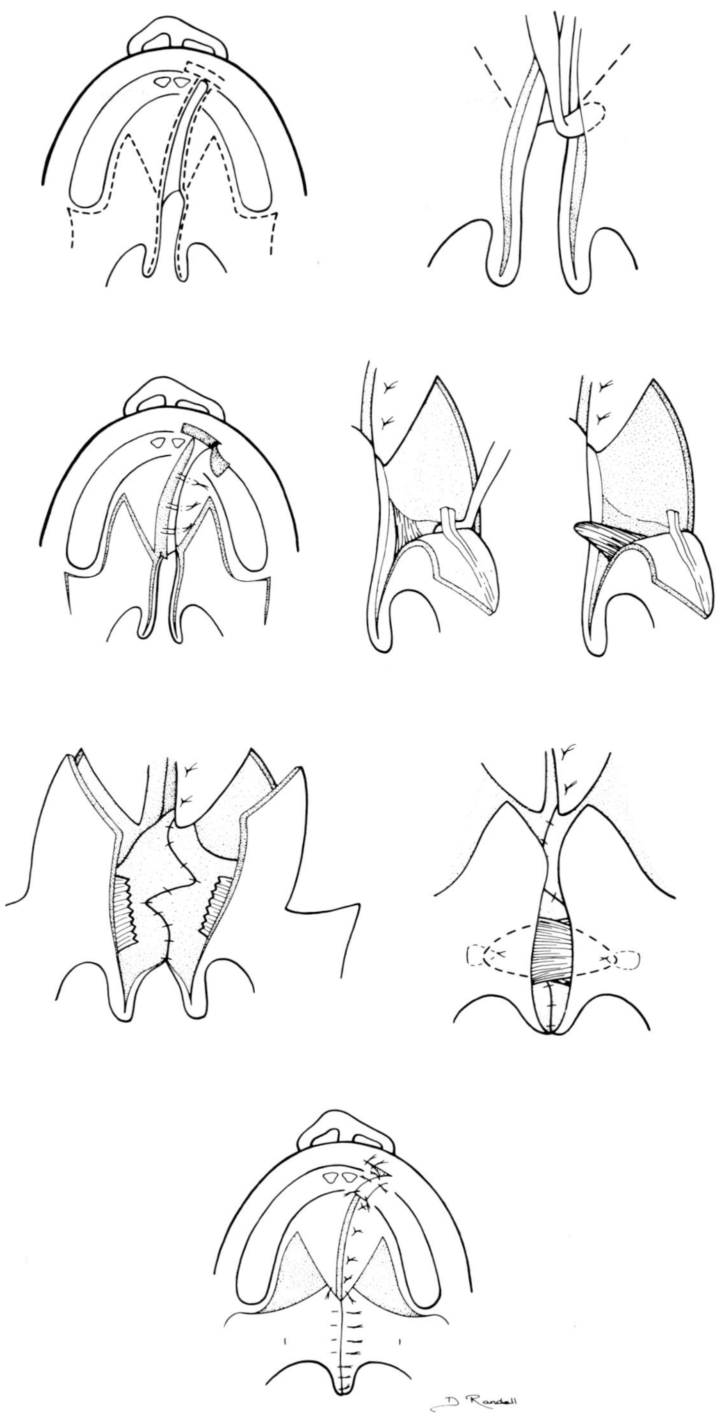

Fig. 20-2. Primary palatal reconstruction using a laterally based buccal sulcus mucosal flap for closure of the alveolus, a vomer flap of mucosa for hard palate closure, a V-Y lengthening of the palate, lengthening of the palatal vessels by stretching them out of the bony canals, dissection of the levator muscle with reorientation and reconstruction in the overlap position, and a Z-plasty lengthening of the nasal mucosa. This closure is usually combined with a primary superiorly based posterior pharyngeal flap of moderate width and lined with a turnover flap of nasal mucosa when the closure is done after 12 months of age. When done before 12 months of age, the primary posterior pharyngeal flap and the V-Y lengthening procedures are omitted.

sertion into the posterior edge of the bony palate and along the medial bony cleft. Next this muscular insertion is separated from the bone, and the dissection is carried out carefully between the muscle and nasal mucosa. In so doing, the levator muscle is completely freed up so it can be repositioned into a much more transverse location and overlapped so as to recreate the "levator sling."[63] The nasal mucosa is lengthened, either with a large Z-plasty or by freeing up flaps from the nasal floor.[11,47] The palate can be lengthened with a V-Y procedure as in the Wardill flaps or Veau incision, or if lengthening is not preferred, the edges can simply be sutured together side to side, as in the Von Langenbeck–Warren operation.[20,26,87] A large flap of mucosa is raised from the exposed portion of the vomer with its base placed superiorly, and an incision is made through the mucosa on the nasal side of the hard palate cleft. The vomer

flap is interdigitated with this flap and secured wtih through-and-through 5-0 chromic catgut suture. This can be done on both sides in bilateral clefts. A buccal sulcus flap of mucosa is raised with the base placed laterally, and rotated into the alveolar cleft to complete closure.

If a primary posterior pharyngeal flap is to be used at the time of the palatel closure, I prefer a superiorly based flap and use only about one half to two thirds of the posterior pharyngeal wall. Parallel incisions are made through the mucosa and muscle down to the prevertebral fascia, and the intervening flap of mucosa and muscle is elevated and cut across inferiorly about 1.5 to 2 cm below the level of the adenoid pad. This is sutured into the nasal side of the soft palate, anterior to the levator muscle reconstruction, and is lined with turnover flaps of nasal mucosa, which are based posteriorly toward the free edge of the palate.

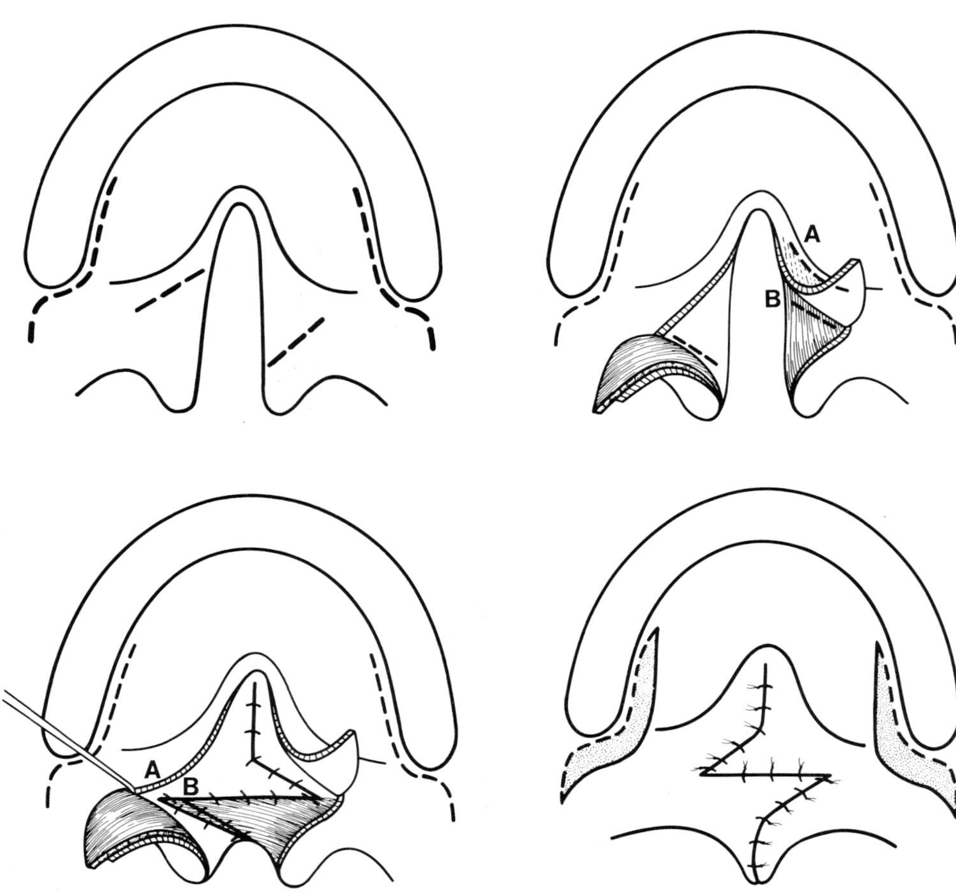

Fig. 20-3. The double-reversing Z-plasty repair of the soft palate described by Furlow.[48] Note that each posteriorly based mucosal flap includes the levator muscle on that side. The muscle *(A)*. extends beyond what can be used in the mucosal flap *(B)*. By reversing the Z-plasty on the nasal mucosa, the opposite levator muscle is included. The operation is simple and allows repositioning and reorientation of the levator muscles with less dissection than in the intravelar veloplasty. It also lengthens the palate and avoids a straight-line closure. It is difficult to do with wide clefts. (From Millard, D.R., Jr.: Cleft craft: bilateral and rare deformities, vol. 2, Boston, 1975, Little, Brown & Co.)

Another ingenious technique for repositioning the levator muscles and adding length to the soft palate at the same time has been described by Furlow[48] (Fig. 20-3). He calls this a double-reversing Z-plasty. A large Z-plasty is designed on the oral mucosa of the soft palate. In raising the flaps the levator muscle is included in the Z-plasty flap whose base is oriented posteriorly, so this flap includes oral mucosa and levator muscle. Its opposite flap includes just oral mucosa. A similar Z-plasty is made in the nasal mucosa, but it is oriented in the reverse direction so the flap based posteriorly is on the opposite side and includes the other levator muscles. I now prefer this technique because it is quick and easy and requires less dissection around the levator muscle. It can be used at 3 months of age and in older children. It can be combined with a primary posterior pharyngeal flap. The lining mucosal flap from the nasal mucosa is taken posterior to the Z-plasty.

I prefer to use 3-0 chromic catgut for primary closure of the pharyngeal donor site and through-and-through sutures to secure the posterior pharyngeal flap in place, 4-0 chromic catgut on the reconstruction of the levator muscle, and 5-0 chromic catgut on the remaining mucosal closure. These sutures should not be tied too tightly, but just tight enough to achieve approximation so as not to necrose tissue. The lateral relaxing incisions are left entirely open and will close spontaneously in a very short period of time.

A No. 18 nasopharyngeal airway is a good precaution, and a heavy suture can be placed as a tongue stitch to help maintain the airway. These children are not routinely given antibiotics; as previously mentioned, myringotomies are usually carried out at the time of the palatal surgery. In the immediate postoperative period they are given small amounts of clear liquids by mouth. Their diet is increased to full liquids (anything that is liquid and all pureed food, including soft and squashy materials such as junket, custard, gelatin, ice cream, etc.) within 24 to 48 hours of surgery. They are hospitalized until they have an adequate oral intake and are free of fever, which is usually 3 to 5 days. Feedings are offered from a cup or the side of a spoon.[39] Sucking and blowing and the use of straws or a bottle are avoided. Arm restraints are maintained for a period of 3 weeks, at which time, the patients are given an unrestricted diet with unrestricted activity. In addition, the mothers are carefully instructed not only on the use of a completely normal diet, but also as normal activities as possible with virtually no restrictions.[14] Speech stimulation is encouraged by simply urging parents and siblings to talk with the child even if the child is just "babbling." Daily efforts are soon made to increase their vocabulary using picture books and magazines. Sucking and blowing exercises are then encouraged using toys such as whistles, mouth organs, drinking through a straw, blowing bubbles, or using a soap bubble pipe. The ears are reexamined within 3 to 4 months of surgery, and the child is seen again in 6 to 12 months for a postoperative evaluation.[52]

Postoperative follow-up

This examination includes inspection of the surgical repair, teeth, ears, and general pediatric conditions, but by far the most important evaluation has to do with speech.

Before the examination I ask the parent how the child's speech is developing, what sounds are said well, which ones cause trouble, whether there are any ear problems, and whether they have noticed any leakage of liquids into the nose such as chocolate milk or ice cream.

I believe that the best evaluation is achieved by listening to the child's relaxed conversational speech. An invaluable way of doing this is simply to buy an inexpensive metal lunch box, and fill it with cheap plastic toys. Considerable tact is necessary to get the child to talk, and the physician may have to leave the room and listen outside the door. At times, if the physician engages the mother in active conversation, the child will keep trying to "butt-in" and be heard as well.

I listen for what sounds the child can say well, with particular attention to stop plosive sounds such as /p/, /t/, and /k/, the production of continuants (sibilants) such as /s/, and /sh/, and blends such as /st/ and /sl/. I also listen for hypernasality (the excessive nasal resonance heard on the vowel sounds) or hyponasality (which is just the opposite, or the denasalized sounds of an obstructed nasal airway). In addition, "nasal escape" may be heard, which is the sound of air leaking into the nose on sounds such as /s/ and /sh/. Normally this should not occur. It is important to note whether any of these, if present, is slight or severe, constant or inconsistent.[20,52,77,78]

Speech can be classified into four categories. The first is good, crisp speech without evidence of misarticulation (except those errors commensurate with age) or hypernasality or nasal air escape. This is evidence of good velopharyngeal function. The third category is clear-cut VPI with obvious hyernasality and difficulty building up intraoral air pressure for anterior consonant sounds, both stop plosives and continuants. Usually nasal air escape is also noted. The second is a category between these two extremes, with partial or inconsistent incompetence. In my experience this second category is by far the most difficult to treat. The fourth is the classification of *indeterminate* for those children who either refuse to speak or for one reason or another cannot be adequately examined.[63]

Having used these four categories of assessment with a battery of testing modalities, including the trained ear of the plastic surgeon and the speech pathologist, as well as radiographic analysis, pressure studies, sound spectrographic examinations, and comparing the evaluation with the eventual disposition of the child, there is no question that the trained ear is by far the most accurate of any of these methods of measuring palatal function.[44]

The patient in category one, with evdience of good velopharyngeal function and the usual sequential development of speech, probably does not need any further testing. It is unlikely for a patient to fall out of this category, although an occasional patient who is achieving good velopharyngeal closure at an early age will lose this ability with growth and deepening of the pharynx, as well as with atrophy of the adenoid pad.[83]

In the third category, with clear-cut VPI it is obvious that something must be done without delay. Again, in these patients there is little need for lengthy documentation. Confirmation of VPI radiographyically might be important for record and medicolegal purposes, but delay for intricate testing and ''trial'' speech therapy are not indicated. In the patient between these two extremes, those in category two, with partial or inconsistent palatal competence (or incompetence), it is advisable to study the situation in considerably more depth. Trial speech therapy, the temporary use of a palatal lift prosthesis, or simply repeat examinations might be indicated. Although it is more difficult to be sure that secondary palatal surgery is indicated in such a patient, it is helpful to know that these patients usually do well with almost any kind of surgical or prosthetic supplement. The reason is simply that they need much more additional valving to be competent.

The child in category four, in whom it has not been possible to determine which of the previously mentioned categories best fits the condition, should be seen frequently and examined carefully until the appropriate category can be determined.

Direct observation of the palatal mechanism by fiberoptic or cystoscopic nasopharyngoscopy has added a whole new dimension to the study of VPI. In the hands of an expert it will show far more than any of the other tests can demonstrate, but it is almost impossible to use in a 2- to 4-year-old child. However, it is invaluable in the older child, unusual situations, and for evaluating function after a pharyngoplasty.*

SECONDARY PALATAL PROCEDURES

Secondary palatal procedures lie in three main categories: those associated with incompetence of the valving mechanism in the velopharyngeal area; those concerned with nasal fistulae of the soft palate, hard palate, or alveolar area; and those needing osteotomies to improve the upper dental arch and occlusion with the mandible. Of these, I believe the most important has to do with VPI and should be searched for within 6 months of the initial surgery. The methods for testing have already been described and of course are detailed and documented by the speech pathologist, although I strongly believe that surgeons doing this type of surgery should be as familiar and capable of testing for palatal competence as the hand surgeon who is testing for hand function.

In the face of severe incompetence there is no way, in my opinion, that speech therapy can overcome such a deficit,

nor is there a need for extensive testing. This type of problem must be addressed right away to make the palate more efficient, and for me the most dependable approach is to use a posterior pharyngeal flap. A palatal lift prosthesis obturator with an extension from a dental palate might achieve competence, but in the severe case, I usually do not rely on this approach. Prolonged dependence on a denture with an added obturator has the problem of putting added strain on the teeth used for retention and the problem of what to do in patients who eventually lose these key teeth.[14,41,63,85]

In the patient with less severe or inconsistent incompetence the situation is quite different. Under these circumstances a number of approaches can be used successfully, and I think it is important to study these patients much more carefully and completely in order to decide which is the best approach. These studies can include speech testing, radiologic studies, including videotapes of both the lateral and base views, nasopharyngoscopy and testing of nasal airflow, plus testing the patient's ability to build up intraoral air pressure to sustain a constant volume of air during maximal breathing capacity. However, many of these tests require a high degree of cooperation on the part of the patient and simply cannot be done by a child who is only 3 or 4 years of age.[24,25,53,73]

Adequate speech training can overcome some deficiencies, but in my experience, if hypernasality is a significant part of the defect, speech therapy alone can seldom overcome the problem.[89] A palatal lift prosthesis or an extension with a pharyngeal obturator might suffice, and if there is good motion of the palate and only a small degree of incompetence, these or a posterior pharyngeal implant might also be considered.[2,4,20] Fortunately, if the deficiency is not great, a high degree of success can be expected with most of these approaches. In fact, in almost any group of plastic surgeons doing much of this type of work it is usual to find that each has its own particular approach to this type of patient and each seems to be achieving a very good degree of success regardless of the approach.* However, it is important not to delay the definitive treatment for these patients, since the results appear to be far better if initiated at an early age.

Most of my experience with pharyngoplasties has been with the use of either the superiorly or inferiorly based posterior pharyngeal flap, and these will be described in detail, although as noted earlier, those using other methods of handling VPI appear to be achieving an equal degree of success.[21,57,62,88] The posterior pharyngeal flap procedure is not a very difficult operation and has a high degree of safety with few complications and a high degree of success. In two retrospective series and one prospective series designed to compare the results obtained with the superiorly based posterior pharyngeal flap as opposed to the inferiorly based flap, all authors believed that they could not detect a sig-

---

*References 7, 8, 14, 43, 49, 53, 60, 66, 74-76, and 84.

*References 14, 26, 28, 36, 51, 56, and 57.

nificant difference, although in this country, the superiorly based flap is far more frequently used.[86]

The superiorly based flap appears to be located in a more normal position for velopharyngeal closure, but I find the superiorly based posterior pharyngeal flap more difficult to constrict than the inferiorly based flap (Fig. 20-4). Also I often have to reincise the soft palate in the midline in order to obtain a high placement of the superiorly based flap. In a palate that already has good motion, I am reluctant to add another surgical scar in the muscle and prefer to use an inferiorly based flap. I find construction on an inferiorly based flap to be an easier operation and useful in those patients with very poor exposure in the posterior pharyngeal area, such as children with limited jaw excursion, those with the Pierre Robin syndrome or the Treacher Collins' syndrome, or those with conditions such as cardiac anom-

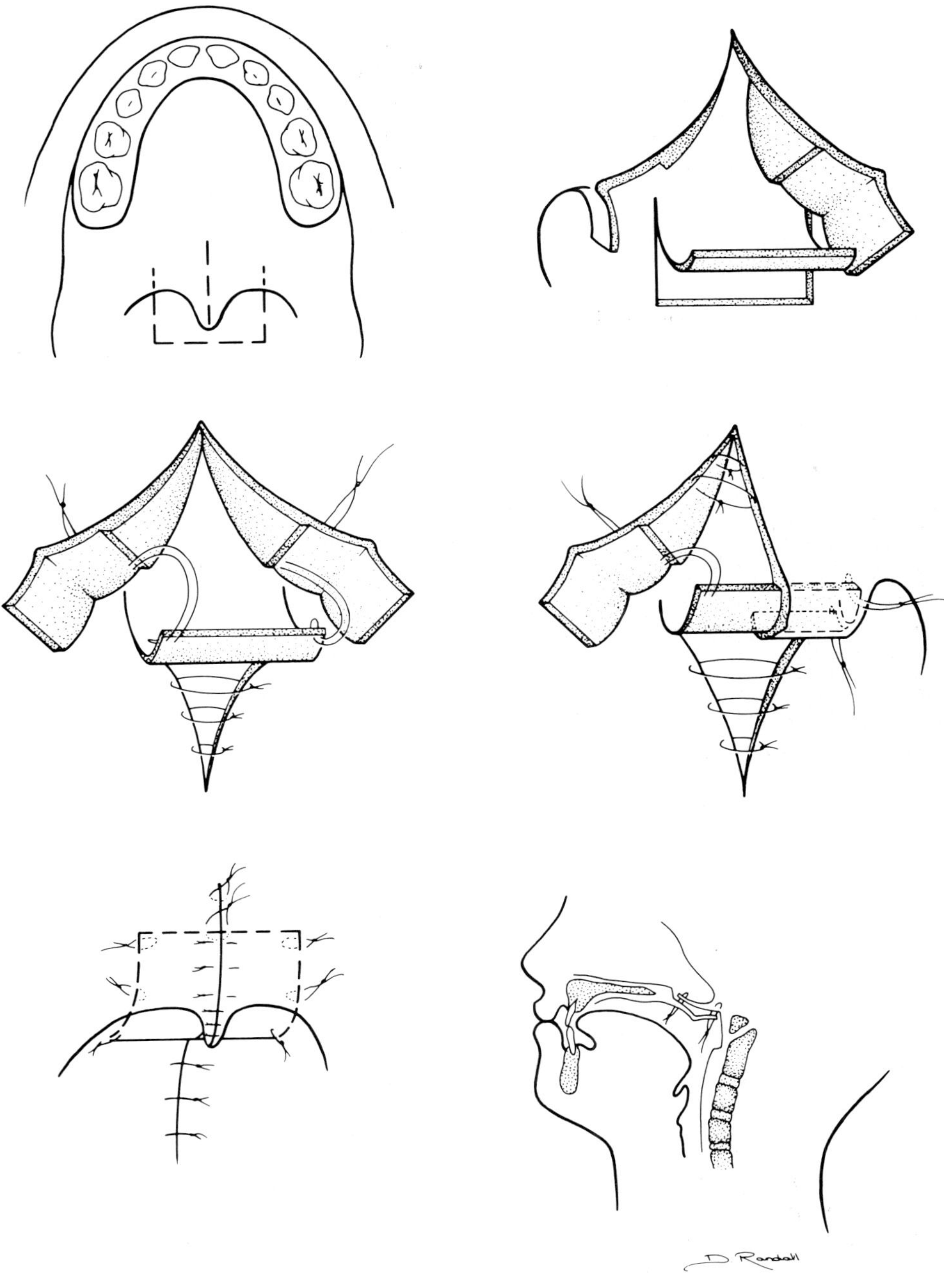

Fig. 20-4. A superiorly based posterior pharyngeal flap lined with turnover flaps of nasal mucosa. Usually the soft palate incision has to be reopened for adequate access, but not to the extent shown in these illustrations (necessary for clarification). The width of the flap will vary, depending on the age of the patient and the local findings.

alies, which can make them poor anesthetic risks.[21] I prefer to line both of these flaps with turnover flaps of mucosa from the soft palate. I also prefer to close the donor sites from side-to-side, although others prefer to leave the donor site open.

Should the findings at surgery or the initial operative report indicate that no reconstruction of the levator palati muscles has been carried out, one will often find that these two muscles are still attached to the posterior edge of the hard palate, in which case it is worthwhile to carry out a reconstruction and repositioning of these muscles at the same time a pharyngoplasty is done.[12]

A lengthening operation at the time of a secondary procedure is usually not done unless there is a severe amount of palatal shortening. In the older child, it appears that the amount of lengthening that can be obtained is really not very much. Perhaps those using the island flap technique for maintaining length in the soft palate believe otherwise. Again, I believe that if a lengthening operation is done, it should be supplemented with a posterior pharyngeal flap or at least with reconstruction of the levator muscle at the same time.

The results obtained with horizontally placed pharyngeal flaps[36] or the palatopharyngeal muscle[28,56] are all good, but I am not sure that any one is better than any other. Certainly in this particular area it is extremely difficult to obtain any kind of objective data. This is understandable because the overall results depend on a tremendous number of variables, such as how severe does the defect have to be before recommending a secondary procedure, who did the original surgery, who is doing the secondary surgery, at what age, how much scar is present, and what are the criteria for measuring the results?

Most palatal perforations leak mouth contents into the nose, and, if they are large, they can interfere with speech. Small perforations will not usually affect speech but constitute a hygiene problem and can cause an occasional embarrassing leakage of oral liquids into the nose.* Those located anteriorly can sometimes be covered by a dental plate or obturator, and I believe this is preferred for those patients in whom multiple surgical procedures have already failed. Otherwise surgical closure of even the larger fistulae can be achieved, provided the adjacent tissue can be adequately mobilized. Most of the time this is a good example of a small defect requiring a large operation. A rather sizable adjacent pedicle flap of tissue needs to be raised and rotated into the defect, with care being taken not to put this under tension and to avoid interference with the blood supply, giving attention to incisions from previous surgical procedures. As previously mentioned, a buccal sulcus mucosal flap based laterally is a good source of tissue for closing alveolar defects. I find the most difficult fistulae to close are those directly behind the premaxilla in bilateral clefts.

Pedicle flaps of tissue from the dorsum of the tongue, buccal mucosa, and a turndown pedicle of nasal septum using mucosa on one side for oral closure, the intervening cartilage for stiffness, and mucosa on the other side for nasal closure can be helpful.[13,22] There appears to be little reason today for bringing in pedicle tissue from a distance.

The surgery on alveolar segments for arch collapse and severe malocclusion really falls outside of the strict interpretation of palatal defects, but these problems are usually seen with other palatal problems and will be discussed here. These patients also must be carefully evaluated by an orthodontist and often by an oral surgeon so that planning for the eventual occlusion will be complete.* As previously mentioned one of the more difficult problems to treat is the vertical deficiency seen in the bony segments adjacent to the cleft. Bone grafts can be used for bridging alveolar clefts, if adequate coverage can be found. They will give adjacent teeth an additional matrix for stabilization and function well to stabilize a freely movable or "floating" premaxillary segment in bilateral clefts.[1,5] Unfortunately, much of the surgery to reposition alveolar segments, particularly those operations designed to shift the entire maxilla in patients with clefts, is frequently followed by a discouraging amount of relapse. Accordingly, when a severe Class III malocclusion is present, it is often more desirable to reposition the mandible as with a sliding osteotomy or segmental osteotomy to bring the jaws into better occlusion rather than to rely on repositioning the maxilla. At times it is necessary to do both.

CONCLUSIONS

Surgery for the child with a cleft of the palate is demanding and complex. It requires not only insight into the surgical problems, but also an understanding of the problems in speech and dentistry. These have been discussed sequentially along with specific surgical techniques and possible complications.

---

*References 19, 27, 29, 42, 55, 68, and 72.

---

*References 9, 14, 23, 26, 34, and 71.

REFERENCES

1. Backdahl, M., Nordin, K.E., Nylen, B., and Strombeck, J.O.: Bone grafting to the maxillary defect in cleft lip and palate by the method of Backdahl and Nordin. In Broadbent, T.R., editor: Transactions of the Third International Congress of Plastic Surgery (1963), Amsterdam, 1964, Excerpta Medica Foundation, International Congress Series No. 66.
2. Blocksma, R.: Correction of velopharyngeal insufficiency by silastic pharyngeal implant, Plast. Reconstr. Surg. **31:**268, 1963.
3. Blocksma, R., Leuz, C.A. and Beernink, J.H.: A study of deformity following cleft palate repair in patients with normal lip and alveolus, Cleft Palate J.**12:**390, 1975.
4. Bluestone, C.D., Musgrave, R.H., McWilliams, B.J., and Crozier, P.A.: Teflon injection pharyngoplasty, Cleft Palate J. **5:**19, 1968.
5. Brauer, R.O., and Cronin, T.D.: Maxillary orthopaedics and bone grafting in cleft palate. In Converse, J.M., editor: Reconstructive plastic surgery, Philadelphia, 1964, W.B. Saunders Co.

CHAPTER 21

The velopharyngeal portal: anatomy, physiology, and the management of incompetence

DONALD SERAFIN and JOHN E. RISKI

In normal speech production expired air is briefly constricted or obstructed by a series of competent muscular valves. The valves include the larynx, velopharyngeal structures, and oral articulators. The velopharyngeal valve normally couples the nasal cavity to the vocal tract for the nasal consonants /m/, /nn/, and /ng/. Also in normal speech velopharyngeal closure separates the nasal cavity from the vocal tract for the remaining consonants and vowels.(See Chapter 16.) A VPI will result when velopharyngeal closure does not occur appropriately. Under this condition speech is characterized by hypernasality, nasal air emission, and unusual misarticulations such as the glottal stop and pharyngeal fricative sound substitutions. [7]

A VPI may result from any of several deviant conditions. Calnan's classification system[7] has been modified to facilitate the categorization of possible causes of velopharyngeal dysfunction. If a VPI is detected, a cause must be sought, the severity ascertained, and treatment instituted.

Since a VPI may have an anatomic or a neuromuscular origin, an understanding of the anatomy and physiology of the velopharyngeal port is a prerequisite to a discussion of the management of an incompetent velopharyngeal valve.

ANATOMY
Osseous anatomy

The external base of the skull, when viewed inferiorly, has several distinctive features[15] (Fig. 21-1). The alveolar arch of the maxilla is readily seen surrounding the hard palate anteriorly and laterally. The bony palate has two sutures; a longitudinal suture separates the bilateral maxillary and palatine processes, and a transverse suture is located

between the maxillary and palatine parts. Opposite the second molar in the palatine bone bilaterally is the greater palatine foramen, through which the greater palatine nerve and artery emerge and course anteriorly, supplying the mucoperiosteum. More posteriorly in the palatine bone are two smaller bilateral foramen, through which exit the lesser palatine nerves and arteries that course posteriorly. The longitudinal suture terminates anteriorly at the incisive foramen, through which the nasopalatine nerves, branches of the pterygopalatine ganglion, emerge onto the hard palate. When lines are drawn bilaterally from the incisive foramen to a point between the lateral incisors and canine teeth, the enclosed area represents the premaxillary segment. Embryologically it is formed by a downward growth of the medial nasal process, which fuses with the lateral maxillary processes.[30]

The medial and lateral pterygoid plates are attached posteriorly to the maxillary tuberosity. They originate from the body and greater wing of the sphenoid bone. The medial pterygoid plate has two diverging edges that contain the scaphoid fossa from which anterior fibers of the tensor muscle of the palatine curtain originate. Inferiorly to this fossa is the hamulus around which the tendon of the tensor muscle courses medially to terminate in the aponeurosis of the soft palate. From the scaphoid fossa posteriorly, the tensor muscle originates posterolaterally from the cartilaginous portion of the eustachian canal and the sphenoid spine. At the base and immediately posterior to the pterygoid plates is the oval foramen, through which exits the fifth cranial nerve. Posterolaterally is the foramen spinosum, which contains the middle meningeal artery. Posteromedially are the petrous

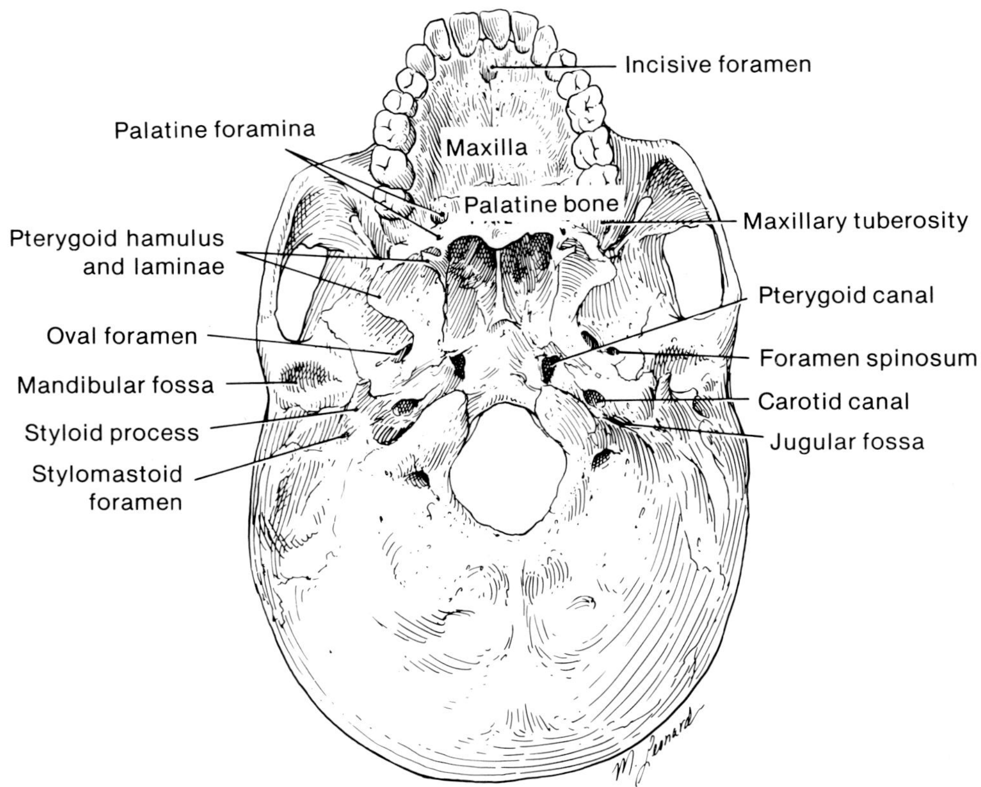

Fig. 21-1. Osseous anatomy at the base of the skull. *MAX*, Maxillae; *PAL*, palate.

portions of the temporal bone, which give origin to the fibers of the levator veli palatini muscle.

Soft palate

The soft palate is a fibromuscular structure extending from the palatine processes of the hard palate, posteriorly terminating in the uvula (Fig. 21-2). The anterior one third is composed of a fibroaponeurotic portion into which inserts bilaterally the tensor muscle of the palatine curtain.[15] The posterior two thirds are muscular, the majority of which consists of fibers from the levator veli palatini muscle (Fig. 21-3). The palatopharyngeal muscle encompasses the levator with fibers demonstrated on both the superior (nasopharyngeal) and inferior (oropharyngeal) surface. Also present on the inferior surface are fibers of the palatoglossus muscle.[5] The muscle of the uvula consists of a small bundle of longitudinally arranged fibers between the palatoglossus and levator muscles.

Skeletal Muscles
Tensor muscle of the palatine curtain

The origin and insertion of this muscle have been described previously. Although it has been described as a tensor muscle of the palatal aponeurosis, this has not been clearly demonstrated. It has been shown, however, that by

its origin from the isthmus of the cartilaginous portion of the estachian tube, contraction results in eustachian tube clearance. Some fibers have common origin with fibers of the tensor muscle of the tympanic membrane, a muscle acting on the malleus to adjust middle ear pressure. Both of these muscles, unlike other muscles of the velopharyngeal mechanism are innervated by the mandibular branch of the fifth cranial nerve.

Levator veli palatini

The origin of this muscle has been described previously. It is generally agreed that from its origin it passes inferior to the eustachian tube and medial to the torus tubarius. It lacks attachment to the eustachian tube and inserts into the velum. Contraction elevates the soft palate superiorly and posteriorly toward the posterior pharyngeal wall. It displaces the torus medially, posteriorly, and superiorly.[8] Thus it appears that the levator veli palatini could be solely responsible for both velar and lateral pharyngeal wall closure during speech.[9]

Palatopharyngeal muscle

The insertion of the palatopharyngeal muscle is closely interwoven with fibers of the levator muscle. Fibers of this muscle course inferiorly, laterally, and posteriorly, becom-

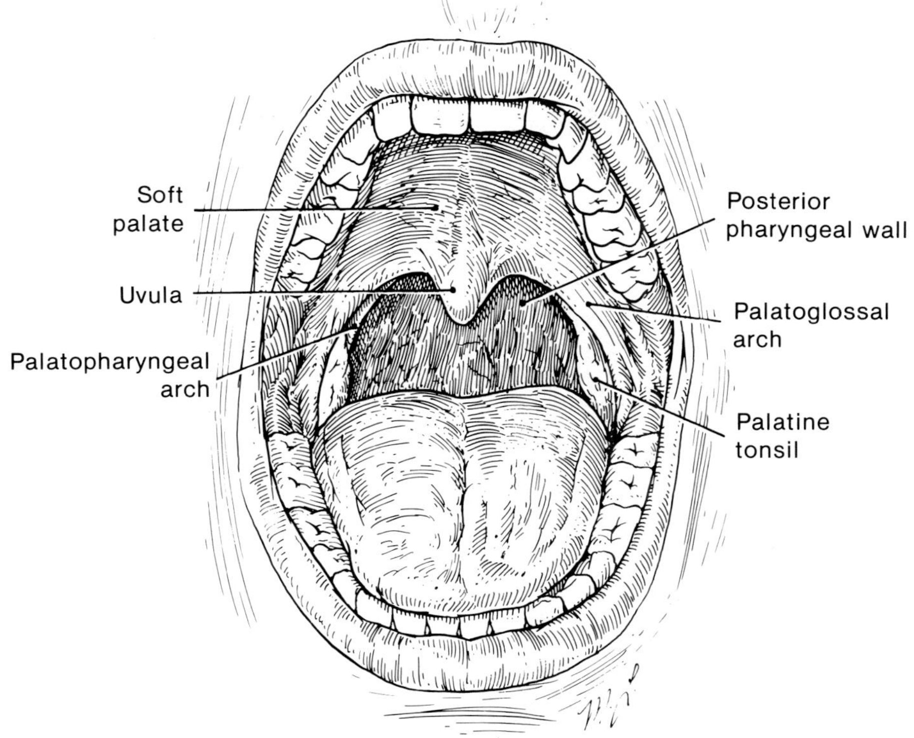

Fig. 21-2. Anatomic landmarks of the oropharynx.

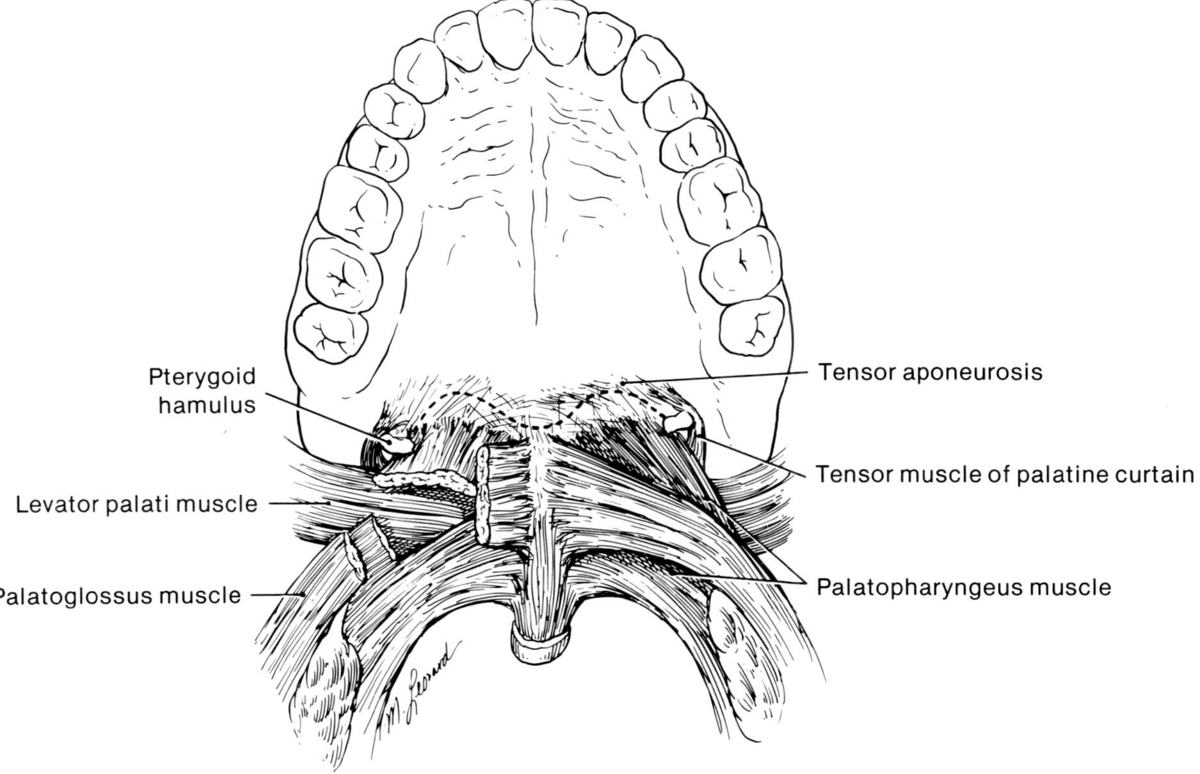

Fig. 21-3. Muscles of the soft palate.

ing indistinguishable from fibers of the superior pharyngeal constrictor muscle. Intraorally its fibers constitute the posterior tonsillar pillar (Fig. 21-2). The muscle appears to function as a velar depressor or oropharyngeal elevator-constrictor and has a more physiologic role in swallowing than in phonation.[9] This is supported by research electromyography (EMG) evidence.[11]

Superior pharyngeal constrictor muscle

The superior pharyngeal constrictor muscle originates from the posterior pharyngeal raphe from the level of the cranial base to the oropharynx (Fig. 21-4). It then courses laterally and anteriorly, inserting into the velum and hamulus superiorly and the pterygomandibular raphe and mandible more inferiorly. The most superior fibers inserting into the velum and hamulus can be identified intraorally, inferior to the velum.[24] This thickened band, when present posteriorly, has been termed *the sphincter of Willis*.[33] Anatomically it has been identified as Passavant's ridge. It is the site opposite the atlas where the nasal cylindric epithelium changes into stratified epithelium of the oropharnyx. It would appear that contraction of the superior pharyngeal constrictor muscle results in medial or medial and anterior motion of the lateral pharyngeal walls. This function is more consistent with the act of swallowing than speech.[9]

Palatoglossus muscle

The palatoglossus muscle originates from the tongue and inserts into the velum inferolaterally. Intraorally its fibers constitute the anterior pillar of the tonsil (Fig. 21-2). It is a depressor of the velum and functions in the act or swallowing by pulling the velum downward and forward.[9] The muscle also elevates the posterior third of the tongue in the formation of /k/, /g/, and /ng/ sounds according to EMG studies.

Innervation
Motor nerves

With the exception of the tensor muscle of the palatine curtain (and tympanic membrane), which is innervated by the mandibular branch of the fifth cranial nerve, all other muscles are innervated through the pharyngeal plexus. The motor fibers of the plexus probably reach it from the vagus nerve. These motor fibers are in reality cranial or bulbar rootlets of the eleventh cranial nerve.[15]

Sensory nerves

Sensation to the palate is provided by the pterygopalatine ganglion and its terminal branches: (1) nasopalatine, (2) greater palatine, and (3) lesser palatine nerves (Fig. 21-5).[15] This ganglion receives fibers predominantly from the

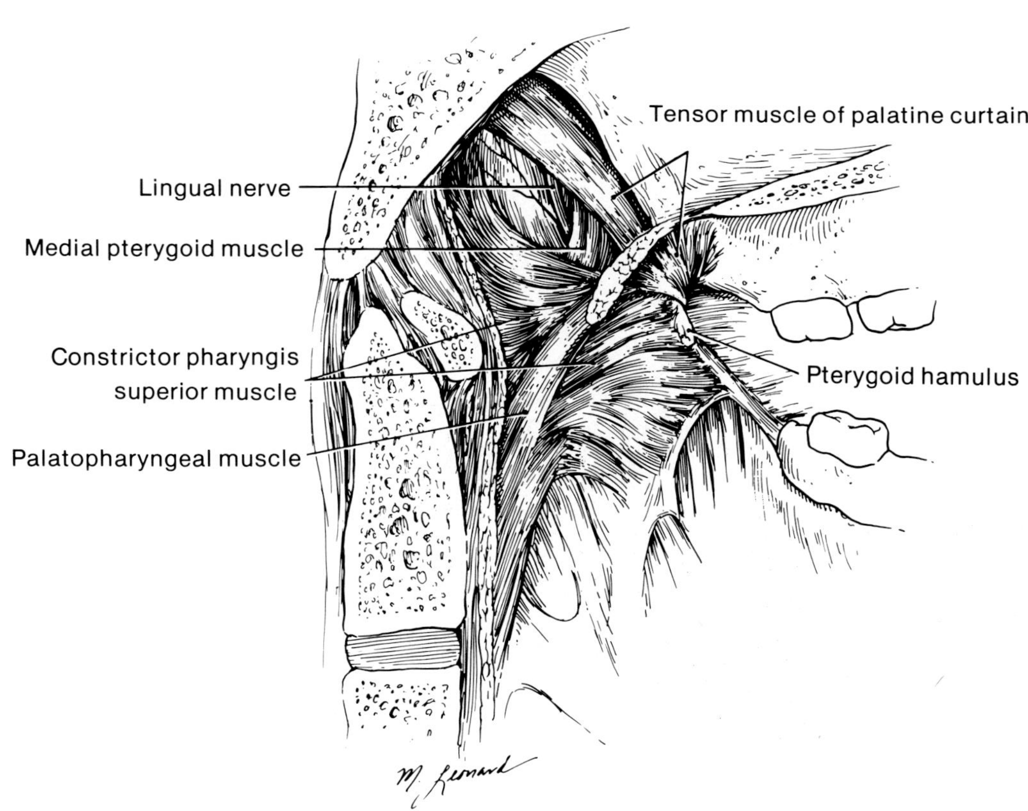

Fig. 21-4. Origin and insertion of the muscles of the nasopharynx.

maxillary nerve but may also receive fibers from the facial nerve (through the greater petrosal nerve) and fibers of the upper spinal nerves (through the nerve of the pterygoid canal, the vidian nerve).

PHYSIOLOGY

Considerable evidence has now accumulated to demonstrate a basic difference in function of the velopharyngeal mechanism between the act of swallowing and speech. During speech the soft palate is elevated superiorly and posteriorly against the posterior pharyngeal walls, whereas the lateral pharyngeal walls are displaced medically and posteriorly.[8,27,28] It appears that lateral pharyngeal wall motion during speech occurs superiorly at the level of the torus tubarius.[1,2,5,8] Both velar elevation and superior lateral wall

motion appear to be related predominantly to contraction of the levator veli palatini. In swallowing, however, the superior and middle pharyngeal constrictor muscles, more inferiorly, are involved in closure. Further discussion of velopharyngeal closure patterns for speech can be found in Chapter 16.

During phonation the velum lengthens and contacts the posterior pharyngeal wall at or slightly below the palatal plane, whereas the high point of the velum is 4 to 5 mm superior to the point of contact.[4,13] Investigators have demonstrated that the height of velar elevation depends on the sound being produced and on phonetic context.[3]

As outlined previously, Passavant's ridge, which is demonstrated in patients with cleft palate, appears to represent superior fibers of the superior constrictor muscle. Although

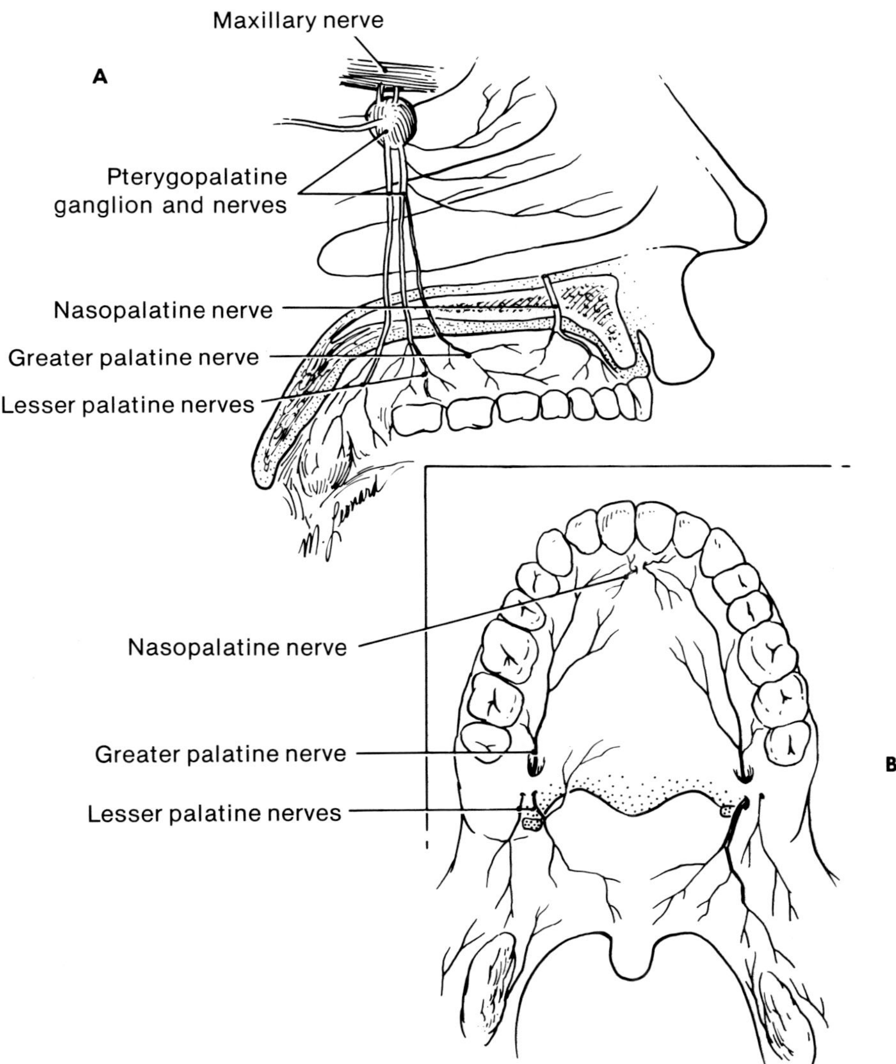

Fig. 21-5. Sensory nerve innervation of the hard **(A)** and soft **(B)** palate.

Passavant in 1863[22] and 1869[23] ascribed contraction to normal velopharyngeal closure, this theory subsequently has been disproven. It is now well documented that Passavant's ridge is a compensatory mechanism to effect velopharyngeal closure in patients with cleft palate.[6,8]

SURGICAL MANAGEMENT

Surgical treatment to establish velopharyngeal competence was introduced in 1876 by Schoenborn,[25] who described an inferiorly based pharyngeal flap for palatal closure. Ten years later in 1886 he described a superiorly based pharyngeal flap.[26] Both inferiorly and superiorly based flaps were used to augment deficient palatal tissue resulting from congenital clefts.

Dorrance[10] in 1925 described his technique of palatal closure and pushback. Mucoperiosteal flaps were raised on either side of the cleft. Emphasis was placed on fracturing the hamulus process, converting the function of the tensor muscle into that of a levator muscle.

Wardill[32] in 1937 described palatal closure of complete clefts using a four-flap technique. If necessary, the greater palatine arteries were cut, the hamulus fractured, and the posterior flaps detached from the hard palate. Veau flaps were employed from the vomer to close the nasopharyngeal mucosa.[31] A pharyngoplasty also was performed before palatal closure, resulting in a " . . . marked reduction in the diameters of the nasopharynx."[32]

The concept of reduction of the cross-section in diameter of the posterior pharynx, however, was not new. Gersuny[12] in 1900 described the injection of petroleum jelly into the uvula and adjacent soft palate to improve the quality or speech. Hagerty[14] used both autogenous and homogenous cartilage grafts to augment the posterior pharyngeal wall.

Hynes[17] in 1950 described his technique of using mucomuscular flaps bilaterally from the posterior pharyngeal wall. These flaps were then transferred medially in a transverse position, producing a ridge above the level of Passavant's ridge.

The concept of transposing mucomuscular flaps to function as a dynamic sphincter was further expanded by Orticochea[20,21] in 1963. Superiorly based flaps consisting of a segment of the palatopharyngeal muscle were placed behind an inferiorly based mucomuscular posterior pharyngeal flap. Although some critics argue against the dynamic nature of the sphincter, none disagree with its obturating effect.

In surgical literature controversy still exists as to the relative value of an inferiorly based or a superiorly based pharyngeal flap for the treatment of VPI. There appears to be little controversy, however, that once created, the flap is adynamic and functions primarily as an obturator. In some instances the tethering effect of a scarred adynamic flap may actually inhibit velar movement. Research in this area has demonstrated that medial movement of the lateral pharyngeal walls is essential to successful closure.[8,19,29] Controversy was recreated after Orticochea's introduction of a dynamic pharyngoplasty in 1963.[20] To date the dynamic nature of the palatopharyngeal mucomuscular flaps has not been resolved. An obturating effect, however, does result which appears to be relatively stable with the passage of time postoperatively. Fibrosis, contracture, and tethering of the soft palate appear to be more predominant in superior- and inferior-based flaps.

THE TRIPLE-FLAP PHARYNGOPLASTY: OPERATIVE TECHNIQUE

The pharyngoplasty described by Orticochea[20,21] serves as the basic design with some additional important modifications (Fig. 21-6). A Dingman or Dot mouth gag and cheek retractor provide exposure. A Lane endotracheal tube is employed during inhalation anesthesia. The head is hyperextended, and a roll is placed under the shoulders. This provides optimal visualization of the posterior pharynx. This position is also one that places the flaps under the greatest tension. After removal of the mouth gag and repositioning of the head and neck to a more neutral position, the newly constructed pharyngoplasty appears to relocate to a more superior position under less tension.

Review of present data indicates that the pharyngoplasty should be constructed at or above the palatal plane. This superior location approximates the contact point of the soft palate and posterior pharyngeal wall noted in normal speech. As a general rule, the pharyngoplasty is placed as superior as possible. An important landmark for placement of the posterior wall pharyngeal flap is the tubercle of the first cervical vertebra, the atlas. Also at this level one can usually detect a transition from the stratified squamous epithelium of the oropharynx to the pseudostratified ciliated columnar epithelium of the nasopharynx. Varying amounts of adenoidal tissue in the nasopharynx can also be identified. At times this may be excessive.

If the soft palate is short or the adenoidal pad is low, a midline superior-based pharyngeal flap is designed as described by Jackson (Fig. 21-6, *A*).[16,18] This facilitates high or superior placement of the pharyngoplasty. However, if the zone of mucosal transition is high and the palate of adequate length, an inferiorly based posterior pharyngeal flap may be constructed (Fig. 21-6, *B*). This flap, as indicated by Orticochea,[20,21] should be 2×1 cm long. In contradistinction to Orticochea, who indicated that the location of the flap be at the middle or lower pole of the tonsil,[21] it should be placed in a more superior location as described previously.

Lateral, superiorly based mucomuscular flaps are created, incorporating as much as possible of the palatopharyngeal muscles (Fig. 21-6, *C* to *E*). As indicated earlier, this muscle has no role in phonation but acts as a palatal depressor during swallowing. No detectable functional loss ensues when this muscle is detached from the posterior pharyngeal wall inferiorly and reattached more superiorly. The posterior pillar of the tonsil is the external landmark of

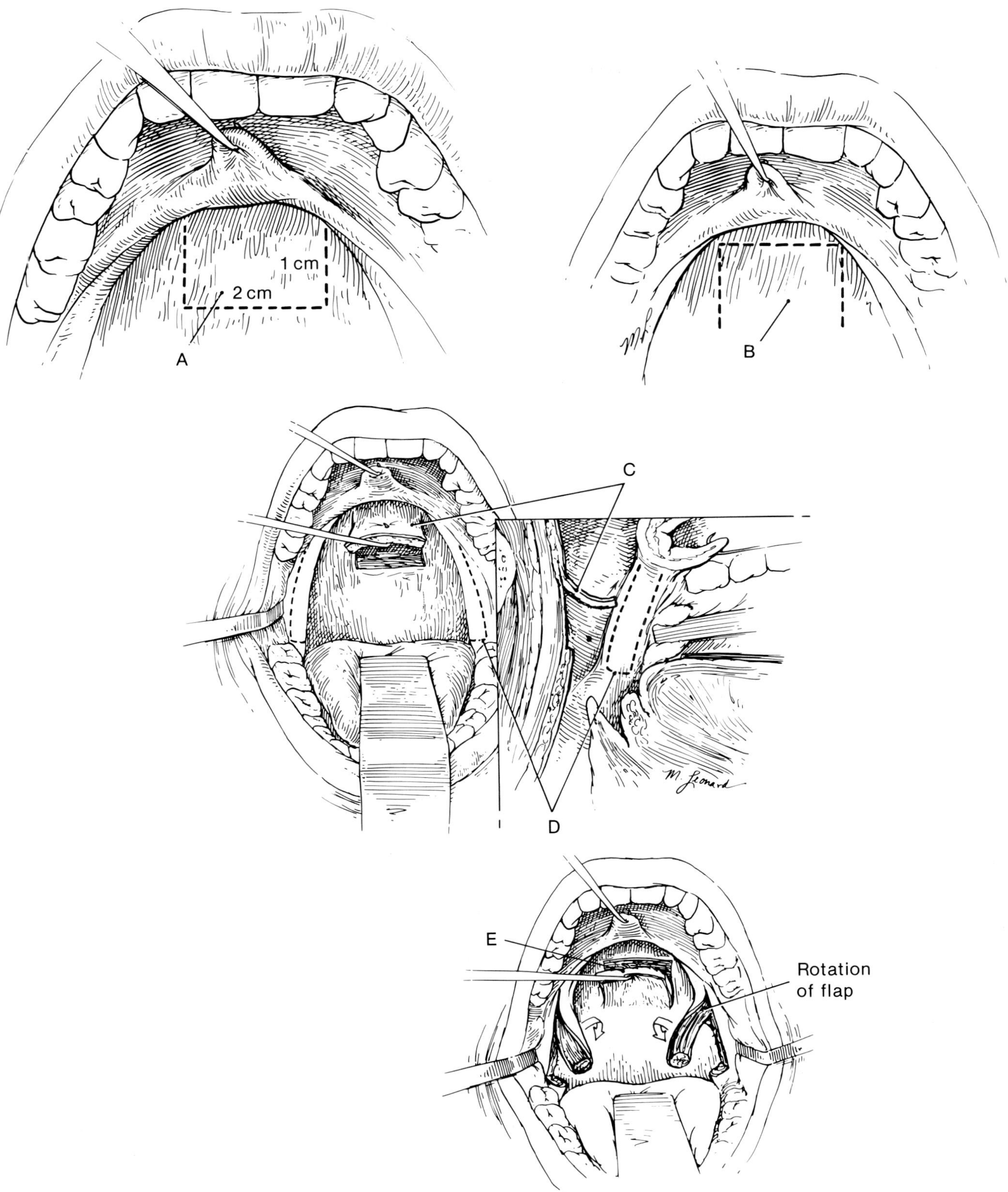

Fig. 21-6. Triple-flap pharyngoplasty. **A,** Superior-based posterior pharyngeal flap. **B,** Inferior-based posterior pharyngeal flap. **C** and **D,** Dissection of bilateral superior-based palatopharyngeal flaps with a superior-based pharyngeal flap. **E,** Dissection and rotation of palatopharyngeal flaps with an inferior-based pharyngeal flap.

Continued.

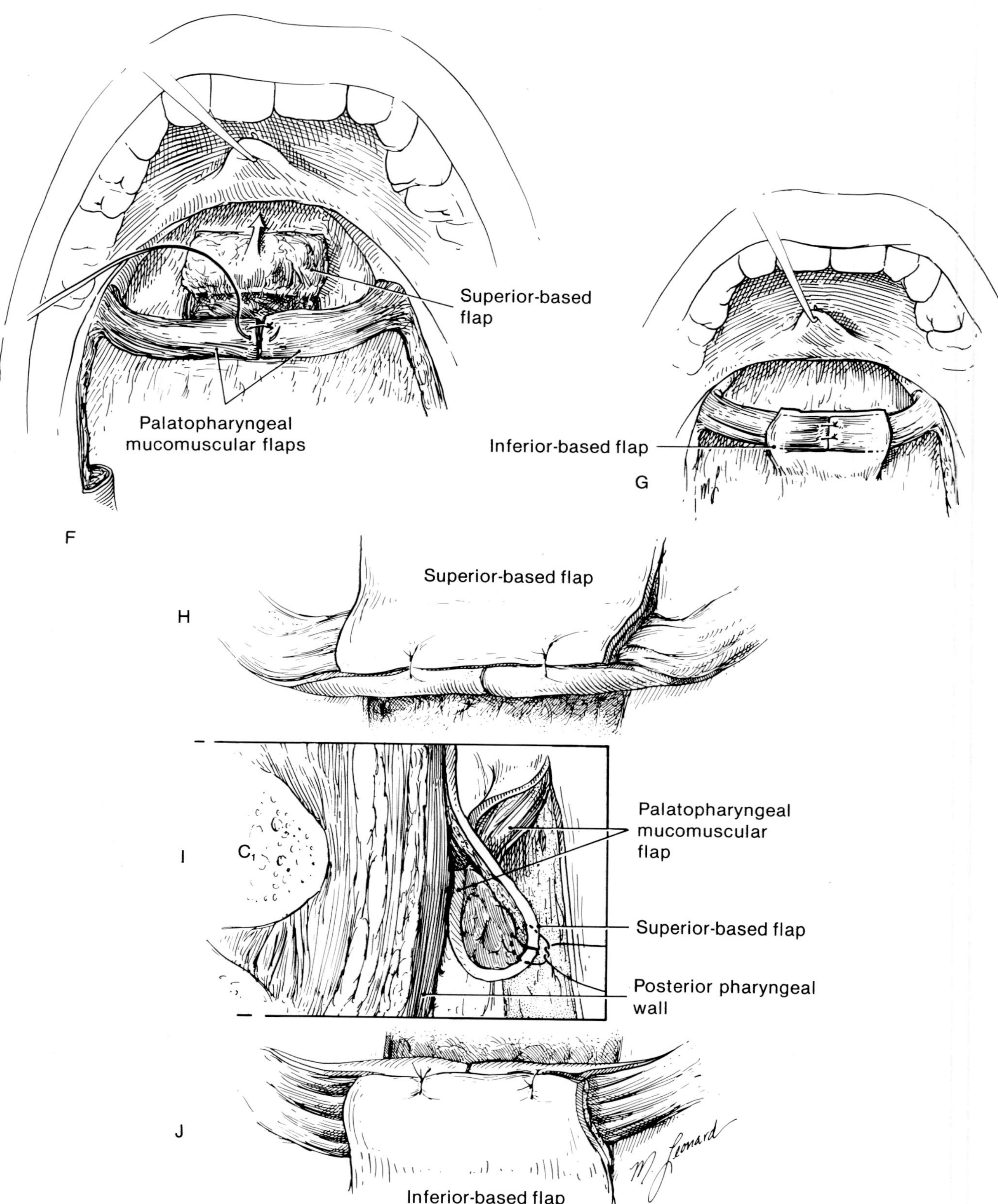

Fig. 21-6, cont'd. F, Insertion of palatopharyngeal flaps with a superior-based pharyngeal flap. **G,** Insertion of palatopharyngeal flaps with an inferior-based pharyngeal flap. **H,** Approximation of the three flaps with a superior-based pharyngeal flap. **I,** Lateral view of a superior-based pharyngeal flap. Note the creation of a pseudo-Passavant pad. **J,** Approximation of three flaps with an inferior-based pharyngeal flap.

this muscle unit. An incision is first made at the junction of the posterior tonsillar pillar. On rare occasions, this groove is obliterated by enlarged tonsils, making a tonsillectomy a requirement before dissection of the lateral superiorly based mucomuscular flap. These flaps are made wide enough to incorporate as much of the palatopharyngeal muscle as possible, while maintaining a bridge or mucosa between these lateral flaps and the midline posterior pharyngeal flap. This bridge permits more rapid epithelialization of the raw surfaces and minimizes the fibrous scar contracture. The flaps are made as long as possible with extension to the base of the tongue. This facilitates approximation more superiorly with minimal tension. Wide flaps incorporating considerable muscle mass maintain the blood supply to the mucomuscular segment and probably its innervation. Considerable controversy still exists as to whether the transposed superiorly based flaps function as a dynamic sphincter or whether the contraction perceived is transmitted from the surrounding pharyngeal and palatal musculature. There is certainly no disagreement that the pharyngoplasty has a considerable obturating effect.

After dissection, all three flaps are approximated in the midline (Fig. 21-6, *F* and *G*). First the two lateral superiorly based flaps are approximated in an end-to-end fashion, making sure that the sutures include both muscle and mucosa. If a superior-based midline flap is selected, the mucomuscular sling is placed beneath this flap, raw surface in contact with raw surface. The medial margins of the lateral flaps are thus approximated to the distal margin of the base of this flap. In addition to the sling effect, a protruding ridge is created on the posterior pharyngeal wall at the level of velar elevation during phonation (Fig. 21-6, *H* to *J*). This augments velar function by reducing the velar excursion necessary for contact and enhances the obturating effect. Thus a ''surgical Passavant's ridge'' is created. If an inferiorly based posterior pharyngeal flap is selected, the lateral margins of the two superiorly based flaps are sutured to the distal end, and the medial margins of the two flaps are sutured to its base. A similar ridge, as described earlier, results on the posterior pharyngeal wall.

Hospitalization after this procedure is usually brief, approximately 3 days. Liquids are begun within 24 hours. Immediate improvement in hypernasality and nasal air escape is apparent. Actually hyponasality immediately after surgery suggests normal resonance when operative edema and contracture have stabilized.

EVALUATION OF PRESENT SERIES

From 1976 to 1978 the pharyngoplasty was performed as described by Orticochea.[20] Intraoral examination revealed that the pharyngoplasty was generally low (in the oropharynx), speech results were less than desirable. In 1978 the surgical procedure was modified. The purpose of the modification was to produce a static pharyngoplasty on the posterior pharyngeal wall that would take advantage of active velar elevation. The height of velar elevation and the attempted point of contact were identified using lateral radiography (Fig. 21-7). The height of velar elevation was determined relative to the atlas of the first cervical vertebra, and the flaps were inserted relative to this landmark. The purpose of this analysis is to assess the efficacy of this modification.

The series included 28 patients (11 male, 17 female) whose primary complaints were hypernasality due to VPI (Table 21-1). A tape recording of a speech sample was made for each patient before and after surgery to assess oral-nasal resonance. In addition, lateral radiographs using either cinefluoroscopy or still radiographs) were obtained to assess velopharyngeal port function.

Preoperatively all 28 patients were rated as hypernasal (Table 21-2). Postoperatively resonance improved in all patients; however, 10 (36%) were rated as moderately hypernasal, 17 (61%) had normal oral-nasal resonance, and 1 (3%) was hyponasal.

The preoperative radiographic examination revealed that none of the patients had better than an inconsistent touch closure during speech attempts (Table 21-3). Postoperatively

Table 21-1. VPI in the present series

Cause	Number of patients
Deep nasopharynx*	13
Submucous cleft	3
Cleft lip and palate	9
Cleft palate only	3
TOTAL	28

*Assessed radiographically.

Table 21-2. Comparison of preoperative and postoperative resonance

Rating	Preoperative resonance	Postoperative resonance
Severe nasality	21 (75%)	0
Mild to moderate nasality	7 (25%)	10 (36%)
Normal resonance	0	17 (61%)
Hyponasality	0	1 (3%)
TOTAL	28	28

Table 21-3. Measurements of the velopharyngeal gap using lateral radiography*

Velopharyngeal gap (mm)	Preoperative measurement (mm)	Postoperative measurement (mm)
Closure	0	12
Touch closure to 2	11	8
3 to 5	10	3
5	3	1
TOTAL	24	24

*Four radiographs were not available for analysis.

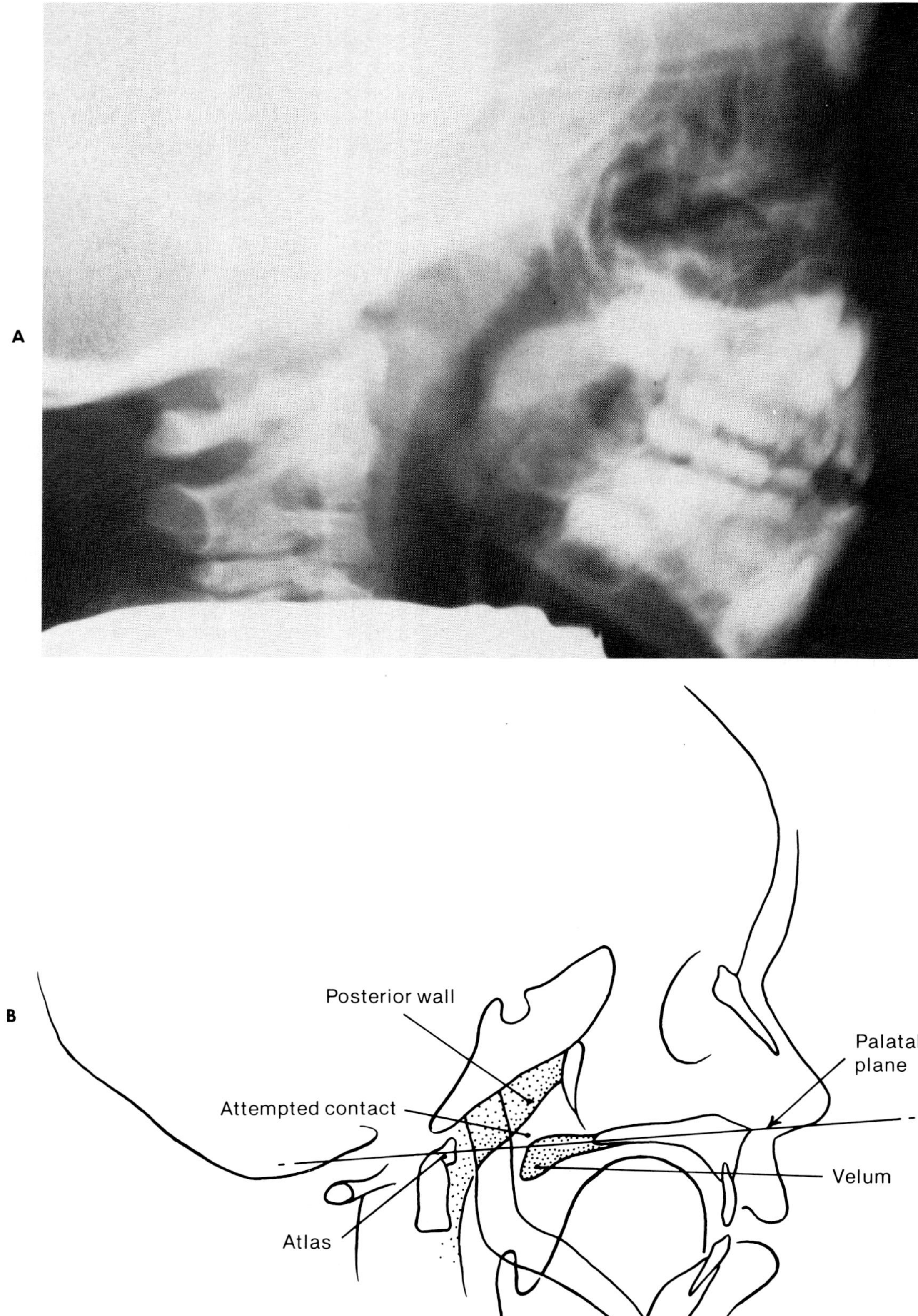

Fig. 21-7. A, Lateral radiograph demonstrating VPI during phonation. **B,** Tracings of a lateral radiograph depicting the palatal plane and point of attempted contact at the posterior pharyngeal wall with reference to the atlas.

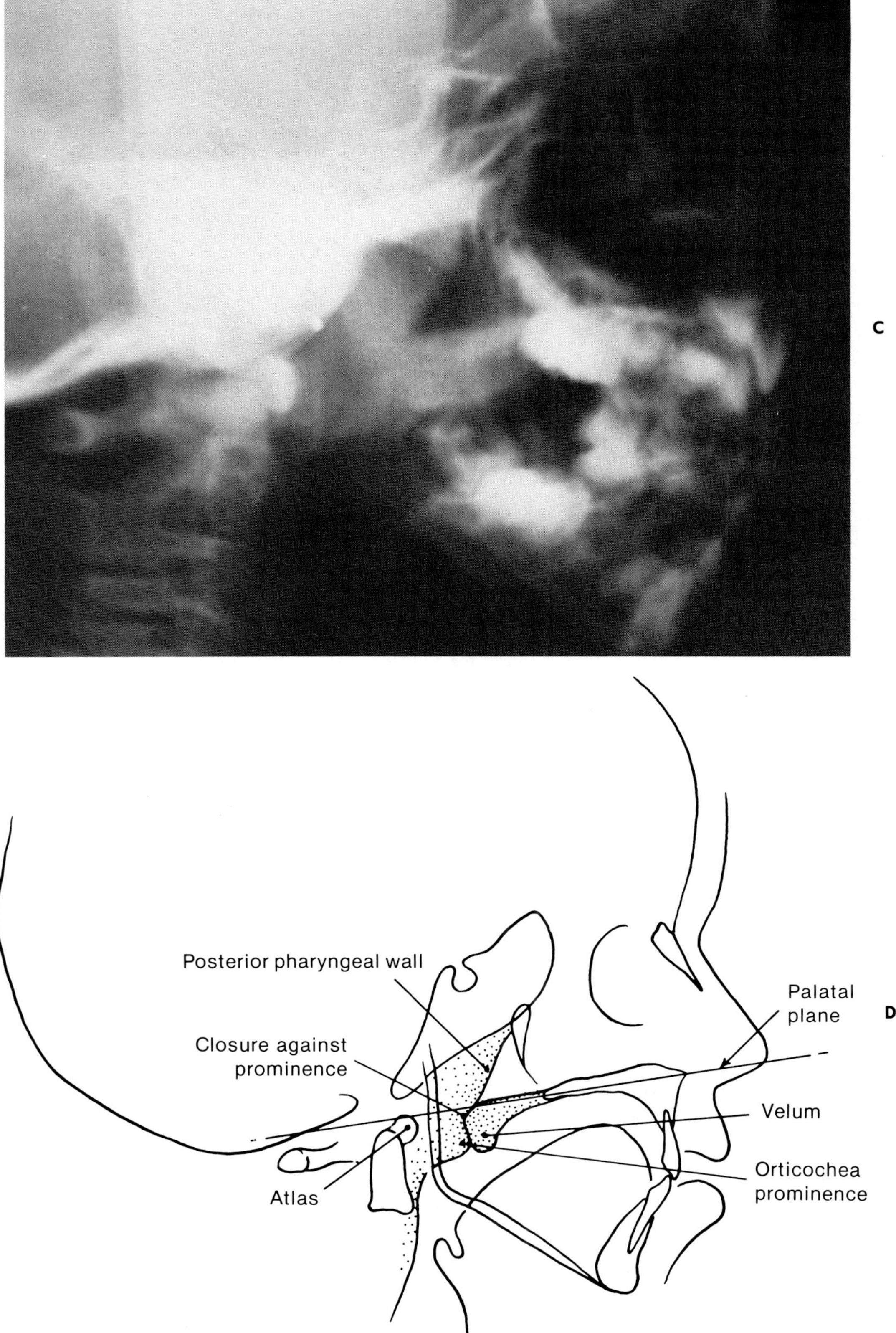

Fig. 21-7, cont'd. C, Postoperative lateral radiograph after Orticochea pharyngoplasty. Note the velopharyngeal closure during sustained phonation. **D,** Tracings of a lateral radiograph demonstrating closure of the velum against the Orticochea prominence. Note the position of the prominence to the atlas.

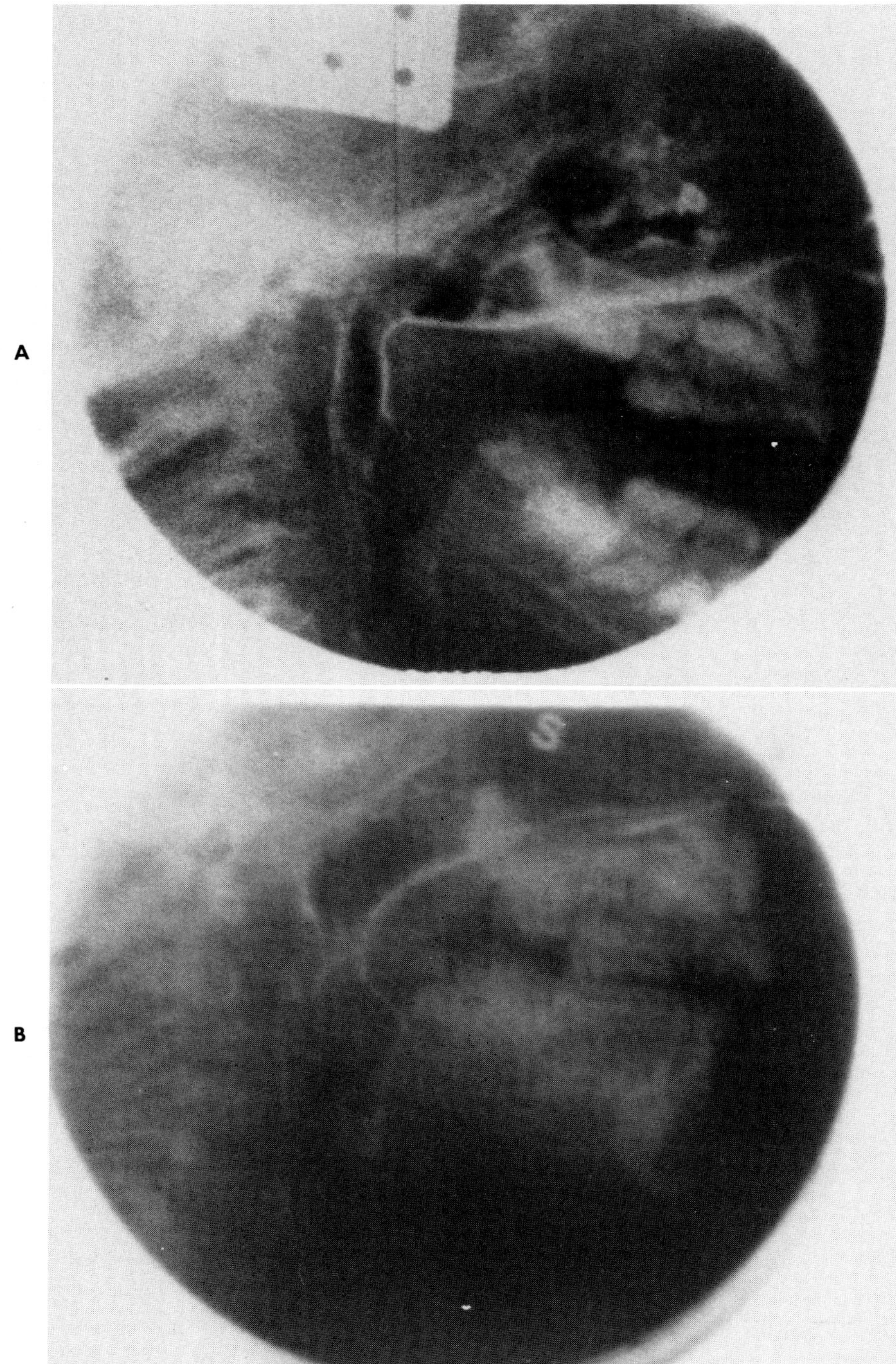

Fig. 21-8. A, Preoperative cineradiograph depicting a 5 mm velopharyngeal gap on sustained phonation. **B,** Lateral cineradiograph demonstrating the velopharyngeal port postoperatively at rest.

14 (50%) of the patients had velar contact against the ridge of the pharyngoplasty. All patients exhibited some narrowing of the anteroposterior dimensions of the nasopharynx postoperatively. Patients with low-based pharyngoplasties had less narrowing than patients with pharyngoplasties placed at or near the point of attempted velopharyngeal closure.

Velar activity as observed radiographically was unchanged postoperatively. Thus a preoperative assessment of velar elevation is predictive of postoperative velar activity. Moreover, the Orticochea pharyngoplasty did not impair or impede velar elevation in any of the patients.

The resolution of hypernasality was directly related to the level of flap insertion relative to the height of velar elevation (Table 21-4). Seven of the eight patients with the pharyn-

goplasty placed at the point of attempted velopharyngeal closure had normal oral-nasal resonance balance. Oral examination of the one patient with a residual mild hypernasality revealed that the palatopharyngeal flaps were not brought to the midline. Thus there was a small midline defect. In contrast, 8 of the 17 patients in whom the flap insertion was below the velar elevation had residual hypernasality.

The tubercle of the atlas was a useful landmark for flap insertion (Table 21-4). All of the 9 patients with flaps inserted at or near the level of the atlas had normal resonance. In contrast, only 6 of 16 patients with flaps placed below the level of the atlas had normal resonance. Fig. 21-8 depicts the preoperative and postoperative radiographic studies of a 5-year-old girl who had a congenital palatal insufficiency due to an exceptionally deep nasopharynx. Preoperative studies (Fig. 21-8, *A*) demonstrated a velum that elevated actively to a level at and just below the atlas. However, a velopharyngeal gap of 5 mm remained, and speech was severely hypernasal.

Fig. 21-8, *B*, demonstrates the velopharyngeal port postoperatively at rest. The prominence of Orticochea pharyngoplasties is between the first and second cervical vertebrae. In Fig. 21-8, *C*, the velum elevates actively, and the distal third of the velum makes a firm contact with the prominence of the pharyngoplasty. Postoperatively resonance was normal.

Table 21-4. Relationship of the atlas and the level of flap placement to resonance*

Rating	Below atlas	At or above atlas
Severe nasality	0	0
Mild to moderate nasality	9	0
Normal resonance	6	9
Hyponasality	1	0
TOTAL	16	9

*Three radiographs were not available for analysis.

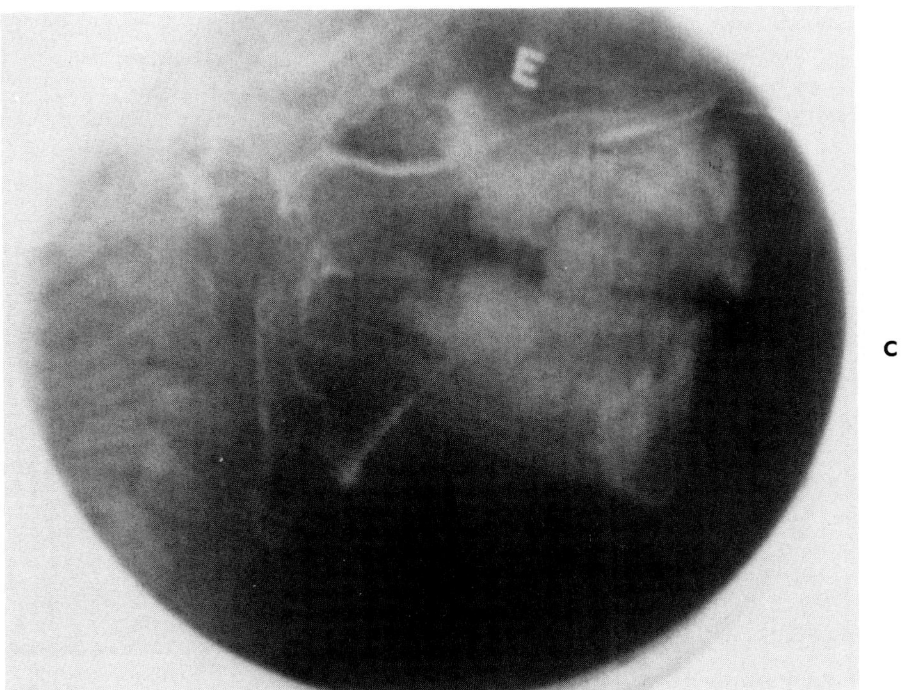

Fig. 21-8, cont'd. C, Postoperative lateral cineradiograph after Orticochea pharyngoplasty demonstrating velopharyngeal competence during sustained phonation.

SUMMARY AND CONCLUSIONS

VPI occurs in approximately 25% to 30% of patients after cleft palate repair. It also may be associated with an intact palate or the following disorders:

Anatomic defects
    Congenital defects
        Cleft palate
        Submucous cleft palate
        Absence of a portion of the velopharyngeal mechanism
        Short palate
        Recessed pharynx
    Acquired defects
        Trauma
        Disease
        Postoperative cleft palate closure
        Postoperative adenoidectomy
Neuromuscular defects
    Neurologic defects
        Nuclear and peripheral nerve paresis
        Supranuclear area
        Cortical area
    Muscular defects
        Agenesis
        Atony

VPI is manifested by an alteration of resonance, oral breath pressure, and articulation. It is now well accepted that both successful diagnosis and treatment must involve careful evaluation of the total velopharyngeal mechanism. Understanding the degree and pattern of posterior and lateral pharyngeal side wall motion is most important. In addition, documenting the level and degree of velar contact during speech to both posterior and lateral pharyngeal walls is essential. The various methods employed during speech evaluation were discussed in Chapter 16. Lateral radiographs, cinefluoroscopy and base view fluoroscopy provide the additional data necessary to quantitate the degree of VPI. Nasal endoscopy also is an important diagnostic tool to evaluate dynamic patterns and the degree of closure of the velopharyngeal portal.

Patients with limited posterior wall, lateral wall, and velar movement are poor candidates for surgery. Movement of these structures is most important to achieve a satisfactory result. If surgical management is selected, however, the triple-flap pharyngoplasty is more likely to give a better result. Patients with good lateral wall movement can be successfully treated with either a superiorly or inferiorly based flap. These patients also can be treated with a triple-flap pharyngoplasty. Patients with limited posterior and lateral wall motion but with good velar motion are generally poor candidates for either superior- or inferior-based pharyngeal flaps. Unless these flaps remain broad, limited lateral wall function cannot obturate the lateral portals (Fig. 21-9). In patients with a relatively short, immobile palate, similar flaps may actually hinder palatal movement by a restricting, tethering effect. It is in this group of patients (i.e., those with limited lateral and posterior walls but good velar movement) that the pharyngoplasty previously described is most indicated. This procedure provides a long-lasting obturating effect with minimal restriction of movement of either the pharynx or soft palate. This obturating effect is enhanced in patients with active velar movement. The ridge created surgically by the three flaps also augments this obturating effect.

Several technical considerations are paramount to success. Whether an inferior- or superior-based posterior pharyngeal flap is employed, it must be placed in a superior location, approximating the location of velar contact. All three flaps must be approximated without tension to minimize postoperative disruption. If dynamic function does occur after flap transposition, then both blood supply and innervation to the palatopharyngeal muscles must be preserved with broad-based flaps. Scar contracture is mini-

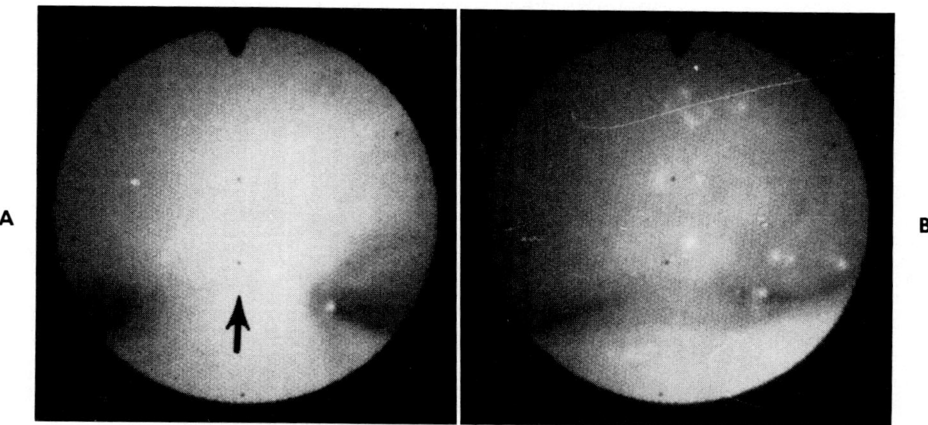

Fig. 21-9. A, View of a superior pharyngeal flap at rest *(arrow)* using nasal endoscopy. **B,** A coronal-type closure pattern with little mesial movement at the lateral pharyngeal walls. Note that a residual velopharyngeal gap remains. This patient would have been more appropriately managed with the Orticochea pharyngoplasty as described in the text.

mized by mucosal closure, if possible, avoiding tension. In addition, the maintenance of a mucosal bridge between the more central posterior pharyngeal flap and the two lateral flaps is important.

The operative procedure is successful if these principles are adhered to. It can be performed with minimal patient morbidity at all ages. Using the method just described, velopharyngeal competence can be restored without violation of an intact soft palate.

Analysis of the present series demonstrates that this modification of the Orticochea pharyngoplasty is a viable and useful addition to the surgeon's armamentarium of pharyngoplasties.

Our evaluation of patients has been enhanced by the discussion and comments of the attending staff of the Division of Plastic and Maxillofacial Surgery at the Duke University Medical Center in Durham, North Carolina. The attending staff includes Dr. Nicholas Georgiade, Chairman; Dr. Ronald Riefkohl; Dr. William Barwick, and Dr. Gregory Georgiade.

REFERENCES

1. Bloomer, H.: Observations on the palatopharyngeal action with special reference to speech, swallowing and blowing, Cleft Palate Bull. **2:**2, 1952.
2. Bloomer, H.: Observations on palatopharyngeal movements in speech and deglutition, J. Speech Hear. Disord. **18:**230, 1953.
3. Bzoch, K.R.: Variations in velopharyngeal valving: the factor of vowel changes, Cleft Palate J. **5:**211, 1968.
4. Bzoch, K.R., Graber, T.M., and Aoba, T.: A study of normal velopharyngeal valving for speech, Cleft Palate Bull. **9:**3, 1959.
5. Calnan, J.: Movements of the soft palate, Br. J. Plast. Surg. **5:**286, 1953.
6. Calnan, J.: Modern views on Passavant's ridge, Br. J. Plast. Surg. **10:**89, 1957.
7. Calnan, J.: Surgery for speech. In Calnan, J., editor: Recent advances in plastic surgery, Edinburgh, 1976, Churchill Livingstone.
8. Dickson, D.R.: Anatomy of the normal velopharyngeal mechanism, Clin. Plast. Surg. **2:**235, 1975.
9. Dickson, D.R., Grant, J.C.B., Sicher, H., et al.: Status of research in cleft palate. I. Anatomy and physiology, Cleft Palate J. **11:**471, 1974.
10. Dorrance, G.M.: Lengthening the soft palate in cleft palate operations, Ann. Surg. **82:**208, 1925.
11. Fritzell, B.: The velopharyngeal muscles in speech: an electromyographic and cinéradiographic study, Acta Otolaryngol. Suppl. **250:**1, 1969.
12. Gersuny, R.: Ueber cine subcutane Prothese, Zeithschrift F. Heilk. Wien Leipz. N.F. **1:**199, 1900.
13. Graber, T.M., Bzoch, K.R., and Aoba, T.: A functional study of the palatal and pharyngeal structures, Angle Orthod. **29:**30, 1959.
14. Hagerty, R.F., and Hill, M.J.: Cartilage pharyngoplasty in cleft palate patients, Surg. Gynecol. Obstet. **112:**350, 1961.
15. Hollinshead, W.H.: Anatomy for surgeons, vol. 1, The head and neck, ed. 2, New York, 1968, Harper & Row, Publishers, Inc.
16. Huskie, C.F., and Jackson, I.T.: The sphincter pharyngoplasty—a new approach to the speech problems of velopharyngeal incompetence, Br. J. Disord. Commun. **12:**31, 1977.
17. Hynes, W.: Pharyngoplasty by muscle transplantation, Br. J. Plast. Surg. **3:**128, 1950.
18. Jackson, I.T., and Silverton, J.S.: The sphincter pharyngoplasty as a secondary procedure in cleft palates, Plast. Reconstr. Surg. **59:**518, 1977.
19. Morris, H.L., and Spriestersbach, D.C.: The pharyngeal flap as a speech mechanism, Plast. Reconstr. Surg. **39:**66, 1967.
20. Orticochea, M.: Construction of a dynamic muscle sphincter in cleft palates, Plast. Reconstr. Surg. **41:**323, 1968.
21. Orticochea, M.: Results of the dynamic muscle sphincter operation in cleft palates, Br. J. Plast. Surg. **23:**108, 1970.
22. Passavant, P.G.: Ueber die verschliessung des schlundes beim sprechen, Frankfurt, 1863, J.D. Sauerländer.
23. Passavant, P.G.: Ueber die Verschliessung des Schlundes beim sprechen, Virchows Archiv. **46:**1, 1869.
24. Ruding, R.: Cleft palate anatomic and surgical considerations, Plast. Reconstr. Surg. **33:**132, 1964.
25. Schoenborn, K.: Ueber eine neue methode der Staphylorrhaphie, Verh. Dtsch. Ges. Chir. **4:**235, 1876; Arch. Klin. Chir. Berl. **19:**527, 1876.
26. Schoenborn, K.: Vorstellung eines Falles Staphyloplastik, Verh. Dtsch. Ges. Chir. **15:**57, 1886.
27. Skolnick, M.L.: Video velopharyngography in patients with nasal speech, with emphasis on lateral pharyngeal motion in velopharyngeal closure, Radiology **93:**747, 1969.
28. Skolnick, M.L.: Videofluoroscopic examination of the velopharyngeal portal during phonation in lateral and base projections—a new technique for studying the mechanics of closure, Cleft Palate J. **7:**803, 1970.
29. Skolnick, M.L., and McCall, G.N.: Velopharyngeal competence and incompetence following pharyngeal flap surgery: videofluoroscopic study in multiple projections, Cleft Palate J. **9:**1, 1972.
30. Stark, R.B.: Development of the face, Surg. Gynecol. Obstet. **137:**403, 1973.
31. Veau, V.E.: Division palatine: anatomie, chirurgie, phonétique, Paris, 1931, Masson et Cie.
32. Wardill, W.E.M.: The technique of operation for cleft palate, Br. J. Surg. **25:**117, 1937.
33. Whillis, J.: Note on muscles of palate and superior constrictor, J. Anat. **65:**92, 1930.

CHAPTER 22

Cleft lip nasal deformity

WILLIAM C. TRIER

The recognition of the abnormal anatomy of clefts of the primary palate has resulted in significant improvement in primary and secondary repair of the lip, but has failed to provide a proportional degree of improvement in the associated nasal deformity. Unfortunately, although this has been pointed out by a number of surgeons for at least the past 60 years, success in lip repair continues to surpass by far success in cleft lip nasal repair or reconstruction. Padgett's statement of the problem cannot be improved on: "A good repair of a cleft lip and the accompanying nasal deformity is the more important in relation to the ultimate end result and often the most difficult to accomplish. Certainly the operation does not attain the dignity of an art until the nostrils are similar and properly balanced, although the lip may be a perfect cupid's bow."[80]

In all fairness to the many surgeons who have struggled to correct the nasal deformity secondary to cleft lip, two important differences, other than the obvious, exist between the lip and nose. First, the pathologic anatomy of the cleft lip nasal deformity has simply not been as well studied as has the abnormal anatomy of the lip. Second, the prominence of a nose, compared to the lip lying in its shadow, makes any deformity or even characteristic more noticeable.

DEVELOPMENTAL ANATOMY

Studies of the development of the facial area have focused on the primary palate, which is the initial separation between the anterior oral and nasal cavities, rather than on the development of the medial and lateral nasal processes, or prominences, that will form the nose. At least three hypotheses regarding the primary palate have been reviewed by Ross and Johnston[92]: mesenchymal penetration, epithelial invagination, and merging. These studies concentrate on the area between the medial and lateral nasal processes and not on the processes themselves. Later studies by Johnston, Hassell, and Brown[43] conclude that the primary palate is formed by fusion of the medial and lateral nasal processes as their epithelial surfaces absorb and that the area of fusion is then penetrated with mesenchyme. Recent studies by Millicovsky, Ambrose, and Johnston[68] compare the developing primary palate in a strain of mice in which 36% of the offspring spontaneously develop clefts of the primary palate with the same area in a strain of mice resistant to clefts of the primary palate and show intrinsic differences in this area between the two strains of mice. In the cleft strain there is wide separation between medial and lateral nasal prominences due to orientation of the medial nasal prominence parallel to the midsagittal plane of the face. In the resistant strain the medial process diverges from the midsagittal plane toward the lateral nasal prominence. In addition, there is an inherent difference in surface epithelial activity in an area at the bottom of the nasal pit between the two strains; the surface epithelium in the spontaneous cleft strain failing to undergo recognizable changes preparatory to fusion of medial and lateral prominences (Fig. 22-1).

Stark and Kaplan,[101] in studies of human embryos with clefts, have also observed differences in the thickness of ectoderm between the cleft and noncleft side of the primitive nose, suggesting deficiency of ectoderm that is unreinforced by mesenchyme.

In noting that cartilage provides support for the tissues of the face in early embryonic development, Avery[4] reported that cartilage in embryos with clefts was deficient, appeared later, and developed more slowly than embryos without clefts.

Despite studies suggesting an intrinsic defect or deficiency, however, a large number of investigators believe cleft lip nasal deformity is due to malposition of essentially normally developed structures.

Studies by Peyton and Ritchie,[84] Coupe and Subtelny,[23] and Atherton[3] suggest that the nasal deformity in clefts of the primary palate is a consequence of displacement of the

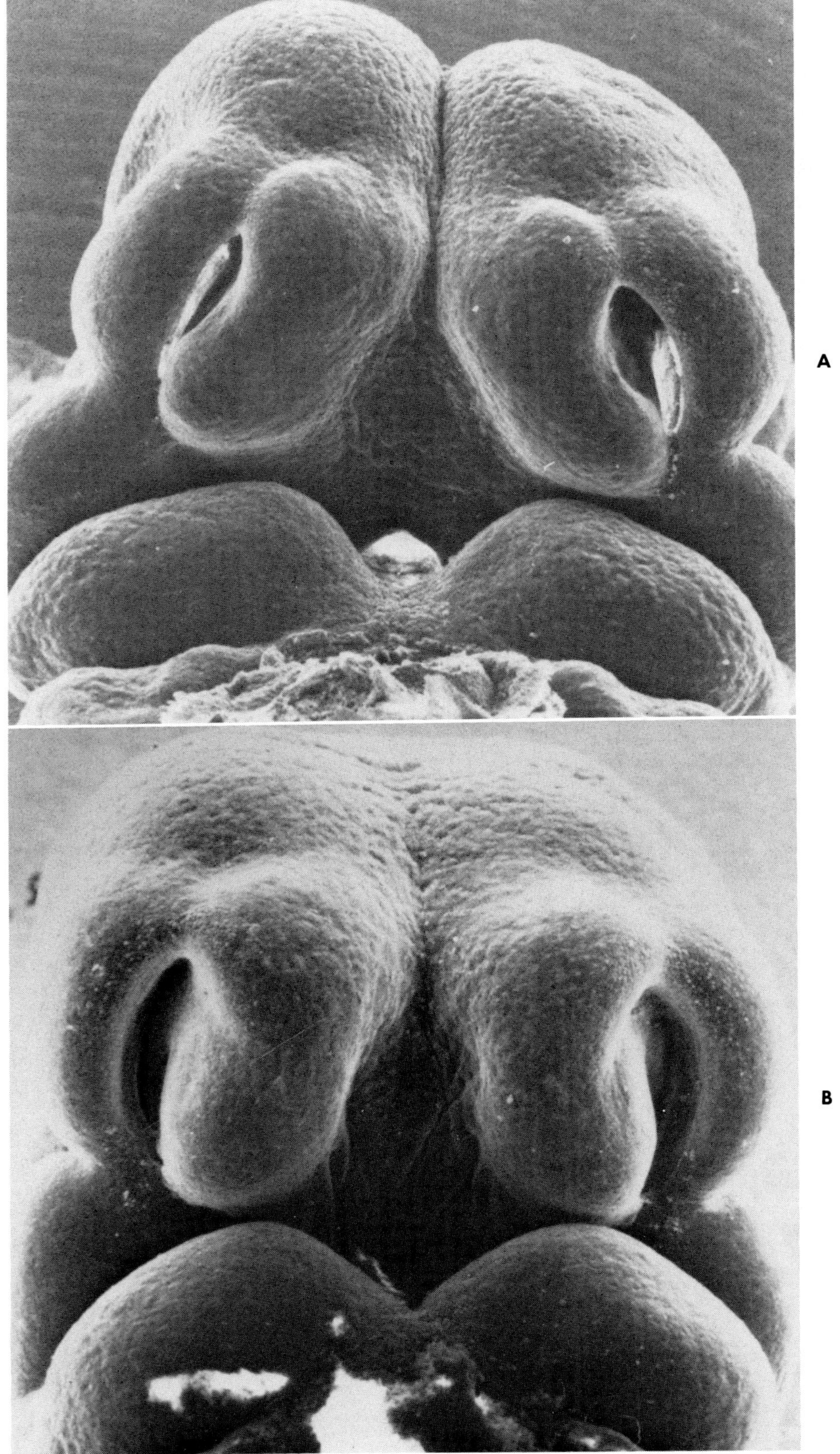

Fig. 22-1. Developmental alterations in mice susceptible to cleft. **A,** Divergence of medial nasal prominence toward lateral nasal prominence in mice resistant to clefts of the primary palate. **B,** Parallel orientation of medial nasal prominences with noticeable gap between medial and lateral nasal prominences in a strain of mice susceptible to clefts of the primary palate. (From Millicovsky, G., Ambrose, L.J.H., and Johnston, M.C.: J. Anat. **164:**29, 1982.)   *Continued.*

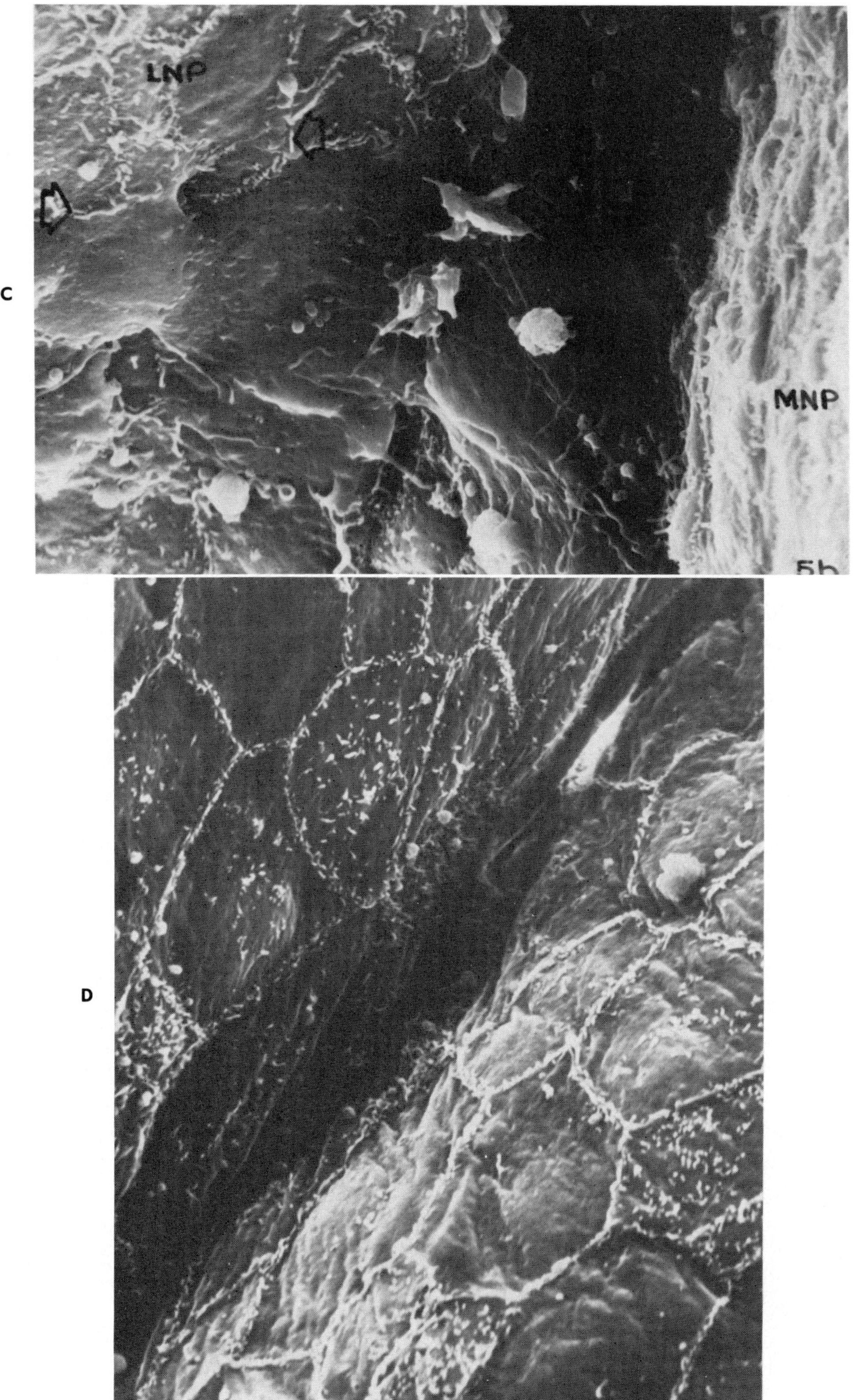

Fig. 22-1, cont'd. C, Epithelial changes in the area of fusion of medial nasal prominence *(MNP* and lateral nasal prominence *(LNP)* of a mouse strain resistant to clefts of the primary palate. Note the disappearance of rows of microvilli at the margins of peridermal cells. **D,** Same area in a mouse strain susceptible to cleft lip showing absence of change in the epithelium.

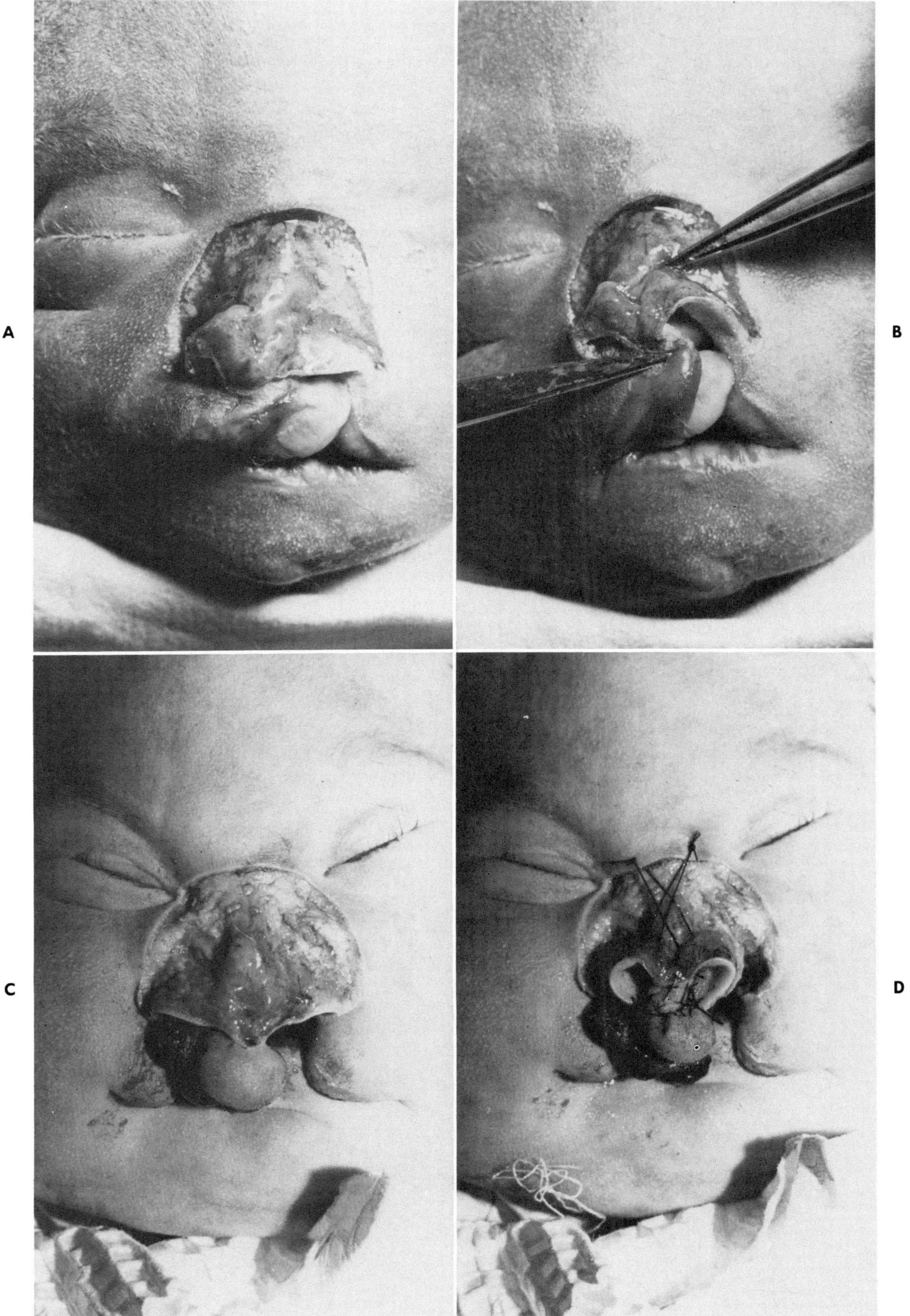

Fig. 22-2. Dissected noses of stillborn infants with unilateral and bilateral cleft lip. **A,** Downward displacement of the left, cleft-side alar cartilage with increased length of nose evident on the cleft side. **B,** Effect of elevation alone on restoring position and shape of alar cartilage (forceps are maintaining cleft-side alar cartilage in some degree of overcorrection). **C,** Downward displacement of both alar cartilages, coupled with lack of columellar development. **D,** Effect of forked flap columellar lengthening and alar cartilage suspension (McComb's technique) to reproduce a columella and correctly position and shape the alar cartilages. (Courtesy Dr. Harold McComb.)

cartilaginous components of the nasal capsule, due chiefly to the faulty position of the underlying maxilla on the cleft side secondary to a lack of orbicular muscle continuity. The tripod hypothesis of Converse, Hogan, and Barton[20] is a similar explanation for the typical deformity in the cleft lip nose.

Pigott and Millard[86] stated that the described mesenchymal deficiency to be found in clefts of the primary palate is in areas lateral to the nasooptic furrow and not in the nasal prominences. Tange and Ohmori[109] had reached their conclusions after carrying out comparative measurements between the cleft and noncleft sides in the unilateral cleft lip nasal deformity.

Studies by Pruzansky[91] and Aduss and Pruzansky[1] of infants with cleft lip and palate before lip repair suggested both intrinsic defects in the developing primary palate on the cleft side and also secondary defects resulting from maxillary malposition. These defects were lessened by improvements in maxillary position after lip repair. For example, they noted a smaller inferior turbinate on the cleft side that lacked the normal scroll-like structure of a normal turbinate.

Pfeifer[85] noted a smaller maxillary sinus on the cleft side, but dated the altered anatomy on the cleft side to the period when the cleft was formed.

Latham's work[47] supported this view, noting that at the time of cleft formation the face was symmetric, but after cleft formation it becomes asymmetric, shortening in both vertical and anteroposterior directions. This is due to deformity of the nasal septum that occurs as a result of loss of bone and muscle continuity. Latham's work suggests that the septum adversely affects the premaxillary-maxillary area and either directly or through maxillary deformity affects the developing nose.

Almost every clinical study of cleft lip nasal deformities cites the 1949 paper of Huffman and Lierle[40] in which the authors ascribe the deformity to faulty position of structures rather than abnormal development of structures. Their paper makes it quite clear that anatomic observations were based on the clinical study of patients preoperatively and in the operating room and analysis of patients' photographs and moulages. Huffman and Lierle concluded that the cleft lip nasal deformity was due to structures of the nose being held in abnormal position, rather than an intrinsic defect in the developing nose.

McComb[58] has had the opportunity recently to dissect the noses of stillborn infants with unilateral and bilateral cleft lips. The dissection shows downward rotation and displacement of the alar cartilage on the cleft side in the unilateral cleft lip that can be corrected simply by elevating the displaced alar cartilage (Fig. 22-2). In the dissected bilateral cleft lip nose, both alar cartilages are rotated downward, but are held in malposition additionally by lack of development of the columella. McComb[56] demonstrated in the dissected nose the effective preliminary forked flap columellar lengthening followed by elevation and suspension of both alar cartilages at the time of primary lip repair.

Nasal deformity in infants with repaired or unrepaired lip clefts also suggests intrinsic anatomic defects (Fig. 22-3). Furthermore, nasal deformities typical of the cleft lip nose

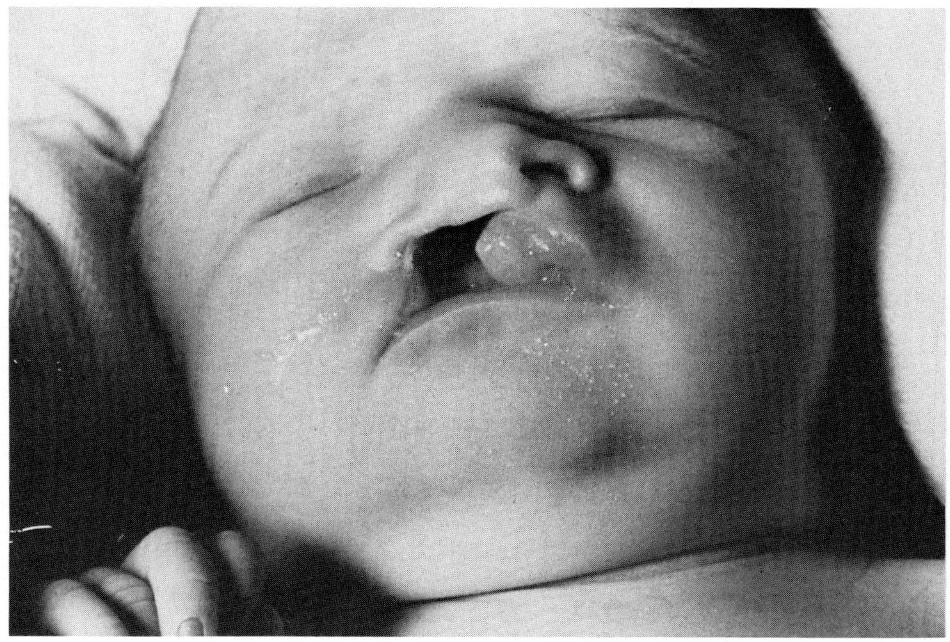

Fig. 22-3. Complete unilateral cleft of the primary and secondary palate. Note diminutive size of the alar base and ala on the cleft side compared to the noncleft side.

in patients with ''normal lips''[16] suggest intrinsic abnormal nasal anatomy. An intact maxillary alveolus and normal muscle continuity make it doubtful that structural alteration could be responsible for the nasal deformity in patients without overt clefts. It must also be acknowledged that the presence of a cleft lip with lack of orbicular muscle continuity and interruption of alveolar segments will cause malposition of normally developed nasal structures.

There are intrinsic deficiencies of soft tissues that are actually defects secondary to remodeling of tissue as a result of changing underlying skeletal relationships. An example is the loss of skin and underlying subcutaneous tissue and fascia that occurs in the adducted thumb after median nerve division and results in loss of the thumb–index finger web. It is therefore possible in the 7 prenatal months after the occurrence of the cleft of the primary palate that remodeling of skin and underlying soft tissue surrounding the supporting skeleton may fully account for what is certainly a very real deficiency of soft tissue at birth.

Studies of human embryos at all stages of development, from the earliest development of the primary palate to birth, and dissection and measurement of the dimensions and bulk

of supporting structures themselves will be needed to determine whether the nasal deformity and lip deformity are due to an intrinsic deficiency or are normal but malpositioned structures or a combination of the two. Reasons for finding the answer are not entirely academic. If the deformity is secondary to malposition and progressive, an important additional reason would exist for intrauterine repair when technically feasible, in addition to the more obvious advantage of the absence of scar in the area of repair.

ANATOMY OF THE NOSE

A traditional knowledge of the anatomy of both the ''normal'' nose and the nose of a patient with a cleft lip is important to the surgeon in order to anesthetize the nose, accurately recognize and dissect nasal structures, and be able to predict the effects of surgical manipulation. The surface, or contour, anatomy of the nose is equally, if not more, important in analyzing the deformity. It is essential to know why a nose appears abnormal before one can correct the deformity.

Brown and McDowell[14] have used the term *contour anatomy* to describe the external features of the nose. They have

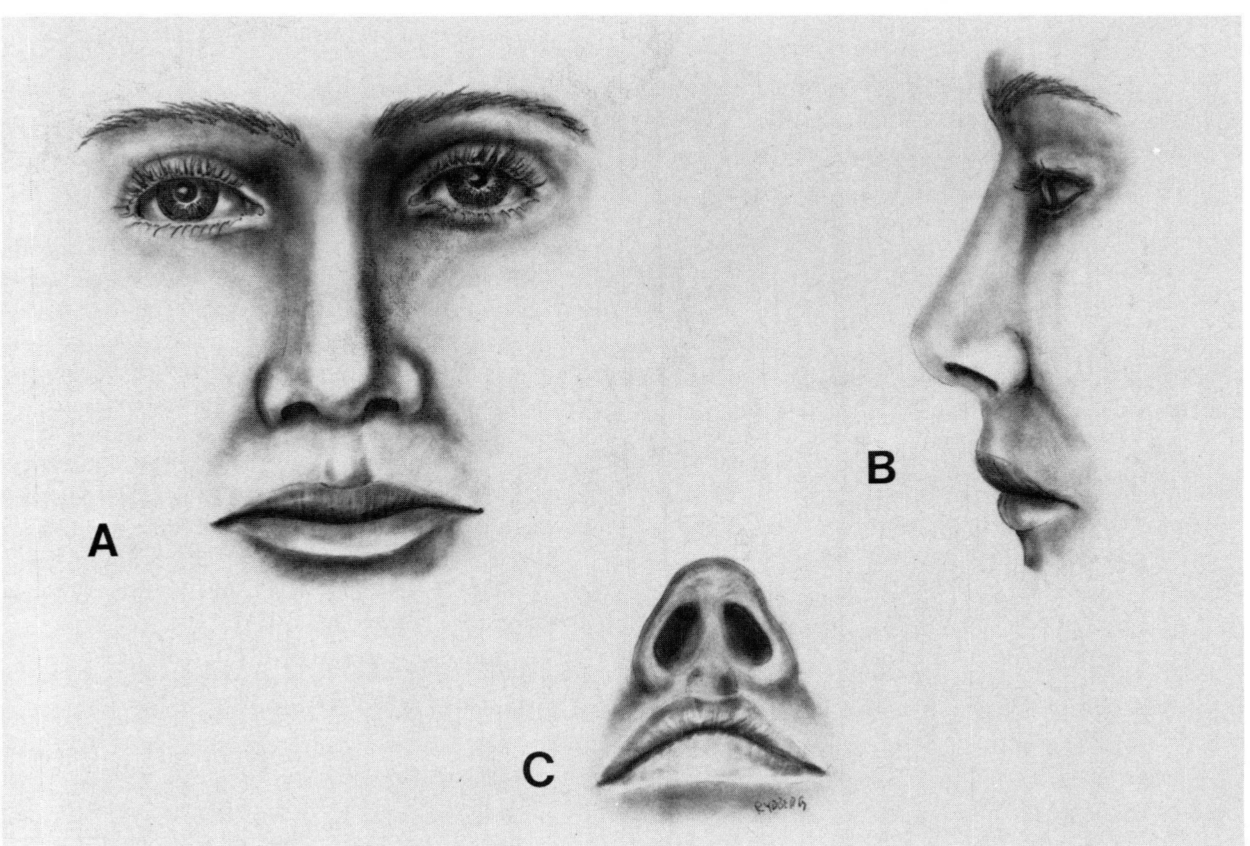

Fig. 22-4. A, Esthetically attractive nose. Graceful planes of the orbit are continued into lateral nasal walls. Note how the alar arches rise symmetrically from a more caudal columella. **B,** Lateral view showing tip projection. The tip plane and columella are parallel and below the alar border. **C,** Base, or tip-up, view showing elliptic, symmetric nostrils inclined toward the nasal tip.

noted that although ideal angles and proportions of noses may be desirable, there are wide variations in normal. Furthermore, nasal appearance is influenced by the appearance of other features of the face "such as prominence of the chin, recession of the forehead, tilt of the upper lip, and length of the middle third of the face."[14]

Sheen and Sheen[97] have artistically analyzed surface anatomy of the esthetically attractive nose stressing the smooth, flowing planes that are extensions of superior and medial

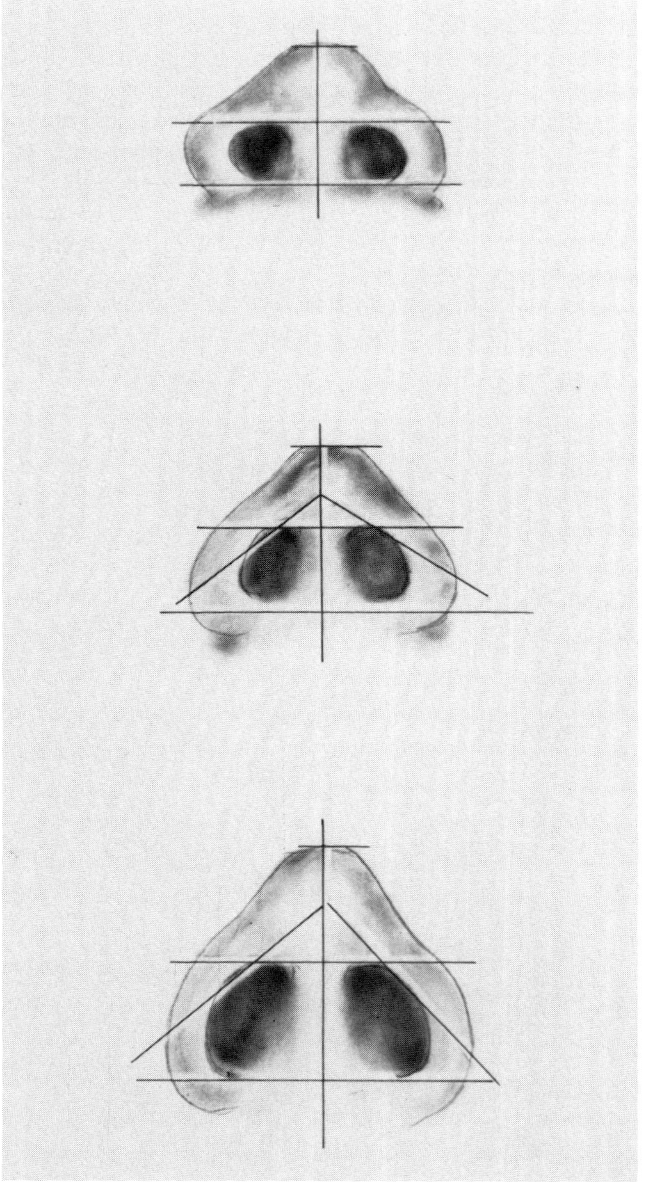

Fig. 22-5. Change in the base or tip-up, view of the nose from infancy to adulthood. *Top,* Infant; *center,* child; *bottom,* adult. (From Pigott, R.W., and Millard, D.R.: Correction of the bilateral cleft lip nasal deformity. In Grable, W.C., Rosenstein, S.W., and Bzoch, K.R., editors: Cleft lip and palate: surgical, dental, and speech aspects, Boston, 1971, Little, Brown & Co.)

orbital features (Fig. 22-4, *A*). As the planes extend caudally in the nose, they diverge and dorsally rise to the domes of the alar cartilages, the nasal tip, and highest projection of the nasal dorsum. As did Brown and McDowell,[14,15] Sheen and Sheen emphasized the esthetic importance of the nasal tip plane when viewed in profile, lying between dorsal and columellar planes (Fig. 22-4, *B*). Adequate tip projection not only requires the support of alar dome arches, but also depends on a sufficiently long columella, as noted by Pigott and Millard.[86] When viewed from the side the columella should be visible parallel to the alar border on each side and lying 2 to 3 mm caudal to the alar margins. The columella is distinct also when viewed full face, lying caudal to the alar arches that rise in curving bilateral arches (Fig. 22-4).

Nostril orifices in the adult should be elliptic and incline medially toward the nasal tip, with the largest dimension of each nostril orifice not less than the height of the nasal lobule or greater than two times the height of the lobule (Fig. 22-4, *C*). However, Pigott and Millard[86] point out the changing proportion of columella length to nasal tip projection; it is less than 1:2 in the infant, but greater than 1:2 in the adult. They also note that the orientation of nostril orifices in relation to the midsagittal line of the columella changes from roughly parallel in the infant to 45 degrees in the adult (Fig. 22-5).

The topographic characteristics of the nose are determined by the osteocartilaginous skeleton, on which the soft tissue of the nose is draped; the bony nose; upper and lower cartilaginous portions of the nasal skeleton; and the bony and cartilaginous septum. The bony nose consists of paired nasal bones resting on the frontal processes of the maxilla and articulating above with the frontal bone. Within the caudal border of the nasal bones and overlapping for a distance of up to 1 cm is the upper cartilaginous vault, consisting of the paired triangular cartilages. These are continuous with the midline septal or quadrangular cartilage in their cephalad portion and caudally are attached to the septum by fibrous connective tissue.[73] The base, or caudal, surface of the nasal pyramid is supported by the paired alar cartilages. The medial, or vertical, crura are joined by the membranous septum to the caudal end of the cartilaginous septum, whereas the lateral crura, overlapping the caudal portions of the lateral cartilages, support the nasal alae.

PRIMARY UNILATERAL CLEFT LIP NASAL DEFORMITY

The nasal deformity in unilateral cleft lip is marked by obvious asymmetry (Fig. 22-3). The entire cleft side of the nose is inferiorly displaced and rotated inferolaterally. Tip projection is decreased on the cleft side, and the bulk of the alar cartilage is deficient when compared with the normal side. The columella, which is short on the cleft side, lies at an angle with the base toward the normal side along with the tip of the nose and caudal end of the deviated septum.

The ala joins the columella at an obtuse angle, and in wide complete clefts the alar border may run almost straight laterally from columella to alar base where it joins the cheek, also at an obtuse angle. The alar base is usually everted on the cleft side. In incomplete clefts the nostril floor is wide on the cleft side, and the circumference of the entire nostril border is increased. The nostril sill is usually rudimentary and often has a central depression.

Reconstruction techniques

Whether cleft lip nasal deformity is caused by malposition of normal structures or is the result of inherent deficiencies in nasal development or both and depending on the severity of the original deformity, much secondary deformity can be prevented by primary lip repair that includes simultaneous nasal correction, as well as lip repair that does not add to the nasal deformity. The rotation-advancement repair as originally described and further perfected by Millard,[62] provides the greatest opportunity for nasal correction. In particular, the preservation of all conceivable useful tissue, lengthening of the cleft-side columella, addition of tissue for lateral vestibular lining, restoration of lip muscle continuity, and proper positioning of the alar base flap provide reconstruction of the nostril sill and floor (Fig. 22-6). Adequate cleft-side tip projection, elimination of vestibular webbing, prevention of alar buckling, and suitable acuteness of the alar-columellar junction may not be possible to accomplish with primary repair.

PRIMARY BILATERAL CLEFT LIP NASAL DEFORMITY

The extent and nature of the bilateral cleft lip nasal deformity is directly related to the degree of the complete or incomplete cleft and whether or not the cleft of the lip is symmetric or asymmetric. The nasal deformity in complete bilateral cleft lip is characterized by symmetry of the nose, but little or no length to the columella, a broad and flattened nasal tip, flaring of the alae with eversion of alar bases, and shortness of the entire nose (Fig. 22-7). Although the columella may vary in length in the bilateral incomplete cleft lip, it is still shorter than normal. This shortness will be intensified by lip repair when the prolabium is incorporated into the lip as its central or philtral portion, which is the correct choice, but one that temporarily at least increases the nasal deformity.

Asymmetric bilateral clefts of the lip quite naturally are accompanied by asymmetric nasal deformities. In my opinion, one indication for a lip adhesion is the asymmetric bilateral cleft lip. A lip adhesion on the completely cleft side makes symmetric repair of the lip cleft easier and also sets the stage for greater symmetry in nasal correction.

Reconstruction techniques

A sound plan for bilateral cleft lip repair should incorporate correction of the nasal deformity. In the bilateral cleft lip, however, the soundest plan requires a minimum of two stages for primary correction of the nasal deformity. Mil-

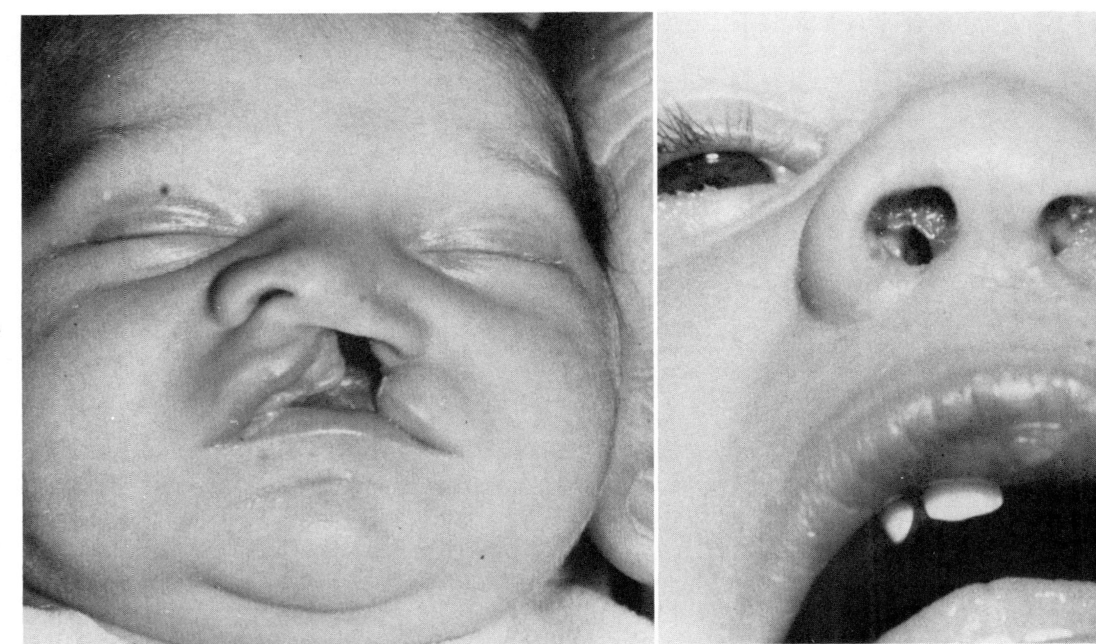

Fig. 22-6. A, Wide complete unilateral cleft of the primary and secondary palate after significant alveolar cleft. **B,** Appearance after initial lip adhesion and later rotation-advancement repair with primary nasal reconstruction. Note the decreased bulk of the ala on the cleft side and slight alar buckling.

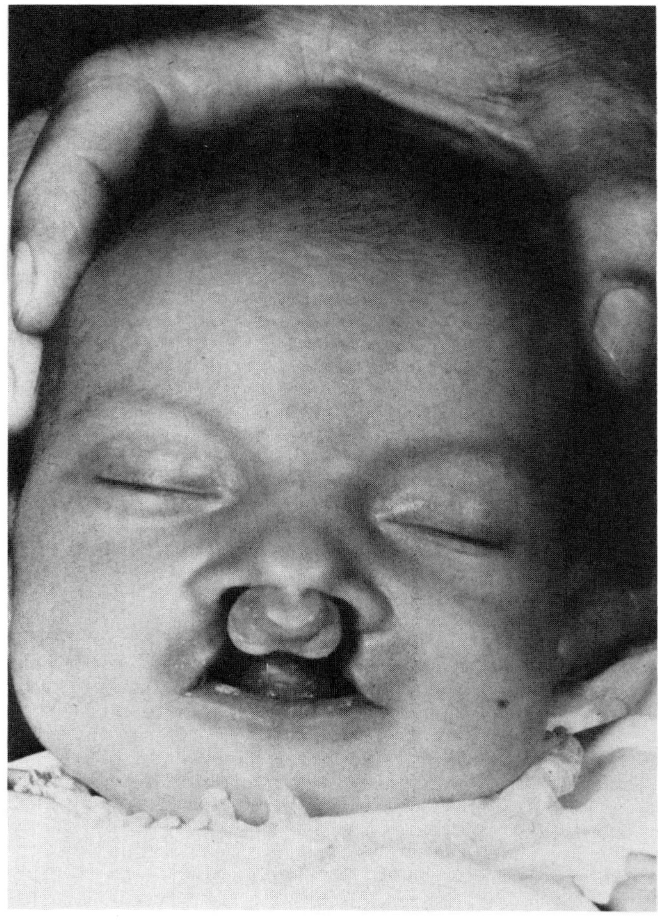

Fig. 22-7. Complete bilateral cleft of the primary and secondary palate. The nose is symmetric, but short. The columella is essentially absent, and the nasal tip is broad and displaced caudally. Alar borders run transversely from the bases of the columella to the alar bases.

lard's technique for bilateral cleft lip repair offers the greatest opportunity for significant and lasting nasal correction.[65] Prolabial skin and subcutaneous tissue that are not needed for a philtrum are "banked" for subsequent columellar lengthening. Alar bases are positioned accurately, and muscle continuity across the full width of the upper lip is provided. Columellar lengthening at the time of repair of the secondary palate provides an adequate soft tissue envelope in which the cartilaginous armature of the nose may grow without restriction. Conservation of all available tissue, especially in locations where the appearance of the tissue is critical (e.g., lip skin used where it is visible), is of major importance (Fig. 22-8).

SECONDARY CLEFT LIP NASAL DEFORMITY
Unilateral deformity

So much depends on the severity of the original cleft lip and associated nasal defect and sophistication and skill of the original surgeon that it is difficult to characterize secondary unilateral cleft lip nasal deformity. In general it represents degrees of severity that are typical of the unrepaired cleft: eversion of the alar base, inadequate projection of the nasal tip on the cleft side, a smaller alar cartilage, webbing between the ala and columella, a shorter columella on the cleft side, and deflection of the caudal end of the septum to the normal side (Fig. 22-9). Areas of both omission and commission may add further deformity, such as absence of the nostril floor, faulty positioning of the alar base and the tip of the alar base flap, and, one of the most difficult defects to reconstruct, an excessively small and constricted nostril due to excision of the lip and nose elements. Correction of malposition of the lip and nose elements requires accurate analysis and proper placement of tissue elements. An abuse of tissue requires correct analysis also, but the less satisfactory replacement of tissue by flaps or grafts.

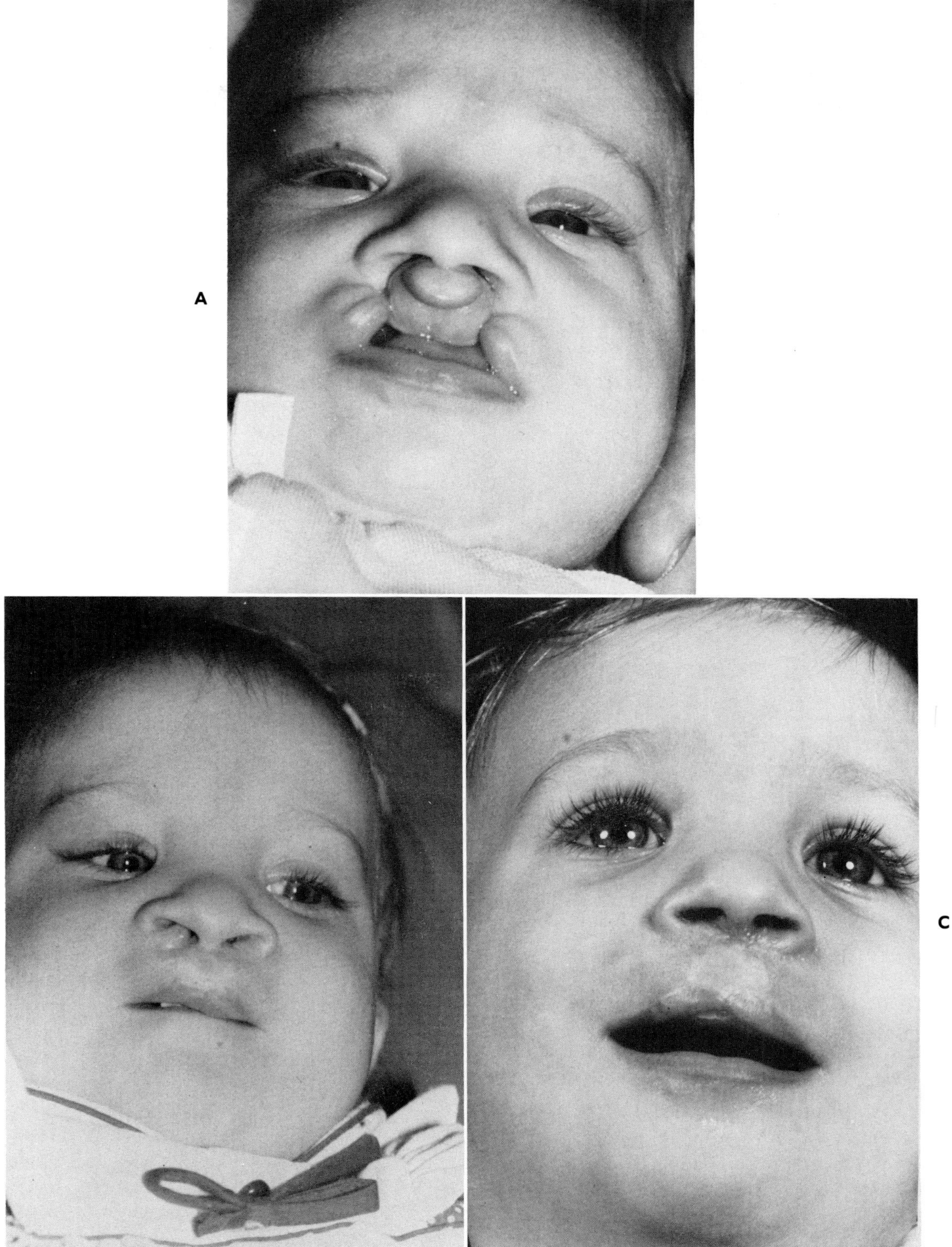

Fig. 22-8. A, Complete bilateral cleft of the primary and secondary palate with narrow alveolar clefts. **B,** The lip has been repaired with narrowing of the prolabium and rotation of lateral prolabial flaps into nostril floors. Muscle continuity across the central lip and a full-depth labial sulcus have been provided. Note the short columella. **C,** The columella has been lengthened at the time of palate repair at 16 months of age.

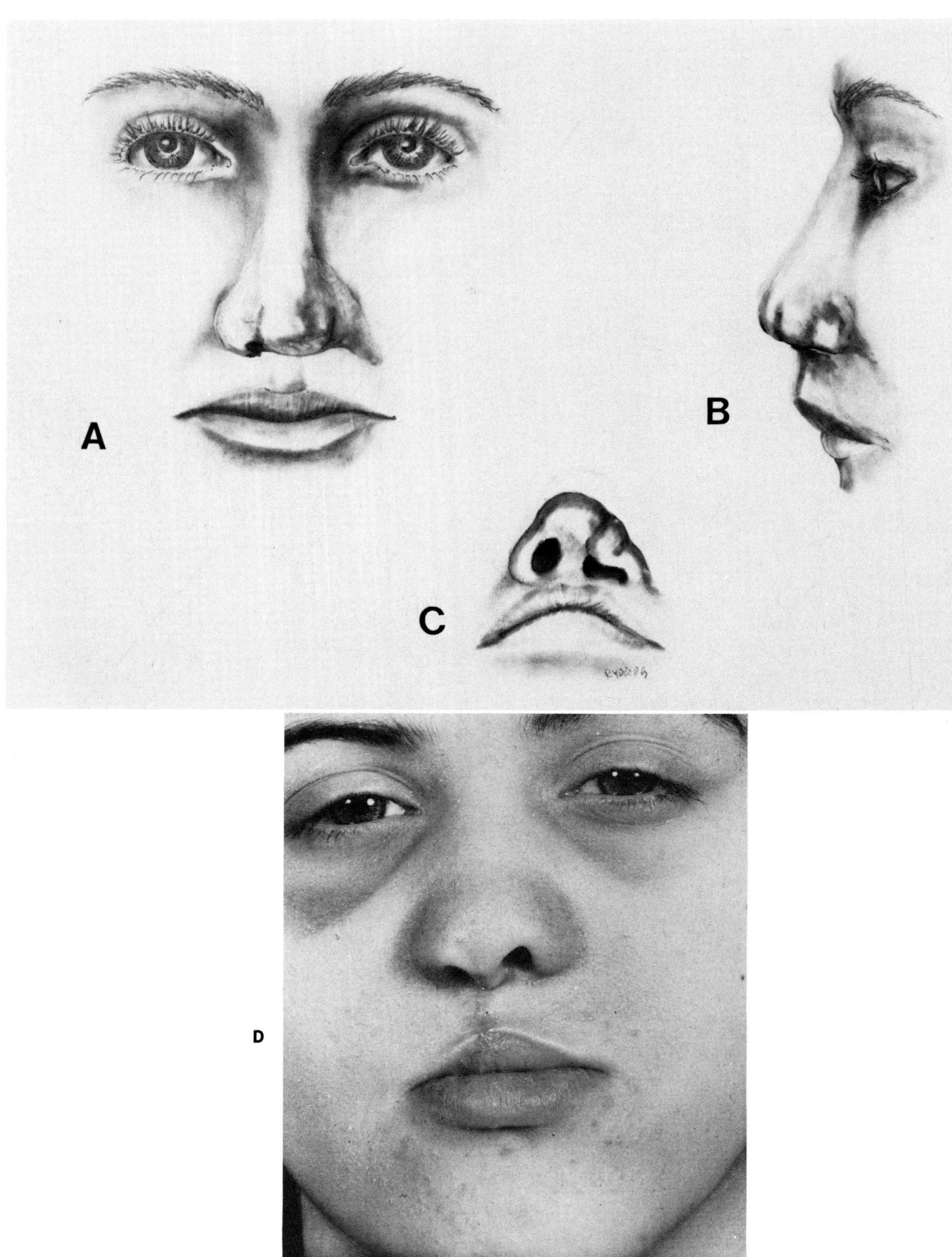

Fig. 22-9. Secondary unilateral cleft lip nasal deformity. **A,** Asymmetry is shown by the displaced highlight and lower alar border on the cleft side. **B,** Loss of tip projection on the cleft side (would be better seen on three-quarter view). **C,** Horizontal orientation of the nostril, deviation of the columella, and obliquity of the alar-cheek junction. **D,** Severe secondary unilateral deformity of both the lip and nose.

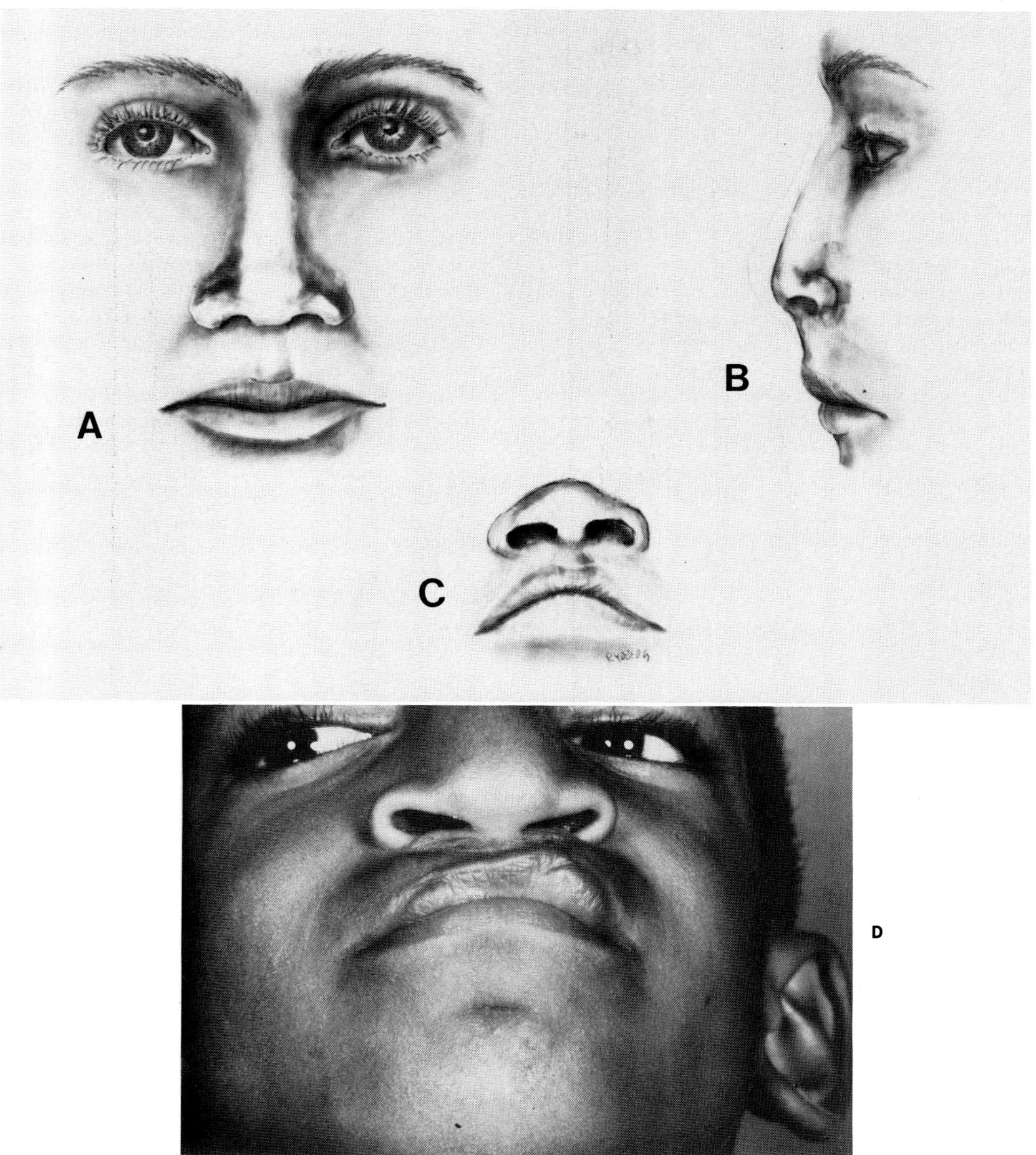

Fig. 22-10. Secondary bilateral cleft lip nasal deformity. **A,** The tip of the nose is displaced caudally due to the short columella and lateral and superior pull of the alar bases. **B,** Snubbed tip and short columella. **C,** Obtuse angle between the columella and alar borders and transverse orientation of the nostrils. **D,** Severe secondary bilateral deformity of lip and nose. Lip is asymmetric. Although nose is severely stigmatized, it is quite symmetric.

Bilateral deformity

The most obvious secondary nasal deformity in bilateral cleft lip is shortness of the columella, with snubbing of the nasal tip, increased breadth of the tip, and eversion of the alar bases (Fig. 22-10). Again surgical errors or oversights may add asymmetry, deficiency of tissue, or malposition of lip and nose elements to the underlying defect.

Reconstruction techniques

Although patients with secondary cleft lip nasal deformity should have significantly lesser degrees of the unilateral or bilateral deformity that is typical of the primary cleft, needless sacrifice of tissue, placement of structures in incorrect positions, and possible complications may obscure and make more severe the underlying basic pathologic anatomy.

Furthermore, simple limitations imposed by a deficiency of soft tissue or still existing deformity of the underlying maxilla may add vestibular webbing, retroposition of the alar base, inward buckling of the ala and deficiency of the alar base, and unilateral or bilateral shortness of the entire lateral nasal wall to the primary stigmata of the unrepaired cleft.

ANALYSIS OF UNILATERAL CLEFT LIP NASAL DEFORMITY AND RECONSTRUCTION TECHNIQUES

Blair and Letterman,[10] in commenting on Webster's search for the originator of the cross-lip flap or "switched lower lip flap for upper lip reconstruction" facetiously explained, "how these ancients steal our thoughts!" They were referring to the fact that Sabattini had performed such a procedure in 1837, although Stein in 1848 and Abbe in 1898 had been generally credited with origination of the procedure. Stein's flap was an upper lip flap to reconstruct a lower lip defect, and I do not know the nature of Sabattini's flap. Abbe's was clearly the first described for reconstruction of the upper lip in a patient with a repaired bilateral cleft lip. Similarly, credit for observation of the particular features of the secondary cleft lip nasal deformity and credit for described techniques for their correction are shared by many surgeons. The serious student of correction of cleft lip nasal deformity should be thoroughly familiar with Millard's beautiful history and critical analysis of the techniques used by many surgeons, past and present, as well as the techniques used by Millard.[66]

Blair in 1925[8] noted the almost uniform increased width of the nostril on the cleft side and that the ala remained or returned to its abnormal relationship to the maxilla in patients with clefts instead of having a close relationship between the alae, premaxilla, and columella as in the normal nose. Berkeley[5] believed the deformity was due to incomplete rotation of the alar cartilage. As noted previously, whether the deformity is due to displacement of the affected maxilla[38] or maxillary deficiency[36,104] or both,[19,53,59] Blair[8] believed that if uncorrected, additional deformities, including loss of the transverse ridge of the nostril floor, abnormal direction of the long axis of the nostril, flattening of the tip on the cleft side, flattening or inward buckling of the ala, deviation of the caudal septum to the noncleft side, and caudal displacement of the cleft-side alar border would occur. Blair[8] and later Brown and McDowell[13] noted the possibility of nostril construction due to surgical loss of tissue. Brown and McDowell[13] also noted the common deformity of vestibular webbing, described much more recently by Uchida.[110]

Skoog,[98] Malek,[53] and Sawhney[94] suggested that the nasal deformity was due to loss of orbicular muscle continuity, whereas Spira, Hardy, and Gerow,[100] Schwenzer,[96] and Sawhney[94] advanced hypoplasia of the lateral crus of the cartilage as a cause of the nasal deformity. Onizuka[79] believed nostril asymmetry was due in part to absence of alar base fullness on the affected side. Schwenzer[96] suggested that both the severity of the original cleft and the effects of previous surgery were directly proportional to the degree of deformity. McComb[58] believed the cleft side of the nose to be longer than the noncleft side, and Ariyan and Krizek[2] believed exactly the opposite.

Blair[8] initially carried out medial and superior rotation of the alar base to correct the abnormal orientation of the nostril orifice. A number of surgeons* have reported various techniques for rotation of the alar base to eliminate the broad, transverse nostril aperture.

In 1931 Blair and Brown[9] reported the technique of vertical columellar division with upward advancement of the columella on the cleft side. Gillies and Kilner[38] reported their extension of this principle (unfortunately incorrectly illustrated initially) (Fig. 22-11, *A*), and Straith reported a similar procedure by Erickson.[105] Berkeley[6] not only described a more extensive rotation upward and medially of the entire cleft-side half of the nose in the secondary cleft lip nasal deformity, but also advocated such a radical rotation in cleft nose correction (Fig. 22-11, *B*). Wilkie,[114] Morel-Fatio,[69] Velazquez and Ortiz-Monasterio[111] advocated the same technique. Instead of rotating the nostril floor into the columella, Hugo and Tumbusch[41] and Neuner[74] incorporated lip skin and scar into the distal end of the columellar flap to provide the needed additional tissue for lengthening of the columella on the cleft side. Unlike the other authors, Dibbell's procedure[28] (Fig. 22-11, *C*) rotated only the nostril periphery rather than half of the columella and the tip of the nose in the area of the dome of the alar cartilage on the cleft side.

Although better surgery, good orthodontic treatment, and orthognathic surgery have proven far better means of correcting the retruded maxilla and nose and Class III malocclusion, Gillies and Kilner[38] had also reported use of buccal inlay skin grafts and appliances to provide adequate nasal projection.

---

*References 2, 12, 13, 27, 28, 36, 75, 77, 103, and 105.

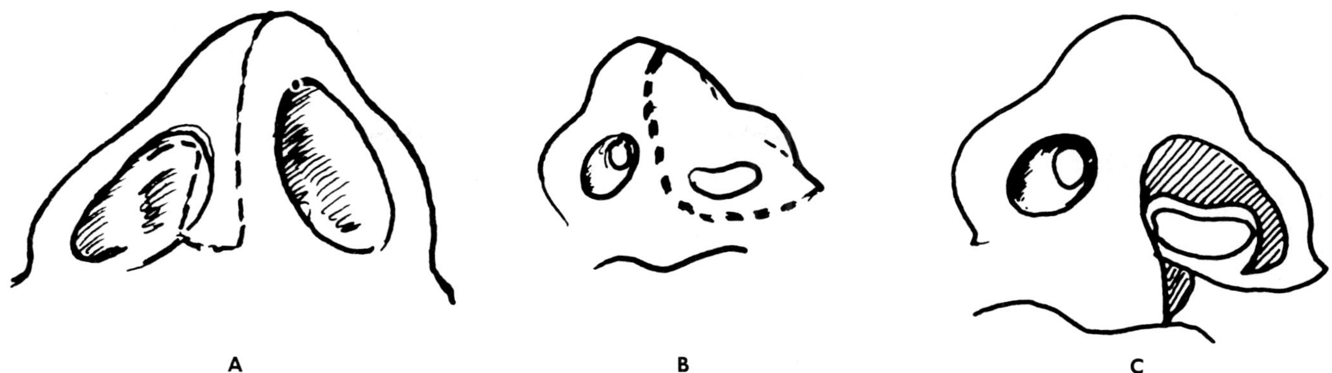

Fig. 22-11. Advancement of half of the columella and nostril rotation principle first reported by Blair and Brown in 1931.[9] **A,** Technique of Gillies and Kilner.[38] (The original artist incorrectly carried the incision to the normal side over the tip of the nose.) **B,** Royster–Berkeley–Ortiz-Monasterio rotation including the alar base, nostril floor, half of the columella, and the cleft-side dome. **C,** Dibbell rotation[28] with an incision around the periphery of the nostril and excision of skin from the alar web and lip. Later excision, when needed, allows closure of the defect created lateral to the alar base.

The location of incisions through which to dissect, expose, and reposition the alar cartilages has been a matter of continuing controversy, as has been the question of whether or not to excise external nasal skin. Various intranasal incisions have been described by Gillies and Kilner,[38] Steffensen,[102] DeKleine,[26] Broadbent and Woolf,[12] Schwenzer,[96] Sawhney,[94] Nishimura and Ogino,[76] and Millard.[64] It seems fair to say that the less severe the deformity, the more likely it is that intranasal incisions alone will permit adequate nasal tip correction, despite the warnings by Brown and McDowell,[13,14] Wynn,[117,118] Elsah,[32] and Schwenzer[96] to use a more limited access.

Certainly adequate access for dissection of alar cartilages from vestibular and external skin has been stressed as a major requirement for reconstruction of alar deformity by McIndoe as early as 1938[59] and emphasized more recently by Broadbent and Woolf.[12] Pedicles of alar cartilage, bipedicle by Lamont,[46] Potter,[87] Stenström,[104] Nishimura and Ogino,[75] and Prado and DiGeronimo[90] outlined by rim and intercartilaginous incisions are advanced upward and medially sutured to the vertical crus of the normal alar cartilage. Farrior[36] and Spina[99] used medially based unipedicle flaps for the same purpose. Millard[67] freed the medial three quarters of the cleft-side alar cartilage and, with the cartilage based laterally, placed the freed portion into a pocket at the nasal tip. Alar flaps that have been switched from one side to the other for tip reconstruction have been reported by Whitlow and Constable,[116] Broadbent and Woolf,[12] Wynn,[118] and McComb.[58]

The better exposure has appeared to justify external incisions, especially in more severe deformities, using the ''flying bird,''[29,33,37,60,100] midline columella,[53,77] and upsilon[113] patterns and a simple stab wound at the nasal tip,[75] so that sutures could be placed more precisely.

Brown and McDowell,[13] Millard,[64] and Marcks et al.[55]

caution that excision of skin should rarely, if ever, be performed. Certainly injudicious skin excisions may result in a less common but severe deformity, constriction of the nostril on the cleft side. Brown and McDowell[14] have reported skin grafts and perialar cheek flaps to fill the defect in the nostril floor after lateral alar base displacement, whereas Farrior[36] has reported laterally directed V-Y advancement to widen the nostril floor.

A shortage of skin because of intrinsic tissue deficiency or remodeling of skin over displaced cartilage support may appear clinically. Excision of skin from the cleft side has been recommended by Straith[105] Blair,[8] DeKleine,[26] Crikelair, Ju, and Symonds,[24] and most recently by Dibbell[28] (Fig. 22-11, *C*). Potter,[87] McIndoe and Rees,[60] Uchida,[110] and Schwenzer[96] have reported a less noticeable access to the alar cartilage by a reflection of a columellar flap from low on the columella or at the base of the columella where it joins the lip.

The difference of opinion regarding preservation or excision of tissue has been demonstrated by treatment of the alar-columellar web. In Millard's earlier technique,[67] and as reported by Ariyan and Krizek,[2] simple excision of vestibular and external skin and interposed alar cartilage has been carried out. As early as 1946 Straith[106] corrected the alar-columellar web by Z-plasty. Musgrave and Dupertuis in 1960,[72] Millard in 1964,[65] and Sawhney in 1976[94] excised cartilage from the web alone, leaving covering and lining skin for remodeling. The principle of conservation of tissue exemplified by conversion of external skin to lining skin in treatment of the alar-columellar web has been reported again by Millard,[67] but a variety of techniques using this principle have been reported by Tajima and Maruyama,[108] Kernahan, Bauer, and Harris,[44] Ogino and Ishida,[78] and Isshiki, Sawade, and Tamura.[42] In even more distant use of alar-columellar tissue, Onizuka[79] has rotated a flap of web tissue

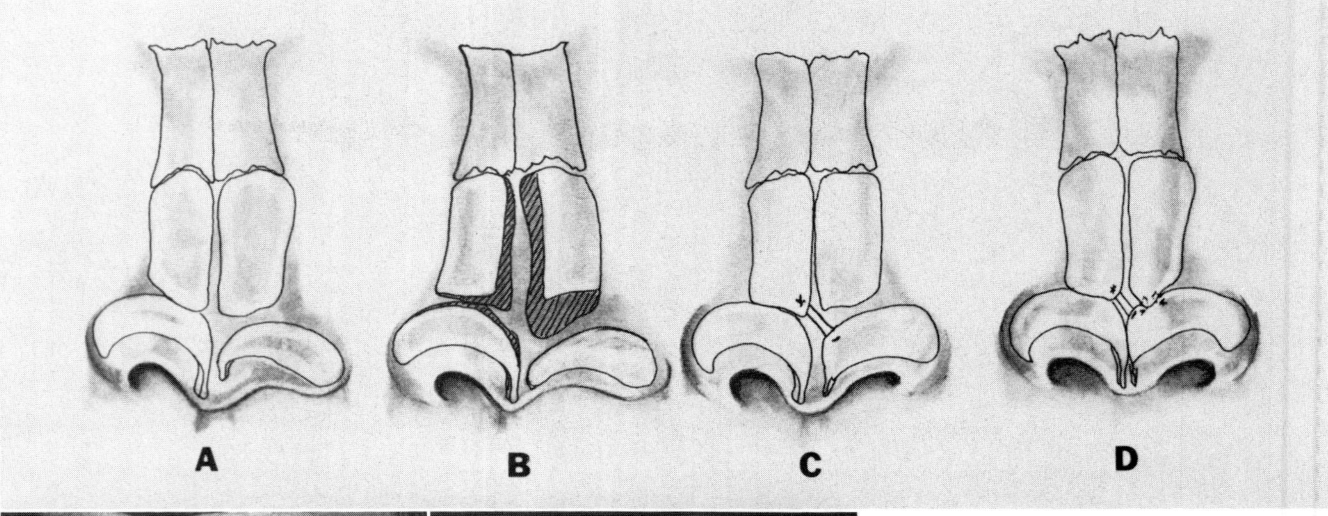

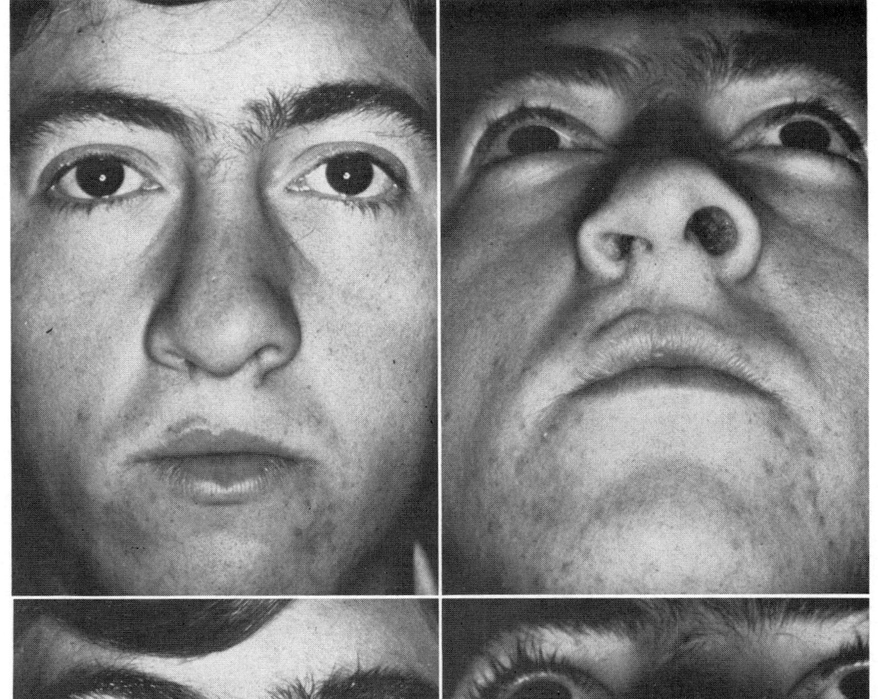

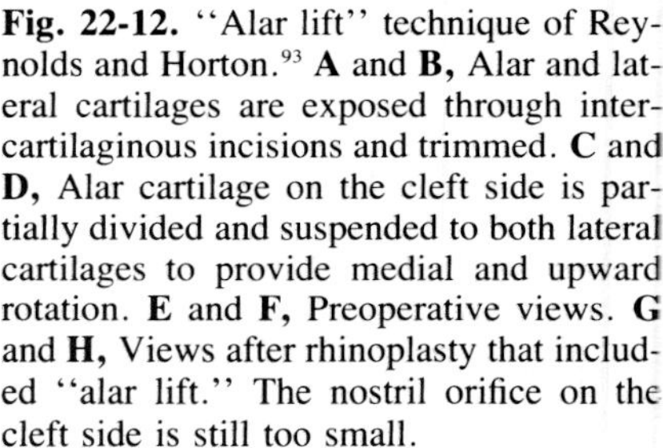

Fig. 22-12. "Alar lift" technique of Reynolds and Horton.[93] **A** and **B,** Alar and lateral cartilages are exposed through intercartilaginous incisions and trimmed. **C** and **D,** Alar cartilage on the cleft side is partially divided and suspended to both lateral cartilages to provide medial and upward rotation. **E** and **F,** Preoperative views. **G** and **H,** Views after rhinoplasty that included "alar lift." The nostril orifice on the cleft side is still too small.

into the base of the columella, whereas Elsah[32] has reported transfer of the flap to produce greater tip projection.

Depending on the surgeon's analysis of either excessive length or shortness of the cleft-side nasal wall and ala, techniques have been chosen to shorten the wall[57,58] in raising the ala by mattress sutures to the nasion or by excision of alar cartilage and the membranous septum on that side.

Abnormal vertical and anteroposterior positions of the alar base have been dealt with in a number of ways. Farrior,[36] Longacre et al.,[50] Hugo and Tumbusch,[41] and Schwenzer[96] reported the use of autogenous bone or cartilage grafts beneath the alar base. Maisels[52] used a composite graft from the normal to the cleft alar base. Ariyan and Krizek[2] raised the ala by cutting it free and placing it on a de-epithelialized base at the proper level and along with Spina[99] sought symmetry of alar bases by appropriate alar base excision, when necessary, on the normal side. Cosman and Crikelair[22] reported the use of a dermal-fat flap in the nostril floor.

As noted previously, vestibular webbing may cause both nasal obstruction on the cleft side and also inward buckling of the ala. This has been corrected by Brown and Mc-Dowell[14] and Stenström[103] by V-Y advancement. Z-plasties have been used by O-Connor, McGregor, and Tolleth,[77] Uchida,[110] and Ariyan and Krizek[2] to achieve the same result.

A number of techniques deal with the inferior displacement of the alar cartilage and correction by suspension or fixation of the ala to the lateral cartilages (Fig. 22-12).* Stenström in 1966[107] reported reshaping of the alar cartilage by a suspension suture around the alar cartilages alone.

The problem of adequate and symmetric nasal projection both for the tip and dorsum has brought forth a number of solutions. Cartilage grafts have been reported by Lamont,[46] DeKleine,[26] and Straith, Straith, and Lawson.[107] Millard[64] has reported the septal cartilage strut for good tip projection, Falces and Gorney[35] use the ''gull-wing'' conchal cartilage graft, and Dibbell[28] uses the ''Bowie knife'' costal cartilage graft. Chait[17] has recently described the C-shaped costal cartilage graft. Neuner[74] Nishimura and Ogino,[75] and Ecker[29] have also reported use of cartilage grafts for improved nasal tip projection.

The need for improved, but less dramatic, correction of inadequate nasal projection by the use of alar cartilages or both alar and lateral cartilages divided lateral to the vertical crus or septum with the medial segments turned up and sutured together back to back was first reported by Kazanjian and later by Straith.[109] Carter,[16] however, had reported a similar technique in 1914. Asymmetry of the nasal tip has been treated by onlay cartilage grafts using excised unneeded portions of the normal alar cartilage.[64,72,99,104]

Pap[81] believed that all deformities of the lip and nose should be corrected simultaneously and combined with osteoplastic rhinoplasty. All experienced authors have reported the use of standard rhinoplastic, septoplastic, and septec-

---

*References 2, 44, 51, 78, 93, 98, 100, 103, and 108.

tomy procedures for correction of the upper nasal deformity and for correction of nasal obstruction due to deformity of the septum. As in the lower nose, the asymmetric upper nose requires modification of techniques to achieve symmetry.

ANALYSIS OF SECONDARY BILATERAL CLEFT LIP NASAL DEFORMITY AND TECHNIQUES FOR RECONSTRUCTION

Pigott and Millard[86] have credited Stenström and Öberg with elucidation of the mechanism of the nasal deformity in bilateral cleft lip. Stenström[103] and Öberg had demonstrated that lateral traction on the alar bases had produced lowering of the alar arch characteristic of the nasal deformity secondary to cleft lip. Pigott and Millard, however, went on to say that traction upward, backward, and laterally on the freed lateral ends of the alar cartilages exactly reproduced the nasal deformity seen in complete bilateral cleft lip. Whether this is due to failure of forward and downward growth of the maxilla on either side, excessive forward positioning of the premaxilla, unrestrained by lack of its attachment to the lateral segments,[48] or a combination of both is not certain.

These findings suggest that the early observations of Blair and Brown,[9] in which premaxillary setback was responsible for snubbing of the nose, were not correct as far as the nasal deformity was concerned, but certainly were responsible for later Class III malocclusion. Latham and Workman's study[48] also appeared to refute Pegram's contention[82] that the short columella in bilateral cleft lip is due to incomplete caudal development of the medial nasal prominences.

Pruzansky[91] believed the bilateral cleft lip nasal deformity to be secondary to an overgrowth or excess of mesoderm at the premaxillary-vomerine suture due to lack of restraint on this area by the absence of the obicular muscle.

Both Potter[89] and McComb[57,58] believed that bilateral cleft lip repair with incorporation of the prolabium into the lip was responsible for the bilateral cleft lip nasal deformity, and for this reason McComb believed the deformity could be prevented by lengthening the columella before lip repair. Straith[105] and Pelliciari[83] believed that if the entire prolabium was advanced forward into the nose to lengthen the columella, a long, tight, and narrow upper lip would result; this is certainly true in secondary columellar lengthening with use of the entire prolabium. As might be expected, since absence of the columella is the most obvious deformity of the nose in patients with bilateral cleft lip, the great majority of papers deal with columellar lengthening.

According to McComb,[57,58] the typical bilateral cleft lip nasal deformity could be prevented by advancing the columella with bilateral quadrilateral forked flaps from the lateral portions of the prolabium at 6 weeks of age (Fig. 22-2, *D*). Millard[67] initially attempted primary forked flap columellar lengthening at the time of lip repair. Because of needed compromises in achieving an anatomically sound lip repair and to protect the vascularity of the prolabium to be left in the lip, he has abandoned primary columellar lengthening at the time of lip repair.

Gillies and Kilner[38] in 1932 reported lengthening of the columella by a V-shaped flap from the prolabium, and Brown and McDowell[14] and Potter[89] reported the use of the trefoil, or Gensoul, flap with the lateral projections of the flap being inset into the sides of the columella. The arguments concerning the shifting of bearded lip skin into the columella was answered by Brown and Mcdowell's admonition[13] that if the proposed flap requires shaving, it should be left in the lip (Fig. 22-13).

Erich and Kragh[34] reported a combined procedure to lengthen the columella and shorten the excessively long lip (specifically when lateral lip elements had been brought below the prolabium) by designing a prolabial stellate flap with lateral darts, the bases of which equaled the length of the planned columella. Unfortunately, closure of the lip resulted in a T-shaped scar with the vertical limb of the T in the center.

As noted in the review of techniques for correction of unilateral cleft lip nasal deformities, Z-plasties of the alar-columellar web as described by Straith[106] provided at least the appearance of columellar lengthening.

Pelliciari,[83] Pegram,[82] Meade,[61] and Musgrave[70] all reported lengthening of the columella by composite grafts of skin and cartilage or ear lobule. Marcks et al.,[55] Skoog,[98] and Lejour and DeMey[49] transposed flaps of lip skin into the columella; however, Lejour and DeMey expressed considerable dissatisfaction with this technique.

Secondary forked flap columellar lengthening was reported in 1958 by Millard[63] and subsequently by Stark and Kaplan[101] and Wray.[116] In the patient with a wide prolabium, muscle continuity, and an adequate upper labial sulcus, bi-

lateral forked flap columellar lengthening improves the appearance of the prolabium and locates the scars in the position of the philtral ridges.

Although Carter[16] in 1914 and Converse[18] in 1957 reported the use of flaps from the wide nostril floors of a patient with a bilateral cleft lip nasal deformity, these flaps were elevated as bilateral unipedicle flaps based on the columella and were sutured together to provide columella advancement. Both Carter and Converse then closed the defects in the nostril floors by medial advancement of the alar bases (Fig. 22-14). It was Cronin,[25] however, who reported columellar lengthening using bilateral bipedicle flaps that included the columellar base, nostril floor, an alar base in single units that in one medial and upward stroke corrected alar flare, and the wide nostril floor and short columella. Gorney and Rosenberg[39] modified Cronin's technique by raising bilateral sleeves of skin and mucoperichondrium and rotating them upward and medially and also added a cartilage strut for better nasal tip projection.

Brauer and Foerster[11] (Fig. 22-15), to avoid encircling of the prolabium by scar, reported lengthening of the columella at its other end, the nasal tip, by essentially raising columellar-alar margin flaps as forked flaps, suturing them to each other, and thus raising and narrowing the tip of the nose. Like the other columellar lengthening procedures that depend on the joining of two flaps in the midline to add the needed length, which is really V-Y advancement, Brauer and Foerster's technique put the V-Y flap at the other end of the columella. Similar V-Y advancements were reported as early as 1950 by Blair and Letterman[10] and in 1971 by Ecker.

Morel-Fatio and Lalardrie[69] and Edgerton[30] have reported V-Y lengthening at the tip also, but incision lines across the alar border in the area of the alar-columellar junctions where

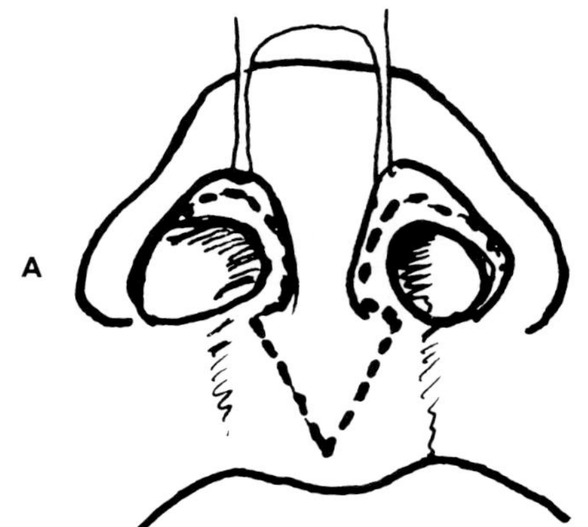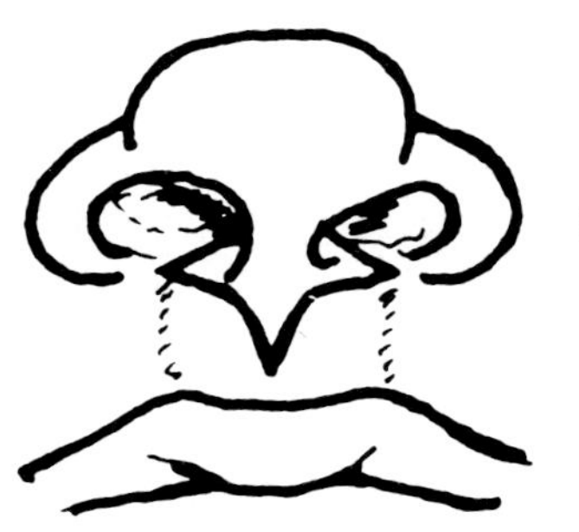

Fig. 22-13. A, Lengthening of the columella with a flap from the prolabium. A triangular flap was reported by Gillies and Kilner in 1932.[38] **B,** Trefoil, or Gensoul, flap with lateral darts to lengthen the sides of the columella and membranous septum. Erich and Kragh[34] deliberately widened the base of the darts to shorten the lip when it was too long.

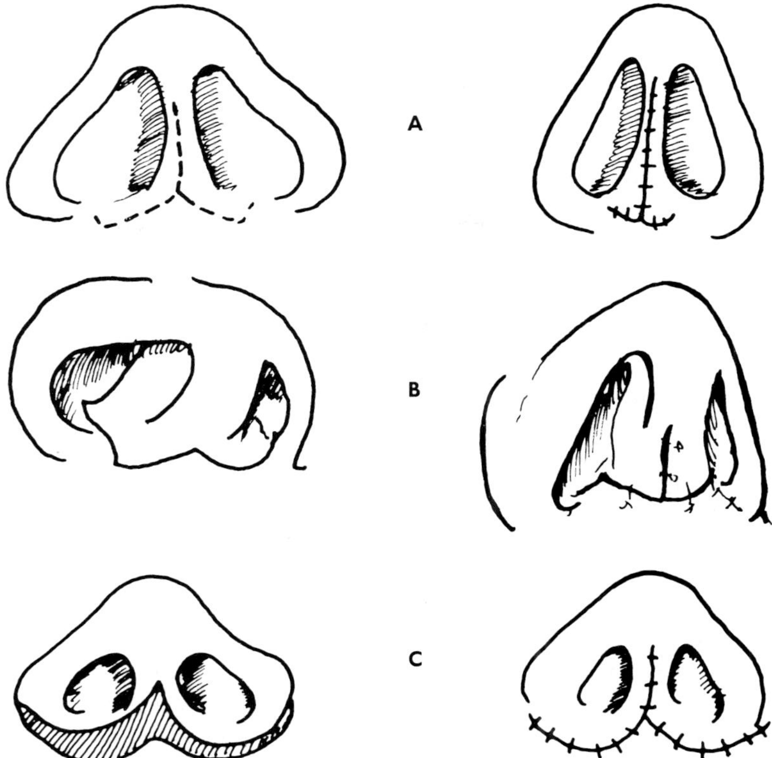

Fig. 22-14. Use of nostril floor tissue to lengthen columella. **A,** Advancement of nostril floor flaps into the columella and a secondary medial alar base shift to close the defect. **B,** Identical technique described by Converse in 1957.[18] **C,** Cronin's columellar advancement[25] with bases of the columella, nostril floors, and alar bases shifted as bipedicle flaps that correct columellar shortness, excessive width of nostril floors, flaring, and eversion of alar bases. (**A** from Davis, J.S.: Plastic surgery: its principles and practice, Philadelphia, 1919, P. Blakiston's Son & Co.)

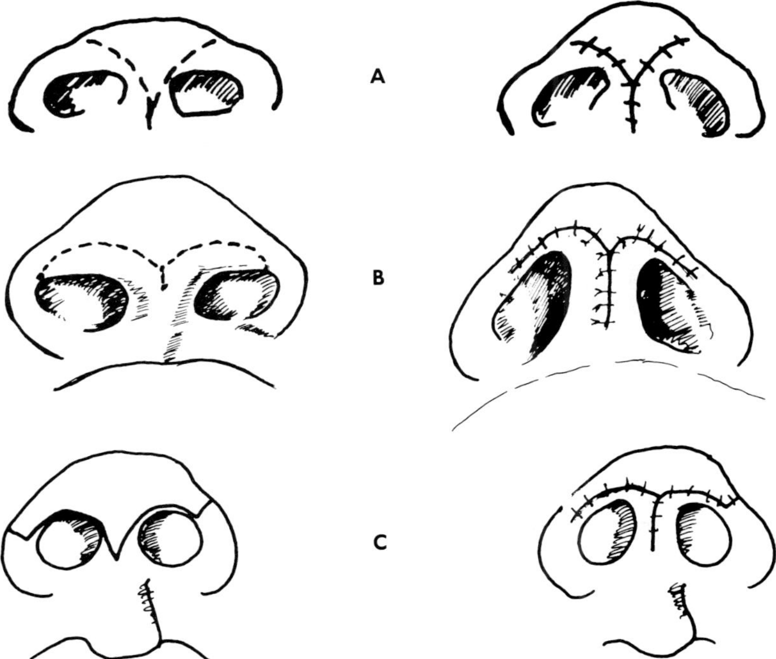

Fig. 22-15. V-Y advancement at the tip end of the nose to raise and narrow the tip and lengthen the columella. **A,** ''Bat-wing'' advancement of Blair and Letterman.[10] **B,** The technique of Brauer and Foerster[11] may be desirable when the nostril floors are narrow and the alar bases are in a good position. **C,** Technique of Ecker.[29]

they are obvious compared with scars in the nostril floor or at either medial or lateral junction of the nostril floor with the columella or ala respectively.

Blair and Letterman[10] excise a diamond-shaped portion of skin from the center of the columella to narrow and lengthen it (by the pantograph principle).

A number of authors lengthen the columella with the prolabium, but reconstruct the upper lip with a full-thickness flap from the lower lip. Although Blair and Letterman[10] first reported this in 1950, it appears that in only 3 of the 15 cases were the cross-lip flaps done at the time of columellar lengthening. The other 12 first had a trefoil flap and subsequently an Abbe flap. Von Deilen,[112] Musgrave,[70] Converse et al.,[19,20] and Malek[53] have all used the Abbe flap to replace the prolabium advanced into the columella.

Correction of deformities of the nostril floor and alar bases has been reported by alar base excisions,[14] transposition of nostril floor flaps to perialar positions to narrow the nostril floors,[21] and raising of the alar bases by bone grafts.[51] DeKleine[26] excised overhanging alar cartilage and skin through rim incisions.

Potter[88,89] reported an improvement in the appearance of the nose by excision of the premaxilla. Along with Schwenzer,[96] he also advocated raising of a columellar flap to correct the bifid tip frequently associated with bilateral cleft lip nasal deformity.[87]

Elevation of the dorsal profile of the entire nose or provision of adequate tip projection has been accomplished by a number of authors using bone and cartilage grafts. Among these were Lamont[46] and Von Deilen,[112] Straith, Straith, and Lawson,[107] and Falces and Gorney,[35] who used the gull-wing conchal cartilage graft also for unilateral cleft lip nasal deformity. Schwenzer[96] reported the use of cartilage grafts and Neuner in 1975[74] reported the use of the excised nasal hump as an autogenous graft. Dibbell[28] used the ''Bowie knife'' costal cartilage graft in the bilateral deformity also. Before insertion of a cartilage graft, DeKleine[26] excised an ellipse of skin and subjacent subcutaneous tissue from the nasal tip to narrow it and provide tip projection.

GENERAL CONSIDERATIONS
IN NASAL REVISION
Prevention of secondary nasal deformity

As noted in the discussion on correction of the nasal deformity at the time of primary lip repair, equal consideration of basic principles and techniques and equal conservation of tissue are essential, even though an equal degree of dissection of both the lip and nose is not warranted. Planning for the long-term consequences of repair is mandatory. Deficiencies of both lip and nose tissue may prevent ideal reconstruction, but the surgeon must at least place all of the available tissue in the correct location at the time of primary repair, even though correction may not persist due to gravity, growth, and stretching of the scar. Failure to lengthen the columella with the C-flap and to advance half

of the columella and membranous septum upward in the rotation-advancement repair will make attainment of later columella and tip symmetry more difficult, if not impossible, to achieve. Sacrifice of alar base tissue or portions of the C-flap may result in a constricted nostril, one of the most difficult problems to correct satisfactorily. For these and other reasons I believe that the rotation-advancement repair, incorporating all of Millard's superb refinements[66] of his own magnificently conceived operation,[62] is the operation of choice for unilateral cleft lip repair.

In the bilateral cleft lip, failure to narrow the prolabium to its proper width, preserve lateral prolabial flaps for an adequate nostril floor, and provide orbicular muscle continuity and a full-length labial sulcus will require later performance of these steps in lip repair with a consequent delay in nasal reconstruction. Even worse, needless sacrifice of tissue or use of valuable prolabial skin for lip sulcus lining may result in an irreparable loss of badly needed tissue.

Brown and McDowell[14] suggested columellar lengthening by the age of 4 years. Earlier advancement, even if it must be repeated, seems desirable, and certainly delays in reconstruction with an inadequate soft tissue envelope for the developing supporting cartilaginous skeleton of the nose may make bone or cartilage grafts mandatory to complete reconstruction at a later time.

Musgrave and Bremner[71] have pointed out the risk of infection in infants and children undergoing cleft and palate surgery. Unrecognized upper respiratory tract infections that arise during or immediately after lip repair have been complicated by streptococcal infection; patients undergoing lip and palate surgery complicated by such infections had a 33% incidence of wound complications. For this reason the administration of antibiotics effective against β-hemolytic streptococci in the immediate preoperative period and intraoperatively seems justified.

Incorporation of correction of nasal deformity
into the treatment plan

Despite well-planned and well-executed attempts at the time of the primary lip repair, some residual nasal deformity will usually remain and require later revision. There are important principles to guide the timing of nasal revision. First, infants, children, and adolescents should undergo as few hospital admissions for surgery as possible. Second, surgery of cleft lip and palate should be performed when the patient is physiologically, functionally, and psychologically ready so that the best possible result can be attained.

Patients with cleft lip and cleft palate usually have pedodontic and orthodontic treatment and frequently undergo speech therapy and otolaryngologic, prosthodontic, and oral surgical treatment. As many surgical procedures as possible should be performed in the same hospital admission and under the same anesthetic. Adequate communication and collaboration in planning and performing the proposed surgical treatment are essential.

Although opinions vary as to whether or not septal and upper nasal surgery should be carried out before the attainment of adult growth, there seems to be no valid reason to delay revision of the lower nose. Therefore surgery on the columella, alae, nostril floors, and entire lower third of the nose should be performed at the time of other surgery and certainly in the preschool period. The stigmata of the cleft lip nasal deformity, in any event, are chiefly apparent in the lower third of the nose. Upper nose deformity, including asymmetry, lateral deviation, or dorsal prominence, although not insignificant problems, are common in the population at large and are not typical of a congenital deformity. Many surgeons perform the classic osteoplastic rhinoplasty under topical and local anesthesia. Lower third nasal correction often can be performed better under general anesthesia, which may be chosen because of other planned surgery or the age of the patient.

TECHNIQUES FOR CORRECTION OF THE CLEFT LIP NASAL DEFORMITY
The unilateral deformity

One obvious advantage in analysis of the unilateral cleft lip nasal deformity is the ability to compare the cleft side to the noncleft or "normal" side. However, the "normal" side may possess ethnic, familial, or acquired characteristics that are quite apart from characteristics secondary to unilateral cleft lip.

It is important to determine whether or not there are obvious deficiencies of tissue such as absence of the alar base, absent tissue at the area of the nasal tip, or a deficient nostril floor or constriction of the nostril. Is there significant displacement of approximated tissue, such as placement of the alar base well within the floor of the nostril or inadequate rotation and upward advancement and rotation of the C-flap into the columella and nostril floor? It is likely that significant past surgical displacement of nasal structures will also be accompanied by significant errors in the primary lip repair. These may include absence of muscle continuity, shortness of the lip, and a severe whistling deformity of the vermilion so that the incisor teeth are fully exposed even when not smiling. If such deformities exist, take down of the entire lip should be performed with provision of a full-length labial sulcus, reconstruction of the orbicular muscle, and a rotation-advancement repair of the skin and tissue superficial to the muscle. This will allow formation of a C-flap for columellar lengthening and nostril floor reconstruction that must include correct positioning of the alar base.

If initial lip repair was performed using a straight-line type of repair or a rotation-advancement repair, revision of the lip is quite straightforward. If initial repair was by the Tennison or LeMesurier technique, however, repeat repair of the lip is more difficult because of the position of the inferiorly placed lip flap and scars crossing into the philtral area. Wilson[115] has converted Tennison and LeMesurier repairs into rotation-advancement repairs by moving the medial portion of the lip above the inferior flap into a C-flap. In the grossly deficient and tight lip, which is rarely seen now, re-creation of the defect with release of nasal structures and repair of the lip with an Abbe flap can be the only choice.

Despite correct planning and execution of lip repair and avoidance of gross displacement of nasal structures, correction may either not be achieved or may not be maintained because of failure to advance the columella on the cleft side sufficently or the alar base far enough medially or failure to position the ala so that its free border corresponds exactly with that on the noncleft side. The L-flap of Millard may not have been used to supplement vestibular lining, or other details of repair may have been overlooked.

A well-repaired lip with a secondary nasal deformity, such as inferior and lateral displacement of the alar cartilage, transverse orientation of the nostril orifice depression of the alar dome, an alar-columellar web, inward buckling of the ala with vestibular webbing, obliquity of the alar-cheek angle, and a short columella, requires a reconstruction technique that will correct all of these abnormalities. One technique is an upward and medial rotation of the entire cleft side of the nose. It is difficult to accomplish this purely through intranasal incisions.

Although adequate and accurate correction is readily achieved with the technique proposed by Royster and popularized by Berkeley[6] and Velazquez and Ortiz-Monasterio[111] (Fig. 22-16), most surgeons simply cannot bear to extend a midcolumellar incision over the tip of the nose to the area between alar and lateral cartilage on the cleft side. I have only used this technique recently in patients who had previously undergone attempted primary or secondary correction by external rotation of half of the nose in which adequate rotation could not be achieved.

Dibbell recently reported[28] correction of the unilateral cleft lip nasal deformity by incisions that lie at the border of the nostril aperture, including excision of skin from the alar-columellar web and lip to close the defect resulting from medial rotation of the alar base. This method seems to possess all of the advantages of the Royster–Berkeley–Ortiz-Monasterio rotation, but leaves much less noticeable scars (Fig. 22-17). The procedures described by Tajima and Maruyama[108] and modified by Kernahan, Bauer, and Harris[44] do provide good correction of the alar-columellar web and have the theoretic advantage of preserving skin in the area rather than excising it. However, they simply do not provide as adequate projection or correction of the alar-cheek angle in the more severe nasal deformity (Fig. 22-18). Dibbell[28] suggests that certain techniques achieve better results in some ethnic groups than others.

Black[7] corrected unilateral and bilateral secondary cleft lip nasal deformities through a combination of rim and upper labial sulcus incisions that permit degloving of the lower nasal cartilaginous skeleton and precise dissection and ap-

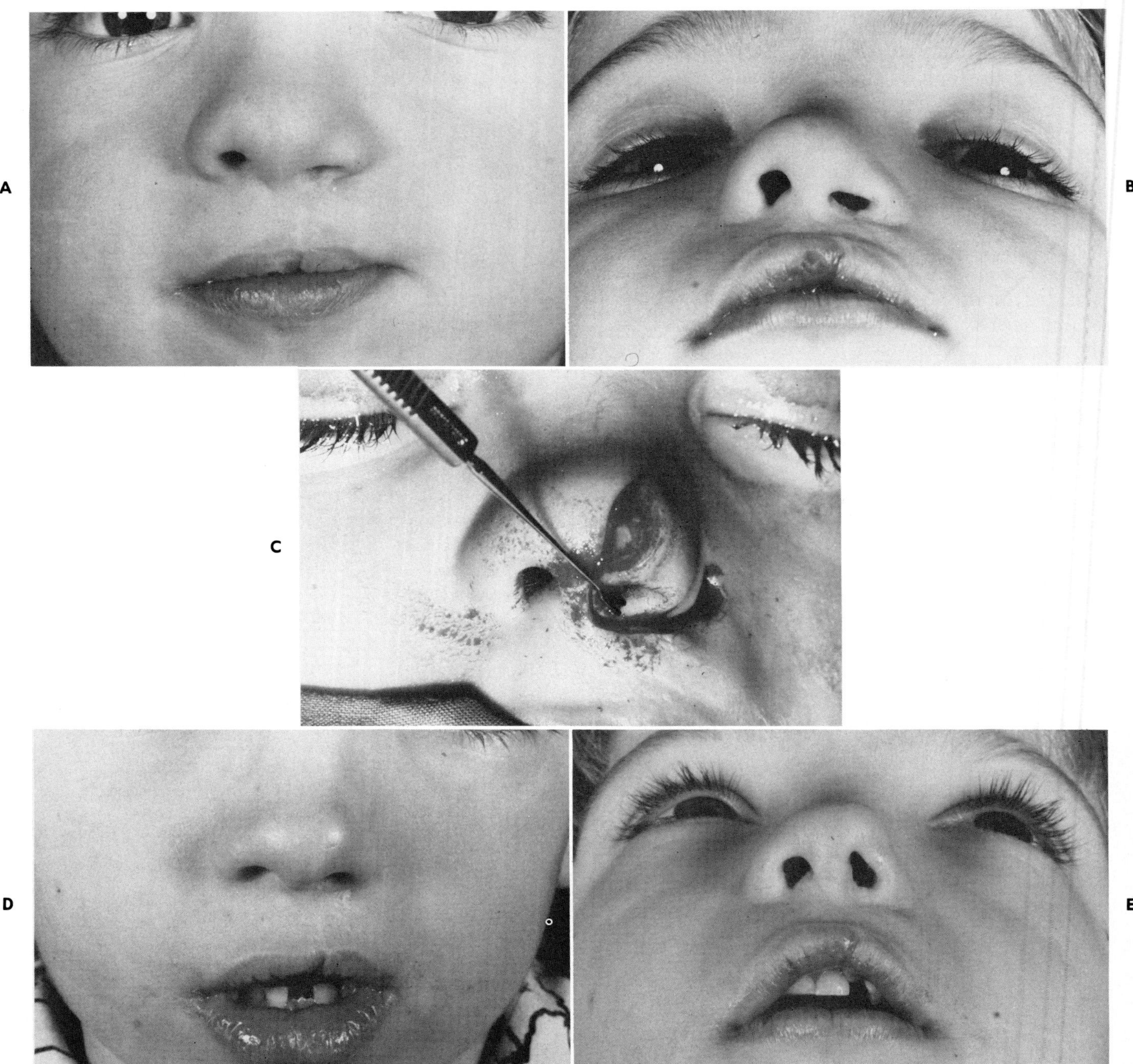

Fig. 22-16. Royster–Berkeley–Ortiz-Monasterio rotation. **A** and **B,** Slumped tip and alar border and a wide nostril floor. **C,** The entire ''sleeve'' of the cleft-side nostril with covering skin being rotated medially and upward. **D** and **E,** Note the tip highlights on the same level and the change in tip projection and nostril orientation in the tip-up view.

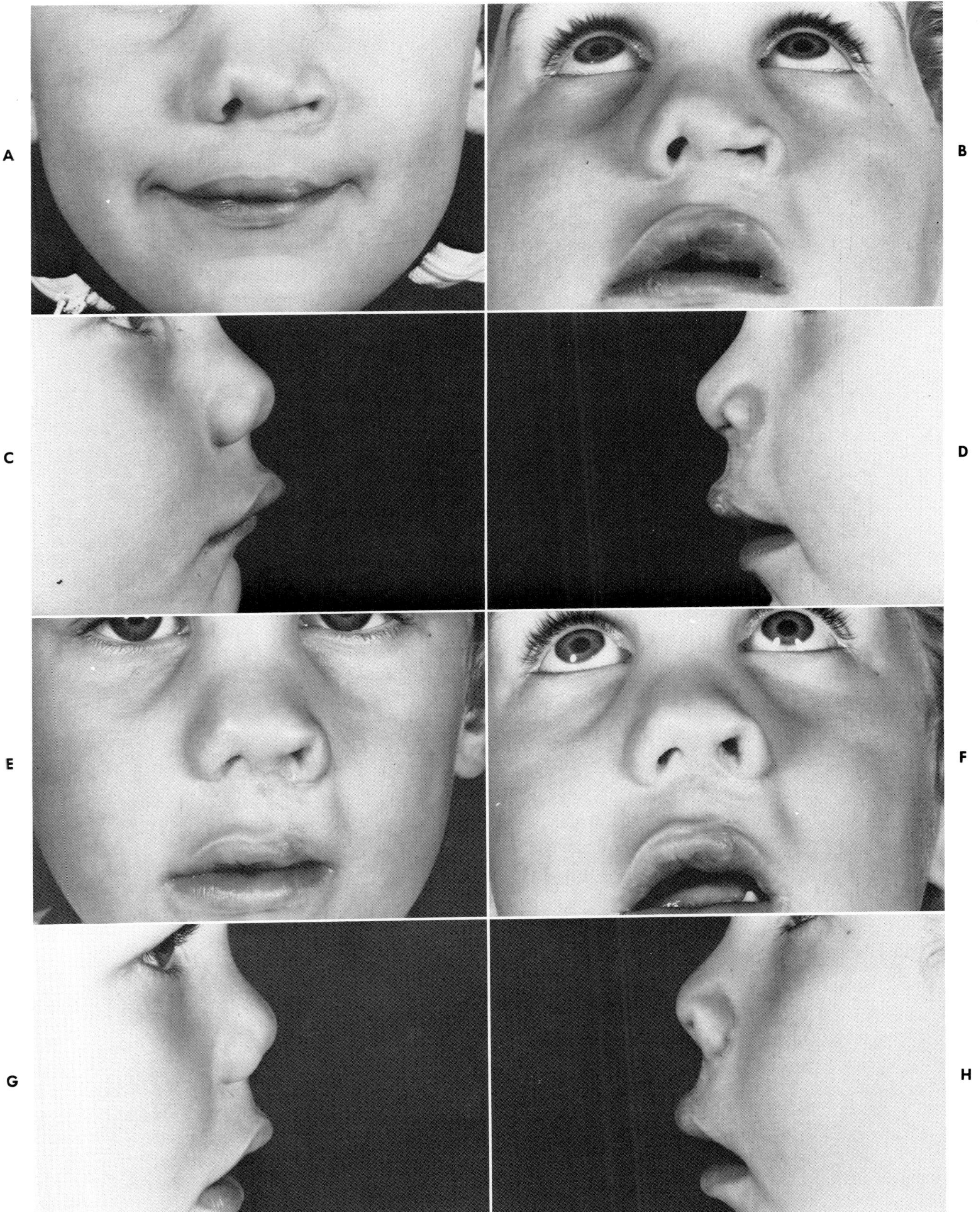

Fig. 22-17. Nasal tip revision by Dibbell's technique.[28] **A** to **D,** Typical secondary unilateral cleft lip deformity. **E** to **H,** Early postoperative views. Note tip highlights at the same approximate level, symmetry of nostril orientation, and elimination of alar buckling.

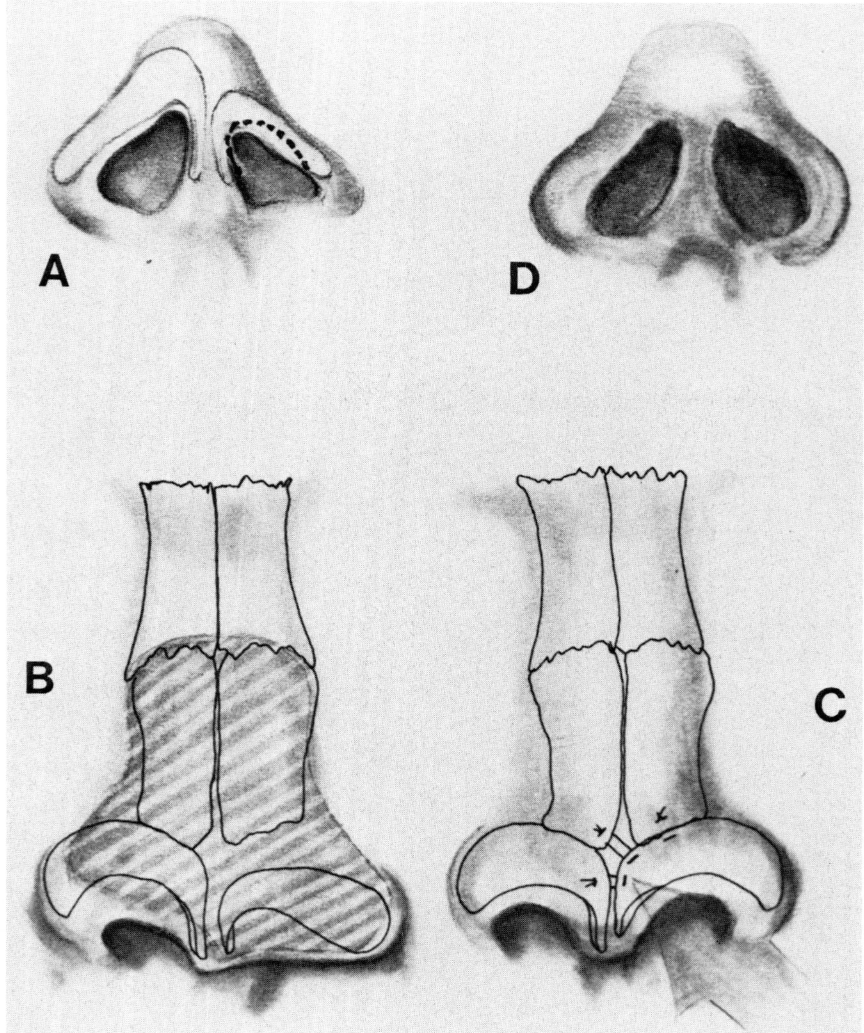

Fig. 22-18. Reverse-U correction of the alar-columellar web. **A** to **D,** Reverse-U incision drawn over the alar-columellar web to convert external skin into vestibular skin. Inferiorly displaced and laterally rotated alar cartilage (**C**) is sutured to normal alar and lateral cartilages and to the cleft-side lateral cartilage. Modifications of this technique proposed by Kernahan, Bauer, and Harris[44] are helpful in performing the procedure.

proximation of alar cartilages under direct vision (Fig. 22-19). No skin is excised, and the covering is simply replaced over the corrected cartilage framework to remodel.

Isolated features of the unilateral cleft lip nasal deformity, such as eversion of the alar base, an increased width of the nostril floor, alar-columellar webbing, vestibular webbing, or possibly a combination of two of these defects, may be corrected by any of the previously cited limited techniques.

Either in childhood or at the time needed and desired, rhinoplasty is performed. Musgrave's technique[70] of inserting tiered cartilage grafts obtained from excess alar cartilage

removed in tip rhinoplasty on the noncleft side provides an excellent means of correcting residual loss of tip projection on the cleft side.

Less frequent and typical deformities require special reconstructive techniques. A constricted nostril or a nostril without an adequate floor may require transposition of a perialar flap. Partial excision of the normal alar base may be indicated to match a modest deficiency of alar base on the cleft side. When there is a severely deficient alar base on the cleft side, it may be best to reconstruct the deformity with a composite graft from the normal to the cleft side or

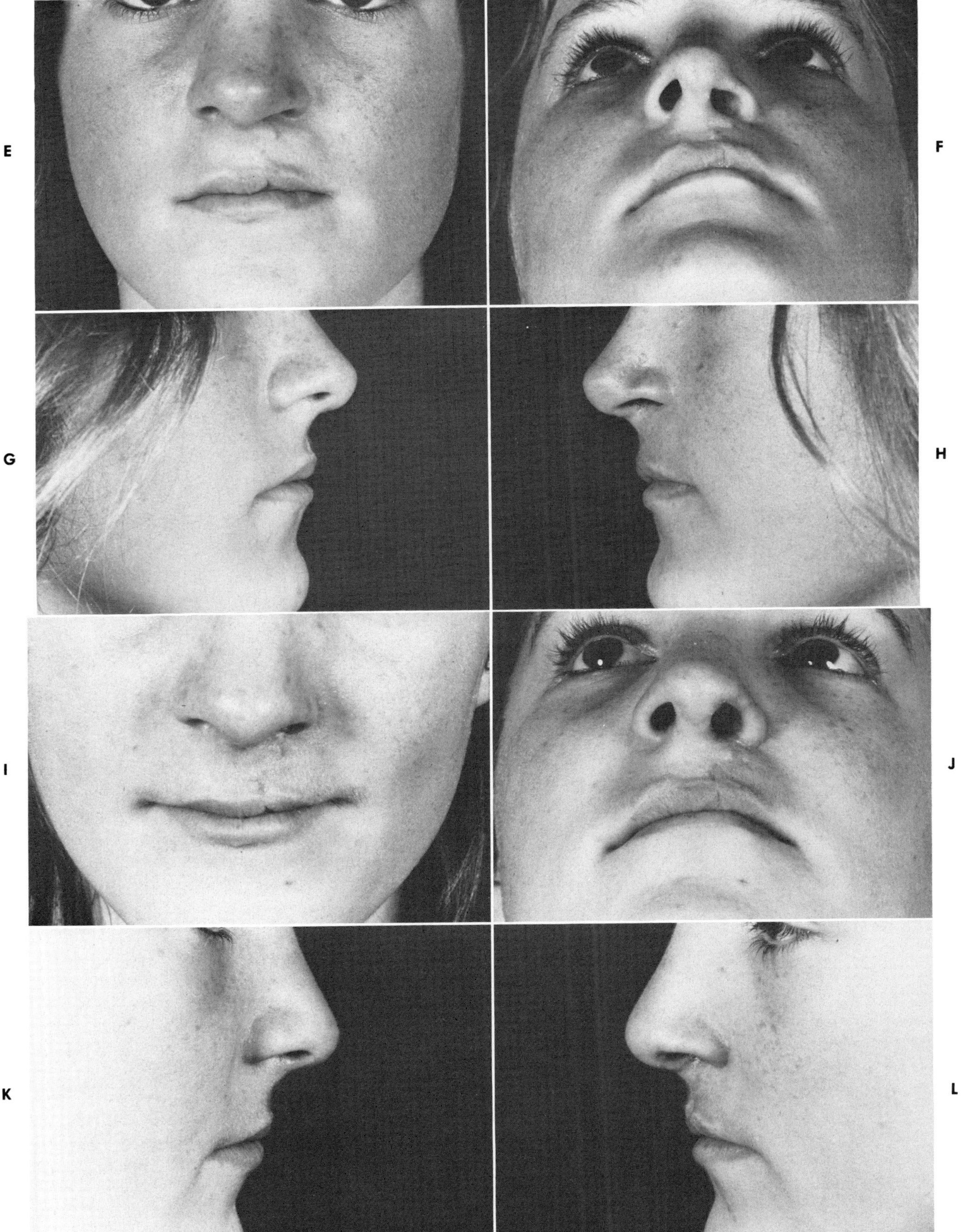

Fig. 22-18, cont'd. E to **H,** Preoperative views. **I** to **L,** The alar base has also been moved medially and rotated internally.

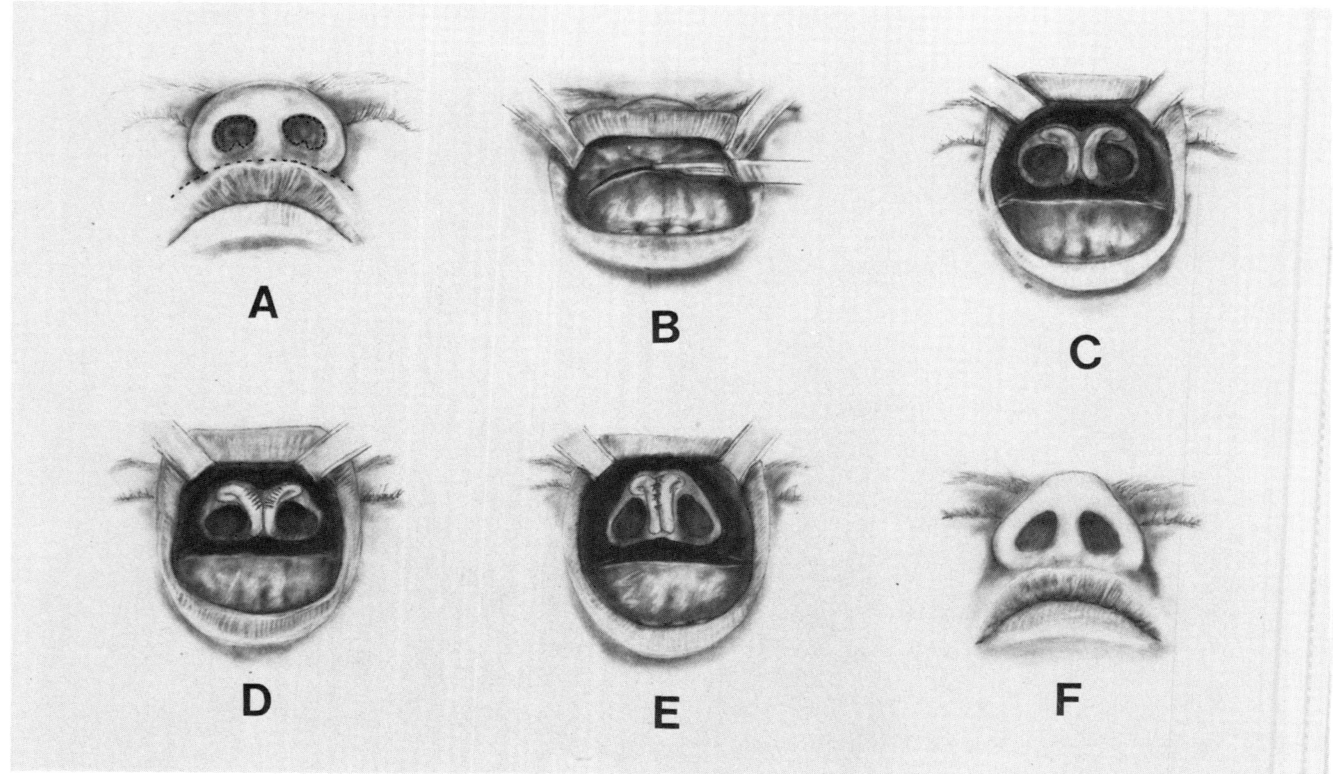

Fig. 22-19. Black's technique[7] for cartilage correction without skin excision or shifting. **A,** Rim incisions with V-flaps in the nostril floor and upper labial sulcus incision. **B,** Upper labial sulcus incision. **C,** Sleeves of nasal vestibules and alar cartilages exposed by a degloving technique. **D,** Scoring of alar cartilages. **E,** Suture approximation of dome areas of the alar cartilages to lengthen the columella and raise and narrow the tip. **F,** Redraped skin over the revised cartilage framework.

by insertion of a nasolabial flap under the alar base on the cleft side.[31] Inadequate support of the alar base requires insertion of bone beneath the base at the time of alveolar bone grafting.

Septal surgery

Deviation of the caudal end of the nasal septum toward the normal side is an almost constant feature of the unilateral cleft lip nasal deformity. Septoplasty should be performed with scoring of cartilage on the normal, concave side beneath elevated mucoperichondrial flaps, and the septum should be freed along the floor of the nose to permit the deviated septum to return to the midline. Spurs of septal cartilage or an obstructing septum posteriorly should be resected by the usual techniques to provide an adequate airway bilaterally.

The upper nose

Deformity of the upper nose and the tip should be corrected by standard rhinoplastic techniques, perferably in adolescence, when the patient desires such correction. Since the upper nose is almost always asymmetric, equalization of the height of the nasal walls must be achieved in lateral

and medial osteotomies to make the sides of the nose symmetric and position the nose in the midline (Fig. 22-20).

Although correction of a deformity of the lower third of the nose can and should be corrected at the time of other surgery, such as closure of an alveolar cleft and alveolar bone grafting, formal and definitive rhinoplasty should not be carried out before surgical maxillary advancement, maxillary expansion, or repositioning, since these procedures may significantly alter the esthetic relationship of the nose to the face. The increased nasal projection that may occur after maxillary advancement may eliminate the need for a bone or cartilage graft to the nose. For this reason Schendel and Delaire[95] have combined lip and nose revision with orthognathic surgery. Although cartilage or bone grafts may still be required,[28,35,39,64] satisfactory nasal projection is frequently obtained by raising the dorsal profile and tip, narrowing the bony nose, and nasal tip correction. An alternative technique is the lateral division of alar and lateral cartilages with back-to-back sutures[106] (Fig. 22-21).

The bilateral deformity

There is usually one advantage in dealing with the bilateral cleft lip nasal deformity—symmetry. Asymmetry also

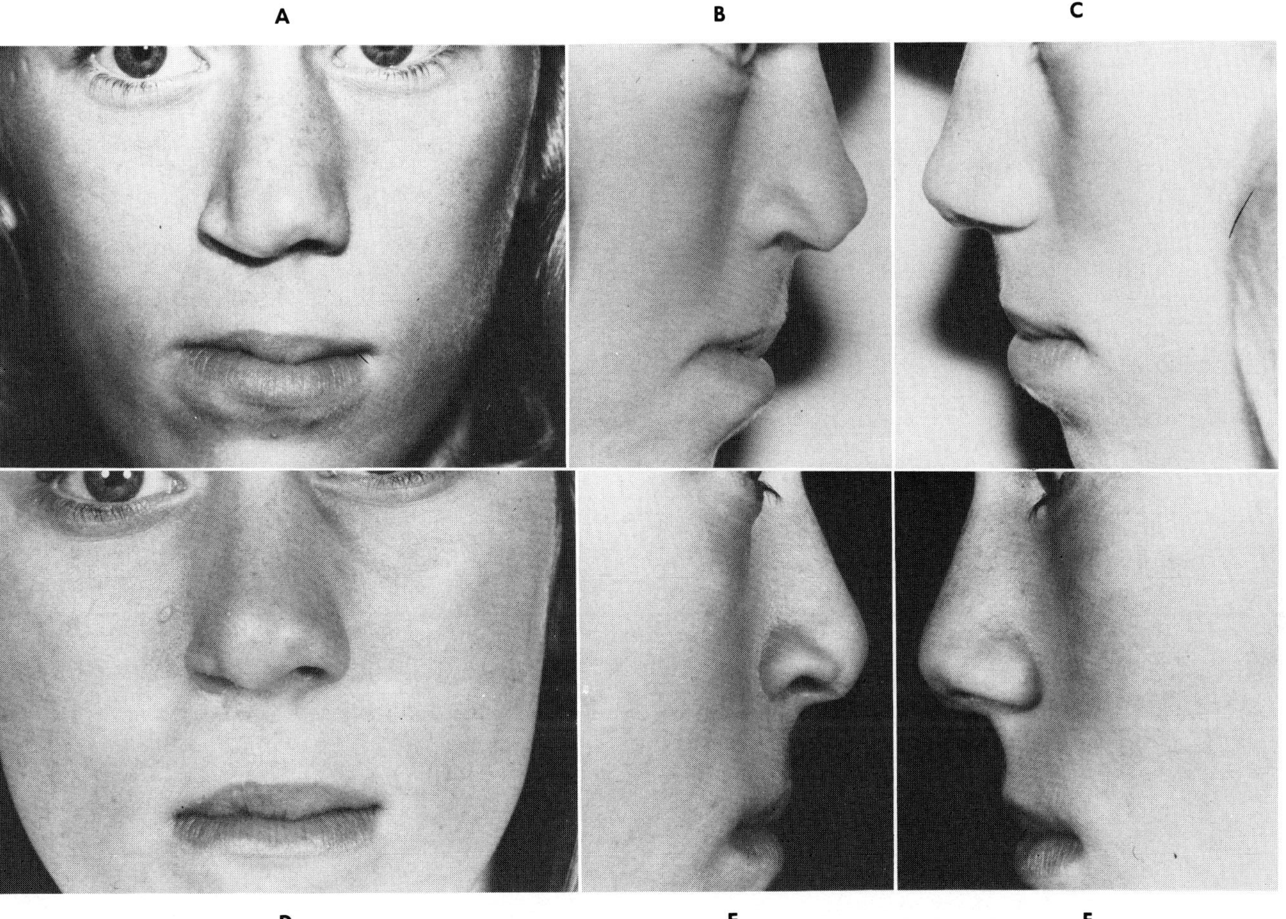

Fig. 22-20. Rhinoplasty for correction of the upper nose and tip revision by an intranasal incision. **A** to **C,** Preoperative views. The upper nose is broad with slight dorsal prominence. Note significant slumping of alar dome and alar border. **D** to **F,** Postoperative views. Good symmetry of tip highlights, but still some alar webbing.

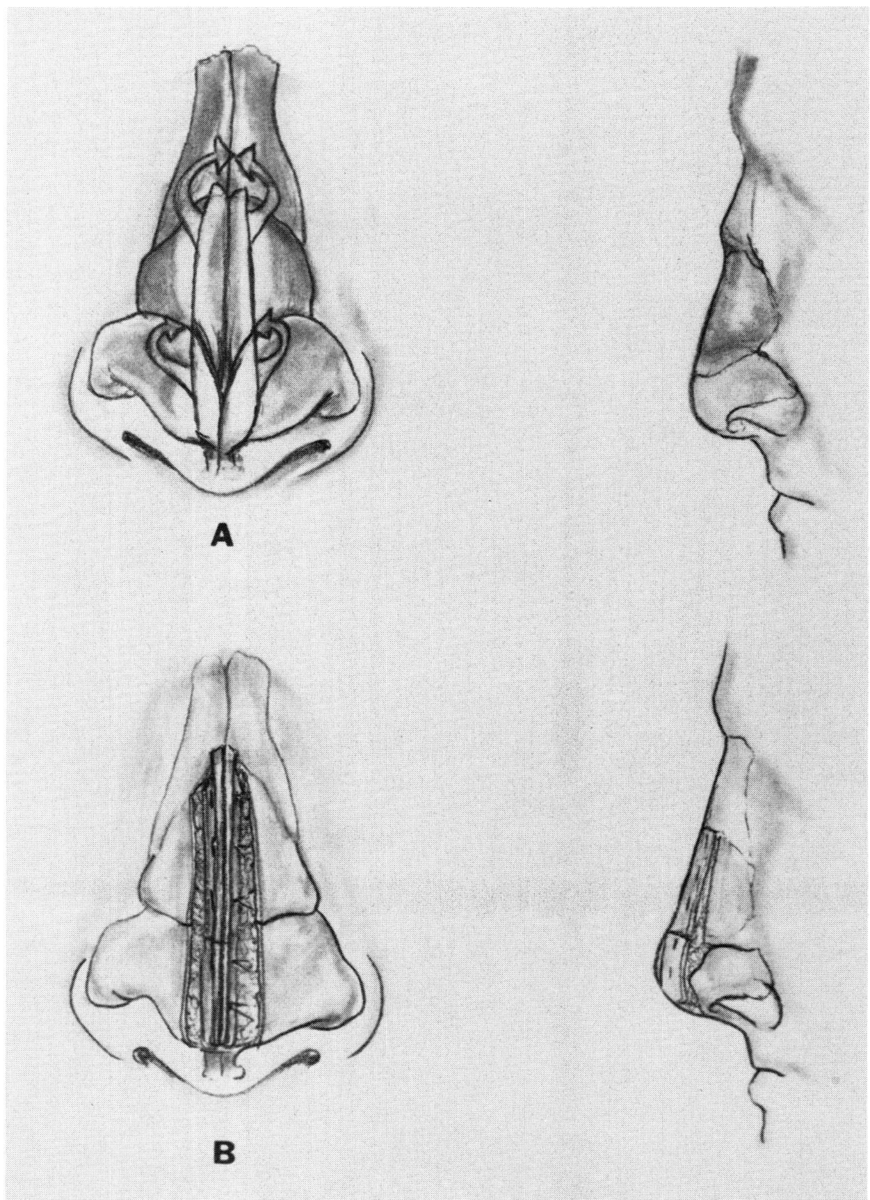

Fig. 22-21. Use of medial portions of alar and lateral cartilages to raise the dorsal profile. **A** and **B,** Lateral and alar cartilages are divided lateral to the septum and domes respectively and turned up back to back and sutured.

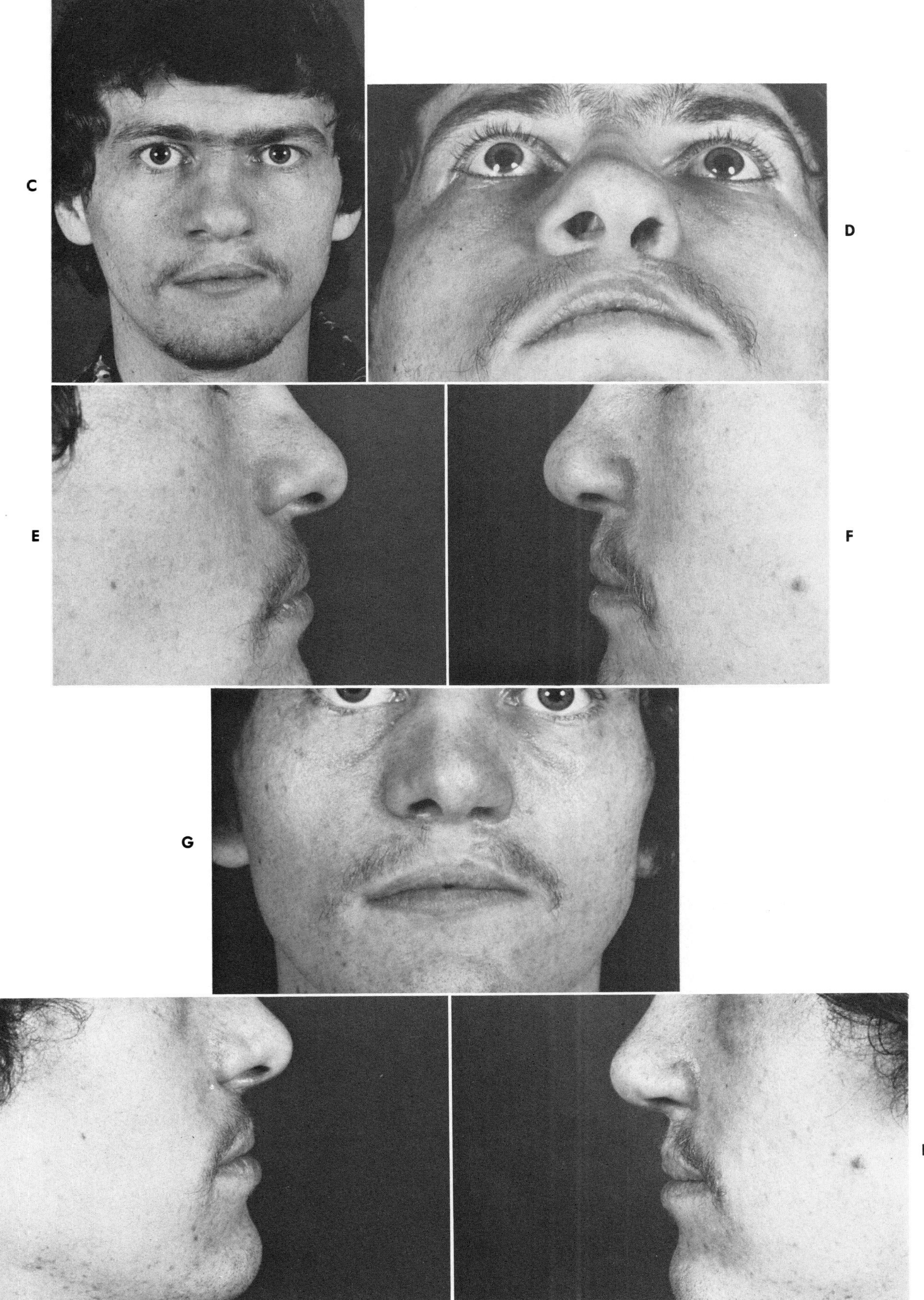

Fig. 22-21, cont'd. C to **F,** Preoperative views. **G** to **I,** Postoperative views after rhinoplasty and raising of the dorsal profile.

may be a component of the bilateral deformity because of asymmetry of the original bilateral cleft (complete on one side, incomplete on the other) or failure to achieve symmetry in staged repair of the two sides.

As in the unilateral cleft, the surgeon should first determine whether or not there are gross deficiencies of the lip and nose that mandate complete reconstruction of both the lip and nose. Absent nostril floors, lack of orbicular muscle continuity, absence of the labial sulcus beneath the prolabium, excessive width of the prolabium, and a significant shortness of the central portion of the lip require take down of the lip repair.

It is strongly recommended that Millard's technique[65,66] for bilateral synchronous lip repair be used. The central prolabium must almost always be narrowed, the lateral prolabial flaps should be rotated into the nostril floors, and the mucous membrane and muscle flaps should be dissected and joined beneath the central prolabial flap to provide muscle continuity and a full-depth upper labial sulcus. The alar bases, lateral prolabial flaps, and lateral lip elements must be approximated to reconstruct nostril floors. Even though vermilion of the lateral lip elements has commonly been discarded at the time of previous unsatisfactory primary repair, narrowing of the prolabium to its correct width may permit discard of the relatively unsatisfactory prolabial vermilion and reconstruction of the entire vermilion from that remaining in the lateral lip elements.

As in the unilateral cleft lip nasal deformity, satisfactory primary or previous lip repair may have been carried out, leading to secondary nasal deformity. Most commonly the deformity consists of inadequate columellar length with snubbing of the nasal tip. Flaring or eversion of the alar bases, bilateral alar-columellar webbing, an increased width of the nasal tip, and loss of nasal tip projection are also typical findings. The actual shortness of the columella may not be obvious to the patient or family, but is responsible for loss of tip projection and obliquity and webbing of the angle between the lip and columella. In these patients columellar lengthening by Cronin's technique[25] provides adequate columellar length and allows correction of alar flaring and eversion (Fig. 22-22). Needed undermining of nasal skin permits excision of fibrous tissue between the alar domes before approximation of the medial crura of the alar cartilages.

Less frequently in bilateral cleft lip nasal deformity the nostril floors are narrow and the alar bases are in excellent position, but the columella is short and the nasal tip is broad and snubbed. Instead of columellar lengthening by Cronin's technique,[25] which would significantly decrease the diameter and size of the nostril apertures and provide inadequate tissue for columellar lengthening, Brauer and Foerster's technique[11] leaves nostril floors and alar bases in position, but narrows and elevates the nasal tip and lengthens the columella with bilateral alar margin flaps (Fig. 22-23).

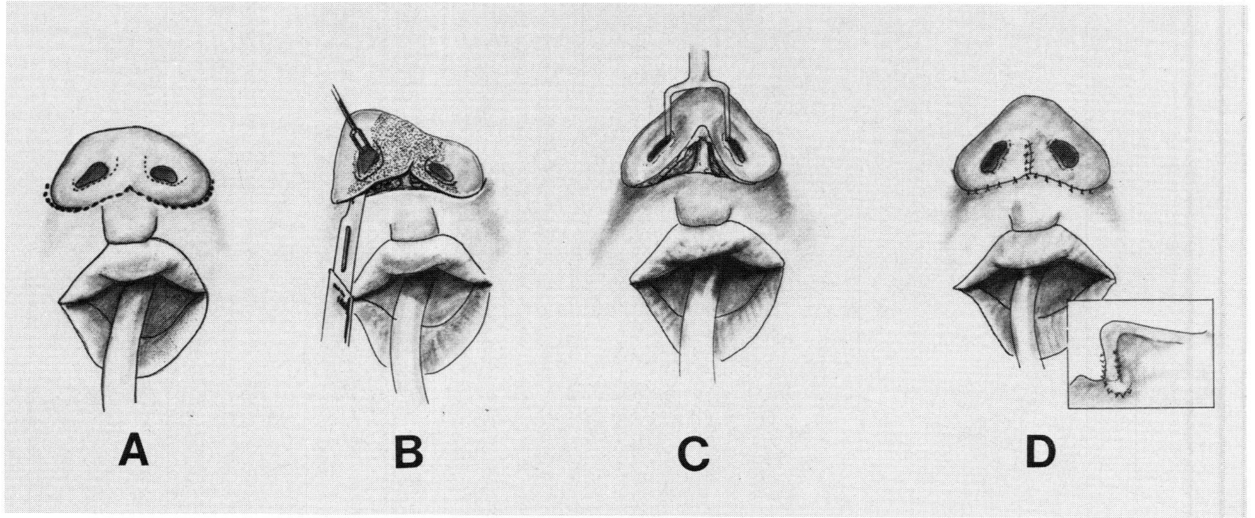

Fig. 22-22. Columellar lengthening by Cronin's technique.[25] **A** and **B,** Bipedicle flaps of columellar bases, nostril floors, and alar bases are outlined and elevated. Membranous septum incisions should reach to the past point of alar domes. Skin over the lower half of the nose should be elevated to allow unimpeded advancement of the tip. **C** and **D,** Skin hook elevation demonstrates V-Y advancement with conversion of width into height, and the vertical limb of the Y is lengthened. **E** to **H,** Appearance of the lip and nose after bilateral synchronous lip repair with "banking" of forked flaps and provision of a full-depth labial sulcus and muscle continuity. **I** to **L,** Significant change in the base of the nose after columellar lengthening at the time of palate repair. Note length of the columella in relation to the lobule and also change in the orientation of the nostrils.

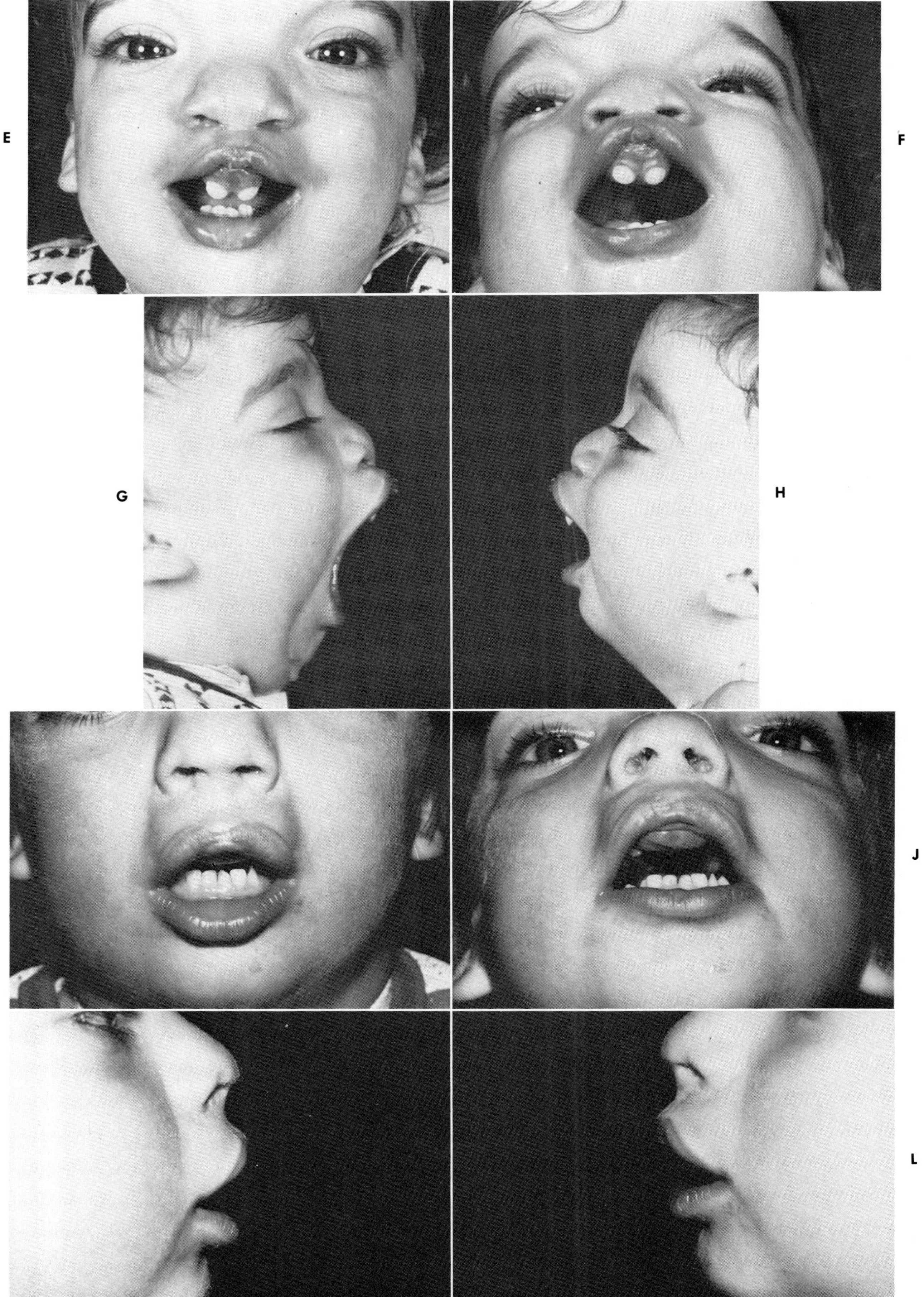

Fig. 22-22, cont'd. For legend see opposite page.

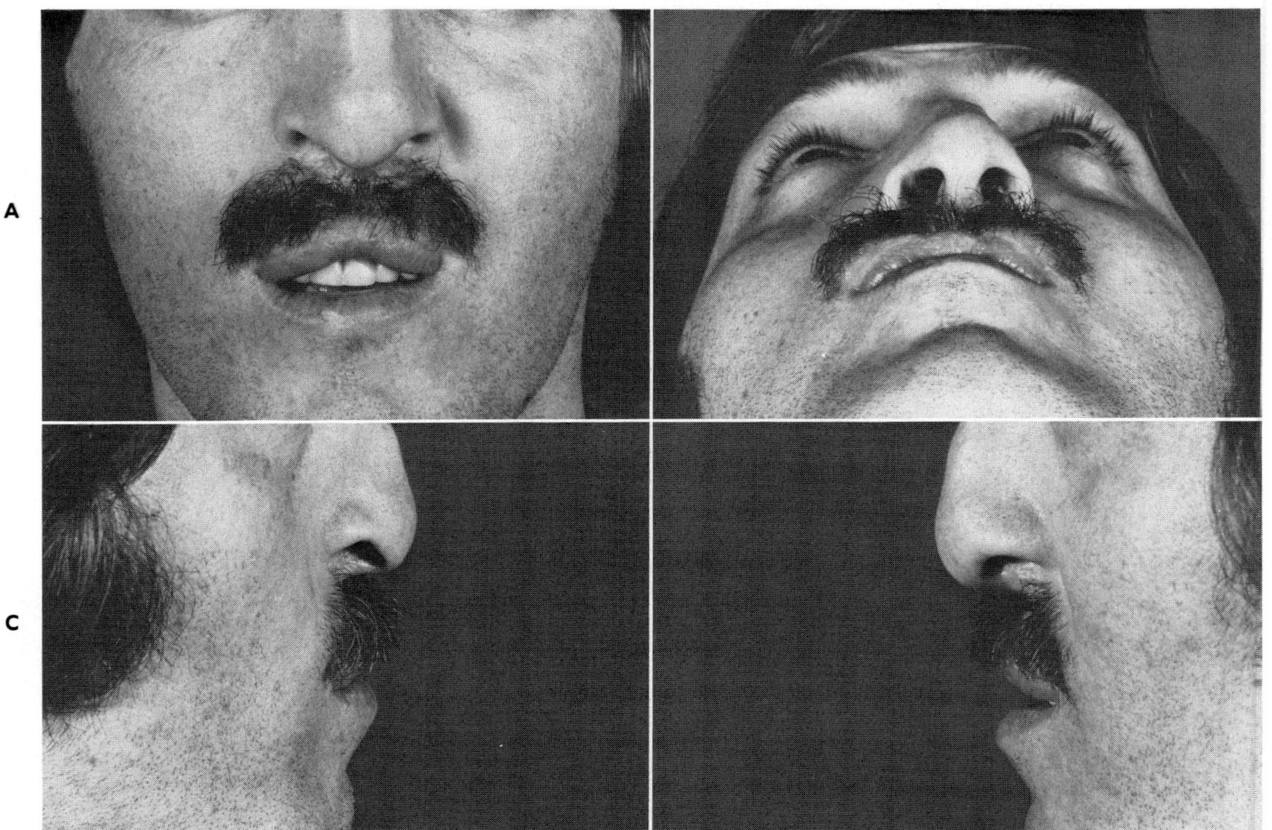

Fig. 22-23. Columellar lengthening at the other end. **A** to **D,** A short columella causing a snubbed tip and an apparent dorsal hump in the profile view. The alar bases are in good position. **E** to **G,** V-Y advancement of the nasal tip by the technique of Brauer and Foerster.[11] **H** to **K,** Columellar lengthening has allowed the tip to move up over the septal tip. Redundant skin of the columella in profile views should be secondarily revised.

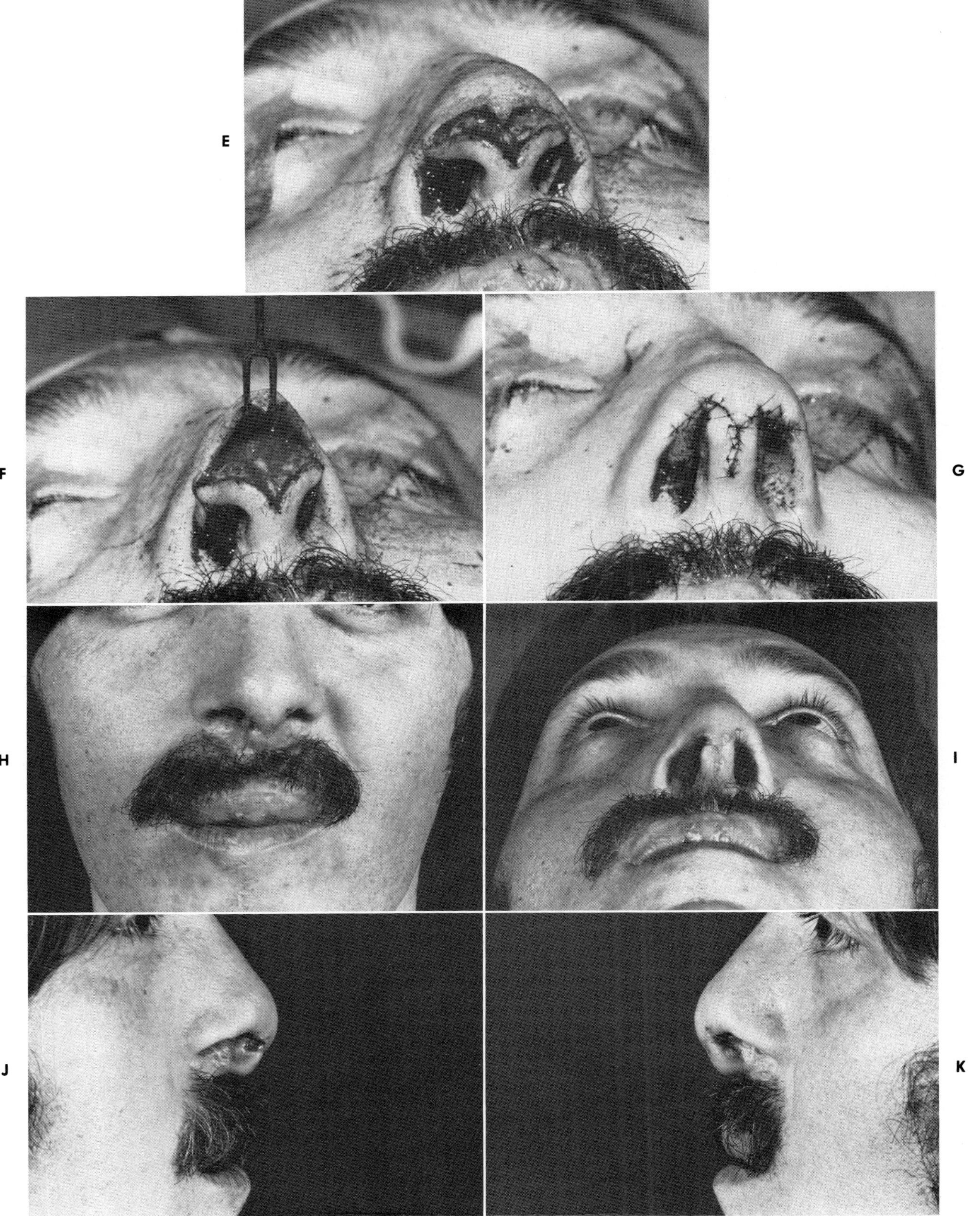

Fig. 22-23, cont'd. For legend see opposite page.

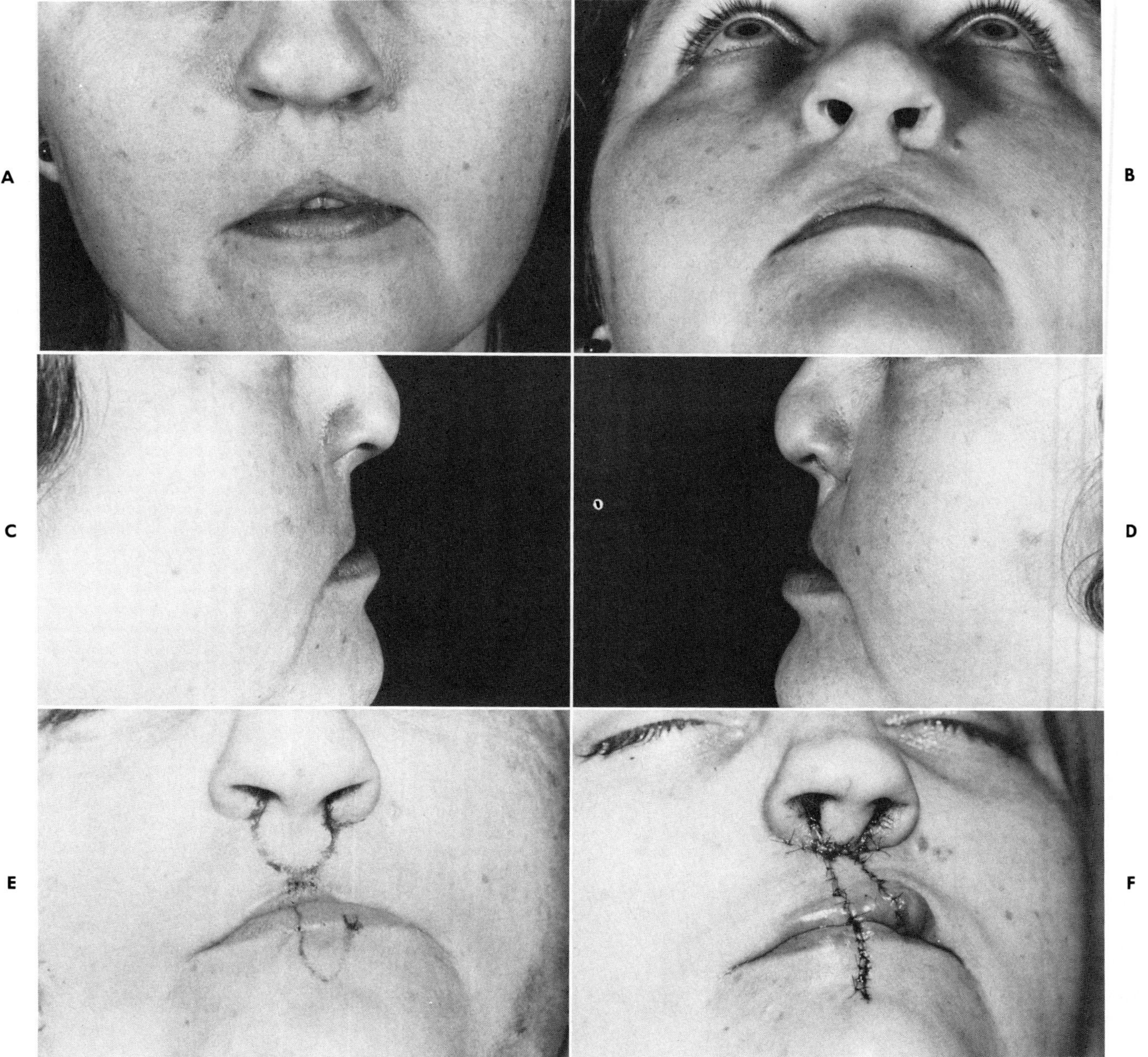

Fig. 22-24. Prolabial advancement into the columella with transfer of an Abbe flap. **A** to **D,** Preoperative views showing short, tight, and retruded lip with a short columella, but with narrow nostril floors and well-positioned alar bases. **E** to **F,** Design and transfer of a shield-shaped central Abbe flap with columellar elongation using the prolabium.

Fortunately a decreasing number of patients have a short columella, narrow nostril floors, and well-positioned alar bases but a tight, retruded, and long upper lip. By contrast, the lower lip protrudes with a relative excess of tissue. These patients should have advancement of the prolabium into the columella and immediate transfer of a central and shield-shaped Abbe flap (Fig. 22-24).

Mention must also be made of special and unusual de-fects, which are similar to those in the unilateral cleft lip nasal deformity. Some of the same reconstructive procedures mentioned previously must be used.

Septal surgery

Septoplasty, or septal resection, may be required to provide adequate nasal airways in patients with bilateral cleft lip as in patients with unilateral cleft lip.

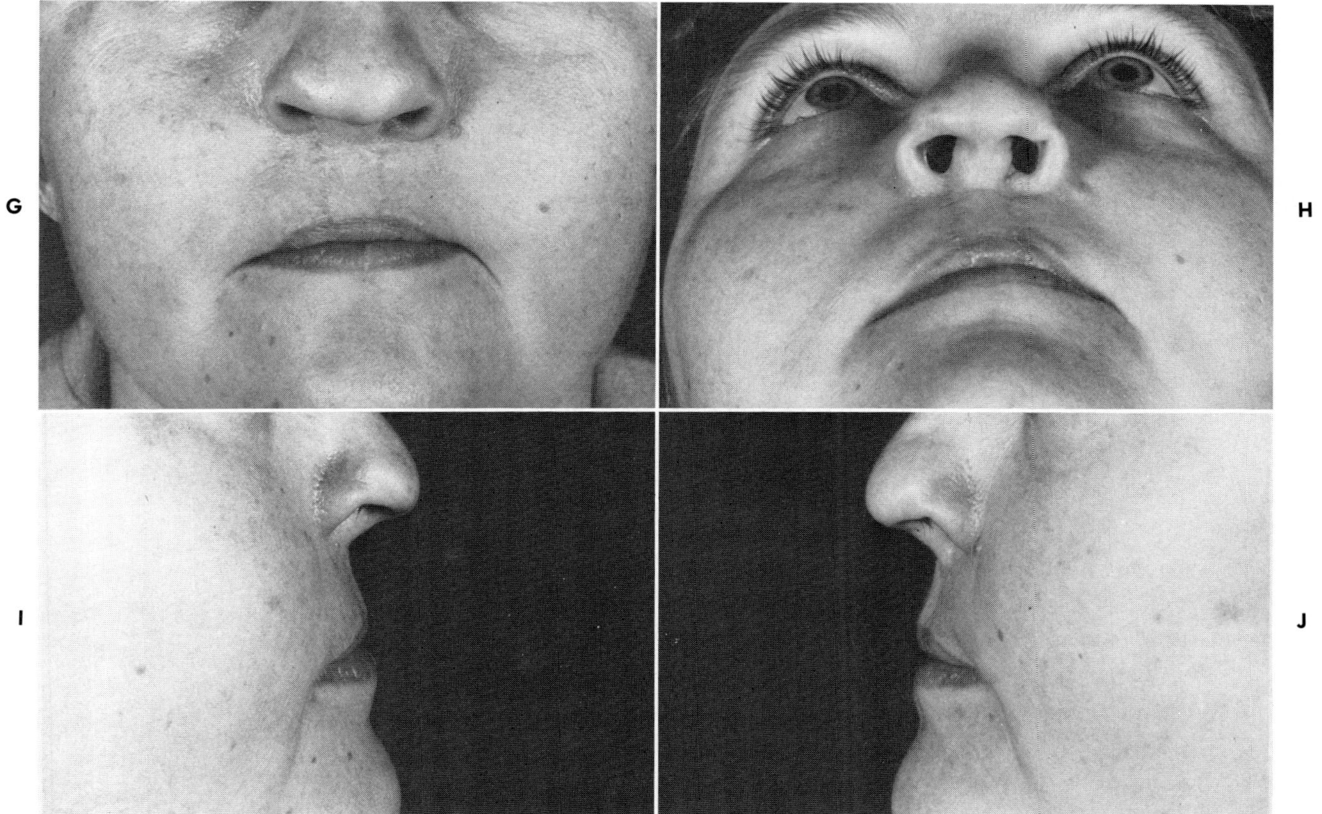

Fig. 22-24, cont'd. G to **J,** The lip is now full and of proper length, as is the columella. Note correction of the snubbed tip.

The upper nose

Classic rhinoplasty techniques may be required in adolescence to correct the upper nasal deformity and, as in the unilateral deformity, should be postponed if orthognathic surgery is planned or likely. The nose of the adolescent or adult with a bilateral cleft lip is frequently too broad and a true dorsal hump is often present, as distinguished from the middle or upper nasal dorsal convexity caused by snubbing of the nasal tip as a result of columellar shortness and lateral retraction of the alar bases.

SUMMARY AND CONCLUSIONS

Major secondary nasal deformity in patients with unilateral and bilateral cleft lip and palate may be avoided by correctly planned and well-executed primary repair of the lip cleft and associated nasal deformity.

Nasal reconstruction in patients with major defects of the lip should be carried out at the time of lip reconstruction or after lip reconstruction. Major deformities of the lower nose alone should be repaired, preferably in the preschool period and at the time other surgery is performed.

Relatively minor deformities can be corrected at the time of rhinoplasty, when this is performed in adolescence at the completion of surgical habilitation.

REFERENCES

1. Aduss, H., and Pruzansky, S.: The nasal cavity in complete unilateral cleft lip and palate, Arch. Otolaryngol. **85:**53, 1967.
2. Ariyan, S., and Krizek, T.J.: A simplified technique for correction of the cleft lip nasal deformity, Ann. Plast. Surg. **1:**568, 1978.
3. Atherton, J.D.: A descriptive anatomy of the face in human fetuses with unilateral cleft lip and palate, Cleft Palate J. **4:**104, 1967.
4. Avery, J.K.: The nasal capsule in cleft palate, Anat. Anz. Suppl. **109:**722, 1962.
5. Berkeley, W.T.: The cleft-lip nose, Plast. Reconstr. Surg. **23:**567, 1969.
6. Berkeley, W.T.: Correction of secondary cleft-lip nasal deformities, Plast. Reconstr. Surg. **44:**234, 1969.
7. Black, P.W.: The cleft-lip nose deformity—a definitive repair, Presented at the annual meeting of the American Association of Plastic Surgeons, Colorado Springs, Colo., May 17, 1982.
8. Blair, V.P.: Nasal deformities associated with congenital cleft of the lip, J.A.M.A. **84:**185, 1925.
9. Blair, V.P., and Brown, J.B.: Nasal abnormalities, fancied and real; the reaction of the patient: their attempted correction, Surg. Gynecol. Obstet. **53:**797, 1931.
10. Blair, V.P., and Letterman, G.S.: The role of the switched lower lip flap in upper lip restorations, Plast. Reconstr. Surg. **5:**1, 1950.
11. Brauer, R.O., and Foerster, D.W.: Another method to lengthen the

columella in the double cleft patient, Plast. Reconstr. Surg. **38:**27, 1966.

12. Broadbent, T.R., and Woolf, R.M.: Correction of cleft lip nasal deformity. In Georgiade, N.G., and Hagerty, R.F., editors; Symposium on management of cleft lip and palate and associated deformities, St. Louis, 1974, The C.V. Mosby Co.
13. Brown, J.B., and McDowell, F.: Secondary repair of cleft lips and their nasal deformities, Ann. Surg. **114:**101, 1941.
14. Brown, J.B., and McDowell, F.: Plastic surgery of the nose, St. Louis, 1951, The C.V. Mosby Co.
15. Brown, R.F.: A reappraisal of the cleft-lip nose with the report of a case, Br. J. Plast. Surg. **17:**168, 1964.
16. Carter, W.W.: The correction of nasal deformities by mechanical replacement and the transplantation of bone (with lantern demonstration), N.Y. State J. Med. **14:**517, 1914.
17. Chait, L.A.: The "C" costal cartilage graft in reconstruction of the unilateral cleft lip nose, Br. J. Plast. Surg. **34:**169, 1981.
18. Converse, J.M.: Corrective surgery of the nasal tip, Laryngoscope **67:**16, 1957.
19. Converse, J.M., Hogan, V.M., and Dupuis, C.-C.: Combined nose-lip repair in bilateral complete cleft-lip deformities, Plast. Reconstr. Surg. **45:**109, 1970.
20. Converse, J.M., Hogan, V.M., and Barton, F.E.: Secondary deformities of cleft lip, cleft lip and nose, and cleft palate. In Converse, J.M., editor: Reconstructive plastic surgery, Philadelphia, 1977, W.B. Saunders Co.
21. Converse, J.M., Horowitz, S.L., Guy, C.L., and Wood-Smith, D.: Surgical-orthodontic correction in the bilateral cleft lip, Cleft Palate J. **1:**153, 1964.
22. Cosman, B., and Crikelair, G.F.: Reconstruction of the unilateral cleft lip nasal deformity, Cleft Palate J. **2:**95, 1965.
23. Coupe, T.B., and Subtelny, J.D.: Cleft palate—deficiency or displacement of tissue, Plast. Reconstr. Surg. **26:**600, 1960.
24. Crikelair, G.F., Ju, D.M.C., and Symonds, F.C.: A method for ala plasty in cleft lip nasal deformities, Plast. Reconstr. Surg. **24:**588, 1959.
25. Cronin, T.D.: Lengthening columella by use of skin from nasal floor and alae, Plast. Reconstr. Surg. **21:**417, 1958.
26. DeKleine, E.H.: Nasal tip reconstructions through external incisions, Plast. Reconstr. Surg. **15:**502, 1955.
27. Dibbell, D.G.: A cartilaginous columellar strut in cleft lip rhinoplasties, Br. J. Plast. Surg. **29:**247, 1976.
28. Dibbell, D.G.: Cleft lip nasal reconstruction: correcting the classic unilateral defect, Plast. Reconstr. Surg. **69:**264, 1982.
29. Ecker, H.A.: A direct approach to the more severely deformed cleft lip nose, Plast. Reconstr. Surg. **67:**369, 1981.
30. Edgerton, M.T.: Surgical lengthening of the external nose to correct congenital or traumatic arrest of nasal growth (an operation of value in treating nasal deformities of cleft lip and palate), Plast. Reconstr. Surg. **38:**320, 1966.
31. Edgerton, M.T., and Marsh, J.L.: Uses of the nasolabial flap in the correction of cleft lip nasal deformities, Plast. Reconstr. Surg. **60:**56, 1977.
32. Elsah, N.I.: A new method for correction of cleft lip nasal deformities, Cleft Palate J. **11:**214, 1974.
33. Erich, J.B.: A technic for correcting a flat nostril in cases of repaired harelip, Plast. Reconstr. Surg. **12:**320, 1953.
34. Erich, J.B., and Kragh, L.V.: Technique for lengthening the columella in cases of repaired bilateral harelip, Minn. Med. **42:**1592, 1959.
35. Falces, E., and Gorney, M.: Use of ear cartilage grafts for nasal tip reconstruction, Plast. Reconstr. Surg. **50:**147, 1972.
36. Farrior, R.T.: The problem of the unilateral cleft-lip nose: a composite operation for revision of the secondary deformity, Laryngoscope **72:**289, 1962.
37. Gelbke, H.: The nostril problem in unilateral harelips and its surgical management, Plast. Reconstr. Surg. **18:**65, 1956.
38. Gillies, H., and Kilner, T.P.: Hare-lip: operations for the correction of secondary deformities, Lancet **2:**1369, 1932.
39. Gorney, M., and Rosenberg, H.L.: Centripetal rotation-advancement for cleft lip nasal dformities, Ann. Plast. Surg. **2:**374, 1979.
40. Huffman, W.C., and Lierle, D.M.: Studies on the pathologic anatomy of the unilateral hare-lip nose, Plast. Reconstr. Surg. **4:**225, 1949.
41. Hugo, N.E., and Tumbusch, W.T.: Repair of the unilateral cleft lip nasal deformities, Cleft Palate J. **8:**257, 1971.
42. Isshiki, N., Sawade, M., and Tamura, N.: Correction of alar deformity in cleft lip by marginal incision, Ann. Plast. Surg. **5:**58, 1980.
43. Johnston, M.D., Hassell, J.R., and Brown, K.S.: The embryology of cleft lip and cleft palate, Clin. Plast. Surg. **2:**195, 1975.
44. Kernahan, D.A., Bauer, B.S., and Harris, G.D.: Experience with the Tajima procedure in primary and secondary repair in unilateral cleft lip nasal deformity, Plast. Reconstr. Surg. **66:**46, 1980.
45. Lamont, E.S.: Reparative plastic surgery of secondary cleft lip and nasal deformities, Surg. Gynecol. Obstet. **80:**422, 1945.
46. Lamont, E.S.: Plastic surgery in reconstructing the primary cleft lip and nasal deformity, Am. J. Surg. **86:**200, 1953.
47. Latham, R.A.: Developmental deficiencies of the vertical and anteroposterior dimensions in the unilateral cleft lip and palate deformity. In Georgiade, N.G., and Hagerty, R.F., editors: Symposium on management of cleft lip and palate and associated deformities, St. Louis, 1974, The C.V. Mosby Co.
48. Latham, R.A., and Workman, C.: Anatomy of the philtrum and columella: the soft tissue deformity in bilateral cleft lip and palate. In Georgiade, N.G., and Hagerty, R.F., editors: Symposium on management of cleft lip and palate and associated deformities, St. Louis, 1974, The C.V. Mosby Co.
49. Lejour, M., and DeMey, A.: Primary lengthening of the columella in bilateral clefts of the lip, Cleft Palate J. **19:**113, 1982.
50. Longacre, J.J., Halak, D.B., Munick, L.H., et al.: A new approach to the correction of the nasal deformity following cleft lip repair, Plast. Reconstr. Surg. **38:**555, 1966.
51. Lowenthal, G.: Secondary surgical treatment of intranasal deformities of the unilateral cleft palate nose, Laryngoscope **91:**1641, 1981.
52. Maisels, D.O.: The alar base composite graft in cleft lip noses, Br. J. Plast. Surg. **31:**220, 1978.
53. Malek, R.: Nasal deformities and their treatment in secondary repair of cleft lip patients, Scand. J. Plast. Reconstr. Surg. **8:**136, 1974.
54. Marcks, K.M., Trevaskis, A.E., Berg, E.M., and Puchner, G.: Nasal defects associated with cleft lip deformity, Plast. Reconstr. Surg. **34:**176, 1964.
55. Marcks, K.M., Trevaskis, A.E., and Payne, M.J.: Elongation of columella by flap transfer and z-plasty, Plast. Reconstr. Surg. **20:**466, 1957.
56. McComb, H.: Primary repair of the bilateral cleft lip nose, Br. J. Plast. Surg. **28:**262, 1975.
57. McComb, H.: Treatment of the unilateral cleft lip nose, Plast. Reconstr. Surg. **55:**596, 1975.
58. McComb, H.: Personal communication, 1982.
59. McIndoe, A.H.: Correction of alar deformity in cleft lip, Lancet **1:**607, 1938.
60. McIndoe, A.H., and Rees, T.D.: Synchronous repair of secondary deformities in cleft lip and nose, Plast. Reconstr. Surg. **24:**150, 1969.
61. Meade, R.J.: Composite ear grafts for construction of columella, Plast. Reconstr. Surg. **23:**134, 1959.
62. Millard, D.R.: A primary camouflage of the unilateral harelook. In Transactions of the First Congress of the International Society of Plastic Surgeons, Baltimore, 1957, Williams & Wilkins.
63. Millard, D.R.: Columella lengthening by a forked flap, Plast. Reconstr. Surg. **22:**454, 1958.
64. Millard, D.R.: The unilateral cleft lip nose, Plast. Reconstr. Surg. **34:**169, 1964.
65. Millard, D.R.: Lengthening the columella. In Georgiade, N.G., and Hagerty, R.F., editors: Symposium on management of cleft lip and palate and associated deformities, St. Louis, 1974, The C.V. Mosby Co.
66. Millard, D.R.: Cleft craft: the evolution of its surgery, Boston, 1976, Little, Brown & Co.
67. Millard, D.R.: Earlier correction of the unilateral cleft lip nose, Plast. Reconstr. Surg. **70:**64, 1982.
68. Millicovsky, G., Ambrose, L.J.H., and Johnston, M.C.: Developmental alterations associated with spontaneous cleft lip and palate in CL/Fr mice, J. Anat. **164:**29, 1982.

69. Morel-Fatio, G., and Lalardrie, J.P.: External nasal approach in the correction of major morphologic sequelae of the cleft lip nose, Plast. Reconstr. Surg. **38**:116, 1966.
70. Musgrave, R.H.: Surgery of nasal deformities associated with cleft lip, Plast. Reconstr. Surg. **28**:261, 1961.
71. Musgrave, R.H., and Bremner, J.C.: Complications of cleft palate surgery, Plast. Reconstr. Surg. **26**:180, 1960.
72. Musgrave, R.H., and Dupertuis, S.M.: Revision of the unilateral cleft lip nostril, Plast. Reconstr. Surg. **25**:223, 1960.
73. Natvig, P., Sether, L.A., Gingrass, R.P., and Gardner, W.D.: Anatomical details of the osseous-cartilaginous framework of the nose, Plast. Reconstr. Surg. **48**:528, 1971.
74. Neuner, O.: Corrective plastic surgery of the cleft nose, J. Maxillofac. Surg. **1**:50, 1975.
75. Nishimura, Y., and Ogino, Y.: The use of two v-flaps for secondary correction of the cleft lip nose, Plast. Reconstr. Surg. **60**:390, 1977.
76. Nishimura, Y., and Ogino, Y.: Autogenous septal cartilage graft in the correction of cleft lip nasal deformity, Br. J. Plast. Surg. **31**:222, 1978.
77. O'Connor, G.B., McGregor, M.W., and Tolleth, H.: The nasal problem in cleft lips, Surg. Gynecol. Obstet. **116**:503, 1963.
78. Ogino, Y., and Ishida, H.: Secondary repair of the cleft-lip nose, Ann. Plast. Surg. **4**:469, 1980.
79. Onizuka, T.: Repair of columella base deformity in unilateral cleft lip, Br. J. Plast. Surg. **25**:33, 1972.
80. Padgett, E.C.: Repair of harelip and accompanying nasal deformity, J. Kans. Med. Soc. **30**:143, 1929.
81. Pap, G.: Simultaneous secondary repair of the nasolabial deformity complex in unilateral cleft lip, Br. J. Plast. Surg. **8**:320, 1956.
82. Pegram, M.: Repair of congenital short columella: a preliminary report, Plast. Reconstr. Surg. **14**:305, 1954.
83. Pelliciari, D.D.: Columella and nasal tip reconstruction using multiple composite free grafts, Plast. Reconstr. Surg. **4**:98, 1949.
84. Peyton, W.T., and Ritchie, H.P.: Quantitative studies on congenital clefts of the lip, Arch. Surg. **33**:1046, 1936.
85. Pfeifer, G.: Morphology of the formation of clefts as a basis for treatment. In Schuchardt, K., editor: Treatment of patients with clefts of lip and alveolus and palate, Stuttgart, 1966, Georg Thieme.
86. Pigott, R.W., and Millard, D.R.: Correction of the bilateral cleft lip nasal deformity. In Grabb, W.C., Rosenstein, S.W., and Bzoch, K.R., editors: Cleft lip and palate: surgical, dental, and speech aspects, Boston, 1971, Little, Brown & Co.
87. Potter, J.: Some nasal tip deformities due to alar cartilage abnormalities, Plast. Reconstr. Surg. **13**:358, 1954.
88. Potter, J.: The nasal tip in bilateral hare lip, Br. J. Plast. Surg. **21**:173, 1968.
89. Potter, J.: The nasal tip in bilateral and unilateral harelip, Ann. Plast. Surg. **6**:85, 1981.
90. Prado, F.A., and DiGeronimo, E.M.: Correction of the deformed alae secondary to cleft lip, Plast. Reconstr. Surg. **69**:541, 1982.
91. Pruzansky, S.: The growth of the premaxillary-vomerine complex in complete bilateral cleft lip and palate, Tandlaegebladet (Kobenhavn) **75**:1157, 1971.
92. Ross, R B., and Johnston, M.C.: Normal embryonic development of the face. In Cleft lip and palate, Baltimore, 1972, Williams & Wilkins.
93. Reynolds, J.R., and Horton, C.E.: An alar lift procedure in cleft lip rhinoplasty, Plast. Reconstr. Surg. **35**:377, 1965.
94. Sawhney, C.P.: Nasal deformity in unilateral cleft lip, Cleft Palate J. **13**:291, 1976.
95. Schendel, S.A., and Delaire, J.: Functional musculoskeletal correction of secondary unilateral cleft lip deformities: combined lip-nose correction and LeFort I osteotomy, J. Maxillofac. Surg. **9**:108, 1981.
96. Schwenzer, N.: Correction of noses associated with clefts of lip and palate, J. Maxillofac. Surg. **1**:91, 1975.
97. Sheen, J.H., ad Sheen, A.P.: Aesthetic rhinoplasty, St. Louis, 1978, The C.V. Mosby Co.
98. Skoog, T.: Repair of unilateral cleft lip deformity: maxilla, nose, and lip, Scand. J. Plast. Reconstr. Surg. **3**:109, 1969.
99. Spina, V.: Repair of unilateral cleft lip-nose, Cleft Palate J. **5**:356, 1968.
100. Spira, M., Hardy, S.B., and Gerow, F.J.: Correction of nasal deformities accompanying unilateral cleft lip, Cleft Palate J. **7**:112, 1970.
101. Stark, R.B., and Kaplan, J.M.: Development of the cleft lip nose, Plast. Reconstr. Surg. **51**:413, 1973.
102. Steffensen, W.H.: A method for repair of the unilateral cleft lip, Plast. Reconstr. Surg. **4**:144, 1949.
103. Stenström, S.J.: The alar cartilage and the nasal deformity in unilateral cleft lip, Plast. Reconstr. Surg. **38**:223, 1966.
104. Stenström, S.J., and Öberg, T.R.H.: The nasal deformity in unilateral cleft lip, Plast. Reconstr. Surg. **28**:295, 1961.
105. Straith, C.L.: Reconstructions about the nasal tip, Surg. Gynecol. Obstet. **62**:73, 1936.
106. Straith, C.L.: Elongation of the nasal columella, Plast. Reconstr. Surg. **1**:79, 1946.
107. Straith, C.L., Straith, R.E., and Lawson, J.M.: Reconstruction of the harelip nose, Plast. Reconstr. Surg. **20**:455, 1957.
108. Tajima, S., and Maruyama, M.: Reverse-U incision for secondary repair of cleft lip nose, Plast. Reconstr. Surg. **60**:256, 1977.
109. Tange, I., and Ohmori, S.: Qualitative analysis of the configuration of the unilateral cleft lip, Proceedings of the Third International Congress of Plastic Surgery, Amsterdam, 1964, Excerpta Medica Foundation.
110. Uchida, J.: A new approach to the correction of cleft-lip nasal deformities, Plast. Reconstr. Surg. **47**:454, 1971.
111. Velazquez, J.M., and Ortiz-Monasterio, F.: Primary simultaneous correction of the lip and nose in the unilateral cleft lip. Plast. Reconstr. Surg. **54**:558, 1974.
112. Von Deilen, A.W.: Some aspects in the secondary repair of cleft lip, palate and nasal deformities (with case report), Plast. Reconstr. Surg. **10**:460, 1952.
113. Whitlow, D.R., and Constable, J.D.: Crossed alar wing procedure for correction of late deformity in the unilateral cleft lip nose, Plast. Reconstr. Surg. **52**:38, 1973.
114. Wilkie, T.F.: The "alar shift" revisited, Br. J. Plast. Surg. **22**:70, 1969.
115. Wilson, L.F.: Personal communication, 1981.
116. Wray, R.C.: Secondary correction of nasal abnormalities associated with cleft lip, J. Oral Surg. **34**:113, 1976.
117. Wynn, S.K.: Primary nostril reconstruction in complete cleft lips, Plast. Reconstr. Surg. **49**:56, 1972.
118. Wynn, S.K.: Correction of secondary cleft lip and nasal deformities. In Georgiade, N.G., and Hagerty, R.F., editors: Symposium on management of cleft lip and palate and associated deformities, St. Louis, 1974, The C.V. Mosby Co.

CHAPTER 23

Secondary reconstructive procedures for patients with clefts

SAMUEL STAL and MELVIN SPIRA

"Trifles make perfection, and perfection is no trifle."
MICHELANGELO, 1475-1564

A wide variety of deformities can occur after repair of the cleft lip.[33] Fortunately, the Tennison[60] repair introduced in 1952 and the Millard[37] repair, which followed a short time later, along with other procedures,[6] have provided us with improved techniques that generally allow the growth and development of a relatively normal-looking lip. Adequate length, appropriate muscle closure, a cupid's bow with a well-defined vermilion ridge, a natural-appearing philtrum, and symmetry of the nose, particularly of the nostrils, are hallmarks of excellence in cleft lip surgery. Residual deformities that involve all segments of the lip are still seen; repair of these must be considered during the growth years.

Before any revisionary surgery, preoperative evaluation should include an assessment of the patient's general health status, previous surgical procedures, evaluation of the occlusion, appropriate photographs, and radiographs. The only rule regarding timing of treatment of any of these deformities is that surgical correction is considered in the year before the child's entering school when peer associations and pressures begin to concern both the child and parents. Commonly the deformities are multiple and not amenable to correction in a single operative procedure; the surgical goals of both the patient and family must be considered when evolving a treatment plan. In general, the severe secondary lip deformity is corrected first, both in unilateral cleft lip and bilateral cleft, in which it is combined with columella advancement. The correction of occlusal deformities is usually undertaken later, with treatment invariably requiring orthodontics and, in severe malocclusions, surgery. Nasal deformity correction is most often done after adolescence, except when severe and accompanied by gross airway ob-

struction, in which case surgery may be done as early as the age of 7 or 8 years.[4]

NORMAL LIP ANATOMY

We must define the esthetics of the normal lip to evaluate the appearance of a repaired cleft lip. Only with a careful anatomic analysis of the deformity can we hope to achieve a natural-looking structure.

A pleasing nose has symmetric alar arches supported by a straight columella and septum. The entire nasal complex is balanced on equally symmetric nasal floors and nostril sills. The normal length of the upper lip, with the mandible in a rest position, is such that 2 mm of the mucosal edge of the maxillary incisor teeth will be exposed. The lip, with its intact orbicular muscle, has a central philtral dimple in a hollow between prominent projecting columns (in an adult this is 0.8 to 1.2 cm). A well-formed, curved cupid's bow with its midline pouting tubercle is set off by a projecting white roll at the vermilion mucocutaneous junction. The natural relationship of the lips is that of the upper lip over and slightly in front of the lower (Fig. 23-1).

UNILATERAL CLEFT LIP

It is difficult to separate the nose from the lip in evaluating the unilateral cleft lip. Therefore a minor lip deformity is usually corrected at the time of rhinoplasty and is not considered a separate surgical procedure.

Cupid's bow and vermilion deformities

The most common deformity seen relates to a deficiency in the cupid's bow. This may be associated with a mismatch of the vermilion margin and an attenuated or absent vermilion ridge. Not infrequently, a notching deformity of the vermilion of the lip may be an associated condition (Fig. 23-2).

When the cupid's bow portion of the vermilion is totally absent, reconstruction should be considered with a small modified Abbe flap (Fig. 23-10). In addition to providing both a vermilion and vermilion ridge sufficient to reshape the bow on the cleft side, this flap will also give a "pout" to the lip, mimicking the normal tubercle.

When a vertical deficiency exists lateral to the cleft, actual excision of skin to match the height and shape of the cupid's bow on the normal side can be carried out with the advancement of subjacent vermilion, as in a vermilionectomy (Fig. 23-3).[49]

In select cases where the lip is short but of sufficient width, the lower third of the lip repair can be taken down and redone to correct a wide cupid's bow by excising the spread scar and extraneous vermilion and then reapproximating the lateral and medial lip elements (Fig. 23-18).

Small notching defects in the lower border of the lip vermilion can be corrected when an adequate cupid's bow is present by simple Z-plasty (Fig. 23-4). Care should be taken not to rotate "wet" vermilion from inside the lip to "dry" vermilion on the external surface.

Construction of the white roll of the vermilion ridge still

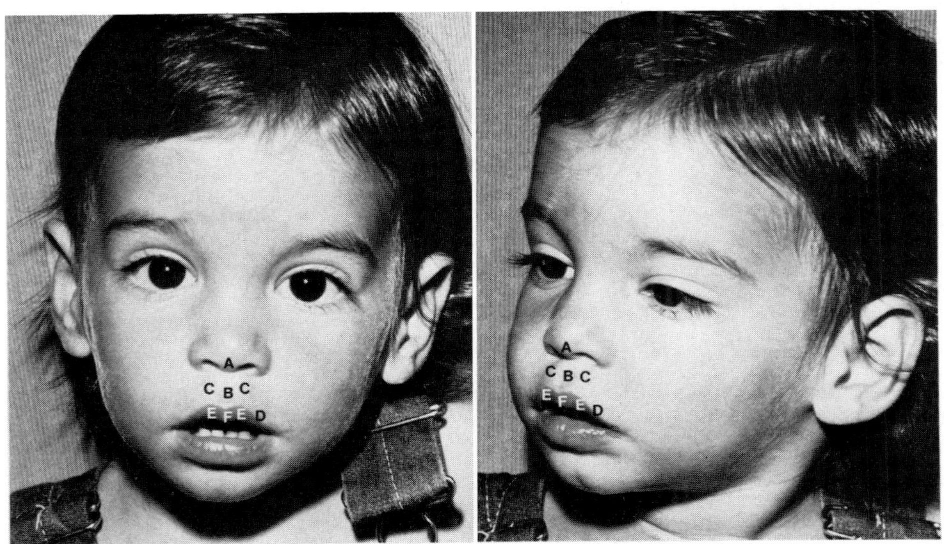

Fig. 23-1. Normal anatomy of the lip. *A*, Columella; *B*, dimple of philtrum; *C*, column of philtrum; *D*, vermilion ridge, or white roll; *E*, cupid's bow; *F*, tubercle.

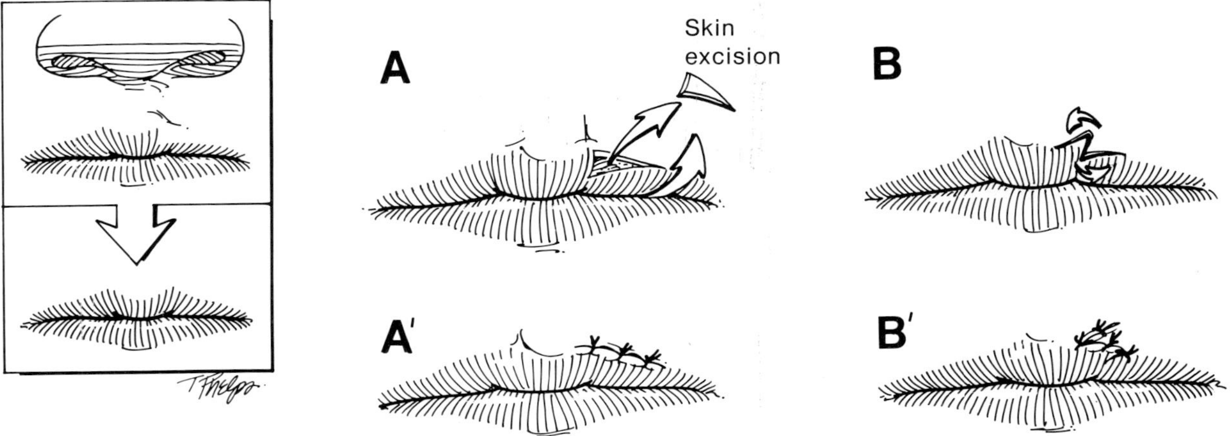

Fig. 23-2. Minimal malalignment of the vermilion ridge. **A,** Excision of skin and advancement of mucosa. Slight overcorrection is advisable. **B,** Repositioning segments with Z-plasty.

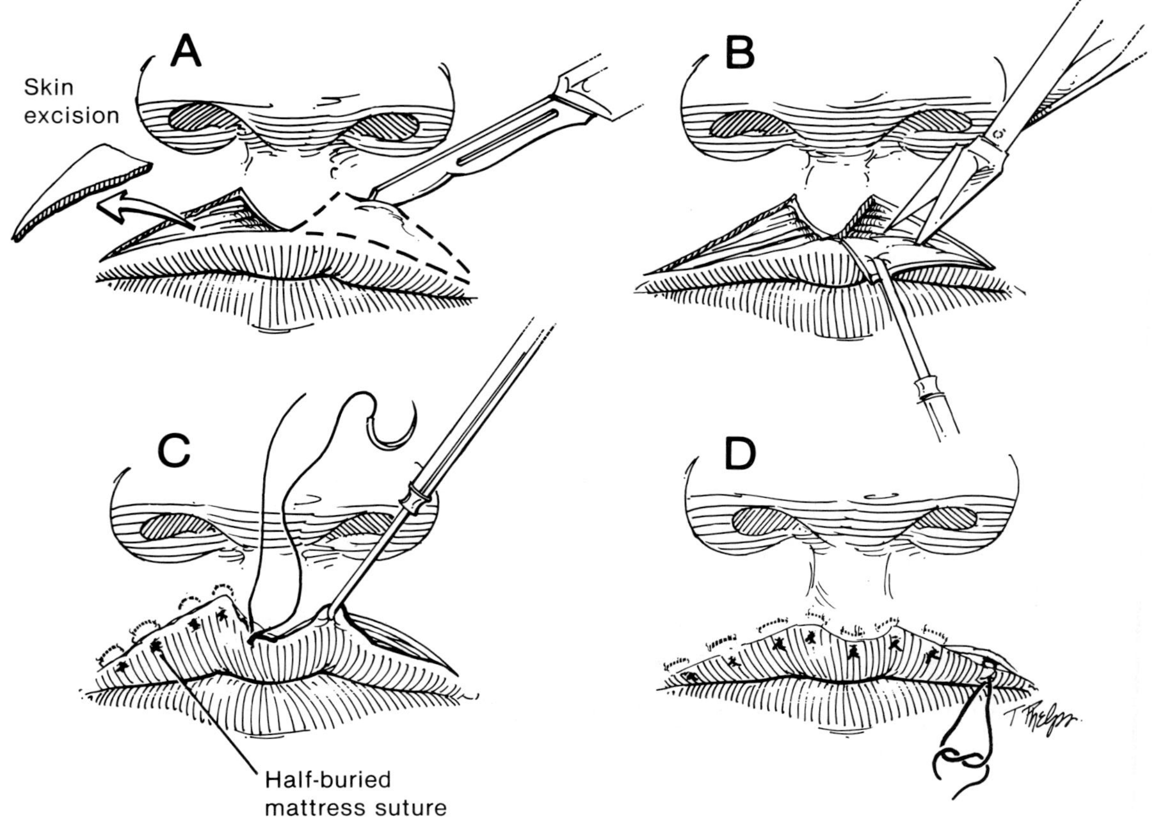

Fig. 23-3. Creation of a cupid's bow. **A,** Excision of skin simulating arches of a cupid's bow. **B,** Mucosal undermining. **C,** Mucosal cephalic advancement. **D,** Closure with half-buried horizontal mattress sutures.

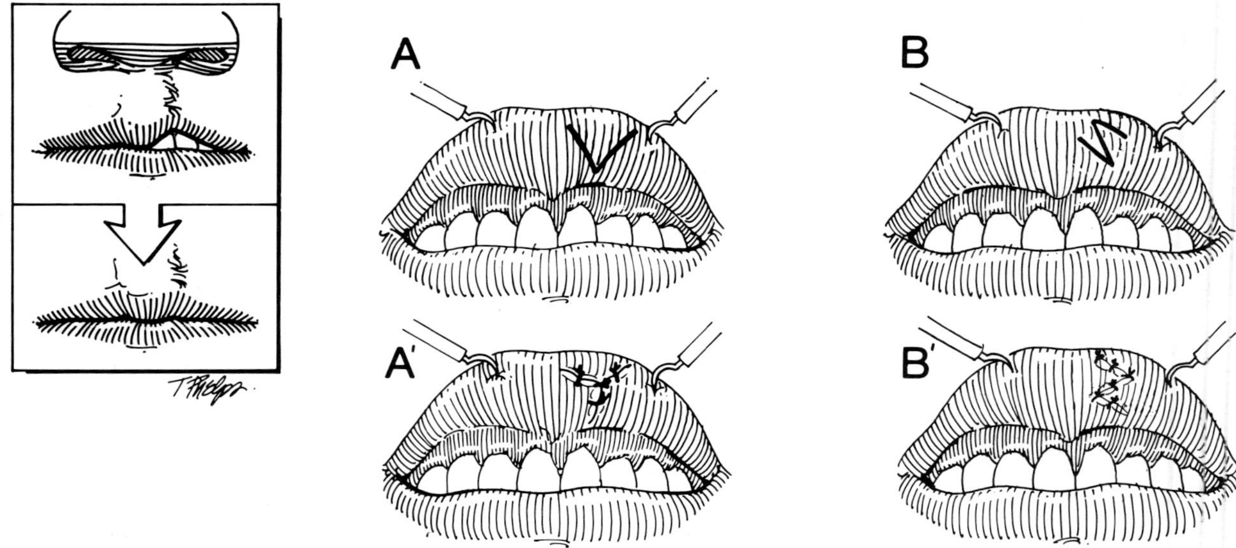

Fig. 23-4. Correction of lower vermilion notching. **A,** Minor deformity corrected by V-Y advancement of the mucosa from within with sufficient undermining. **B,** Deformity also can be corrected with Z-plasty using the lateral mucosa.

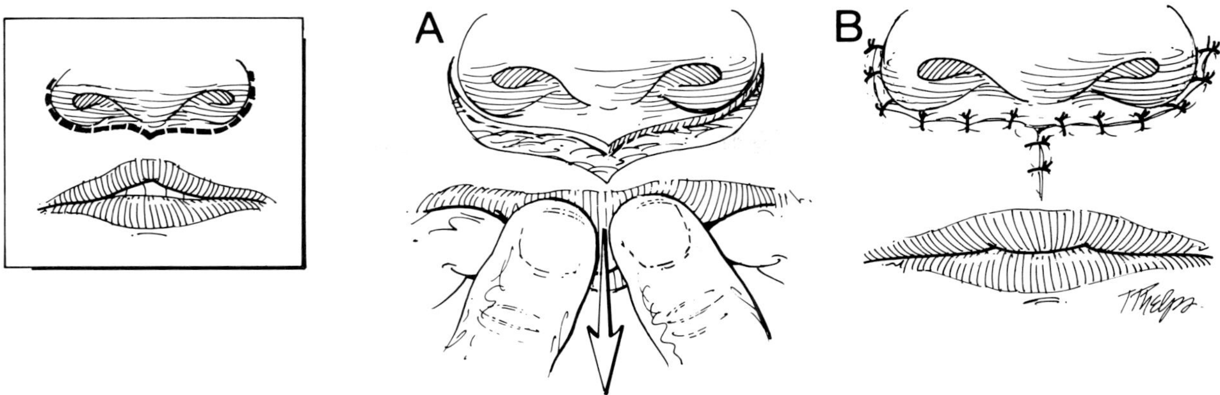

Fig. 23-5. Lengthening the short upper lip. **A,** Outline of perialar incisions. **B,** V-Y advancement medially and caudally to achieve lengthening of the lip.

remains a surgical enigma. Implantation of small strips of free dermal grafts of this tissue from the lower lip and dermabrasion have been employed in an effort to create elevation and slight color change. Artificial collagen (Zyderm) has been suggested as a possible alternate treatment in the hope that it might provide projection at the vermilion ridge site sufficient to highlight the area and provide the illusion of elevation and a white roll.

When the entire upper lip vermilion is thin, correction can be in the form of a transverse mucosal muscular flap from the lower lip[23] if there is sufficient donor tissue or a dermal fat graft can be placed in a prepared submucosal tunnel to provide bulk for the upper lip, both in the vertical and transverse dimensions. A modest degree of overcorrection is required at the time of implantation.

Short lip

The problem of a short lip on the cleft side after unilateral cleft lip repair usually can be handled with a through-and-through Z-plasty; this will be especially effective if a Millard repair was done or if the Millard repair can be redone to secure additional downward rotation and advancement. If a Tennison repair or some modification thereof was performed, the repair can be taken down and additional length provided by increasing the width of the base of the triangular flap. All techniques designed to provide additional length to the lip are predicated on the lip's being of sufficient width and flexibility to provide the additional tissue necessary to secure the desired length (Fig. 23-5). Occasionally, lip shortness may be secondary to scarring and labial mucosa deficiencies; correction in the form of V-Y advancements and internal Z-plasties is usually not adequate. In the case of severe mucosal shortness, either a free graft or a lateral buccal flap to provide additional tissue in the sulcus may be required; this would be an unusual situation in unilateral clefts. Here, too, the Abbe flap may be useful when the

shortness is in both the lateral and vertical dimensions and a composite of tissue is needed.

Long lip

A common finding after Tennison repair of the incomplete cleft lip is the excessively long lip. At the time of the original repair, this is usually provided for by the resection of a triangular composite of skin, subcutaneous tissue, and underlying muscle at the base of the nose. When the lip is long, secondary correction is truly difficult and, as a general rule, overcorrection is required to secure a satisfactory result.[63] With associated vermilion deformity, opening the entire lip from the base of the nose through the vermilion, excising an adequate tissue composite at the base of the nose along the nostril floor, extending the incision around the base of the ala, and then repairing the defect as in an original lip repair can usually provide great improvement. Care must be taken to anchor the lateral lip to the periosteum of the piriform aperture (Fig. 23-6). Occasionally, because of the difficulties associated with correction of the excessively long lip after unilateral cleft lip repair, consideration has been given to the employment of a fascial sling between the lip and piriform aperture to support the lip and maintain the shortening achieved at surgery. Simple resection of tissue can cause deformity, a pulling down of the base of the ala on the cleft side, and, although the distance between the vermilion and nose may measure the same as on the normal side, the lower border of the cleft side will appear long. There is a tendency for these lips to lengthen after what appears to be an adequate initial surgical correction.

BILATERAL CLEFT LIP

The number and severity of the deformities associated with bilateral cleft lip repair are greater than those seen after unilateral cleft lip repair. Patients frequently have multiple deformities that lend themselves to simultaneous correction.

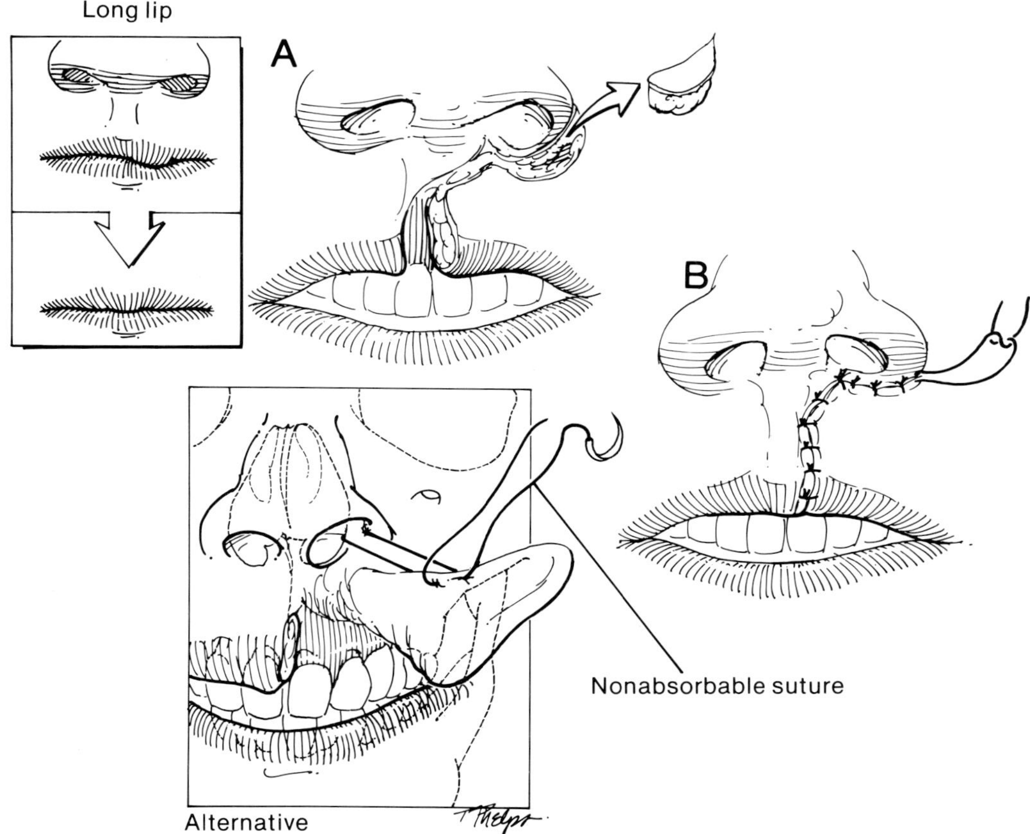

Fig. 23-6. Repair of the unilateral long lip. **A,** Revision of lip repair with excision of perialar composite. **B,** The lip is closed in three layers with an anchor to the piriform aperture with a nonabsorbable suture or fascia.

In an effort to simplify the problem, we will describe the defects observed after bilateral cleft lip repair and the various techniques employed for their correction.

Vermilion deficiencies

The most common deformity seen in the vermilion of a bilateral cleft lip is the "whistle deformity," or central notching defect. A variety of techniques have been proposed for its correction,[36,56] including the double V-Y advancement described by Robinson, Ketchum, and Masters[54] (Fig. 23-7). Hogan and Converse[25] described a larger V-Y advancement in which the entire labial sulcus is released and the labial mucosa and vermilion advanced medially and inferiorly to give an internal vertical scar. Previous operative procedures and resultant scarring often limit the amount of correction achieved with this procedure (Fig. 23-8).

Kapetansky[31] has successfully employed triangular vermilion muscle (Fig. 23-9), which is mobilized with the underlying orbicular muscle and advanced medially to provide tissue where it is absent in the central portion of the lip. This procedure has been modified by Juri, Juri, and De Antueno[30] (Fig. 23-9) to accentuate a central tubercle by rotating inferiorly the medial side and base of the vermilion mucosal muscular flaps.

A free composite graft from the central lower lip, originally described by Flanagin,[19] has been employed where a deficiency of 1 cm or less exists. The take of these small composite flaps is at best tenuous; in our opinion they are useful only where minimal deficiency exists and where there is inadequate vermilion on either side of the deformity to provide sufficient tissue for its correction.

The vermilion cross-lip flap, a variation of the Abbe full-composite lip switch, also has been used successfully for the correction of this problem.[27] Initially described by Gillies[22] and Millard[23] and subsequently by Kawamoto,[32] it is best employed where the lateral elements in the vermilion are thin and tissue available for medial advancement is inadequate (Fig. 23-10). The tongue flap will be discussed elsewhere.

Finally, when the whistle deformity is relative and secondary to the excessive amount of vermilion laterally, not to central vermilion deficiency, simple transverse wedge excisions can be considered.

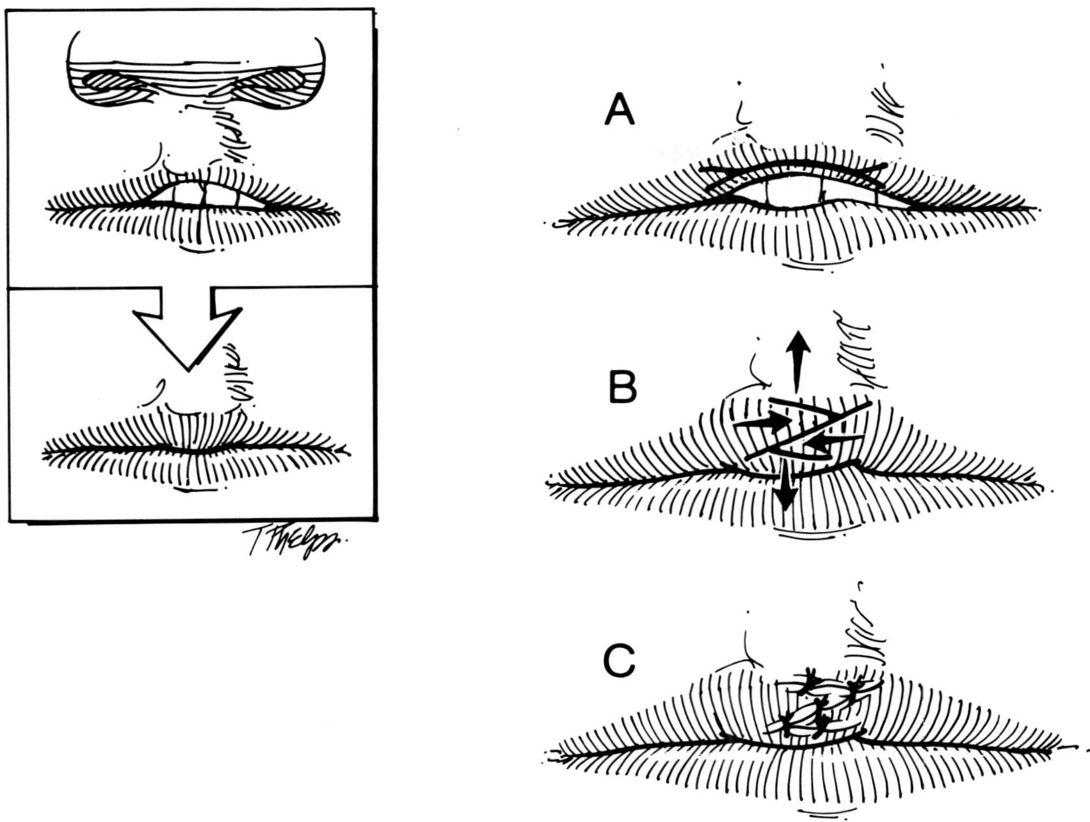

Fig. 23-7. Notching of the lower vermilion border. **A,** Outline of the flaps after the lip is everted. **B,** and **C,** Correction of the deformity with medial advancement of the flaps. (Modified from Robinson, D.W., Ketchum, L.D., and Masters, F.W.: Plast. Reconstr. Surg. **46:**241, 1970.)

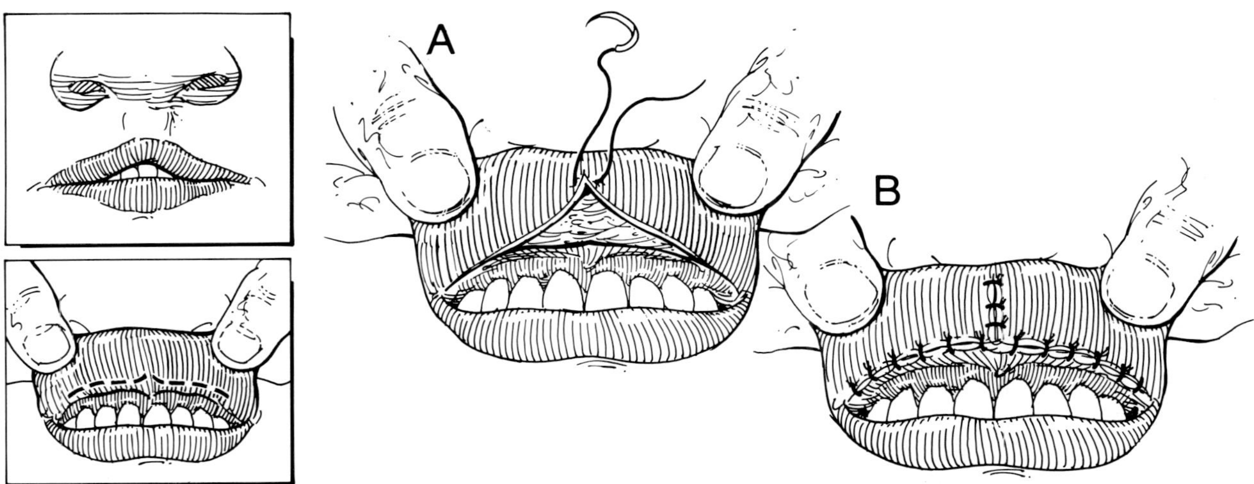

Fig. 23-8. Correction of a whistle deformity. *Top inset,* Midline whistle deformity. *Bottom inset,* With the lip everted, an incision is made, preserving an adequate mucosal cuff for closure. **A,** V-Y advancement cephalically. **B,** After closure. (From Converse, J.M. Hagan, V.M., and Barton, F.E.: Secondary deformities of cleft lip, cleft lip and nose, and cleft palate. In Converse, J.M.: Reconstructive plastic surgery, vol. 4, Philadelphia, 1977, W.B. Saunders Co.)

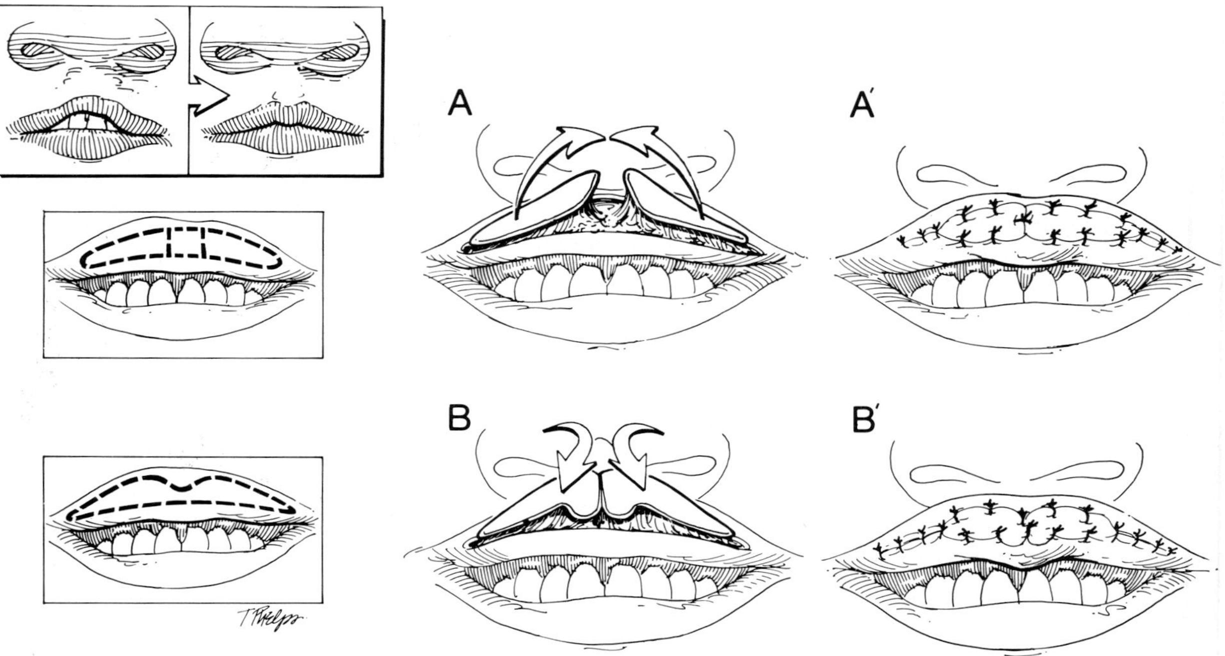

Fig. 23-9. Pendulum flaps for whistling deformities in bilateral cleft lips. **A,** Deficiency of central vermilion after primary repair of a bilateral cleft lip. Creation of lateral island flaps (pyramids, with vermilion at the bases) with intact subcutaneous pedicles. **A′,** Flaps are rotated medially together as a pendulum to meet in the prolabium. **B,** Modification of the pendulum technique[30] using thicker lateral flaps with greater skeletalization of the flaps. **B′,** Flaps turned in caudally at the central lip line to better reconstruct the center tubercle. (Modified from Kapetansky, D.I.: Plast. Reconstr. Surg. **47:**321, 1971.)

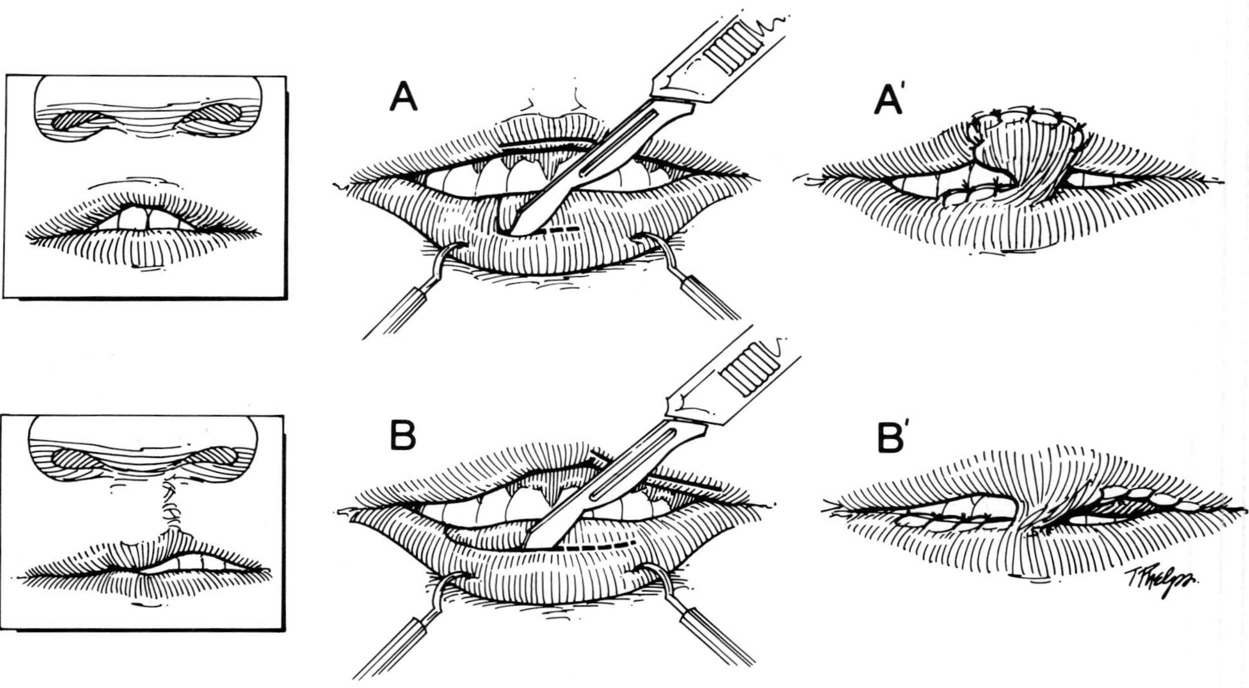

Fig. 23-10. Cross-lip vermilion flaps for correction of defects of the vermilion. **A,** Central defect corrected using a mucosal flap from the inner surface of the lower lip. **A′,** Tissue is left attached for 7 to 10 days; the donor site is closed primarily. **B,** For lateral defects a flap from the contralateral side of the lower lip, which is wedge shaped, is raised and rotated 150 degrees and inset into the atrophic upper lip through a horizontal incision. **B′,** Flap inset and defect primarily closed. (**A** modified from Gillies, H., and Millard, D.R.: The principles and art of plastic surgery, Vol. 1, Boston, 1957, Little, Brown & Co.; **B** modified from Kawamoto, H.K.: Plast. Reconstr. Surg. **6:**35, 1979.)

Absent or deformed cupid's bow

Construction of a cupid's bow represents a true challenge to the plastic surgeon. A variety of techniques have been proposed. Simple skin excision in the shape of a cupid's bow with forward advancement of the mucosa, as in a vermilionectomy, and as described for the unilateral cleft lip, sacrifices the vermilion ridge; it is not a popular procedure (Fig. 23-3).

The method described by Vecchione[62] appears to provide a well-proportioned cupid's bow and a vermilion ridge. This technique seems particularly useful in lighter skinned individuals. It requires that a full-thickness skin graft be placed immediately above the newly created depression between the height of bows, which is a potential problem in darker skinned patients. The technique is particularly noteworthy for its ability to recreate a central philtral dimple (Fig. 23-11).

Absent philtrum

The absence of a philtrum is one of the signs of bilateral cleft lip repair. A variety of techniques have been proposed for construction of a philtrum.

O'Connor and McGregor[43,44] have used a method in which the prolabial skin and subcutaneous tissue are elevated as an inferiorly based flap. Three parallel incisions, extending from the base of the nose to the vermilion, are made in the underlying tissue. Two tubes of subcutaneous tissue and underlying muscle are thus created, sutured together, and

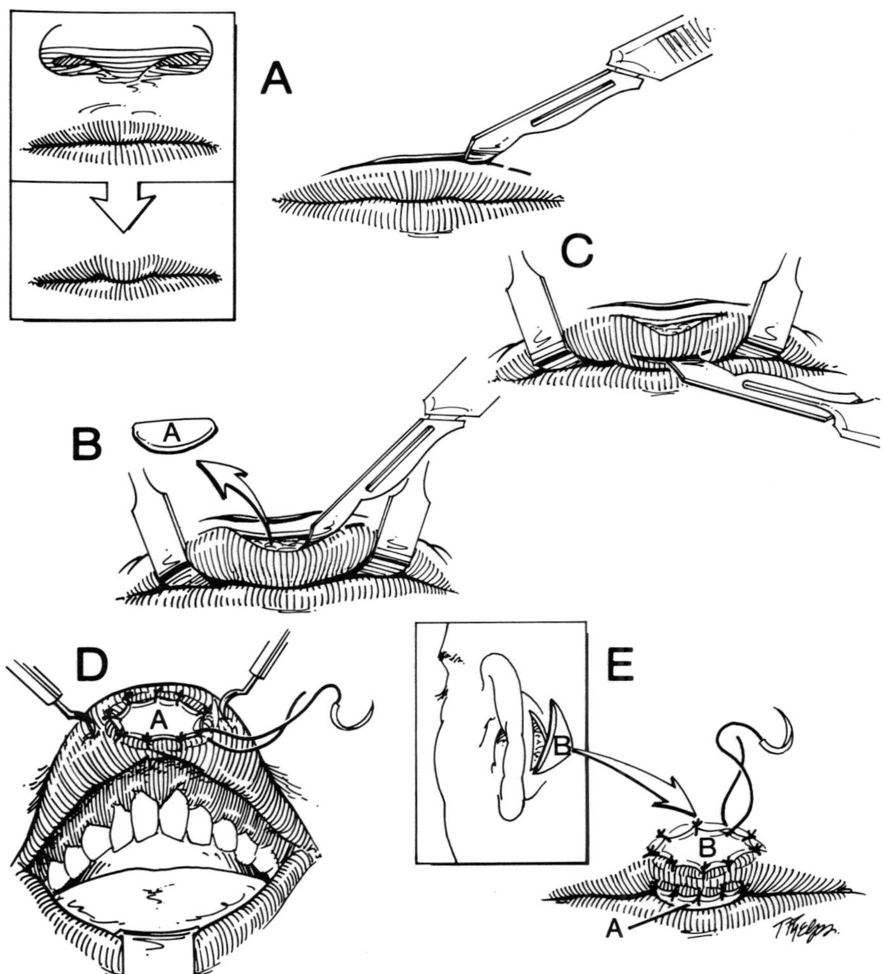

Fig. 23-11. Construction of a cupid's bow. *Inset,* After primary repair the lip often lacks a central concave white roll, philtral dimple, priminent tubercle, and peaked philtral ridges. **A,** Resection of the central vermilion and incision for the cupid's peak, preserving the vermilion white roll. **B,** The white roll is retracted inferiorly as a bucket handle below the new philtral dimple created through resection of muscle and scar. **C,** An incision is made for the new tubercle. **D,** The resected central vermilion is sutured as a composite to develop a new tubercle. **E,** A full-thickness graft is sutured to the depth of the philtral depression. (Modified from Vecchione, T.R.: Plast. Reconstr. Surg. **65:**830, 1980.)

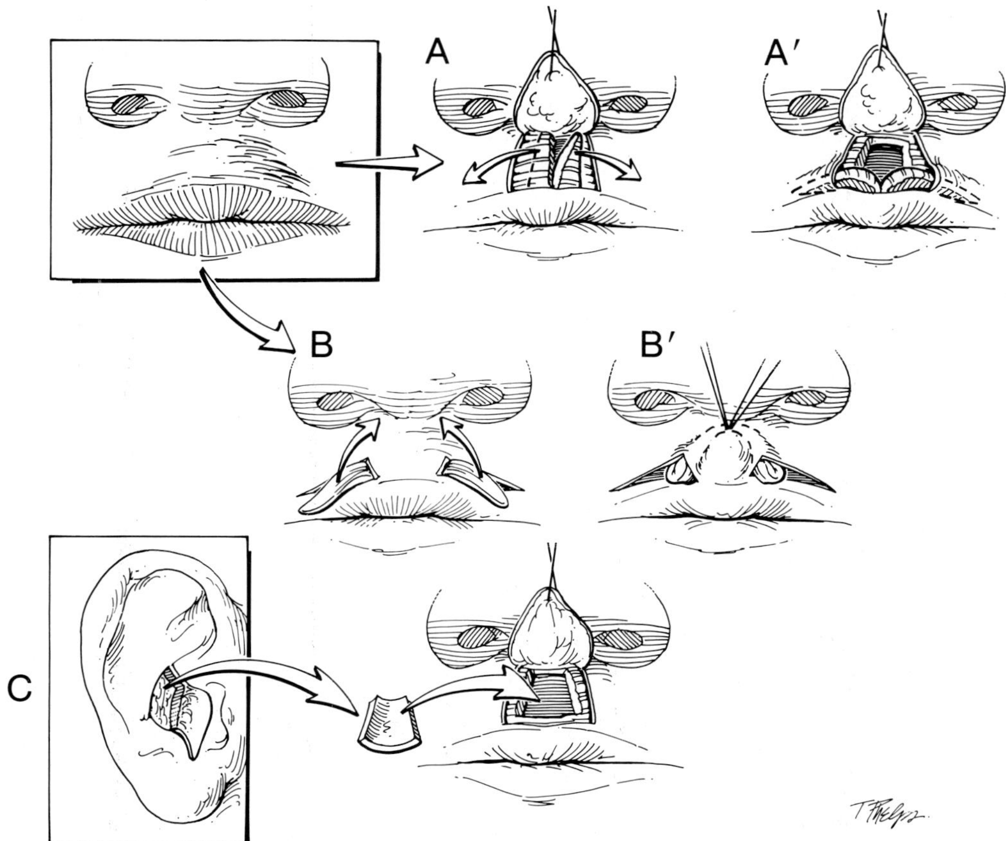

Fig. 23-12. Re-creation of the philtrum to give an illusion of a column and dimple. **A,** Elevation of prolabial skin and development of subcutaneous flaps based inferiorly. These flaps are rotated downward into position in the lateral vermilion border, **A',** The illusion of a philtral dimple is created by closing skin over the central concavity. **B,** Development of soft tissue flaps from the mucocutaneous junction. **B',** The flaps are rotated superiorly through prepared subcutaneous tunnels to simulate prominent philtral columns. **C,** An auricular cartilage graft is buried subcutaneously to give the illusion of a concave philtrum. (**A** modified from O'Connor, G.B., and McGregor, M.W.: Am. J. Surg. **95:**227, 1958; **B** modified from Millard, D.R., Jr.: Cleft craft: the evolution of its surgery, vol. 1, The unilateral deformity, Boston, 1980, Little, Brown & Co.; **C** modified from Neuner O.: Secondary correction of cleft lip and palate. In Sanvenero-Rosselli, G., and Boggio-Robutti, G., editors: Transactions of the Fourth International Congress of Plastic and Reconstructive Surgery, Amsterdam, 1967, Excerpta Medica Foundation.)

fitted laterally beneath the skin at the site of the proposed new vermilion ridges to give the required projection (Fig. 23-12).

When there is adequate length to the lip, both in the skin and vermilion, Millard's modification[40] may have real possibilities. This technique employs medially based de-epithelialized flaps that are taken from just above the vermilion ridge of the upper lip, turned medially and upward, and buried in a tunnel created where the planned philtrum columns are designed (Fig. 23-12).

Neuner[42] and Schmid[55] have described the use of a free composite tissue graft. In this technique skin and cartilage are taken from the ear and inserted into the central lip in an effort to create a natural-appearing philtrum (Fig. 23-12).

Onizuka[47,48] created a philtrum by rolling the underlying tissue laterally from the normal side to the site of the defect to deepen the trough between the philtral ridges and give projection to the philtral column on the cleft side. Although designed for the unilateral cleft, this technique can be modified to treat the bilateral deformity (Fig. 23-13).

The vermilion flap reconstruction described by Peterson, Ellenber, and Carroll[50] appears to be a modification of the Abbe procedure. This method will not only provide adequate tissue for the cupid's bow, but gives the illusion of a trough and a more natural-appearing philtrum.

Tight lip

A tight lip is not an uncommon deformity and represents a true deficiency of tissue that is correctable primarily by

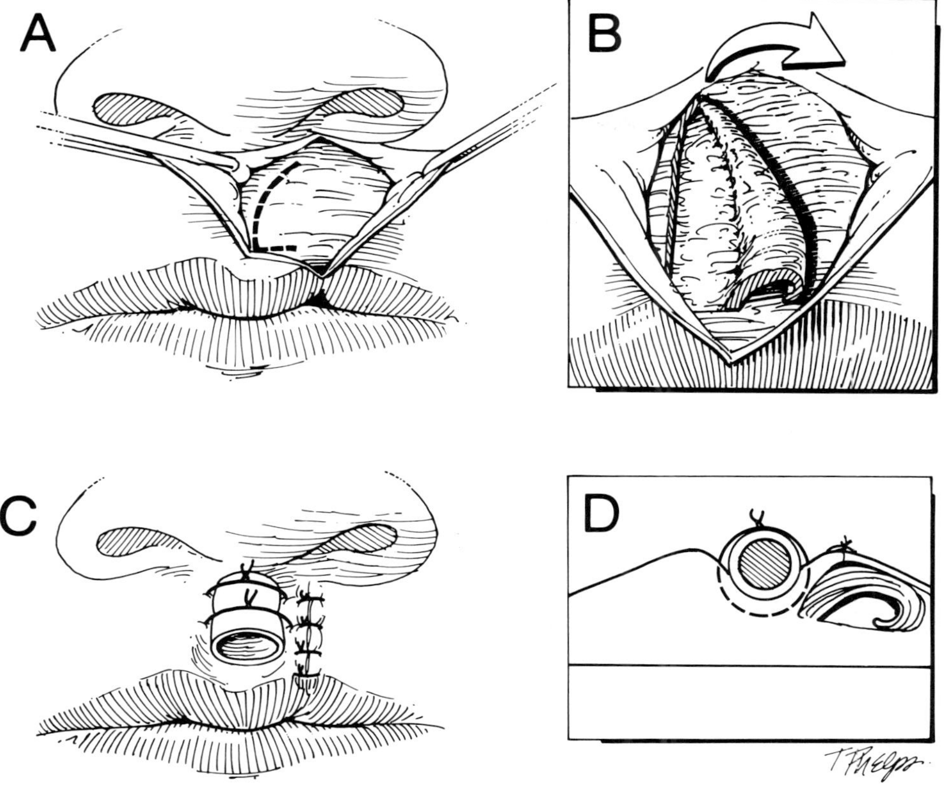

Fig. 23-13. Creation of a philtrum in the unilateral cleft lip. **A** and **B,** A layer of subcutaneous tissue and muscle from the normal side is rolled over the cleft side. **C** and **D,** The defect is splinted with the bolus, giving a philtral dimple column on the cleft side. (Modified from Onizuka, T.: Plast. Reconstr. Surg. **56:**522, 1975.)

use of the Abbe lip-switch flap.[34] This flap has been well described by others, including Garrett and Musgrave,[20] and has found a particular niche in the armamentarium of cleft lip surgeons for correction of the tight lip. A number of modifications have been described by Cannon,[10] Jackson,[29] Hogan and Converse,[25] and Converse et al.[11] In addition to simply providing skin and vermilion to the lip, the Abbe flap brings additional muscle, which Jackson[29] has shown to be effective in improving orbicular muscle function. It will reduce the thickness and projection of the lower lip to further camouflage any deficiencies in the upper lip (Fig. 23-14). The procedure is rarely carried out before school age and, as a rule, the child is older and more cooperative. A few general principles should be mentioned. The actual size of the deficiency must be carefully assessed. Determination of a V- or M-shaped donor flap depends on whether the entire vertical dimension of the lip is to be augmented (M-shaped flap) or whether the primary deficiency exists transversely in the vermilion ridge and lower lip skin area (V-shaped flap). Regardless of where the deficiency is believed to exist, central placement of the Abbe flap is important for symmetry and ideally should represent the philtral portion of the lip rather than the lateral elements. In an

effort to secure a philtral dimple, surgeons have used such techniques as suturing the subcutaneous tissue of the flap to the underlying maxillary periosteum with subsequent ear cartilage graft augmentations for philtral ridges. DePalma, Leavitt, and Hardy[14] have shown that in the absence of complications sensation and orbicular motor function will return within a 2-year period. The flap has an excellent inset and generally can be divided within 2 weeks. Minor touch-ups or scar revisions are generally required at a later date.

Long lip

The bilateral cleft lip repair employed by Barsky[2] and others has frequently resulted in an excessively long lip after growth. A radical revision, to include excision of the inferior lateral flaps located between the original prolabium and the vermilion, is required.[24]

Wide lip

When muscle is deficient in the original prolabium or there has been a failure to unite the muscle of the lateral lip on either side at the time of repair, a characteristic deformity may result in patients with bilateral cleft lips. Hypertrophy, bulging, or excessive fullness in the lateral upper

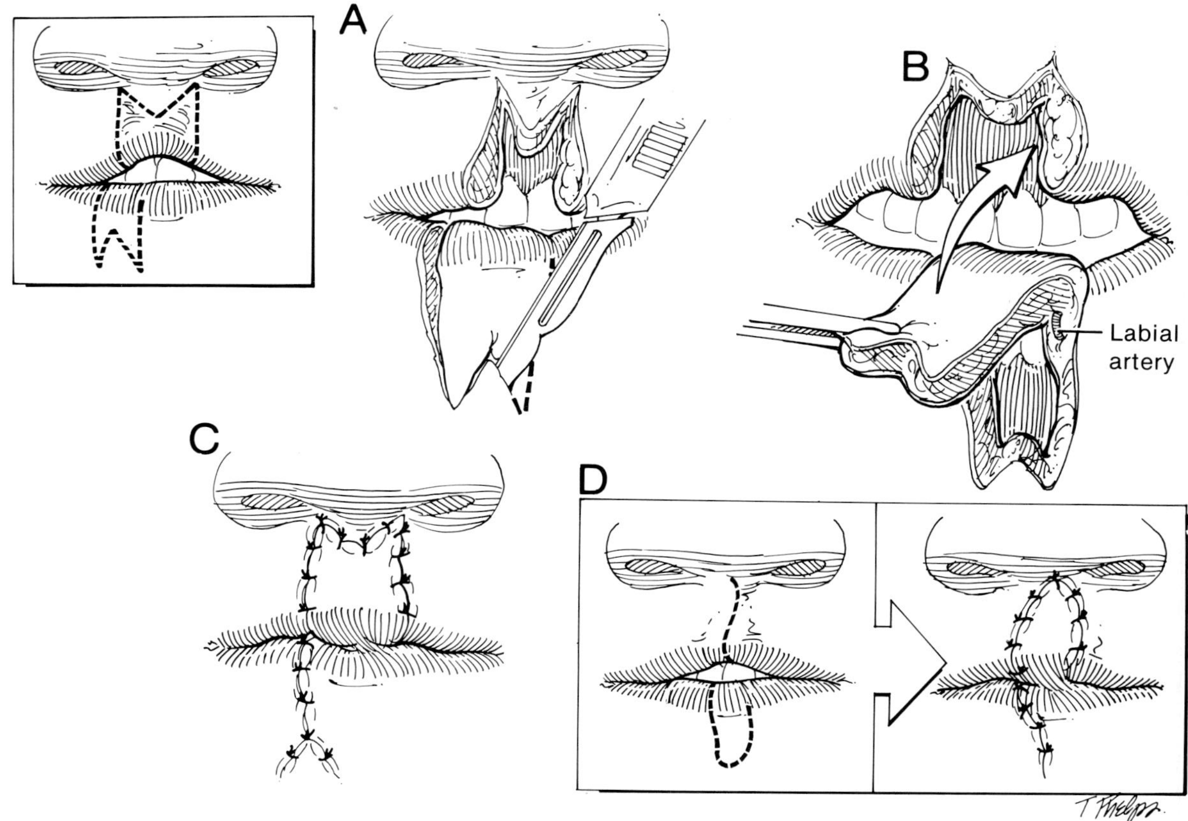

Fig. 23-14. Treatment of the tight lip with an Abbe flap. **A,** After excision of the redundant nonfunctional philtrum in the bilateral cleft lip, and M-shaped flap is devised from the lower lip. **B,** The flap is off center to facilitate rotation. **C,** The donor area is closed primarily and the flap is inset in. **D,** A V-shaped flap may be used in the unilateral cleft lip but must be placed in the midline.

lip may be minimally obtrusive in repose, but becomes more noticeable with smiling or whistling. Fara and Smahel[18] have provided a clear anatomic description of the deficiencies of muscle associated with the unilateral and bilateral cleft lip deformity. Randall, Whitaker, and LaRossa[53] provided an additional explanation of the anatomy of this area and made suggestions for restitution of the orbicular muscle and correction of secondary deformities. In general, when dealing with the unilateral or bilateral cleft lip, the muscle fibers, which are vertically oriented before repair, must be dissected free, brought down, transferred across the philtral area, and sutured together or plicated to restore horizontal continuity (Fig. 23-15).[46] Reduction of the wide prolabium in conjunction with correction of the bulging lateral lip is a procedure that can be combined with columella advancement in the bilateral cleft lip deformity.

Tight or scarred labial sulcus

Inadequacies in the vermilion secondary to tightness and scarring in the labial sulcus may be corrected by either one of two methods.

Falcone[17] described release of the central prolabium and deepening of the labial sulcus in a secondary repair of the bilateral cleft lip. This technique employs a superiorly based flap of alveolar mucosa that is dissected upward and inset at a higher level to deepen the sulcus, allowing the denuded alveolar bone to either epithelialize spontaneously or be grafted (Fig. 23-16).

Horton et al.[26] modified the V-Y advancement combined with a Z-plasty and employed buccal mucosa as a full-thickness graft to provide additional depth to the sulcus (Fig. 23-16).

The tight sulcus also can be released during bone grafting or maxillary osteotomies.

Scar deformities

Scars can widen and become discolored; men may develop the additional problem of absence of hair in the scar line. Revision of the scars by excision and primary closure can effect considerable improvement. The scar tissue should not be discarded because it frequently can be employed as a buried graft to give additional projection to the philtral ridge (Fig. 23-17). When verticle shortening of the scar causes elevation of the height of the cupid's bow on one

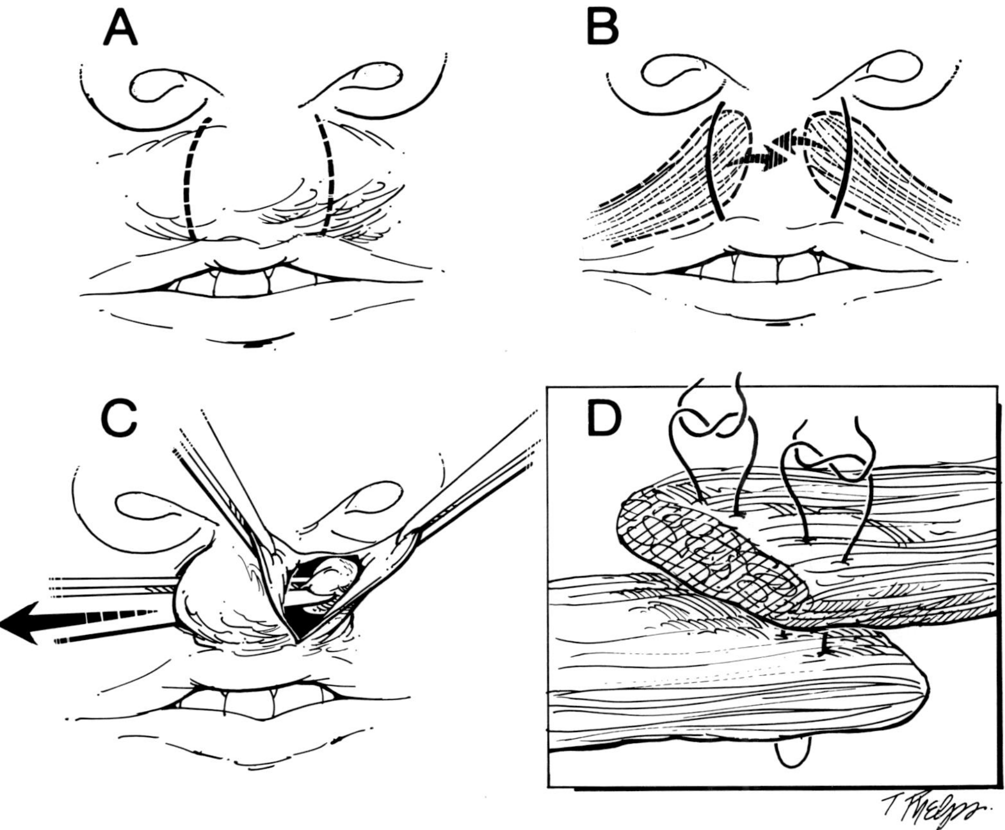

Fig. 23-15. Reorientation and approximation of muscle fibers. **A,** Characteristic muscle bulge when the patient smiles. **B,** An abnormal attachment of muscle fibers must be dissected. **C** and **D,** Through lip incisions the muscle is freed and plicated. (Modified from Puckett, C.L., Reinisch, J.F., and Werner, R.S.: Cleft Palate J. **17:**34, 1980.)

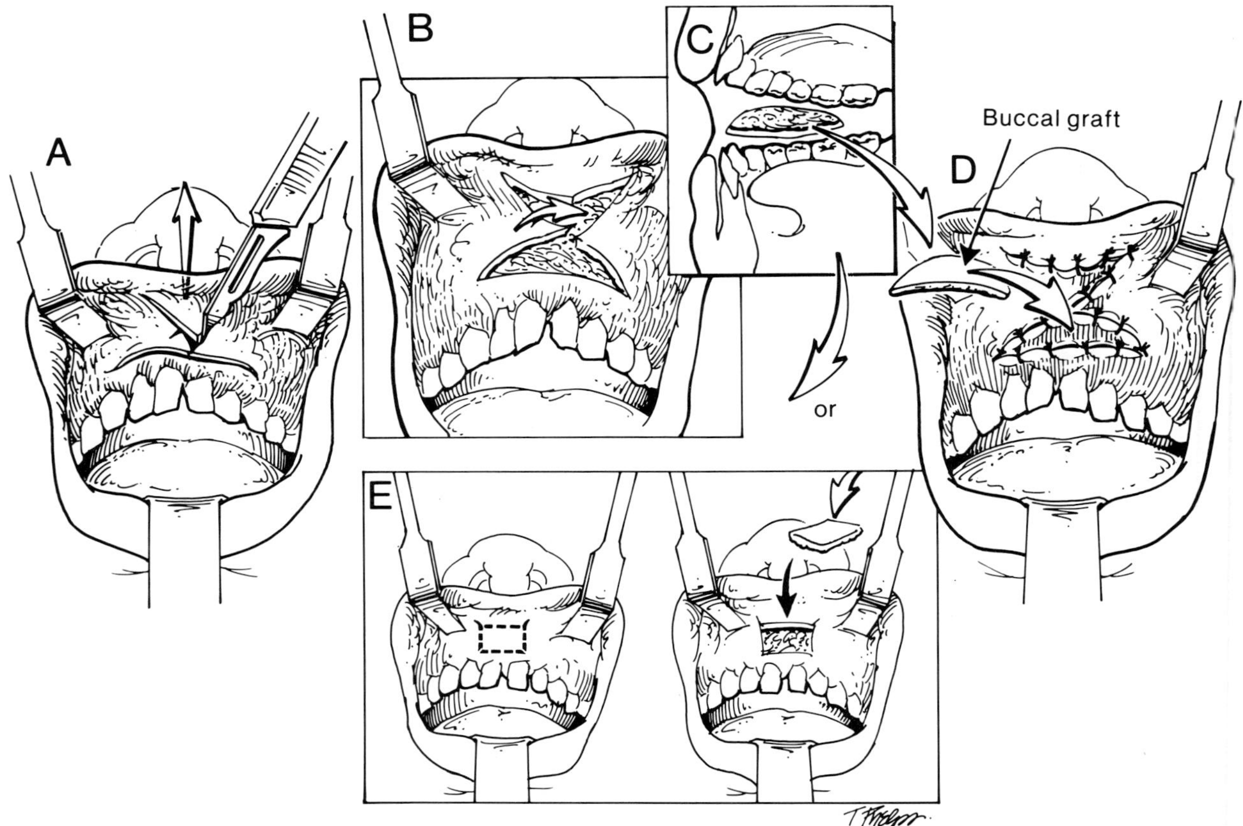

Fig. 23-16. Secondary correction of upper sulcus scarring and adhesions. **A,** Incisions shown to correct a short central segment of the upper lip using a V-Z advancement. **B,** V-Z advancement undermining the flap widely. **C,** A mucous membrane graft is removed from the buccal area. **D,** The graft is sutured to the exposed alveolar ridge. **E,** Outline of gingival mucosal flaps leaving exposed periosteum. The flap is advanced upward, releasing the adhesion. The defect may be grafted or left to spontaneously epithelialize. (Modified from Horton, C.E., Adamson, J.E., Mladick, R.A., and Taddeo, R.J.: Plast. Reconstr. Surg. **45:**31, 1970.)

side of the cleft or the other, a simple skin Z-plasty or diamond-shaped excision could be considered (Fig. 23-18). Dermabrasion for this problem is generally of limited usefulness. In rare cases in men, a temporal vascular island flap to bring hair-bearing tissue from the scalp to the upper lip can be used in an effort to resurface a deeply scarred, deformed area and to camouflage other deficiencies in the bilateral cleft lip repair.

SUMMARY OF SECONDARY CORRECTION OF CLEFT LIP REPAIRS

1. Consider early, preschool correction of the lip when the deformity is severe.

2. In the unilateral lip deformity two of the most difficult problems to correct, *cupid's bow deficiency* and an *excessively long lip,* can be avoided by an adequate primary repair. Both the Millard and Tennison repairs tend to preserve a natural cupid's bow in the resultant lip repair. In the incomplete cleft lip, deliberate slight shortening of the lip on the repaired side will counteract the tendency for the lateral lip to lengthen, especially with growth.

3. Recognize a *comparative tissue deficit* as opposed to a *true tissue deficiency*; local tissue rearrangement can be effective for correcting the former, whereas pedicle flaps or free grafts are needed for the latter.

4. *V-Y advancements are of limited usefulness,* particularly when previous surgical procedures have scarred the operative site.

5. *Notching defects are best treated by Z-plasty* rather than by excision and primary closure.

6. In the correction of secondary deformities, *slight to moderate overcorrection* is called for, particularly when building a tissue projection (e.g., philtral ridge, cupid's bow, or vermilion ridge).

7. The isolated deformity after cleft lip repair is rare; *multiple defects are frequently present* and their treatment should be in an *orderly fashion.* The possible exception is an excessively long lateral lip after unilateral repair of an incomplete cleft lip. A tissue excess in one site can frequently be used to rebuild a deficiency elsewhere and even *apparent excess tissue should not be discarded* until it is certain that it cannot be used.

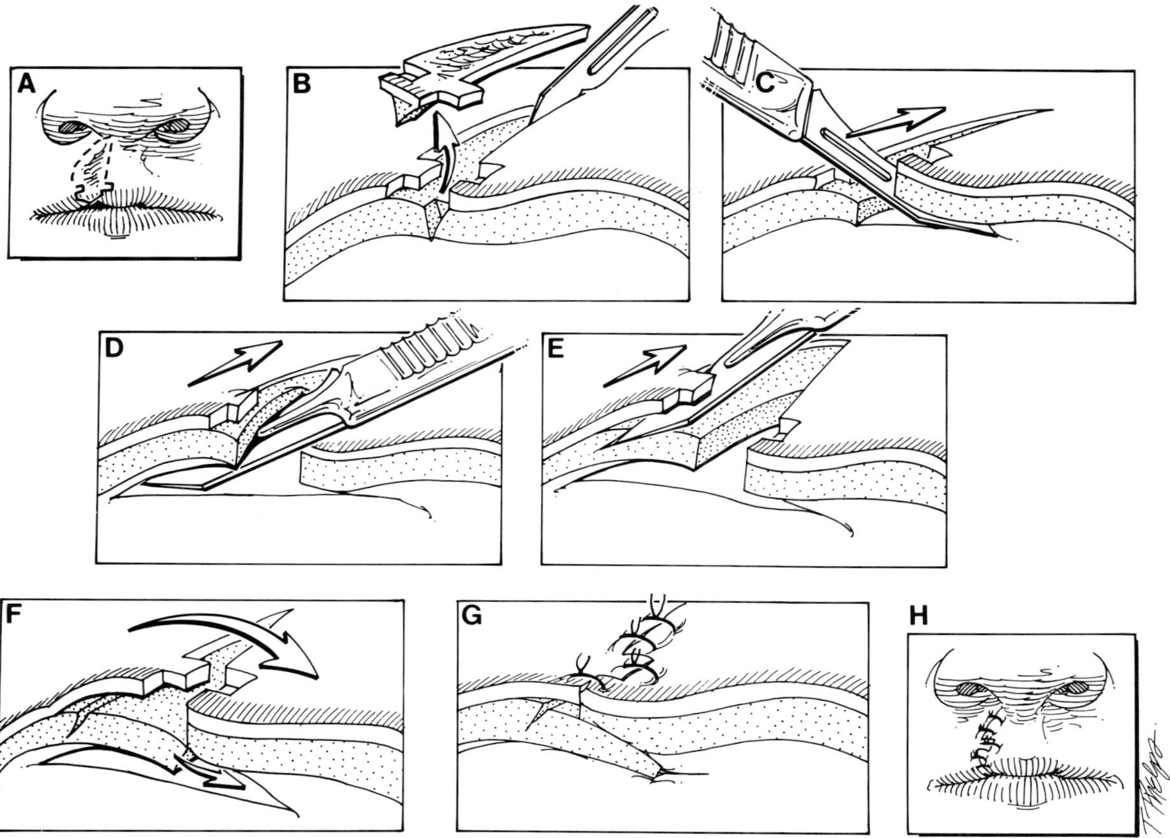

Fig. 23-17. Scar revision with "vest-over-pants" dermal closure. **A,** Scar hypertrophy. **B,** The epithelial component of the scar is excised. **C,** The underlying dermis is incised and preserved. **D,** The plane is elevated between the dermis and subcutaneous layer. **E,** The epidermis on one side is elevated over the dermal flap. **F,** The dermal flap is buried under the contralateral dermis. **G,** Closure is complete. **H,** The scar is narrowed with a greater projection due to increased bulk.

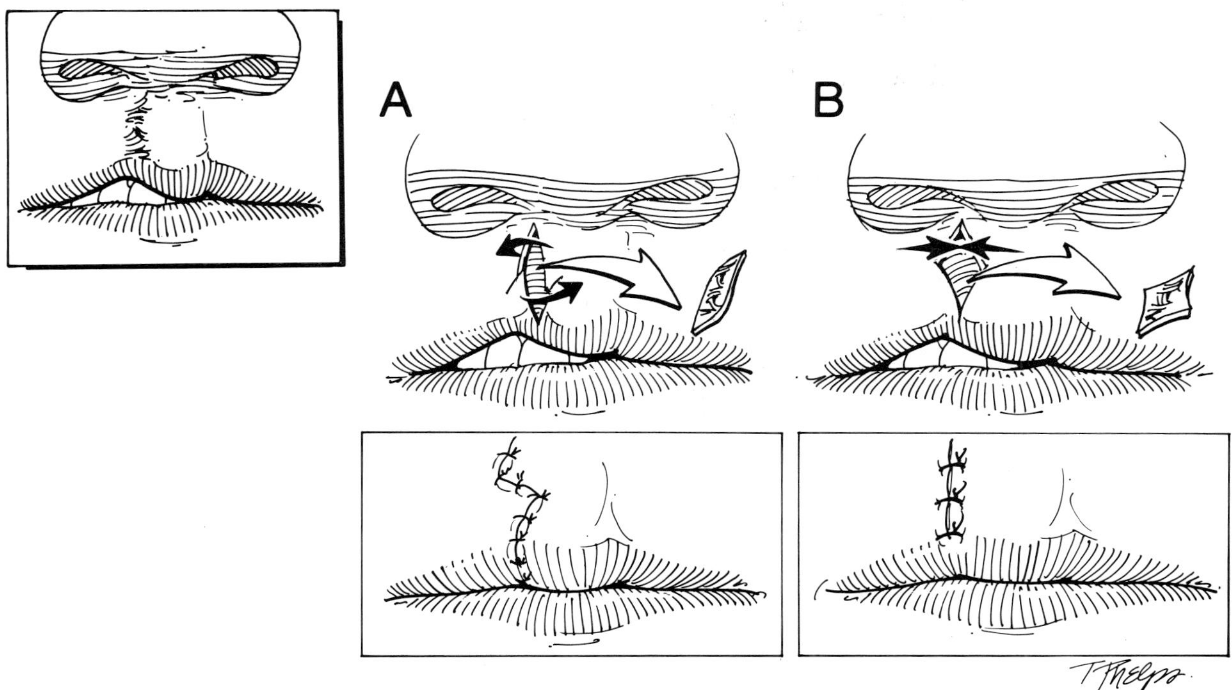

Fig. 23-18. Scar revision. **A,** Excising the scar epithelium and increasing the length with Z-plasty. **B,** Diamond-shaped resection of scar epithelium and primary closure.

REPAIR OF ORONASAL FISTULAE

The most commonly seen defect in the hard palate after cleft palate repair is the fistula. The fistula may be located either anterior to the alveolar ridge, where it is referred to as an *oronasal fistula,* or posteriorly on the palate, where it is called simply a *palatal fistula.*[45] Most fistulae are small and are noted within a few weeks after primary repair. Sometimes they cause regurgitation of food through the nose; however, speech generally is not affected by smaller fistulae. Occasionally, fistulae of varying sizes will result from orthodontic treatment or after rapid expansion of the dental arches in an effort to obtain an improved functional occlusion.

The timing of treatment of oronasal fistulae can vary considerably. When the fistula is small and of no functional significance, closure can be delayed for several years. Small fistulae tend to close spontaneously with growth or at least become nonfunctional. With simple oronasal fistulae anterior to the alveolar arch, closure can be done at the time of the secondary lip surgery. Frequently, correction of the cleft lip-nose deformity is required, and closure of the fistula can be undertaken at that time.

Escape of fluid and food through the nose can be a source of embarrassment, calling for closure at a preschool age. A large defect that affects speech should also be repaired before the child starts school.

Anterior alveolar palatal fistulae

Fistulae of the anterior alveolar palate are generally repaired when secondary lip revision is undertaken or in conjunction with bone grafting to the alveolar sulcus. If bone grafting is performed to fill in a significant alveolar arch deficiency in the area of the cleft, a two-layer closure is mandatory. Usually a turnover flap can be employed to line the nasal side of the defect, with bone inserted as required to bridge any defect or fill any deficiency in contour. A long buccal flap, based medially and turned around to cover the bone or provide an oral closure to the defect, involves the fewest complications (Fig. 23-23). In some cases, when the labial sulcus mucosa is quite loose, a sliding advancement flap based laterally will cover the oral side. The local tissue is often deeply scarred, and a simple purse-string closure is impossible. It should be stressed that a two-layer closure is essential and that flaps must be made larger than the defect to minimize tension.

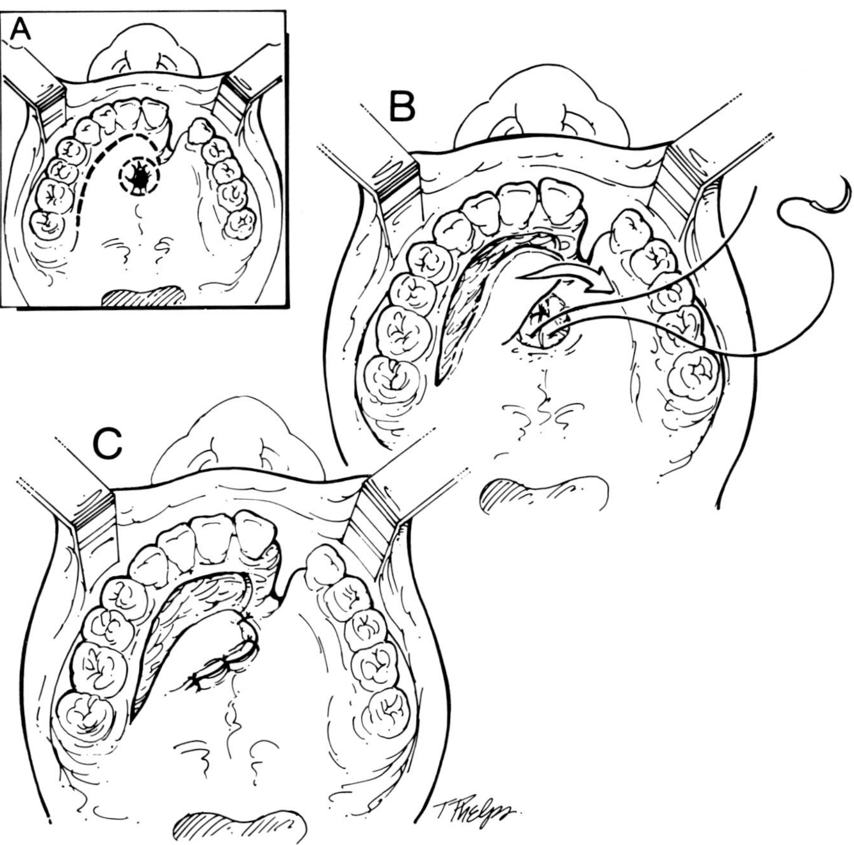

Fig. 23-19. Closure of a hard palate fistula. **A,** Local adjacent tissue with turnover flap or purse-string closure for the nasal layer. **B,** Mucoperiosteal rotation advancement flaps serving as an oral cover. **C,** The denuded portion of the palate is left to reepithelialize.

Palatal fistulae

Palatal fistulae may vary from 2 or 3 mm in size to 1 cm or larger. The patient will have had previous attempts at repair with the entire palate being scarred, stiff, and immobile. A double-layer closure, consisting of a simple turnover flap from the side of the palate with the least tissue and a larger rotation flap from the opposite side to provide the oral closure is adequate for a small fistula (Fig. 23-19). In most repairs a palate pack, consisting of gauze impregnated with tetracycline (Achromycin), is inserted and held in place with transpalatal 0 silk sutures.

When the defect is longitudinal, a modification of the Von Langenbeck procedure with two flaps can provide adequate tissue for closure. This type of defect is usually seen after rapid arch expansion, and closure is accompanied by wedge-type bone grafting. When the fistula is quite small, a purse-string closure for the nasal side can be done in which sutures are brought through the nose with a threaded probe (Fig. 23-20). In larger defects the use of buccal sulcus flaps brought through the nasal fossa onto the defect in the hard palate to provide nasal lining must be considered (Fig. 23-21). This entails the use of the palate tissue for the closure on the oral side.

For larger defects, particularly when previous attempts at closure have failed, the tongue flap should be considered. A large fistula and short palate might require repair using a pharyngeal flap. Both the tongue and pharyngeal flap procedures are described elsewhere.

Finally, when the patient is literally crippled by the fistula and repeated unsuccessful attempts have been made at closure, a prosthesis such as a properly fitting obturator can be helpful. Some patients require a prosthesis to replace teeth that were lost because of the original cleft or through dental caries or periodontal disease. The prosthesis can serve two functions: to replace the missing teeth and close the fistula. In some instances it can be used with a posterior extension (lift) to provide improved velopharyngeal competency.

Summary of repair of oronasal fistulae

1. An oronasal fistula may allow regurgitation of food through the nose but generally does not interfere with the development of good speech, except when the defect is very large.

2. An oronasal fistula located anterior to the alveolar arch in the labial sulcus should be corrected at the time of bone grafting if the latter is planned.

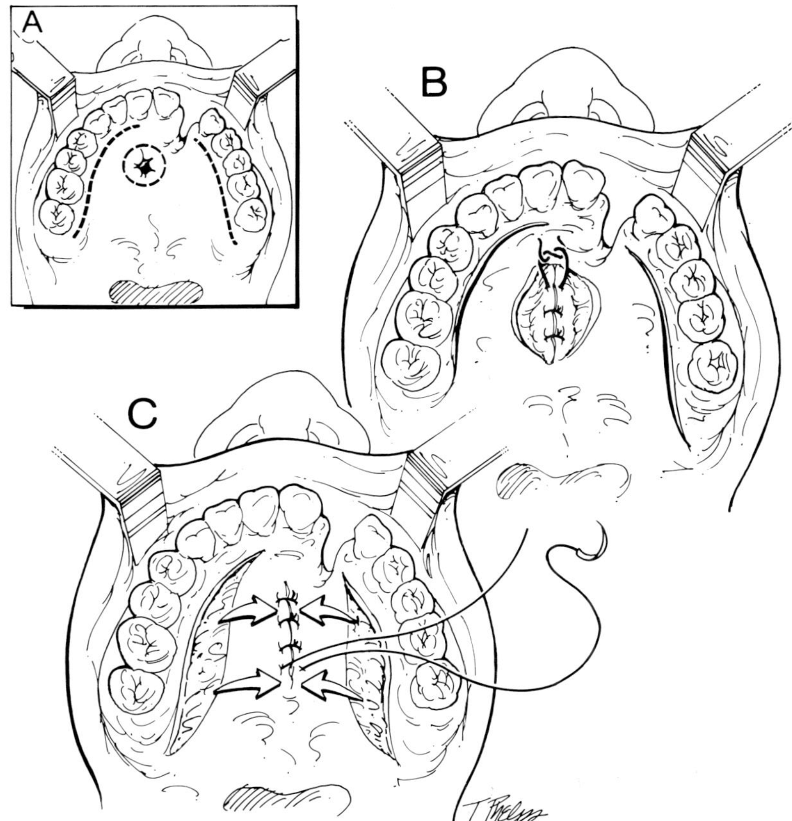

Fig. 23-20. Closure of a midpalatal defect, **A,** Purse-string closure of adjacent tissue to achieve a nasal layer. **B** and **C,** Mobilization of von Langenbeck flaps for oral coverage.

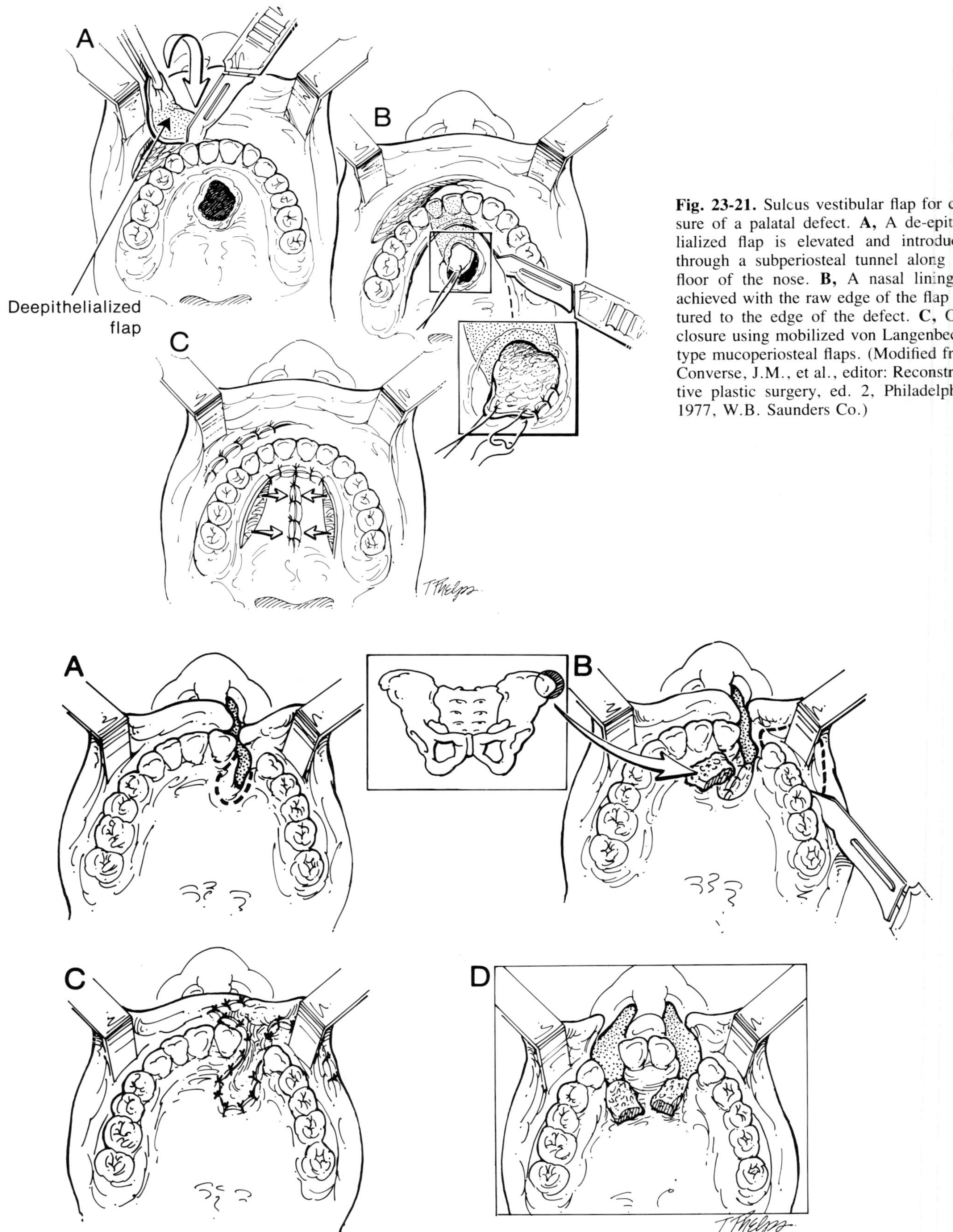

Fig. 23-21. Sulcus vestibular flap for closure of a palatal defect. **A,** A de-epithelialized flap is elevated and introduced through a subperiosteal tunnel along the floor of the nose. **B,** A nasal lining is achieved with the raw edge of the flap sutured to the edge of the defect. **C,** Oral closure using mobilized von Langenbeck–type mucoperiosteal flaps. (Modified from Converse, J.M., et al., editor: Reconstructive plastic surgery, ed. 2, Philadelphia, 1977, W.B. Saunders Co.)

Fig. 23-22. Closure of an alveolar cleft. **A,** Local tissue is turned down as inner mucosal flaps. **B,** Cancellous bone is used as an inlay graft, and a buccal flap is developed for the outer lining. **C,** After two-layer closure. **D,** The same technique is applied to stabilize the premaxilla in a bilateral cleft.

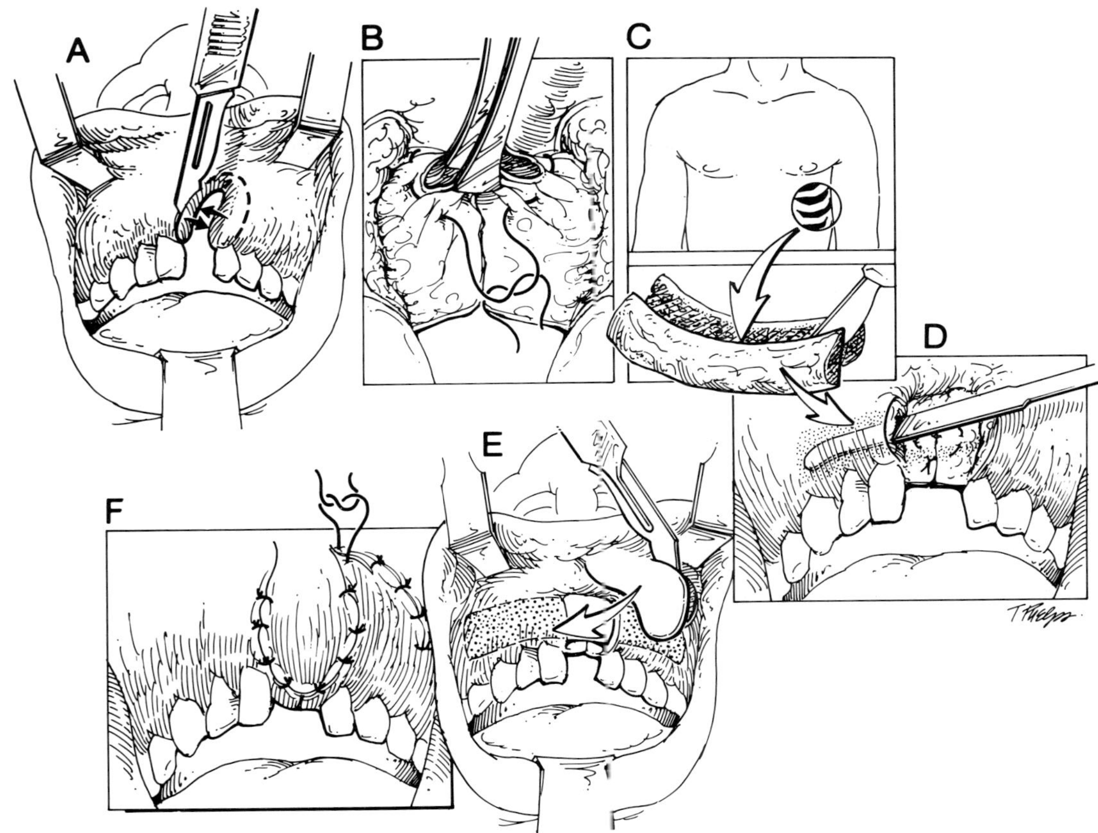

Fig. 23-23. Onlay bone graft to an alveolar cleft. **A,** Outline of local flaps for the inner layer. **B,** The purse-string suture technique is used for closure. **C,** The rib graft is split using a Beaver blade. **D,** A pocket for the graft is made. **E,** The natural curvature of the rib is used for an onlay graft with the buccal flap developed for coverage. **F,** The buccal flap in place with the donor site closed.

3. At the time of surgery the palatal defect may appear considerably larger than it did in the preoperative evaluation.

4. Local flaps are employed to close a palatal fistula. The flaps must be made significantly larger than the defect and planned so as to be mobile. Mucoperiosteum is stiff and does not lend itself to either transposition or suturing.

5. A two-layer closure is ideal, but a single-layer strong closure, with a large flap, is preferred to a double-layer closure that is attenuated and tight.

6. Patients who have had repeated attempted fistula closure with failure are best treated by prosthodontists.

BONE GRAFTING AND MAXILLARY OSTEOTOMIES

Secondary bone grafting in the patient with a cleft lip or palate is generally employed in two situations, the most common of which involves the patient with a bilateral cleft of the primary and secondary palate. Frequently the premaxillary segment is unstable, and orthodontic treatment, which is invariably required in this group of patients, is more difficult to carry out in the presence of a mobile premaxillary segment.

When a bony deficiency in the alveolar arch occurs, cancellous bone grafting can be employed to fill in the defect, not only to provide alveolar arch continuity but also to provide an onlay graft for additional contour when maxillary hypoplasia exists (Fig. 23-22). When a bony deficiency is present, the permanent teeth erupting adjacent to the cleft may have inadequate bony support, and early bone loss around these teeth due to peridontal disease invariably contributes to the overall dental problem. Again, when the defect is significant, fixed bridgework should be considered, since the long-term use of a removable prosthetic appliance puts excessive stress on the teeth adjacent to the defect. The resultant forces cause hypermobility of the involved teeth, loss of periodontal support and finally failure to support the appliance. It should be emphasized that when there is localized maxillary hypoplasia at the base of the nose on the cleft side, onlay bone grafting is essential to provide an adequate foundation on which to build up the nasal base.

The question of timing of this procedure is controversial. We believe that in the unilateral cleft it is best to wait until the patient is prepubescent, that is ages 8 to 11, before grafting is carried out. At this time any anterior alveolar deficiency that manifests itself in loss of lip contour or depression of the labial elements can be considered during the procedure. With an inlay bone graft for the actual defect and an onlay graft for restoration of contour deficiency, the technique employing a split rib graft is seen in Fig. 23-23. This technique can be incorporated with nasal reconstruction as advocated by Gerow, Stal, and Spira[21] with the three bone grafts articulating, thus giving better projection and stability (Fig. 23-24).

In patients with bilateral clefts in whom the premaxilla is unstable, the age of operation depends on the degree of deformity, as well as the philosophy of those participating in the treatment. The plastic surgeon, in conjunction with the orthodontist, will usually elect to stabilize the premaxilla in the immediate preschool period when the deciduous dentition has fully erupted. In rare cases, this procedure may be carried out in combination with a vomer setback when there is gross protrusion of the premaxillary component. Grafting for premaxillary stabilization also can be carried out in the prepubertal period, shortly before eruption of the canines. The technique for closure of the bilateral defect is similar to closure for the unilateral defect with a circum-

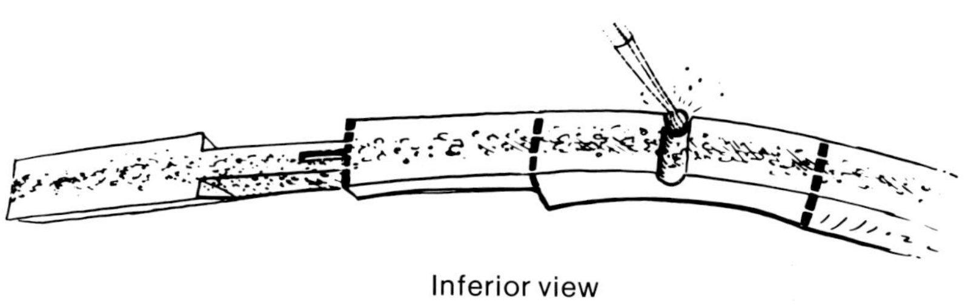

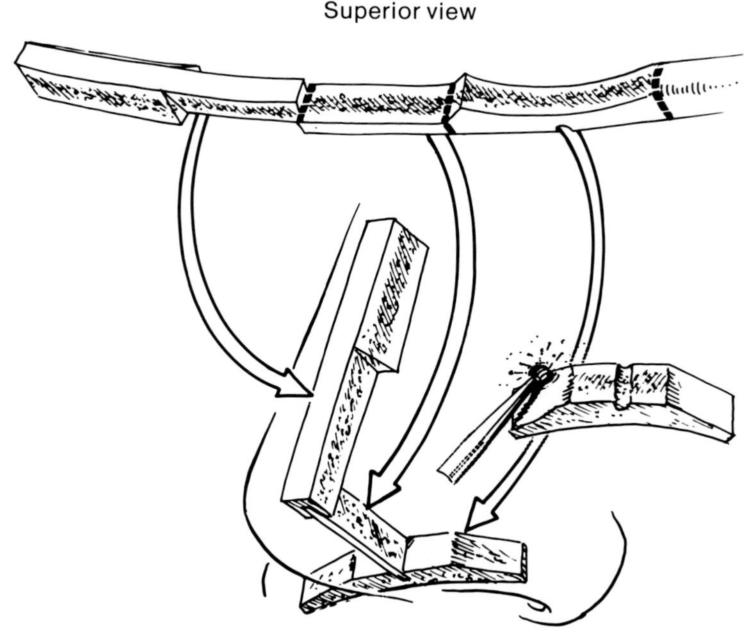

Fig. 23-24. "Totem pole bone graft." A single rib is used to create three articulating segments to onlay and augment the premaxilla and nose. (Modified from Gerow, F.J., Stal, S., and Spira, M.: The totem pole rib graft reconstruction of the nose, Ann. Plast. Surg. **11:**273, 1983.)

ferential turn-in or purse-string–type suture flap being employed for the nasal lining and medially based buccal sulcus mucosal flaps for the oral side (Fig. 23-22). The donor site for the bone graft varies with the preference of the surgeon. In most patients the rib is convenient; however, if the scar is objectionable, the iliac crest can be used. Another bone graft donor site that has been favored is the anterior tibial crest. This donor site reportedly is associated with minimal morbidity, an acceptable scar, and accessibility. Also commonly used because of its easy access and proximity is the calvaria graft, either as outer table or the diploic bone.[28] It has been suggested that this bone will vascularize more rapidly in the recipient site (Fig. 23-25).

In most instances maxillary hypoplasia is localized at the base of the nose on the cleft side secondary to inadequate growth or combined with lateral anterior arch collapse. When this is the case, osteotomies usually are not necessary, and orthodontic correction of the occlusal deficiency, combined with inlay-onlay bone grafting, will restore adequate contour to the lip and base of the nose to reduce the associated nasal deformity. In the wide unilateral cleft lip-palate deformity, an associated lateral arch collapse may be so severe that it is not amenable to routine orthodontic treatment. This requires an approach through a labial buccal incision, exposing the maxilla above the apices of the teeth with the unilateral transverse osteotomy through the max-

illary sinus, through the base of the lateral nasal wall at least 3 mm above the floor of the nasal fossa. This necessitates adequate mobilization of the collapsed arch segment to bring it down and buccally into occlusion with the mandibular teeth. Immobilization for the usual 6-week period can be avoided with a more sophisticated technique using an appropriate acrylic bite plate that is wired to the intermaxillary dentition and stabilizes the mobilized side.

In both unilateral and bilateral cleft palates in which deformity is severe and associated with maxillary retrusion, more classic orthognathic surgery in the form of a LeFort I transverse maxillary osteotomy is needed to totally mobilize the maxilla. The maxillary dentition should be stabilized with cap splints or a fixed appliance before surgery. It may then be brought forward and downward, if vertical height is needed to improve facial contour into more satisfactory occlusion with the mandibular dentition (Fig. 23-26). In such cases bone grafting is required to fill the gap between the stable malar-maxillary complex above and the mobilized maxilla below, as well as to provide a buttress between the maxillary tuberosity and the pterygoid plates. Immobilization of the osteotomized segment with intermaxillary fixation is usually for a minimum of 8 weeks, and elastic bandages are invariably worn at night to maintain advancement achieved at surgery. Relapse and recurrence of the deformity are not uncommon.[3]

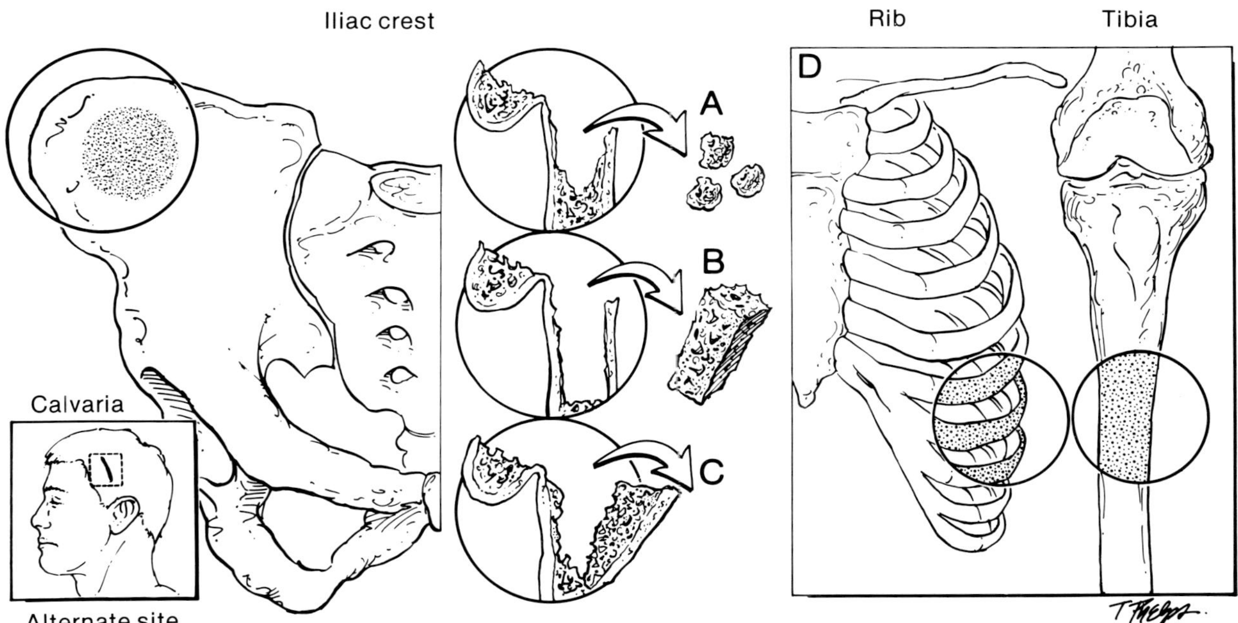

Fig. 23-25. Bone graft sites. The inner table of the iliac crest can be removed, preserving contour and muscle insertion. It can be removed as cancellous bone chips **(A)**, a cancellous bone block **(B)**, or a composite of cortical and cancellous bone **(C)**. Ribs 6, 7, and 8 can be taken from an inframammary incision with good exposure. A solid block can easily be removed from the anterior tibia. The calvaria is a good site because of easy accessibility.

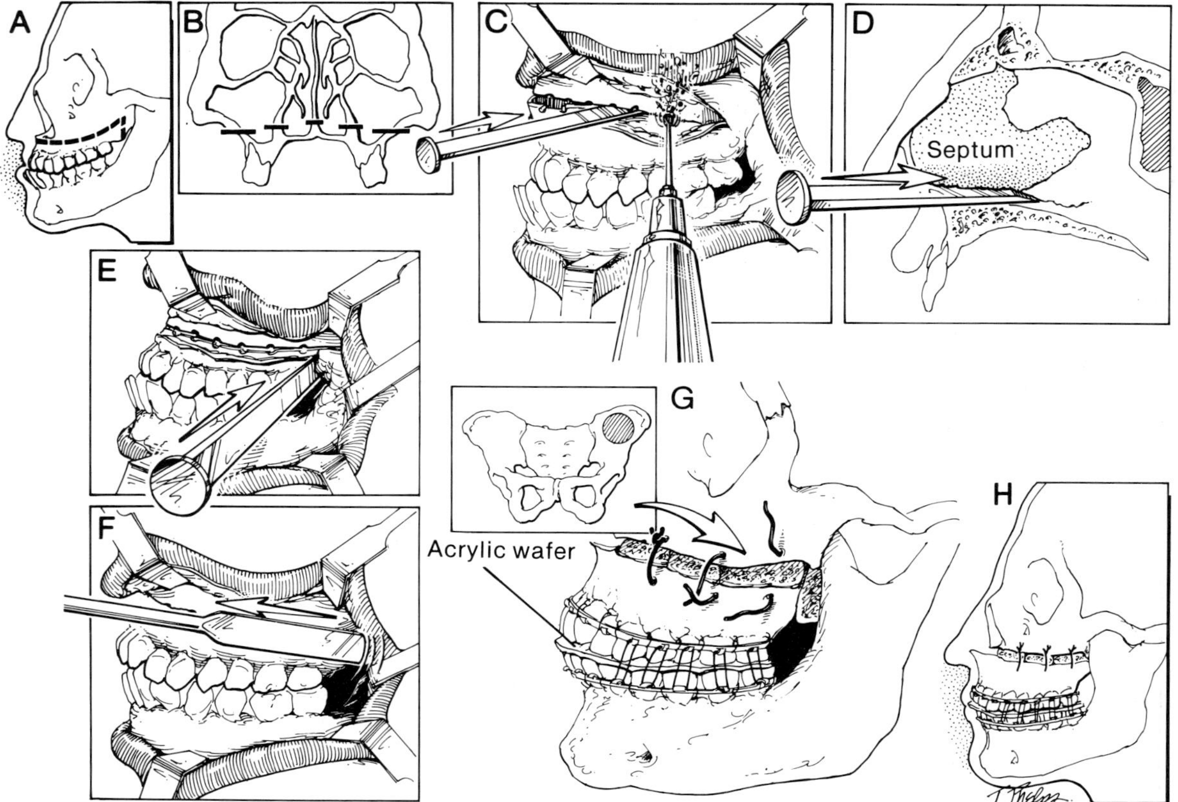

Fig. 23-26. A LeFort I osteotomy for midface advancement. **A** and **B,** The level of osteotomy cuts are outlined. **C,** The initial round bur holes on the lateral surface of the maxilla are joined by an osteotome cut. **D,** The septum is detached from the roof of the maxilla and vomer with an osteotome. **E,** The osteotome divides the maxillary tuberosity from the pterygoid plates. **F,** Impaction forceps are employed to totally mobilize the maxilla. **G,** Bone grafts are usually taken from the inner surface of the iliac bone and employed as an interpositional graft between the malar complex above to immobilize the maxilla below and pterygoid process posteriorly. **H,** Occlusion after reduction.

Summary of bone grafting alveolar defects and maxillary osteotomies

1. *Presurgical and postsurgical orthodontic treatment* is the rule rather than the exception if full and permanent correction of the dentition is to be achieved and arch and maxillary form are to be attained.[57]

2. *Nasal intubation is mandatory,* and a nasogastric tube is always inserted at the time of surgery. Extubation is carried out when the patient is fully awake, frequently the next day, and the nasogastric tube is removed at 48 to 72 hours.

3. When correcting an alveolar arch defect or stabilizing a premaxilla, one must provide for a *two-layer closure* with a local turn-in flap to provide nasal lining and a bed for the graft with some type of buccal mucoperiosteal flap for the oral cover and closure.

4. *LeFort I transverse maxillary osteotomy* to correct protrusion in a cleft palate deformity is a far more difficult procedure than the treatment of simple midface hypoplasia, as in Binder's syndrome. Arch stability and horizontal maxillary continuity during the operative procedure are best achieved and maintained by a cemented (fixed) expansion-type appliance or cap splints. A history of repeated palatal operations, with associated extensive scarring, compounds the deformity and difficulty encountered at the time of surgery.

5. The amount of *bone is more frequently underestimated* than overestimated. Slight but definite overcorrection is desirable in each instance.

6. In calculating postoperative soft tissue changes secondary to bony movement, a *1 cm advancement of bone is usually accompanied by half as much protrusion of the lip.*

7. Total *bony stability may require up to 12 weeks in intermaxillary fixation,* followed by several weeks of wearing elastic bandages at night if relapse is to be avoided.

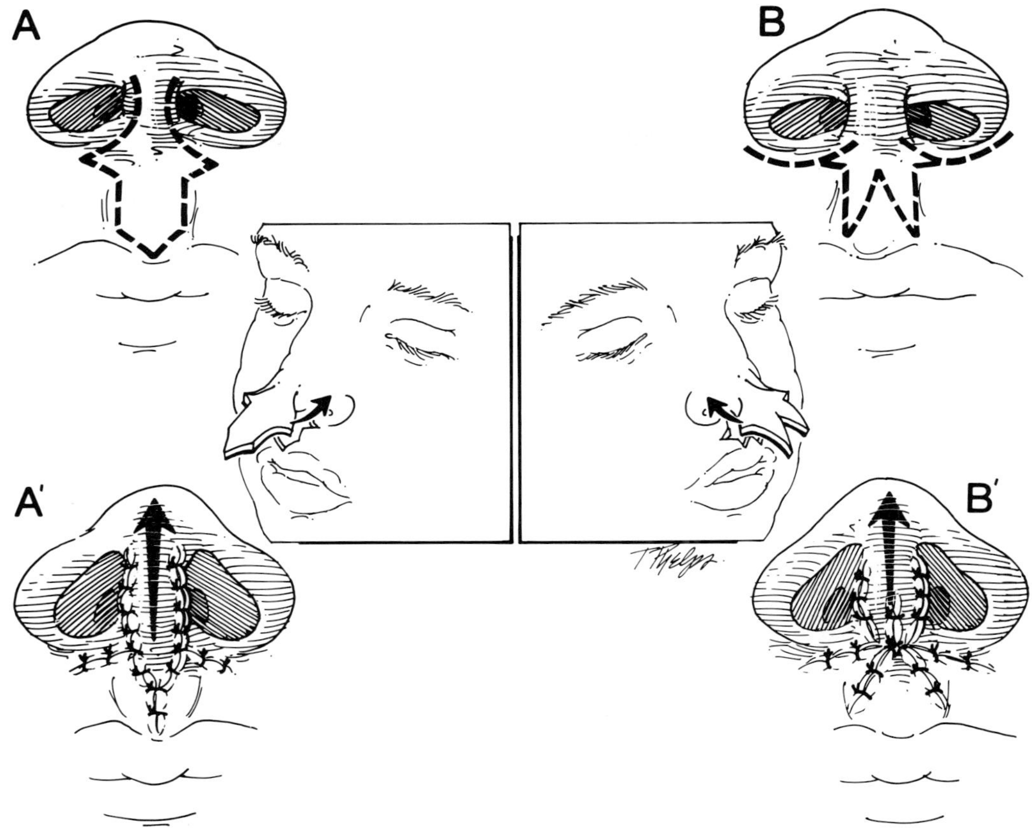

Fig. 23-27. Columella lengthening using tissue from the lip. **A,** Outline of the advancement flap using prolabial skin. **A',** Effective lengthening with a midline scar. **B,** Outline of forked flaps and alar release incisions. **B',** Effective lengthening with a narrowed philtrum and scars in a more anatomic position. (Modified from Brown, J.B., and McDowell, F.: Ann. Surg. **114:**101, 1941.)

COLUMELLA LENGTHENING

The problems associated with the columella relate primarily to the bilateral cleft lip deformity. In the wide bilateral cleft lip, the associated columella deformity is usually short, severe, and noticeable. There is no consesus relative to timing of an operative procedure to correct the columella deficiency, but it is our opinion that early release of the tip cartilage by some type of columella reconstruction is preferable to waiting until the patient reaches adolescence to advance the short columella and perform definitive nasal correction. The question of whether or not release of the aforementioned structures might permit the full growth potential of these tissues to occur is debatable. Although little can be done for the bilateral cleft lip nose at the time of the original lip repair, our impressions that columella advancement can be carried out at a preschool age and that such timing is probably in the best interest of the patient.

When the surgeon is faced with reconstruction of a very short columella, a source of tissue for the reconstructive effort generally falls into three categories. The following sites have been employed for this purpose: the upper lip, nasal structure, and nasal skin.

Upper lip

Prolabial tissue can be used if the patient is a girl and particularly when an Abbe flap is also required to give additional dimension and appropriate contour to a short tight upper lip. The technique for moving the prolabium into the columella is basically a V-Y advancement with several variations. The original procedure described by Lexer[35] of lengthening the columella is an operation that was improved on by Brown and McDowell[9] with their development of a philtral flap (Fig. 23-27). Their procedure included V-Y advancement of the central portion of the upper lip and used lateral wings of the flap to lengthen the columella to a more reasonable size. In boys all techniques employing prolabial tissue to augment columella length have the decided disadvantage of moving hair-bearing tissue from the upper lip into the nose where it causes yet another deformity.

Forked flaps, or some modification thereof, as originally

described by Trauner,[61] have been used effectively in columella augmentation.[51,52] In the original procedure superiorly based vertical flaps from the upper lip were rotated bilaterally and inset transversely into the base of the columella to provide *additional length*. Millard[38,39] combined forked flaps developed from either side of the prolabium, along with vestibular-based flaps, to provide elongation of the columella and to simultaneously narrow the nasal floors (Fig. 23-27).

Nasal structure

The floor of the nose in these patients tends to be wide and has been employed by a number of surgeons to lengthen the columella by raising bilateral flaps from the nasal floor and advancing them medially and forward into the columella and nose.[2,12,13,25] Cronin's technique [12,13] creates a bipedicle flap that is carried around the base of the ala to the base of the nasolabial fold, with the entire floor of the nose undermined and the lateral components advanced medially (Fig.

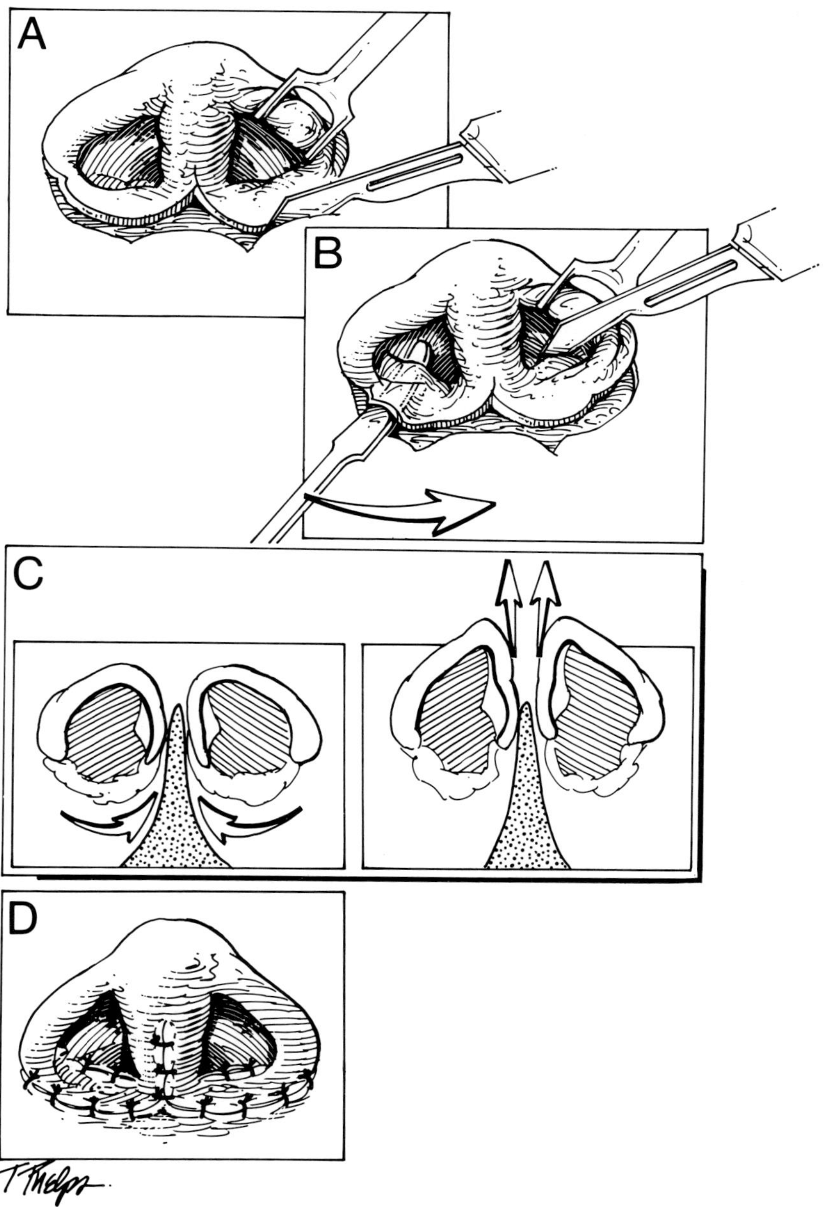

Fig. 23-28. Columella lengthening using nasal tissue. **A,** Creation of bipedicle flaps at the base of the nose. **B,** The entire floor of the nose is released and undermined. **C,** This release allows medial advancement of lateral components. **D,** Effective lengthening can be combined with a bone graft or suture of the medial crura. (Modified from Cronin, T.D.: Plast. Reconstr. Surg. **21:**417, 1958.)

23-28). This technique, combined with wedge resections from the upper lip, gives the necessary columella length. The technique usually combines suturing the medial crura of the lower lateral cartilages together to provide additional stability and support to the columella, as well as to narrow the nasal tip.

Nasal skin shifting by external incision

Numerous operations exist,[58] beginning with a V-incision in the tip, which is then moved upward and closed as a V-Y advancement. Brauer and Foerster[7] have described a through-and-through ''flying bird'' incision employing the alar rims, which are moved medially to give the columella length and tip projection. This technique has the advantage of using tissue that is normally in excess (Fig. 23-29). Although the columella is lengthened a somewhat peculiar configuration of the nostrils results from this procedure, giving it limited applicability. A simple Z-plasty is advocated by Straith, Straith, and Lawson[59] as generally effective only in the most minimally short columellas. In most bilateral cleft lip noses, the nasal bridge and tip are very broad. This factor has been employed by Dieffenbach[15] and later by Morel-Fatio[41] as a reverse V-Y advancement to provide additional length to the columella. Edgerton, Carson, and McKnelly[16] modified the technique with the addition of gull-wing flaps from the lateral nasal skin to provide further augmentation (Fig. 23-30).

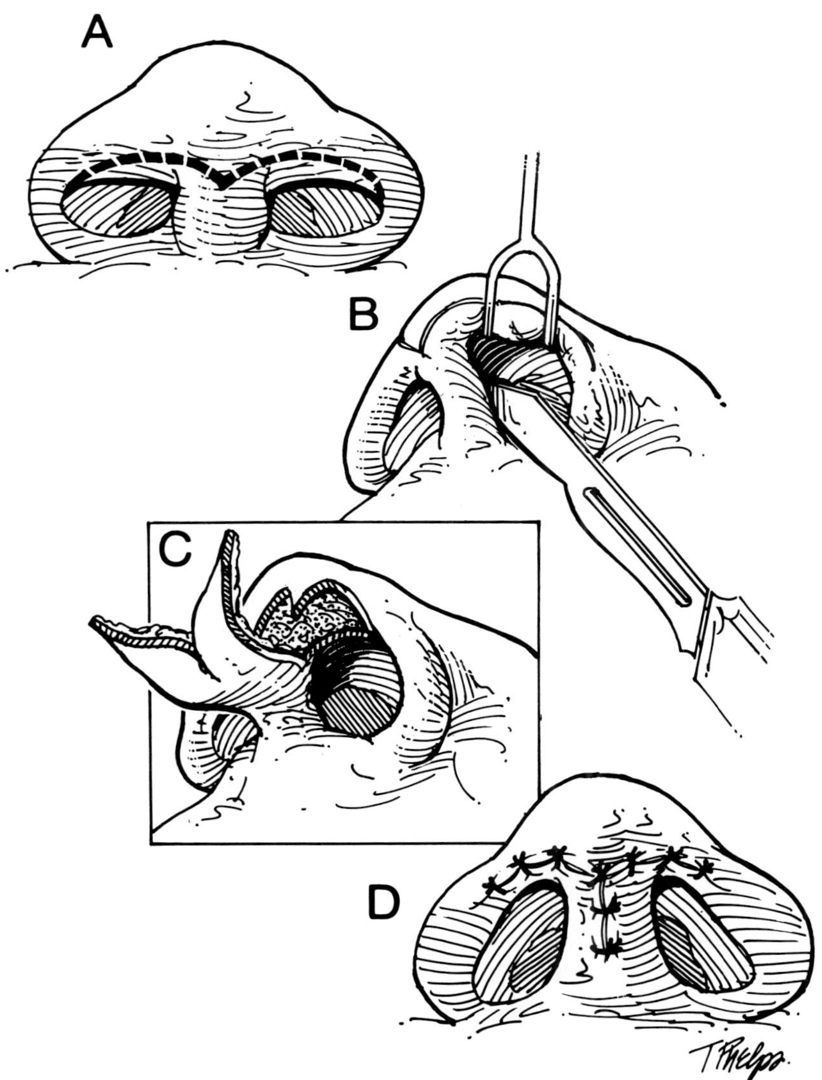

Fig. 23-29. Columella lengthening. **A,** Outline of a ''flying bird'' incision. **B,** The columella is freed with an incision in the membranous septum. **C,** Columella flap after release. **D,** Effective lengthening using the upper alar skin. (Modified from Brauer, R.O., and Foerster, D.W.: Plast. Reconstr. Surg. **38:**27, 1966.)

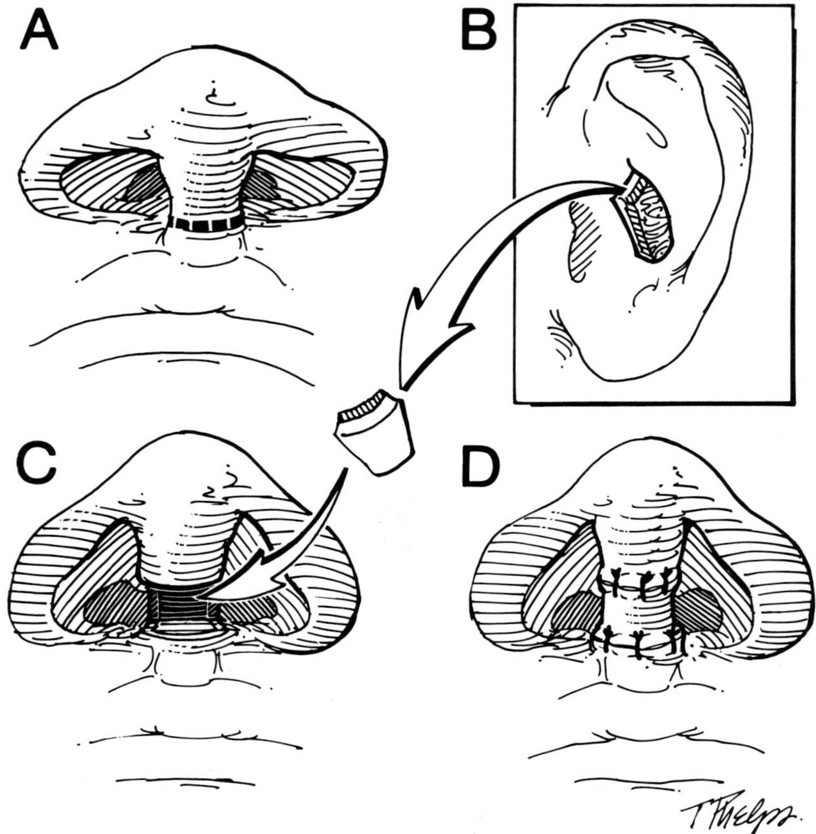

Fig. 23-30. Columella lengthening using a composite graft. **A,** A full-thickness incision is outlined. **B,** Auricle donor site. **C** and **D,** A composite graft is placed in the defect after release, thus lengthening the columella.

Summary of columella lengthening

1. In the severe deformity an operative procedure in the preschool child should be considered. *Early release of the lower lateral cartilages by columella lengthening* and lateral release by narrowing the nostril base will allow a more natural growth pattern.

2. *When the upper lip is tight or scarred,* particularly in girls, a combined procedure using the *prolabium as a modified V-Y advancement* into the columella for additional columella length and an *Abbe lip-switch flap* to fill the defect left by release of the lip and prolabial advancement provides a bulk of tissue that is generally soft, unscarred, and of adequate size. An additional advantage to this technique is that a comparative excess of tissue in the lower lip is removed, providing a more harmonious relationship between upper and lower lip size.

3. In columella reconstruction, additional *tip support should be provided, either by a cartilaginous strut or a bonegraft,* whenever feasible.

4. Patients will invariably accept an external scar if the overall form of the nose is good or improved.

5. When other deformities exist, such as a large oronasal fistula, consideration should be given to repairing the fistula at the same time as columella advancement.

6. *Overcorrection* is to be emphasized, especially in surgical procedures involving lengthening the columella to provide tip projection.

SUMMARY AND CONCLUSIONS

Deformities in patients with clefts are multiple and are usually not amenable to correction in a single operative procedure. Both unilateral and bilateral clefts are frequently repaired in the neonatal period. In a bilateral cleft repair is often combined with columella advancement. The correction of occlusal deformities is usually undertaken later, with treatment invariably requiring orthodontics and, in severe malocclusion, surgery. Nasal tip deformities associated with a short columella may be corrected in the preschool period. Nasal deformities requiring osteotomies are most often done after adolescence.

Secondary corrective procedures after cleft lip repair may be necessary. Deformities of the lip are best corrected in the preschool period. In the unilateral cleft lip two of the most difficult problems, cupid's bow deficiency and an excessively long lip, can usually be avoided by an adequate primary repair. When the cupid's bow portion of the vermilion is totally absent, reconstruction should be considered with a small modified Abbe flap. If a vertical deficiency exists lateral to the cleft, vermilion advancement on the side of the defect can be carried out. Small notching defects in the lower border of the lip vermilion are best reconstructed by simple Z-plasty. Correction of a long lip may be difficult. Correction involves opening the entire lip from the base of the nose through the vermilion, excising an adequate tissue composite at the base of the nose along the nostril floor, extending the incision around the base of the ala, and then repairing the defect as in an original lip repair.

Any oronasal fistulae located anterior to the alveolar arch in the labial sulcus should be corrected at the time of bone grafting if it is planned. Palatal fistulae are best closed with a two-layered closure employing local flaps. Larger defects may require a tongue flap.

Presurgical and postsurgical orthodontic treatment is the rule rather than the exception in patients with clefts. In performing a bone graft to either the alveolar arch defect or in stabilizing the premaxilla, one must provide for a two-layer closure. Osteotomies may be required to correct protrusion and occlusion. In calculating postoperative soft tissue changes secondary to bony movement, a 1 cm advancement of bone is usually accompanied by half as much protrusion of the lip. In the severe deformity early release of the lower lateral cartilages by columella lengthening and lateral release by narrowing the nostril base will allow a more natural growth pattern. This is often performed in the preschool period. When the upper lip is tight or scarred and the columella is short, the prolabium may be advanced in a V-Y fashion into the columella and an Abbe lip-switch flap employed to fill the defect. In columella reconstruction, whenever possible, additional tip support should be provided either by a cartilage strut or a bone graft.

REFERENCES

1. Abbe, R.: A new plastic operation for the relief of deformity due to double harelip, Med. Rec. N.Y. **53:**477, 1898.
2. Barsky, A.L.: Principles and practice of plastic surgery, Baltimore, 1950, Williams & Wilkins.
3. Bell, W.H., Profitt, W.R., Jacobs, J., et al.: Maxillary and midface deformity. In Bell, W., et al., editors: Surgical correction of dentofacial deformities, vol. 2, Philadelphia, 1980, W.B. Saunders Co.
4. Bernstein, L.: Secondary reconstructive procedures for cleft lip and nose, Trans Am. Acad. Ophthalmol. **71:**71, 1967.
5. Bloomquist, D.S.: Bone grafting in dentofacial defects. In Bell, W., et al., editors: Surgical correction of dentofacial deformities, vol. 1, Philadelphia, 1980, W.B. Saunders Co.
6. Brauer, R.O.: Lengthening the columella. In Georgiade, N.G., and Hagerty, R.F., editors: Symposium on management of cleft lip and palate and associated deformities, St. Louis, 1974, The C.V. Mosby Co.
7. Brauer, R.O., and Foerster, D.W.: Another method to lengthen the columella in the bilateral cleft lip, Plast. Reconstr. Surg. **38:**27, 1966.
8. Broadbent, T.R.: The badly scarred bilateral cleft lip: total resurfacing, Plast. Reconstr. Surg. **20:**485, 1966.
9. Brown, J.B., and McDowell, F.: Secondary repair of cleft lips and their nasal deformities, Ann. Surg. **114:**101, 1941.
10. Cannon, B.: The split vermilion bordered lip flap, Surg. Gynecol. Obstet. **73:**94, 1941.
11. Converse, J.M., et al., editor: Reconstructive plastic surgery, ed. 2, Philadelphia, 1977, W.B. Saunders Co.
12. Cronin, T.D.: Lengthening columella by use of skin from the nasal floor and alae, Plast. Reconstr. Surg. **21:**417, 1958.
13. Cronin, T.D., and Upton, J.: Lengthening of the short columella associated with bilateral cleft lip, Ann. Plast. Surg. **1:**75, 1978.
14. DePalma, A.T., Leavitt, L.H., and Hardy, S.B.: Electromyography in full thickness lip rotation between upper and lower lips, Plast. Reconstr. Surg. **21:**448, 1958.
15. Dieffenbach, J.F. Quoted by Axhauser, G.: Technik und Ergebnisse der Spaltplastiken, Munich, 1952, Hauser.
16. Edgerton, M.T., Carson, M.D., and McKnelly, L.D.: Lengthening of the short columella by skin flaps from the nasal tip and dorsum, Plast. Reconstr. Surg. **40:**343, 1967.
17. Falcone, A.E.: Release of the adherent prolabium and deepening of the labial sulcus in the secondary repair of bilateral cleft lips, Plast. Reconstr. Surg. **38:**42, 1966.
18. Fara, M., and Smahel, J.: Postoperative follow-up of restitution procedures in the orbicularis oris muscle after operation for complete bilateral cleft of the lip, Plast. Reconstr. Surg. **40:**13, 1967.
19. Flanagin, W.S.: Free composite grafts from lower to upper lip, Plast. Reconstr. Surg. **17:**376, 1956.
20. Garrett, W.S., and Musgrave, R.H.: The Abbe flap: a twenty-year cumulative experience. In Georgiade, N.G., and Hagerty, R.F., editors: Symposium on management of cleft lip and palate and associated deformities, St. Louis, 1974, The C.V. Mosby Co.
21. Gerow, F.J., Stal, S., and Spira, M.: The totem pole rib graft reconstruction of the nose, Ann. Plast. Surg. **11:**273, 1983.
22. Gillies, H., and Kilner, T.P.: Harelip: operations for the correction of secondary deformities, Lancet **2:**1369, 1932.
23. Gillies, H., and Millard, D.R.: The principles and art of plastic surgery, vol. 1, Boston, 1957, Little, Brown & Co.
24. Harding, R.L.: Secondary repair of bilateral cleft lips. In Grabb, W.C., Rosenstein, S.W., and Bzoch, K.R., editors: Cleft lip and palate, Boston, 1971, Little, Brown & Co.
25. Hogan, V.M., and Converse, J.M.: Secondary deformities of unilateral cleft lip and nose. In Grabb, W.C., Rosenstein, S.W., and Bzoch, K.R., editors: Cleft lip and palate, Boston, 1971, Little, Brown & Co.
26. Horton, C.E., Adamson, J.E., Mladick, R.A., and Taddeo, R.J.: The upper lip sulcus in cleft lips, Plast. Reconstr. Surg. **45:**31, 1970.
27. Hovey, L.M.: Secondary unilateral cleft lip repair: Combining rotation-advancement principles with a cross-lip muscle-vermilion flap, Ann. Plast. Surg. **3:**241, 1979.
28. Jackson, I.T., Scheker, L.R., Vandervord, J.G., and McLennan, J.G.: Bone marrow grafting in the secondary closure of alveolar-palatal defects in children, Br. J. Plast. Surg. **34:**422, 1981.
29. Jackson, I.T., and Soutar, D.S.: The sandwich Abbe flap in secondary cleft lip deformity, Plast. Reconstr. Surg. **66:**38, 1980.
30. Juri, J., Juri, D., and De Antueno, J.: A modification of Kapetansky technique for repair of whistling deformities of the upper lip, Plast. Reconstr. Surg. **57:**70, 1976.
31. Kapetansky, D.I.: Double pendulum flaps for whistling deformities in bilateral cleft lips, Plast. Reconstr. Surg. **47:**321, 1971.
32. Kawamoto, H.K.: Correction of major defects of the vermilion with cross-lip vermilion flap, Plast. Reconstr. Surg. **6:**35, 1979.
33. Lamont, E.S.: Reparative surgery of cleft lip and nasal deformities, Surg. Gynecol. Obstet. **80:**422, 1945.
34. Lehman, J.A., Jr.: The dynamic Abbe flap, Ann. Plast. Surg. **3:**401, 1979.
35. Lexer, E.: Der plastische Ersatz des septum cutaneum, Dtsch. Z. Chir. **81:**560, 1906.
36. Masters, F.W., and Craft, P.D.: Corrections of ''notch'' or ''whistling'' deformities of the lip. In Georgiade, N.G., and Hagerty, R.F., editors: Symposium on management of cleft lip and palate and associated deformities, St. Louis, 1974, The C.V. Mosby Co.
37. Millard, D.R.: A primary camouflage of the unilateral harelip, Transactions of the First International Congress of Plastic Surgery (1955), Baltimore, 1957, Williams & Wilkins.
38. Millard, D.R., Jr.: Columellar lengthening by a forked flap, Plast. Reconstr. Surg. **22:**454, 1958.

39. Millard, D.R.: Lengthening the columella. In Georgiade, N.G., and Hagerty, R.F., editors: Symposium on management of cleft lip and palate and associated deformities, St. Louis, 1974, The C.V. Mosby Co.
40. Millard, D.R., Jr.: Cleft craft: the evolution of its surgery, vol. 1, The unilateral deformity, Boston, 1980, Little, Brown & Co.
41. Morel-Fatio, D., and Lalardrie, J.P.: External nasal approach in the correction of major morphologic sequelae of the cleft lip nose, Plast. Reconstr. Surg. 38:116, 1966.
42. Neuner, O.: Secondary correction of cleft lip and plate. In Sanvenero-Rosselli, G., and Boggio-Robutti, editors: Transactions of the Fourth International Congress of Plastic Surgery, Amsterdam, 1967, Excerpta Medica Foundation.
43. O'Connor G.B., and McGregor, M.W.: Surgical formation of the philtrum and the cutaneous upsweep, Am. J. Surg. 95:227, 1958.
44. O'Connor, G.B., et al.: Advancement of soft tissue to correct mild mid-facial retrusion, Plast. Reconstr. Surg. 52:42, 1973.
45. Oneal, R.M.: Oronasal fistulas. In Grabb, W.C., Rosenstein, S.W., and Bzock, K.R., editors: Cleft lip and palate, Boston, 1971, Little, Brown & Co.
46. Oneal, R.M., Greer, D.M., Jr., and Novel, G.L.: Secondary correction of bilateral cleft lip deformities with Millard's midline muscular closure, Plast. Reconstr. Surg. 54:45, 1974.
47. Onizuka, T.: Philtrum formation in the secondary cleft lip repair, Plast. Reconstr. Surg. 56:522, 1975.
48. Onizuka, T., et al.: A new method to create a philtrum in secondary cleft lip repairs, 62:842, 1978.
49. Perko, M.A.: Secondary lip correction in unilateral cleft lips, J. Maxillofac. Surg. 5:245, 1977.
50. Peterson, R.A., Ellenber, A.H., and Carroll, D.B.: Vermilion flap reconstruction of bilateral cleft lip deformities (a modification of the Abbe procedure), Plast. Reconstr. Surg. 38:109, 1966.
51. Pigott, R.W., and Millard, D.R., Jr.: Correction of the bilateral cleft lip nasal defect. In Grabb, W.C., Rosenstein, S.W., and Bzoch, K.R., editors: Cleft lip and palate, Boston, 1971, Little, Brown & Co.
52. Puckett, C.L., Reinisch, J.F., and Werner, R.S.: Late correction of orbicularis discontinuity in bilateral cleft lip deformity, Cleft Palate J. 17:34, 1980.
53. Randall, P., Whitaker, L.A., and LaRossa, D.: The importance of muscle reconstruction in primary and secondary cleft lip repair, Plast. Reconstr. Surg. 54:316, 1974.
54. Robinson, D.W., Ketchum, L.D., and Masters, F.W.: Double V-Y procedure for whistling deformity in repaired cleft lips, Plast. Reconstr. Surg. 46:241, 1970.
55. Schmid, E.: The use of auricular cartilage and composite grafts in reconstruction of the upper lip, with special reference to construction of the philtrum. In Broadbent, T.R., editor: Transactions of the Third International Congress of Plastic Surgery, Amsterdam, 1963, Excerpta Medica Foundation.
56. Smith, J.W.: Clinical experiences with the vermilion bordered lip flap, Plast. Reconstr. Surg. 27:527, 1961.
57. Spira, M., Findlay, S., Hardy, S.B., and Gerow, F.J.: Early maxillary orthopedics in cleft palate patients: a clinical report, Cleft Palate J. 6:461, 1969.
58. Spira, M., Hardy, S.B., and Gerow, F.J.: Correction of nasal deformities accompanying unilateral cleft lip, Cleft Palate J. 7:112, 1970.
59. Straith, C.L., Straith, R.E., and Lawson, J.M.: Reconstruction of the harelip nose, Plast. Reconstr. Surg. 20:455, 1957.
60. Tennison, C.W.: The repair of the unilateral cleft lip by stencil method, Plast. Reconstr. Surg. 9:115, 1952.
61. Trauner, R.: Correction of nose deformities during first operation of unilateral harelips. In Skoog, T., editor: Transactions of the First International Congress of Plastic and Reconstructive Surgery, Baltimore, 1957, Williams & Wilkins.
62. Vecchione, T.R.: Construction of the cupid's bow, Plast. Reconstr. Surg. 65:830, 1980.
63. Webster, J.P.: Crescentic peri-alar cheek excision for upper lip flap advancement with a short history of upper lip repair, Plast. Reconstr. Surg. 16:434, 1955.

CHAPTER 24

Orthodontic treatment in craniofacial anomalies

PETER J. COCCARO

The initial examination of a patient with a craniofacial abnormality involves a thorough inspection of the oral cavity, including all the soft and hard tissues. Routine screening for dental caries, missing teeth, and characteristics of the gingiva, tongue, and palatal and pharyngeal structures is essential. Clinical and radiographic assessment of any existing jaw disparities and the status of the accompanying dental malocclusion should be recorded. A general history of any medical problems involving breathing, eating, and swallowing are vital to underlying etiologic factors responsible for open bite and speech-associated disorders. Deviations in palatal architecture and development may be closely identified with both of these problems. A history of the patient, including problems during growth and development and the age and onset of the condition under study, should be recorded.

TREATMENT OF CLEFT LIP AND PALATE

Orthodontists' services may be necessary throughout the formative years for children with a cleft lip and palate.[3,27,31-33] Knowledge of growth and development of the jaws and dentition is linked with treatment procedures to counter the adverse impact the defect may have had on the maxilla and developing dentition. Special areas of interest to the orthodontist are (1) skeletal structures (maxilla, mandible, and cranium), (2) dentoalveolar structures (teeth and alveolar processes), and (3) the relationship of dentoalveolar structures to skeletal structures. The same may be true for other types of craniofacial deformities.

Nature of the cleft

The cleft appears more often in the dentoalveolar area where the developing lateral incisor would normally be located (between the maxillary central incisor and the canine). In all types of cleft lip and palate, except in the lip and alveolar group, the defect involves the premaxilla, palatal processes of the maxilla, and horizontal processes of the palatine bone. Disruption of the continuity of the bony palate contributes to the abnormality in muscle attachment and function, resulting in constriction of the palate and an accompanying malocclusion[5] (Fig. 24-1).

Although it is generally accepted that the forces exerted by the repaired lip musculature may displace the maxillary segments medially,[21,28] it is an established fact that early orthodontic treatment can effectively reposition malpositioned segments. As a result, the maldeveloped and displaced segments are not only improved in their position, but contribute toward the correction of the existing crossbite malocclusion.[3,19,33,34]

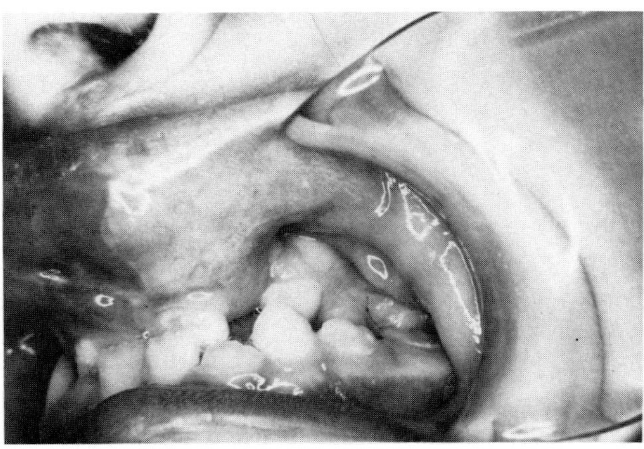

Fig. 24-1. Severe constriction of maxillary segments in a patient bilateral cleft lip and palate.

Philosophies of treatment

Two orthodontic treatment philosophies prevail for the child with cleft lip and palate. One philosophy is to defer treatment as long as possible and align the dental arches and supportive bone in a definitive one-stage treatment regimen after the permanent teeth have erupted. The other is to treat the problems early as they become evident.

Several periods of treatment are sometimes necessary for a given patient, beginning with deciduous teeth and extending trhough the mixed dentition to include all of the permanent teeth. These stages of treatment are followed by inevitable long periods of retention.

Advocates of the early treatment philosophy cite three basic reasons for orthodontic treatment procedures to be pursued on a continuing basis from childhood to adulthood. The first reason stems from the fact that there are usually displaced and/or deficient palatal segments. In addition, the palatal deformity carries with it abnormalities of the teeth that can create severe problems of malocclusion (Fig. 24-1). The second reason is that the growth of impacted palatal segments is adversely affected (Fig. 24-2). The third reason is the need to maintain the gains made in palatodental corrections and palatal growth. Results achieved at an early age need long periods of retention because of the high tendency for relapse of the displaced palatal segments.

On the other hand, children appear to tolerate a malocclusion such as crossbite very well. In the absence of a functional problem many orthodontists decide not to treat early, thus avoiding long periods of retention. However, some partial treatment is often undertaken for specific problems such as rotated incisors that interfere with a pleasing cosmetic affect.

Since variations are noted in all types of clefts, each case should be analyzed on an individual basis. The orthodontic approach, whether involving early or deferred treatment, should employ treatment procedures designed to bring the deformed arch within normal limits by adulthood (Fig. 24-2).

Skeletal characteristics of the maxilla

It is generally accepted that the maxilla in children with cleft lip and palate is deficient in the vertical and horizontal dimensions.[16,20,29] This may vary with the severity of the cleft. Clinical and radiographic observations indicate that there are morphologic differences in the character of the palatal defect from one patient to another within specific cleft palate categories and between the different types.

One of the major clinical features common to many cleft lip and palates is the distorted and constricted maxillary arch. McNeil,[23] Nordin,[25] and others believe that a constriction of the maxilla cannot be avoided after lip surgery. Pruzansky and Aduss[28] have shown that other factors are

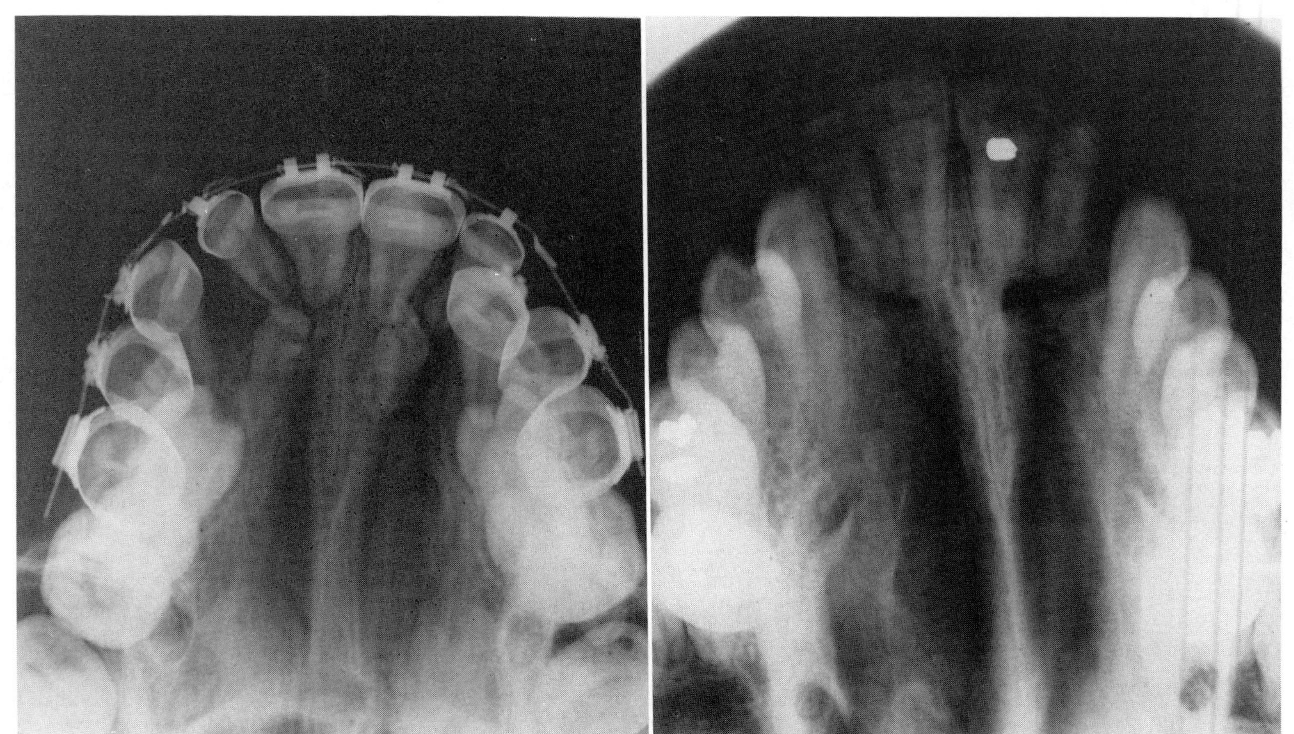

Fig. 24-2. Occlusal radiographic view of the changing character of the palatal segments and dental alignment resulting from orthodontic treatment.

responsible for collapse of the arch. Whether it is due to a molding effect of the lip after surgery or not, collapse of the arch is a skeletal factor orthodontists have to face up to in patients with cleft palate (Fig. 24-3). Since both displacement and deficiency of tissue are associated with cleft palates, the anatomic defect should be adequately defined as early as possible. Coupe and Subtelny[12] showed a deficiency of hard palate tissue in all types of clefts involving the hard palate. The deficiency was greatest in bilateral clefts.

Early management of the skeletal problem

Early orthodontic correction in the child with a cleft lip and palate has been recommended by many orthodontists in this country and is still widely practiced. It may be initiated after the eruption of all deciduous teeth, at approximately 3 years of age. [3,5,31-33]

The advantages of early treatment are believed to be many, particularly in the areas of function, esthetics, speech, and the improved anatomic relationships of parts that create the foundation to support the surgically reconstructed lip. Repositioning displaced palatal segments of the maxilla depends on the presence of sound teeth, both primary and permanent.

Early orthodontics in the mixed dentition does not preclude the need for orthodontics at a later age. Correction of skeletal and dental abnormalities is usually undertaken as soon as they become apparent. Although removable expansion appliances may be used, full banding and arch wires are usually the appliances of choice. Palatal segments are rotated laterally and anteriorly to improve arch form, and irregularities in the dentition can be corrected at the same time (Fig. 24-4).

Close observation should be continued until all the permanent teeth have fully erupted into the oral cavity. The final phases of orthodontic positioning of the permanent teeth should be complete by later adolescence.

The goals of early treatment involve correction of the arch form by way of repositioning impacted palatal segments; in later phases treatment focuses more on correcting dental irregularities. In some cases the need to establish a balance between arch form and the number and size of teeth exists. As a result the extraction of certain teeth may be in order.

Effects of orthodontics

As an apparent result of early treatment, favorable growth is believed to be encouraged within the malpositioned palatal segments. With a more normal appearing dental arch, the alveolar and palatal surfaces of the maxilla may reflect a growth expression that is directly related to the new and favorable position of the segments. Positive changes in maxillary dental arch form and the morphologic appearance of the alveolar process at the cleft site are believed to be closely correlated with early orthodontic therapy.

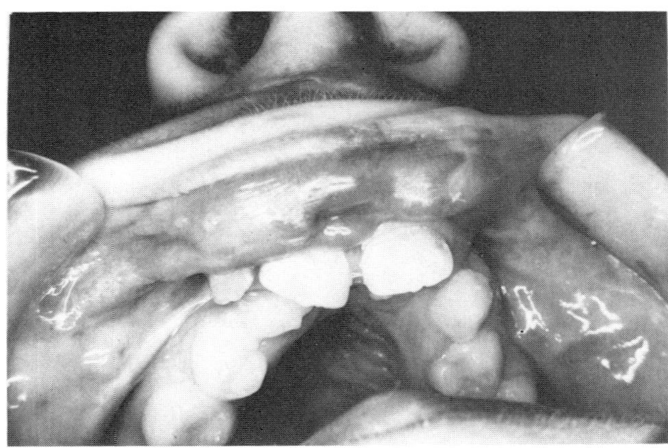

Fig. 24-3. Medially collapsed palatal segments and blocked out and impacted premaxilla.

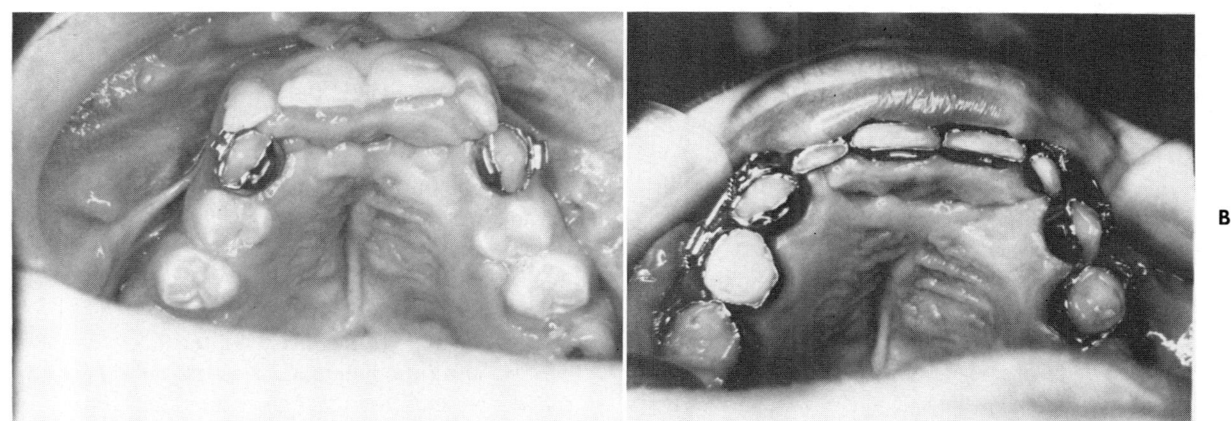

Fig. 24-4. A, Slight collapse of palatal segments during the transitional period of dental development. **B,** Improvements in maxillary arch form and dental alignment with orthodontic treatment.

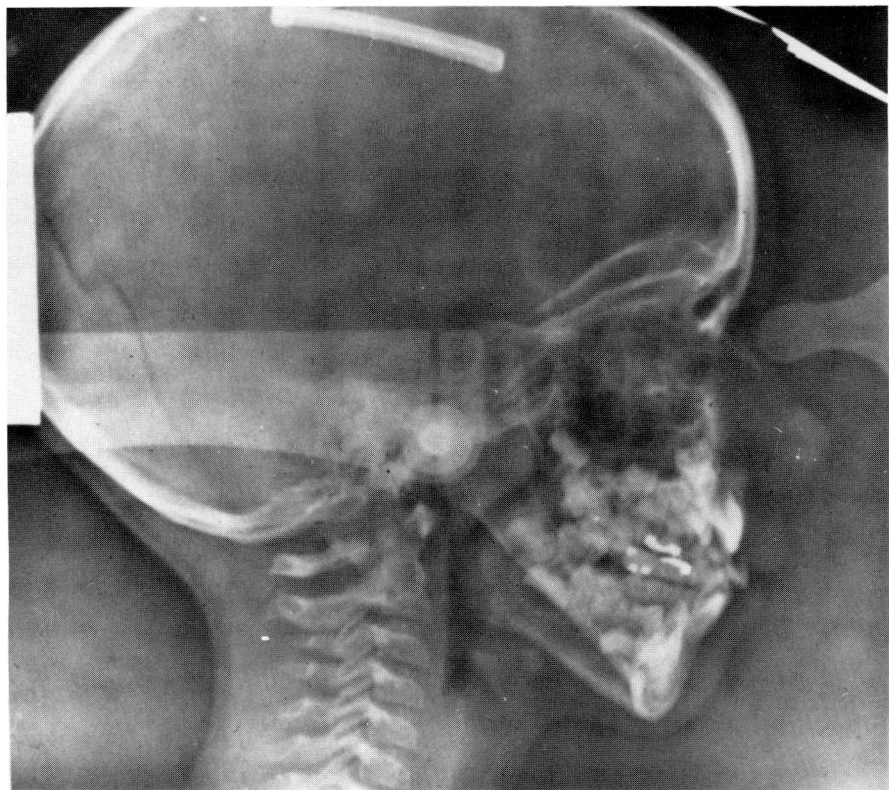

Fig. 24-5. Lateral cephalometric radiograph of a patient with hemifacial microsomia at 5 years of age. Observe the significant disparity in ramus height from the affected to the unaffected side.

TREATMENT OF HEMIFACIAL MICROSOMIA
Nature of the problem

Of all the anatomic structures that may be involved in patients with hemifacial microsomia, the one that has the greatest adverse impact on facial symmetry is the anomaly of the mandible on the affected side.[7] Malformations of the mandible reflect a wide range of variability, from no apparent discernible effect to a complete agenesis of the condyle and ramus. Accompanying the various mandibular anomalies are alterations in mandibular position associated with growth disparities between the affected and unaffected sides (Fig. 24-5). As a result, facial asymmetry and varying degrees of severe malocclusion are common findings in these patients. In addition to mandibular deformities, there is also a generalized hypoplasia of the dentoalveolar process of the maxilla noted on the affected side. This contributes to the abnormal cant of the occlusal plane and the higher dentoalveolar and occlusal levels commonly seen on the affected side of the maxilla. Such a finding tends to reflect an underdevelopment of the alveolar process and the infraeruption of the accompanying dentition. It may be assumed that failure of the mandible to achieve maximal vertical growth on the abnormal side and produce the needed interocclusal space limits the downward growth of the maxilla, dentition, and alveolar processes.[9,10]

PHILOSOPHY OF TREATMENT

Falkowski[14] inserted an iliac crest graft so that soft tissue would not be deprived of the essential functional and physiologic stimuli. The more localized nature of the deformity as seen in the acquired asymmetry may give a better prognosis when functional therapy is established at an early age.[3]

Parker[26] reports a bone graft in a 13-year-old girl. The earlier the bone graft can be inserted, the better it will be as far as maxillary growth is concerned, if it is believed, as Kazanjian[17] suggested, that the deficient growth of the mandible on the affected side will also limit maxillary growth on that side. If the hypothesis that the maxilla and accompanying dentoalveolar processes depend on the growth and lowering of the mandible is correct, then early functional therapy should be feasible to mechanically produce the space and favorably alter the structure of the mandible.

Skeletal character of mandible

Condylar growth sets the stage for the resulting morphologic pattern of mandibular development via activity of the appropriate muscles attached to the ramus, body, and symphysis of the mandible.[2,13]

In condylar growth deficiency the actual cause of the prenatal dysplasia is unknown. The effect on the mandible is one of overall reduction in size on the affected side with significant alteration of the muscular actions.[4] Mandibular development is determined by function, which in turn affects bone remodeling.[1]

According to Moss,[24] the growth of any mandibular skeletal unit is secondary and adaptive to changes in the functional matrix. Growth in length and the overall development of the mandible depend on the process of bone remodeling, and this is affected by the functional matrix. This matrix leads the directions of growth of the mandible and answers special needs at various times by apposition and deposition of bone.

Normal bone growth and maintenance of osseous form are primarily a reflection of the functional demands made on the ligaments and muscles of the temporomandibular joint.

Treatment

Immediate restoration of normal function is desirable for the growing child because normal bone growth and maintenance of osseous form are primarily a reflection of the mechanical requirements of the structures needed to carry out the function of mastication.

Thus a more critical analysis of the nature of mandibular deformities and their postnatal patterns of growth are an integral part of the overall diagnosis and treatment plan for patients with a first and second branchial arch anomaly.[7,10,13,36] This appears to be in conflict with the general concept that childhood mandibular deformities be deferred until mandibular growth directed by the presumed growth center is complete.

The orthodontist should address this kind of reasoning and determine the best course of treatment. The beneficial impact resulting from orofunctional therapy plus full orthodontic treatment at a later stage is intimately associated with the future decision for surgical planning. The impact of surgery at different age levels should be an important consideration and should be tempered with the full knowledge of the growth potentials of the mandible in question. Orthodontists should use their skills to improve mandibular position and enhance the growth potential of the mandible with obvious growth disparities.

Functional therapy affects changes in the structure of the condyle, as well as other processes of the mandible.[18,30] It is indicated when the status of the functional components of the temporomandibular joint warrant such treatment procedures. Thus functional therapy should be employed above and beyond the routine orthodontic procedures to improve dental balance and alignment within each arch. The final resolution in some of these skeletal anomalies, however, is to be obtained through surgery.[8,10,11,18]

TREATMENT OF CRANIOFACIAL SYNOSTOSIS
Nature of the malformation

Despite the early release of prematurely closed cranial sutures, midfacial hypoplasia becomes increasingly apparent with growth and development. The maxilla is hypo-

plastic and has failed to achieve normal dimensions in width, height, and depth. More important, it has failed to relocate anteriorly and inferiorly to a satisfactory degree. As a result, there is a "dished in" facial appearance with (pseudo) facial prognathism that is more related to the deformity in the maxilla than an abnormality within the mandible. It would appear that lack of normal growth at the site of the transverse palatine suture is highly suggestive of a premature closure of the suture. It precludes essential movement of the palatal processes of the maxilla away from the horizontal processes of the palatine bone. As a result, the normal process of bone apposition that follows from such movement at the site of the transverse palatine suture is retarded or absent in these cases. To add to the progressive facial prognathic profile is the active ongoing growth discernible in the mandible. This will vary depending on the character of growth inherent in the mandible for each patient.[36] Failure of the maxilla to move away from the cranial base also produces problems in development for nasopharyngeal height and depth, resulting in little if any patency of the velopharyngeal isthmus. Difficulty in nasal respiration contributes to mouth breathing. Furthermore, the deficient maxilla creates an imbalance between the developing dentition and the accompanying arch length and form. Thus skeletal and dental structures are severely affected and combine to produce a severe dental malocclusion.[15]

Philosophy of orthodontic treatment

The need for early and continuous orthodontic treatment is closely allied to the obvious growth abnormalities within the maxillary complex. The secondary impact it has on the imbalance between tooth material and arch length makes early intervention essential. The lack of space in the dental arch becomes quite apparent about the time of the erupting maxillary first permanent molars; blocked out or impacted first and second premolars are not an uncommon finding in these patients. Hence, most of these patients would profit by a serial extraction treatment program that would provide the essential balance needed between tooth material and arch length. The removal of primary maxillary and mandibular first molars plus their permanent successors (first premolars) bilaterally should be routine, particularly in light of our knowledge about growth and development of the abnormally retrusive maxilla.

Effects of treatment

Since the skeletal disparities between the developing maxilla and mandible are so great, it becomes obvious that orthodontics alone cannot correct the extremes in malocclusion seen in these patients. Thus early orthodontic treatment procedures should be directed toward creating a balance between the number and size of the teeth and the existing arch length. Good dental alignment and arch form are helpful to establish before surgery, but this is not always practical or feasible. Preoperative orthodontic treatment is carried out to maximize the beneficial effects resulting from the LeFort III surgical procedure.[35] Orthodontic appliances also provide necessary fixation after the osteotomies, an important function in the whole process of the surgical experience.

After a plan of analysis using cephalometric radiographs and dental models, determinations are made regarding the type of movement and the amount of relocation of the maxilla anteriorly and inferiorly.[6,9-11] An acrylic wafer is used to dictate positioning of the maxilla. If satisfactory orthodontic treatment has been accomplished, good dental interdigitation may occasionally be achieved in the operating room to permit intermaxillary fixation of the osteotomized maxilla to the mandible.

Skeletal characteristics of the maxilla

The maxilla is hypoplastic, as it is in patients with cleft lip and palate, but differs with respect to growth and development. Growth abnormalities associated with craniofacial synostosis are due to failure of growth expression at important facial sutural sites, whereas in cleft lips palates there is a deficiency of hard and soft palatal tissue. In the presence of deficient and distorted palatal segments, there still is a growth pattern not unlike that noted for normal persons. This is not true for patients with craniofacial synostosis, in whom the growth pattern for the maxilla has been interrupted. This is translated into differences in respiration and speech between the two groups. For patients with craniofacial synostosis breathing is difficult through the nasal portal and speech may be hyponasal; patients with clefts have above-average patency within the velopharyngeal isthmus, creating no breathing problems, but a potential for hypernasal speech.[6,15,22]

Management of skeletal problems

Orthodontic treatment is reserved for correcting dental irregularities. The skeletal aspects inherent in craniofacial

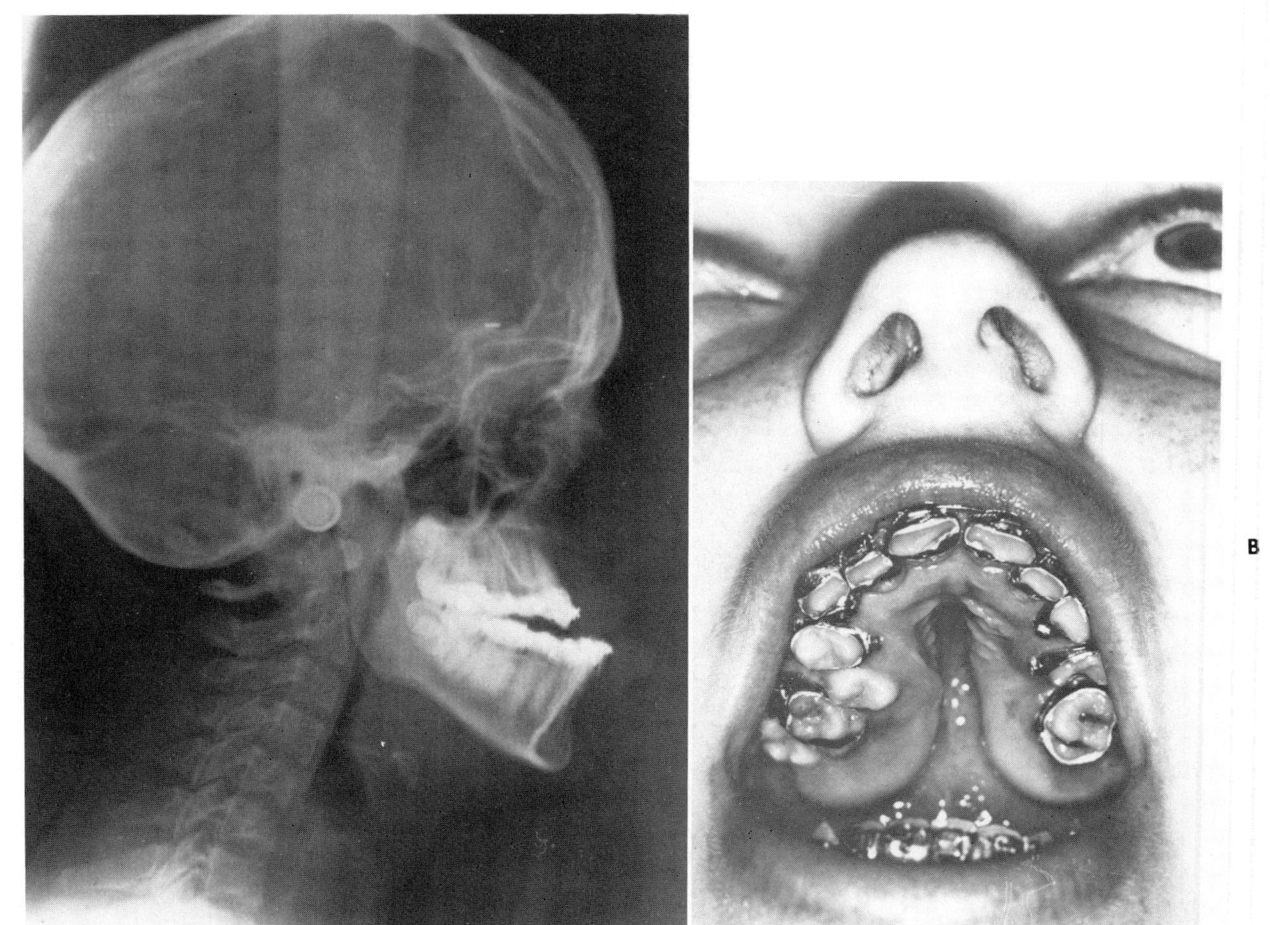

Fig. 24-6. A, Lateral cephalometric radiograph of a 13-year-old girl with Crouzon's disease. Note the dramatic impact of the hypoplastic maxilla on the skeletal and soft tissue profile and its effect in producing an abnormal pharyngeal height and depth. **B,** Byzantine arch commonly seen in patients with craniofacial synostosis. Note the fibromatous character of the gingivopalatal tissue.

synostosis have to be resolved through severe and radical cranial and facial surgery that often involves a neurosurgeon and plastic surgeon.[35] Orthodontists working closely with such a team can be effective in diagnostic treatment planning and presurgical orthodontics. They can contribute professional skills in the operating room by manipulation and positioning the osteotomized maxilla into a satisfactory relationship with the mandible. They can also apply intermaxillary fixation at that time to secure the positions established. Surgery is essential to free up the maxilla within the frontoorbitomaxillary regions. The patient is left in intermaxillary fixation for at least 10 weeks, preferably 12. Liquid diets are essential.

Case report

A 12-year-old girl with a diagnosis of Crouzon's disease exhibited all the clinical symptoms commonly seen in patients with craniofacial synostosis. The characteristic retrusive frontal bone and midfacial region combined to reduce the bony orbital dimensions. As a result, there was severe exophthalmos and a prominent prognathic facial profile. The retrusive maxilla failed to move away from the cranial base in a satisfactory downward and forward manner and created nasopharyngeal height and depth dimensions that were notably abnormal (Fig. 24-6). Difficulty in breathing through the nasal portal made it necessary for the child to breathe through her mouth.

The hypoplastic maxilla was deficient in its skeletal base development and produced disparities in the balance between the dental arch length and tooth material. Crowded and blocked out developing permanent teeth were inevitable and necessitated extraction of permanent premolars (right and left) (Fig. 24-6). This was an essential part of the presurgical orthodontic treatment plan needed to provide space within the dental arch for the eruption of the remaining permanent teeth. The dental arches were rounded out, and satisfactory occlusal levels were established within both jaws. Expansion forces were employed in the upper arch to ensure the needed space for the remaining teeth. This is important because of the severe deficiency of dental arch length in this syndrome. To attempt to reduce the great disparity that is prevalent anteroposteriorly, extraction of premolars in the lower arch was followed by a period of retracting the mandibular incisors (Fig. 24-7). Hence treatment of the dentition was directed to dental alignment and dental arch form that would permit a satisfactory interdental relationship when the jaws were brought together after the LeFort III maxillary advancement surgical procedure.[10,11,35]

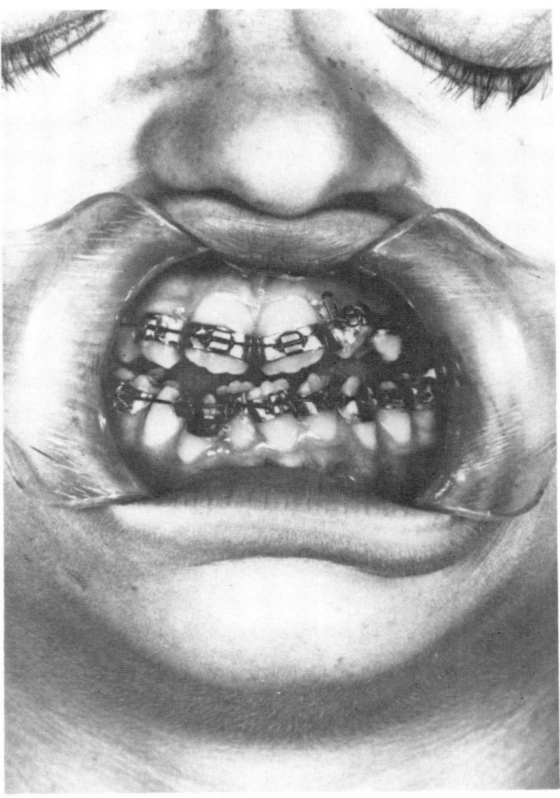

Fig. 24-7. Dental occlusion shows severe crowding of the dentition and a Class III malocclusion that is directly related to the skeletal abnormality in the upper face.

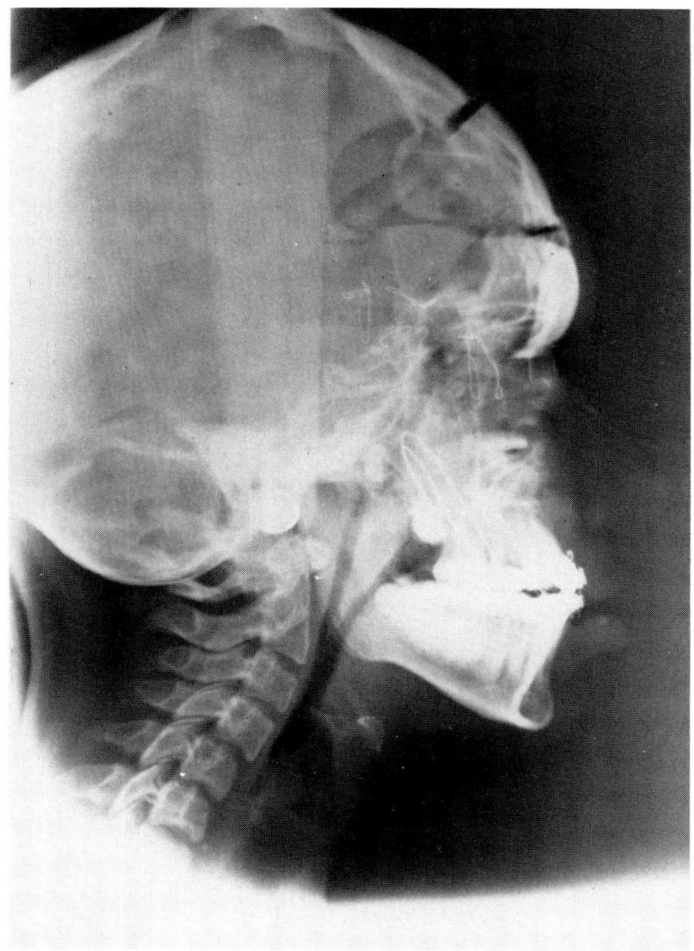

Fig. 24-8. Lateral cephalometric radiograph showing improvement in skeletal, dental, and soft tissue relationships for the patient after a frontoorbitomaxillary surgical advancement procedure.

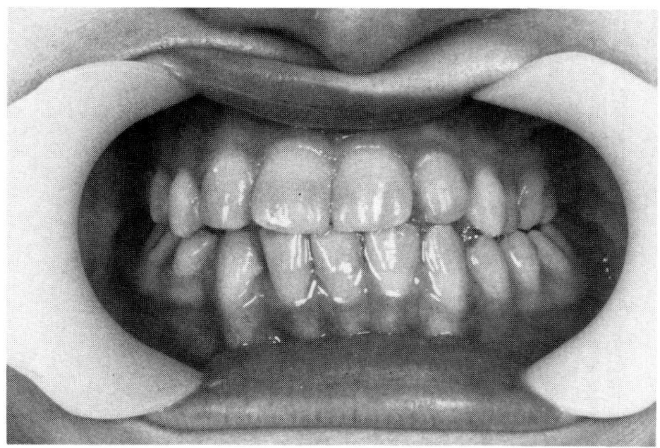

Fig. 24-9. Dental occlusion after the combined surgical and orthodontic treatment procedures.

After the satisfactory period of presurgical orthodontics, a frontoorbitomaxillary surgical procedure was performed. The neurosurgeon carried out the preliminary intracranial procedures, providing the plastic surgeon with ready access to the anterior cranial fossa. The essential osteotomies within the anterior cranial fossa and bony orbit and at the junction of the maxillary tuberosity and pterygoid plates permitted the movement to relocate the frontoorbitomaxillary regions of the upper and middle face to the desired inferior and anteroposterior levels (Fig. 24-8).

The treatment provided the necessary skeletal and dental corrective procedures needed to resolve all involved dental areas (Fig. 24-9). Surgical procedures were effective in improving orbital dimensions and reducing the severity of exophthalmos and the prognathic facial appearance (Fig. 24-10). Follow-up studies show that there is a high degree of stability for the osteotomized maxilla (Fig. 24-11).

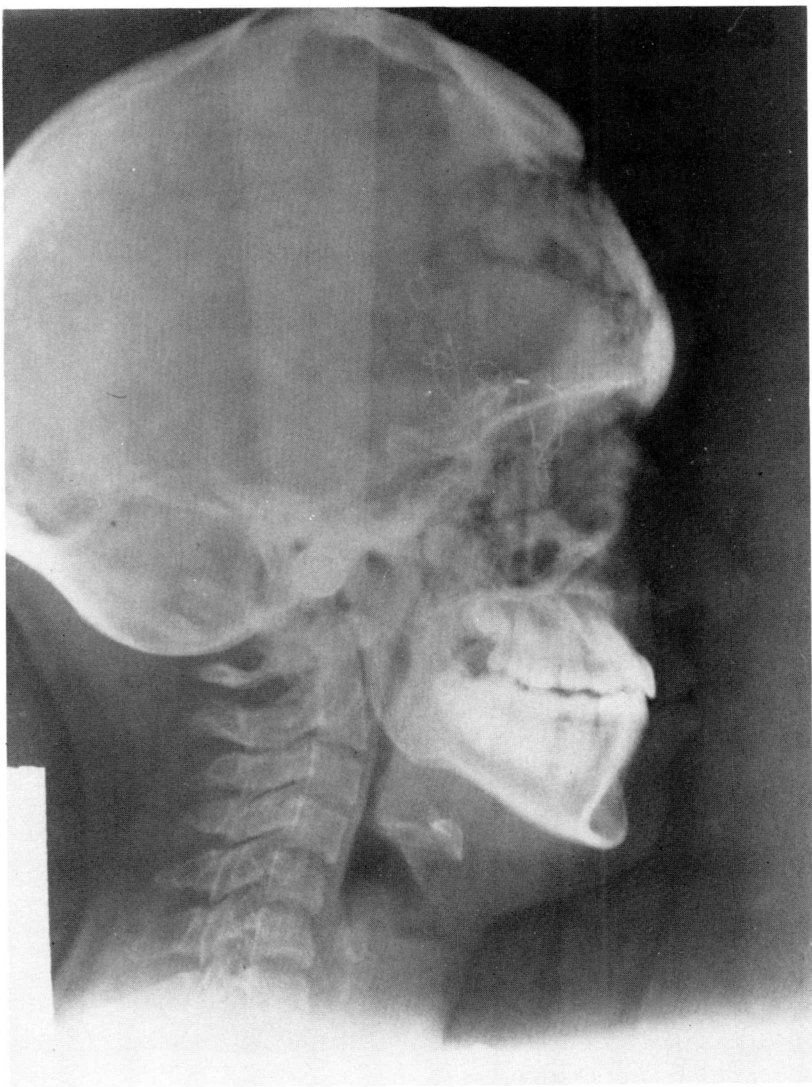

Fig. 24-10. Facial improvement after additional orthodontic treatment.

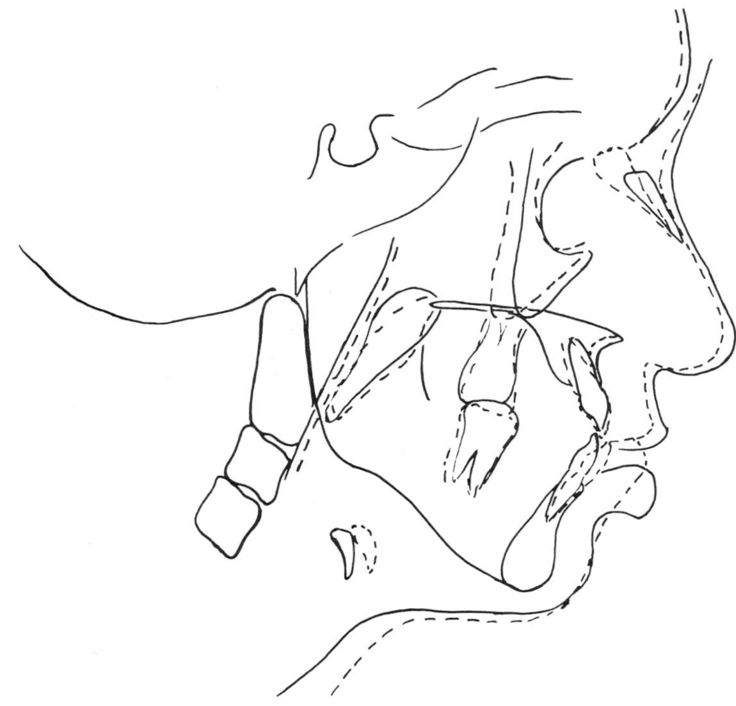

Fig. 24-11. Superimposed tracings of lateral cephalometric radiographs. A high degree of maxillary stability is possible after osteotomies of the maxilla. *Black line,* Postoperative appearance; *broken line,* postoperative appearance after 1 year.

SUMMARY AND CONCLUSIONS

The patient with craniofacial dysplasia requires coordinated, multidisciplinary treatment planning for optimal care. Knowledge of growth and development and the characteristics of specific syndromes are necessary prerequisites for successful management. The timing of treatment depends on the nature of the deformity and the overall goals of treatment.

For the patient with cleft lip and palate, an early orthodontic treatment approach has been stressed; however, this involves expansion of the dental arches and long-term retention. The patient with hemifacial microsomia has a deformity of the mandible and, in most instances, some distortion of the cant of the maxillary dental base. Early restoration of normal function in the dental arches is recommended. Later, surgery of the affected parts is the procedure of choice.

The patient with craniofacial synostosis is a candidate for early surgery to advance the midface area. Such surgery produces dramatic improvements in facial profile and provides improved nasopharyngeal dimensions for speaking and breathing.

REFERENCES

1. Becker, M.H., Coccaro, P.J., and Converse, J.M.: Antegonial notching of the mandible: an often overlooked mandibular deformity in congenital and acquired disorders, Radiology **121:**149, 1976.
2. Bosma, J.F.: Form and function in the infant's mouth and pharynx. In Bosma, J.F., editor: Third symposium on oral sensation and perception, the mouth of the infant, Springfield, Ill. 1972, Charles C Thomas, Publisher.
3. Coccaro, P.J.: Orthodontics in cleft palate children: a continuing process, Cleft Palate J. **6:**495, 1969.
4. Coccaro, P.J., Becker, M.H., and Converse, J.M.: Clinical radiographic variations in hemifacial microsomia, Birth Defects **11:**314, 1975.
5. Coccaro, P.J., and Valauri, A.J.: Orthodontics in cleft lip and palate children. In Converse, J.M., editor: Reconstructive plastic surgery: principles and procedures in correction, reconstruction and transplantation, ed. 2, Philadelphia, 1977, W.B. Saunders Co.
6. Converse, J.M., and Coccaro, P.J.: Diagnosis and treatment of maxillomandibular dysplasias, Am. J. Orthod. **68:**625, 1975.
7. Converse, J.M., Coccaro, P.J., Becker, M., and Wood-Smith, D.: On hemifacial microsomia: the first and second branchial arch syndrome, Plast. Reconstr. Surg. **51:**268, 1973.
8. Converse, J.M., Horowitz, S.L., Coccaro, P.J., and Wood-Smith, D.: The corrective treatment of the skeletal asymmetry in hemifacial microsomia, Plast. Reconstr. Surg. **52:**221, 1973.
9. Converse, J.M., Kawamoto, H.K., Wood-Smith, D., et al.: Deformities of the jaws. In Converse, J.M., editor: Reconstructive plastic surgery: principles and procedures in correction, reconstruction and transplantation, ed. 2, Philadelphia, 1977, W.B. Saunders Co.
10. Converse, J.M., McCarthy, J.G., Wood-Smith, D., and Coccaro, P.J.: Craniofacial microsomia. In Converse, J.M., editor: Reconstructive plastic surgery: principles and procedures in correction, reconstruction and transplantation, ed. 2, Philadelphia, 1977, W.B. Saunders Co.
11. Converse, J.M., Wood-Smith, D., McCarthy, J.G., and Coccaro, P.J.: Craniofacial surgery, Clin. Plast. Surg. **1:**499, 1974.
12. Coupe, T.B., and Subtelny, J.D.: Deficiency or displacement of tissue, Plast. Reconstr. Surg. **30:**426, 1962.
13. Engel, M.B., and Brodie, A.G.: Condylar growth and mandibular deformities, Surgery **22:**976, 1947.

14. Falkowski, S.: Czafsopismo. **7:**7, 1954.
15. Firmin, F., Coccaro, P.J., and Converse, J.M.: Cephalometric analysis in diagnosis and treatment planning of craniofacial dysostoses, Plast. Reconstr. Surg. **54:**300, 1974.
16. Graber, T.M.: A study of the congenital cleft palate deformity, doctoral thesis, Chicago, 1950, Northwestern University.
17. Kazanjian, V.H.: Jaw reconstruction, Am. J. Surg. **43:**249, 1939.
18. Knowles, C.C.: Cephalometric treatment planning and analysis of maxillary growth following bone grafting to the ramus in hemifacial microsomia, Dent. Pract. **17:**28, 1966.
19. Matthews, D., and Grossman, W.: Restoration of the collapsed maxillary arch by rapid expansion and bone grafting, Cleft Palate J. **1:**430, 1964.
20. Mazaheri, M., Harding, R.L., Cooper, J.A., and Meier, J.A.: Changes in arch form and dimensions of cleft patients, Am. J. Orthod. **60:**19, 1971.
21. Mazaheri, M., Harding, R.L., and Nanda, S.: The effect of surgery on maxillary growth and cleft width, Plast. Reconstr. Surg. **40:**22, 1967.
22. McCarthy, J.G., Coccaro, P.J., and Schwartz, M.D.: Velopharyngeal function following maxillary advancement, Plast. Reconstr. Surg. **64:**180, 1979.
23. McNeill, C.K.: Congenital oral deformities, Br. Dent. J. **101:**191, 1956.
24. Moss, M.L.: The functional matrix. In Kraus, B., and Riedel, R., editors: Vistas in orthodontics, Philadelphia, 1962, Lea & Febiger.
25. Nordin, D.E.: Treatment of primary total cleft palate deformity: preoperative orthopaedic correction of the displaced components of the upper jaw in infants, followed by bone grafting to the alveolar process clefts. In Hallet, G.M.: Trans. Eur. Orthod. Soc., The Hague, 1957.
26. Parker, C.D.: A case of marked asymmetry of the face due to a unilateral condylar hypoplasia, Dent. Pract. **13:**82, 1962.
27. Pruzansky, S.: The role of the orthodontist in a cleft palate team, Plast. Reconstr. Surg. **14:**10, 1954.
28. Pruzansky, S., and Aduss, H.: Prevalence of arch collapse and malocclusion in complete unilateral cleft lip and palate, Trans. Eur. Orthod. Soc. **1:**16, 1967.
29. Ross, R.B., and Johnston, M.C.: Cleft lip and palate, Baltimore, 1972, The Williams & Wilkins Co.
30. Smeets, H.J.: Orthodontic treatment of unilateral hypoplasia of the mandible, Br. Dent. J. **123:**170, 1967.
31. Subtelny, J.: The significance of early orthodontia in cleft palate habilitative planning, J. Speech Hear. Disord. **20:**135, 1955.
32. Subtelny, J.: Importance of early orthodontic treatment in cleft palate planning, Angle Orthod. **27:**148, 1957.
33. Subtelny, J.D.: Orthodontic treatment of cleft lip and palate: birth to adulthood, Angle Orthod. **36:**273, 1966.
34. Subtelny, J.D., and Brodie, A.G.: Analysis of orthodontic expansion in unilateral cleft lip and palate patients, Am. J. Orthod. **40:**686, 1954.
35. Tessier, P.: The definitive plastic surgical treatment of the severe facial deformities of craniofacial dysostosis: Crouzon's and Apert's diseases, Plast. Reconstr. Surg. **48:**419, 1971.
36. Walker, G.F.: Summary of a research report on the analysis of craniofacial growth, N. Z. Dent. J. **63:**31, 1967.

CHAPTER 25

Rare craniofacial clefts

JOSEPH G. McCARTHY and BARRY M. ZIDE

The person with a congenital facial deformity enters the world with a "spoiled identity."[9] By virtue of the disfigurement's visibility, the individual is reduced, in the perception of others and himself, from a whole and valued person to a tainted, discounted one. On the basis of the original stigma, society tends to impute a wide range of additional imperfections, thus geometrically extending the discreditation. In addition, the feeling of failure that exists for the mother and father must be considered. The sense of frustration has been described as a "chronic sorrow" that pervades the existence of parents with a mentally or physically deformed child.[17] It is not unusual to observe patients with severe facial deformity who demonstrate normal intellectual functioning and yet have been institutionalized and treated as retardates because of their physical stigmata. Patients with craniofacial clefts have a higher incidence of associated mental retardation, and the social deprivations and impairments in interpersonal functioning further weaken daily functioning.

Craniofacial clefts present much confusion for the clinician because of the myriad patterns of clinical expression. The clefts may be unilateral or bilateral, incomplete or complete. Since craniofacial clefts are rare, the number of clinical studies is limited, and there is a paucity of data relating to classification, incidence, and pathology.

CLASSIFICATION

For decades a diverse group of specialists have treated patients with rare craniofacial deformities; they described the patients according to their own special area of interest. However, severe craniofacial clefts with a conglomeration of deformities defy categorization. As one surgeon has stated, "How do you describe what is left of the glass after it shatters on the floor?"

To date, attempts at classification have had similar basic deficiencies. The American Association of Cleft Palate Rehabilitation (AACPR) divided craniofacial clefts into four major groups: (1) mandibular process clefts, (2) nasoocular clefts, (3) oroocular clefts, and (4) oroaural clefts.[11] This classification system was imprecise; it dealt only with surface anatomy, giving no consideration to the underlying skeletal pathologic condition. In addition, the system omitted the major midfacial clefts and the Treacher Collins' syndrome.

Boo-Chai[2] noted the deficiencies of this classification in his description of the oroocular cleft, which he subdivided into two types. The first type extends in a cephalic direction, from a point just lateral to the cupid's bow to a point medial to the infraorbital foramen; the other, which is rare, begins in a more lateral position on the upper lip and passes cephalad to a point lateral to the infraorbital foramen. The bony cleft spares the piriform aperture as it passes from the premolar teeth to the infraorbital rim.

Karfik[12] presented the following revised classfication of rare craniofacial clefts based on embryologic and morphologic criteria:

Group A Rhinencephalic disorders
    A1 Axial (frontonasal) problems
    A2 Paraxial (e.g., oroocular clefts) disorders
Group B Branchiogenic disorders
    B1 Lateral olocephalic (e.g., unilateral craniofacial microsomia) disorders
    B2 Medial axial (e.g., midline cleft of lower lip) disorders
Group C Ophthalmoorbital disorders (e.g., microphthalmos, upper-eyelid colobomata)
Group D Craniocephalic disorders (e.g., Apert's syndrome)
Group E Atypical facial disorders (e.g., hemiatrophy)

Tessier[22] categorized medial facial clefts into two broad groups: (1) those involving a tissue deficiency (Fig. 25-1) and (2) those having a normal or excess amount of tissue with an associated malformation (Fig. 25-2). The deficiency

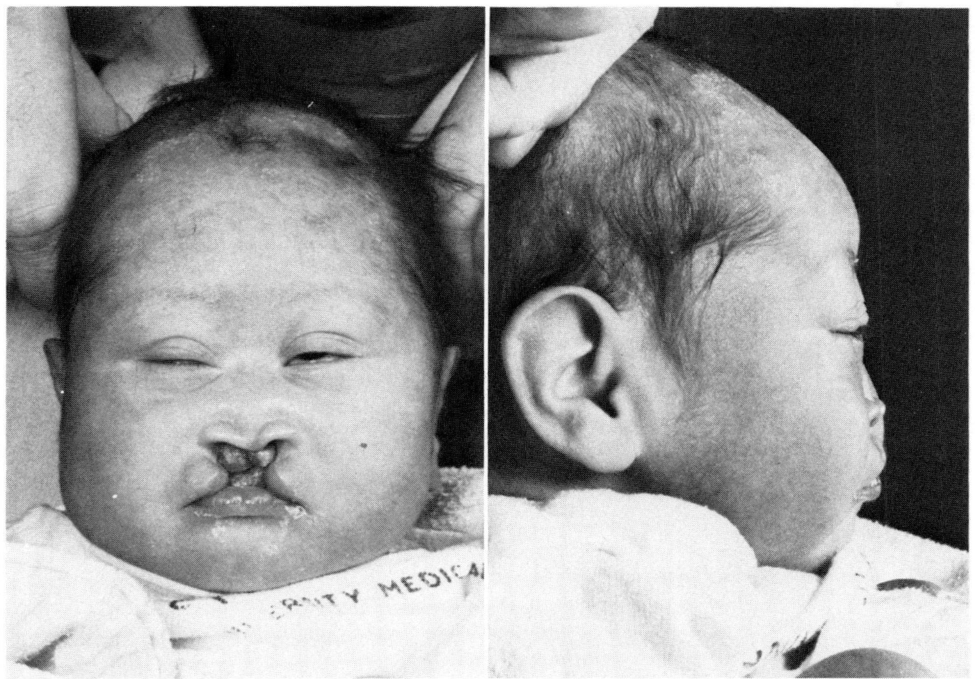

Fig. 25-1. Deficiency cleft. Note the hypotelorism, loss of nasal support, and median cleft lip.

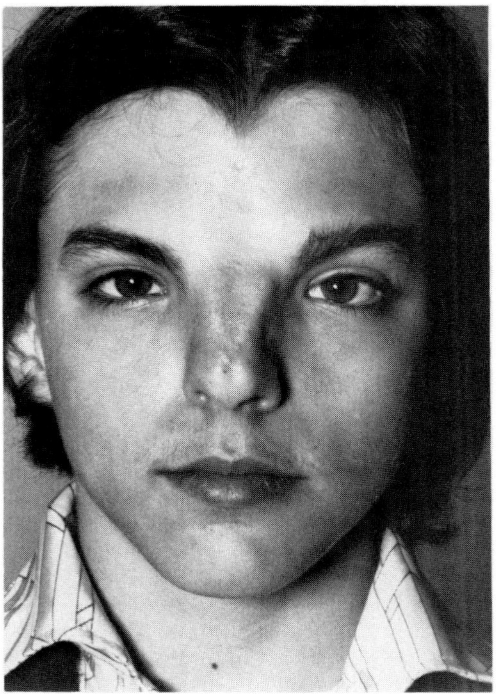

Fig. 25-2. Excess cleft. Note the hypertelorism, bifid nose, and hair peak.

clefts, called *arrhinencephaly** malformations, are caused by an underlying developmental arrest in cleavage of the forebrain. DeMyer,[7,8] proposed the term *holoprosencephaly* to denote the fact that the prosencephalon remains "holistic" (Figs. 25-3 and 25-4). There are five types of holoprosencephalic deformities: (1) cyclopia, (2) cebocephaly, (3) ethmocephaly, (4) orbital hypotelorism with median cleft lip, and (5) orbital hypotelorism with hypoplastic intermaxillary segment (bilateral cleft lip and a flat nose). All of these infants have some degree of orbital hypotelorism[3] and microcephaly.

DeMyer[7,8] has termed malformations with normal or excess midline tissue *median cleft face syndrome*. The correlation between the distorted face and the underlying prosencephalon is minimal. The spectrum of anomalies varies from a slight midline notch of the upper lip to severe orbital hypertelorism.

---

*The term *arrhinencephaly*, is derived from the rhinencephalon or primitive nosebrain, designates failure of the telencephalon to subdivide into cerebral hemispheres. This term is not entirely accurate. Although the olfactory bulbs are lacking, the rhinencephalon is present. The basic defect seems to be a failure of the rostral brain to develop a cleft in the midline.

The following seven features may be associated with this syndrome:

1. Orbital hypertelorism
2. V-shaped frontal hairline
3. Bifid cranium
4. Median cleft of the upper lip
5. Medial cleft of the premaxilla
6. Median cleft of the palate
7. Primary telecanthus

The probability of mental retardation is low when orbital hypertelorism is combined with one or more of the other six features. However, the chances of retardation increase when an extreme form of orbital hypertelorism is the sole anomaly or when extracephalic anomalies coexist. The term *frontonasal dysplasia* has been proposed by Sedano et al.,[20] who consider it to be at the opposite end of the spectrum from holoproscencephaly. The designation FND-EC has been devised for those patients with frontonasal dysplasia and associated extracephalic deformities.[19]

The Tessier classification

Although the Tessier system[22] is neither foolproof nor complete, its strengths are that it is based on anatomic stud-

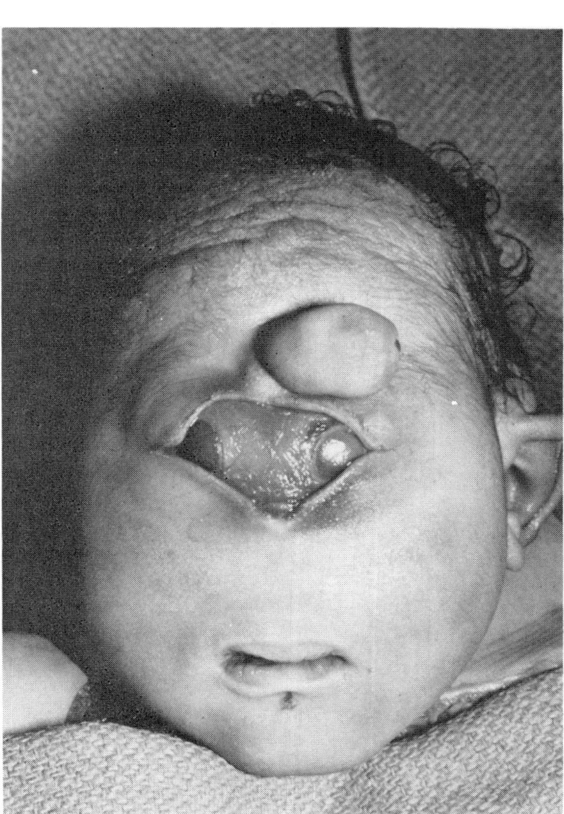

Fig. 25-3. Cyclopia. Hypotelorism of the most extreme type is demonstrated. The midline proboscis represents rudimentary nose formation.

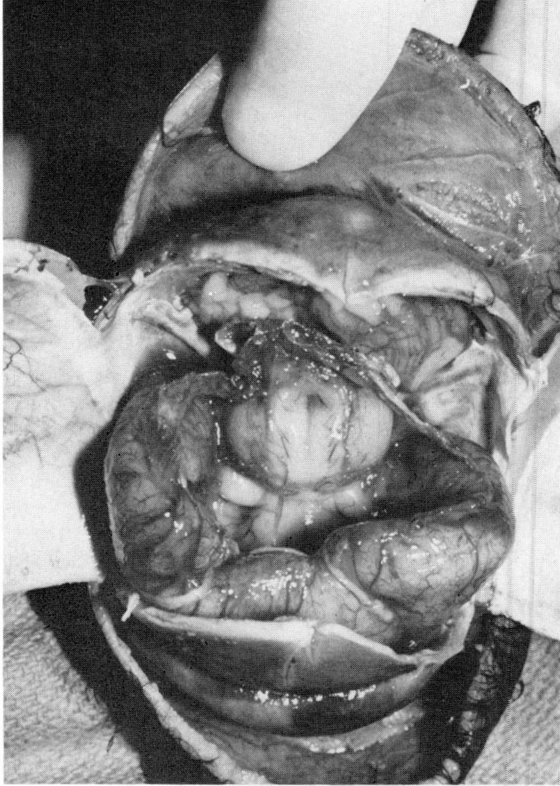

Fig. 25-4. Holoprosencephaly. Cleavage into the cerebral hemispheres does not occur when the brain remains "holistic" (autopsy specimen).

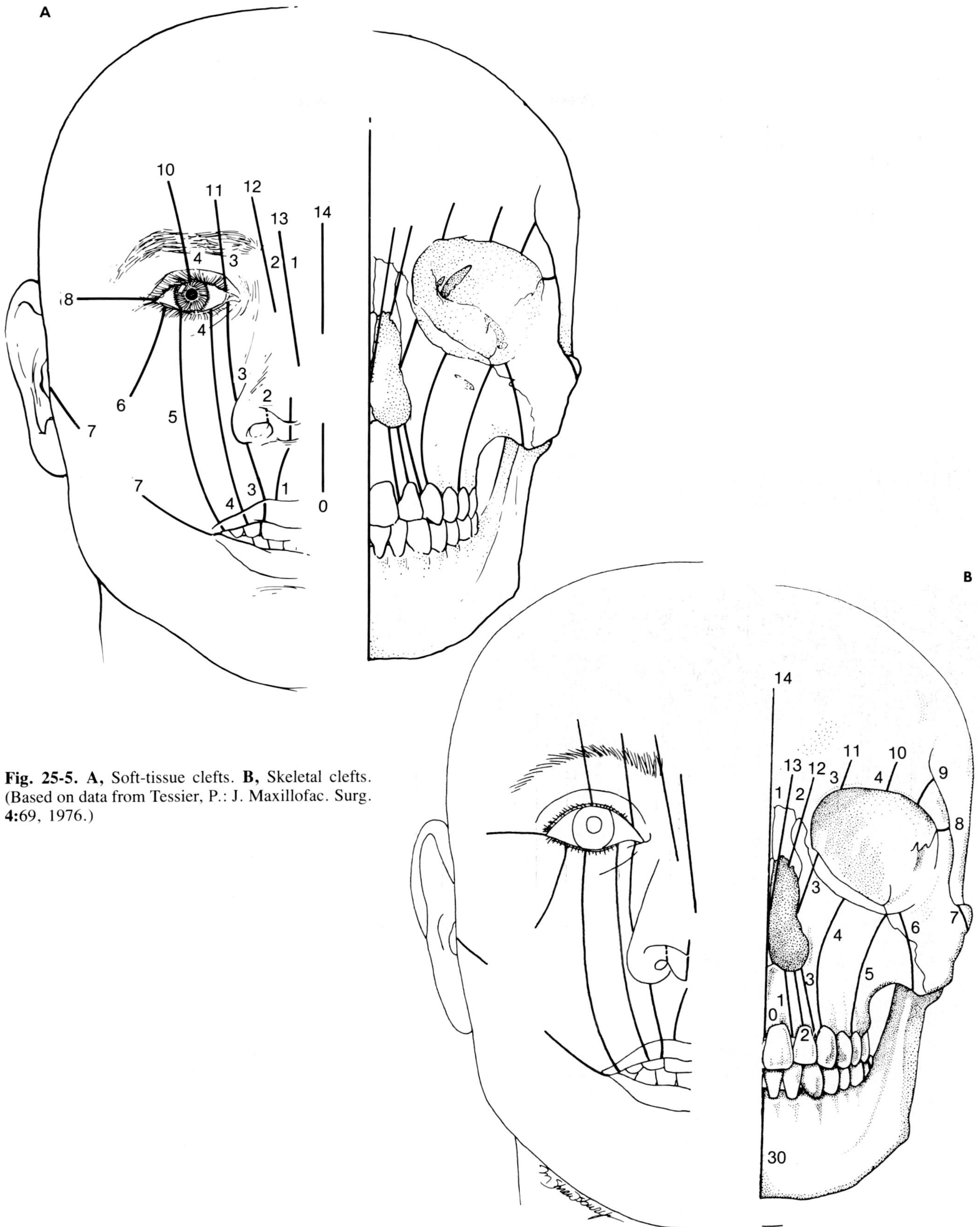

Fig. 25-5. A, Soft-tissue clefts. **B,** Skeletal clefts. (Based on data from Tessier, P.: J. Maxillofac. Surg. **4:**69, 1976.)

ies, and it can be easily and meaningfully used by the clinician. In this system the clefts are numbered from 0 to 14 and extend circumferentially around the orbit along constant planes from the lips to the cranium (Fig. 25-5). Those which are ''northbound'' extend through the upper eyelid and are considered to be cranial in nature. The ''southbound'' clefts, which are designated as facial, pass through the lower eyelid. The eye is the horizontal anatomic zone that separates the cranial from the facial clefts. Athough the clefts appear to follow certain time zones around the orbit, the embryonic processes do not coincide with the north-south pathways. The combination cranial and facial (craniofacial) clefts usually add up to 14; that is, a number 1 facial cleft is usually seen in combination with a number 13 cranial cleft, a number 2 facial with a number 12 cranial cleft, and so on.

The section that follows discusses the separate clefts as combinations, but *they do not always occur that way in reality.* Numbers 12, 13, and 14 clefts are most commonly associated with orbital hypertelorism, although numbers 9, 10, and 11 clefts can produce splaying of the orbits when there is sufficient disorganization.

Tessier[21] has classified orbital hypertelorism according to the radiographic distance recorded between the dacryons (the junction of the frontal, ethmoid, and lacrimal bones). The interorbital distance ranges between 22 to 28 mm in adult females and 24 to 32 mm by age 12. In the females the curve levels off at approximately 13 years, but in males

the interorbital distance continues to increase until age 21.[6] According to the Tessier classification[21] orbital hypertelorism can be divided into three groups:

Interorbital distance

First degree	30 to 34 mm
Second degree	34 to 40 mm
Third degree	40 mm

It should be emphasized that other measurements, such as interpupillary distance, can be misleading. Interpupillary distance can be falsely increased by exotropia, which is common in patients with orbital hypertelorism. Frequently the faces suggest the appearance of hypertelorism even when the radiographic interorbital distance is within normal range; this is ''illusory'' or ''pseudohypertelorism'' (Fig. 25-6). The illusion of hypertelorism may be caused by lateral displacement of the medial canthi, since pseudohypertelorism is commonly seen with orbital fractures (posttraumatic telecanthus), a flat nasal radix, blepharophimosis, widely spread eyebrows, or epicanthal folds.

The principal anatomic abnormality associated with the increase in interorbital distance is the horizontal widening of the ethmoid labryinth.[5] The increase in width of the ethmoidal sinuses is localized to the anterior part of the ethmoid bones and does not usually affect the posterior ethmoidal or sphenoidal sinuses. Although the roof of the ethmoidal sinuses may be enlarged, the cribriform plate is usually not significantly enlarged. Thus a combined intra-

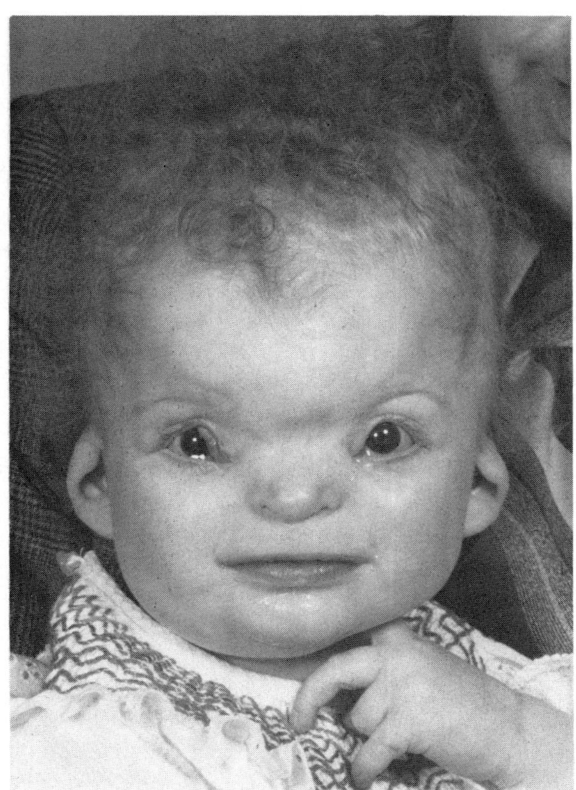

Fig. 25-6. Illusory hypertelorism. The bony interorbital distance (radiographic) is normal; a midline lipoma has produced telecanthus.

cranial-extracranial surgical procedure for the correction of orbital hypertelorism with preservation of the cribriform plate and olfactory nerves has been possible.

In the orbital hypertelorism syndromes the olfactory grooves may be enlarged and rounded, the crista galli absent or duplicated, but the sphenoid bone, including that portion between the optic foramina, usually shows no abnormalities. The latter finding by Tessier, that the optic canals were in normal position or minimally widened, encouraged surgical mobilization of the orbits to within 8 mm of the apex without fear of damage to the optic nerves.

The angle of divergence of the axis of each orbit from the midsagittal plane is approximately 25 degrees in the normal person but can increase to 60 degrees with severe hypertelorism. In the most severe cases the lateral wall of the orbit is reduced in the anteroposterior dimension; the lateral orbital rim may even be absent.

FEATURES OF RARE CRANIOFACIAL CLEFTS
Clefts 0 to14

This group includes median cleft face syndrome, holo-prosencephaly, and frontonasal dysplasia.

Incidence: Hypotelorism is rare; frontonasal dysplasia is seen more commonly.

Basic anatomic characteristics: May involve hyperplasia or hypoplasia (Figs. 25-1 and 25-2).

Chin and mandible
Unusual part of this syndrome; called cleft number 30 by Tessier (Fig. 25-7).

Lower lip, alveolus, and tongue
1. Notch in the lower lip, mandible, tongue, neck, hyoid bone, and sternum have been reported.
2. The tongue may be bifid.
3. The lower alveolus cleft passes between the central incisors.

Upper lip
1. True median cleft.
2. Occasionally the frenulum is duplicated.
3. In the hypoplasia type the philtrum may be absent.

Alveolus and palate
1. The cleft passes between the central incisors.
2. The cleft may continue posteriorly as cleft palate.
3. If hypoplastic, the premaxilla may not form.

Nose
1. Bifid (Fig. 25-8).
2. Wide columella.
3. Nostrils may be deformed asymmetrically.

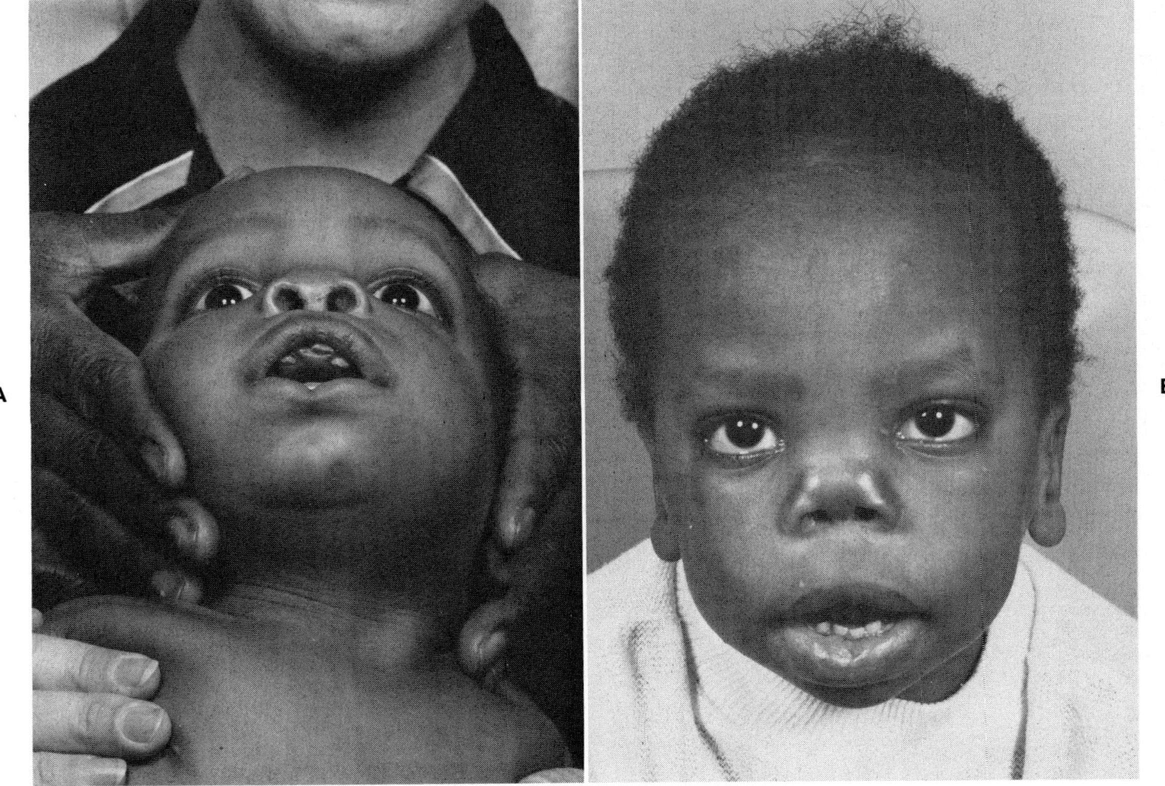

Fig. 25-7. A, Cleft number 30 showing midline cleft of the lower lip. Note the associated number 0 cleft. **B,** appearance after surgical correction of the lower lip.

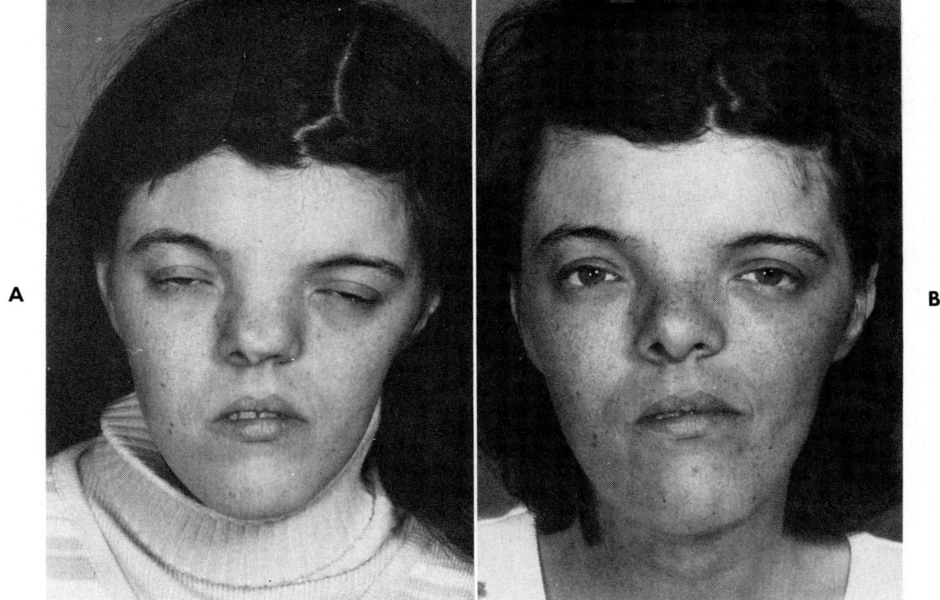

Fig. 25-8. A, Preoperative appearance of hypertelorism and a bifid nose. **B,** The excess nasal skin was resected and an autogenous bone graft placed on the nasal dorsum. Because of only minimal hypertelorism, orbital surgery was not performed.

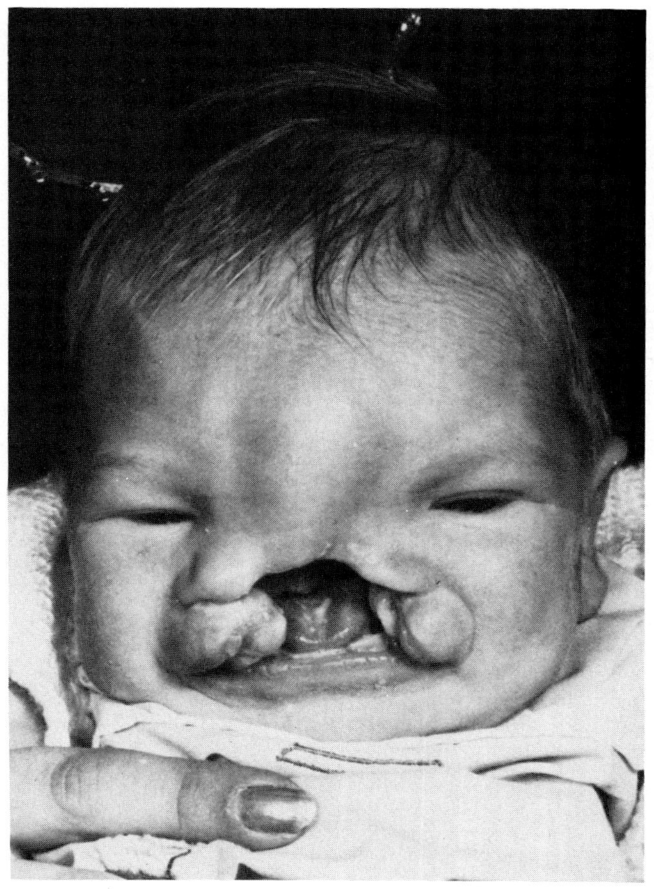

Fig. 25-9. Orbital hypertelorism and frontal encephalocele.

4. Upper lateral cartilages may be displaced, laterally or distorted.
5. The radix is broad; bones may be hyperplastic.
6. The septum is thick and double.
7. In the hypoplasia type, the columella may be small, flat, or absent.
   Cartilages may be hypoplastic or aplastic.
   Proboscis or arrhinia (absent nose) may be present.
   Septum may be aplastic.

Cranium with hypertelorism

1. Orbits are displaced by the bifid cranium or frontal encephalocele (Fig. 25-9).
2. Increased distance between the olfactory grooves.
3. The crista galli is widened, duplicated, or absent.
4. The cribriform plate is displaced downward.
5. Flattened frontal bone; indistinct glabella.

Cranium with hypotelorism

1. The cranium is microcephalic or trigonocephalic.
2. Associated holoprosencephaly malformations such as cyclopia and cebocephaly are present.

Clefts 1 to 13

Included in this category are proboscis lateralis, some cases of nasal hemiatrophy, and other cases previously grouped with frontonasal dysplasia and median cleft face syndrome.

Incidence: This cleft is rare and usually occurs in association with other clefts.

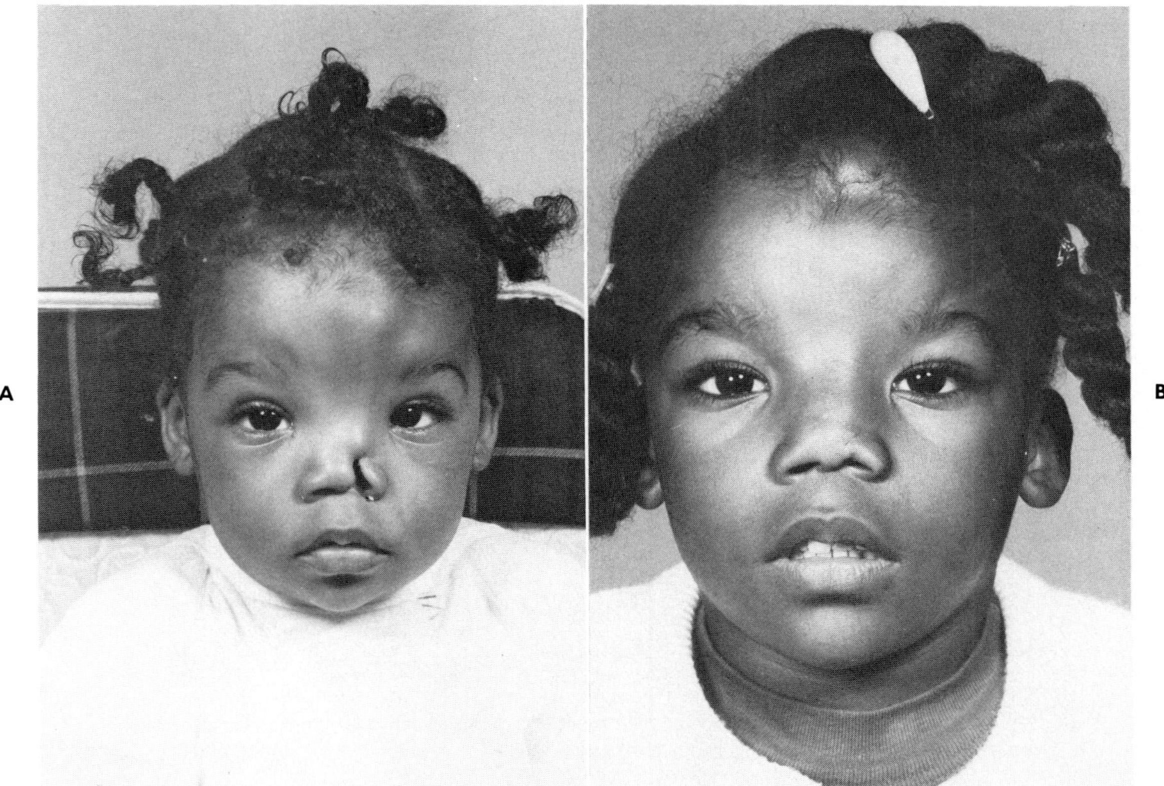

Fig. 25-10. A, Cleft number 2 extending through the alar rim. Note the cranial extension. **B,** Cleft number 2. The alar rim was transposed as a laterally based flap, and a cheek-nasal flap was inferiorly displaced. The frontal encephalocele was reduced and a bone graft placed in the defect.

Basic anatomic characteristics

Upper lip

1. The cleft begins at the cupid's bow and continues in a cephalic direction (Fig. 25-5).

Alveolus and nose

1. Notch in the nostril dome.
2. The septum is not involved.
3. A bony cleft passes between the central and lateral incisors, through the piriform aperture lateral to the anterior nasal spine, and through the nasal bone or nasofrontal junction and ethmoid bone.

Orbital and cranial region

1. Medial canthi are not involved, but orbital dystopia (vertical displacement) can occur.
2. The medial eyebrow is dystopic, since the cleft extends into the forehead-glabella area as in cleft number 13.
3. Hypertelorism.

Clefts 2 to 12

The nasoocular, paraxial, oblique facial, and nasomaxillary clefts (Fig. 25-10) are found in this group.

Incidence: Extremely rare.

Basic anatomic characteristics: The cleft lies at the union of the medial nasal and lateral nasal maxillary processes. Complete, incomplete, unilateral, and lateral forms can coexist.

Lip, alveolus, and nose

1. The lip cleft lies in the region of the common cleft lip.
2. The cleft passes through the midportion of the alar rim.
3. The lateral aspect of the nose is flattened.
4. The nasal bridge is flattened.
5. The bony cleft continues cephalad from a point between the lateral incisor and canine to the lateral piriform aperture. The frontal process of the maxilla is usually uninvolved.

Orbital region

1. Hypertelorism may be present.
2. Medial canthal dystopia (inferior displacement of the canthus).
3. Hypoplastic and displaced medial canthal tendon.
4. The cleft continues cephalad to the medial third of the upper eyelid, eyebrow, and frontal region.

Cranium

1. May cause orbital hypertelorism by traversing the ethmoidal labyrinth.

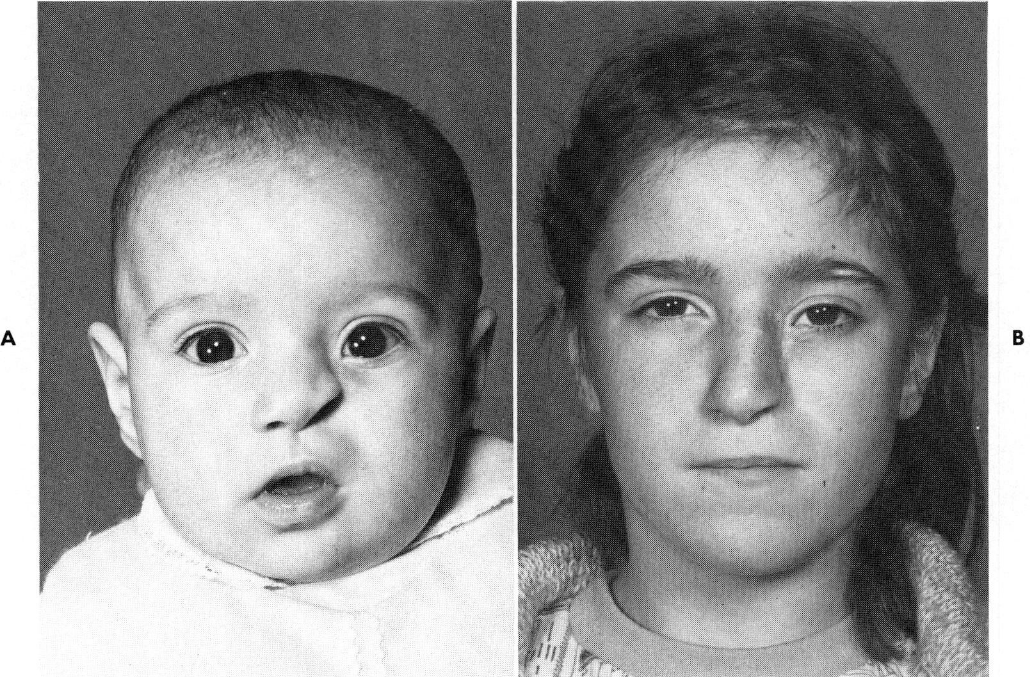

Fig. 25-11. **A,** Preoperative appearance of cleft number 3. **B,** The entire left side of the nose was elevated and transposed inferiorly. A full-thickness skin graft was placed in the dorsal defect.

2. May pass lateral to the ethmoid bone, producing a cleft in the medial third of the eyebrow and orbital rim.

Clefts 3 to 11

This category includes the nasoocular, paraxial, oblique facial, and nasomaxillary clefts (Fig. 25-11).

Incidence: More common than clefts 1 and 2.

Basic anatomic characteristics: The cleft lies at the union of the medial nasal, lateral nasal, and maxillary processes. Complete, incomplete, unilateral, and bilateral forms can coexist.

Lip and alveolus

Similar to common clefts of the lip and palate.

Nose

1. The cleft passes through the alar base (varies from a notch to a complete cleft).
2. The distance between the alar base and medial canthus is shortened.
3. The bony cleft continues cephalad from a point between the lateral incisor and canine to the lateral aspect of the piriform aperture. The nose and maxillary sinus may be unseparated. The frontal process of the maxilla is disrupted at the lacrimal groove.

Orbital region

1. The nasolacrimal system is disturbed. The lower canaliculus is beyond repair.

2. Medial canthal dystopia.
3. Lower-eyelid coloboma medial to punctum.
4. Hypoplastic and inferiorly displaced medial canthal tendon.
5. Possible microphthalmos.
6. The cleft continues cephalad to the medial third of the upper eyelid, eyebrow, and frontal region (Fig. 25-11).

Cranium

1. May produce hypertelorism by traversing the ethmoidal labyrinth.
2. May pass lateral to the ethmoid bone, producing a cleft in the medial third of the eyebrow and orbital rim.

COMMENT: The asymmetric nonmidline clefts are extremely difficult to correct. There is a considerable shortage of bony skeleton as well as soft tissue. Bone grafts are thus required to support the orbit and reconstruct the gaping skeleton. Skin flap coverage must be supplemented with mucosa from the nasal floor or septum. Extensive undermining is necessary to obtain the necessary soft-tissue coverage. The nasolacrimal apparatus, which is susceptible to recurrent infection, is best resected. A medial canthopexy is necessary to correct the dystopia. The globe must be protected unless there is microphthalmos.

Clefts 4 to 10

This group consists of oroocular, paraxial, and vertical facial clefts (Fig. 25-12).

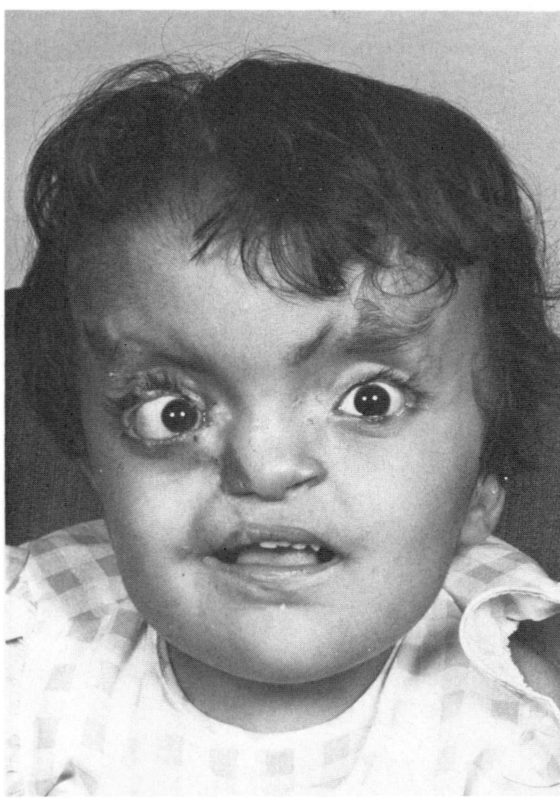

Fig. 25-12. Cleft number 4. The ala is tilted. A cleft extends cephalad through the medial brow (number 10 or 11 cleft). Cleft number 4, right. A discolored composite graft has resulted after reconstruction of the alar base. The nasolacrimal apparatus is affected. The cleft extends cephalad to the number 10 and 11 regions.

Incidence: Rare.
Basic anatomic characteristics
Lip and alveolus
1. The cleft is lateral to the cupid's philtral ridge (actually midway between the commissure and philtral column).
2. The cleft passes between the lateral incisor and canine.

Nose
The cleft does not pass through the nose or piriform aperture, but does cause tilting of the ala because of deficiency of the adjacent soft tissue and skeleton.

Cheek
1. The cleft passes lateral to the ala and terminates at a point medial to the punctum.
2. The bony cleft continues upward through the anterior wall of the maxillary sinus but lateral to the nasal wall.

Periorbital region
1. The nasolacrimal canal and sac are normal.
2. The globe usually is present, but some degree of hypoplasia may occur.

3. Coloboma of the upper eyelid.
4. The midportion of orbital rim is cleaved; the medial portion of orbital rim and floor may be involved.

Cranium
1. The cleft continues through the medial third of upper eyelid, eyebrow, and frontal bone.
2. The eyebrow is disrupted in the middle third.
3. The bony cleft continues upward from the midportion of the orbital rim through the midorbital roof and frontal bone.
4. A frontoorbital encephalocele is often present.
5. The cleft causes the orbit to be laterally and inferiorly displaced.

Clefts 5 to 9

Incidence: Number 5 is the rarest oblique facial cleft.
Basic anatomic characteristics (Fig. 25-5)
Lip and alveolus
1. The lip cleft is located medial to the commissure.
2. The skeletal cleft begins posterior to the canine in the premolar area.

Cheek and maxilla
1. The cleft courses upward across the lateral cheek to end between the middle and lateral third of the eyelid.
2. The vertical distance between the mouth and eyelid is decreased.
3. The bony cleft traverses the maxilla lateral to the infraorbital foramen to enter the orbit.
4. The orbital contents may prolapse into the maxillary sinus.

Periorbital region
1. Microphthalmos is frequent.
2. The bony cleft passes through the inferolateral orbital rim and orbital floor.
3. The cranial extension of the cleft continues at the junction of the medial and lateral third of the upper eyelid.

Cranium
The bony cleft at the superolateral rim of the orbit continues to the frontal bone.

Cleft 6

This category includes the incomplete form of Treacher Collins' syndrome. The complete form has clefts 6, 7, and 8 (Fig. 25-13).
Incidence: Common.
Genetic basis: Autosomal dominant.
Basic anatomic characteristics
Lip and alveolus
Not involved.

Malar area
1. Skin depression over the deficient malar bone.
2. The malar bone is present but hypoplastic.

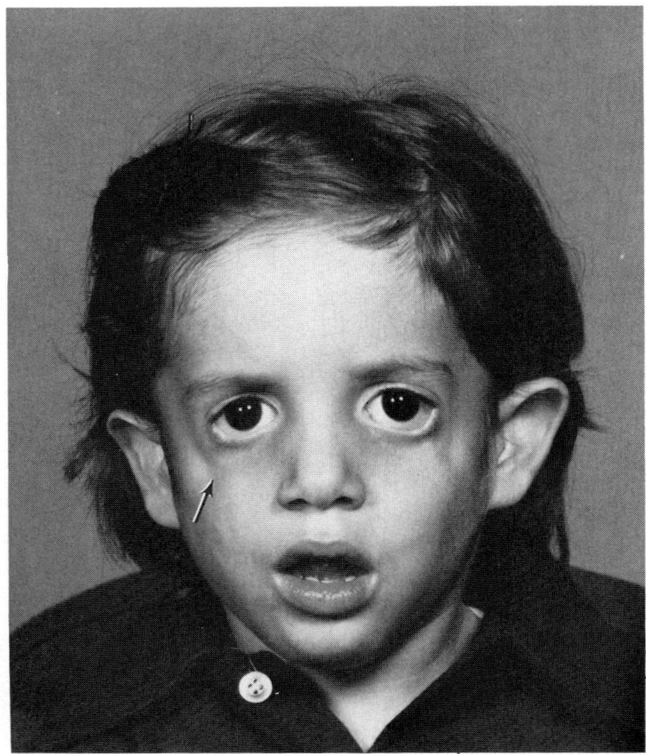

Fig. 25-13. Cleft number 6: Treacher Collins' syndrome. Note the zygomatic hypoplasia *(arrow)*, lower eyelid coloboma, and antimongoloid obliquity of the palpebral fissure.

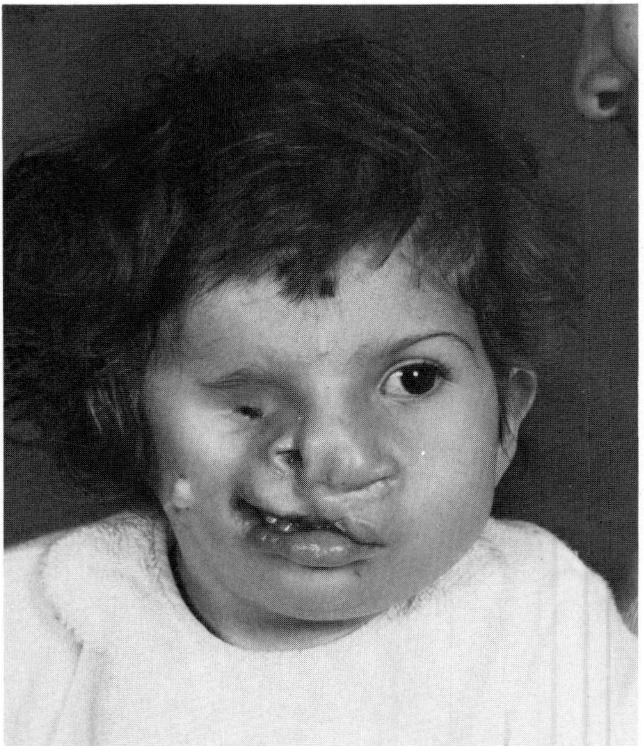

Fig. 25-14. Cleft number 7 with associated cleft numbers 0 and 2. Note the transverse cleft at the oral commissure. Anophthalmos of microphthalmos often accompanies cleft number 7.

3. The cleft is located at the zygomaticomaxillary suture up to and including the inferolateral orbital rim. The orbital rim has a teardrop rather than a circular configuration.
4. The zygomatic arch is intact.
5. A prong of sideburn points anteriorly on the cheek.

Periorbital region
1. The orbital floor is deficient.
2. Antimongoloid slant of palpebral fissure.
3. Lower lateral eyelid coloboma with a short orbital septum.
4. Deficient eyelashes in the medial third of the lower eyelid.

COMMENT: The basic treatment for this cleft follows:
1. Bone grafting to augment the hypoplastic malar-zygomatic area. Often this must be performed more than once.
2. Lateral canthopexy to correct the antimongoloid slant.
3. Surgical procedures to correct the coloboma (e.g., tarso-conjunctival flap, scleral grafts, and transposition flaps from the upper lid).
4. A procedure to augment the soft tissue (e.g., dermis-fat graft).
5. Rhinoplasty.
6. Mandible or chin advancement.

Skeletal augmentation should take precedence over soft tissue reconstruction. An otologic evaluation may include an audiogram or temporal bone tomography.

Cleft 7

This group is made up of unilateral craniofacial microsoma, first and second branchial arch syndrome, otomandibular dysostosis, transverse or lateral facial clefts, unilateral facial agenesis, and otomandibular-auricular syndrome (Figs. 25-14 and 25-15).

Incidence: Most common of rare clefts; 1 in 3000 to 5500 births. May be bilateral in approximately 7% to 12% of the cases.

Genetic basis: Weak, probably sporadic occurrences, but some families have more than one member involved; Goldenhar's syndrome, a variant with epibulbar dermoids and vertebral anomalies, which may have an autosomal dominant transmission.

The clinical expression varies greatly. Occasionally minimal facial asymmetry is present; the mandibular component may be visualized only by radiographic study. The cleft is transverse and commonly there can be considerable soft tissue deficiency. The point is often understated in evaluating these patients.

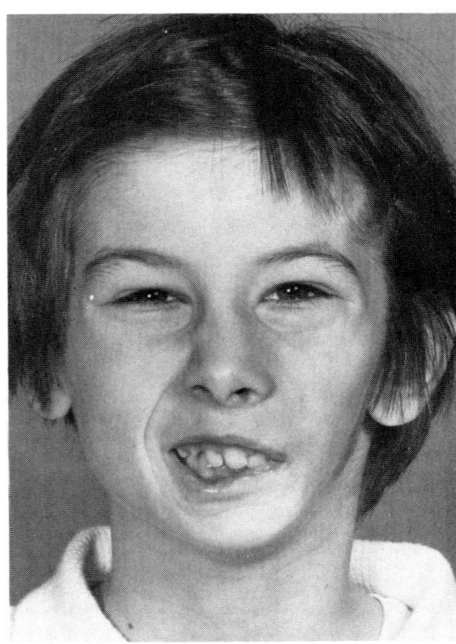

Fig. 25-15. Cleft number 7. Facial paralysis is frequently associated with this cleft.

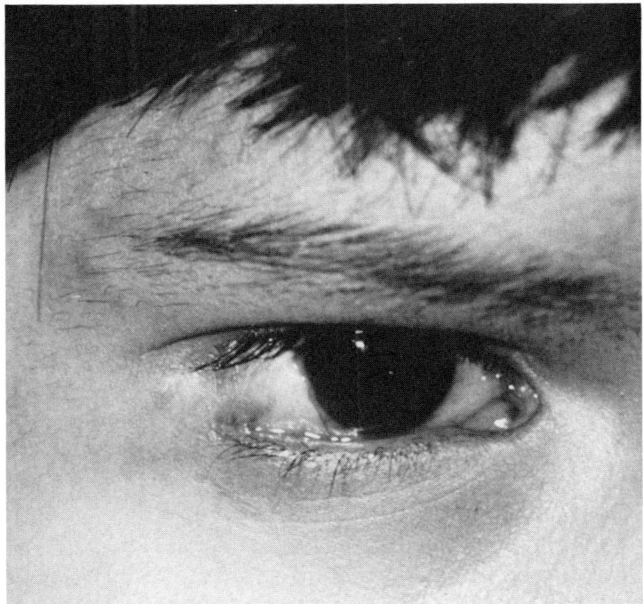

Fig. 25-16. Cleft number 8. This cleft does not occur in isolation.

Basic anatomic characteristics

Lip

Transverse cleft at the commissure; may extend along the cheek to the tragus of the helix (between the maxillary and mandibular processes of the developing first branchial arch).

Mandible

1. Varying degrees of hypoplasia of the condyle, ramus, and body. This degree of bony deficiency cannot be adequately explained by the cleft theory, since there is no specific transverse bony cleft.
2. All cases of external auditory canal and auricular hypoplasia with middle ear deformity have mandibular changes on the affected side.

Side of face

1. The soft tissue deficiency varies.
2. There may be hypoplasia of the parotid gland, parotid duct, tongue, or soft palate.
3. Occasional fifth or seventh cranial nerve palsies occur, but any cranial nerve may be affected (Fig. 25-15).
4. Muscles of mastication (pterygoid, masseter, and temporalis) may be hypoplastic. The muscular influence on the bony development is evident
5. Bony involvement other than that of the mandible.
   a. Hypoplasia of the maxilla.
   b. Hypoplasia of the temporal bone and pterygoid processes.
   c. Zygomatic deficiency leads to drooping of the superolateral angle of the orbit; Tessier[22] speculated that the cleft is located at the zygomaticotemporal suture.

Ear

1. Microtia and skin tags in varying degrees.
2. The mastoid processes may be small or acellular.
3. Malformations of external ossicles.
4. The extent of the ear deformity does not parallel that of mandibular deformity.

COMMENTS: The mandibular deformity of unilateral craniofacial microsomia is the most obvious defect. The condyle may be flattened, small, or absent. The ramus may be short or absent, and the body of the mandible curves superiorly to join the ramus on the shortened side. The gonial angle is obtuse. With growth and development the facial asymmetry is progressive. The disparity causes the mandible to deviate toward the affected side. The cant of the occlusal plane (which is higher on the affected side) is caused by the short hypoplastic ramus and by hypoplasia of the zygoma, maxilla, and alveolar process on the affected side. Downward growth of the maxilla on the affected side is hindered by the vertically restricted ramus. The condyle and ramus are often medially displaced, a finding that results in crossbite (i.e., the mandibular arch is lingual to the maxillary dentition). The effect of hypoplastic development of the masticatory muscles on the abnormal side may cause aberrant movements of the mandible. Protrusive opening lateral movements are affected. When the mouth is opened, the mandible shifts to the affected side because of the minimal or absent contribution of the affected pterygoid muscle.

Cleft 8

This category includes the lateral orbital and ophthalmic commissural clefts (Fig. 25-16).

Incidence: Rare, seen only in association with other clefts, usually in unilateral craniofacial microsomia.

Basic anatomic characteristics: The cleft begins at the lateral canthal region and extends in a temporal direction. The skin over the lateral orbital rim may extend onto the conjunctiva and cover the sclera laterally. Vision is not affected unless a severe underlying orbital deficiency is present.

Bony cleft: Located at the frontozygomatic suture.

PREOPERATIVE ASSESSMENT FOR PATIENTS WITH RARE CRANIOFACIAL CLEFTS

Before surgery a baseline psychometric evaluation is helpful to gain insight into the patient's image of self and body. The entire family often requires psychologic counseing in preparation for the long-term treatment of a deformed child. Longitudinal studies also ensure that postoperative changes in attitude can be recorded. Some patients who have accommodated to a deformed appearance for many years have difficulty in dealing with their newer, less disfigured face after surgery. Counseling thus plays an important role for the patient and the immediate family.

The genetics group should always examine the patient and family members. Family members are examined for the following reasons: (1) to establish a definitive diagnosis, (2) to determine if a genetic cause is involved, (3) to ascertain whether the disorder exists within the family, and (4) to assess the risks of recurrence and the possibility of mutations.

All patients have an ophthalmologic evaluation on entry into the craniofacial anomalies program. Preliminary eye data consist of an assessment of visual acuity and refraction, biomicroscopy of the anterior segment (cilia, lids, conjunctiva, cornea, anterior chamber, and iris), direct and indirect ophthalmoscopy of the posterior segment, and evaluation of the lacrimal apparatus. When indicated, an orthoptist evaluates ocular mobility.

Photographs, cephalograms, and a CT scan are obtained for baseline documentation and observation of growth patterns. CT is invaluable; it can be used to document lateral deviation of the orbits, the position of the ethmoid complex, the presence of intracranial malformations such as ventricular anomalies.

SUMMARY AND CONCLUSIONS

Although many classifications of rare craniofacial clefts have been described, the Tessier system is unique in that it is based on anatomic studies which can be easily and meaningfully used by the clinician. The clefts are numbered from 0 to 14 and extend circumferentially around the orbit along constant planes from the lips to the cranium. The orbit is a horizontal anatomic zone that separates the cranial from the facial defects.

In the Tessier classification system, numbers 12, 13, and 14 clefts are most commonly associated with orbital hypertelorism. Orbital hypertelorism can be subclassified into three groups: first, second, and third degree. Third-degree hypertelorism involves those patients with an interorbital distance greater than 40 mm. The principal anatomic abnormality associated with an increase in interorbital distance is the horizontal widening of the ethmoid labyrinth.

In this chapter craniofacial clefts are grouped according to similarity and for descriptive purposes. For example, numbers 0 to 14, 1 to 13, 2 to 12, 3 to 11, 4 to 10, and 5 to 9 are combined. Numbers 6, 7, and 8 clefts usually occur separately.

The 0 to 14 cleft combination includes the median cleft face syndrome, holoprosencephaly, and frontonasal dysplasia. Numbers 1 to 13 include proboscis lateralis, some cases of nasal hemiatrophy, and other cases previously associated with frontonasal dysplasia and the median cleft face syndrome. Numbers 2 to 12 include nasoocular, paraxial, oblique facial, and nasomaxillary clefts. Clefts numbered 3 to 11 were previously called nasoocular, paraxial, oblique facial, and nasomaxillary clefts. Numbers 4 to 10 include oroocular, paraxial, and vertical facial clefts. Numbers 5 to 9 are the rarest of the oblique facial clefts. Cleft number 6 includes the incomplete form of the Treacher Collins syndrome; the complete form of this syndrome has numbers 6, 7, and 8 clefts. Cleft number 7 is associated with unilateral craniofacial microsomia, the first and second branchial arch syndrome, otomandibular dysostosis, transverse or lateral facial clefts, unilateral facial agenesis, and the otomandibular-auricular syndrome. Cleft number 8 includes a lateral orbital cleft and ophthalmic commissural cleft.

In the substance of the text the incidence, genetic basis (when known), and basic anatomic characteristics of each of the facial clefts or combinations are indicated.

Before surgery a baseline psychometric evaluation is helpful to gain insight into the patient's image of self and body. The clinical genetics team should always examine the patient and the family members. All patients are required to have an ophthalmologic examination as well. Photographs, cephalograms, and a CT scan are obtained for baseline documentation and observation of growth patterns.

REFERENCES

1. Boo-Chai, K.: The transverse facial cleft: its repair, Br. J. Plast. Surg. **22:**119, 1969.
2. Boo-Chai, K.: The oblique facial cleft: a report of 2 cases and a review of 41 cases, Br. J. Plast. Surg. **23:**352, 1970.
3. Converse, J.M., McCarthy, J.G., and Wood-Smith, D.: Orbital hypotelorism: pathogenesis, associated faciocerebral anomalies, surgical correction, Plast. Reconstr. Surg. **56:**389, 1975.
4. Converse, J.M., McCarthy, J.G., and Wood-Smith, D., editors: Symposium on diagnosis and treatment of craniofacial anomalies, vol. 20, St. Louis, 1979, The C.V. Mosby Co.
5. Converse, J.M., Ransohoff, J., Mathews, E.S., et al.: Ocular hy-

pertelorism and pseudohypertelorism: advances in surgical treatment, Plast. Reconstr. Surg. **45:**1, 1970.

6. Currarino, G., and Silverman, F.N.: Orbital hypotelorism, arrhinencephaly and trigonocephaly, Radiology **74:**206, 1960.

7. DeMyer, W., and Zeman, W.: Alobar holoprosencephaly (arrhinencephaly) with median cleft lip and palate: clinical, electroencephalographic and nosologic considerations, Confin. Neurol. **23:**1, 1963.

8. DeMyer, W., Zeman, W., and Palmar, C.G.: The face predicts the brain: diagnostic significance of median facial anomalies for holoprosencephaly (arrhinencephaly), Pediatrics **34:**256, 1964.

9. Goffman, E.: Stigma: notes on the management of spoiled identity, Englewood Cliffs, N.J., 1963, Prentice-Hall, Inc.

10. Hansman, C.: Growth of interorbital distance and skull thickness as observed in roentgenographic measurements, Radiology **86:**87, 1966.

11. Harkins, C.S., Berlin, A., Harding, R.L., et al.: A classification of cleft lip and cleft palate, Plast. Reconstr. Surg. **29:**31, 1962.

12. Karfik, V.: Oblique facial cleft, Transactions of the Fourth International Congress of Plastic and Reconstructive Surgery (1967), Amsterdam, 1969. Excerpta Medica Foundation.

13. Kawamoto, H.K.: The kaleidoscopic world of rare craniofacial clefts: order out of chaos (Tessier classification), Clin. Plast. Surg. **3:**529, 1976.

14. Kawamoto, H.K., Wang, M.H., and Macomber, W.B.: Rare craniofacial clefts. In Converse, J.M., editor: Reconstructive plastic surgery: principles and procedures in correction, reconstruction, and transplantation, vol. 4, Philadelphia, 1977, W.B. Saunders Co.

15. McCarthy, J.G.: The concept of a craniofacial anomalies center, Clin. Plast. Surg. **3:**611, 1976.

16. Obwegeser, H.L.: Correction of the skeletal anomalies of Otomandibular dysostosis, J. Maxillofac. Surg. **2:**73, 1974.

17. Olshansky, S.: Chronic sorrow: a response to having a mentally defective child, Social Casework **43:**190, 1962.

18. Poswillo, D.E.: Otomandibular deformity: pathogenesis as a guide to reconstruction, J. Maxillofac. Surg. **2:**64, 1974.

19. Reich, E.W., Cox, R.P., McCarthy, J.G., et al.: A new heritable syndrome with frontonasal dysplasia and associated extracranial anomalies, Proceedings of the Fifth International Conference on Birth Defects, Montreal, Quebec, Aug. 1977.

20. Sedano, H.O., Cohen, M.M., Jr., Jeriasek, J., et al.: Frontonasal dysplasia, J. Pediatr. **76:**906, 1970.

21. Tessier, P.: Orbital hypertelorism. I. Successive surgical attempts, material and methods, causes and mechanisms, Scand. J. Plast. Reconstr. Surg. **6:**135, 1972.

22. Tessier, P.: Anatomical classification of facial, craniofacial and laterofacial clefts, J. Maxillofac. Surg. **4:**69, 1976.

23. Tessier, P., Guiot, G., and Derome, P.: Orbital hypertelorism. II. Definite treatment of orbital hypertelorism by craniofacial or by extracranial osteotomies, Scand. J. Plast. Reconstr. Surg. **7:**39, 1973.

24. Whitaker, L.A., and Katowitz, J.A.: Nasolacrimal apparatus in craniofacial deformity. In Converse, J.M., McCarthy, J.G., and Wood-Smith, D., editors: Symposium on diagnosis and treatment of craniofacial anomalies, vol. 20, St. Louis, 1979, The C.V. Mosby Co.

CHAPTER 26

Craniosynostosis

W. JERRY OAKES

Patients with abnormal head shapes resulting from premature fusion of one or more cranial sutures have been grouped under the term *craniosynostosis* for more than a century. Within this large group is a wide range of abnormality. In one of its mildest forms the patient will be noted to have an exaggerated anteroposterior diameter of the skull and a decreased biparietal distance (scaphocephaly). This presents a social and cosmetic problem but is not believed to represent an abnormality that damages the underlying brain. Much less commonly the infant or child will develop severe restriction of brain growth from multiple suture involvment and have clinical evidence of increased intracranial pressure, blindness, severe developmental delay, or mental retardation. Along this clinical spectrum lies the current patient population, with the majority of children having the more benign expression of the disease process.

For decades neurosurgeons viewed craniosynostosis in terms of the cranial vault sutures only, paying little or no attention to the skull base. Within recent years, however, more interest and clinical attention have been directed to the skull base with a significant increase in our understanding of the problem and an improvement of the therapeutic results. In some instances it is believed that progressive involvement of the adjacent facial sutures has been avoided by early and extensive surgery of the intracranial aspect of the skull base.

The complicated and involved subjects of orbital hypertelorism and craniofacial dysostosis will be discussed in separate chapters. It should simply be noted here that these patients require a multiple-component team approach to their therapy and should not be treated by the interested but single-dimensional soloist.

INCIDENCE

Estimates of the incidence of simple craniosynostosis not secondary to a known metabolic disturbance vary widely.[19] The best data indicate that the incidence is probably between 0.4/1000[49] and 1/1000[89] live births. The other two main categories, genetically determined craniosynostosis, which prominently involves the facial sutures, and secondary craniosynostosis, are much less frequent than primary simple craniosynostosis.

ETIOLOGY AND PATHOLOGIC PROCESS

Virchow[90] is given credit for first using the term craniosynostosis and applying it to patients with abnormal head shapes. He postulated that this occurred because of premature fusion of one or more cranial sutures. He also set down the general tenet of pathologic skull growth with premature fusion of a cranial suture: growth is restricted perpendicular to the direction of the suture and enhanced parallel to it (Fig. 26-1). This assumes that the suture or sutures accepting the compensatory growth are physiologically open and not involved in the synostotic process. Isolated involvement of the sagittal suture most clearly demonstrates these principles, with the affected child developing a long narrow head. The growth perpendicular to the involved suture is limited, giving the head a narrow appearance, and the compensatory growth occurs in the direction of the suture, resulting in a scaphocephalic or "boatlike" appearance.

Our understanding of the underlying mechanism of the premature fusion of a suture has awaited further understanding of the normal growth processes of the skull.[72,81,82,87] It now appears that the dura, or inner periosteum of the skull, is the guiding or directing tissue with regard to skull and suture development. Dural reflections such as the falx cerebri and tentorium cerebelli mark the site of suture formation with ossification occurring between these dural reflections. Pathologic states in which the dural reflections are absent or displaced result in a corresponding absence or displacement of the appropriate suture.[87] Moss has championed the role of the cranial base with its attachment of the dural

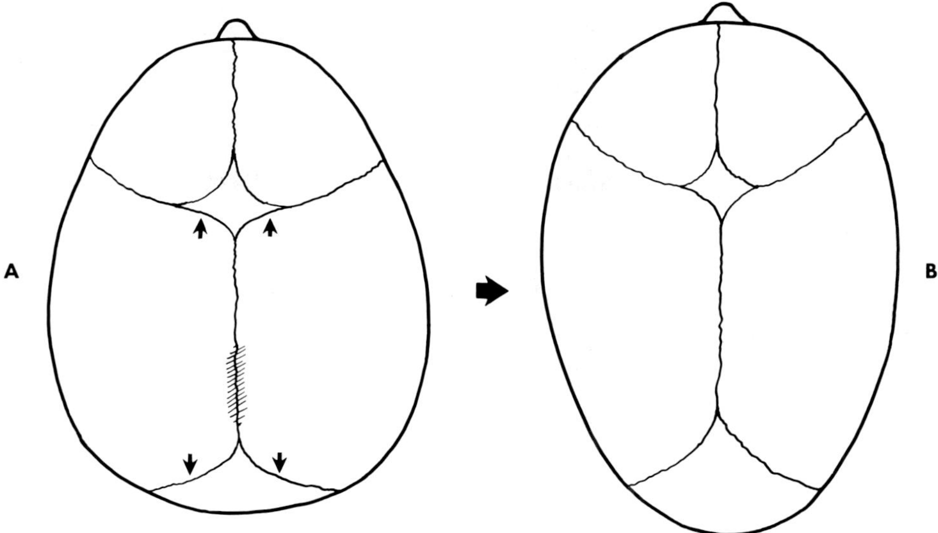

Fig. 26-1. A, Vertex view of fetal skull. During gestation fusion occurs in the posterior aspect of the sagittal suture of the normally shaped fetal skull. As growth continues the fusion enhances growth parallel to the involved suture and restricts growth perpendicular to it. **B,** Vertex view of newborn with scaphocephaly. By the time of delivery the skull shape has been altered by the synostotic process as growth of the skull and brain continue; this elongation may become somewhat more prominent.

reflections as the operative factor in the causation of most craniosynostosis.[71,72,73] Therefore the underlying abnormality in scaphocephaly is a spatially malformed cribriform plate and crista galli, whereas coronal involvement occurs with malformation of the lesser sphenoid wing. On histologic examination the sutures have single and not multiple areas of union. No histologic abnormalities are seen other than the timing of the suture fusion.[1]

Although these observations help explain the mechanisms of the development of the abnormal skull shape, they do not explain the initiating or triggering factors. Clinical observation has helped in this regard. In discussing the etiologic origin of craniosynostosis it is best to divide the patients into two broad categories, primary and secondary craniosynostosis. In the simple primary form of the disease the abnormality of skull configuration is present at birth, although it may be initially difficult to separate from skull molding as a result of passage through the birth canal. Patients within the simple primary group represent an isolated cranial sutural problem that is unassociated with other recognized bony or metabolic abnormalities. Occasionally skull configuration is determined by an ever-increasing number of genetically transmitted diseases. In these patients primary complex craniosynostosis is only part of the total expression of abnormalities. Crouzon's disease and Apert's syndrome are two of the more common problems within this category. Although both have midfacial hypoplasia, their clinical appearances are not identical. In addition, syndactyly is seen with Apert's syndrome. Several recent publications review

our current understanding of the genetically determined form of craniosynostosis.[18,19] Of special importance within the genetically determined form of primary craniosynostosis is the localization of the short arm of the seventh chromosome for the occurrence of premature cranial suture fusion.[25,66] This chromosomal localization may help to open an exciting aspect of the underlying mechanism of these genetically determined disorders.

Within the large group of patients with primary simple craniosynostosis, uterine malformation and its concomitant restriction of fetal head growth is being increasingly recognized as a possible cause of the underlying abnormality.[46,69] Although intrauterine constraint has not been proven to cause craniosynostosis, its clinical association with sagittal,[40] coronal,[39] and metopic[41] premature cranial fusion makes this possiblity intriguing. Uterine abnormalities that are seen with increased frequency in primary simple craniosynostosis include bicornate and septate uteri. Additional support is given to the intrauterine restraint theory by the frequently associated anomalies of other organ systems seen as a restriction of their growth as well. Abnormalities that fall into this category include mandibular asymmetry, overfolding of the helix of the ear, joint contractures, edema of the limbs, pulmonary hypoplasia, and hip dislocation. Within a single infant one or more of these abnormalities will commonly be associated with an abnormal head shape. Simple intrauterine constraint of growth can be easily confused with chromosomal or metabolic disturbances.

Molding of the skull from passage through the birth canal

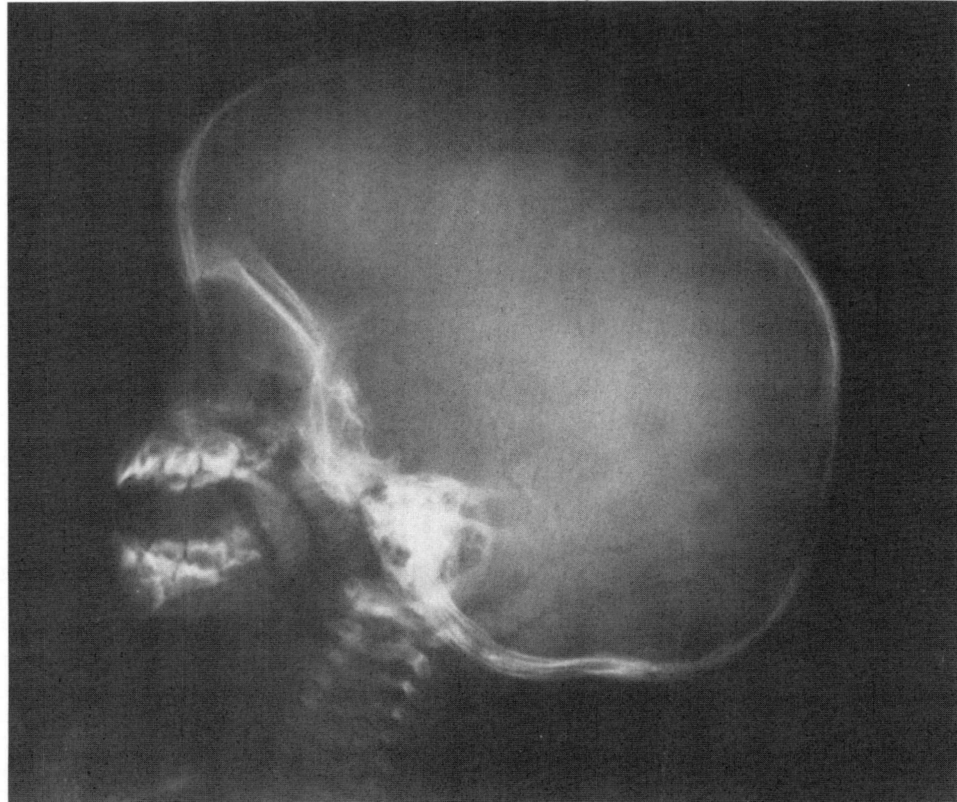

Fig. 26-2. Lateral radiograph of an infant with scaphocephaly and congenital Addison's disease.

is common and is associated with spontaneous correction without any therapeutic intervention. Breech positioning of the head has a particularly high association with a scaphocephalic appearance.[42] This is not associated with a radiographic abnormality of the cranial sutures and shows progressive improvement within the first few days to weeks of life. It is important to differentiate patients with true premature suture fusion from those with compensatory head molding who do not have underlying suture abnormalities.

Secondary cranial suture fusion is a result of the following predisposing events or diseases[27]:

1. Metabolic bone diseases[63,83]
   a. Rickets
   b. Hypophosphatasia
   c. Osteopetrosis
   d. Idiopathic hypercalcemia
   e. Mucopolysaccharidosis
   f. Achondroplasia
   g. Metaphyseal dysostosis
   h. Infantile cortical hyperostosis
2. Cranial trauma with the fracture crossing the suture or causing suture diastasis[44]
3. Rapid intracranial decompression from ventricular shunts for hydrocephalus[6,55]
4. Hematologic disorders
   a. Congenital hemolytic icterus
   b. Polycythemia vera
   c. Sickle cell disease
   d. Thalassemia major
5. Endocrinologic disturbances[23,53,79]
   a. Spontaneously occurring hyperthyroidism
   b. Iatrogenic hyperthyroidism
   c. Congenital adrenal hypoplasia (?) (Fig. 26-2)

Although brain growth can be restricted with any of these generalized disorders, the brain problem seldom becomes a prominent clinical feature because of the serious and frequently fatal effect of the underlying disease on other organ systems.

CLINICAL MANIFESTATIONS
Primary simple craniosynostosis

Patients with the simple primary form of craniosynostosis can be diagnosed at birth from their appearance. The obstetric history is important in these patients, with early descent of the fetus into the mother's lower pelvis or severe pelvic pressure within the last few weeks of pregnancy being common.[39] Early lightening and an abnormal fetal lie also may be present. As previously mentioned, these give support for

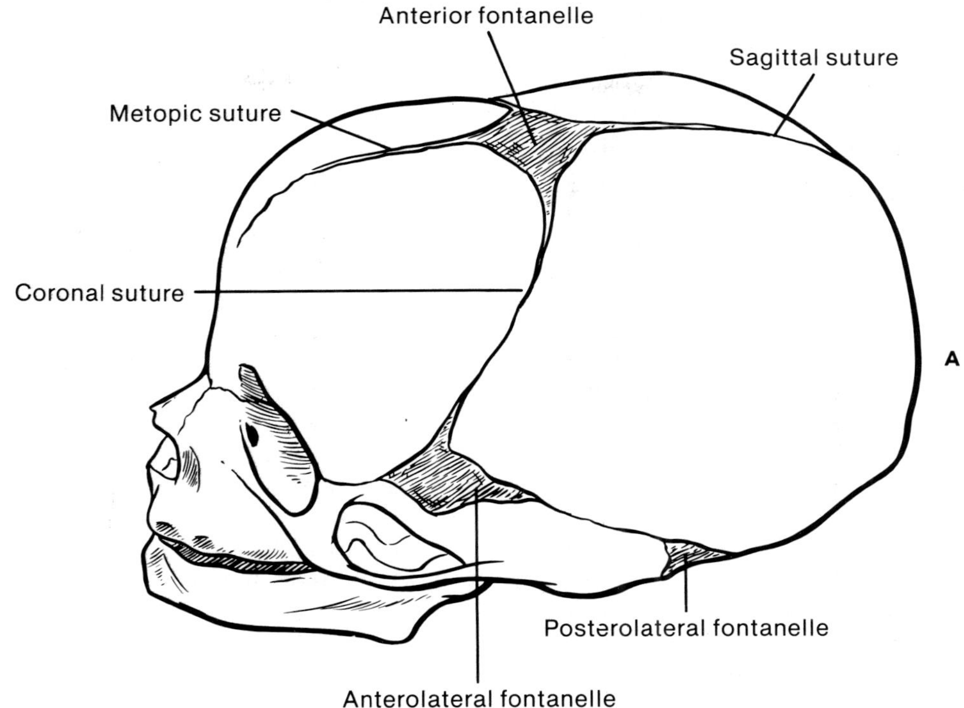

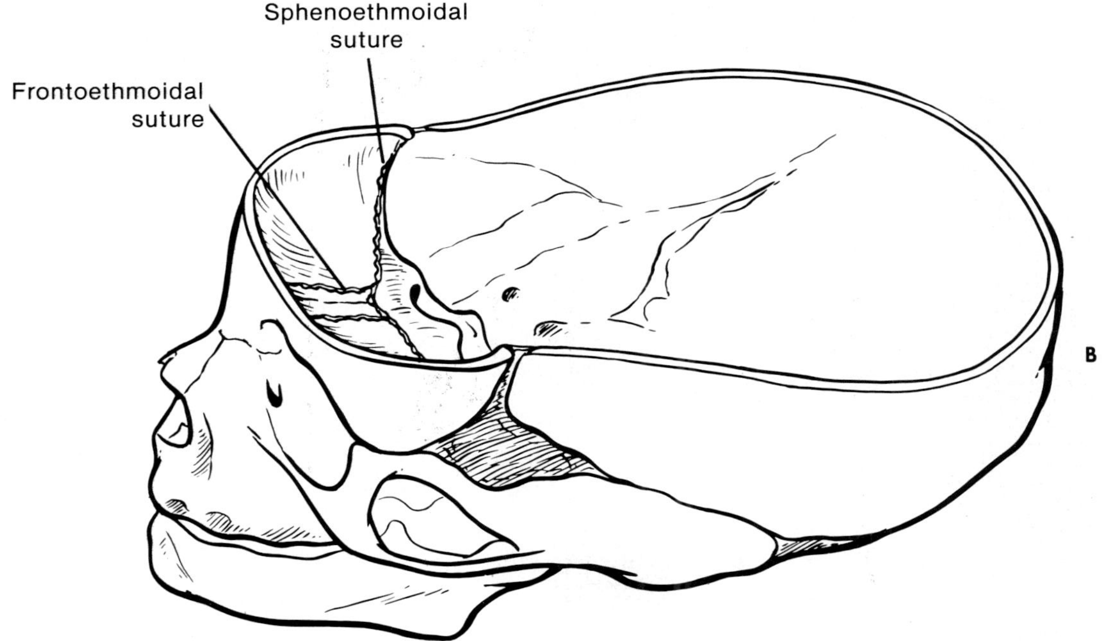

Fig. 26-3. A, Lateral oblique view of the infant's skull showing the major vault sutures and fontanelle. **B,** Internal view of the infant's skull showing the major sutures of the anterior skull base. (From Oakes, W.J., and Wilkins, R.H.: The newborn: neurosurgical considerations. In Filston, H.C.: Surgical problems in children: recognition and referral, St. Louis, 1982, The C.V. Mosby Co.)

the intrauterine constraint theory of development of the problem.[40] Uterine abnormality should be specifically sought, particularly if the mother has a history of spontaneous abortion, retained placenta, or premature labor and delivery.[69] Some structural abnormalities of the uterus (septate uterus) can be surgically corrected and thereby increase the likelihood of survival of subsequent fetuses.[13] Evidence that the surgical correction of uterine abnormalities (metroplasty) will decrease or eliminate a specific individual's tendency to constrain fetal growth and therefore lessen the likelihood of subsequent offspring being born with craniosynostosis has yet to be demonstrated.

The clinical appearance of most patients with primary craniosynostosis can easily be predicted by knowing the extent of involvement of the various cranial sutures and fontanelles (Fig. 26-3). An extensive review of the more than 35 cranial sutures will not be given here; for those interested, reference to a detailed anatomic atlas is suggested.

Scaphocephaly (sagittal suture)

The sagittal suture is most commonly affected as an isolated phenomenon in patients with craniosynostosis. The problem tends to affect boys three or four times more frequently than girls. The patient will have a long thin head with a narrowed biparietal diameter, particularly posteriorly. This deformity is termed *scaphocephaly,* or *dolichocephaly* (Fig. 26-4). When viewed posteriorly the area near the suture appears peaked, and a synostotic ridge may be seen and palpated. The posterior aspect of the sagittal suture is usually affected first and more extensively than the anterior aspect. Once the fusion process begins, it proceeds both anteriorly and posteriorly along the sagittal suture from a single point of origin. The anterior fontanelle is seldom significantly affected, whereas the posterior fontanelle is usually extensively involved. The posterior skull may take on the appearance of a shell with a prominent occipital shelf; frontally the forehead may be bossed (Fig. 26-5). In the sagittal suture of normal newborns both parietal bones will move independently on palpation. With premature closure the parietal bones become fused and lose this mobility. This is best demonstrated by attempting to move the bones near the suture with pressure alternating from one side to the other. The head circumference of scaphocephalic patients also will be greater than the intracranial volume would indicate when plotted on head growth charts derived from infants with normal globular head shapes. Care should be taken not to rely on head circumference alone as an indi-

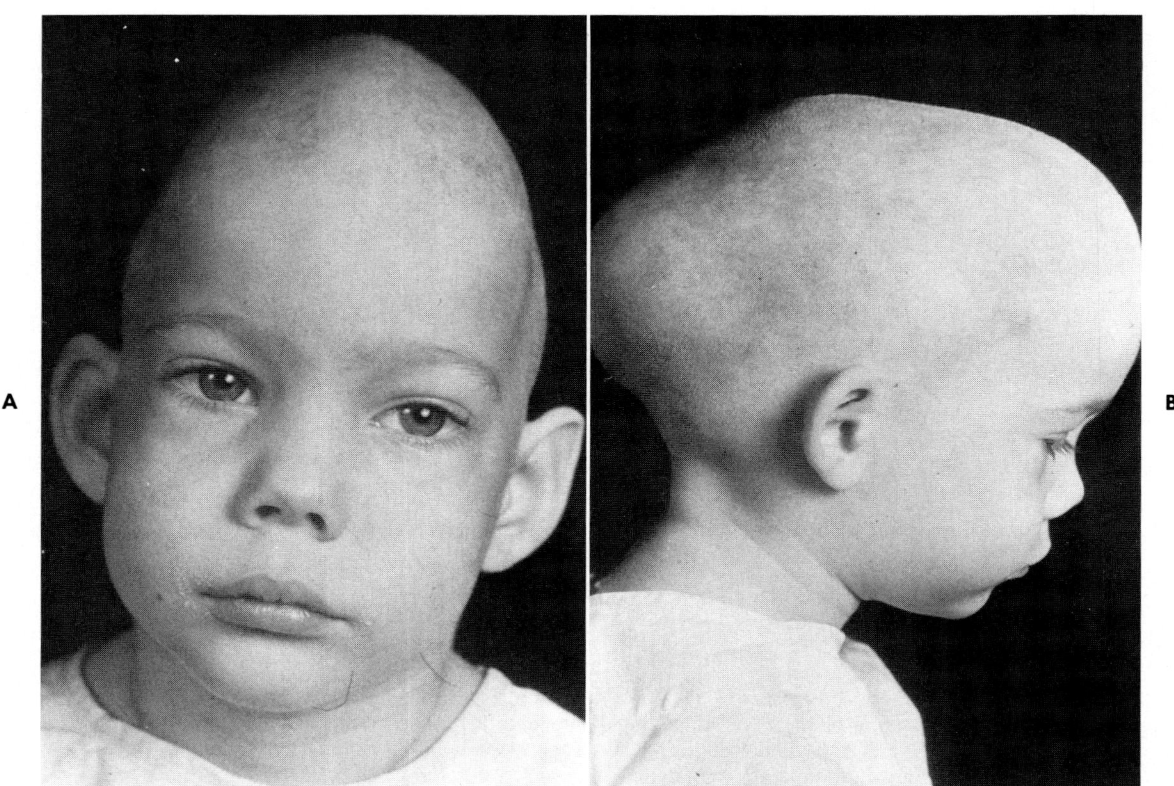

Fig. 26-4. Anterior and lateral views of a 3-year-old boy with scaphocephaly. **A,** Peaked appearance of the vertex. **B,** Shell-like deformity of the occiput.

cation of macrocrania in the presence of scaphocephalic distortion of the skull.

This simple form of craniosynostosis will make up approximately 55% of patients who have an abnormal head shape in a North American neurosurgical practice.[86] This percentage varies somewhat, depending on the degree of acceptability of scaphocephaly to the general population and therefore the referral patterns of pediatricians.

Mental impairment has not been clearly shown to result from restraint of the biparietal growth of the skull. Occasional evidence of increased intracranial pressure, visual impairment from papilledema or optic atrophy, or other congenital anomalies related either to the central nervous system or other organ systems are reported in connection with scaphocephalic patients.[12] It should be emphasized, however, that these are unusual occurrences; in the vast majority of patients with premature closure of the sagittal suture this phenomenon occurs in isolation without serious physiologic sequelae.

Plagiocephaly (coronal and frontosphenoidal sutures)

Plagiocephaly is an oblique or asymmetric development of the skull. This term is applied to processes that unilaterally affect the coronal suture and its basal extension. It is

manifested clinically by flattening of the forehead on the involved side (Fig. 26-6, *A* and *B*). The acuteness of the slope of the forehead may most easily be appreciated by viewing the face from above (Fig. 26-6, *C*) or below. The eye on the involved side may appear proptotic because of the restriction of growth of the orbit. The eyebrow will appear raised due to the bony configuration of the supraorbital rim and forehead. Occasionally the growth of the orbit will be severely restricted, and the globe will project forward onto the infant's cheek (Fig. 26-7). Alternatively the globe may move in and out with relaxation and Valsalva maneuvers. When extreme proptosis is present and the cornea can no longer be kept moist, vision may be lost from drying that occurs in the exposed portion of the globe. In this case referral and treatment take on a more urgent tenor in an attempt to preserve functional vision. Before definitive treatment it is important to keep the cornea moist and free from abrasion.

The position of the palate is noted, as well as evidence of restriction of growth of the midface. Frequently with bilateral involvement the palate develops a high arch, and nasal breathing is restricted.

Whereas the sagittal suture is primarily affected posteriorly, the coronal suture seems to be involved more laterally

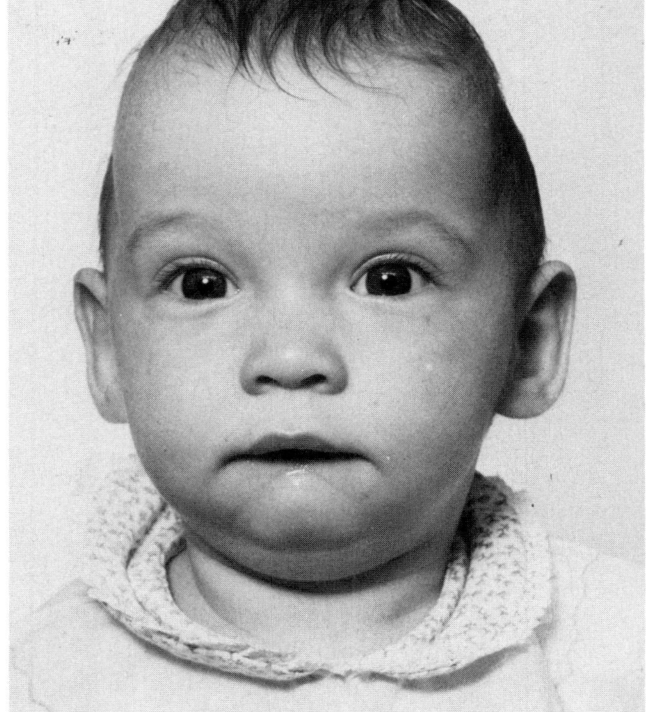

Fig. 26-5. Frontal view of a 5-month-old girl with prominent frontal bossing and scaphocephaly.

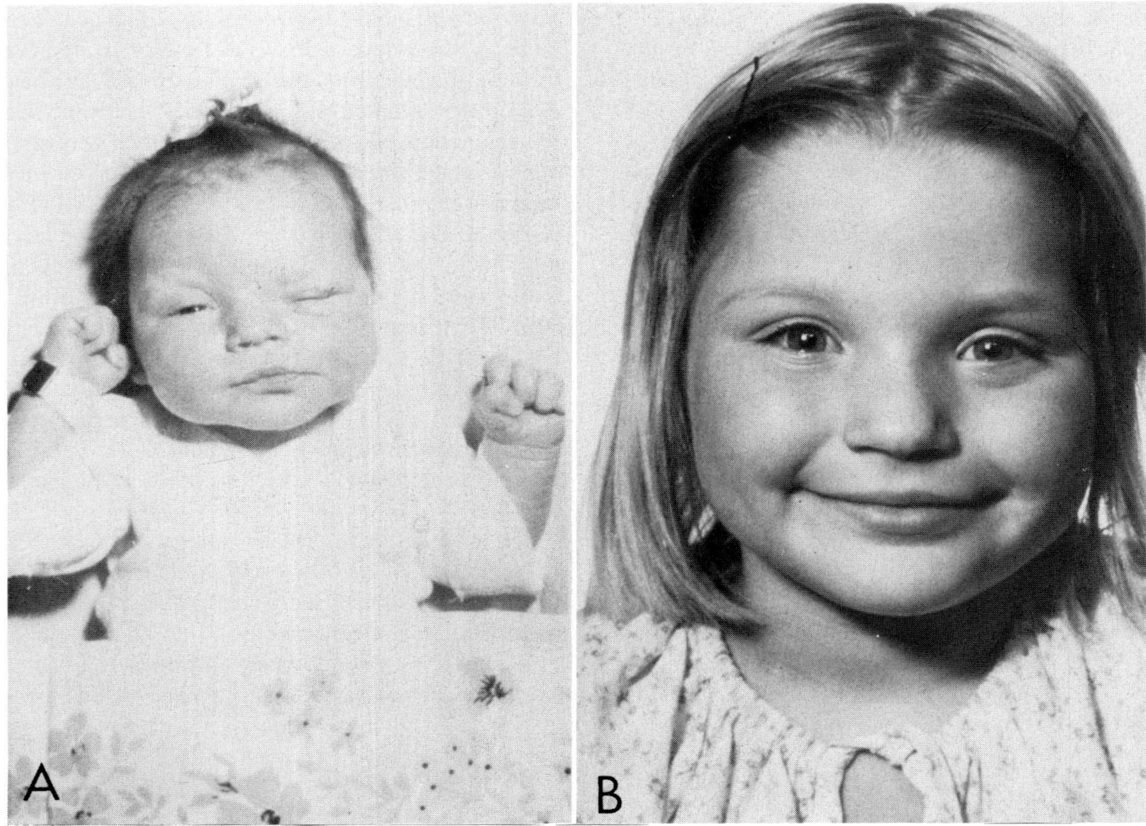

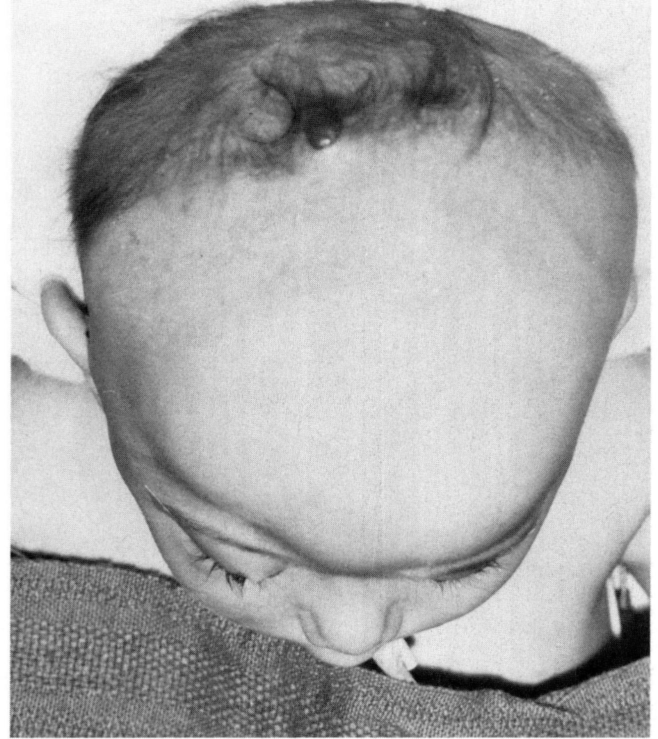

Fig. 26-6. A, Newborn with right-sided plagiocephaly. The involved side appears flattened, and the eyebrow is raised. In this case the eye is partially opened. The left forehead is mildly prominent as a means of compensating for the limited growth in the right anterior fossa. **B,** Four-year follow-up of the same child with good cosmetic result. **C,** Anterior vertex view of another patient with prominent right-sided plagiocephaly. The posterior slope of the forehead can be visualized more easily from this vantage point.

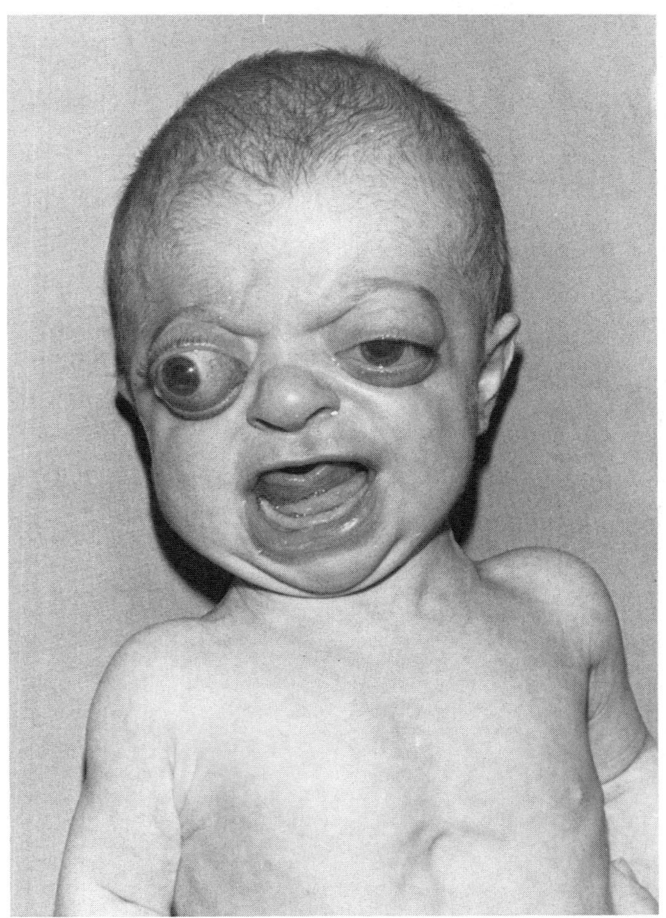

Fig. 26-7. Newborn with Crouzon's disease and generalized restriction of growth of the skull and face. The right orbit is severely hypoplastic, causing proptosis and corneal drying.

with the premature closure process slowly advancing toward the anterior fontanelle and more rapidly along the skull base. As has been pointed out by others[11,47,75] the coronal suture continues under the frontal lobe at the anterior lateral fontanelle. At that point it merges with the frontosphenoidal suture. The frontosphenoidal sutures unite in the midline of the base of the skull and merge with the frontoethmoidal sutures. In unilateral disease of the coronal suture complex, loss of volume in the ipsilateral frontal area is compensated for by developing frontal bossing of the contralateral forehead and expansion of the occipital area on the ipsilateral side. Contralateral forehead expansion may become quite prominent and confuse both parents and inexperienced physicians as to which side of the head represents the pathologic process.

Plagiocephaly is seen less commonly than scaphocephaly, with approximately 10% of most neurosurgical series composed of this problem. The anomaly is also more commonly associated with involvement of other sutures (squamosal, lambdoid, and metopic) than diseases affecting the sagittal suture. Male and female involvement is approximately equal. Palpable ridges along the synostotic suture are less common than in sagittal synostosis, and mobility is more difficult to assess both in the normal and synostotic patient.

Brachycephaly (bilateral coronal and frontosphenoidal sutures)

When both coronal suture complexes are involved the head shape is termed *brachycephaly* (Fig. 26-8). This refers to a short high cranial vault where growth is primarily directed up. Again, the lateral aspect of the suture is usually primarily affected. Typically the childrens' heads are symmetric, with the degree of synostosis being relatively equal on both sides. Evidence of increased intracranial pressure, papilledema, and optic atrophy are all more commonly associated with brachycephaly than either plagiocephaly or scaphocephaly. The incidence of mental retardation also rises sharply when the disease occurs bilaterally. The head circumference in the more circular head of children with brachycephaly is smaller than the intracranial volume expectation. Head circumference measurements should then be interpreted in this light with early radiographic investigation for the presence of hydrocephalus or other cranial anomalies in questionable patients.

Midface hypoplasia may or may not be present in asso-

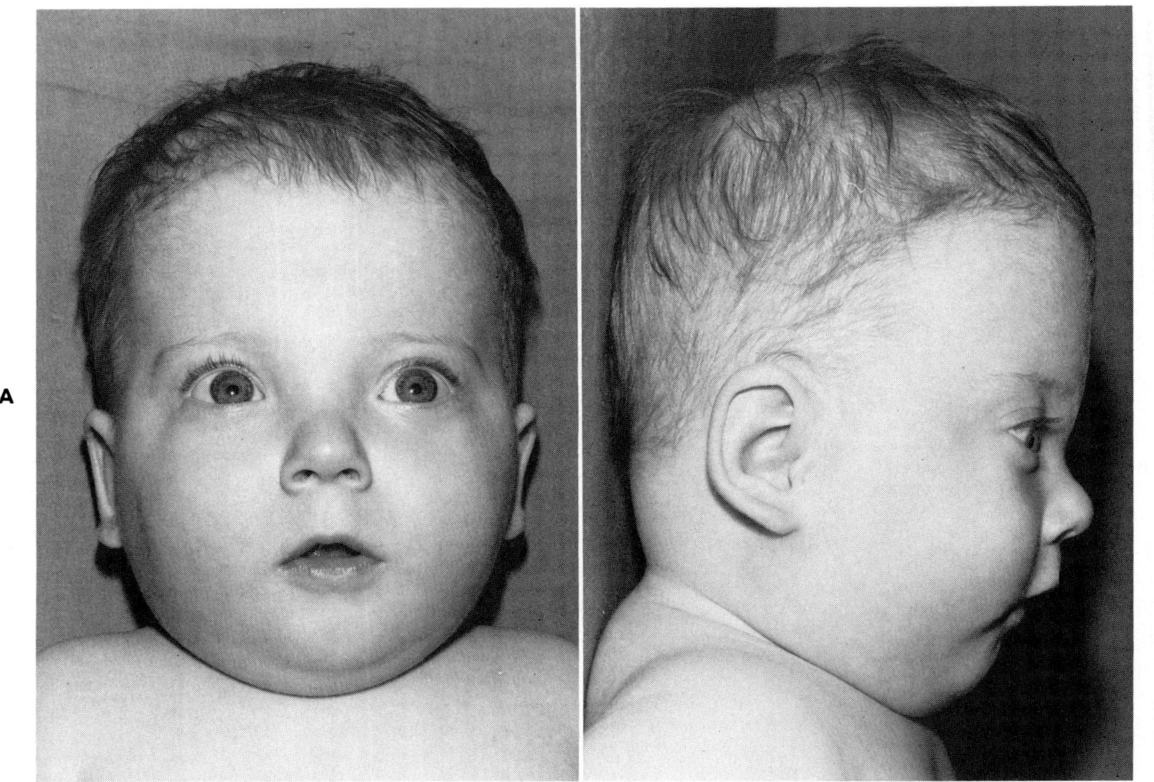

Fig. 26-8. Infant with brachycephaly viewed both frontally **(A)** and laterally **(B).** Since growth is restricted in an anterior posterior plane, the compensatory growth has occurred superiorly, giving the head a vaulted appearance.

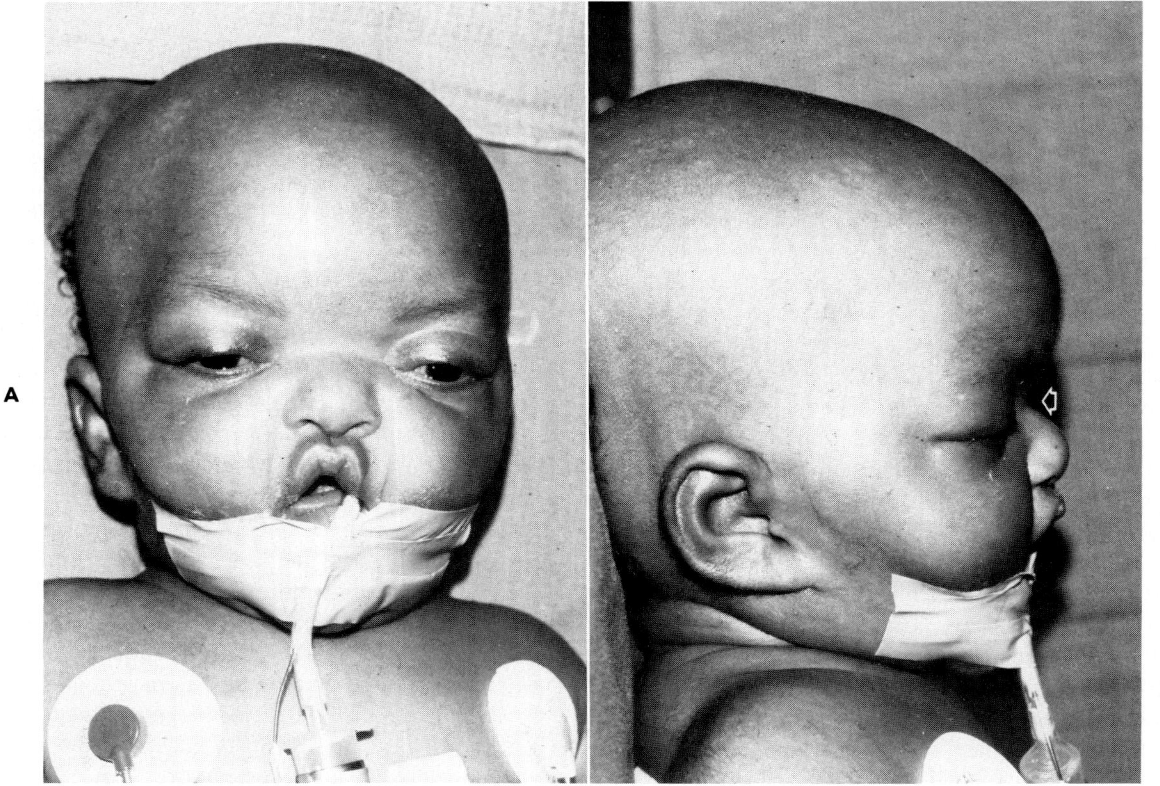

Fig. 26-9. Frontal and lateral views of a child with Crouzon's disease. **A,** The general shape of the vertex is relatively normal. The orbits are hypoplastic, giving the child the appearance of proptosis. **B,** Restriction of growth in the midface is prominent, with a pinching in of the glabella *(arrow)* and maxillae.

ciation with brachycephaly. The incidence of bilateral involvement of the coronal suture complex approaches 10% of patients with craniosynostosis, with many of these patients falling into the subcategories of Crouzon's syndrome and Apert's syndrome in which prominent involvement of facial sutures is seen (Fig. 26-9). Decreased visual acuity and optic atrophy are common in untreated patients, particularly in the presence of the Crouzon's syndrome and Apert's syndrome. Whether this results from chronic papilledema or angulation of the optic nerve as it passes through the deformed optic foramen is still unclear.[2,7]

Trigonocephaly (metopic and frontoethmoidal sutures)

A less common form of craniosynostosis is involvement of the metopic suture with resultant trigonocephaly. This occurs in isolation in less than 5% of patients with craniosynostosis. Infants with trigonocephaly have an easily visible and palpable midfrontal ridge that extends from the anterior fontanelle to the glabella (Fig. 26-10). The interpupillary distance is decreased at the expense of the ethmoid complex. When viewed from above the forehead resembles the keel of a boat with a swept back appearance of both supraorbital ridges. This triangular or egg-shaped configuration is easily recognizable at birth. The intracranial volume of both frontal areas is reduced, and compensatory growth is seen in both parietal areas.

Patients with trigonocephaly are divided into two distinct groups.[5,22] Simple trigonocephaly is unassociated with other facial and central nervous system defects. In other patients the trigonocephalic appearance is associated with or dominated by one of the several forms of arrhinencephaly. In this case the bony abnormality of the forehead is only a superficial indicator of a more serious underlying developmental anomaly. Severity and type of involvement of the underlying brain and eyes vary greatly. In its mildest form the olfactory nerves, bulbs, and tracts will simply fail to

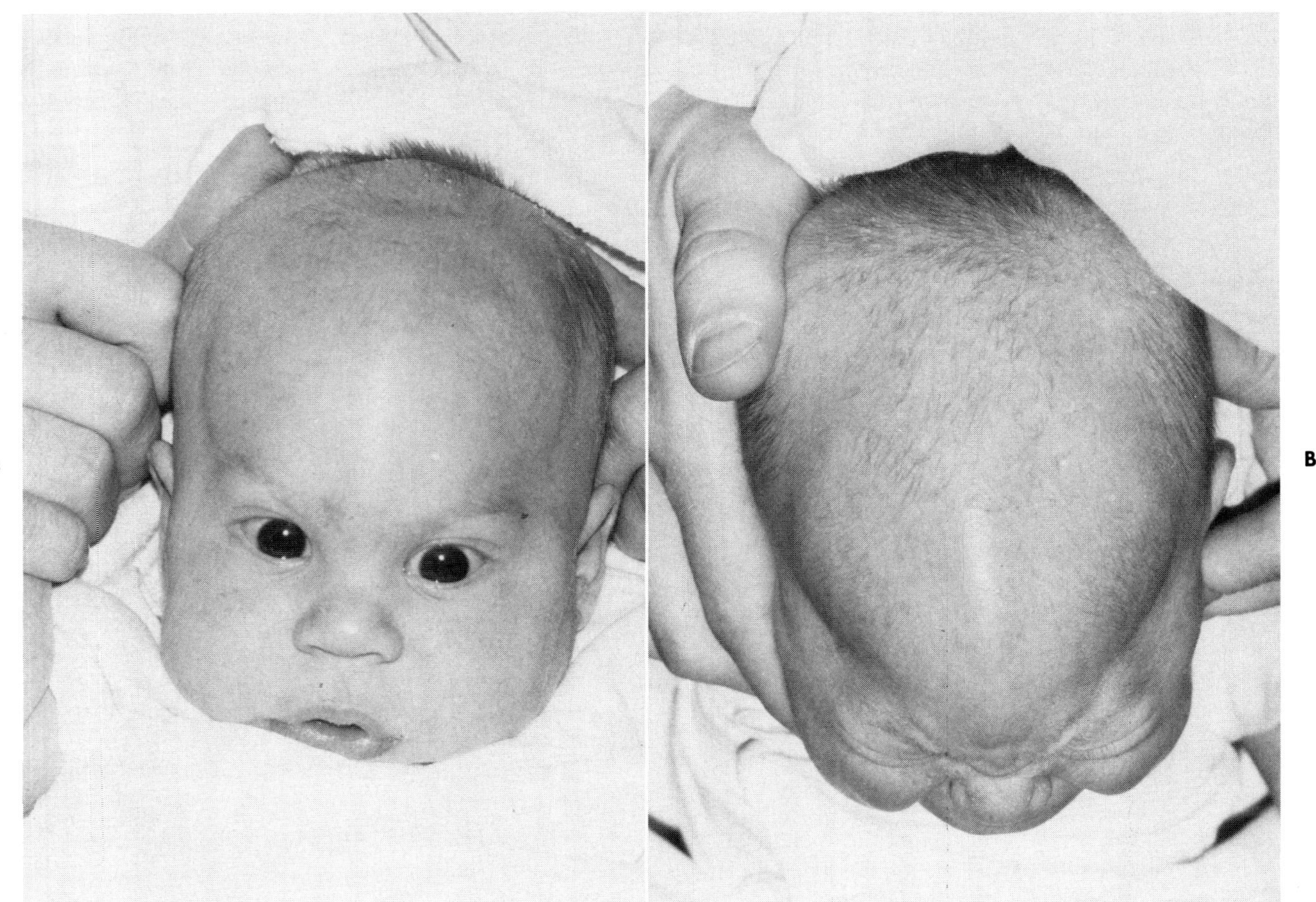

Fig. 26-10. Frontal and vertex view of an infant with trigoenocephaly. **A,** Frontal view demonstrates the hypotelorism and ridge over the metopic suture. Note the general smallness of the anterior fossa. **B,** Vertex view of the same infant again demonstrates the prominent metopic ridge and the lateral slope of both sides of the forehead in the supraorbital region.

develop. This is compatible with normal intelligence and is occasionally found as an incidental autopsy finding. In the severest form the orbits actually fuse medially, forming a single bony area to house the deformed globes. The ventricular system within the forebrain forms a single midline ventricle with fusion of the medial aspect of both frontal areas and failure of development of the falx cerebri. This cyclops appearance in infants is usually associated with a stillborn infant or death shortly after delivery. Other severe anomalies include orbits that are significantly hypoteloric but separated as two distinct orbital structures. Major nasal and frontal lobe dysmorphism also are seen. The nasal and midfacial bony anomalies include absence or distortion of the vomer, ethmoid, maxillae, nasal, and lacrimal bones, as well as the turbinate. A cardinal feature of this entire group of patients remains the absence of the olfactory apparatus. Because of severe damage to the neocortex, early death is common. The most common form of arrhinencephaly and facial anomalies are those associated with median cleft syndrome. A midline cleft in the lip is confluent with a single open nasal cavity. The interpupillary distance is decreased, and the optic foramen may be fused. Along with a cleft in the lip is a midline palatal cleft. Trigonocephalic appearance of the forehead is common. Narrowed carotid arteries may supply the meninges alone. Survival beyond the neonatal period is unlikely. Last, the triangular appearance of the forehead may be associated with lateral cleft lip and palate syndromes.

Most clinical papers addressing the subject of simple trigonocephaly emphasize the limitation of growth in both frontal areas or make no comment as to the natural history of the appearance of the untreated patient.[5,38,86] Because of the stated preference to recommend surgery in these patients, it can be assumed that these authors believe the problem to be ongoing and not self-correcting. This view is the overwhelming consensus both in the surgical[62,68] and the pediatric neurologic literature.[30,32,34]

A conservative approach has recently been advocated in the radiologic literature.[26] Convincing documentation is presented that simple trigonocephaly with radiographic evidence of synostosis affecting the metopic suture will frequently be associated with significant cosmetic improvement without surgical intervention. Resolution or improvement in untreated patients includes improvement in hypotelorism and ethmoidal hypoplasia and dissipation of the ridge overlying the fused metopic suture. Much of the objectionable triangular appearance of the forehead region was lost. This benign natural history questions the current generally accepted practice of surgery, however, the study needs confirmation by other centers. Harwood-Nash[44] takes an intermediate position and believes that the skull deformity may correct itself, but that persistent hypotelorism will necessitate surgical intervention.

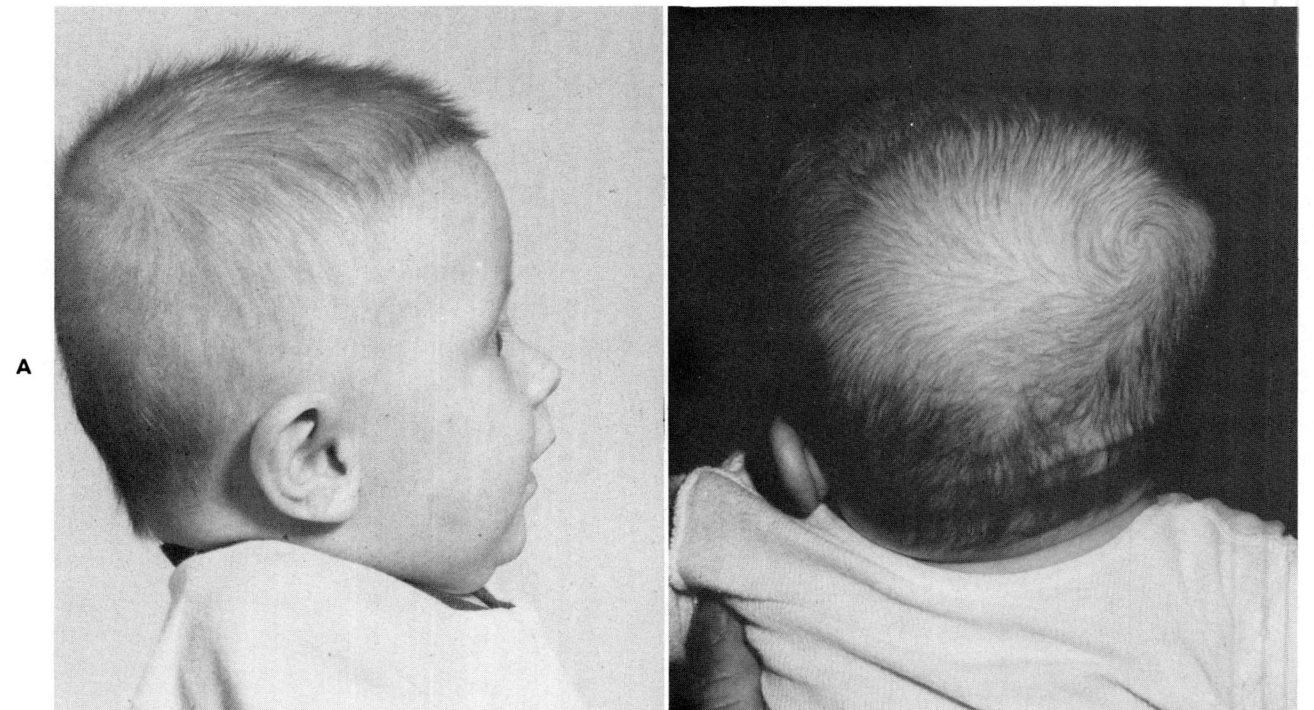

Fig. 26-11. A, Infant with bilateral lambdoid synostosis. The occiput is flat. There is a gentle midline bony groove extending from the posterior fontanelle inferiorly. The skull vault has taken on a tower appearance (turricephaly). **B,** Posterior view of a different infant demonstrating the occipital flattening associated with unilateral lambdoid synostosis.

Plagiocephaly (lambdoid suture)

The lambdoid sutures also may be involved with craniosynostosis either unilaterally or bilaterally. On the side of involvement the occipital area becomes flattened (Fig. 26-11). The unilateral form of the disease is occasionally referred to as *plagiocephaly,* which causes confusion with unilateral coronal and basal suture involvement. In both situations the head develops asymmetrically or obliquely. To avoid confusion it is probably best simply to indicate which sutures are believed to be involved and avoid a single term that describes both clinical entities. Movement of this suture cannot normally be palpated with alternating pressure on each side of the involved suture. Therefore loss of movement is not a reliable clinical sign of fusion. Hypertrophic ridges, which are so commonly seen over affected sagittal and metopic sutures, do not reliably occur with lambdoid synostosis. Although this is said to be the rarest form of single suture fusion,[44] in my experience it occurs about as

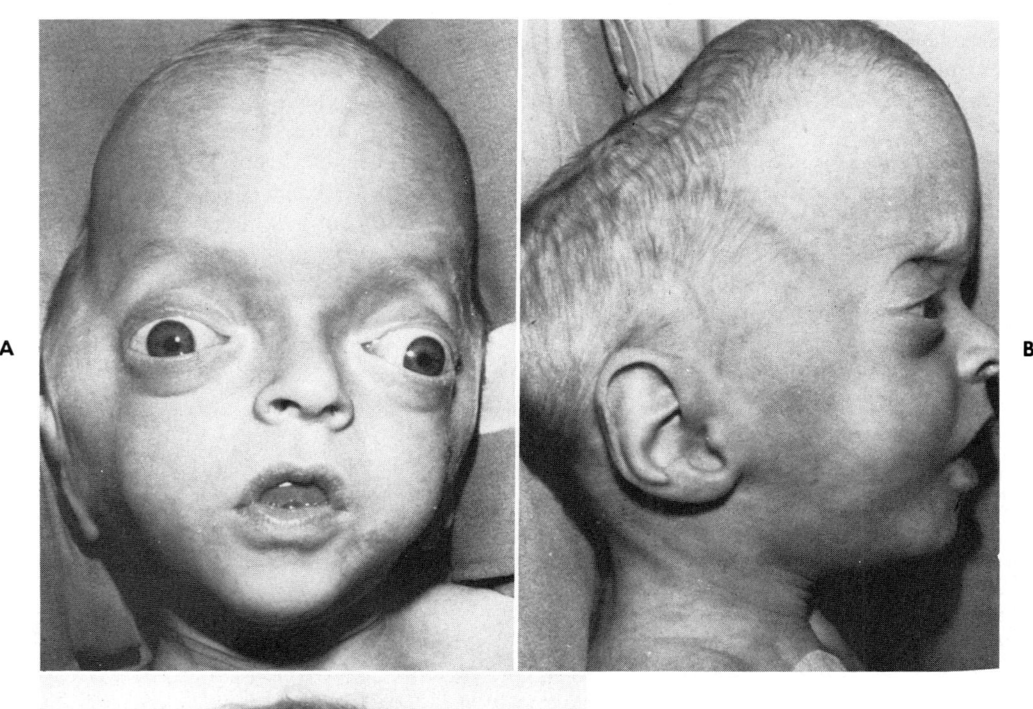

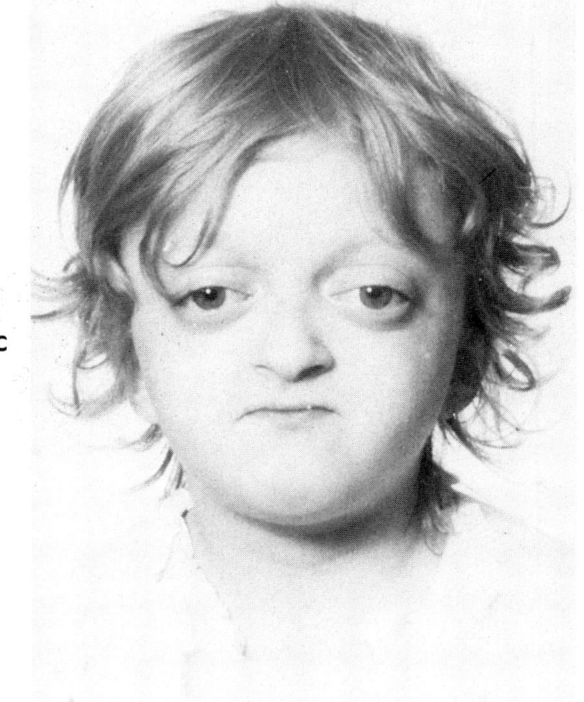

Fig. 26-12. A and **B,** Frontal and lateral views of a 3-month-old child with Crouzon's disease and a cloverleaf skull, or the Kleeblattschädel anomaly. Midface hypoplasia and venous engorgement over the head are apparent. The significant limitation of growth in the posterior aspect of the skull, with all compensatory growth occurring through the partially opened anterior fontanelle, is best visualized on the lateral view. The mother of this child had already become blind from increased intracranial pressure associated with Crouzon's disease. **C,** When a family history was obtained, an asymptomatic 3-year-old sibling was also found. On physical examination this child had Crouzon's disease with bilateral papilledema and a beaten metal appearance to the inner aspect of the skull. (From Oakes, W.J., and Wilkins, R.H.: The newborn: neurosurgical considerations. In Filston, H.C.: Surgical problems in children: recognition and referral, St. Louis, 1982, The C.V. Mosby Co.)

frequently as metopic synostosis, making up approximately 5% of patients.

Turricephaly (bilateral lambdoid sutures)

With bilateral involvement of the lambdoid sutures there is significant restriction of occipital bone growth. The compensatory growth occurs toward the vertex; the head appears flattened over both occipital areas and has a decreased anteroposterior diameter. This cylinder or tower-like appearance is sometimes termed *turricephaly.* The lambdoid suture is frequently involved with a variety of other sutures in complex and frequently unique situations. When bilateral lambdoid involvement does occur, it can be detected by the characteristic flattening of the occipital area and restriction of growth in the posterior aspect of the skull base.

Unilateral lambdoid synostosis creates the mildest cosmetic deformity of all forms of craniosynostosis. The occipital flattening is easily concealed with an appropriately designed hairdo; however, children with this anomaly become embarrassed and shy about their appearance during swimming and on other occasions where the asymmetric skull configuration is revealed.

Multiple suture involvement

Multiple suture involvement with craniosynostosis may cause a variety of skull deformities. Some clinical appearances are characteristic enough to predict suture involvement from simple clinical examination (Kleeblattschädel, or cloverleaf skull, anomaly [Fig. 26-12]), where as others are more unique and require careful clinical and radiographic examination to determine which sutures are involved (Fig. 26-13). With increasing suture involvement and restricted brain growth, increased intracranial pressure, papilledema, optic atrophy, and mental retardation all become significantly more common. With the extensive forms of disease, such as the Kleeblattschädel anomaly, even aggressively treated individuals are at high risk to develop these problems.[28] As more sutures become involved, the indication for surgical intervention changes from cosmetic considerations along to the more pressing problem of the preservation of neurologic function.

The ultimate in craniosynostosis is simultaneous involvement of all cranial sutures, which leaves no areas to accomodate brain growth. The anterior fontanelle is closed, and the skull has a microcephalic appearance with cephalo-

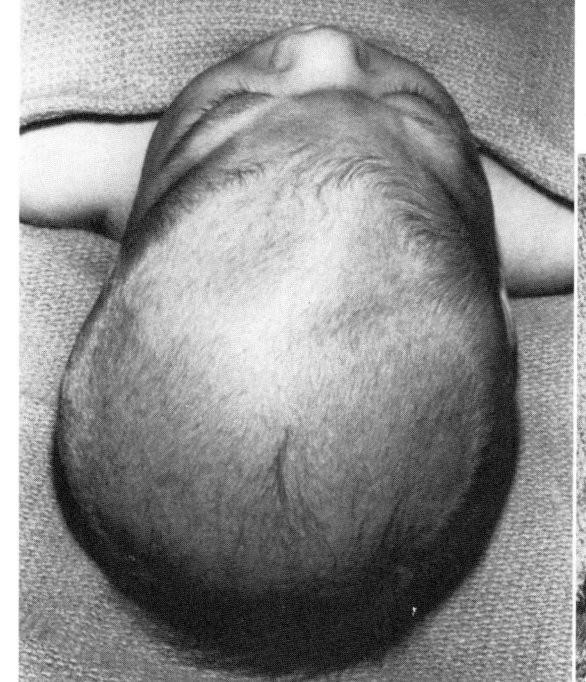
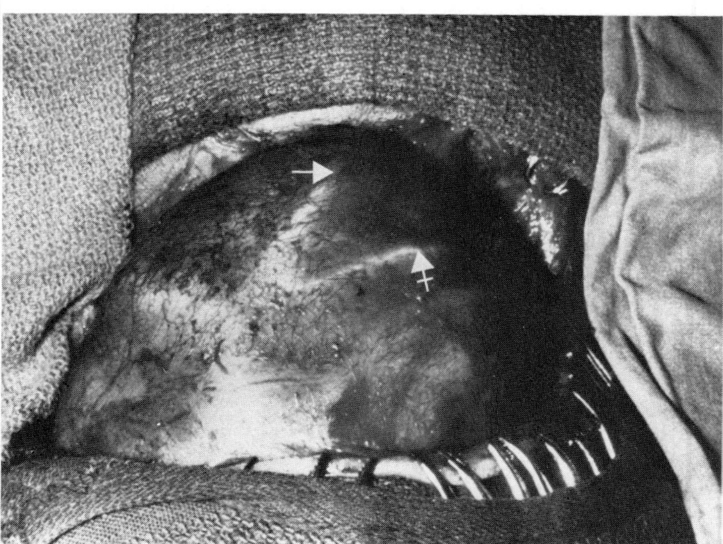

Fig. 26-13. Three-month-old child with an asymmetric head with restriction of growth in the right coronal and frontosphenoidal, inferior metopic, and left frontosphenoidal sutures, with minimal involvement of the coronal suture. **A,** Exaggeration of the supraorbital ridge. **B,** Intraoperative exposure of the child's sutures shows advancement of the right coronal suture to a more anterior position than normal *(hatched arrow)* and right-sided displacement of the metopic suture *(arrow).* (From Oakes, W.J., and Wilkins, R.H.: The newborn: neurosurgical considerations. In Filston, H.C.: Surgical problems in children: recognition and referral, St. Louis, 1982, The C.V. Mosby Co.)

facial disproportion but no other abnormalities of shape. Papilledema, which is so rarely seen in neonates and young infants because of their compensatory ability to decompress increased intracranial pressure through skull expansion, may be seen in this unusual situation. A much more common cause of microcrania, however, is that which develops secondary to limited or poor brain development. The induction growth of the skull in this case occurs at a much lower rate, and there are no signs of increased intracranial pressure or premature sutural fusion on skull radiographs. In both forms of microcrania the anterior fontanelle will close prematurely. Those patients in whom microcrania is secondary to limited induction from the injured or otherewise compromised brain will not benefit from and may be harmed by unnecessary surgical procedures directed at releasing the normal cranial sutures.

Secondary craniosynostosis

All sutures are usually affected simultaneously in patients with the secondary forms of craniosynostosis, producing a small rounded head. If individual sutures are differentially affected, the sagittal and coronal complex are the most frequently involved. Patients with significant involvement and evidence of increased intracranial pressure may demand early neurosurgical intervention if neurologic function is to be preserved.

Evaluation

With few exceptions patients with the simple forms of craniosynostosis can be adequately evaluated with routine skull radiographs. These should include lateral, frontal, Towne, basal, or submentovertex projections. Oblique lateral views may be necessary if the coronal sutures are superimposed and it is desired to see them separately. Confusion arises when superimposed coronal sutures are not recognized and the radiographs are interpreted as showing coronal synostosis. The basal projection is particularly helpful in demonstrating the anterior angulation and constriction of growth in the involved skull base. The angle made between the petrous ridge and sphenoid ridge can easily be assessed and then used for comparison in the postoperative period (Fig. 26-14). Although CT scanning adds significant information about the intracranial contents, this information is not necessary in planning therapy for all but the most

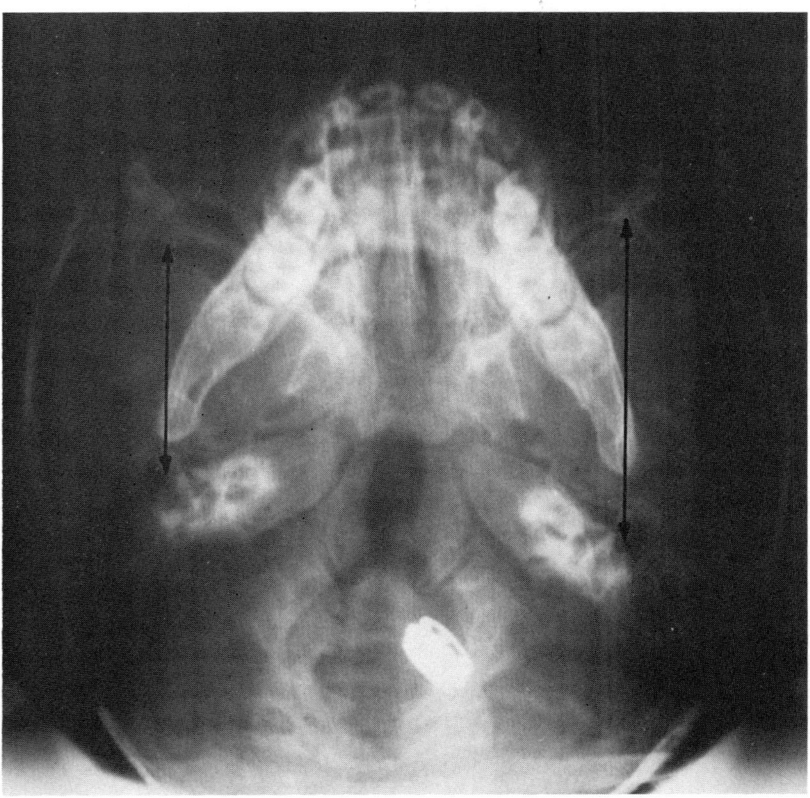

Fig. 26-14. Basal view of a patient with plagiocephaly. The normal angulation between the sphenoid ridge *(top of arrows)* and petrous ridge *(bottom of arrows)* is present on the patient's right side, whereas acute angulation and forward displacement of both the petrous and sphenoid ridge are present on the patient's left.

severely affected infants and children. When hydrocephalus or other developmental anomalies of the central nervous system are suspected, CT scanning adds essential information and is clearly indicated. I make this statement about simple forms of craniosynostosis despite the fact CT scanning using bone windows has significantly increased our understanding of the natural history and development of the underlying disease process. I simply believe that it is difficult to justify the additional expense on a routine basis for patients with simple forms of the disease.

When CT scanning of the brain and skull has been performed in patients with craniosynostosis, evidence of a reversible local pressure increase within the brain directly under the fused suture has been demonstrated.[15] This finding has been seen in the absence of generalized increased intracranial pressure, and it is an important observation that adds support in favor of surgical intervention, even in the simple forms of craniosynostosis.

Bone scanning using technetium[99] has also been employed at some centers to help identify patients with true craniosynostosis when plain skull radiography has been questionable[35,88] I have not found this technique necessary or informative in most patients.

A discussion of the medical evaluation of patients with craniosynostosis secondary to metabolic bone disease or endocrine abnormalities is beyond the scope of this chapter and can easily be found in most standard pediatric texts.

The changes seen in routine skull radiographs are best discussed under the categories of skull changes seen with simple primary craniosynostosis. Isolated involvement of the sagittal suture is easily detected (Fig. 26-15). The skull is symmetrically elongated in an anteroposterior diameter and narrowed in the biparietal distance. The point of primary fusion in the posterior aspect of the sagittal suture can frequently be seen (Fig. 26-16). The shelflike configuration of the posterior aspect of the head and the bifrontal prominence is also easily seen. The palpable ridge over the suture and the peaked appearance near the vertex is visible on appropriately angulated frontal projections (Fig. 26-17). The scaphocephalic appearance can be seen in premature neonates and severely ill infants with little or no spontaneous head movement. In this situation the head passively alternates position from one side to the other. The head does not rest stably on the occiput without some evidence of head control. This forces the neonate into alternating lateral postures of the head and tends to flatten the skull's configuration if sufficient time passes before the development of head control. Radiographically the sutures are open, and the deformity tends to correct itself spontaneously when head control is gained.

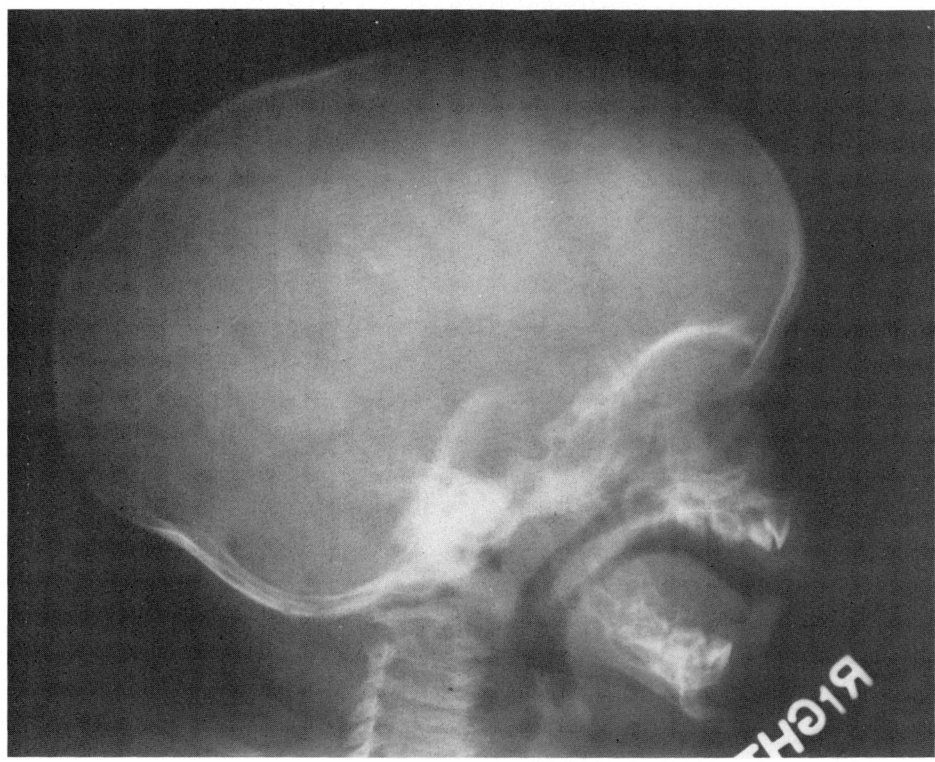

Fig. 26-15. Lateral radiograph of a child with scaphocephaly. The head is elongated in an anteroposterior direction.

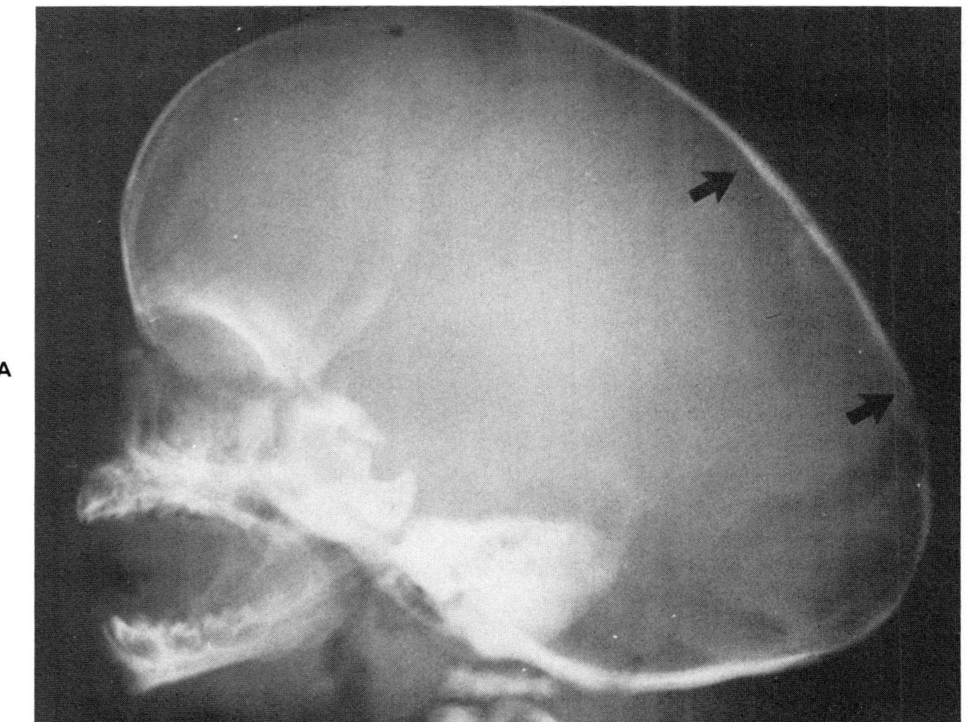

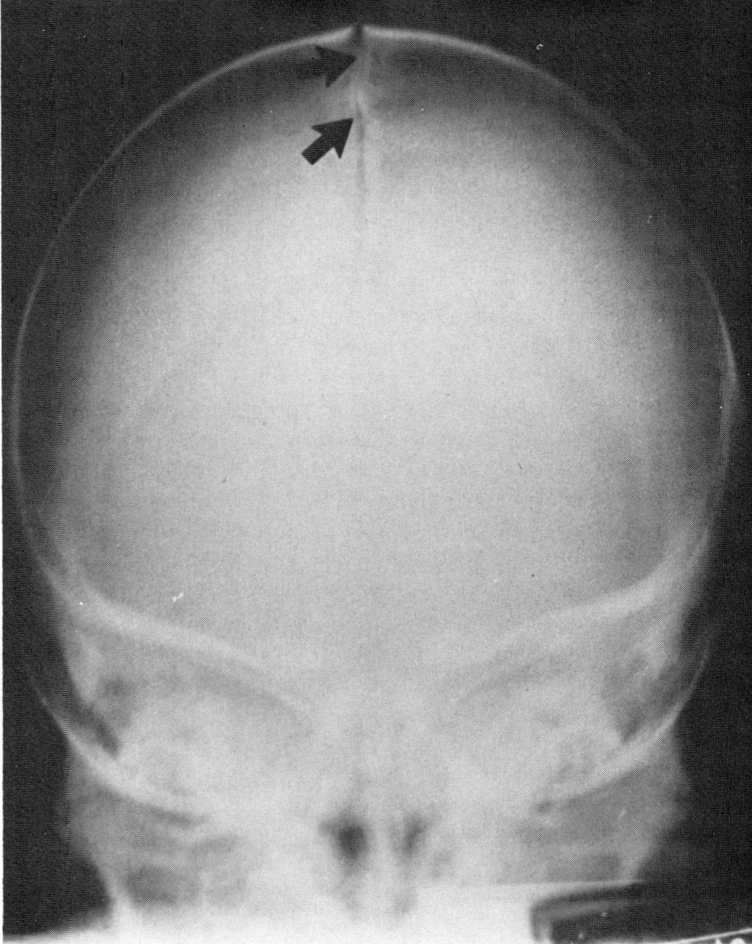

Fig. 26-16. A, Lateral view of an infant with scaphocephaly in whom the primary area of suture closure can be seen in the posterior aspect of the sagittal suture *(arrows)*. **B,** Towne projection of same patient, again showing the area of premature closure *(arrows)* over a limited portion of the involved suture.

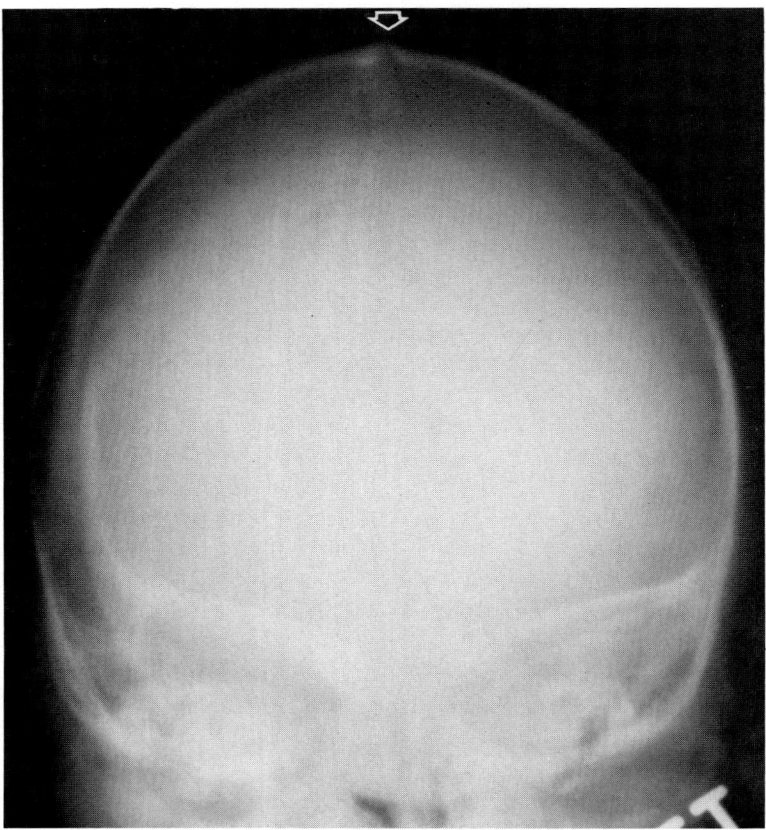

Fig. 26-17. Towne view of another patient with scaphocephaly and a prominent external ridge on the synostotic sagittal suture *(arrow)*.

The determination of radiographic fusion of a suture bears special mention. During the final stages of fusion the entire suture may appear equally involved, but at an earlier stage only a portion of the suture may show changes. The problem of parietal suture fusion has been addressed by others, including Caffey.[14] The earliest radiographic sign of suture fusion is narrowing of the suture with an increase in the bone density adjacent to the narrowing.[48] This occurs at a single spot along the suture and then expands to involve more of the suture. Even when the process involves only a portion of the suture, it is functionally fused as if the entire suture were involved throughout its length. A surer radiographic sign of restricted suture expansion is cranial deformity.[36,56] This is more reliable than sutural narrowing or sclerosis.

The radiographic appearance of patients with plagiocephaly from coronal and frontosphenoidal suture synostosis is also easily detected (Fig. 26-18). The most prominent feature is an elevation and thickening of the lateral aspect of the orbit as it merges with the lateral portion of the sphenoid wing. The oblique elevation of the lateral orbit is termed a *harlequin orbit*. The orbit itself is shallow and the forehead flattened on the involved side. The synostotic process involves the frontosphenoidal suture in the vast majority of infants[85] and sutures of the midface in some patients with tilting of the nasal septum and crista galli to the side of the synostotic involvement. The more medial aspect of the coronal suture near the anterior fontanelle will remain radiographically open in a significant percentage of patients. In this situation the diagnosis does not depend on *total* fusion of the coronal suture; a more reliable radiographic sign is the presence of the affect of the synostotic process on the lateral aspect of the coronal suture complex (harlequin orbit deformity and forehead flattening). In addition, the angle created by the petrous ridge and sphenoid ridge is made more acute by the restriction of growth of the basal sutures[70] (Fig. 26-14).

With bilateral coronal and basal involvement the shortened anteroposterior diameter of the skull and in particular the floor of the anterior fossa is striking (Fig. 26-19). Harlequin orbit deformities appear bilaterally, and both orbits are shortened. The bulk of the anteroposterior diameter shortening is at the expense of the anterior cranial fossa. The basal angle becomes more acute bilaterally, although this may not be exactly symmetric. Since increased intracranial pressure is more common with increasing suture

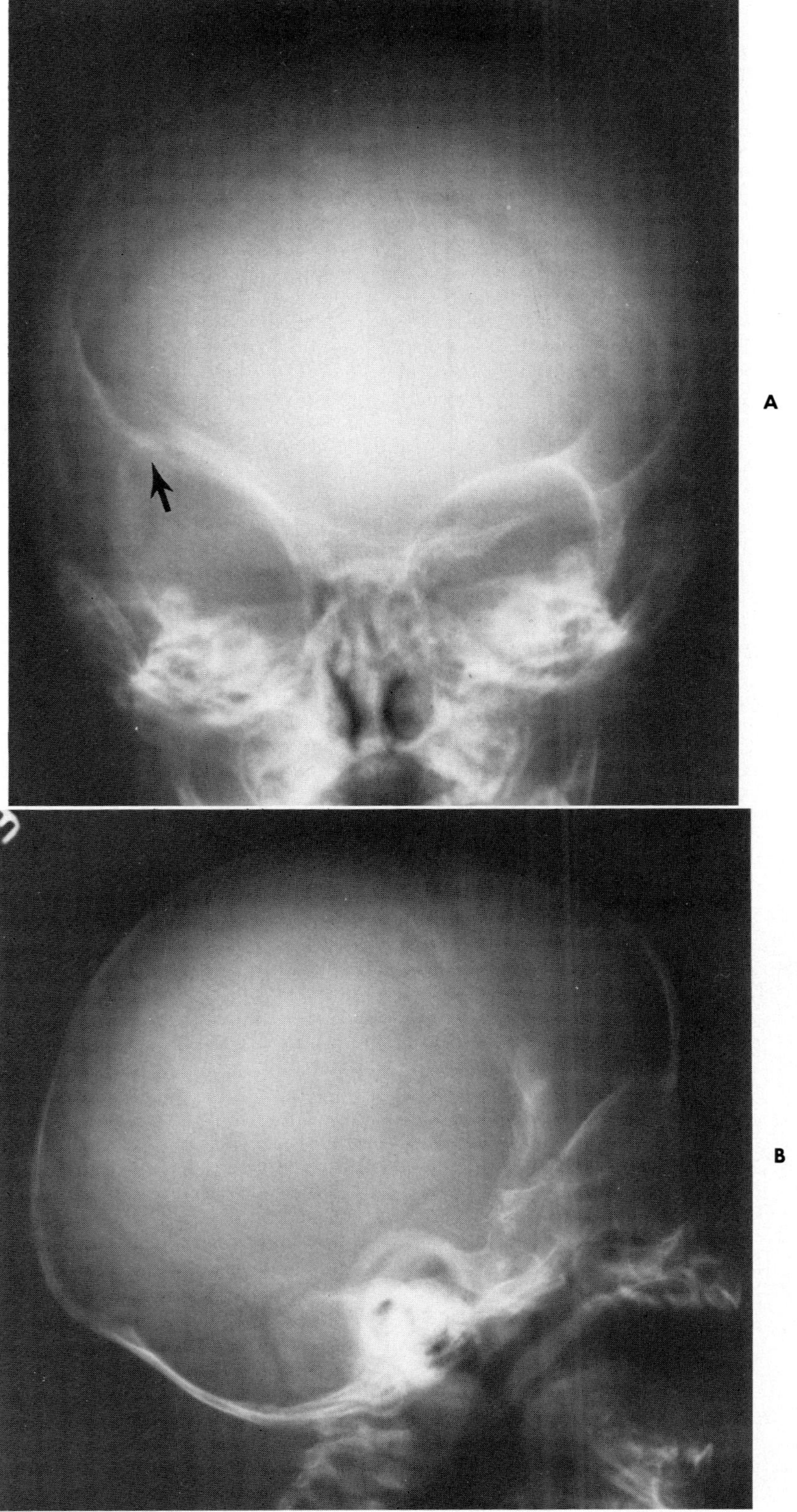

Fig. 26-18. A, Frontal view of a child with plagiocephaly and a harlequin deformity of the orbit *(arrow)*. Thickening of the lateral sphenoid ridge on the involved side can also be seen. **B,** Lateral radiograph of the same patient showing an area of unilateral coronal synostosis with deformity of the orbital roof.

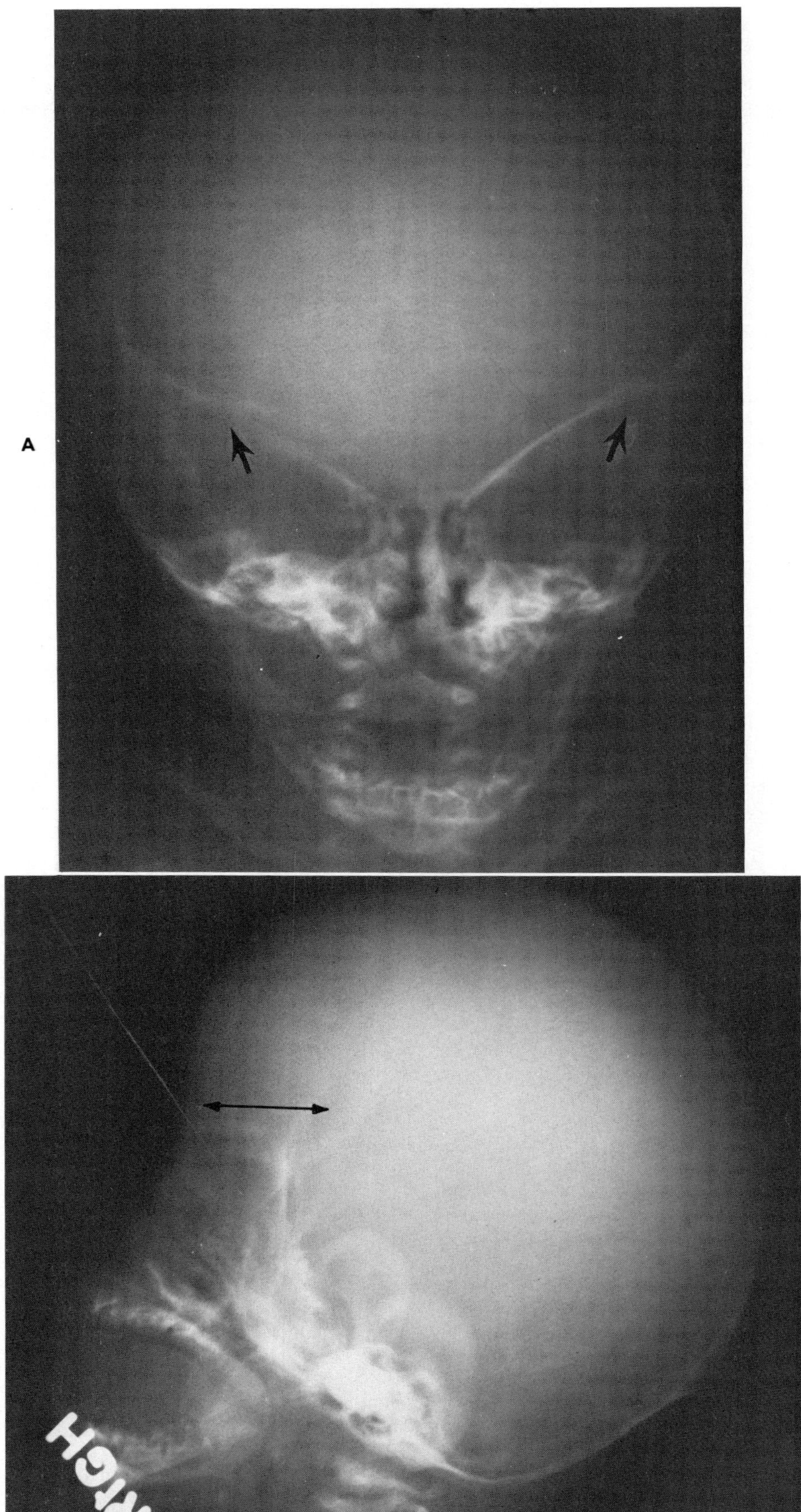

Fig. 26-19. A, Frontal view of a patient with brachiocephaly and bilateral harlequin deformity *(arrows)*. **B,** Lateral view of the same patient demonstrating the notable shortening of the anterior cranial fossa *(arrow)* from involvement of the basal sutures. Midface hypoplasia is also apparent.

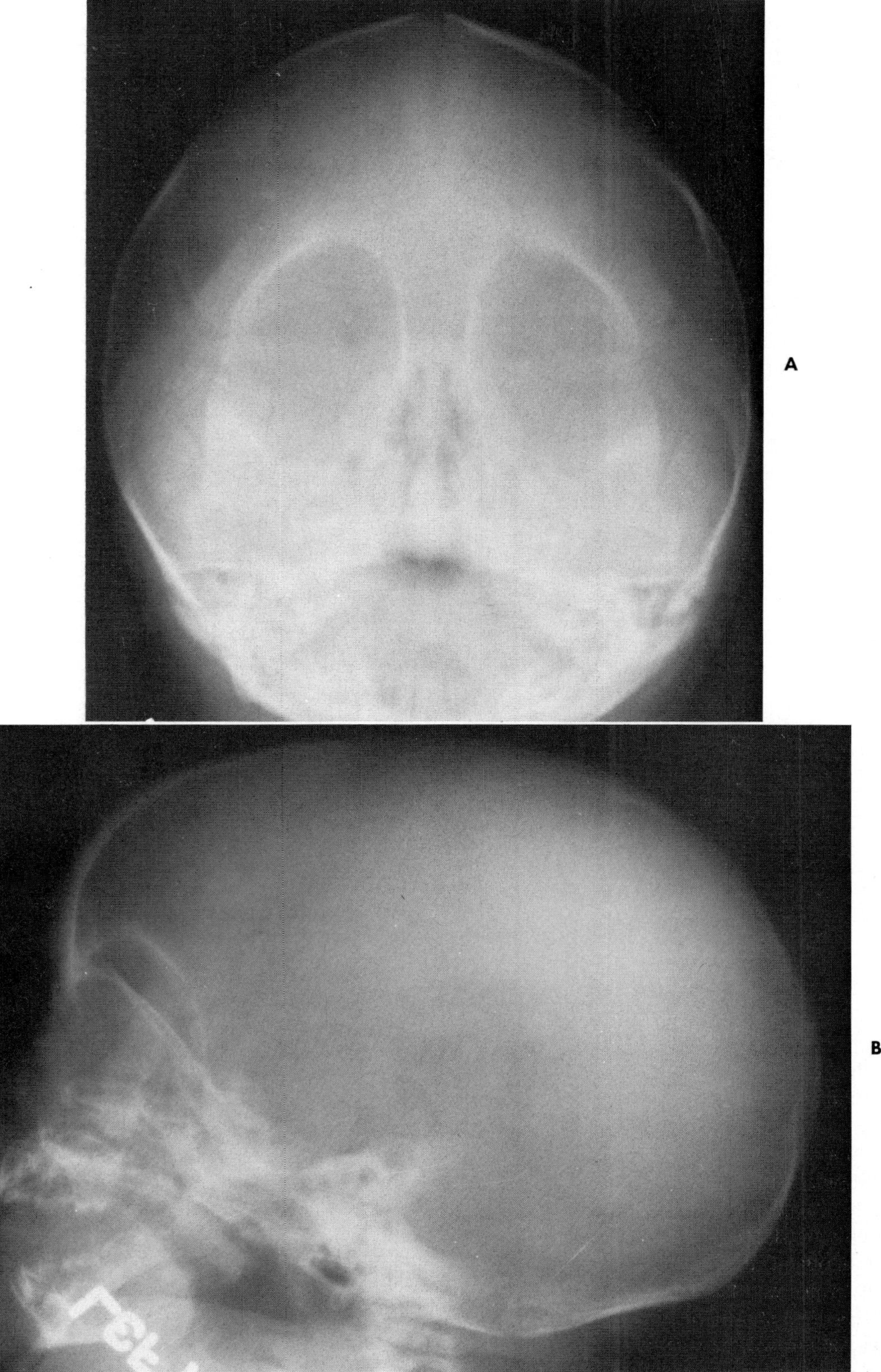

Fig. 26-20. A, Frontal projection of a patient with trigonocephaly. Hypotelorism and prominence of the metopic suture can easily be visualized. In addition, the orbits are deformed with a vector superiorly and medially. **B,** Lateral radiograph of the same patient showing limitation of expansion of the anterior cranial fossa. *Continued.*

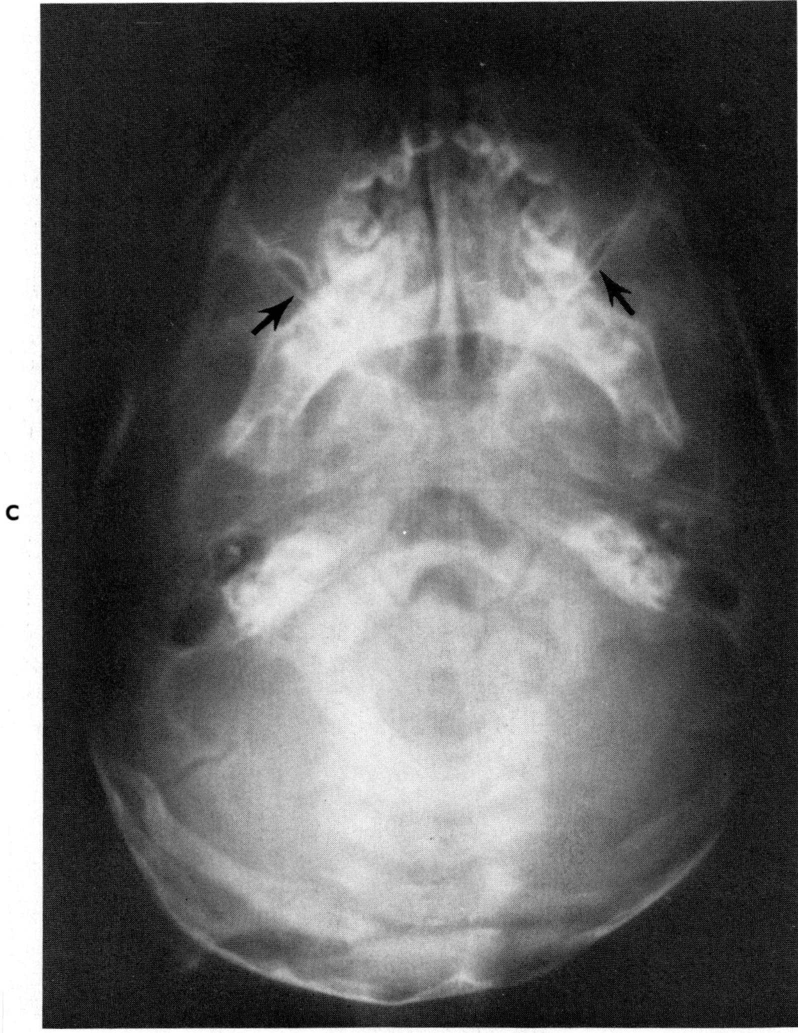

Fig. 26-20, cont'd. C, Basal view of same patient demonstrating hypotelorism with medial displacement of the lateral portion of both orbits *(arrows).*

involvement, the beaten metal appearance on the inner table of the skull is more common with bilateral coronal and basal involvement.

Hypotelorism and premature synostosis with the metopic and frontoethmoidal suture complex results in trigonocephaly with a beaked appearance of the forehead. The orbits are not only displaced medially but also angulated up and toward one another at their superior medial borders (Fig. 26-20). As in coronal and basal suture synostosis, the anterior cranial fossa is shortened and the radiographically visible metopic suture will be sclerotic. The abnormal angulation of the orbits and sphenoid ridges can be most easily visualized in the basal projection. Associated with trigonocephaly in complicated patients is the cleft palate deformity. When holoprosencephaly is suggested by defective development of the crista galli, vomer, or nasal bones,[58] CT scanning is indicated to determine the degree of cerebral dysgenesis.

The radiology of lambdoid synostosis is more confusing and less exact. When flattening of the involved occipital area is associated with narrowing and parasutural sclerosis of the ipsilateral lambdoid suture, the diagnosis is simple (Fig. 26-21). This is also usually associated with asymmetry of the foramen magnum. As emphasized by Harwood-Nash,[44] however, sutures in general and the lambdoid in particular may show varying degrees of radiographic fusion with significant skull deformity. The process of suture fusion and restricted growth is not an all-or-none phenomenon, and gradations of this process are possible. The "sticky lambdoid suture" may be associated with some parasutural sclerosis, usually on the occipital side of the suture with occipital flattening, but without radiographic suture narrowing or fu-

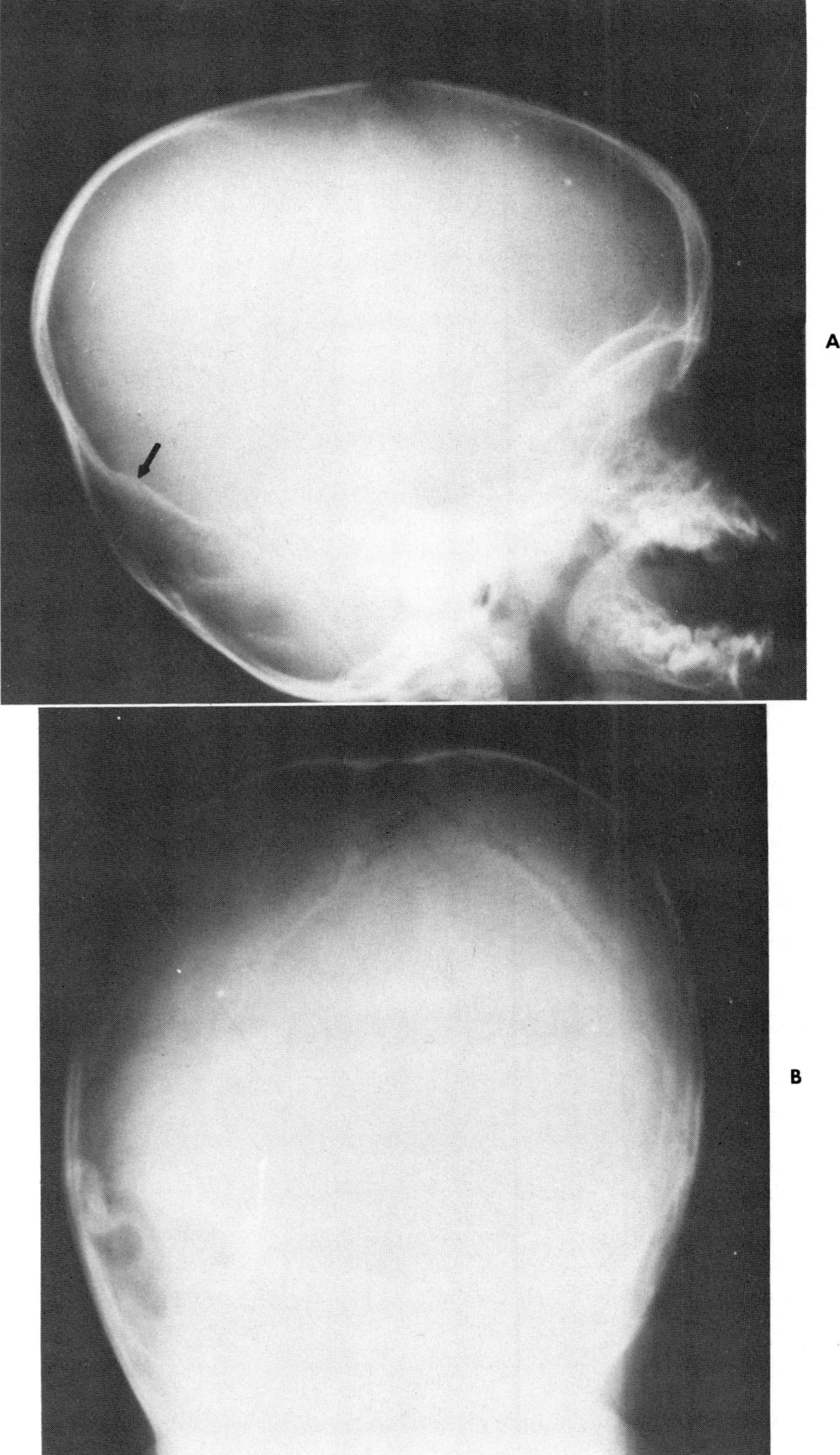

Fig. 26-2l. A, Lateral radiograph of a child with lambdoid synostosis and flattening of the occiput and posterior fossa. The line of sclerosis along the suture can easily be seen *(arrow)*. **B,** Towne view of the same patient demonstrating sclerosis with lateral fusion of the suture. Sclerosis is much more apparent on the occipital side of the suture. The suture remains radiographically open more medially.

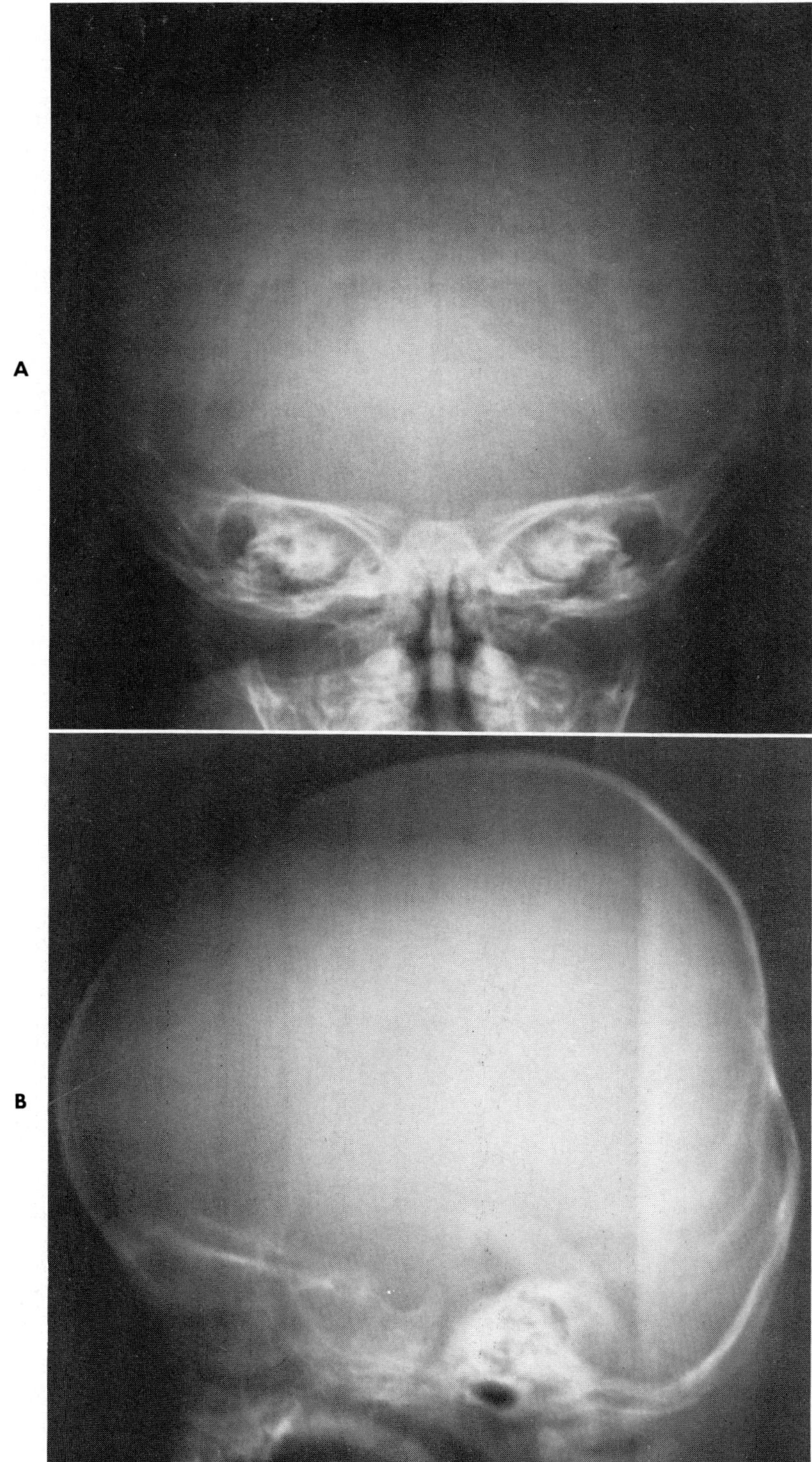

Fig. 26-22. A, Towne view of patient with bilateral lambdoid synostosis. Both lambdoid sutures appear radiographically patent. **B,** Lateral radiograph demonstrates the characteristic skull deformity and radiographic sclerosis. This child's lambdoid sutures were functionally closed, although on the Towne view radiograph, this was not supported.

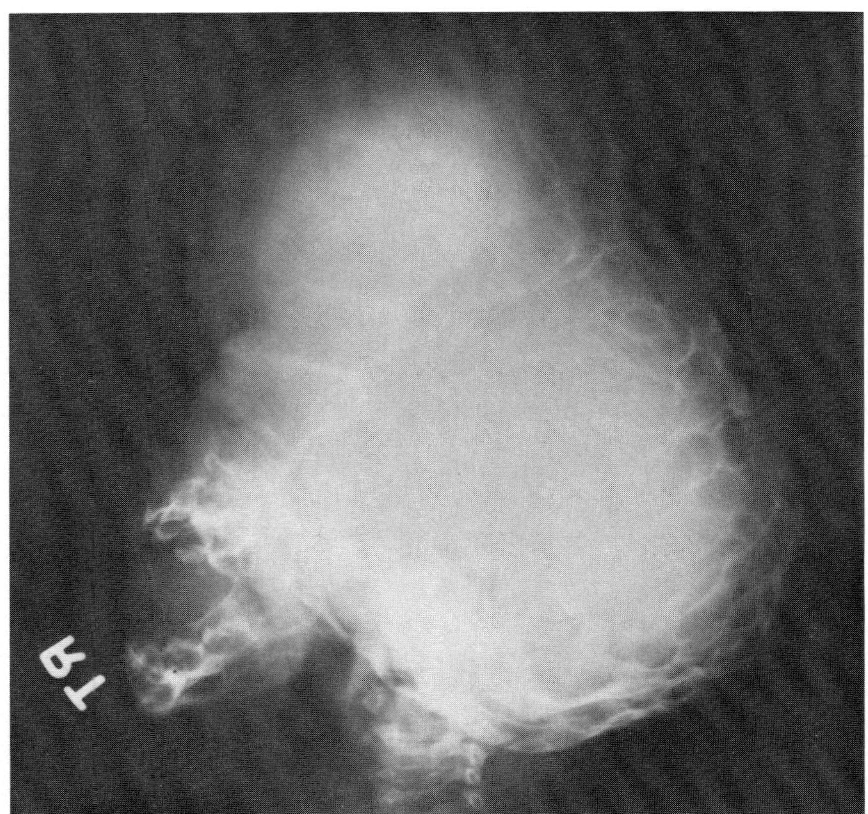

Fig. 26-23. Radiograph of the patient depicted in Fig. 26-12, *A*. The beaten metal appearance of the inner aspect of the parietal and occipital regions is apparent, with compensatory growth occurring through the anterior fontanelle. Severe hypoplasia of the midface is also apparent.

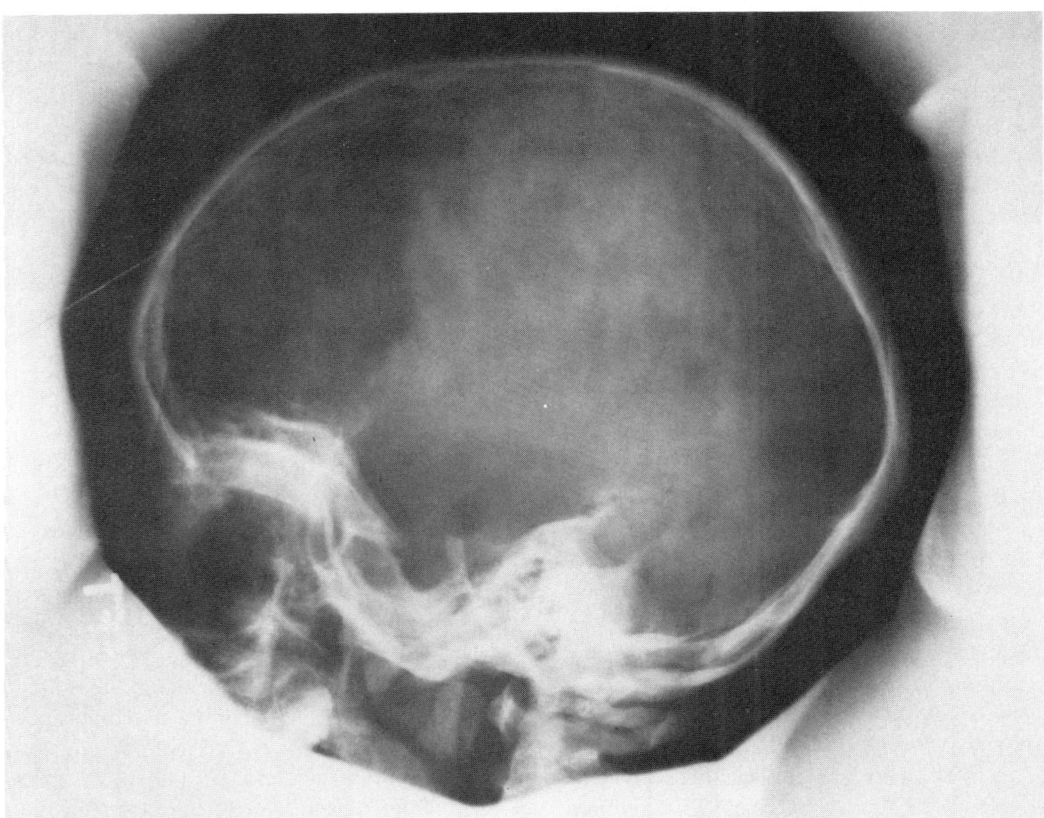

Fig. 26-24. Lateral radiograph of a patient with diffuse craniosynostosis but with preservation of the normal skull configuration. The patient had papilledema and evidence of increased intracranial pressure clinically. The increased density of the orbital rim and petrous apex should be noted. Further evaluation confirmed the child to have cranial metaphyseal dysplasia.

sion (Fig. 26-22). True synostosis of the lambdoid suture is associated with increased brain markings in the area of the synostotic suture, whereas with the "sticky suture" this is not seen. This implies that true radiographic fusion is associated with a more-severe form of restricted brain growth than is the "sticky lambdoid suture."

Lambdoid synostosis that involves both sutures does significantly restrict brain growth and is associated with increased brain markings bilaterally. Although flattening of the occiput can be easily camouflaged with an approprite hairstyle, the bilateral form of the disease should be viewed as more than a cosmetic problem.

Multiple suture involvement from craniosynostosis raises the incidence of radiographic evidence of increased intracranial pressure. A beaten metal appearance of the inner aspect of the skull, grotesque deformity as a means of compensating for rapid brain growth through open suture areas, and erosion of the posterior clinoid processes can all be seen (Fig. 26-23). When multiple sutures are involved, the texture of the bone should be evaluated critically (Fig. 26-24). If questions of an abnormal bony matrix or density of the involved bone are raised, a survey of other areas is indicated.

THERAPEUTIC ALTERNATIVES

Once a diagnosis of primary simple craniosynostosis is made, the therapeutic options are quite limited. If the disease process is restricted in its scope to the sagittal suture, a single coronal and basal suture complex, or a single lambdoid suture, the brain is believed to have a normal potential for development without serious risk of increased intracranial pressure. This situation may appear to represent a purely cosmetic problem, and the potential improvement in appearance with and without surgical intervention may be discussed. Although neurologic and psychologic testing may detect no focal deficit of the brain directly under the synostotic suture, both plain radiographic accentuation of brain markings in the vicinity of the synostotic suture[44] and CT evidence of local pressure increase[15] indicate that adjacent brain may be adversely affected. Pathologic evidence of gliosis or other histologic structural change in the brain under these synostotic sutures have neither been confirmed nor denied in large series. What has been seen is that the developing brain distorts itself to accommodate the area of restriction. Once multiple suture involvement is recognized, the patient's neurologic functional status is jeopardized and the indications for surgical intervention are much stronger.

The psychologic importance of a normal-shaped skull should not be minimized.[8] The stress associated with an abnormal head shape can be severe and has even been believed to be responsible for the development of a duodenal ulcer in childhood.[74] The common and cosmetically mild form of craniosynostosis, scaphocephaly has variously been referred to by young classmates as "bomb brain" or "bullet head."

If untreated in infancy, these children or their parents tend to seek a second medical opinion with regard to correction of the deformity at two distinct times. The first is at the age of 5 or 6, shortly after the child begins attending school. Peer pressure and the stress of acceptance may cause this crisis. A second time is at 12 to 14 years of age, when the patient begins to become more concerned about appearance in anticipation of dating. Recently two children were seen in this clinic within a week of beginning swimming lessons; their unilateral lambdoid synostosis was detected by peers when their wet hair laid flat against their misshapen skulls. Both children vehemently refused to return to any social situation that would require their hair to become wet and to divulge their "secret." Until society and in particular young children develop more acceptance of variations from the norm with regard to head shape, even the mildest forms of craniosynostosis will be associated with anxiety in both parents and patients.

Surgical therapy for cosmetic deformity secondary to craniosynostosis is not universally accepted.[33,45] Much of the objection to surgery is the associated risks. Both the anesthetic and the operative risk for surgical intervention have significantly decreased in the past two decades. Even though these risks are lessened they will never be eliminated. The decision to surgically correct a skull deformity for cosmetic indications alone must always be weighed against potential risks inherent in such procedures. For the family unwilling to accept any risks in exchange for cosmetic improvement, it is totally unjustified to pressure or forcefully persuade them that withholding operation is not a viable alternative. The single factor I believe must be emphasized after a careful discussion with the family is that, if the child's cosmetic defect is accepted and surgery is not performed, this should be a decision based on a thoughtful analysis of the risks and cosmetic benefits. During later emotional and stressful periods when this decision might be questioned no guilt on the part of the parents should be associated with the decision for no surgery.

The skull deformity of craniosynostosis cannot currently be influenced by medications, which make this alternative nonexistent. A recently popularized nonoperative alternative of head molding deserves special comment.[16,17] In infants with torticollis and asymmetric skull development (plagiocephaly that is *not* secondary to craniosynostosis), head shape can be improved or normalized if an appropriately fitted polypropylene helmet is intermittently applied. Unfortunately this form of therpay has not proven successful when true craniosynostosis is present and is not an alternative therapeutic option in the group.

As discussed previously, the natural history of unoperated trigonocephaly secondary to metopic synostosis has recently been questioned.[26] The hypotelorism and forehead deformity were both believed to resolve spontaneously with time. Harwood-Nash and Fitz[44] hold an intermediate view, believing that patients with trigonocephaly should be operated on because although much of the forehead deformity may resolve, the hypotelorism will not. Current opinion favors surgical correction because of the persistent or progressive nature of the skull deformity. It is hoped that these incompatible views will be resolved with further experience with unoperated patients.

Once an informed decision by the parents to accept the risks of surgical intervention has been made, the surgical techniques for each type of repair of craniosynostosis can be split into two categories. The traditional neurosurgical approach has been to resect involved sutures and to rely on continued brain growth and skull expansion to reshape and redirect growth in the area of restriction. This type of operation depends on further growth of the skull; therefore it must be performed early in life, ideally within the first 6 months so that sufficient potential for skull growth remains and the expected cosmetic improvement outweighs the involved risks.[65,80] As the child becomes progressively older, the degree of improvement with this simple type of release operation decreases. Beyond the first year of life operations directed only at resecting synostotic sutures are not justified. Exceptions to this general rule are patients who are operated on not for cosmetic improvement but for the relief of increased intracranial pressure. In this situation operation at any time to preserve vision or eliminate intracranial hypertension is justified.

The alternative class of operation to simple resection of involved sutures is for the surgeon at the operating table to actually change the shape of the skull. This type of operation does not depend on further skull growth and can be performed at any time. In fact, there is significant advantage in waiting for the majority of skull growth to have already occurred before attempting intraoperative repositioning of bony structures. If further growth is anticipated, the degree of correction achieved for a 2-year-old child may become inappropriate as the head continues to enlarge.

The surgical correction of scaphocephaly is the simplest of all forms of craniosynostosis to be significantly influenced with operative therapy. A simple linear craniectomy performed directly through the involved suture[24,68] and adjacent to it[4,62] has been advocated. The bilateral paramedian approach is advocated for fear of injuring the sagittal sinus and causing serious blood loss. An additional factor for consideration is that having performed two parallel craniectomies, the period of time necessary before refusion across the craniectomy site is increased to allow additional time for lateral expansion of the skull. Whichever approach is used, it is important to carry the craniectomy throughout the length of the suture. It should cross both the coronal and lambdoidal junctions. This is especially true of the lambdoid area, since the majority of the skull deformity will be found posteriorly. If the patient is incorrectly positioned (supine) to have their procedure performed, it is difficult to consistently reach the lambdoid suture with the craniectomy. A lateral or prone position is superior in this regard and

allows easy visualization of the entire area of the craniectomy.

Since this type of operation relies heavily on the synostotic suture remaining unfused, two methods have been advocated to retard bony regrowth into the area of the craniectomy. One method is to line the side of the craniectomy with an inert substance to retard the ingrowth of bone from the exposed edge. Since pure polyethylene has been associated with the formation of sarcomas in laboratory animals,[10,77] Silastic is the preferred substance if this technique is to be used. The implantation of any foreign body raises the risk of infection, and the long-term benign character of any substance implanted within the body cannot be assured. These factors question the advisability of implanting a foreign substance if an acceptable alternative is available.

The second method that has been advocated to retard bony regrowth from the dura is by painting the exposed dura with a tissue fixative derived from Zenker's solution.[3,78] In clinical settings this has proven to be effective in retarding bony regrowth into the craniectomy site. Multiple experimental sutides, however, have shown disruption of the blood-brain barrier[60] and damage to the underlying cerebral cortex.[64] Clinically the incidence of seizures after the application of modified Zenker's solution to the exposed dura is high, and this technique can no longer be justified. It is therefore concluded that both methods previously advocated to retard bony regrowth of the craniectomized area carry risks that do not warrant their use today.

Jane et al.,[52] have advocated an alternative technique in infants for the immediate correction of sagittal synostosis (Fig. 26-25). Paramedian sagittal craniectomies are performed in a routine manner but are carried laterally down the coronal suture to the level of the anterolateral fontanelle. The freed midline bone over the sagittal sinus is strutted forward and held in place with medium-gauge wire. This causes an immediate shortening of the anteroposterior skull diameter and biparietal expansion of the skull. It also significantly alters the dural tensions, which have previously been discussed as being the instigating factors causing the underlying premature fusion.[71] Although Jane has not advocated the use of this procedure in infants beyond 1 year of age, I have modified the technique slightly (Fig. 26-26) and included a posterior craniectomy along the lambdoid suture bilaterally. This has been successfully performed in infants as old as 18 months with a gratifying and immediate correction of skull deformity (Fig. 26-27). This is my current preferred method of surgery for scaphocephaly. Cosmetic change is immediate and dramatic, and the procedure incorporates the principles of altering the dural tensions, which enhances continued normal growth of the skull.

Because of severe psychologic stress, remolding of the scaphocephalic skull later in children has occasionally been performed[74] with gratifying results. These procedures are performed in multiple stages and because of their complexity and extensive nature carry increased inherent risks. They

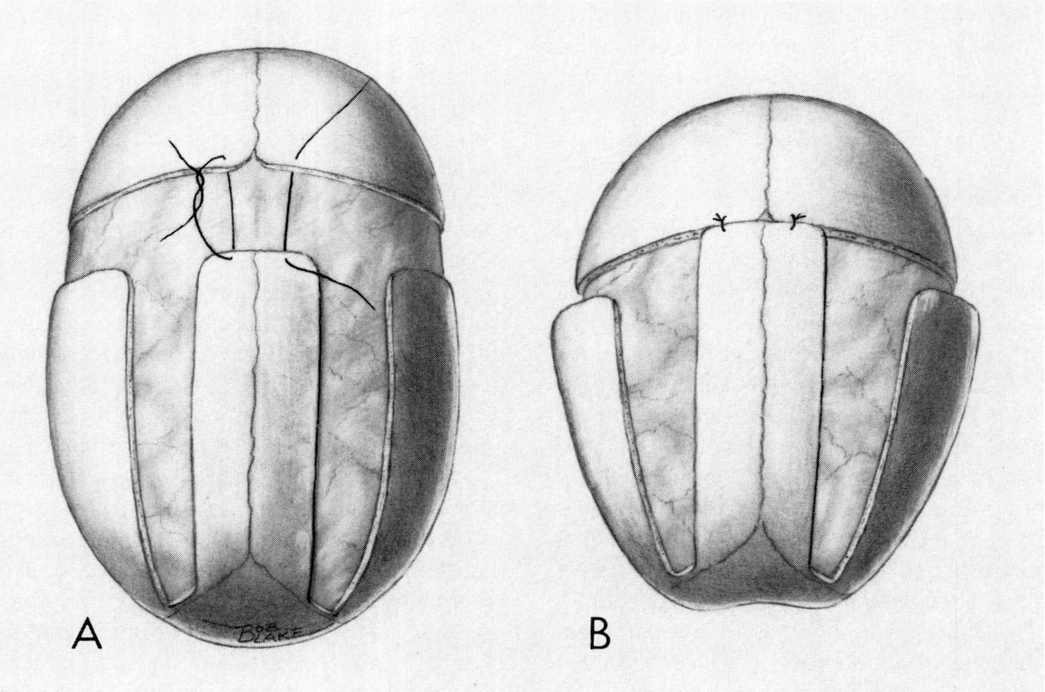

Fig. 26-25. A, Intraoperative view of Jane procedure for scaphocephaly. Paramedian sagittal and coronal craniectomies have been performed and the bone overlying the sagittal suture is in the midst of being repositioned anteriorly. **B,** After repositioning, the head takes on an immediate decrease in anteroposterior diameter with expansion occuring biparietally.

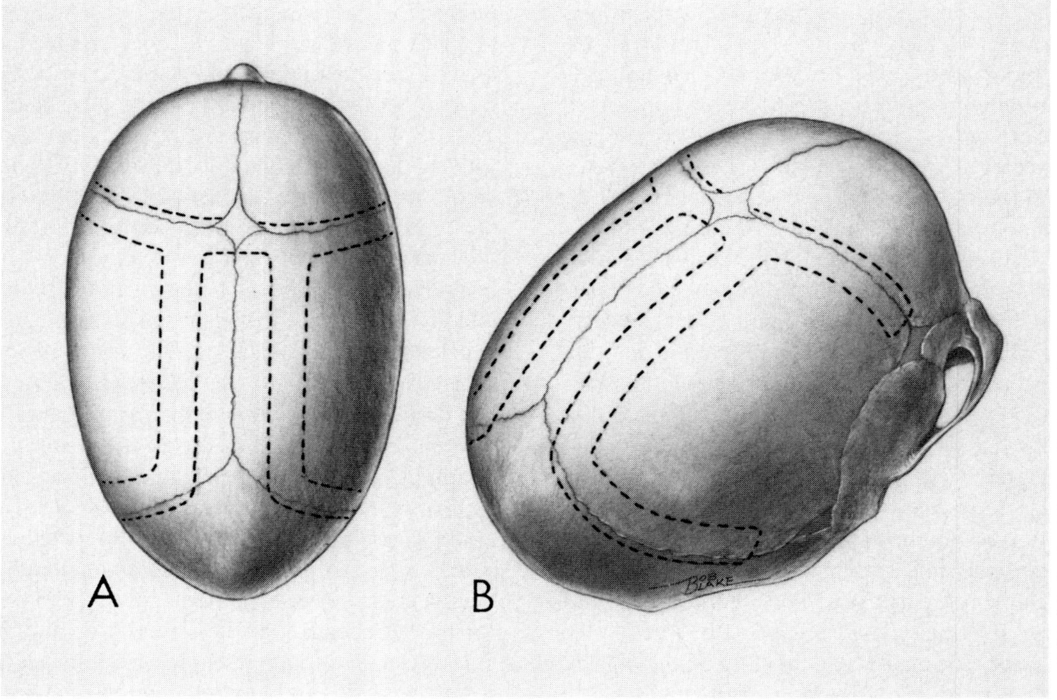

Fig. 26-26. Modified Jane procedure **(A)** with craniectomies performed in a paramedian fashion parallel to the sagittal suture, as well as laterally along coronal and both lambdoid sutures **(B).** This leaves the parietal bone hinged to the skull only by the squamosal suture.

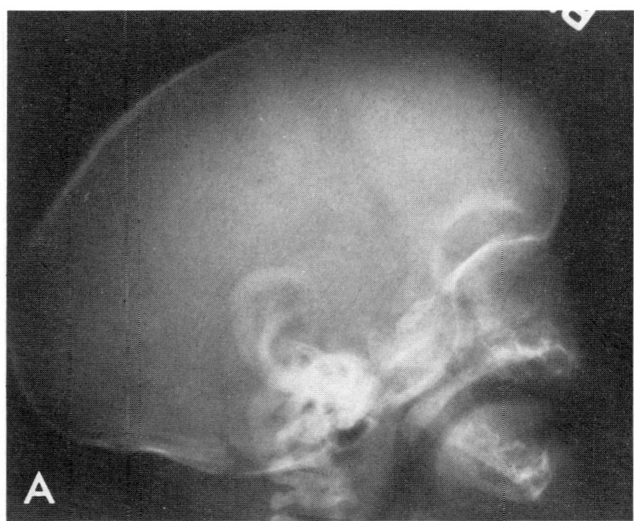

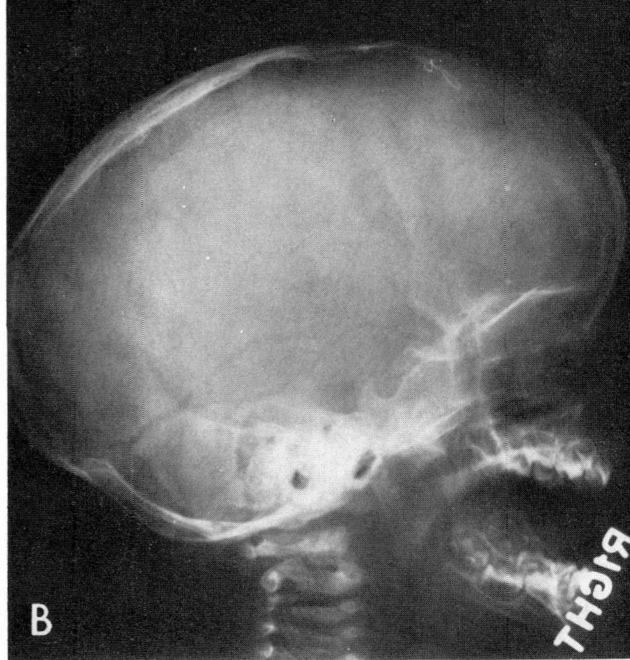

Fig. 26-27. A, Child with scaphocephaly and significant prominence of the occipital area. **B,** Several months after a modified Jane procedure the head has virtually normal configuration.

should be reserved for the older child who is having significant psychologic stress that cannot be adequately relieved by other means.

The surgical procedures devised to treat patients with plagiocephaly from coronal and frontosphenoidal synostosis have changed significantly in the past two decades. The standard procedure of performing a linear craniectomy along the fused coronal suture[61] influenced the child's cosmetic appearance minimally. Armed with the knowledge that the frontosphenoidal suture was routinely involved in the synostotic process[85] and that the coronal sutures formed a continuous circle at the base of the skull with the extension of the frontosphenoidal and posterior frontoethmoidal su-

tures,[11] surgeons began to experiment with more extensive procedures aimed at the base of the skull. To support this conceptual change was the realization that growth perpendicular to the coronal and basal ring was retarded, whereas growth parallel to it was enhanced. This met the cardinal tenets of restricted growth with craniosynostosis. At first it was suggested that the linear craniectomy simply be continued into the frontal bone immediately behind the supraorbital ridge (Fig. 26-28).[24] Then it was suggested that a more extensive craniectomy be performed in the area of the pterion and along the frontosphenoidal suture where much of the dense adhesion between dura and overlying skull is characteristically seen. This would help to discon-

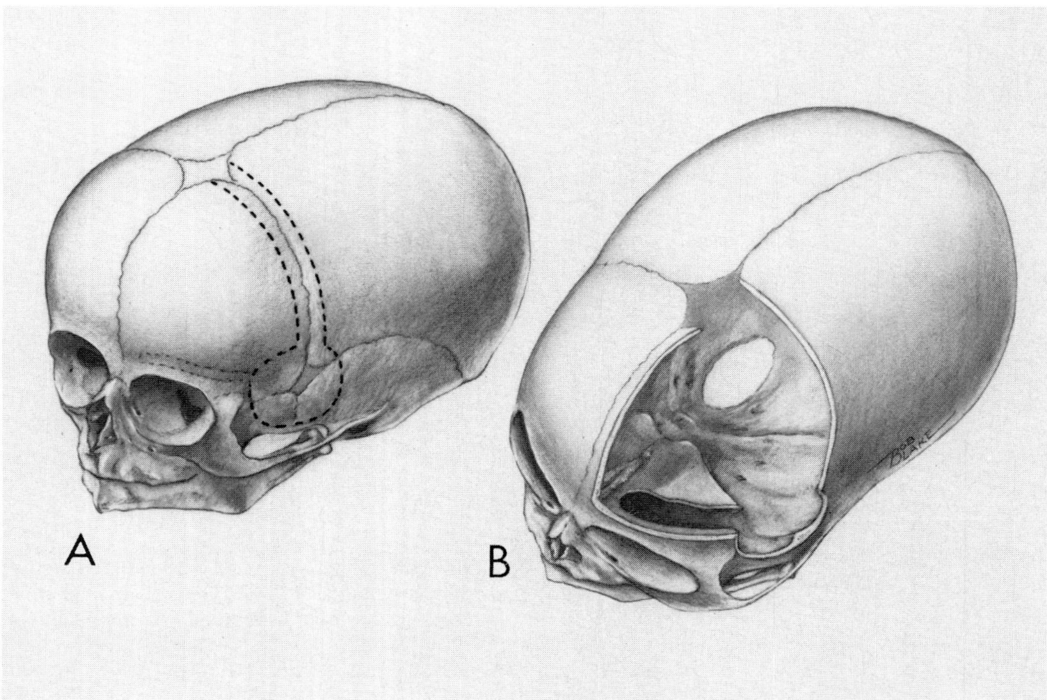

Fig. 26-28. A, Conventional craniectomy for plagiocephaly with removal of the involved coronal suture and the bone around the anterolateral fontanelle. **B,** Removal of the orbital roof immediately behind the superior orbital ridge allowed it to be disconnected from the skull except at its medial attachment and strutted forward.

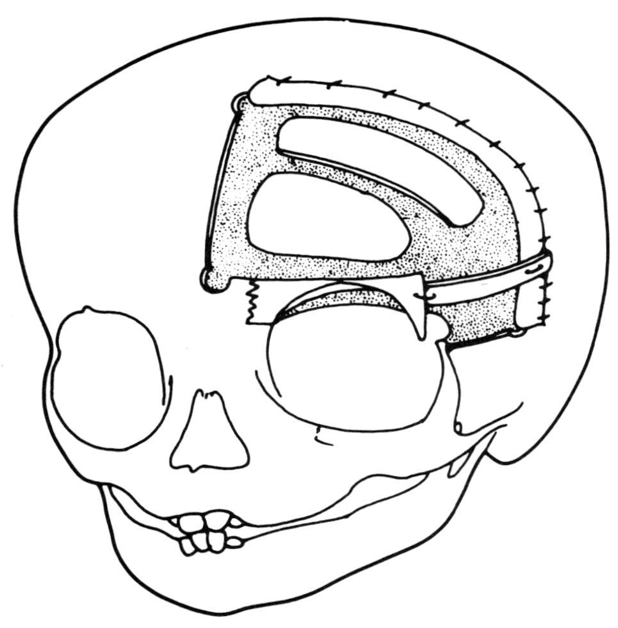

Fig. 26-29. Lateral canthal advancement. (From Hoffman, H.J., and Mohr, G.: J. Neurosurg. **45:**378, 1976.)

nect the foreshortened frontal fossa from the frontal bone but tended to quickly fill in the craniectomy site with new bone formation. Insufficient time of uninhibited growth of the anterior cranial fossae occurred. An alternative approach adopted the two previous innovations, but to prolong the effect of the basal craniectomy, the lateral aspect of the superior orbital ridge was strutted forward with a graft from the posterior aspect of the skull flap (Fig. 26-29). This "lateral canthal advancement" caused an immediate improvement in the infant's appearance and yielded a significantly improved long-term result.[47] The disadvantages of this procedure quickly became apparent. With unilateral involvement, the question of the extent of advancement of the supraorbital ridge was always difficult to judge. If the surgeon was too enthusiastic about building in room for further growth, the infant would appear overcorrected and have a bony prominence along the lateral aspect of the forehead. If corrected an appropriate amount to make the child symmetric at the time of operation, the degree of correction would be inadequate with further growth, necessitating an additional procedure to advance or strut the supraorbital ridge forward. More commonly undercorrection resulted in persistent shortening of the anterior cranial fossa.

Since lateral canthal advancement can be performed in older children and does not rely exclusively on further

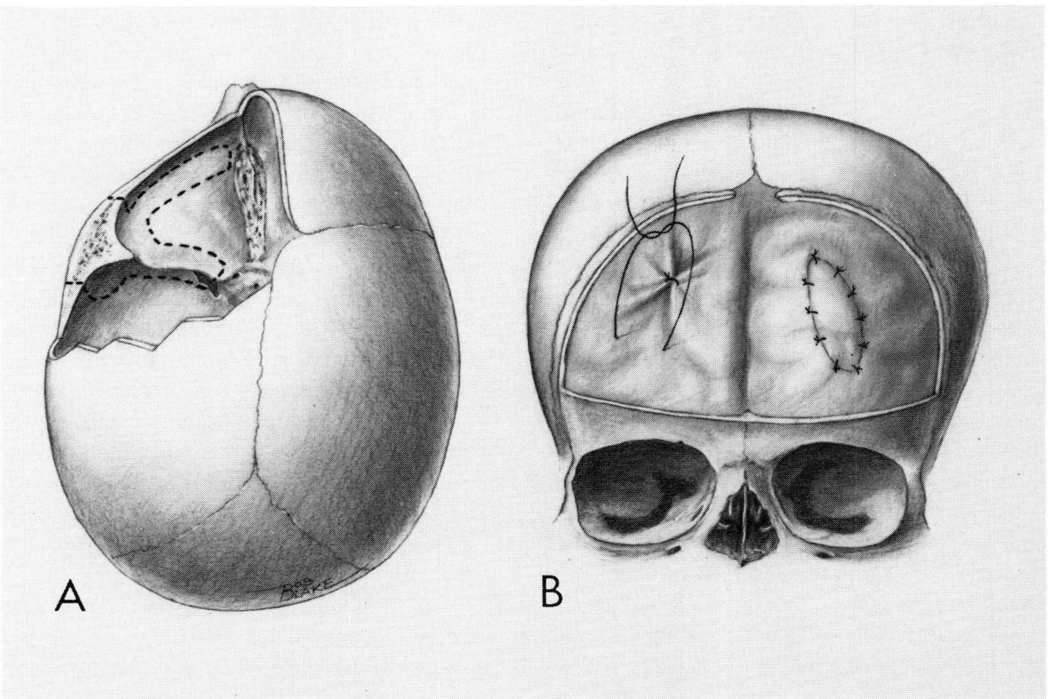

Fig. 26-30. A, Current technique for plagiocephaly involves a frontal craniotomy, which is carried out bilaterally if there is prominent frontal bossing on the uninvolved side. After removal of both frontal bones, the craniectomy on the involved side is carried well inferiorly into the base of the sphenoid ridge. The orbital roof is separated from the superior orbital rim, and the craniectomy is extended medially along the sphenoid ridge to the superior orbital fissure. **B,** Dura on the uninvolved side is plicated, whereas the dura on the side of restricted brain growth is grafted.

growth of the skull, much of the difficulty associated with determining the degree of correction can be avoided by waiting until the child is 3 or 4 years of age and greater than 90% of the expansion of the skull has occurred. The younger the patient, the more difficult it is to determine the degree of advancement, and therefore the less predictable the result.

I agree with Jackson[51] and Mohr et al.[70] that for the best cosmetic results, operation for coronal and basal synostosis should be performed between 1 and 6 months of age to take advantage of subsequent growth of the developing frontal and temporal areas to help reshape the overlying bone. The advance to help accomplish this goal was the recognition that the frontosphenoidal suture could be resected medially.[3,67] In young infants extensive bone removal along the coronal suture, in the area of the pterion, along the frontosphenoidal suture, and the frontal bone immediately behind the supraorbital ridge allow the skull base to reshape itself in a virtually normal configuration. The frontosphenoidal craniectomy is extended medially to include much of the lesser wing of the sphenoid and the lateral and anterior aspect of the greater wing (Fig. 26-30, *A*). When the lateral aspect of the superior orbital fissure is reached, the cra-

niectomy is halted. My initial fear of the development of pulsatile exophthalmos with this extensive procedure on the skull base has not been borne out in fact. The densest attachments between dura and the inner aspect of the skull are usually encountered laterally just beneath the greater sphenoid wing. These pathologically dense adhesions are particularly prominent in infants with Apert's syndrome and in this condition may extend the entire length of the sphenoid ridge. A frontal craniotomy is necessary to fully visualize the medial removal of the sphenoid bone and the craniectomy behind the superior orbital ridge. After the craniectomies, the freed frontal bone flap is secured in position to the underlying dura and not attached to the surrounding bone of the skull. The pericranium over the frontal area is widely resected as an additional precaution to impede bony regrowth.

If the contralateral forehead is particularly prominent and bossed as the result of compensatory growth but uninvolved in the synostosis process, a second frontal craniotomy is carried out on the protuberant side. The dura on this side is plicated to reduce the intracranial volume (Fig. 26-30, *B*) and the dura on the involved side is grafted to allow more room for expansion. This alters the dural tensions significantly and allows proper bony regrowth. No craniectomy of the basal area is required on the side of the frontal bossing.

The procedure of choice in the patient more than 12 months of age with significant plagiocephaly but no evidence of increased intracranial pressure is to perform a lateral canthal advancement when the head circumference reaches 90% of the predicted adult value. This delay is believed to be beneficial to allow a more accurate prediction of the exact position that will yield the best cosmetic results. This procedure yields significant cosmetic improvement[70] but relies on the surgeon and not the growing and developing brain to properly advance the supraorbital ridge.

The same general guidelines can be used in determining the appropriate surgical treatment for brachiocephaly, with early operation on the skull base with dura grafting if the patient is less than 12 months of age at the time of coming to the neurosurgical attention. In the older patient lateral canthal advancement is again employed. It has also been stated that early operation on the skull base may lessen or actually avoid extensive facial involvement with the synostotic process.[29,70] The reliability of this is yet to be proven.

As is more common with bilateral involvement of the coronal and basal suture complex, increased intracranial pressure requires that more intracranial volume be provided immediately at the time of operation. Therefore operations that rely on eventual brain growth are inappropriate in this setting. Traditionally this problem has been solved by removing large sections of both frontal and parietal bones and performing a marcellation procedure.[54] The large sections are split into smaller sections and sutured back into place as a loose fitting bony matrix that provides a suprastructure for the ingrowth of osteoblasts. Because the neonate and young infant have the ability to regenerate large areas of skull, subtotal calvariectomy has also occasionally been advocated.[43] Interestingly, sutures will reform in the appropriate areas as long as the dural integrity has not been violated.[59] This adds support to the argument that the position and behavior of the cranial vertex sutures are directed by the dural tensions formed by its attachment across the skull base.

The surgical approach to trigonocephaly is similar to brachycephaly. Bilateral frontal craniotomies are performed along with the excision of a generous area of pericranium. The bony ridge involving the metopic suture is removed

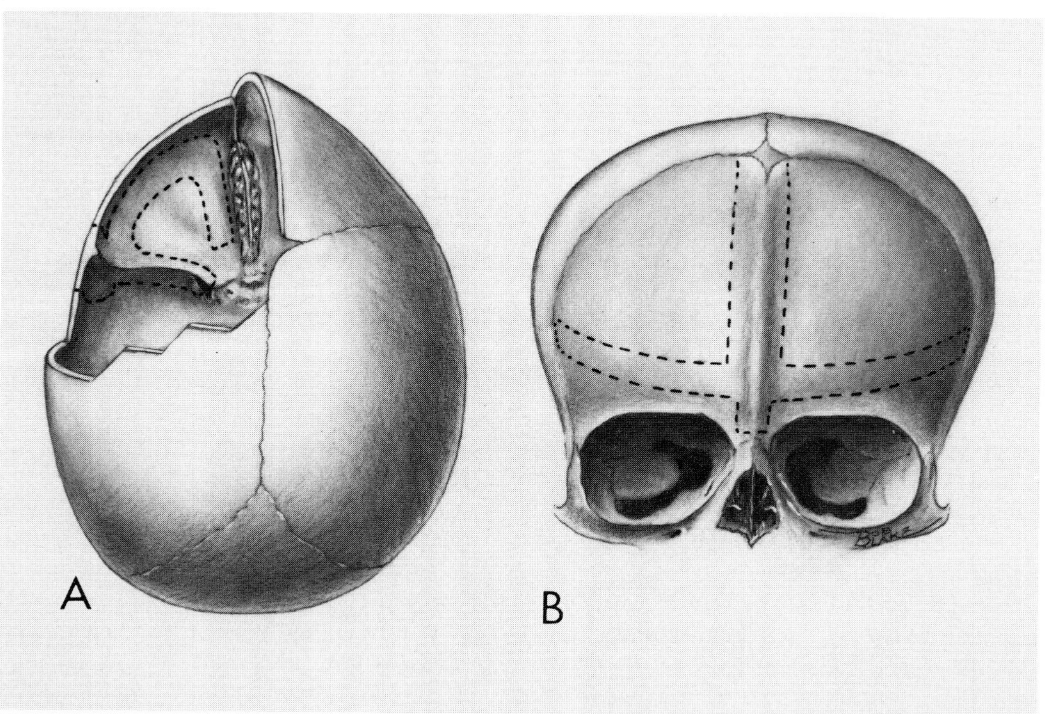

Fig. 26-31. A, Current surgical technique for the treatment of trigonocephaly involves a bifrontal craniotomy with removal of the lateral sphenoid ridge. The sphenoid ridge removal is continued to the superior orbital fissure. The bone of the orbital roof is resected immediately behind the supraorbital ridge and immediately lateral to the cribriform plate. **B,** Removal of the metopic suture with its prominent ridge is carried well down to the bridge of the nose. This allows maximal movement of the bony portions of the lateral orbit and forehead.

from the anterior fontanelle to an area well below the glabella (Fig. 26-31). The supraorbital ridge is freed from its connection to the floor of the anterior cranial fossa but left attached by a green-stick fracture medially. The bone over the pterion is generously removed bilaterally and both frontosphenoidal sutures are resected to the superior orbital fissure. A wide resection of the frontoethomoidal suture immediately lateral to the cribriform plate area is then accomplished. This avoids damage to the olfactory apparatus. A small thin plate of bone then lies free between the undersurface of the frontal lobe and the superior aspect of the periorbita. Both frontal bones are secured to the dura. Their orientation may be changed to maximize the lateral expansion of the anterior cranial fossa.

Lambdoid synostosis, whether it involves one or both sides, is dealt with by simple linear craniectomy (Fig. 26-32). The area of the posterior lateral fontanelle is usually associated with the densest adhesions between the dura and overlying bone and cartilage. This area is resected generously. The craniectomy is then extended caudally toward the foramen magnum.

The more extensive the synostotic process, the more extensive the bony removal that is required. This is particularly true of patients with visual change and evidence of increased intracranial pressure. If the child with extensive craniosynostosis is seen beyond 1 year of age, the regenerative capacity of the skull is limited and subtotal calvariectomy will not be followed by the re-creation of full skull protection. In these older children a King marcellation procedure or bilateral central osteoplastic flaps incorporating portions of both frontal and parietal bones[84] provide the best means for

immediate decompression of the intracranial contents. Careful attention to the possible development of hydrocephalus is necessary in these children.

COMPLICATIONS AND FOLLOW-UP

Of the potential serious complications seen with operation for craniosynostosis intraoperative hemorrhage from the dural venous sinuses is the most serious and feared. Meticulous surgical technique, attention to detail, and experience of the surgeon and surgical team with craniosynostosis surgery can minimize this risk. Shillito and Matson[86] reviewed their experience in Boston from more than 500 patients surgically treated for craniosynostosis. Even though this review was done on patients treated between 1927 and 1966, before many surgical and anesthetic advances, the operative mortality in the entire series was 0.39% and permanent undesirable sequelae occurred in only 0.58%. This impressive achievement is a record worthy of duplication even with our current technology. With proper care and attention, similar statistics should be attainable from any experienced surgical team. This underlines the acceptable morbidity and mortality associated with craniosynostosis surgery.

Although the risk of serious irreversible complications occurring with craniosynostosis surgery is low, it is not and will never be insignificant. The serious nature of the operative procedure must always be carefully and fully explained to the parents during the preoperative conference.

Infection in the operative field is an additional problem that is more common with the more extensive and lengthy procedures outlined previously. Subgaleal hematoma formation is common after cranisoynostosis surgery and has

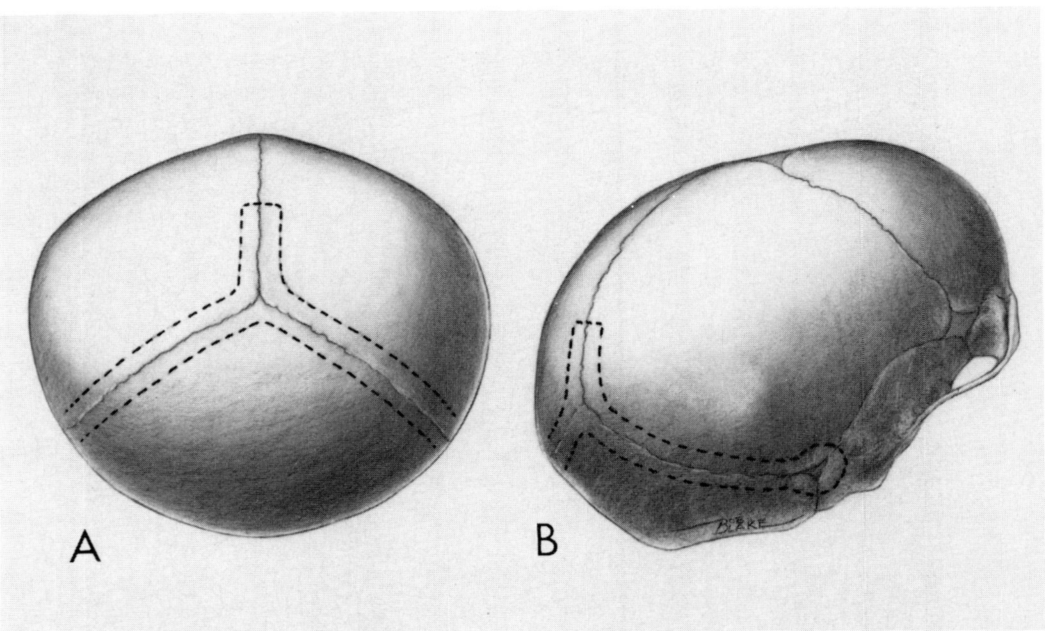

Fig. 26-32. Posterior and oblique view of the skull to demonstrate the current extent of the linear craniectomy for bilateral lambdoid synostosis.

prompted some authors to recommend insertion of a subgaleal drain for 24 to 48 hours after surgery to minimize this occurrence. I do not agree with this judgment and believe that adequate hemostasis is a more acceptable alternative. If infection does occur and a plastic interposition material has been used, reoperation to remove the foreign body is necessary in addition to systemic antibiotics and drainage of the purulent material.

Serious damage to the underlying brain rarely occurs with craniosynostosis surgery if increased intracranial pressure is not present. If papilledema or other evidence of intracranial hypertension is present, the adhesions between the dura and the inner table of the skull, particularly over the fibrous components of the skull can be tenacious. Dural tears occur more frequently, and the integrity of the dural sinuses can be interrupted. If dural tears do occur and CSF is seen at the time of the operation, these must be repaired to avoid CSF cysts occurring in the subgaleal space.

Hydrocephalus can occur after craniosynostosis surgery and may be secondary to intraventricular or extraventricular obstruction to CSF flow.[31] In general the more extensive the synostotic process the more likely is the development of hydrocephalus (Fig. 26-33). When present, the hydrocephalus should be treated with the insertion of a valve-regulated shunting device. If hydrocephalus is diagnosed before craniosynostosis surgery, the shunting procedure should precede the skull surgery to help avoid accumulation of CFS in the subgaleal space, which will escape from small holes in the dura because of the high intradural pressure. Whether the occurrence of subarachnoid hemorrhage from the craniosynostosis surgery is contributory to the postoperative

development of hydrocephalus is speculative but a logical conclusion.

An important aspect of long-term follow-up of patients with craniosynostosis is to ensure that recurrence of the synostosis process at the original suture site or the involvement of additional sutures does not occur.[76] If involvement of adjacent sutures is recognized from follow-up radiographic examinations, additional surgery is indicated. Once increased intracranial pressure develops from multiple suture involvement, eventual mental retardation appears more likely.[76] The incidence of premature formation of a bony bridge across the surgically created craniectomy defect may require reoperation. This was believed to be necessary from 0% to 38% of Shillito and Matson's series[86] and depended greatly on which sutures were initially involved. It is believed that reoperation on scaphocephaly can be avoided by the bony advancement procedure described in the technique section (pp. 429 to 431). This is particularly true when it is understood that the dural tensions have been significantly altered by this procedure and therefore the stimulus for rapid bony ingrowth in the craniectomy site has been ablated. Similar arguments could be advanced to explain the difference in the incidence of reoperation experienced by Shillito and Matson after simple coronal craniectomy and the experience of contemporary surgeons with having less than 5% of patients requiring a second procedure. The opposite of rapid bony ingrowth into the craniectomy site is the occasional older infant or child who undergoes a wide craniectomy and sufficient bone fails to form at the craniectomy site; cranioplasty must be considered. I have no experience with this complication, although it has been reported.[4,86] It

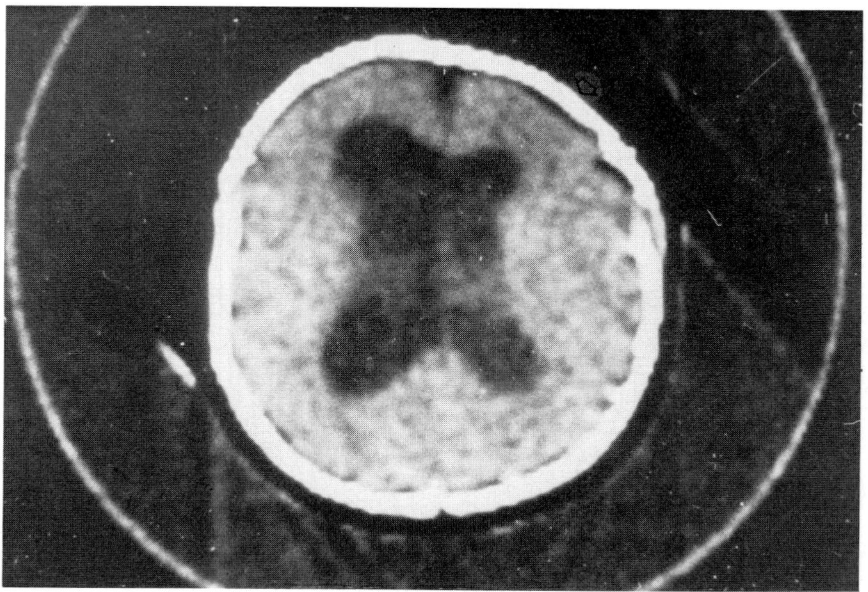

Fig. 26-33. Axial CT scan of a patient with right-sided plagiocephaly *(arrow)*, as well as multiple other suture involvement of the skull base. In addition, the patient has hydrocephalus.

obviously can be avoided by early operation and removing only the bone necessary to allow more physiologic brain growth.

The degree of mental retardation seen with craniosynostosis varies greatly, depending on the extent of the synostotic process and the effectiveness and timing of the therapeutic intervention. Previous estimates of significant increase in the incidence of mental retardation secondary to a single suture have been challenged.[37,45] Hunter and Rudd,[49] in a large comprehensive study of patients with sagittal synostosis with no evidence of coronal involvement, still show 8.9% of patients with IQs less than 80. In half of these patients the lower IQ could be explained easily by a process unrelated to the craniosynostosis; however, this still left almost 4.5% of their patient population in whom craniosynostosis process could possibly be linked to poor intellectual function. The authors do comment that the affected patients had a significantly lower mean birth weight, higher frequency of additional malformations, and later age of performance of operation than the control group. Whether or not isolated synostosis of the sagittal sutures does significantly alter intellectual function continues to be a debatable issue.

When patients with unilateral and bilateral coronal and basal suture involvement were examined by the same authors, even higher rates of retardation were found.[50] They found that 10% of patients with unilateral and 26% with bilateral involvement had IQs less than 80. Most of this increase was believed to be secondary to other major congenital malformations, with the children frequently having "complicated medical histories." These authors also believed that the mental retardation was "uncommon in simple and uncomplicated coronal synostosis." In a less exhaustive study Brenner and Kraus[12] found that 5% of patients with craniosynostosis had mental retardation secondary to the synostotic process and that these patients were much more likely to have extensive disease.

Malformations in other organ systems also can be associated with craniosynostosis, varying in incidence from 22%[49] to 59%.[86] A higher figure occurs in patients with bilateral coronal and basal involvement or in patients with mixed suture involvement. The most frequent major anomalies include congenital heart disease (tetralogy of Fallot, ventricular septal defect, a vascular ring compressing the trachea, a hypoplastic aortic arch, and bicuspid aortic valves), inguinal hernias, esotropia, and extranumerary digits.

Both operated and unoperated patients should receive follow-up examinations. It has been my practice to require clinic visits from postoperative patients every 6 to 12 months through their fifth birthday and to repeat skull radiographic examination yearly, particularly if multiple suture involvement exists. Without clinical indications, CT scanning is not repeated as a portion of the routine follow-up.

The genetic aspects of simple craniosynostosis have been extensively investigated.* Both dominant and recessive inheritance patterns have been described but neither occur in

---

*References 9, 18-21, 49, 50, and 57.

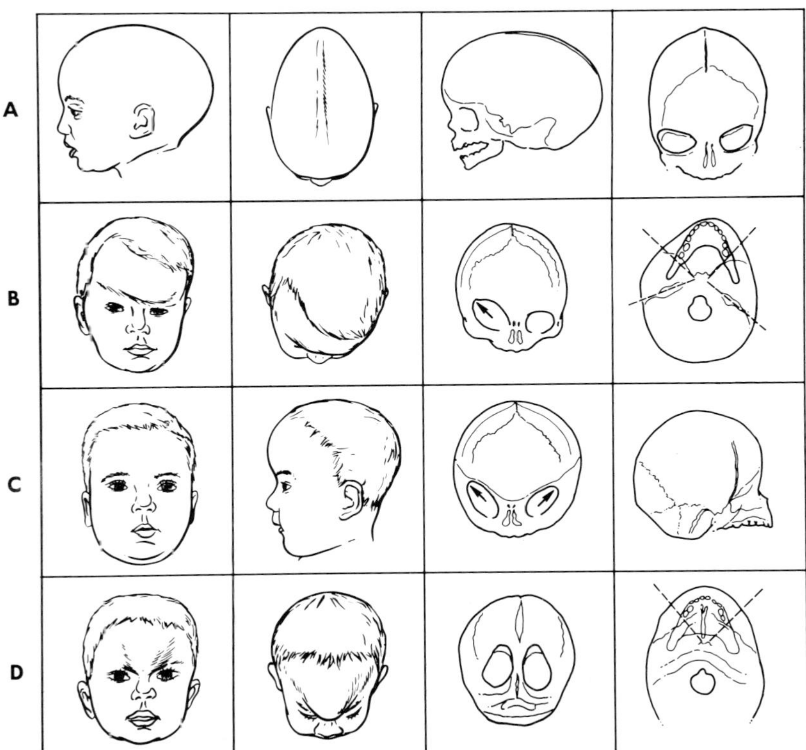

Fig. 26-34. Summary of clinical and radiographic findings of the more common forms of craniosynostosis. **A,** Scaphocephaly (sagittal synostosis). **B,** Plagiocephaly (unilateral coronal and basal synostosis). **C,** Brachycephaly (bilateral coronal and basal synostosis). **D,** Trigonocephaly (metopic synostosis). (From Oakes, W.J., and Wilkins, R.H.: The newborn: neurosurgical considerations. In Filston, H.C.: Surgical problems in children: recognition and referral, St. Louis, 1982, The C.V. Mosby Co.)

a majority of affected patients. A careful family history and review of family photographs is the best method of determining hte inheritance pattern within an individual family. This is necessary before any consideration of genetic counseling for an individual patient.

SUMMARY AND CONCLUSIONS

Patients with the simple forms of craniosynostosis are easily diagnosed at birth or on the first routine postdelivery examination (Fig. 26-34). Molding from the delivery process can be confused with craniosynostosis within the first few days of life, but this process quickly corrects itself so that by the sixth-week follow-up visitation the results of molding should be minimal if present at all. The presumptive diagnosis of craniosynostosis can be easily confirmed by routine skull radiographs (including a basal view), and referral to a neurosurgeon knowledgeable in the evaluation and care of these patients should be made. The unusual patient with extensive craniosynostosis or evidence of increased intracranial pressure should be operated on to preserve intellectual function and vision. Despite early appropriate therapy, many severely affected infants will still remain intellectually dull.

The majority of infants with single suture involvement should have surgery considered in an attempt to improve their cosmetic appearance. Surgery for craniosynostosis is relatively safe and with recent advances are effective in achieving an improved skull shape. Surgery is routinely performed within the first 3 months of life while the growing brain still has the potential to significantly reshape the malformed bone that is not removed at the time of operation. In general the more extensive the operative procedure, the more cosmetically acceptable is the patient's eventual result.

Patients who come to clinical attention after 1 year of age and require therapy must have an operation that allows correction of the bony defect at the operating table and does not rely on future skull growth. These more extensive procedures carry increased operative risks and less cosmetic improvement than those performed early in life. The psychologic consequence of any form of craniosynostosis should not be underestimated in this world of frequent criticism and disagreement over much less than one's head shape.

REFERENCES

1. Albright, A.L., and Byrd, R.P.: Suture pathology in craniosynostosis, J. Neurosurg. **54**:384, 1981.
2. Anderson, B., and Woodhall, B.: Visual loss in primary skull deformities, Trans Am. Acad. Ophthalmol. Otolaryngol. **57**:497, 1953.
3. Anderson, F.M.: Treatment of coronal and metopic synostosis: 107 cases, Neurosurgery **8**:143, 1981.
4. Anderson, F.M., and Geiger, L.: Craniosynostosis, J. Neurosurg. **22**:229, 1965.
5. Anderson, F.M., Gwinn, J.L., and Todt, J.C.: Trigonocephaly, J. Neurosurg. **19**:723, 1962.
6. Anderson, H.: Craniosynostosis as a complication after operation for hydrocephalus, Acta Paediatr. Scand. **55**:192, 1966.
7. Archer, D.B., Gordon, D.S., Maguire, C.J.F., and Gleadhill, C.A.: Ophthalmic aspects of craniosynostosis, Trans. Ophthalmol. Soc. U.K. **94**:172, 1974.
8. Barritt, J., Brooksbank, M., and Simpson, D.: Scaphocephaly: Aesthetic and psychosocial considerations, Dev. Med. Child Neurol. **23**:183, 1981.
9. Bell, H.S., Clare, F.B., and Wentworth, A.F.: Familial scaphocephaly: case reports and technical notes, J. Neurosurg. **18**:239, 1961.
10. Bering, E.A., McLaurin, R.L., Lloyd, J.B., and Ingraham, F.D.: The production of tumors in rats by the implantation of pure polyethylene, Cancer Res. **15**:300, 1955.
11. Bertelsen, T.I.: The premature synostosis of the cranial sutures, Acta Ophthalmol. **51**:1, 1958.
12. Brenner, H., and Kraus, H.: Craniosynostosis, Progr. Neurol. Surg. **4**:429, 1971.
13. Buttram, V.C., Zanotti, L., Acosta, A.A., et al.: Surgical correction of the septate uterus, Fertil. Steril. **25**:373, 1974.
14. Caffey, J.: Pediatric x-ray diagnosis: a textbook for students of pediatrics, surgery, and radiology, Chicago, 1978, Year Book Medical Publishers, Inc.
15. Carmel, P.W., Luken, M.G., and Ascherl, G.F.: Craniosynostosis: computed tomographic evaluation of skull base and calvarial deformities and associated intracranial changes, Neurosurgery, **9**:366, 1981.
16. Clarren, S.K.: Plagiocephaly and torticollis: etiology, natural history, and helmet treatment, J. Pediatr. **98**:92, 1981.
17. Clarren, S.K., Smith, D.W., and Hanson, J.W.: Helmet treatment for plagiocephaly and congenital muscular torticollis, J. Pediatr. **94**:43, 1979.
18. Cohen, M.M.: Genetic perspectives on craniosynostosis and syndromes with craniosynostosis, J. Neurosurg. **47**:886, 1977.
19. Cohen, M.M.: Craniosynostosis and syndromes with craniosynostosis: incidence, genetics, penetrance, variability, and new syndrome updating, Birth Defects **15**(5B):13, 1979.
20. Cohen, M.M.: Perspectives on craniosynostosis, West J. Med. **132**:507, 1980.
21. Cross, H.E., and Opitz, J.M.: Craniosynostosis in the Amish, J. Pediatr. **75**:1037, 1969.
22. Currarino, G., and Silverman, F.N.: Orbital hypotelorism, arrhinencephaly, and trigonocephaly, Radiology **74**:206, 1960.
23. Daneman, D., and Howard, N.J.: Neonatal thyrotoxicosis: intellectual impairment and craniosynostosis in later years, J. Pediatr. **97**:257, 1980.
24. Davis, C.H., Alexander, E., and Kelly, D.L.: Treatment of craniosynostosis, J. Neurosurg. **30**:630, 1969.
25. Dhadial, R.K., and Smith, M.F.: Terminal 7p deletion and 1:7 translocation associated with craniosynostosis, Hum. Genet. **50**:285, 1979.
26. Dominguez, R., Sang Oh, K., Bender, T., and Girdany, B.R.: Uncomplicated trigonocephaly, Radiology **140**:681, 1981.
27. Duggan, C.A., Keener, E.B., and Gay, B.B.: Secondary craniosynostosis, A.J.R. **109**:277, 1970.
28. Eaton, A.P., Sommer, A., and Sayers, M.P.: The Kleeblattschädel anomaly, Birth Defects **11**:238, 1975.
29. Epstein, F., McCarthy, J.G., and Coccaro, P.J.: Prophylatic craniofacial surgery, Child's Brain **5**:204, 1979.
30. Farmer, T.W.: Pediatric neurology, ed. 2, Hagerstown, Md., 1975, Harper & Row, Publishers, Inc.
31. Fishman, M.A., Hogan, G.R., and Dodge, P.R.: The concurrence of hydrocephalus and craniosynostosis, J. Neurosurg. **34**:621, 1971.
32. Ford, F.R.: Diseases of the nervous system in infancy, childhood, and adolescence, ed. 6, Springfield, Ill., 1973, Charles C Thomas, Publisher.
33. Freeman, J.M., and Borkowf, S.: Craniostenosis: review of the literature and report of thirty-four cases, Pediatrics **30**:57, 1962.
34. Gamstorp, I.: Pediatric neurology, New York, 1970, Appleton-Century-Crofts.
35. Gates, G.F., and Dore, E.K.: Detection of craniosynostosis by bone scanning, Radiology **115**:665, 1975.
36. Giuffré, R., Vagnozzi, R., and Savino, S.: Infantile craniosynostosis: clinical, radiological, and surgical considerations based on 100 surgically treated cases, Acta Neurochir. **44**:49, 1978.
37. Gordon, H.: Craniostenosis, Br. Med. J. **109**:292, 1959.
38. Graham, J.M.: Craniostenosis: a new approach to management, Pediatr. Ann. **10**:27, 1981.

39. Graham, J.M., Badura, R.J., and Smith, D.W.: Coronal craniostenosis: fetal head constraint as one possible cause, Pediatrics **65**:995, 1980.
40. Graham, J.M., deSaze, M., and Smith, D.W.: Sagittal craniostenosis: fetal head constraint as one possible cause, J. Pediatr. **95**:747, 1979.
41. Graham, J.M., and Smith, D.W.: Metopic craniostenosis as a consequence of fetal head constraint: two interesting experiments of nature, Pediatrics **65**:1000, 1980.
42. Haberkern, C.M., Smith, D.W., and Jones, K.L.: The breech head and its relevance, Am. J. Dis. Child. **133**:154, 1979.
43. Hanson, J.W., Sayers, M.P., Knopp, L.M., et al.: Subtotal neonatal calvariectomy for severe craniosynostosis, J. Pediatr. **91**:257, 1977.
44. Harwood-Nash, D.C., and Fitz, C.R.: Neuroradiology in infants and children, St. Louis, 1976, The C.V. Mosby Co.
45. Hemple, D.J., Harris, L.E., Svien, H.J., and Holman, C.B.: Craniosynostosis involving the satittal suture only: guilt by association? J. Pediatr. **58**:342, 1961.
46. Higginbottom, M.C., Jones, K.L., and James, H.E.: Intrauterine constraint and craniosynostosis, Neurosurgery, **6**:39, 1980.
47. Hoffman, H.J., and Mohr, G.: Lateral canthal advancement of the supraorbital margin, J. Neurosurg. **45**:376, 1976.
48. Hope, J.W., Spitz, E.B., and Slade, H.W.: The early recognition of premature cranial synostosis, Radiology **65**:183, 1955.
49. Hunter, A.G.W., and Rudd, N.L.: Craniosynostosis: sagittal synostosis: its genetics and associated clinical findings in 214 patients who lacked involvement of the coronal suture(s), Teratology **14**:185, 1976.
50. Hunter, A.G.W., and Rudd, N.L.: Craniosynostosis: coronal synostosis: its familial characteristics and associated clinical findings in 109 patients lacking bilateral polysyndactyly or syndactyly, Teratology **15**:301, 1977.
51. Jackson, I.T.: Aesthetic correction of coronal craniosynostosis, Clin. Plast. Surg. **8**:317, 1981.
52. Jane, J.A., Edgerton, M.T., Futrell, J.W., and Park, T.S.: Immediate correction of sagittal synostosis, J. Neurosurg. **49**:705, 1978.
53. Johnsonbaugh, R.E., Bryan, R.N., Hierlwimmer, R., and Georges, L.P.: Premature craniosynostosis: a common complication of juvenile thyrotoxicosis, J. Pediatr. **93**:188, 1978.
54. King, J.E.J.: Oxycephaly, Ann. Surg. **115**:488, 1942.
55. Kloss, J.L.: Craniosynostosis secondary to ventriculoatrial shunt, Am. J. Dis. Child. **116**:315, 1968.
56. Knudson, H.W., and Flaherty, R.A.: Craniosynostosis, Am. J. Roentgenol. Radium Ther. Nucl. Med. **84**:454, 1960.
57. Kosnik, E.J., Gilbert, G., and Sayers, M.P.: Familial inheritance of coronal craniosynostosis, Dev. Med. Child Neurol. **17**:630, 1975.
58. Kurlander, G.J., DeMyer, W., Campbell, J.A., and Taybi, H.: Roentgenology of holoprosencephaly, Acta Radiol. **5**:25, 1966.
59. Mabbutt, L.W., Kokich, V.G., Moffett, B.C., and Loeser, J.D.: Subtotal neonatal calveriectomy, J. Neurosurg. **51**:691, 1979.
60. Marlin, A.E., Brown, W.E., Huntington, H.W., and Epstein, F.: Effect of the dural application of Zenker's solution on the feline brain, Neurosurgery **6**:45, 1980.
61. Matson, D.D.: Surgical treatment of congenital anomalies of the coronal and metopic sutures, J. Neurosurg. **17**:413, 1960.
62. Matson, D.D.: Neurosurgery of infancy and childhood, ed. 2, Springfield, Ill., 1969, Charles C Thomas, Publisher.
63. McCarthy, J.G., and Reid, C.A.: Craniofacial synostosis in association with vitamin D–resistant rickets, Ann. Plast. Surg. **4**:149, 1980.
64. McComb, J.G., Withers, G.J., and Davis, R.L.: Cortical damage from Zenker's solution applied to the dura mater, Neurosurgery **8**:68, 1981.
65. McLaurin, R.L., and Matson, D.D.: Importance of early surgical treatment of craniosynostosis: review of 36 cases treated during the first six months of life, Pediatrics **10**:637, 1952.
66. McPherson, E., Hall, J.G., and Hickman, R.: Chromosome 7 short deletion and craniosynostosis A 7p-syndrome, Hum. Genet. **35**:117, 1976.
67. Menezes, A.H.: Early correction of anterior cranial base and coronal synostosis, Neurosurgery **5**:381, 1979.
68. Milhorat, T.H.: Pediatric neurosurgery, Philadelphia, 1978, F.A. Davis Co.
69. Miller, M.E., Dunn, P.M., and Smith, D.W.: Uterine malformation and fetal deformation, J. Pediatr. **94**:387, 1979.
70. Mohr, G., Hoffman, H.J., Munro, I.R., et al.: Surgical management of unilateral and bilateral coronal craniosynostosis: 21 years of experience, Neurosurgery **2**:83, 1978.
71. Moss, M.L.: The pathogenesis of premature cranial synostosis in man, Acta Anat. **37**:351, 1959.
72. Moss, M.L.: Inhibition and stimulation of sutural fusion in the rat calvaria, Anat. Rec. **136**:457, 1960.
73. Moss, M.L.: Functional anatomy of cranial synostosis, Child's Brain **1**:22, 1975.
74. Mullan, S.: Late moulding of the scaphocephalic skull, Am. J. Dis. Child. **99**:55, 1960.
75. Nathan, M.H., Collins, V.P., and Collins, L.C.: Premature unilateral synostosis of the coronal sutures, Radiology **86**:433, 1961.
76. Norwood, C.W., Alexander, E., Davis, C.H., and Kelly, D.L.: Recurrent and multiple suture closures after craniectomy for craniosynostosis, J. Neurosurg. **41**:715, 1974.
77. Oppenheimer, B.S., Oppenheimer, E.T., and Stout, A.P.: Sarcomas induced in rodents by imbedding various plastic films, Proc. Soc. Exp. Biol. Med. **79**:366, 1952.
78. Pawl, R.P., and Sugar, O.: Zenker's solution in the surgical treatment of craniosynostosis, J. Neurosurg. **36**:604, 1972.
79. Penfold, J.L., and Simpson, D.A.: Premature craniosynostosis—a complication of thyroid replacement therapy, J. Pediatr. **86**:360, 1975.
80. Persing, J., Babler, W., Winn, H.R., et al.: Age as a critical factor in the success of surgical correction of craniosynostosis, J. Neurosurg. **54**:601, 1981.
81. Persson, K.M., Roy, W.A., Persing, J.A., et al.: Craniofacial growth following experimental craniosynostosis and craniectomy in rabbits, J. Neurosurg. **50**:187, 1979.
82. Pritchard, J.J., Scott, J.H., and Girgis, F.G.: The structure and development of cranial and facial sutures, J. Anat. **90**:73, 1956.
83. Reilly, B.J., Leeming, J.M., and Fraser, D.: Craniosynostosis in the rachitic spectrum, J. Pediatr. **64**:396, 1964.
84. Samra, K.A., And Sorour, O.: Bilateral flap operation for craniosynostosis, J. Neurosurg. **29**:591, 1968.
85. Seeger, J.F., and Gabrielsen, T.O.: Premature closure of the frontosphenoidal suture in synostosis of the coronal suture, Radiology **101**:631, 1971.
86. Shillito, J., and Matson, D.D.: Craniosynostosis: a review of 519 surgical patients, Pediatrics **41**:829, 1968.
87. Smith, D.W., and Tondury, G.: Origin of the calvaria and its sutures, Am. J. Dis. Child. **132**:662, 1978.
88. Tait, M.V., Gilday, D.L., Ash, J.M., et al.: Craniosynostosis: correlation of bone scans, radiographs, and surgical findings, Radiology **133**:615, 1979.
89. Tessier, P.: Relationship of craniostenoses to craniofacial dysostoses, and to faciostenoses, Plast. Reconstr. Surg. **48**:224, 1971.
90. Virchow, R.: Über den Cretinismus, namentlich in Franken, and über pathologische Schädelformen, Verhandl. d. Phys.-Med. Gesellsch. Würzb. **2**:230, 1851.

CHAPTER 27

Craniofacial dysostosis

IAN T. JACKSON

Craniofacial dysostosis is a component of many syndromes: Crouzon's, Apert's, Pfeiffer, Saethre-Chotzen, and Carpenter's syndromes.[11] The basic pathologic condition is one of bicoronal craniosynostosis with involvement of the basal chondrocranium.

In Crouzon's disease[6,7,17] there is maxillary retrusion with a Class III malocclusion. There may or may not be retrusion of the supraorbital-frontal area with brachycephaly. The orbits are shallow, resulting in exorbitism. The infraorbital rim is underdeveloped and lies well behind its normal relationship to the most anterior part of the cornea. When there is frontal and supraorbital involvement, the supraorbital rim lies behind the cornea instead of 1 to 1.5 cm anterior to it as in the normal individual. Frequently there is a high-arched palate. There may be an increase in the interorbital distance, representing true hypertelorism, or telecanthus. The inheritance is autosomal dominant.

In Apert's syndrome[1,2,5] the facial deformity is more complex; almost always there is brachycephaly. Frequently there is an increased intercanthal distance. The nose is short and stubby. There is vertical shortness of the maxilla with an anterior open bite. The palate is high arched, and 25% have palatal clefts. The hands have severe syndactyly with distal phalangeal fusion, forming a mitten hand. The thumb has the typical deformity of the delta phalanx. Although there is metacarpophalangeal movement, there is no mobility beyond these joints. Syndactyly of the toes occurs. Apert's syndrome is an autosomal dominant condition.

The Pfeiffer syndrome[12,25] has many of the features of Apert's syndrome, but the thumbs and great toes are characteristically short, wide, and deviated medially. The inheritance is autosomal dominant.

The Saethre-Chotzen syndrome[4,24,26] is also an autosomal dominant trait. The forehead and occiput are flat, the face is asymmetric, and there is unilateral or bilateral ptosis of the upper eyelids. The nose is beaked, and the palate is high arched. There may be mandibular prognathism and soft tissue syndactyly.

The Carpenter's syndrome[3,8] is an autosomal recessive disorder. It features a tower skull, which may be asymmetric, flat nasal bridge with epicanthal folds, and hypoplastic mandible.

INVESTIGATION

Apart from a general physical examination, face and skull radiology, cephalometry, and dental models are essential. CAT scanning is important to illustrate any intracranial anomalies, especially variations in ventricular size, which would indicate raised intracranial pressure or unsuspected hydrocephalus. Skull and facial bone radiographs may show the "paw marking" of raised intracranial pressure and the anomalous positioning of the sphenoid wings, especially in the presence of a unilateral craniosynostosis (Fig. 27-1). Ophthalmologic examination is important to measure the degree of esotropia or exotropia and to carefully document exorbitism. The orthodontist relies on two main ancillary investigations.

Cephalometry

Cephalometry allows assessment of the degree of maxillary retrusion in relation to the cranial base and its relationship to the position of the mandible. According to the clinical and radiologic findings, an operative plan can be formulated as to the required anterior and downward maxillary movement. An estimate of profile change can be obtained. In addition to its planning and predictive role, the cephalogram is useful in follow-up examinations to assess the presence or absence of relapse and changes due to growth.

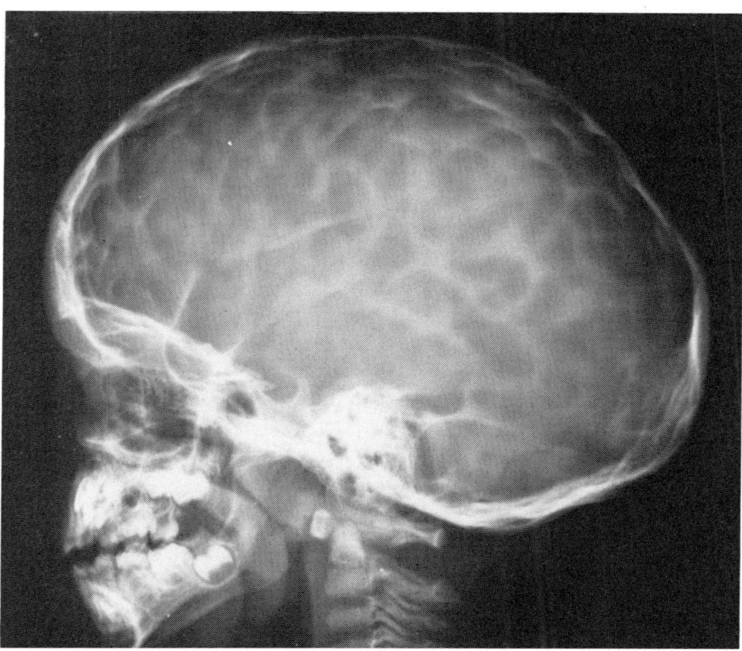

Fig. 27-1. Typical ''paw-marked'' or ''beaten copper'' appearance of the skull with raised intracranial pressure.

Dental study models

Dental study models provide an accurate method of examining tooth position and predicted occlusion. If the latter is unstable, then presurgical orthodontic treatment is instituted and continued until an adequate, stable predicted occlusion is obtained. When articulated and cut, the models can give a fairly accurate idea of the amount of anterior and inferior shift required. The latter is necessary in the presence of an anterior open bite. With the models in the desired occlusion, an acrylic resin bite-guard splint is manufactured that, after the osteotomy, will allow eventual jaw fixation in the estimated ideal occlusion. Dental models are also useful in follow-up to assess relapse and growth changes in the jaws.

General assessment

It is wise to have an ear, nose, and throat examination in patients with craniofacial synostosis to obtain a baseline, since many have nasal obstruction; in addition, some have ear and hearing problems.

If possible, a psychologic profile of the patient should be obtained. This provides a gauge for emotional changes that may take place after surgery. The overall mental and intellectual capabilities of the patient are assessed. These factors are important in deciding whether or not it is reasonable to carry out the surgical procedure.

The geneticist constructs a family genetic profile and gives counseling on the chance of deformity in future chil-dren and on the possibility of the patient's producing deformed children.

A comprehensive pediatric examination is an essential feature of the preoperative workup.

The anesthesiologist will eventually see the patient when surgery has been decided on and will check potential anesthetic problems, such as a small mandible, trismus, large tongue, and stiff neck.

The neurosurgeon, when involved, assesses intracranial risks.

Photographs are taken, and an artist may be enlisted to provide predictive illustrations.

The decision to proceed with surgery is made after a team discussion when all salient facts regarding surgery, and the potential complications have been considered and clearly presented to the parents.

Timing of surgery

In the infant with bicoronal craniosynostosis and maxillary retrusion, a frontal-supraorbital advancement should be performed without delay, usually within the first 3 months. Although this improves supraorbital and frontal contour, in our experience it has little or no effect on the position of the maxilla, despite reports to the contrary.[20]

Evidence suggests that delay of maxillary advancement until adolescence is ideal because mandibular growth has ended, and the permanent dentition is well established. At this time, a definitive advancement will be stable. In contrast, advancement at an early age is more difficult and has only the primary or mixed dentition for fixation and stabilization. More important, the advanced maxilla in the majority of patients shows no tendency to grow in an anterior direction, although there seems to be a variable amount of vertical growth.[16] With mandibular growth and development, maxillary-mandibular disproportion with the recurrence of a Class III malocclusion may be reestablished, and a later LeFort I or III level is required.[13]

Despite this, there are indications for early surgery. These may be emotional, such as parental concern and the inability to accept the child's deformity, or the child may be suffering due to nonacceptance or ridicule from peers. If this course is chosen, the parents must be warned that a later, repeat osteotomy might well be necessary.

There is another aspect of timing to be discussed in the patient who requires frontal, orbital, and maxillary advancement (e.g., those with Apert's syndrome). This may be performed in one procedure, but in view of the problems that have occurred from ascending infection from the nasopharynx with resulting osteomyelitis or meningitis, it is probably safer to split this into a cranial and maxillary procedure, unless there is some pressing reason for doing otherwise.

TREATMENT
Frontal and supraorbital retrusion

The amount of advancement is determined by measuring the relationship of the supraorbital rim to the anterior-most part of the cornea. Normally in whites the rim is 1 to 1.5 cm in front of the cornea; thus the advancement in cases of supraorbital retrusion is frequently in the range of 2 to 2.5 cm. It is rare to have a frontal bone of satisfactory contour to allow advancement, apart from some cases of Crouzon's disease. Thus the preoperative plan frequently incorporates the use of skull from another area to give a more satisfactory frontal reconstruction.[15,28]

The approach is by the classic coronal incision. The bicoronal flap may be raised above or below the periosteum. If the periosteum is left on the skull, it is divided about 1.5 to 2 cm above the supraorbital rims, and the remainder of the dissection proceeds subperiosteally. The dissection is made over the nasal bridge down to the upper part of the nasal bones. The periorbita is dissected from the orbital roof and upper part of the medial orbital wall; the medial canthi are not disturbed. Laterally the periosteum is also elevated over the malar and infraorbital rim. It is important not to disturb the temporal muscle unless absolutely necessary, otherwise one may run the risk of temporal atrophy, which results in obvious temporal concavities. The temporal muscle is thus elevated from the lateral aspect of the lateral orbital wall but not from the temporal fossa.

The periosteum over the frontal area is now incised sagittally in the midline and coronally just in front of the pos-

terior scalp edge; two periosteal flaps can be elevated on the temporal muscle. The muscle may have to be elevated from the skull in its upper part to allow the supraorbital advancement to be performed.

A plan of the projected supraorbital osteotomy and the skull-switch procedure is outlined on the skull. The neurosurgeon places bur holes and raises the frontal bone flap, based on this plan (Fig. 27-2).

As the craniotomy is being performed, spicules of bone on the inner surface of the skull are noted. These will often dive deeply, causing significant invagination of the dura. The practical importance of these formations is that they can deflect the craniotome and cause tears of the dura. These represent indentations of the skull of the gyri, resulting from increased intracranial pressure and cause the "beaten copper" or "paw-marked" appearance of the skull on radiographs (Fig. 27-3).

After removal of the anterior skull, CSF pressure is reduced by spinal drainage and administration of mannitol. This allows for easier brain retraction, less brain trauma, and less risk of cerebral edema. Brain retraction need not be radical, since the anterior cranial fossa osteotomy is made quite far forward.

Initially a cut is made just anterior to the junction of the lateral orbital wall and the middle cranial fossa. The inferior extent of the cut is determined by how much orbital wall is to be advanced; frequently it is taken to the inferior orbital fissure. A horizontal cut is made through the lateral orbital rim at the planned level. A stepped osteotomy is made high on the temporal area with a posteriorly directed horizontal cut and then a vertical cut to the skull edge, resulting from removal of the frontal and temporal bone flap. The length of the step must be such that it will allow the planned advancement and maintain a satisfactory overlap for stabilization. Because of the position of the sphenoid wings, part of this cut may be in the middle cranial fossa, and thus a retractor must be placed laterally, under the sphenoid wing, to retract and protect the temporal lobe (Fig. 27-4, *H*).

The lateral vertical cut is the guideline for the anterior cranial fossa osteotomy. This is taken across the orbital roofs, sometimes through the free margin of the sphenoid wing laterally. It lies in front of the crista galli and its associated dura. When this has been completed, short vertical osteotomies are made in the medial orbital walls. These are joined across the nose by an inverted V osteotomy at the junction of the frontal and nasal bones. It is now possible to mobilize and remove the supraorbital block.

If required, at this stage the periosteum over the anterior surface of the malar bone and maxilla is elevated. Suitably contoured portions of skull can be placed along and anterior to the infraorbital rim to augment this hypoplastic area. There is good evidence to suggest that membranous skull bone shows less tendency to resorb than other types of bone grafts originating from endochondral bone.[27]

Text continued on p. 447.

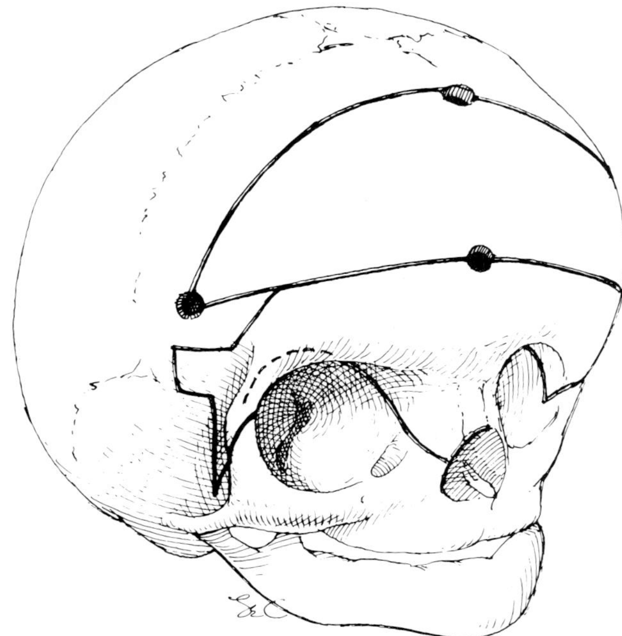

Fig. 27-2. Planned frontal-supraorbital advancement.

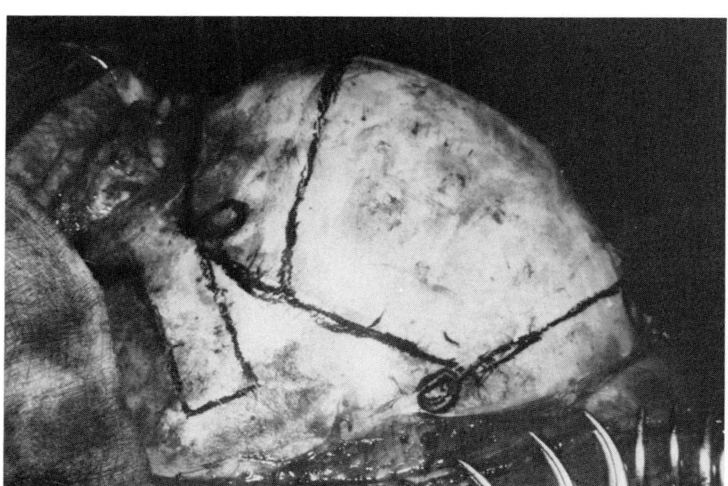

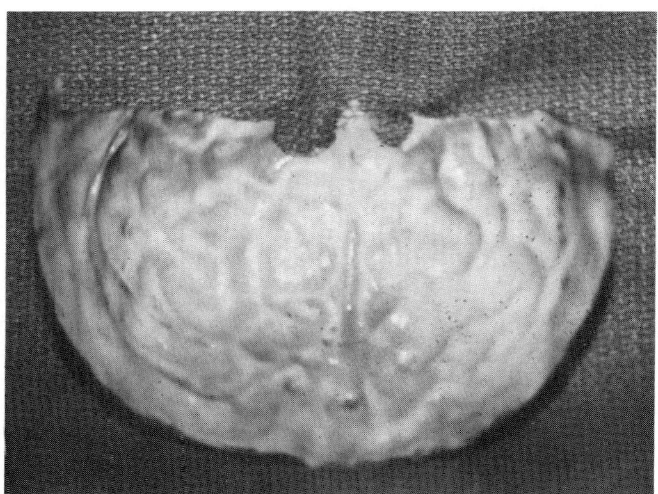

Fig. 27-3. Inner aspect of skull showing gyral indentations.

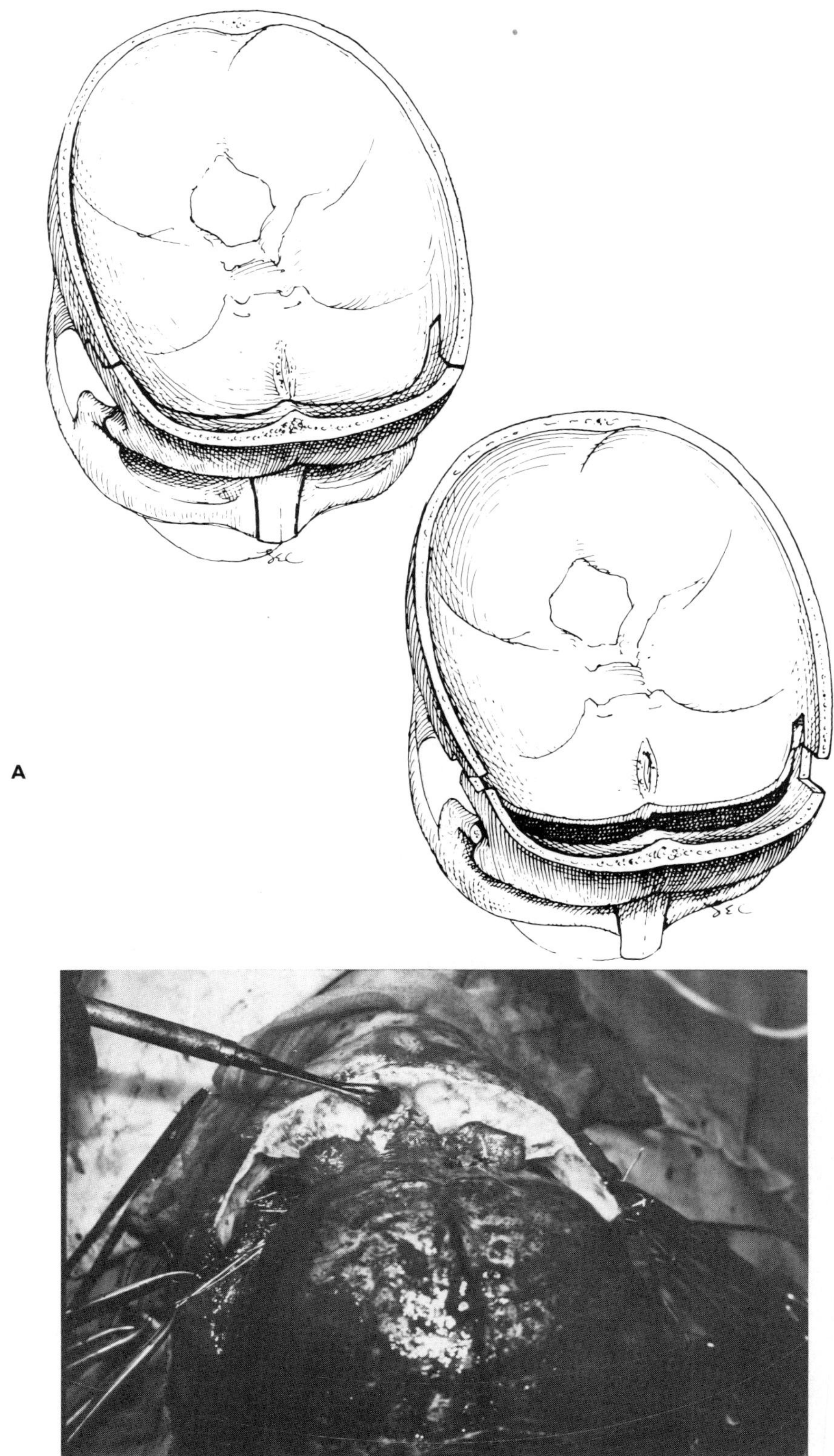

Fig. 27-4. A, Intracranial portion of the osteotomy.

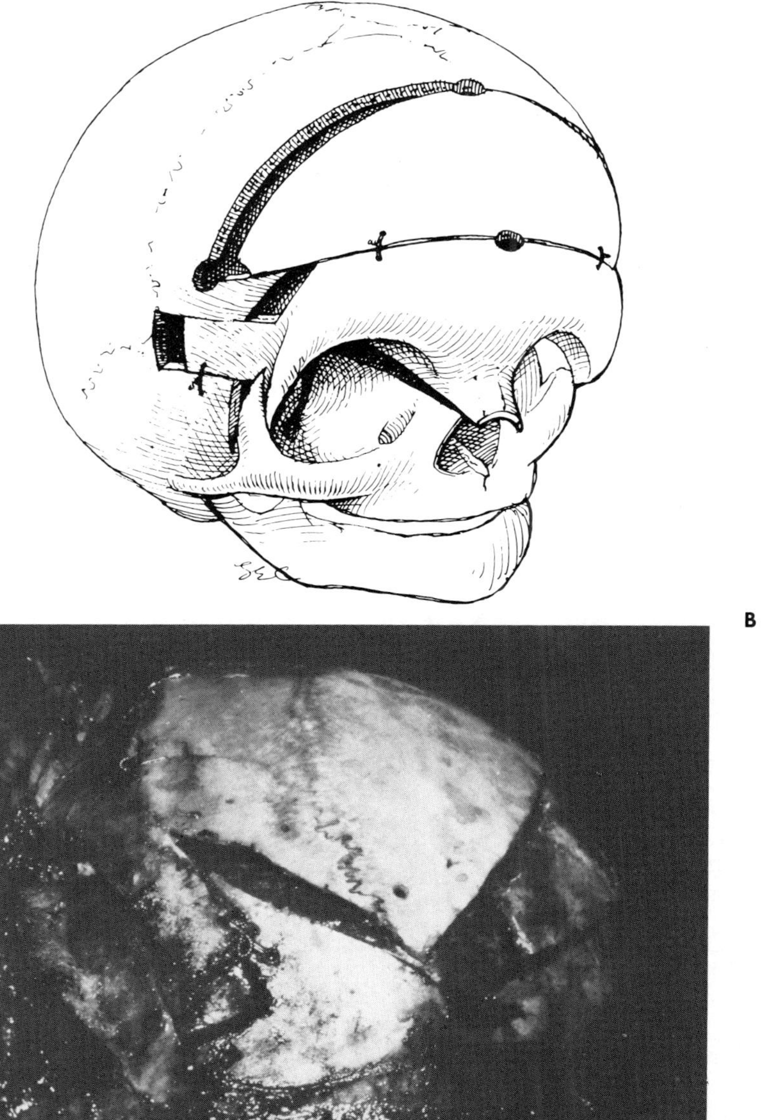

Fig. 27-4, cont'd. B, Frontal-orbital advancement completed.

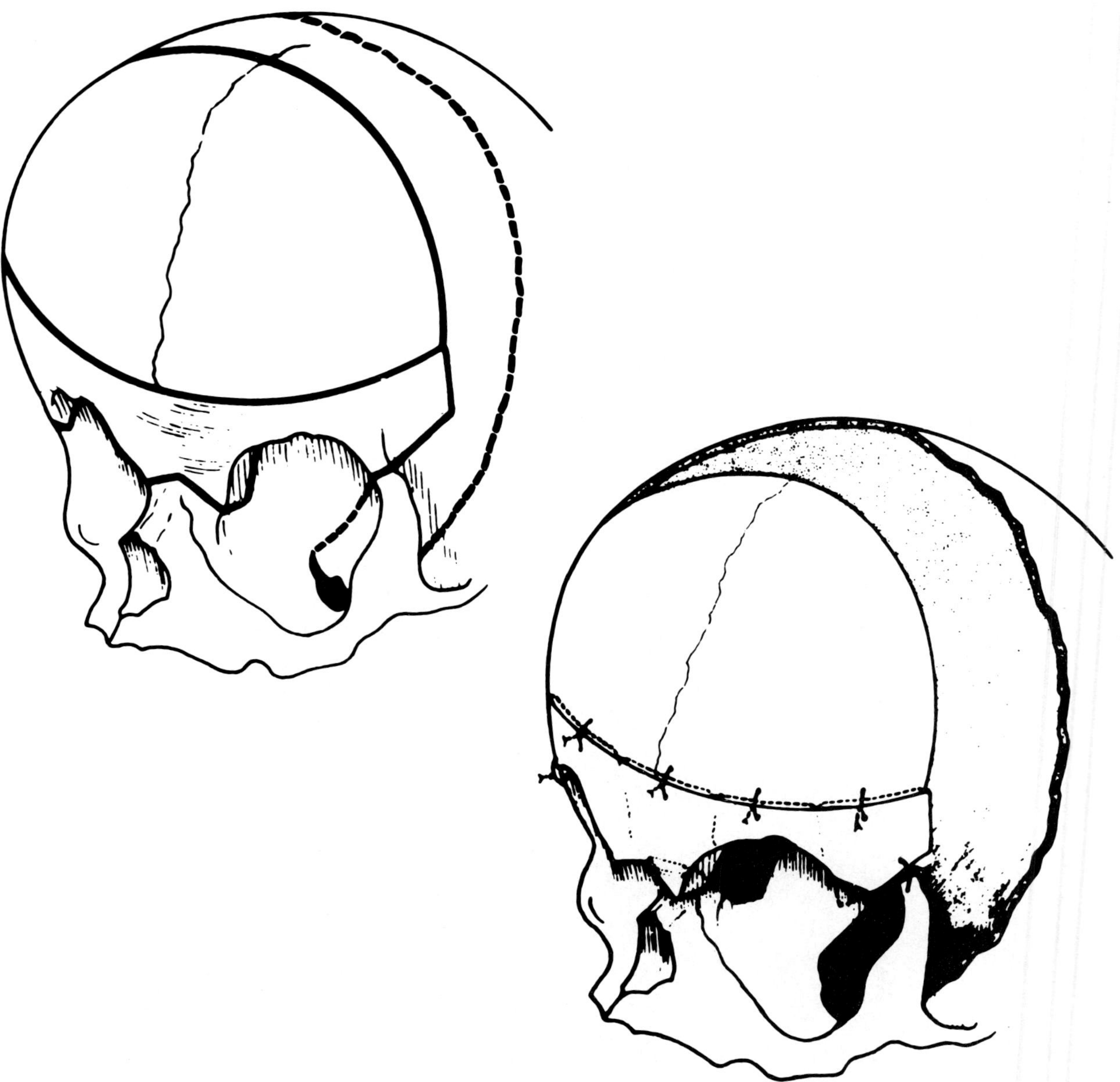

Fig. 27-5. Osteotomies involved in the ''floating forehead'' technique.

If necessary, the supraorbital block is contoured by bending and is advanced as planned. Stable wiring can be achieved medially and laterally. Skull bone grafts are wired into the defects in the lateral orbital wall and temporal areas. The frontal skull plate is now examined. Frequently, simple rotation through 180 degrees gives a satisfactory contour.[14] If not, it may have to be cut up and rearranged to ensure a good appearance.[22] Cranial defects are left open in younger patients. Over age 6 to 8, split skull or bone dust from the bur holes may be used for reconstruction. If possible, distant bone graft donor sites are avoided; this reduces pain and an area of additional blood loss, particularly in infants (Fig. 27-4, *B*).

The lateral canthal ligaments are identified, dissected out, and reattached through drill holes high at the junction of the lateral and superior orbital rims using nonabsorable suture material or wire.

It is frequently necessary to advance the temporal muscle. Previously this was lifted and moved forward; however, for the reasons stated earlier, this technique is no longer used. Instead, the temporal fascia is scored vertically. This allows the muscle to expand, and the anterior defect can be filled with ease. It appears that this has no adverse effect on the vascularity of the temporal muscle.

The pericranium is now replaced and stabilized where possible with nylon or Vicryl sutures. The coronal flap is closed with a running Prolene suture for hemostasis. Two suction drains are used, and a very light dressing of gauze or elastic bandage is applied. This is removed in 3 to 4 days, and the patient usually leaves the hospital in 7 days.

Antibiotic cover, the normal dose of cephalosporin, is given just before surgery, during surgery, and then every 6 hours for 48 hours, when it is discontinued. This regimen is standard in all maxillofacial and craniofacial procedures.

In children under the age of 1 year, the floating forehead technique of Marchac[18,19] is employed. In this technique, after release of the coronal and sphenozygomatic suture lines, the advanced supraorbital area and frontal bone are stabilized on the maxilla medially at the nasal bridge line and laterally at the lateral orbital rim. Posteriorly, there is no attachment to the skull, and a wide defect remains extending down to the inferior orbital fissure. This frontal-orbital block is free to be pushed forward by the expanding brain and thus produce a satisfactory contour (Figs. 27-5 and 27-6).

Maxillary surgery

Maxillary surgery may be performed at the same time as a frontal advancement or later. Sometimes it may be the only procedure required. The osteotomy is performed at the

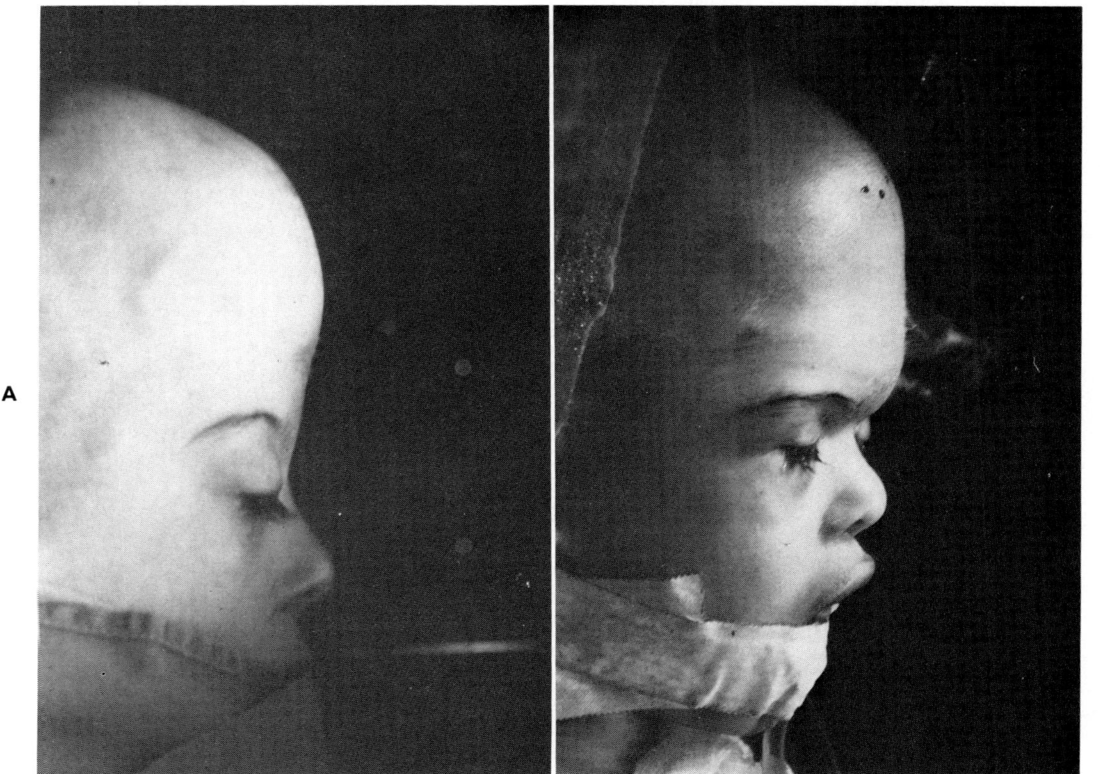

Fig. 27-6. A and **B,** Immediate postoperative appearance in frontal advancement. Note the position of the supraorbital rim to the eyes.   *Continued.*

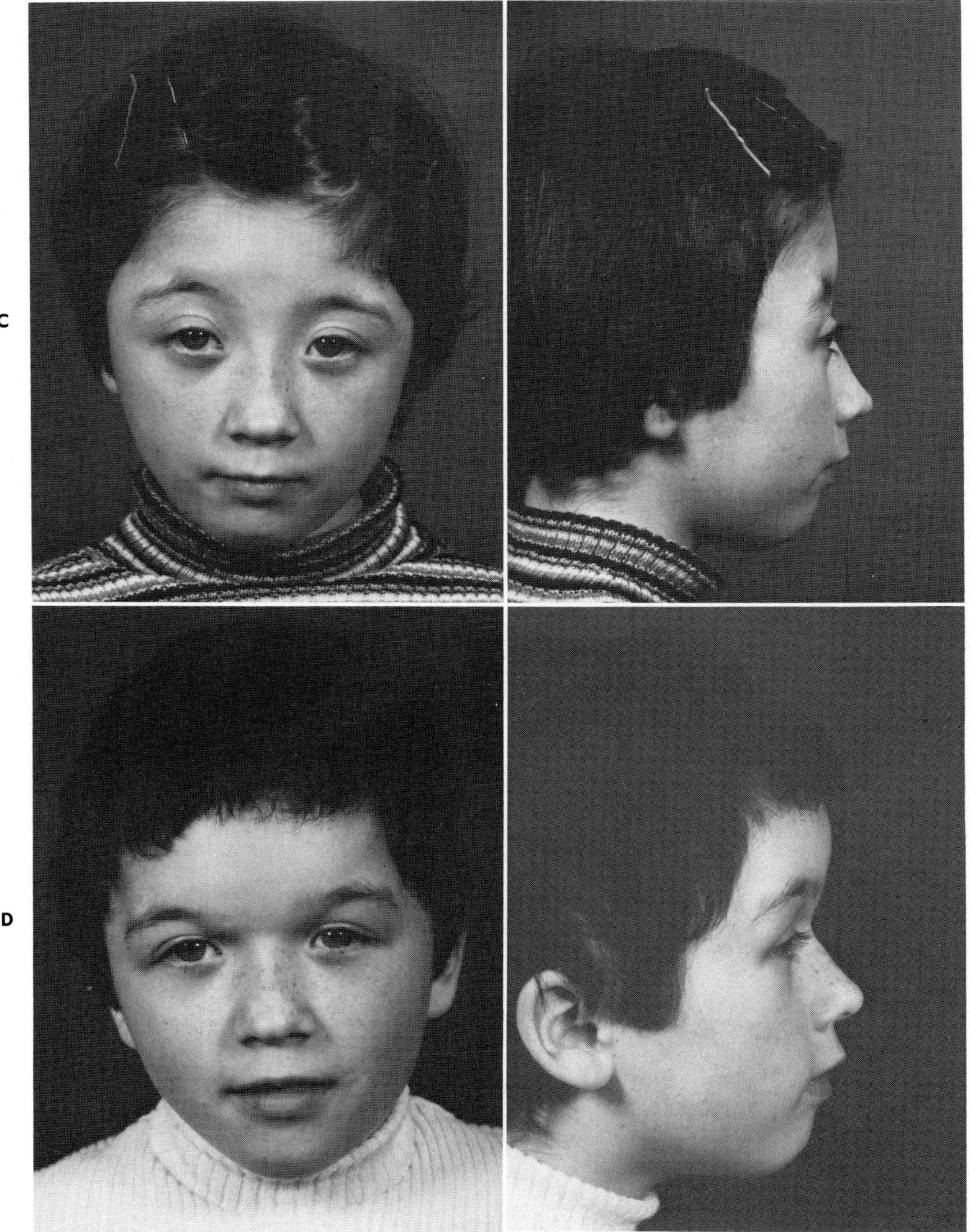

Fig. 27-6, cont'd. C and **D,** Preoperative and postoperative results in frontal advancement.

LeFort III level and varies in its vertical extent, depending on the distribution of the facial deformity.

Tessier I osteotomy

This is the classic osteotomy (Fig. 27-7) described by Tessier in 1967.[29] The first steps in this direction were made by Harold Gillies in 1950.[10] The approach uses the coronal flap, which is raised as described earlier.

At about 2 cm above the supraorbital rims the periosteum is raised, and the periorbital dissection begins. The orbital contents are freed completely from both walls, the roof, and the floor of the orbit. An attempt is made to preserve the

Text continued on p. 453.

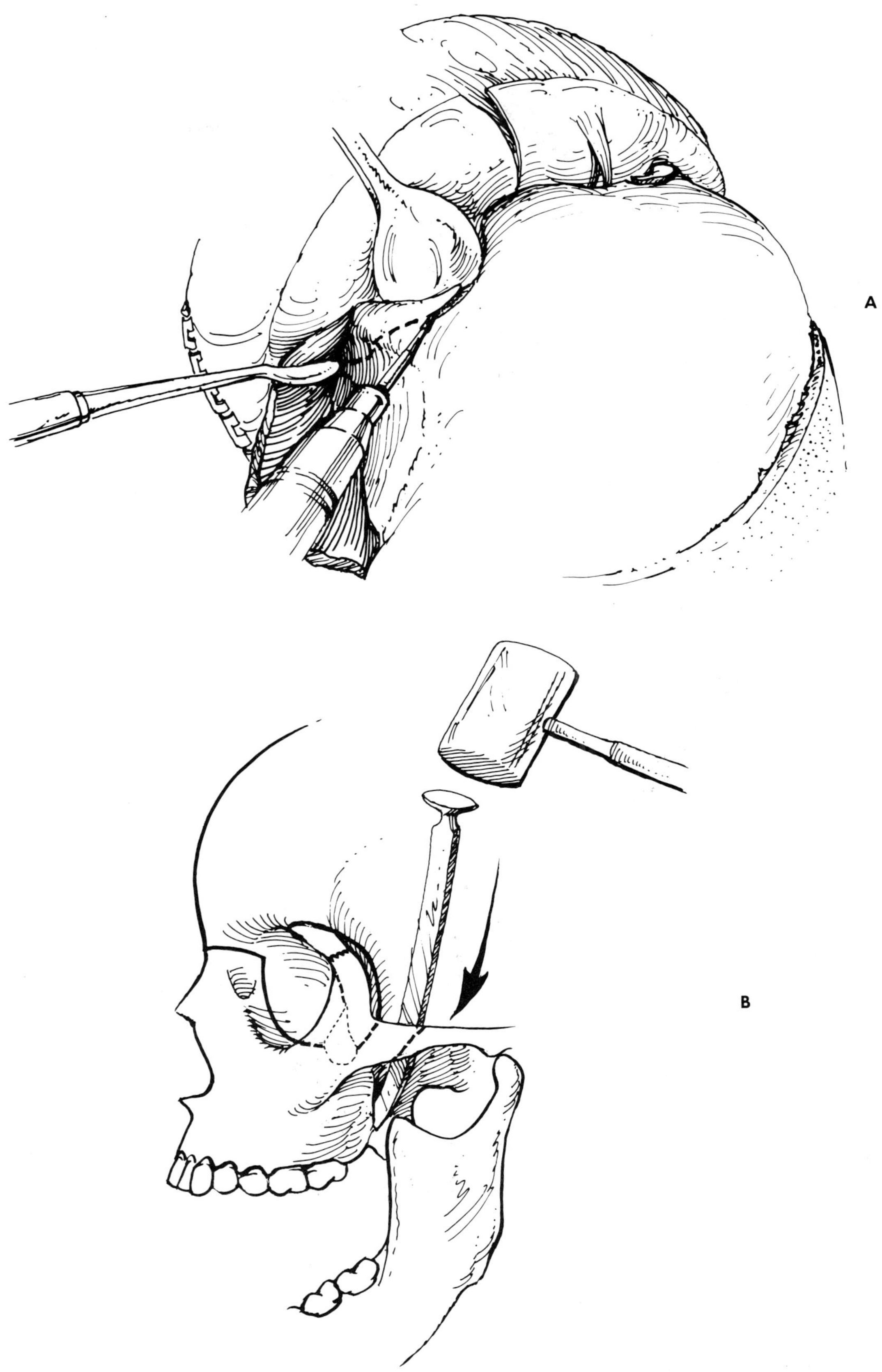

Fig. 27-7. LeFort III (Tessier I) osteotomy. **A,** Lateral orbital wall osteotomy. **B,** Separation of maxillary tuberosities from pterygoid plates.   *Continued.*

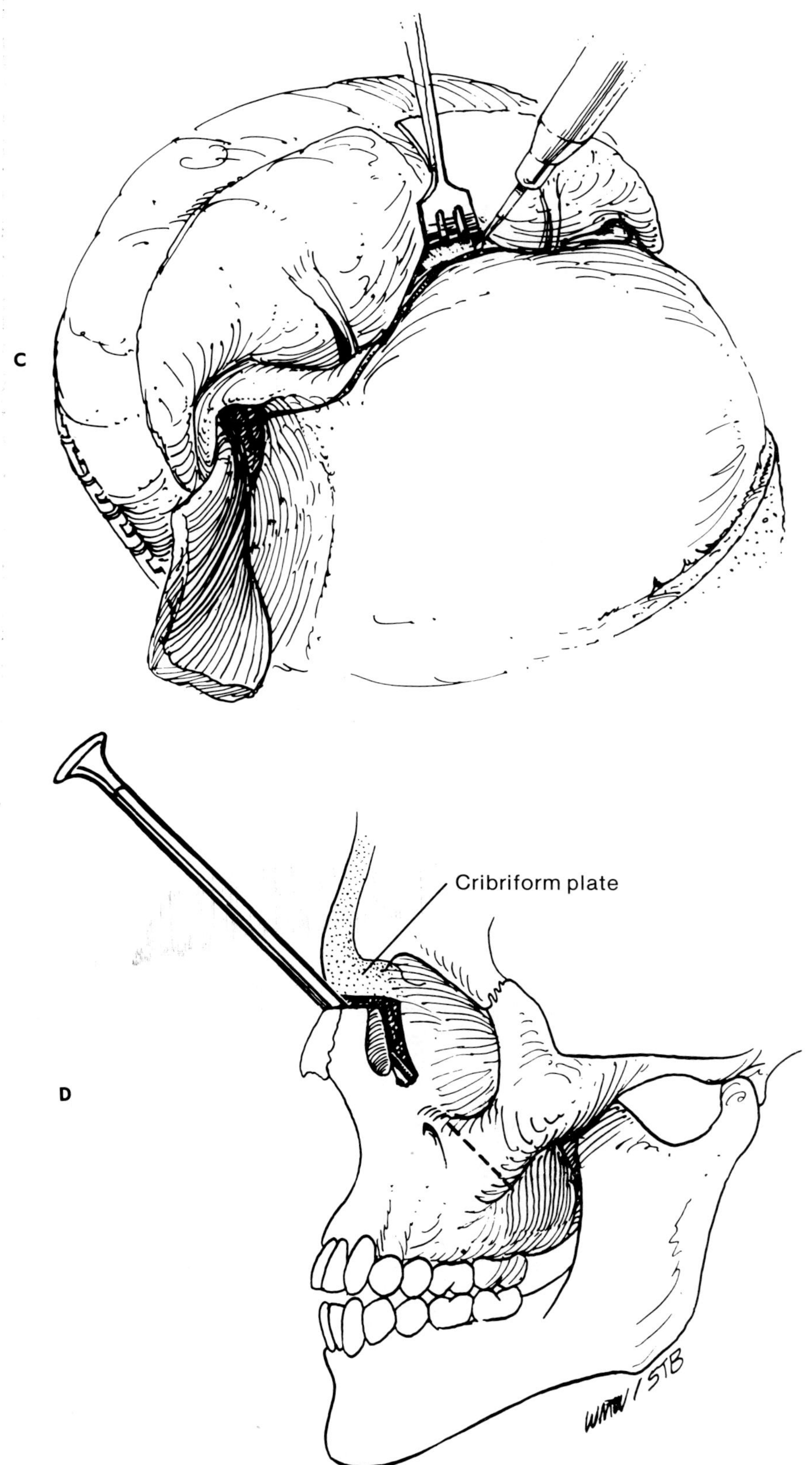

Fig. 27-7, cont'd. C, Osteotomy at the junction of the nose and frontal area. **D,** Osteotome introduced to separate the maxilla from the base of the skull. Dotted line shows direction that should be followed.

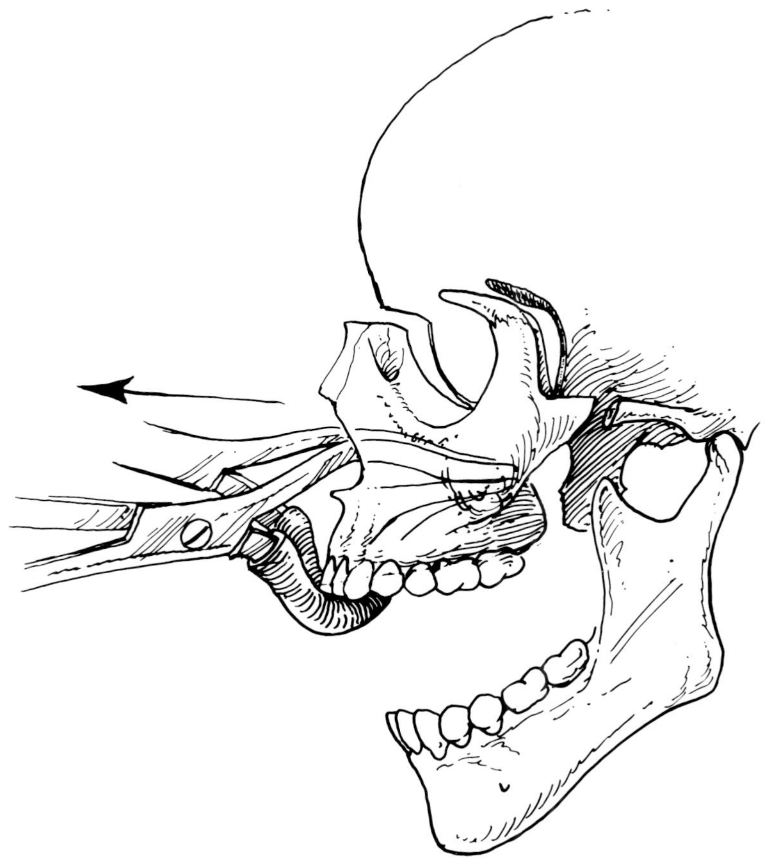

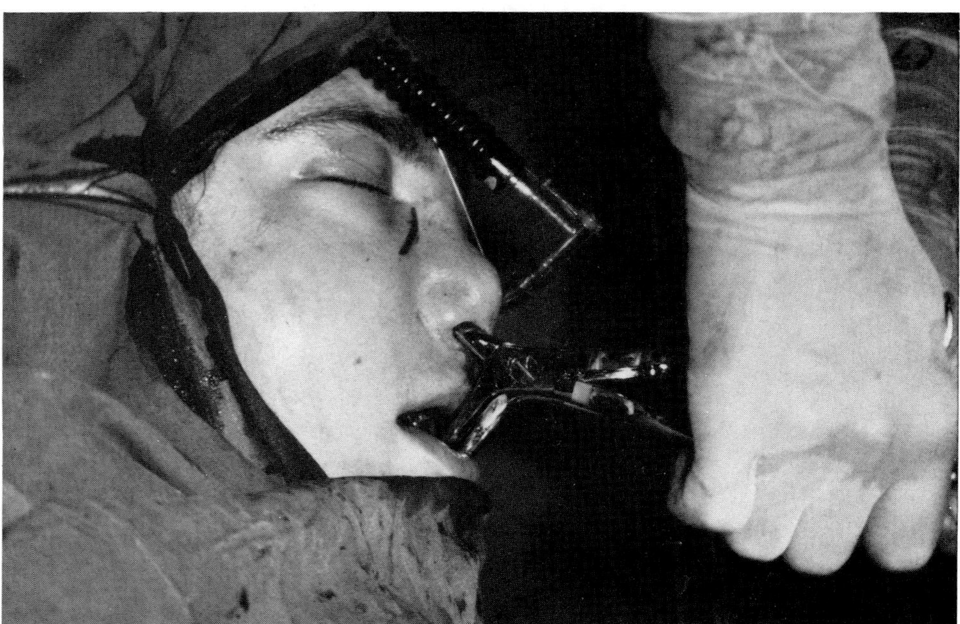

Fig. 27-7, cont'd. E, Forceful mobilization with Rowes' disimpaction forceps.

Continued.

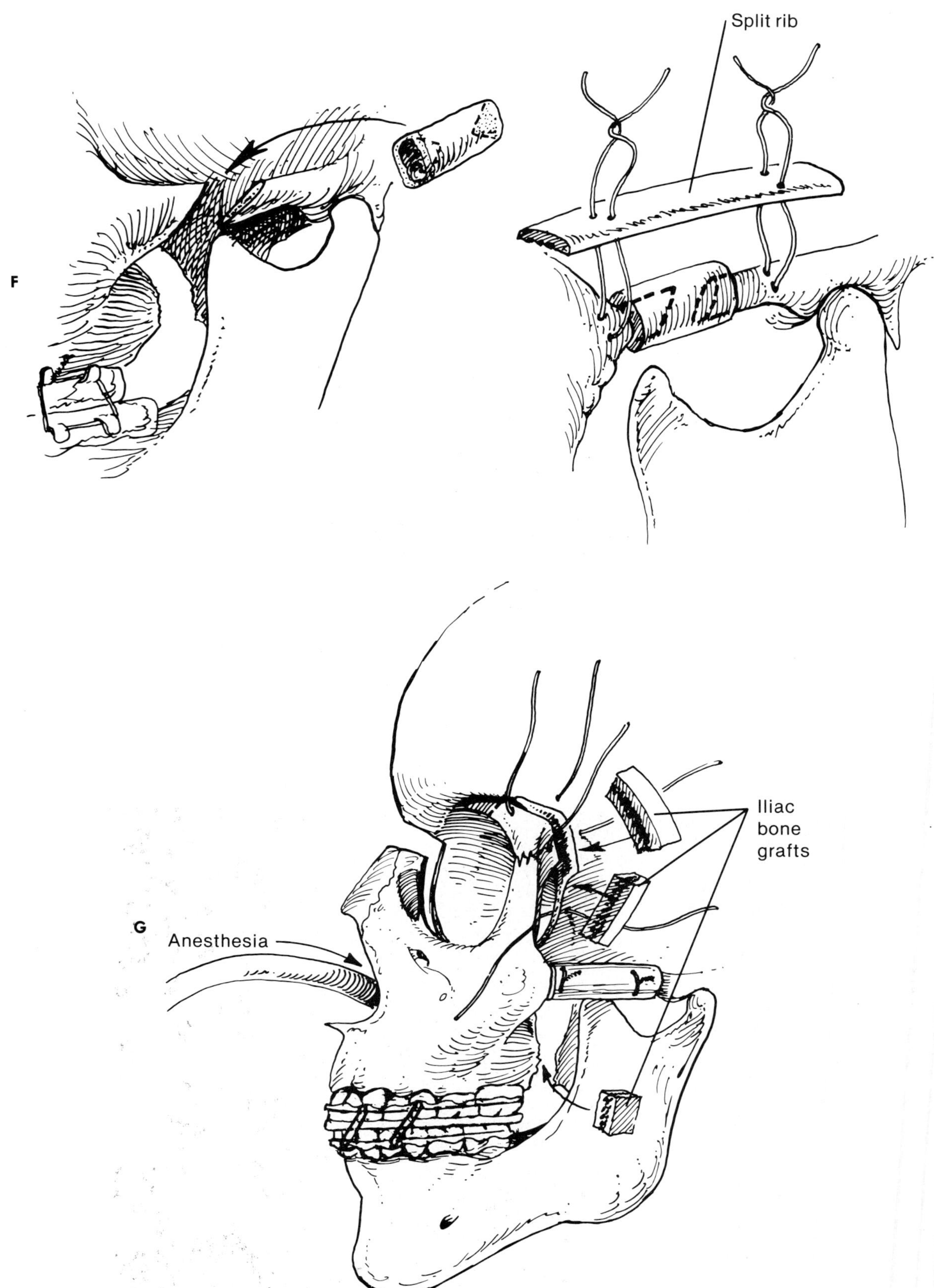

Fig. 27-7, cont'd. F, Method stabilizing zygomatic arch. **G,** Bone grafts inserted into bony defects.

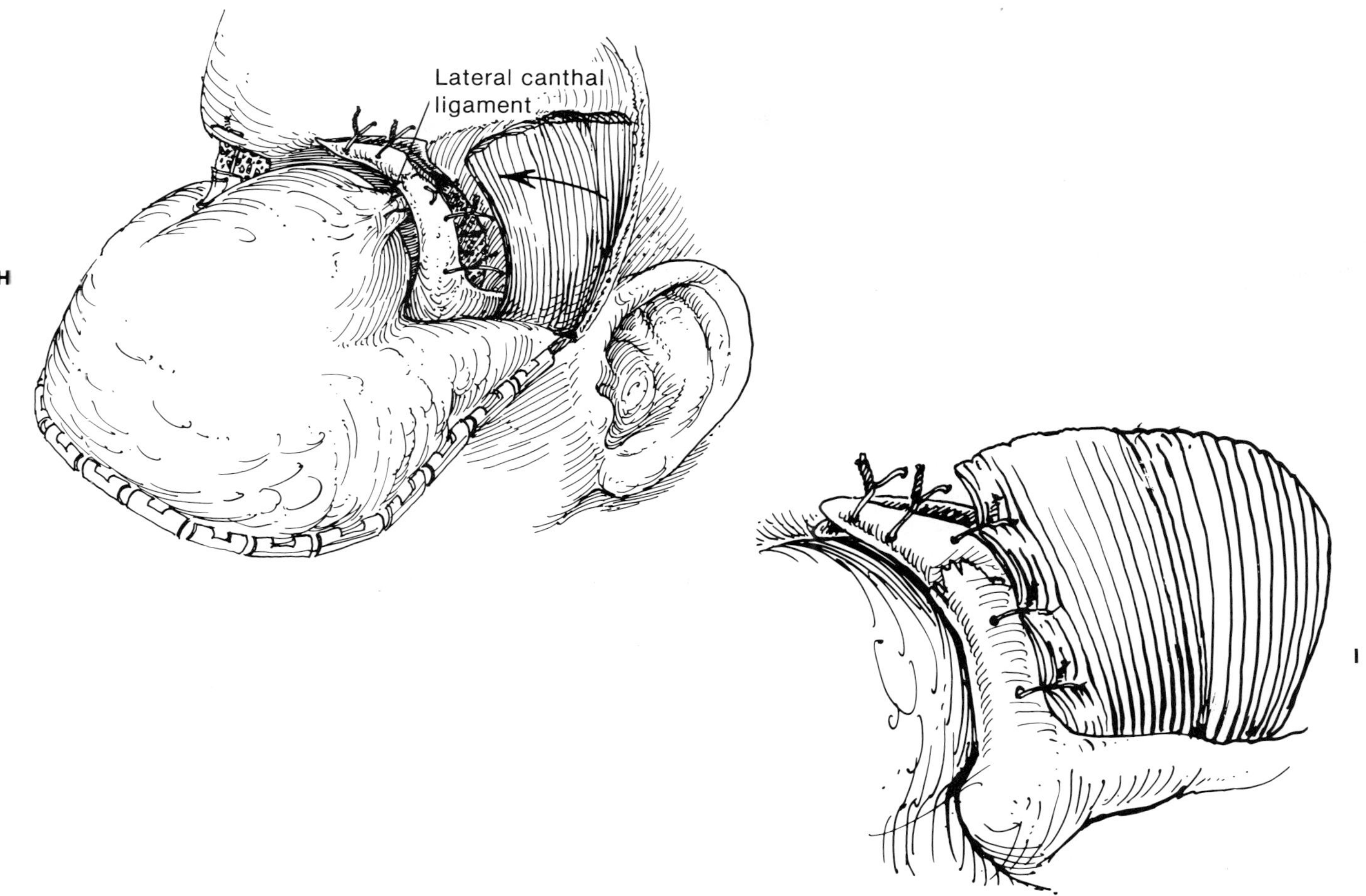

Fig. 27-7, cont'd. H, Attachment of lateral canthal ligament. **I,** Reattachment of temporal muscle.

medial canthal ligament attachment. The skin is elevated over the temporal fascia down to the zygomatic arch. This dissection should stay close to the fascia, otherwise the frontal branch of the facial nerve could be damaged. The temporal muscle is freed from the rim of the lateral wall of the orbit to its junction with the middle cranial fossa. The groove between the tuberosity and the pterygoid plates is identified. Dissection over the anterior surface of the maxilla is unnecessary unless bone grafting in this area is contemplated. There are no external skin or intraoral incisions.

A transverse or curved osteotomy is made high on the lateral orbital wall. It becomes vertical and is taken down to the inferior orbital fissure about 2 to 3 mm anterior to its junction with the middle cranial fossa (Fig. 27-7, *A*). The orbital contents are lifted from the floor of the orbit with a suitable retractor, often a teaspoon, and a bone cut is made across the floor. The zygomatic arch is cut diagonally or in a step fashion, depending on the type of stabilization used. The maxillary tuberosities are now separated from the pter-

ygoid plates using an osteotome directed caudally (Fig. 27-7, *B*). The nasal bridge line is cut transversely, well back onto the medial orbital wall (Fig. 27-7, *C*). This cut now becomes vertical behind the medial canthal ligament and joins the orbital floor cut at its inferior limit.

A curved osteotome is introduced into the nasal bridge cut and directed downward and backward to separate the nasal septum and vomer from the skull base (Fig. 27-7, *D*). Before this, the lateral skull radiograph should be examined to determine the position of the cribriform plate and to ensure that the osteotome cut is made below this level. Another potential complication to be avoided is damage to the endotracheal tube with the osteotome in the nasopharyngeal area. The osteotomy is now completed, and maxillary mobilization commences. This is an important maneuver. Without excellent mobilization, relapse is a real possibility. Mobilization is achieved using Rowes' disimpaction forceps; the first movement is a down fracture, followed by side-to-side and rotatory manipulations. Frequently a finger must be inserted behind the tuberosities to free medial and posterior soft tissue attachments that can prevent total maxillary freeing and advancement. It should now be possible to advance the maxilla with light forward traction; inability to do this calls for further mobilization (Fig. 27-7, *E*).

The acrylic resin bite-guard splint is inserted, the teeth are related as planned, and the jaws are wired together using the bands placed on the teeth preoperatively by the orthodontist. It is convenient to discuss fixation in the very young child at this stage. The maxilla can be placed in the correct position as judged by preoperative splints, then bone grafted and fixed to the skull and zygomatic arch. It may then be left without intermaxillary fixation and the child given a soft diet.

If splints are necessary, the upper one is held in position using a circumpalatal wire taken through the anterior part of the piriform aperture; in this way, tooth buds are not damaged. The mandibular splint is held by circummandibular wires.

The next move is to stabilize the zygomatic arch. This may be done in one of several ways. If the arch is thick, it may have been cut in a step fashion so that as the maxilla slides forward, bony contact is maintained and direct wiring can be carried out. Defects can be bone grafted with the outer table of the skull or ilium. In most children the arch is thin, and this method is not possible. In these children a portion of rib, having the ends cored out with a contouring drill, is inserted between the ends of the arch, which has been cut at an angle. This is usually a stable arrangement. To ensure optimal stability, a split rib is overlaid and wired to both segments of the zygomatic arch. Total stability results (Fig. 27-7, *F*).

The bony defect of the lateral orbital wall and the gap between the tuberosity and pterygoid plates are grafted with a single solid block of the outer table of the skull of ilium. The maxilla is now effectively stabilized. Small bone grafts of the outer table can be placed in the orbital floor and, if necessary, in the nasal bridge line and at the lateral orbital rims to smooth out any step deformities that may occur here (Fig. 27-7, *G*).

In some patients with maxillary hypoplasia, onlay bone grafts are placed on the anterior surface of the maxilla. If the infraorbital rim is very hypoplastic, it is too thin to give optimal support for the lower eyelid; in these cases, a suitably contoured bone graft is wired to the rim to establish normal structure and give better lid support.

The lateral canthi are identified; if there is any difficulty, a hypodermic needle is passed from the skin surface through the periorbita, where it punctures in approximately the region of the canthus. A fine hemostat is placed on the canthal ligament to provide traction; the canthus is pulled up to a position of 1 or 2 o'clock when related to the left orbit and 10 or 11 o'clock on the right orbit. If there is any difficult in performing this maneuver, an inferomedial release of the

periorbita is performed. The canthus can now be elevated with minimal effort. A drill hole is made, and the canthus is wired into position. This may be done in several ways. The simplest and most effective method is to cut the wire at an angle and, using the end as a needle, pass this through the lateral canthal ligament, taking two bites. The lower pass of the wire is taken through the drill hole, and the ligament is positioned by tightening the wire; overcorrection is to be aimed for, since a downward sag of the lateral canthus may occur in the long term (Fig. 27-7, *H*).

The temporal muscle is advanced as described previously. For secure positioning, the temporal fascia is fastened through drill holes to the lateral orbital rim; it is also sutured to the lateral canthus (Fig. 27-7, *I*). The pericranium is sutured to that on the coronal flap to reestablish continuity. The scalp is sutured and dressings applied as described earlier. If there are worries about eye swelling, light pressure dressings may be used (this is rarely necessary). Ice packs also may be used. It is desirable to assess vision as early as possible. Intermaxillary fixation is maintained for 6 to 8 weeks. At this point the wires are removed, but the splint is left in position. Over the next 2 weeks, the patient's occlusion is closely observed. If there is any evidence of relapse, the wires or elastic bands can be reapplied for a further period of fixation. This is rarely necessary if mobilization has been adequate and the bone graft fixation is sound and secure (Fig. 27-8).

Tessier II osteotomy

With experience, it has become obvious that the standard Tessier I/LeFort III osteotomy is not suitable for all patients. Also, the combined frontal advancement/LeFort III procedure is too extensive. There are individuals with retrusion of varying amounts of the lateral portion of the supraorbital rim. Split-rib bone grafting has been used in the past, but variable resorption was a constant problem. To cope with this, a modified intracranial approach has been devised.

A bur hole is made in the temporal area, which exposes the frontal lobe (Fig. 27-9, *A*). The latter can now be freed from the inner aspect of the skull in the extradural plane and retracted as necessary. If a large segment, for example, one half to three fourths, of the supraorbital rim is to be moved, then the bur hole should be enlarged using bone rongeurs to give better exposure.

The standard lateral orbital wall osteotomy is continued up to the frontotemporal area. It is then taken across the frontal bone, with the brain retracted and protected through the bur hole, continues above the supraorbital rim for the required distance, and is brought through the rim. A cut is now made in the orbital roof. This cut is taken to meet the lateral wall osteotomy (Fig. 27-9, *B*). From this point the mobilization, bone grafting, stabilization, and dressing are identical to the Tessier I procedure, apart from one step. The bony discrepancy between the supraorbital rim and the frontal bone should be reduced; this potential step deformity

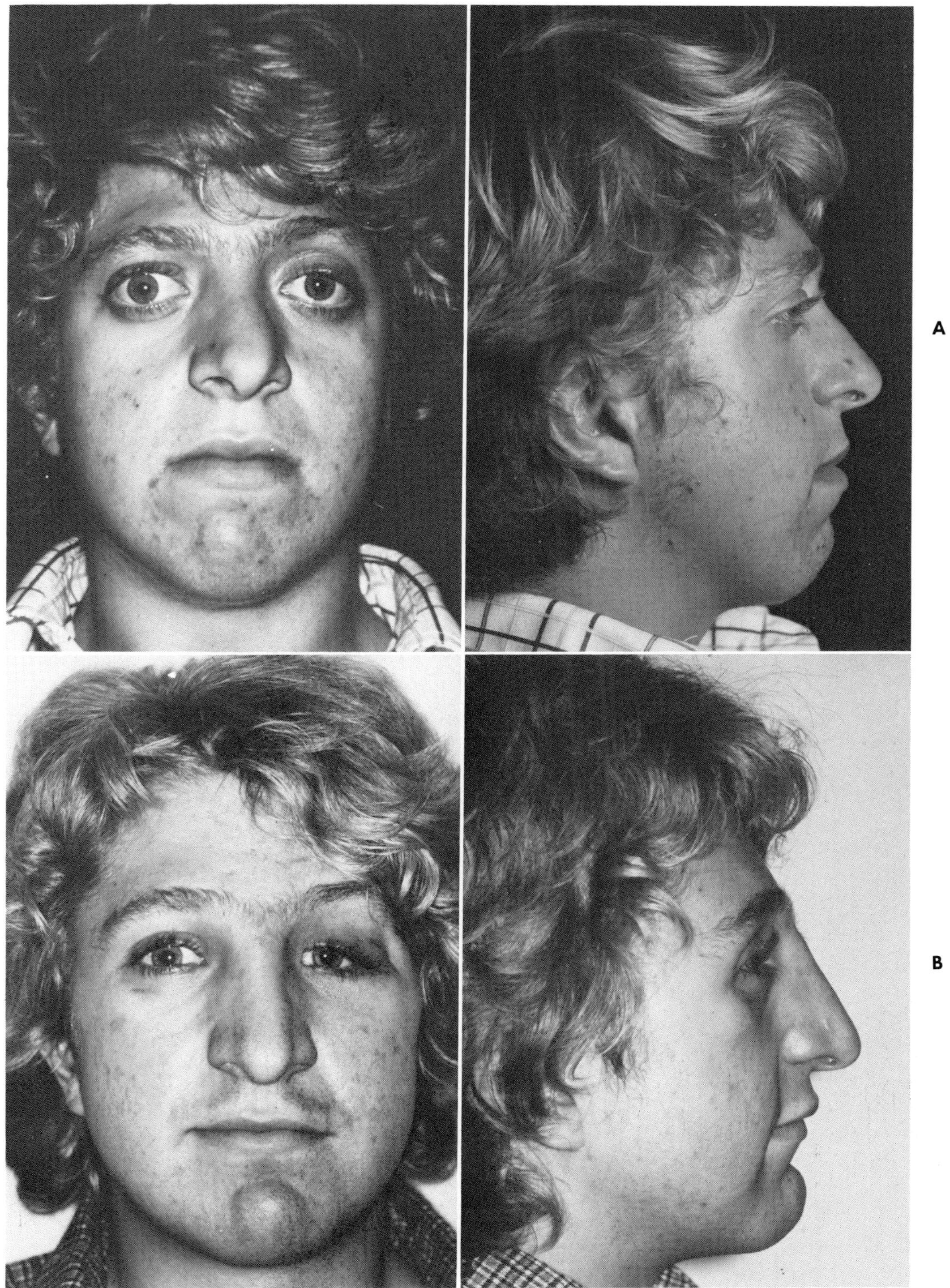

Fig. 27-8. Preoperative **(A)** and postoperative **(B)** results of Crouzon's disease treated with subcranial LeFort III (Tessier I) maxillary osteomy. Note postoperative ptosis of the left eye; this will occasionally occur after a LeFort III osteotomy.

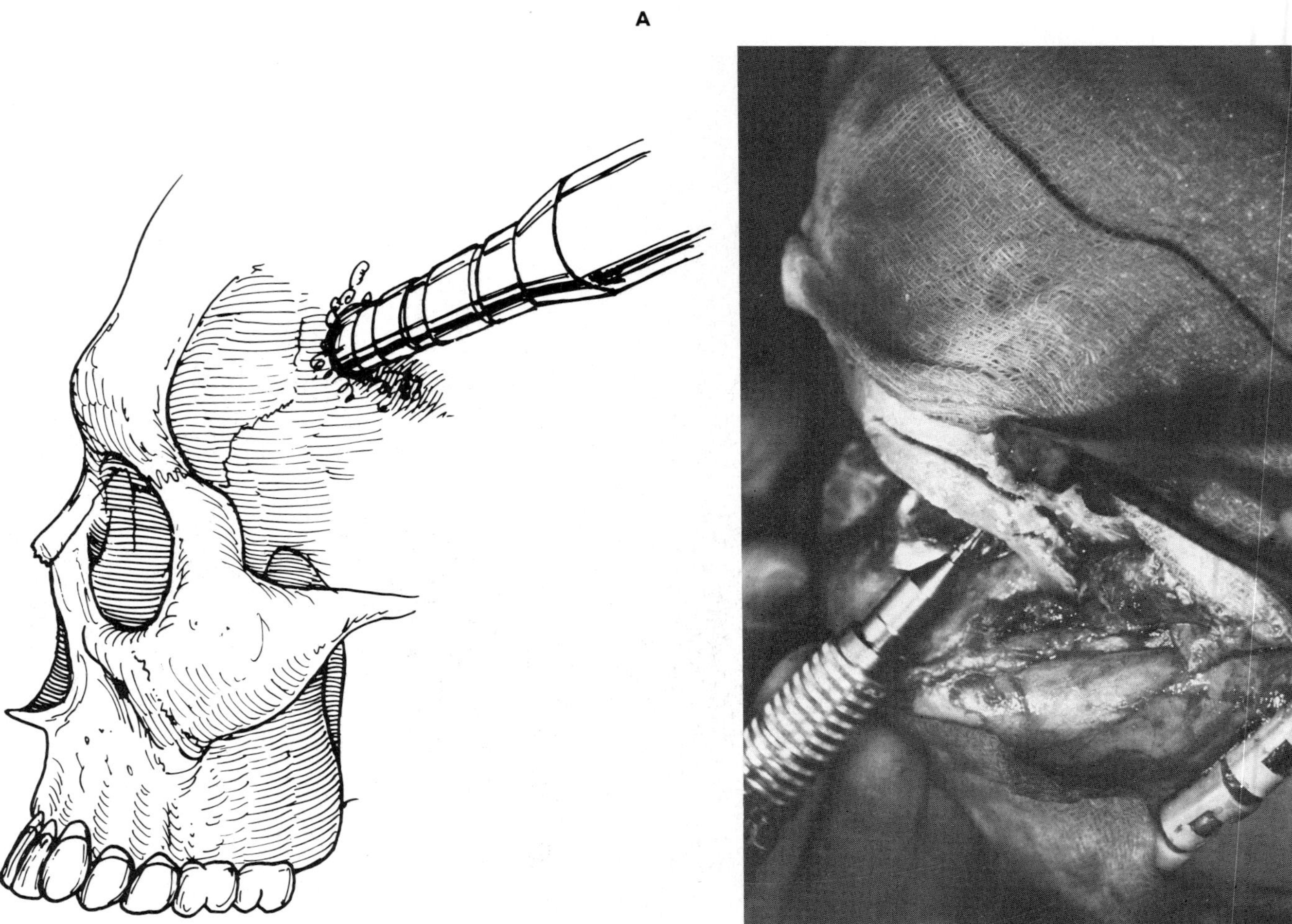

Fig. 27-9. A, Bur hole to gain access to the anterior cranial fossa.

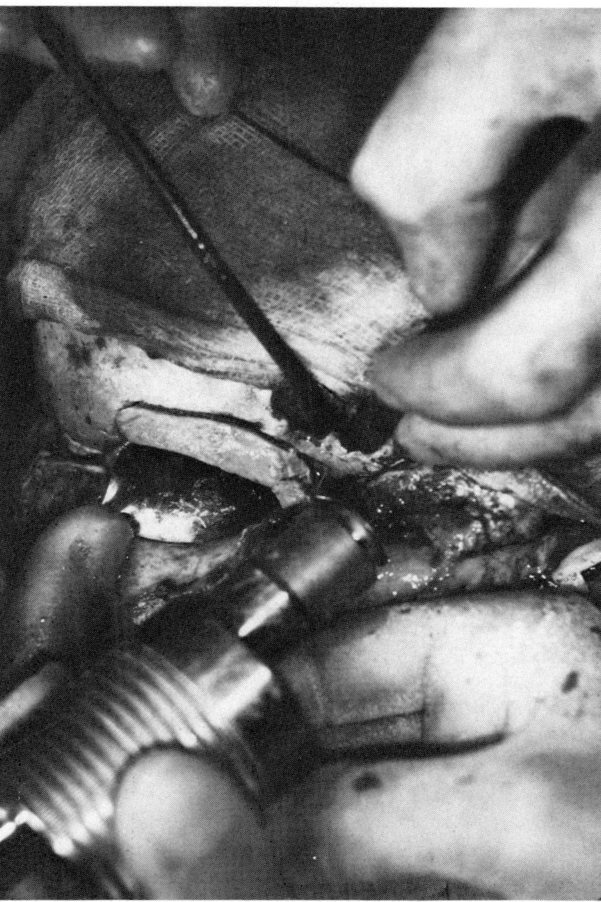

Fig. 27-9, cont'd. B, The frontal lobe is protected while a supraorbital rim osteotomy is being performed.

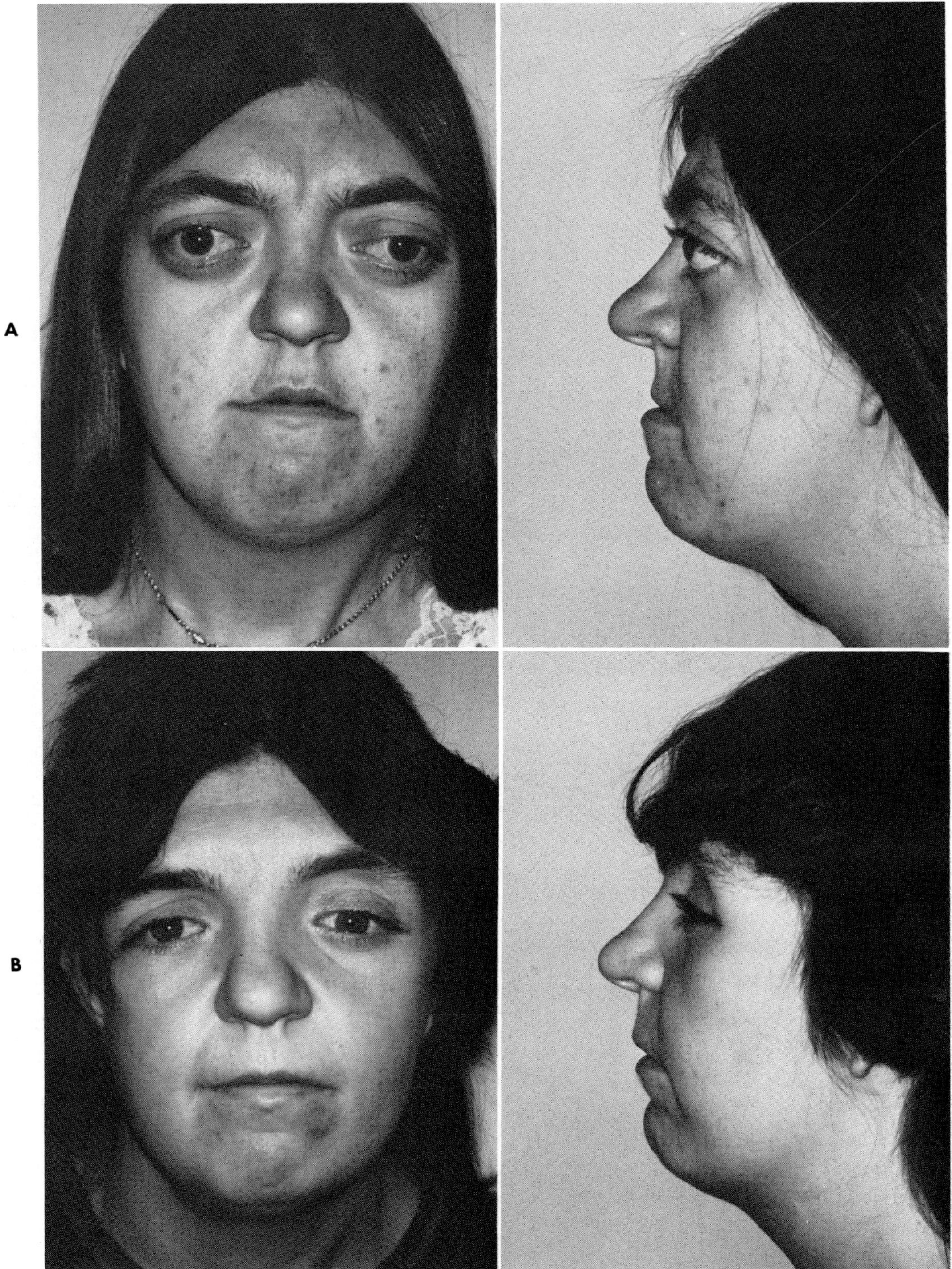

Fig. 27-10. Preoperative **(A)** and postoperative **(B)** results of LeFort III (Tessier II) maxillary advancement for Crouzon's disease.

is bone grafted with a portion of iliac bone contoured to a suitable wedge shape (Fig. 27-10).

Tessier III osteotomy

In this modification, partial self-stabilization is obtained. The variation lies in the temporal area. Here a bur hole is made, and the brain is protected as described previously (Fig. 27-11, *A*). The osteotomy is made in a Z fashion so that the posterior limb locks onto the lateral orbital rim and can be wired in this region. The mobilization must be done with care, and when the maxilla is advanced, it is moved down and forward; otherwise, the anterior Z-plasty limb may be broken off (Fig. 27-11, *B*). Contouring with bone grafts is necessary at the lateral orbital rim. The remainder of the steps are identical to the classic LeFort I procedure (Fig. 27-12).

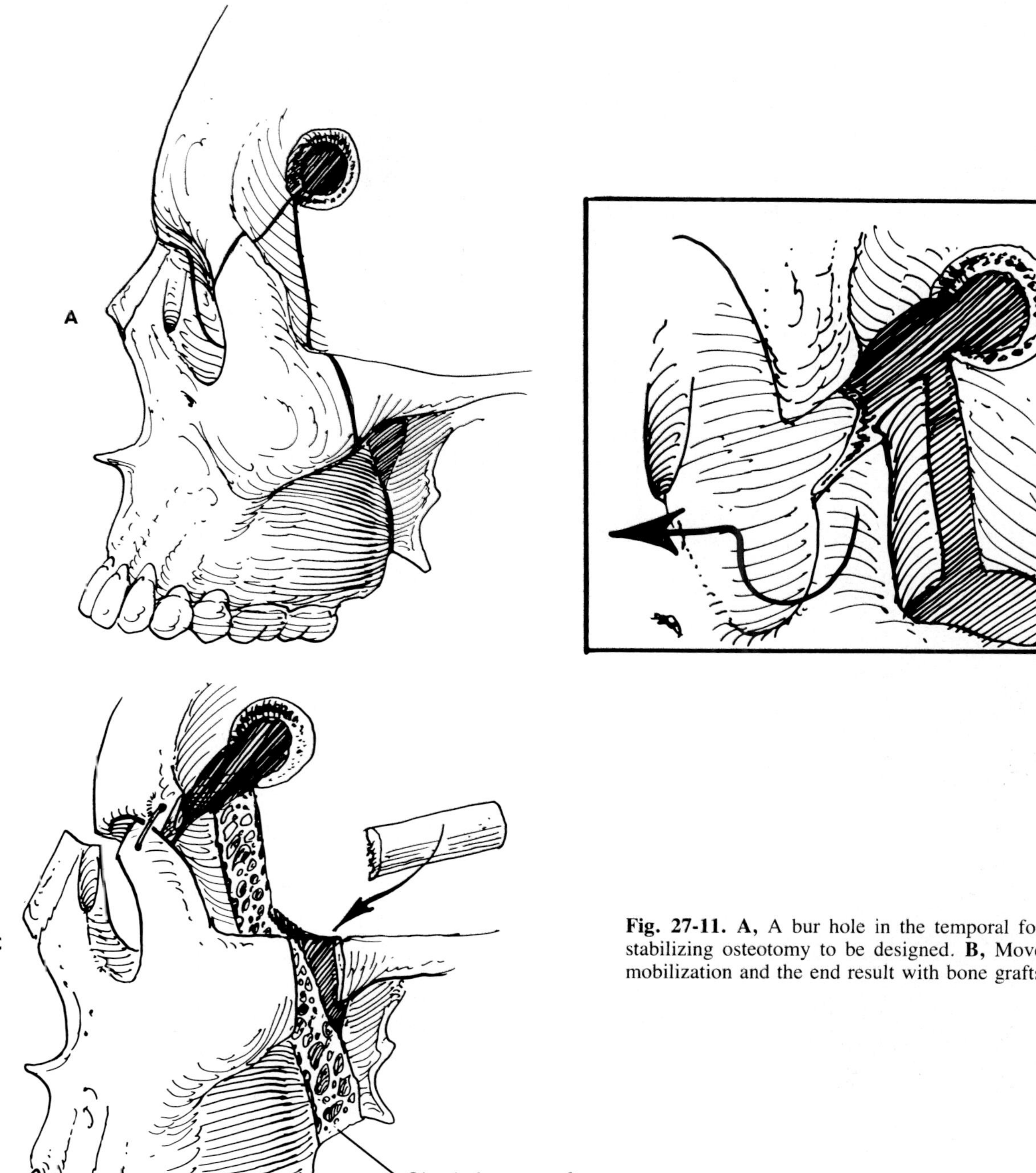

Fig. 27-11. A, A bur hole in the temporal fossa allows a self-stabilizing osteotomy to be designed. **B,** Movement required in mobilization and the end result with bone grafts in place.

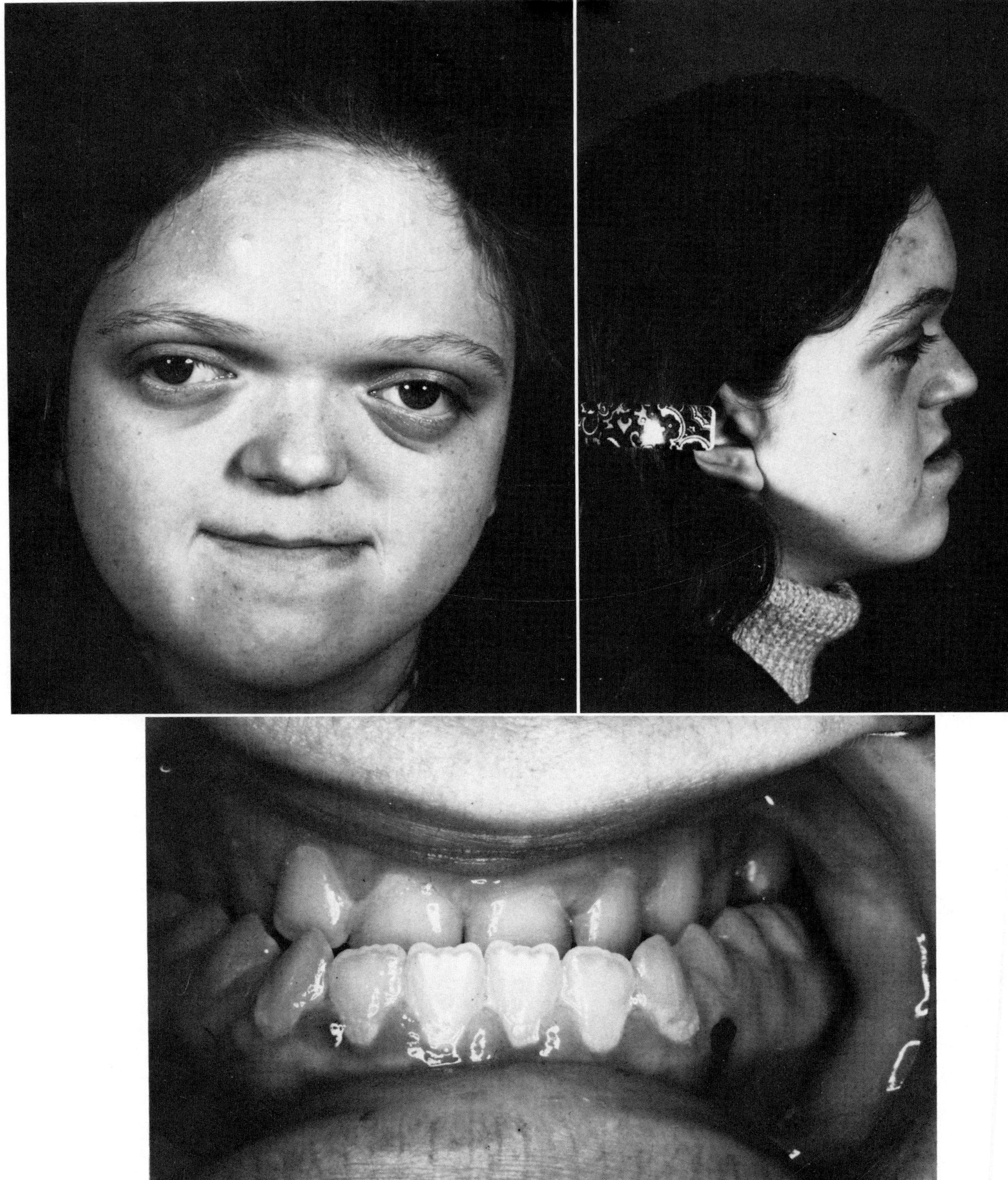

Fig. 27-12. Preoperative **(A)** and postoperative **(B)** results of LeFort III (Tessier III) maxillary advancement for Crouzon's disease.

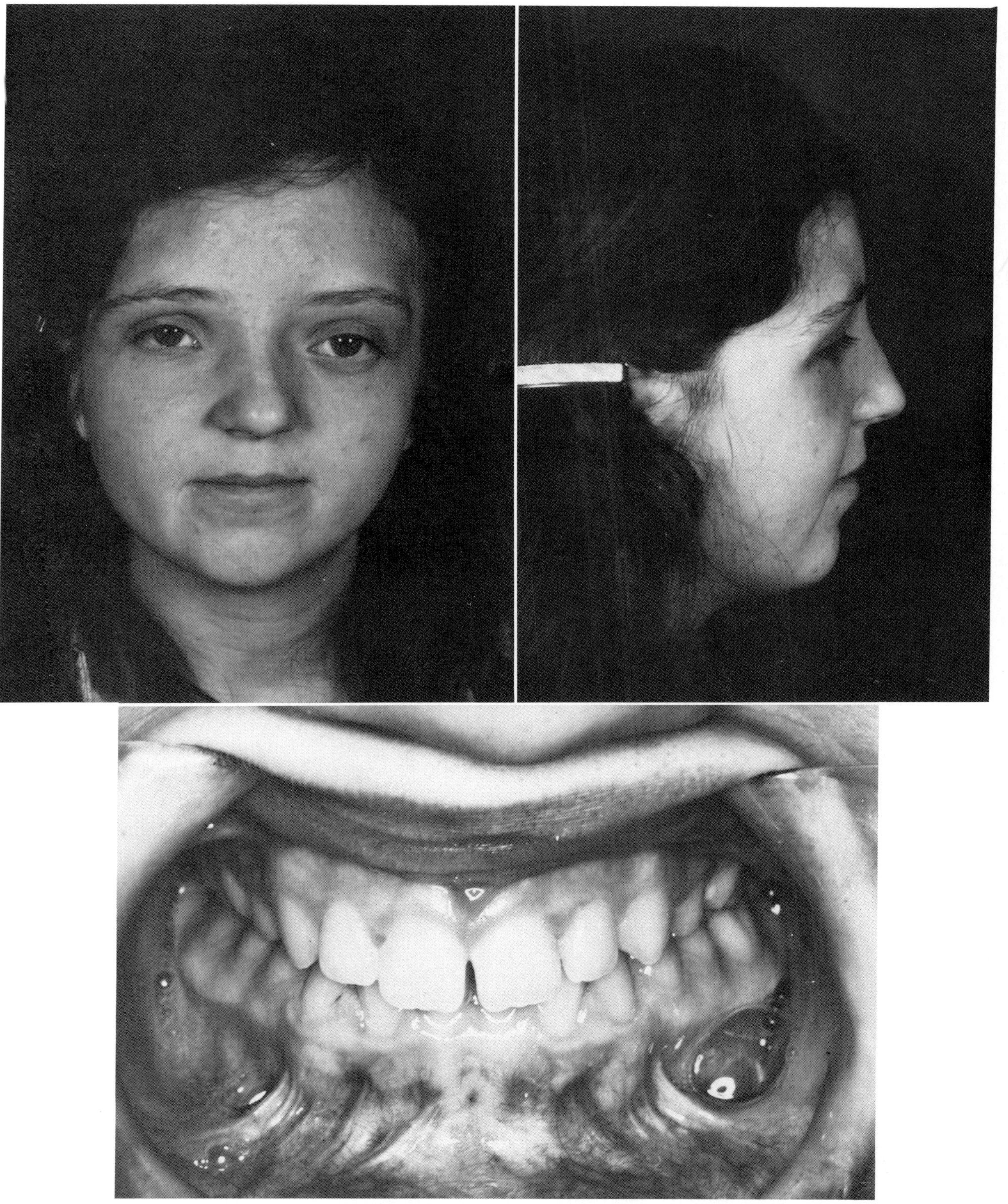

Fig. 27-12, cont'd. For legend see opposite page.

Monobloc advancement (LeFort IV)

Monobloc advancement was described by Ortiz-Monasterio, Fuente-del-Campo, and Carrillo[23] in 1978 but had been used quite extensively by others before.[13] It is used in cases of brachycephaly, where a separate frontal-supraorbital advancement is contraindicated. With brachycephaly there is an overall, uniform retrusion of the face.

An intracranial and extracranial approach is necessary. After removal of the frontal bone flap, a total circumorbital osteotomy is made. The cut on the orbital roof need not be too far back. These orbital roof cuts are joined anterior to the cribriform plate. The lateral orbital wall cuts are brought up to the temporal area, where they are stepped to provide bony overlap for wiring after the advancement. The lateral osteotomy joins the orbital roof osteotomy at its lateral limit. The standard posttuberosity bone cut is made, and the septum is separated from the skull base by introducing an osteotome through the osteotomy in the anterior cranial fossa just anterior to the cribriform plate. This is done with care to prevent overenthusiastic displacement of the orbital contents. Apart from the fixation in the temporal area, the remainder of the maxillary procedure is virtually identical to that described for the standard LeFort III osteotomy. The frontal bone may be advanced with two posterior tongues for fixation, or it may be reconstructed from another portion of skull if the brachycephaly is significant (Fig. 27-13).

The step osteotomy

In some patients, it is necessary to selectively advance the maxilla and orbits, supraorbital rim, and frontal bone. This is best separated into two separate procedures as much as possible.

As in the Tessier I procedure, the maxilla is advanced at a subcranial level into the precalculated position, stabilized, and bone grafted. The patient is prepared and draped again and the personnel scrub and gown. A frontal-supraorbital rim advancement is performed. An attempt is made to leave the floor of the anterior cranial fossa intact in front of the cribriform plate to eliminate a nasopharyngocranial connection. If there is a small gap, a flap of pericranium and occipitofrontal muscle based inferiorly on the supratrochlear vessels is swung down to seal the gap. In doing this over the past 10 years, no infections have occurred in this procedure (Fig. 27-14).

Anterior open bite correction

Anterior open bite correction is handled in essentially three ways. In minor degrees, the whole maxilla may be tilted anteriorly with some posterior impaction. If this is attempted in more significant degrees of anterior open bite, the face is unduly elongated, and the orbits become oval, with displacement of the eyebrows.

In these cases, a simultaneous LeFort III/LeFort I pro-

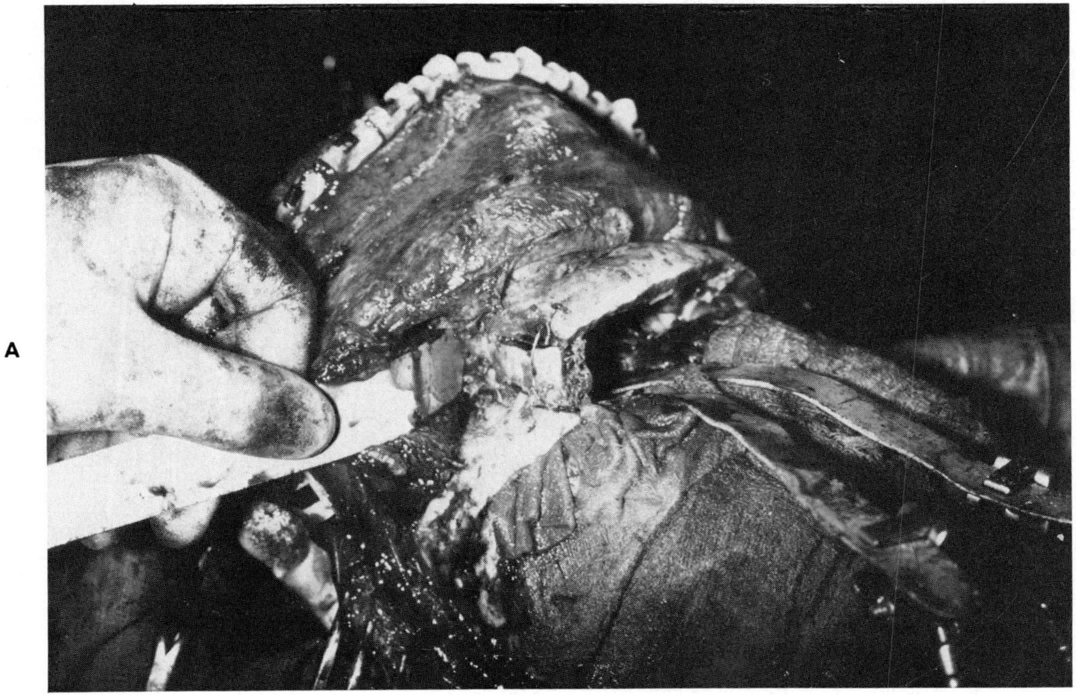

Fig. 27-13. A, LeFort IV osteotomy completed, and bone grafts inserted in temporal area. **B,** Preoperative appearance. **C,** Postoperative results of LeFort IV maxillary advancement.

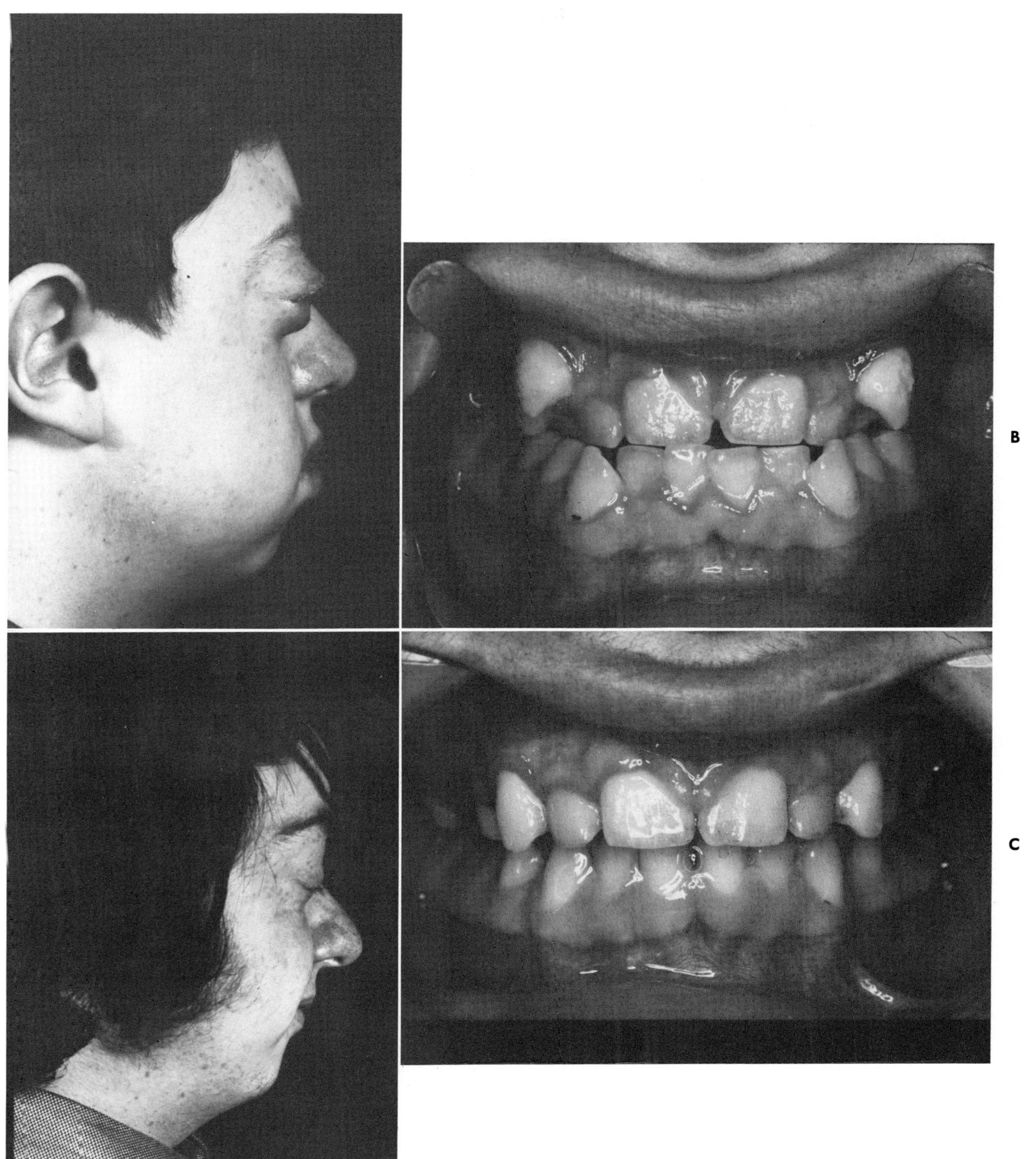

Fig. 27-13, cont'd. For legend see opposite page.

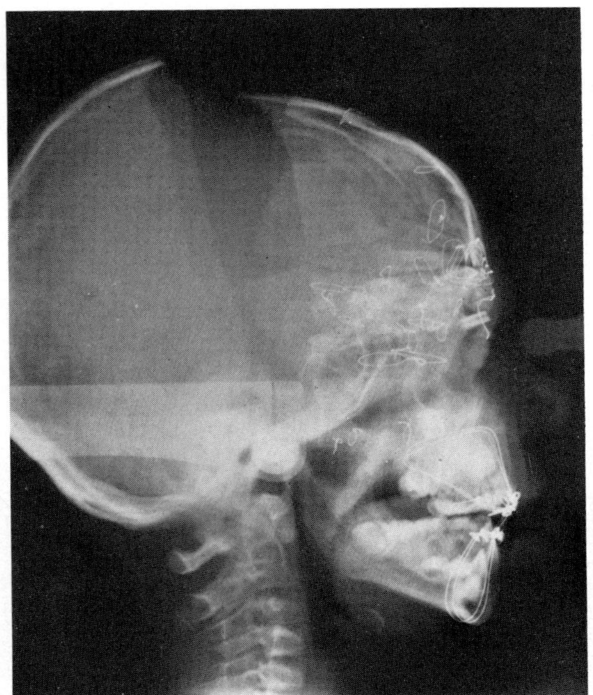

Fig. 27-14. Radiograph showing the step frontal-supraorbital maxillary osteotomy.

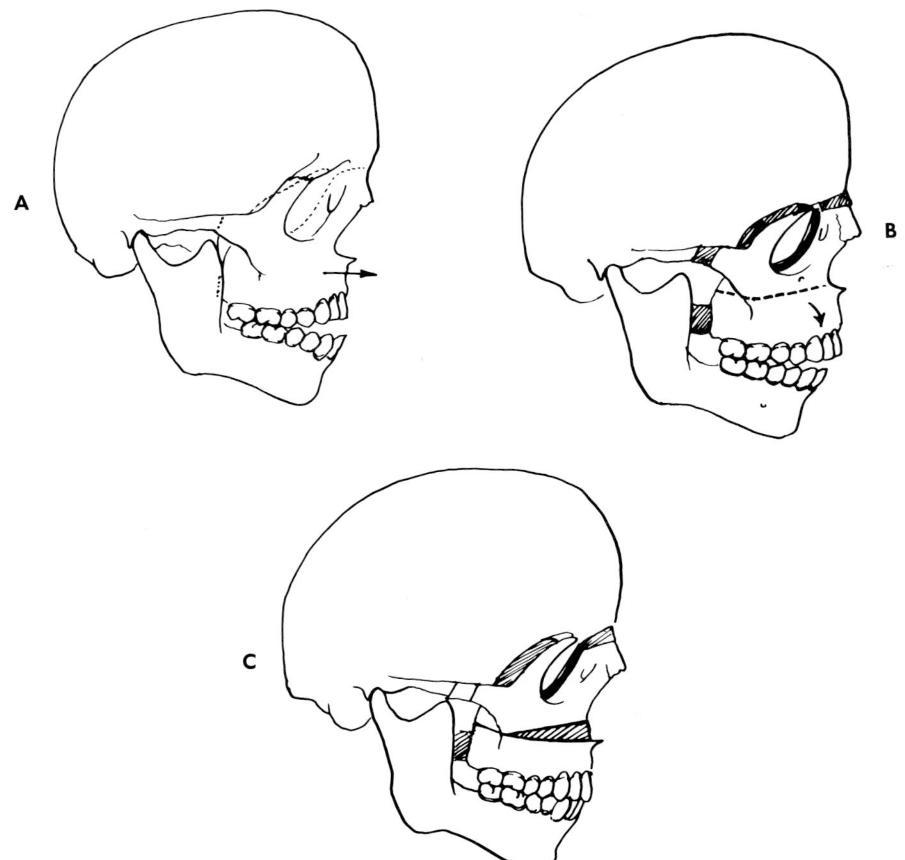

Fig. 27-15. A, Simultaneous LeFort III/LeFort I osteotomy to advance the maxilla and correct the anterior open bite deformity. **B,** Preoperative appearance. **C,** Postoperative results of simultaneous LeFort III and high-level LeFort I osteotomy in Apert's syndrome.

cedure with bone grafting in the transverse osteotomy may be used (Fig. 27-15). Often better results will be obtained by simply advancing the face at the LeFort III level and after everything is stable and healed (usually 6 months), performing a LeFort I osteotomy. To obtain the best possible result, this procedure may have to be segmentalized. It is only applicable to older children with eruption of permanent dentition.

ADDITIONAL SURGICAL PROCEDURES
Nose

At the initial maxillary advancement, the nose is frequently bone grafted. Soft tissue is freed from the skeleton, dissecting from above, and a graft—either rib and costal cartilage or bone—is inserted right to the nasal tip to give definition of that area. The graft is stabilized by wiring to either the glabellar or nasal area, depending on which gives the best profile, using the cantilever principle. Bone chips or cancellous bone fragments are packed around the portion of the graft in relation to the nasal bones to fill up any dead space. Occasionally, after 12 to 18 months, further surgery on the nose may be necessary to narrow the tip and improve the bridge line.

Mandible

It is rarely necessary to advance the mandible in classic cases. If necessary, it should be performed when the child is older. Frequently the chin is retrusive, and an advancement genioplasty is indicated. This cannot be done at an early age because of developing teeth. Only after the secondary dentition has erupted can the genioplasty be safely carried out.

Onlay bone grafting

In come cases supraorbital ridge grafting for augmentation is carried out at the initial procedure. These grafts are wired in position. The anterior surface of the maxilla is frequently grafted because of inherent hypoplasia. Sometimes it is possible to wire the graft in position on the malar area and at the infraorbital rim; on other occasions, a pocket is made and the graft fills the pocket. As stated earlier, the skull is a frequent donor site.

Occasionally, bone graft resorption will occur, necessitating regrafting. It is wise to delay this for 12 to 18 months. A useful technique is to make a very small incision within the temporal hairline and to dissect down over the malar bone and anterior maxilla to create a pocket. Cancellous bone is then taken from the hip by way of a small skin incision, making a drill hole in the crest, and scraping out the graft with a curette. This is then packed into the pocket. This technique gives good graft take with minimal nonessential soft tissue disturbance and little discomfort and scarring.

All of the operative techniques described in this chapter have recently been presented in more detail.[16]

ANESTHETIC CONSIDERATIONS IN MAXILLARY OSTEOTOMIES

Anesthetic considerations may be summed up as establishment and maintenance of the airway; if hypotensive anesthesia can be added to this, it is a most welcome bonus.[9]

The anesthesiologist should carefully assess the patient before surgery to be aware of potential problems. A tracheostomy is rarely if ever indicated, especially since the introduction of the fiberoptic bronchoscope. The endotracheal tube is passed through the nose and secured with tape and sutures. At the time of mobilization of the maxilla, care must be taken by the surgeon to avoid dislocation of the tube. The surgeon should cooperate closely with the anesthesiologist, such as alerting the anesthesiologist to periods of excessive blood loss that may occur during maxillary mobilization or cautioning about vagal overstimulation and bradycardia due to eye retraction.

Careful monitoring of blood loss is mandatory both during surgery and postoperatively; it is unwise to fall behind in blood replacement. To maintain a secure airway postoperatively, the patient is frequently sent to the intensive care area with the nasotracheal tube in place. It is usually possible to remove this the next day. If there is any worry about the adequacy of the airway, the tube can be maintained longer. If it is judged that the patient has swallowed blood and postoperative emesis is anticipated, the passage of a nasogastric tube at the end of the procedure is strongly advocated. This allows gastric aspiration and drainage.

To ensure the best possible patient management, a good line of communication is essential between the surgeon, anesthesiologist, and pediatric nursing staff. If this is established, mishaps are rare.

SUMMARY AND CONCLUSIONS

Since Tessier described the extracranial LeFort III osteotomy, there has been a steady evolution of philosophy with modifications of the procedure: the intracranial-extracranial approach, self-stabilization, and monobloc advancement. With these options, preoperative assessment must be more accurate and sophisticated. This, of course, comes with experience. As the surgery becomes more extensive, so the complications increase. The combined frontal-supraorbital and maxillary procedures have the highest incidence of death and serious infection. The latter will often lead to sequestration and removal of frontal bone and supraorbital rims. When this occurs, it is a disaster of considerable magnitude and requires a complex reconstructive procedure. The reason for complications in this operation is the frontal dead space, which leads directly into the nasopharynx, where the mucosa is usually torn.[30,31]

It is important to mention at this time that the incidence of serious complications is low. (See Table 28-1.) In experienced groups, with reduction of operating time and sophistication of surgical and anesthetic techniques, complication rates are being significantly decreased.

Relapse is always to be considered, but rarely occurs in the well-executed adult osteotomy. In children there is little or no anterior growth after the advancement, thus it may be necessary to repeat the advancement osteotomy when the face is fully grown. At the moment, we do not have enough information about this to make definitive statements. It does, however, raise the question of when to perform surgery. When there are good indications, such as severe deformity, peer problems, corneal exposure, or globe prolapse, surgery should be performed without hesitation, accepting that a repeat procedure may be necessary. With minor degrees of deformity, correction may be postponed until parental pressure demands it.

It is important to be realistic about our achievements in these cases. In minor deformities (craniosynostosis and Crouzon's disease), the results range from good to excellent. In Apert's syndrome and other complex problems, there are frequently disappointments, both for the surgeon and patient. In these cases complications occur for which we have no consistent solutions at the moment. This is most strikingly seen in the lateral canthal area, where downward drift and subsequent antimongoloid slant occur despite vigorous attempts to overcome them during surgery.

Other problems are differences in eye level with diplopia, which is often temporary, and extraocular muscle palsies, which may or may not recover spontaneously. Damage to the sixth cranial nerve with resulting lateral rectus palsy occurs most frequently. Temporary upper lid ptosis is not uncommon; occasionally it does not resolve and requires surgical correction.

Many patients with Crouzon's disease and Apert's syndrome have an increase in the intercanthal distance. Since this is usually not severe, it is probably reasonable to leave it uncorrected. An illusion of narrowing can be created by augmenting the nasal bridge line with a bone graft. In most cases, this is preferable to a surgical reduction of the interchanthal distance because of potential problems.

To summarize the state of the art at the moment, advances have been considerable in terms of reduction of morbidity and mortality. With refinements of technique, results have improved, but in some areas we must strive for better understanding of the problems and provide improvement in results.

REFERENCES

1. Apert, E.: De l'acrocéphalosyndactylie, Bull. Mem. Soc. Med. Hop. Paris **23:**1310, 1906.
2. Buchanan, R.C.: Acrocephalosyndactyly, or Apert's syndrome, Br. J. Plast. Surg. **21:**406, 1968.
3. Carpenter, G.: Case of acrocephaly, with other congenital malformations—autopsy, Proc. R. Soc. Med. **2:**199, 1909.
4. Chotzen, F.: Eine eigenartige familiäre entwicklungsstörung (akrocephalosyndaktylie, dysostosis craniofacialis und hypertelorismus), Mschr. Kinderheilk **55:**97, 1932.
5. Cohen, M.M., Gorlin, R.J., Berkman, M.D., and Feingold, M.: Facial variability in Apert type agrocephalosyndactyly, Birth Defects **7:**143, 1971.
6. Crouzon, O.: Dysostose cranio-faciale héréditaire, Bull. Mem. Soc. Med. Hop. Paris **33:**545, 1912.
7. Dodge,H.W., Wood, M.W., and Kennedy, R.L.J.: Craniofacial dysostosis: Crouzon's disease, Pediatrics **23:**98, 1959.
8. Eaton, A.P., Sommer, A., Kontras, S.B., and Sayers, M.P.: Carpenter syndrome—acrocephalopolysyndactyly type II, Birth Defects **10:**249, 1974.
9. Ferguson, D.J.M., Barker, J., and Jackson, I.T.: Anesthesia for craniofacial osteotomies, Ann. Plast. Surg. (In press.)
10. Gillies, H., and Harrison, S.H.: Operative correction by osteotomy of recessed malar maxillary compound in a case of oxycephaly, Br. J. Plast. Surg. **3:**123, 1950.
11. Goodman, R.M., and Gorlin, R.J.: Atlas of the face in genetic disorders, ed. 2, St. Louis, 1977, The C.V. Mosby Co.
12. Hodach, R.J., Vieskul, C., Gilbert, E.F., et al.: The Pfeiffer syndrome: association with Kleeblattschädel and multiple visceral anomalies, Z. Kinderheilk. **119:**87, 1975.
13. Jackson, I.T.: Midface retrusion. In Whitaker, L.A., and Randall, P., editors: Symposium on reconstruction of jaw deformity, St. Louis, 1978, The C.V. Mosby Co.
14. Jackson, I.T.: Aesthetic correction of coronal craniosynostosis, Clin. Plast. Surg. **8:**317, 1981.
15. Jackson, I.T., Hide, T.A.H., and Barker, D.T.: Transposition cranioplasty to restore forehead contour in craniofacial deformities, Br. J. Plast. Surg. **31:**127, 1978.
16. Jackson, I.T., Munro, I.R., Salyer, K.E., and Whitaker, L.A.: Atlas of craniomaxillofacial surgery, St. Louis, 1982, The C.V. Mosby Co.
17. Jones, K.L., and Cohen, M.M.: The Crouzon syndrome, J. Med. Genet. **10:**398, 1973.
18. Marchac, D.: Early correction of craniofacial deformity (under one year of age). In Jackson, I.T., editor: Recent advances in plastic surgery, ed. 2, Edinburgh, 1981, Churchill Livingstone.
19. Marchac, D., and Renier, D.: "Le front flottant": traitement précoce des facio-craniostenoses, Ann. Chir. Plast. **24:**121, 1979.
20. McCarthy, J.G., Coccaro, P.J., Epstein, F., and Converse, J.M.: Early skeletal release in the infant with craniofacial dysostosis: the role of the sphenozygomatic suture, Plast. Reconstr. Surg. **62:**335, 1978.
21. Munro, I.R.: Personal communication, 1978.
22. Munro, I.R.: Early correction of craniofacial deformities. In Jackson, I.T., editor: Recent advances in plastic surgery, ed. 2, Edinburgh, 1981, Churchill Livingstone.
23. Ortiz-Monasterio, F., Fuente del Campo, A., and Carrillo, A.: Advancement of the orbits and the midface in one piece, combined with frontal repositioning, for the correction of Crouzon's deformities, Plast. Reconstr. Surg. **61:**507, 1978.
24. Pantke, O.A., Cohen, M.M., Witkop, C.J., et al.: The Saethre-Chotzen syndrome, Birth Defects **11:**190, 1975.
25. Pfeiffer, R.A.: Dominant erbliche akrocephalosyndactylie, Z. Kinderheilk. **90:**301, 1964.
26. Saethre, H.M.: Ein beitrag zum turmschädelproblem (pathogenese, erblichkeit und symptomatologie), Dtsch. Z. Nervenheilk **119:**533, 1931.
27. Salyer, K.E.: Recent developments in bone grafting. In Jackson, I.T., editor: Recent advances in plastic surgery, ed. 2, Edinburgh, 1981, Churchill Livingstone.
28. Stricker, M., Montaut, J., Hepner, H., and Flot, F.: Les ostéotomies du crane et de la face, Ann. Chir. Plast. **17:**233, 1972.
29. Tessier, P.: Osteotomies totales de la face: syndrome de Crouzon, syndrome d'Apert, oxycéphalies, scaphocéphalies, turricéphalies, Ann. Chir. Plast. **12:**273, 1967.
30. Whitaker, L.A., Munro, I.R., Jackson, I.T., and Salyer, K.E.: Problems in cranio-facial surgery, J. Maxillofac. Surg. **4:**131, 1976.
31. Whitaker, L.A., Munro, I.R., Salyer, K.E., et al.: Combined report of problems and complications in 793 craniofacial operations, Plast. Reconstr. Surg. **64:**198, 1979.

CHAPTER 28

Orbital hypertelorism

IAN T. JACKSON

The condition of orbital hypertelorism (teleorbitism)[2] is best described as lateralization of the total orbit. In this condition the intercanthal and interpupillary distances are greater than normal (Fig. 28-1). Bony telecanthus is a lateralization of the medial orbital walls, the lateral orbital wall position being unchanged. Here the intercanthal distance is increased, but the interpupillary distance is normal (Fig. 28-2). The most acceptable measure of hypertelorism is the interorbital distance, which will be discussed later.

The primary anatomic abnormality associated with orbital hypertelorism is enlargement of the ethmoidal sinuses, which can be uniform or confined to a particular area. As a result, the orbits rotate laterally, and the optic foramina remain in their normal fixed position. This is not a primary condition but is secondary to other processes; it is frequently a component of other syndromes. It is predominantly a clefting deformity and, according to the position of the cleft, may be symmetric or asymmetric.[16] The nose may be in-

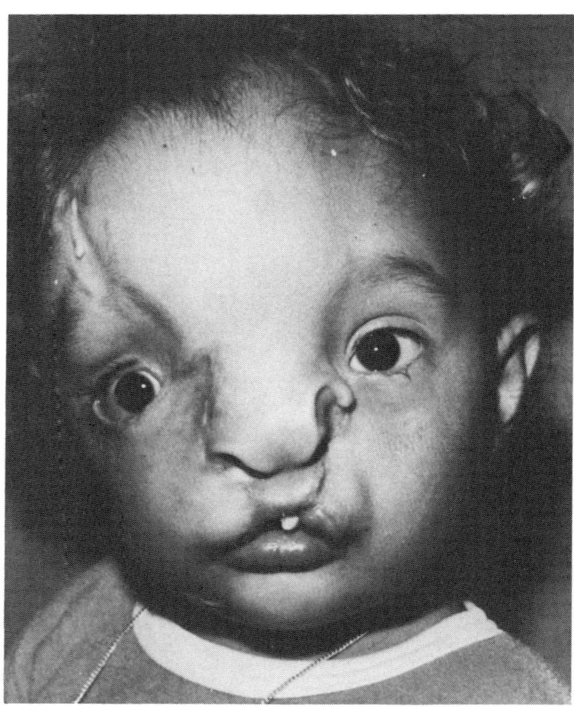

Fig. 28-1. This patient has orbital hypertelorism with an assortment of facial clefts.

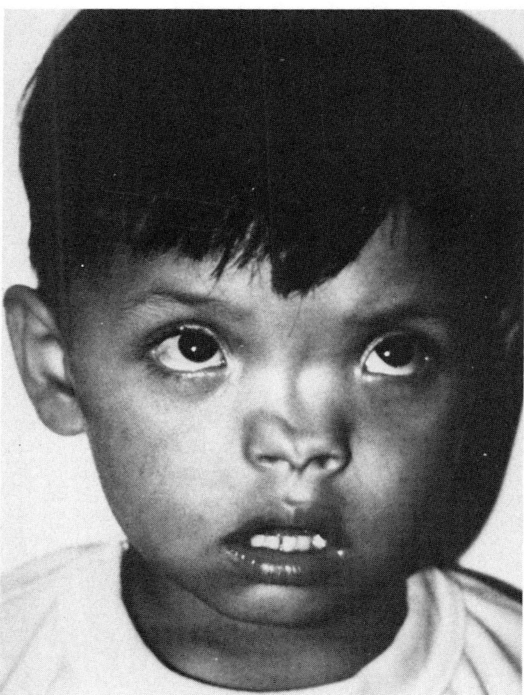

Fig. 28-2. Telecanthus. Only the medial orbital walls are displaced laterally. The lateral orbital walls are in the correct position.

volved slightly, as in the midline cleft, or severely distorted, as in the more lateral cleft. It may occur in association with cleft palate, a midline or basal encephalocele, Crouzon's disease, or Apert's syndrome. When a frontonasal encephalocele is associated with hypertelorism, it arises high in the frontal area; as its origin descends toward the nose, bony telecanthus results.

INVESTIGATIONS

A general pediatric physical examination should be undertaken to determine general health and the presence or absence of other physical anomalies. Clinical examination of the face gives much useful information. The intercanthal and interpupillary distances are noted purely as reference data. The forehead is assessed for symmetry, retrusion, or protrusion. Any angulation, rotation, or horizontal or vertical asymmetry of the orbits is noted. At the same time the palpebral fissures, eyelids, and medial and lateral canthi are studied. The relationship of the maxilla to the mandible is examined, as is occlusion. Intraoral examination confirms or excludes a cleft palate and occasionally a basal encephalocele. Particular attention is paid to the nasal deformity, since this is frequently the most difficult aspect of the condition to correct.

Radiographs of the skull and facial bones provide useful information as to orbital position and shape and the presence of frontal defects. The most important quantitative investigation to perform is a 2 m posteroanterior face radiograph. From this can be determined the interorbital distance, which is defined as the distance between the medial orbital walls at the level of the posterior lacrimal crest. This measures the true extent of the hypertelorism (Fig. 28-3).

A biplanar axial CT scan illustrates the relative orbital displacement, shape, and size and also shows any intracranial anomalies such as enlargement or decrease in size of the ventricles, which would suggest abnormal changes in CSF pressure. Another important feature illustrated by axial CT scans is the variability of ethmoidal sinus enlargement. It is essential for the treatment plan to note whether the enlargement is uniform, posterior, anterior, or central.[6] Tomography was popular in the past but gives little more information then the axial CT scan and exposes the patient to much more irradiation (Fig. 28-4).

Other specialists such as ear, nose, and throat physicians; ophthalmologists; oral surgeons; and psychologists, interview the child and parent. Decisions about the nature and extent of the surgery are made by the plastic surgeon and neurosurgeon. The parents are informed of what is involved, and the nature and incidence of the associated risks are discussed with them.

TREATMENT

The treatment for orbital hypertelorism was pioneered by Paul Tessier[13-15,17,18] and subsequently modified by

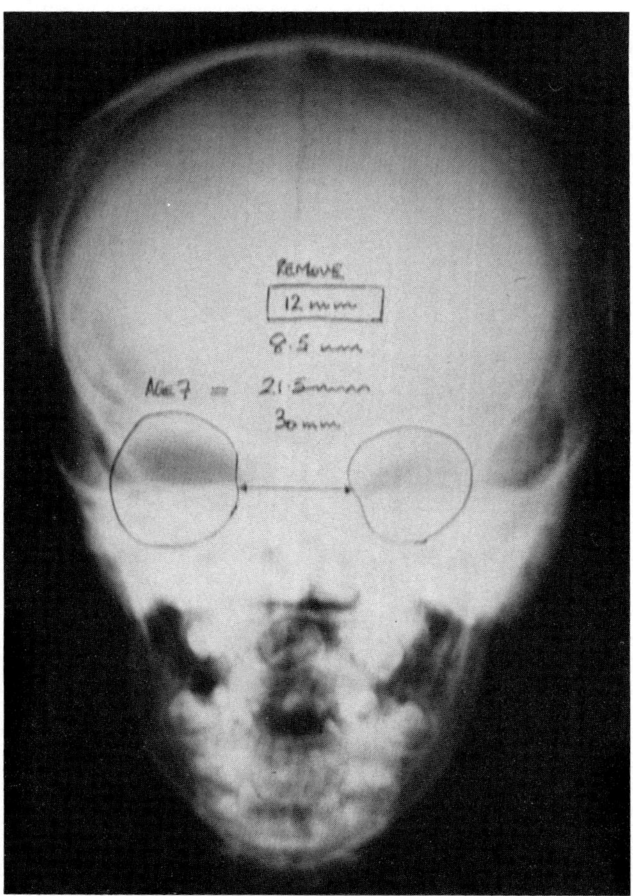

Fig. 28-3. Posteroanterior face radiograph (2 m) allows calculation of excessive interorbital width.

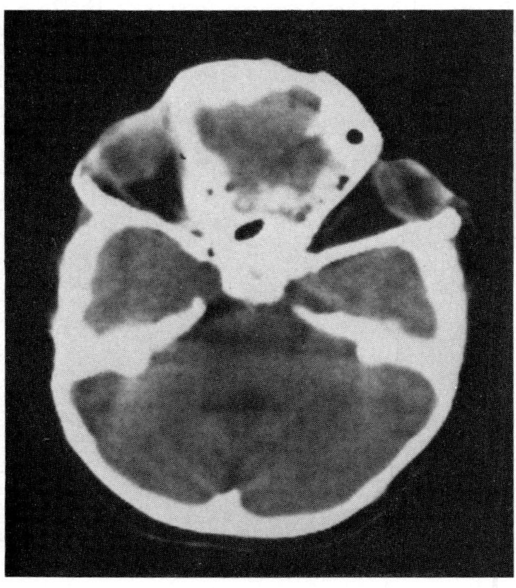

Fig. 28-4. Axial CT scan of hypertelorism.

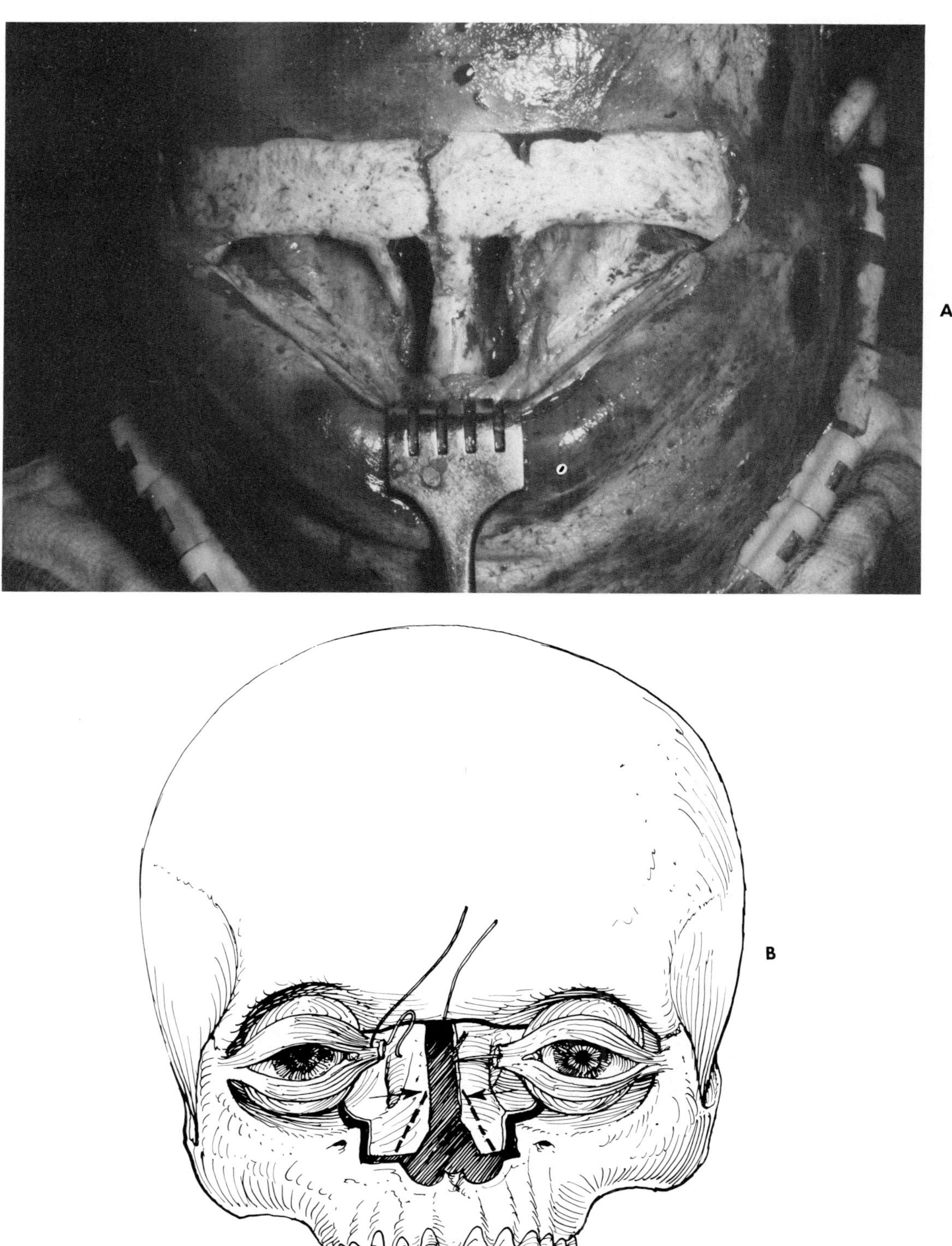

Fig. 28-5. Subcranial hypertelorism correction. **A,** Segments of nasal bones and ethmoidal sinuses have been resected on either side of the nasal septum. **B,** Osteotomy lines. Note that the septum was resected in this case. *Continued.*

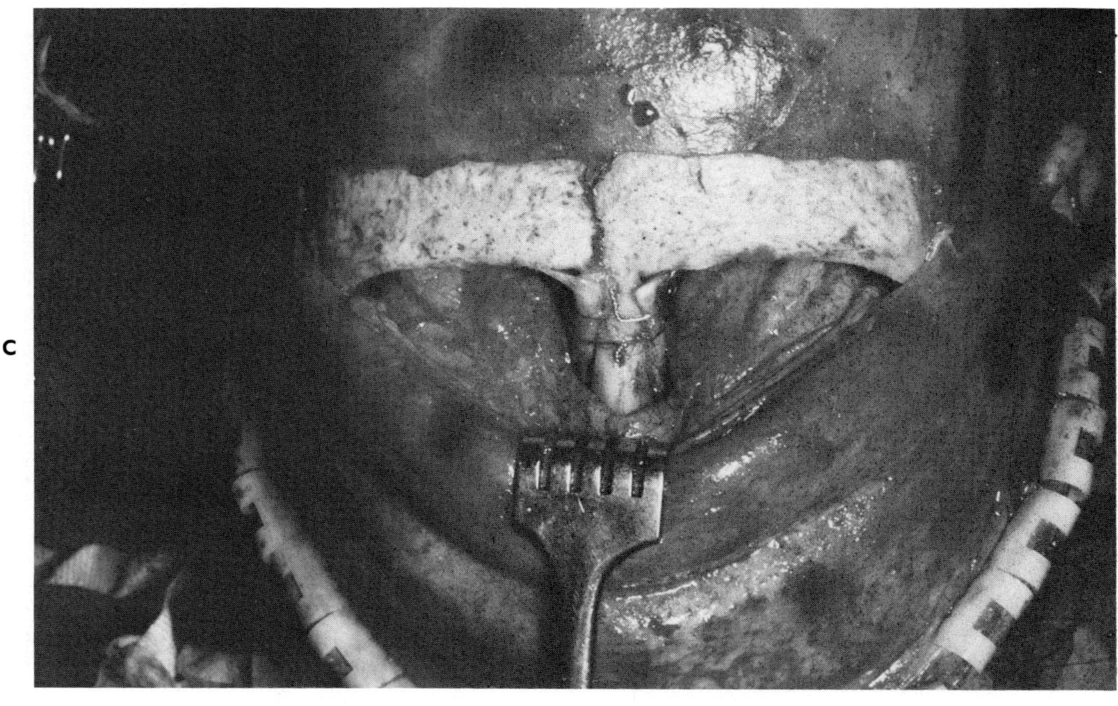

C

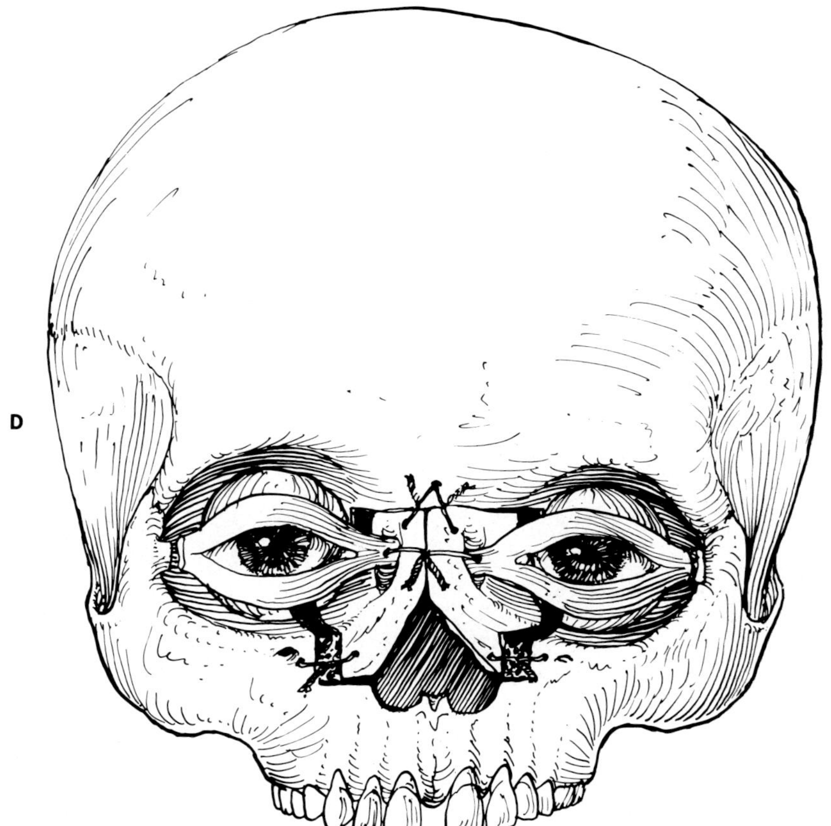

D

Fig. 28-5, cont'd. C, Medial orbital walls moved together. **D,** Interosseous wiring, canthal ligament positioning, and bone grafting.

others.[1,11,12] It may be divided into the subcranial (or extracranial) and transcranial (or intracranial) approaches. The intracranial approach is indicated in moderate to severe cases, which are defined as any having an interorbital distance of more than 30 mm in a child, a cribriform plate that lies below the frontonasal suture, and the presence of an encephalocele. Mild cases, with an interorbital distance of 25 to 30 mm, can be handled by the subcranial approach. In children these measurements are not absolute, since the interorbital distance is 18 mm at 1 year and gradually increases to approximately 25 mm at ages 12 or 13.

The subcranial approach

As stated before, the subcranial approach (Fig. 28-5) is reserved for minor degrees of hypertelorism and telecanthus due to medial bony widening. Presence of the frontal sinus should be carefully noted. It is recommended that a degree of experience in correcting more severe hypertelorism be gained before embarking on this maneuver, since familiarity with the anatomy will obviate serious complications.

The surgical approach is by coronal incision. The dissection continues above the periosteum until a point 1 to 1.5 cm above the supraorbital rim; it then becomes subpericranial. The nasal skeleton is exposed, and the periosteum in the midline from the nasal bone area is divided vertically and the edges separated with scissors. This provides transverse periosteal relaxation and consequently better exposure. Lateral dissection reveals the lateral orbital rim and will eventually expose the zygomatic arch. The temporal muscle is left undisturbed. As the medial wall dissection is performed, the lacrimal sac is located and elevated to ensure effective protection during the osteotomy. The infraorbital rim is exposed medially, and the infraorbital nerve is visualized.

If, as is usual in these patients, the nasal bridge line is satisfactory, it is maintained in its original position, and segments of frontonasal bone on either side are planned to be resected. The amount to be removed can be that which would give an interorbital distance of 15 mm. Often, with experience, one aims for the narrowest bridge line that will be compatible with a stable medial orbital segment capable of medial movement. At the lower edge of the nasal bone, the nasal mucosa is separated from the bone, and, using a narrow periosteal elevator, it is dissected off the inner aspect of the nasal bones until the most superior aspect of the nasal cavity is reached. The planned amount of bone is removed with a drill or oscillating saw. At this point, the nasal mucosa is protected with a retractor. This maneuver unroofs the ethmoidal sinuses. Using bone rongeurs, the mucosa and bony septa of the sinuses are removed completely. The medial wall of the sinuses is carefully identified, since damage here may expose the dura and cause an associated dural tear (Fig. 28-5, *A* and *B*).

After studying the radiographs for a safe position and noting where the ethmoidal sinuses terminate cranially, a transverse cut is made in the glabellar area. It runs laterally until it reaches the supraorbital rim; a bone cut is then taken backward to the posterior portion of the junction of the medial wall and roof of the orbit.

Inferiorly from the level of the nasal floor, a cut is taken laterally below the infraorbital nerve and then vertically to the infraorbital rim. The relationship of this cut to the infraorbital nerve varies with the position of the nerve. A vertical cut is made with a small right-angled oscillating saw far back on the medial orbital wall; this cut joins the previously described superior and inferior osteotomies.

The orbital segments are now capable of being mobilized and will remain in single units if this mobilization is performed carefully. They are wired to one another and to the central nasal strut with two wires. It is unusual to be able to bone graft on the supraorbital rim. If there is a small defect, however, a portion of the outer table of the skull can be taken and wired in place. This is usually possible in the infraorbital rim. If enough bone is available in the resected specimen, this can be used as the graft; if not, cranial bone is used (Fig. 28-5, *C* and *D*). Should the medial canthal ligaments become detached, they must be reattached; this procedure will be described later.

Because of the small medial wall shift in these cases, the orbital volume is only slightly increased, and thus enophthalmos and lateral strain on the medial canthal ligaments are a consideration. A lateral orbital wall osteotomy is then performed. The temporal muscle is elevated from the lateral wall, and an intraorbital vertical osteotomy is made at the junction of the lateral wall and the temporal bone. Using a small right-angled oscillating saw, horizontal cuts are made cranially and caudally at the extreme limits of the wall. It is now moved medially by the desired amount, being wired at the supraorbital and infraorbital rims. The temporal fascia is scored vertically, allowing the muscle to be moved into the defect resulting from the bone shift. The coronal incision is closed with suction drain, and a standard head dressing is applied (Fig. 28-6).

The transcranial approach

The transcranial approach (Fig. 28-7) is employed in moderate and severe degrees of hypertelorism. Through small transverse incisions in the medial canthal area, the medial canthal ligaments are dissected out and tagged with black silk (Fig. 28-7, *A*). This allows for easier identification later in the procedure. The main approach uses a coronal incision. Periosteal elevation is extensive over the zygoma, upper maxilla, and piriform fossa. The temporal muscles are elevated to expose the lateral orbital wall and the anterior part of temporal fossa. An attempt is made to leave the medial and lateral canthal ligaments undisturbed. When there is severe nasal deformity, a midline nasal incision may be employed; however, this should be used with care and always incorporated into an overall plan for nasal recon-

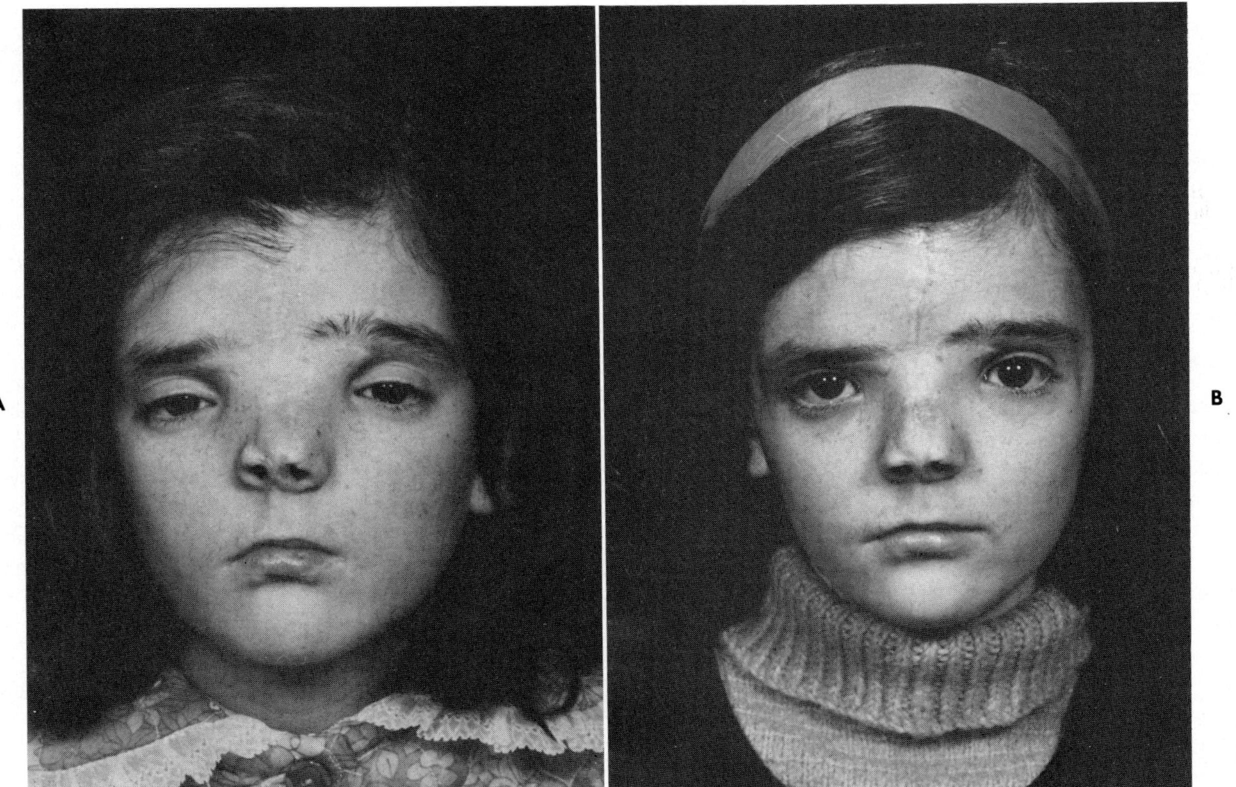

Fig. 28-6. A, Preoperative appearance. **B,** Postoperative result of subcranial hypertelorism correction.

struction. Skin should not be sacrificed until there is absolute certainty that it will not be required, either during this procedure or in the future. A midline vertical forehead incision is unnecessary and should be avoided. The skin of the nose is elevated down to the tip; this is easier if a nasal skin incision has been made. In many of these cases, the nasal bridge line is poor, and thus a total block resection of midline structures is planned. A distance of 15 mm or less is the goal. The nasal mucosa is extensively elevated as described earlier and protected with a retractor as the vertical cuts are made in the nasal area (Fig. 28-7, *B*).

The orbital osteotomy cuts are outlined. These are vertical in the nasal region down to the rim of the piriform aperture and transverse or horizontal in the maxilla from the nasal floor under the infraorbital nerve. At approximately 1 to 1.5 mm above the supraorbital rim, a horizontal line is drawn into the upper portion of the temporal fossa. The lateral osteotomy plane angles anteriorly and downward to where the lateral orbital wall joins the temporal bone; it then runs vertically downward to the inferior orbital fissure. A vertical cut through the anterior zygomaticomalar area will join with the horizontal line on the anterior maxilla. A frontal bone flap is planned in such a way as to leave a 15 mm bar of bone intact above the orbital osteotomy. Plans for vertical

shift of one orbit if there is dystopia are now outlined on the frontal bar, indicating the amount of bone to be excised. If there is to be forehead remodeling, the reconstructive plan is formulated at this time (Fig. 28-7, *C* to *E*).

A standard frontal bone flap is elevated and removed by the neurosurgeon. The anesthesiologist relieves any brain tightness by controlled CSF drainage and intravenous administration of mannitol; the brain is elevated from the anterior cranial fossa. The medial extent of this elevation is the lateral border of the cribriform plate; to proceed beyond this area invites an inevitable dural tear. Posteriorly the frontal lobe is elevated to the edge of the sphenoid wing. Cuts are made in the roofs of the ethmoidal sinuses. The amount of bone to be removed is the same as that to be removed from the corresponding frontonasal area. From the posterior limit of the ethmoidal sinuses, with the orbital contents protected, a transverse osteotomy is made in the orbital roof, ending in the temporal area (Fig. 28-7, *F*). This is now angled forward to the lateral orbital wall. It may be necessary to slip a metal strip retractor under the sphenoid wing to protect the temporal lobe. The vertical cut in the lateral orbital wall is made just anterior to its junction with the temporal bone and continues down to the inferior orbital fissure (Fig. 28-7, *G*). With a retractor in the orbit,

Text continued on p. 479.

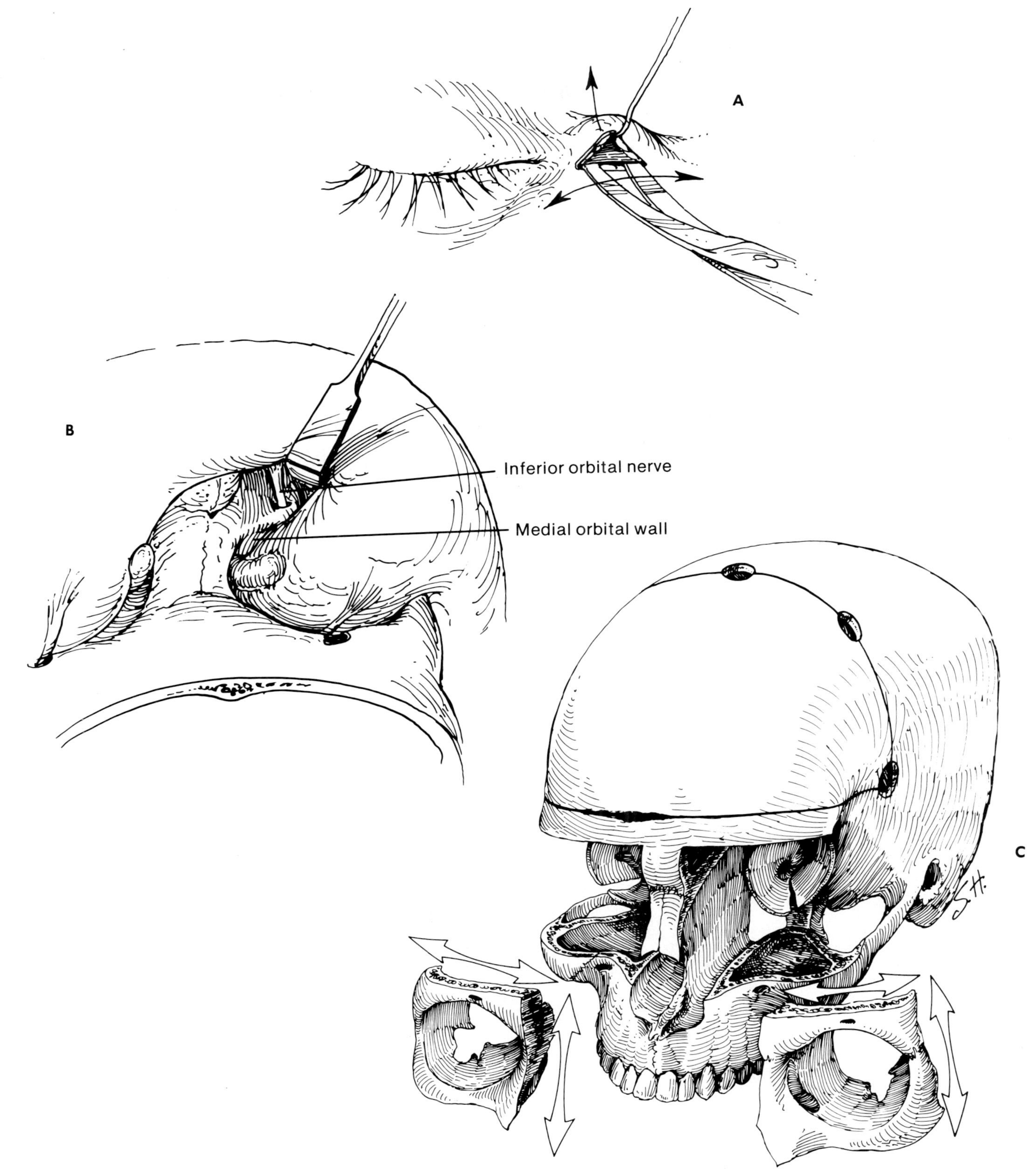

Fig. 28-7. Transcranial hypertelorism correction. **A,** Dissection of medial canthal ligaments. **B,** Extent of dissection. **C,** Cuts that will be made around and within the orbits to allow three-dimensional movements.

Continued.

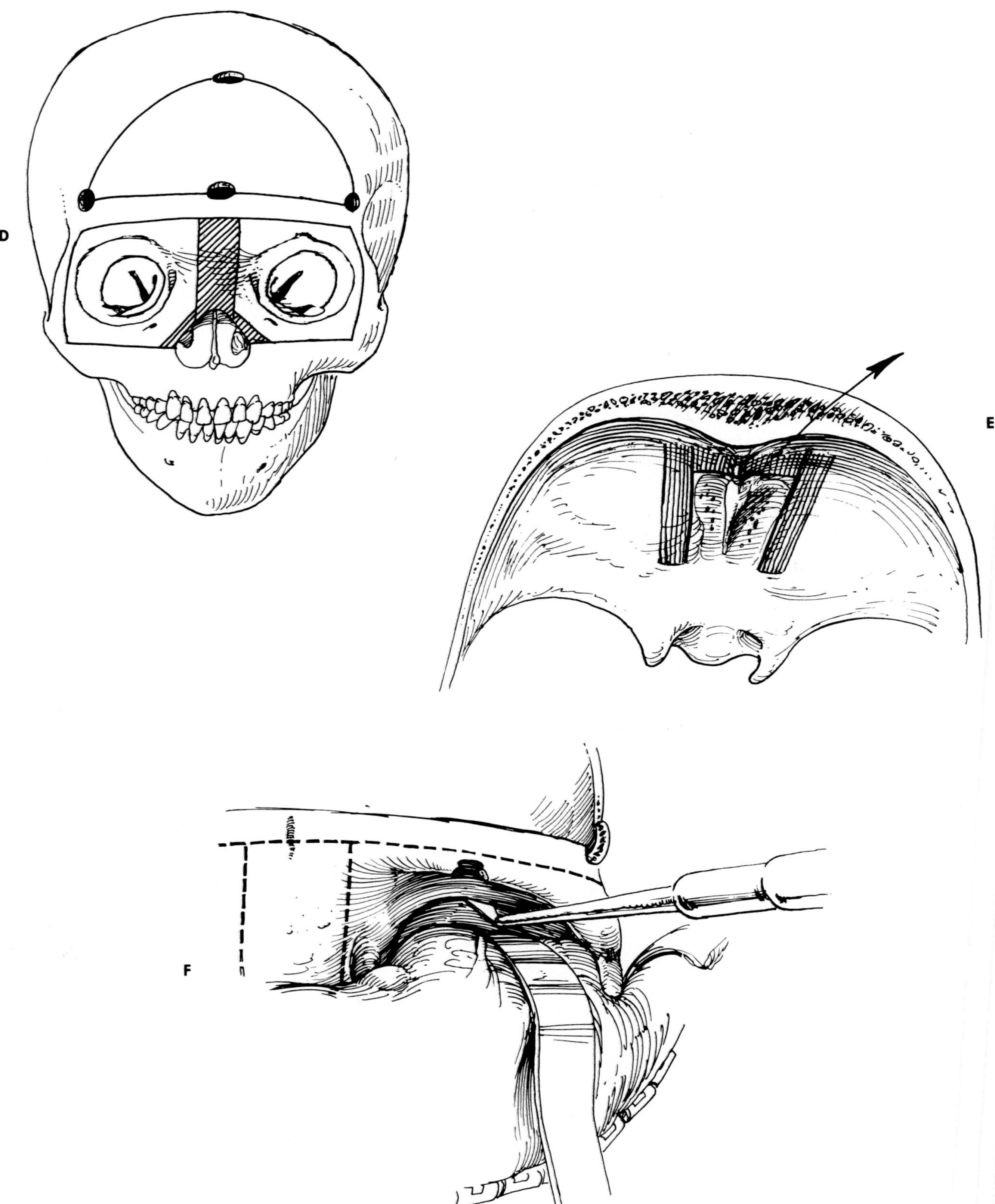

Fig. 28-7, cont'd. D, Shaded areas represent bone to be excised extracranially. **E,** Shaded areas represent bone to be excised intracranially. **F,** Osteotomy of the orbital floor.

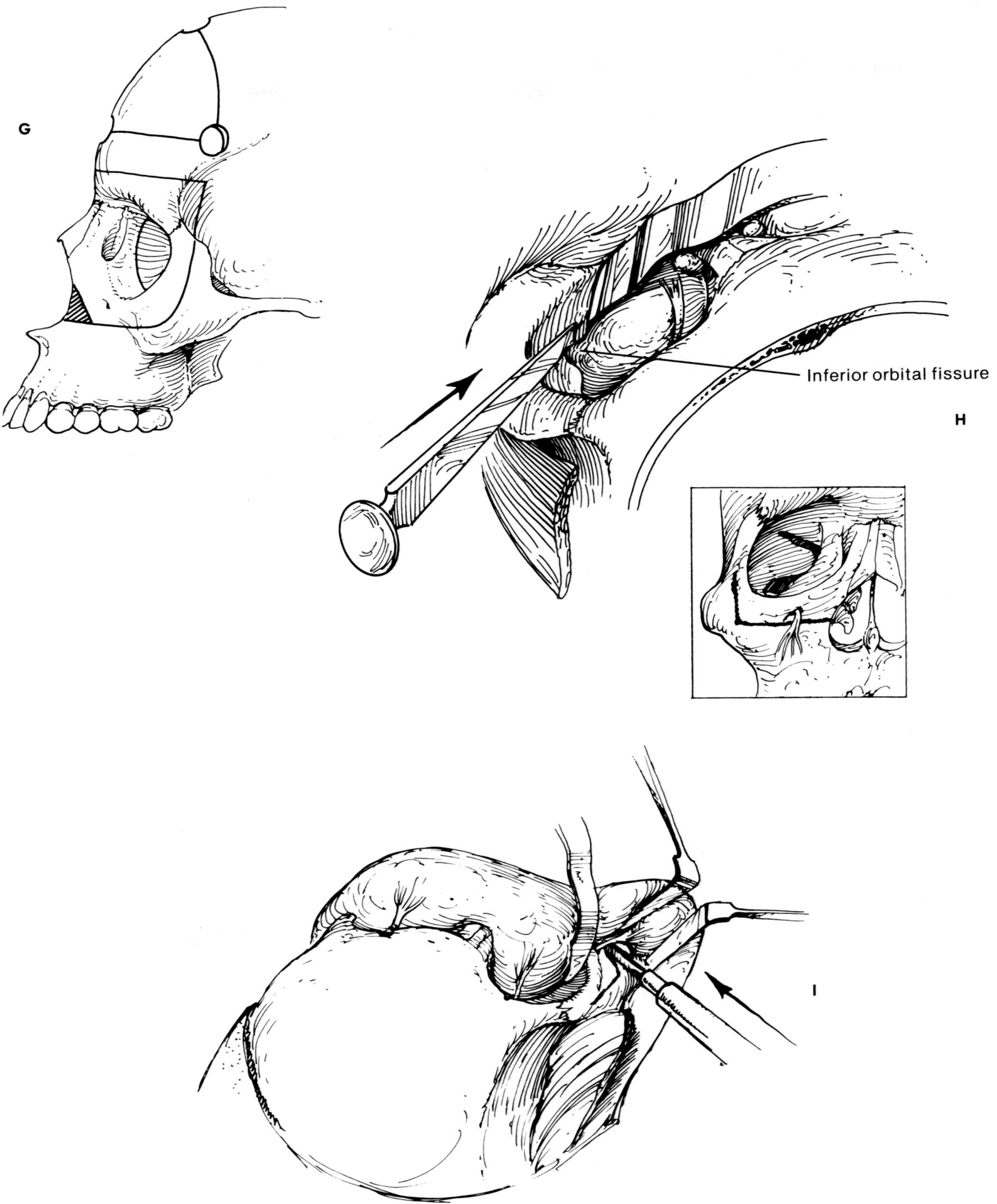

Fig. 28-7, cont'd. G, Osteotomy of the lateral orbital wall and malar region. **H,** Osteotomy of the orbital floor. **I,** Infraorbital osteotomy.

Continued.

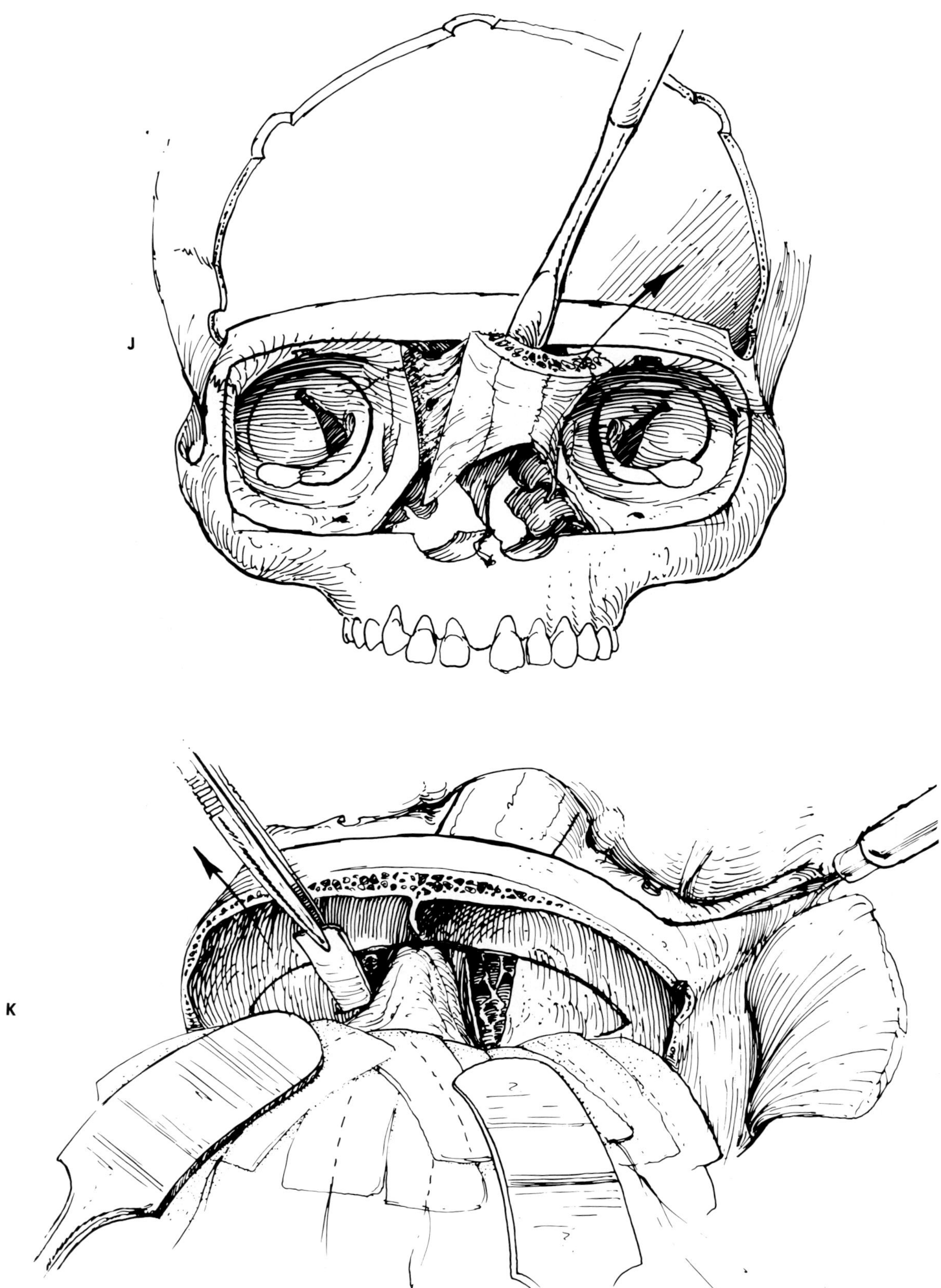

Fig. 28-7, cont'd. J, Removal of the central bone block. **K,** Removal of the roof of the ethmoidal sinuses.

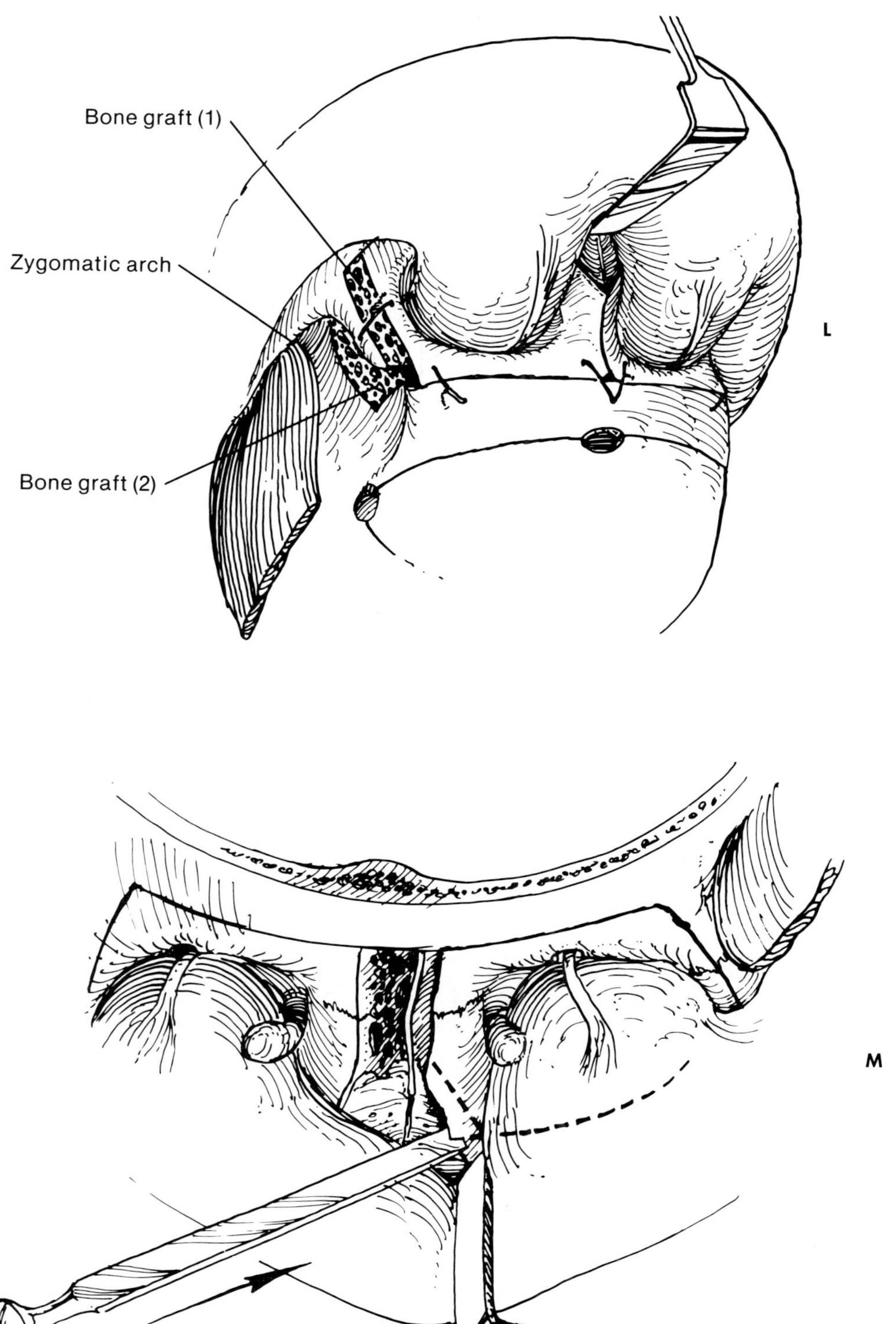

Fig. 28-7, cont'd. L, Placement of bone grafts after the medial orbit shift. **M,** The dotted line illustrates bone to be removed to enlarge the piriform aperture. *Continued.*

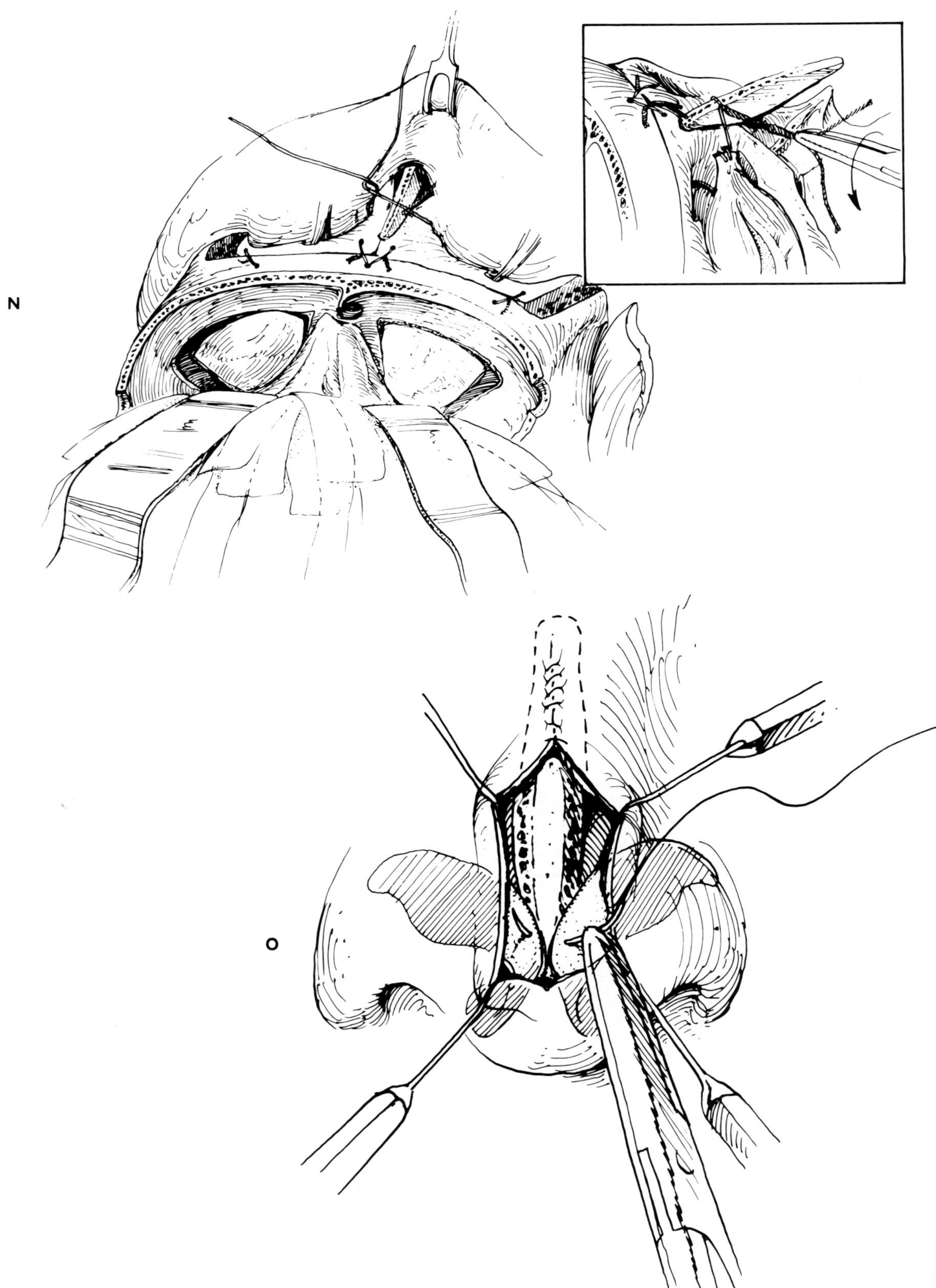

Fig. 28-7, cont'd. N, The orbits have been moved medially and a bone graft inserted *(inset)* to build up the nasal bridge line. **O,** Suturing of the lower lateral nasal cartilages.

the floor is cut across as far posteriorly as possible, taking care to not sever the infraorbital nerve as it lies in its canal just under the orbital floor (Fig. 28-7, *G* and *H*). A vertical cut is made in the malar area and angled horizontally toward the piriform fossa. It will lie below the infraorbital nerve foramen. This cut is best made with a rotating drill or reciprocating saw, the tissues being protected with an Aufricht nasal retractor (Fig. 28-7, *I*).

The lower edge of the frontal bar is cut through from the upper part of the temporal osteotomy. The vertical cuts are completed in the frontonasal area. To complete the intraorbital osteotomy, medial wall vertical cuts are made far back in the orbit, protecting the medial canthal ligaments and lacrimal apparatus.

Using bone rongeurs and protecting the nasal mucosa, the central frontonasal block is removed together with the cartilaginous septum and vomer. The septal mucosa should be maintained intact. Particular care is taken high in the nose to prevent damage to the cribriform plate (Fig. 28-7, *J*). Intracranially, the ethmoidal sinuses are unroofed, and, working from above and below, the sinus contents are totally removed (Fig. 28-7, *K*). If one orbit is to be raised in relation to the other, bone may now be removed from the frontal bar to allow for this. The orbits are mobilized. An osteotome can assist mobilization high in the lateral orbital wall area and medially at the edge of the piriform aperture.

The orbits are stabilized in the midline with a wire from the frontal bar through the medial parts of both orbits. There is further stabilization onto the supraorbital bar. Bone grafts from the skull or iliac crest are inserted into the lateral wall defects and wired securely (Fig. 28-7, *L*). Large defects in the orbital walls or floor may be bone grafted; this is rarely necessary, however.

Enlargement of the piriform aperture is achieved by removal of bone from the medial edge of the advanced orbits (Fig. 28-7, *M*). A bone graft is constructed from a rib, iliac crest, or skull; inserted into a prefashioned hole in the glabellar area; and wired onto the newly created nasal bone area (Fig. 28-7, *N*). Depending on the nasal deformity, the lower lateral cartliages may be sutured together above or below the tip of the bone graft (Fig. 28-7, *O*).

Management of the medial canthal ligament

Management of the medial canthal ligament is so important as to be considered separately. On some occasions, it is preserved in its original attached position and no separate maneuver is necessary.

If the medial orbital wall is well developed, the ligament can be wired directly to the wall *before* the orbits are moved together. On movement of the orbits, the medial canthus lies in the correct position.

If the medial wall is thin, repositioning of the canthus is done after the orbits have been stabilized in their new position. Two drill holes are made from the thickest portion of the midline bone down to where the ligament is to be inserted. In this area a small portion of bone can be removed to allow satisfactory seating of the medial canthal ligament. The ligament is identified by the black thread previously

Text continued on p. 485.

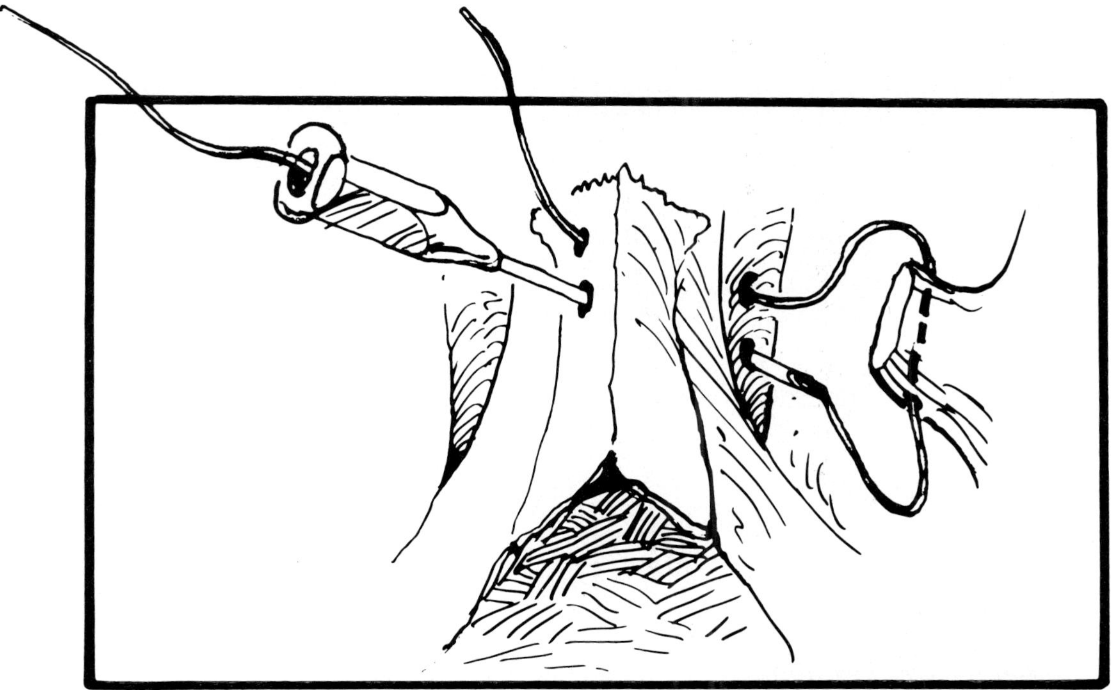

Fig. 28-8. Suggested method of medial canthal ligament fixation (there are other alternatives).

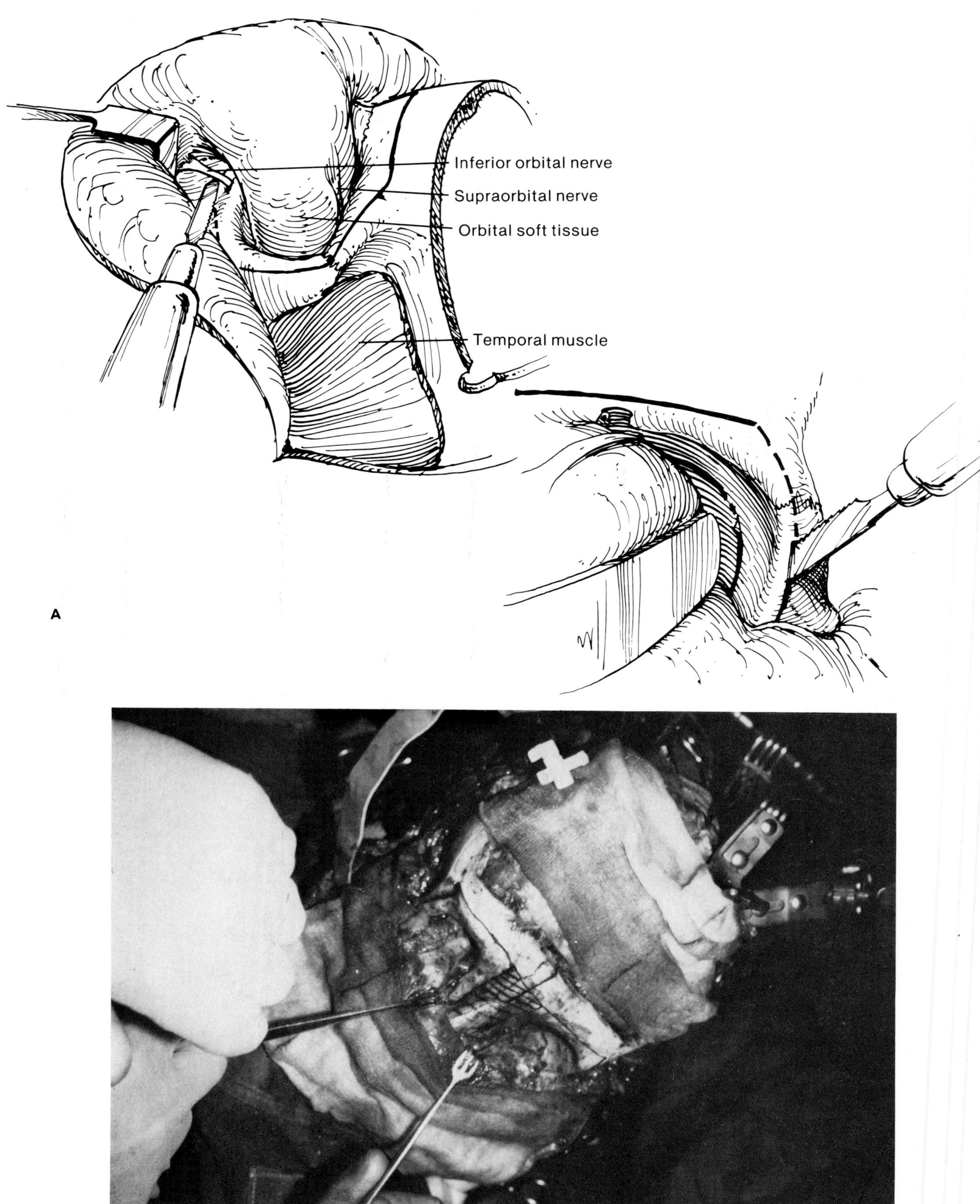

Fig. 28-9. A, Plan for sagittal split of the lateral orbital wall.

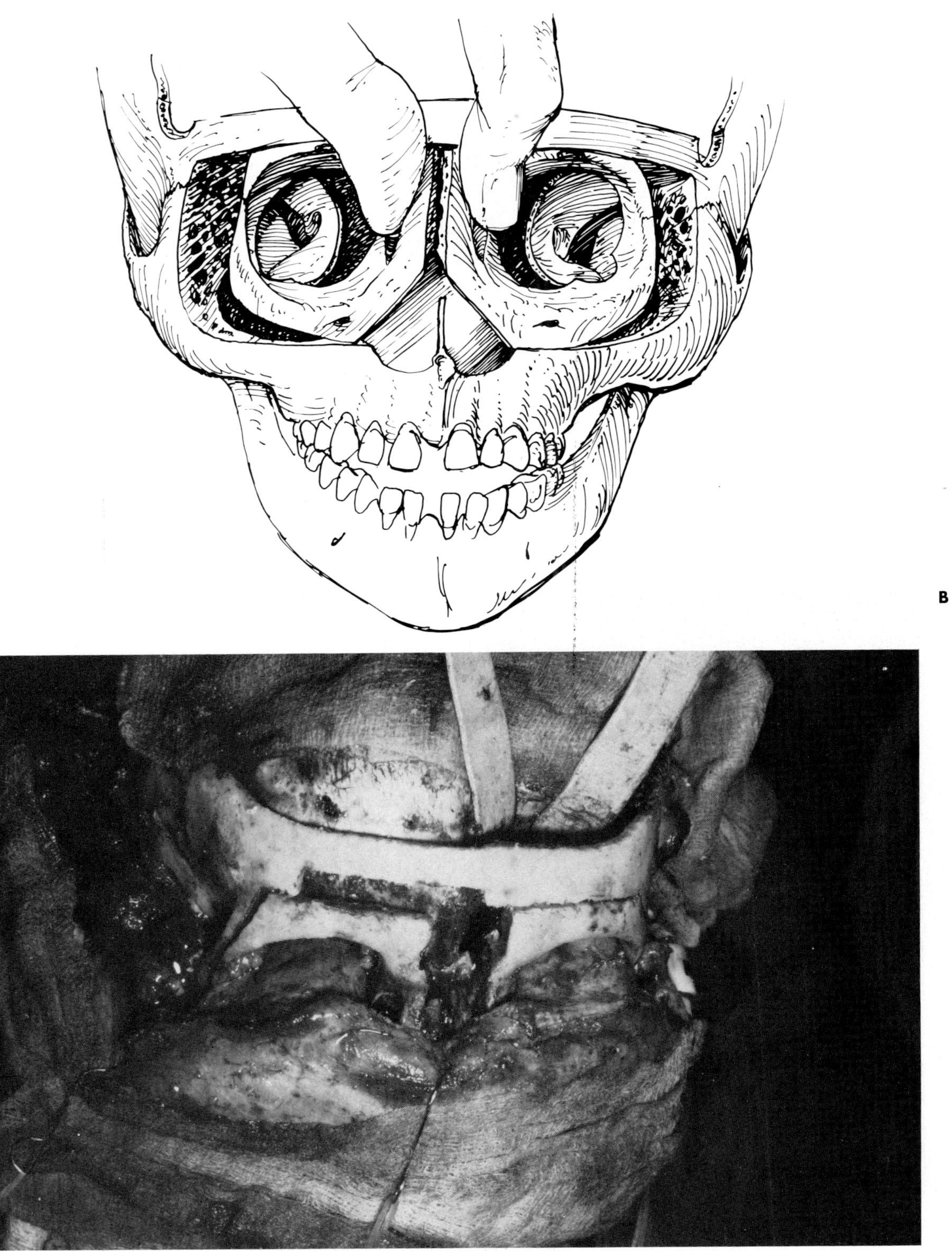

Fig. 28-9, cont'd. B, Medial shift of the orbits after sagittal split of the lateral orbital walls.

Continued.

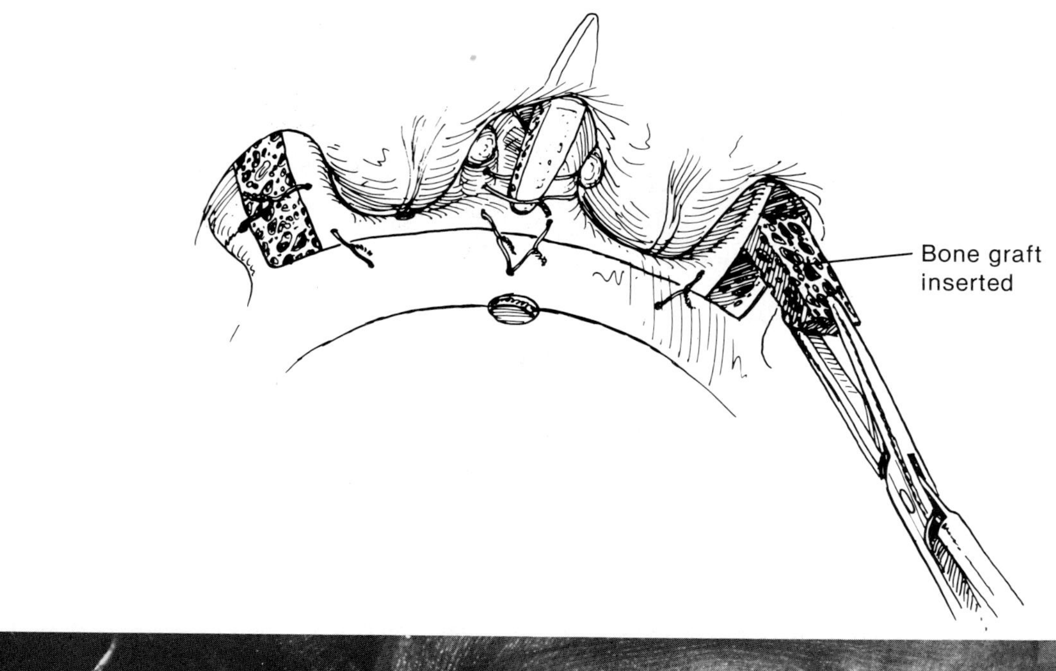

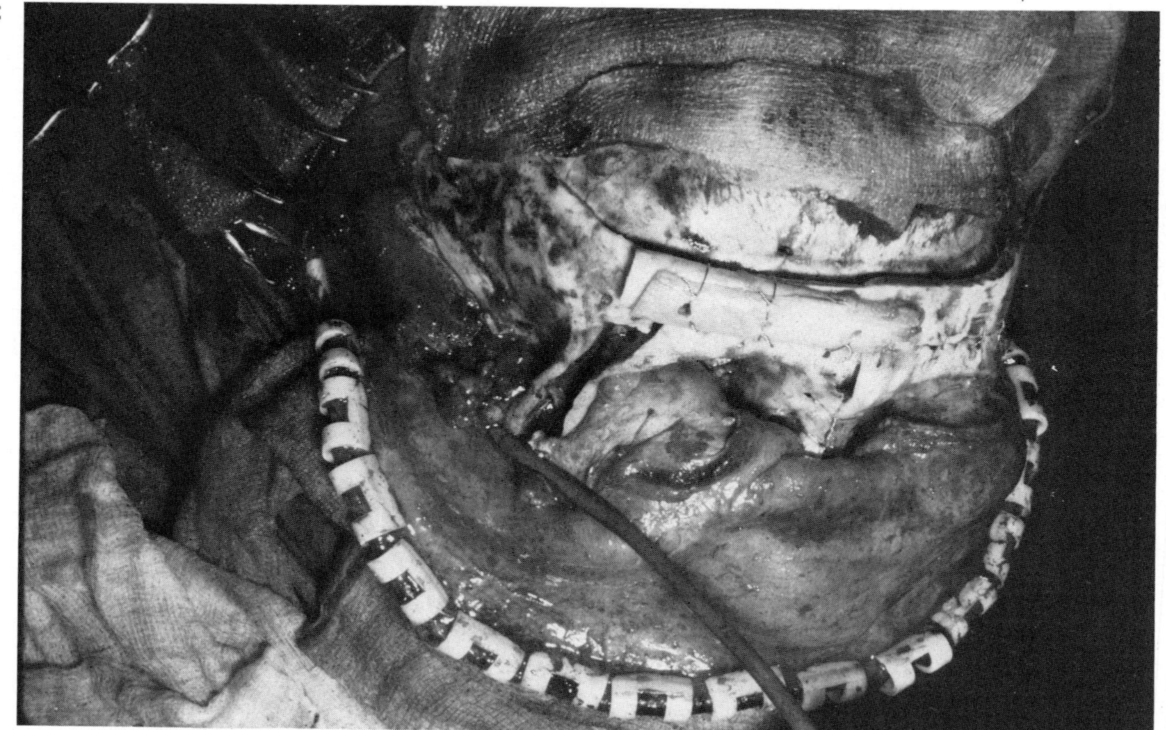

Fig. 28-9, cont'd. C, Placement of bone graft after medial shift of the orbits.

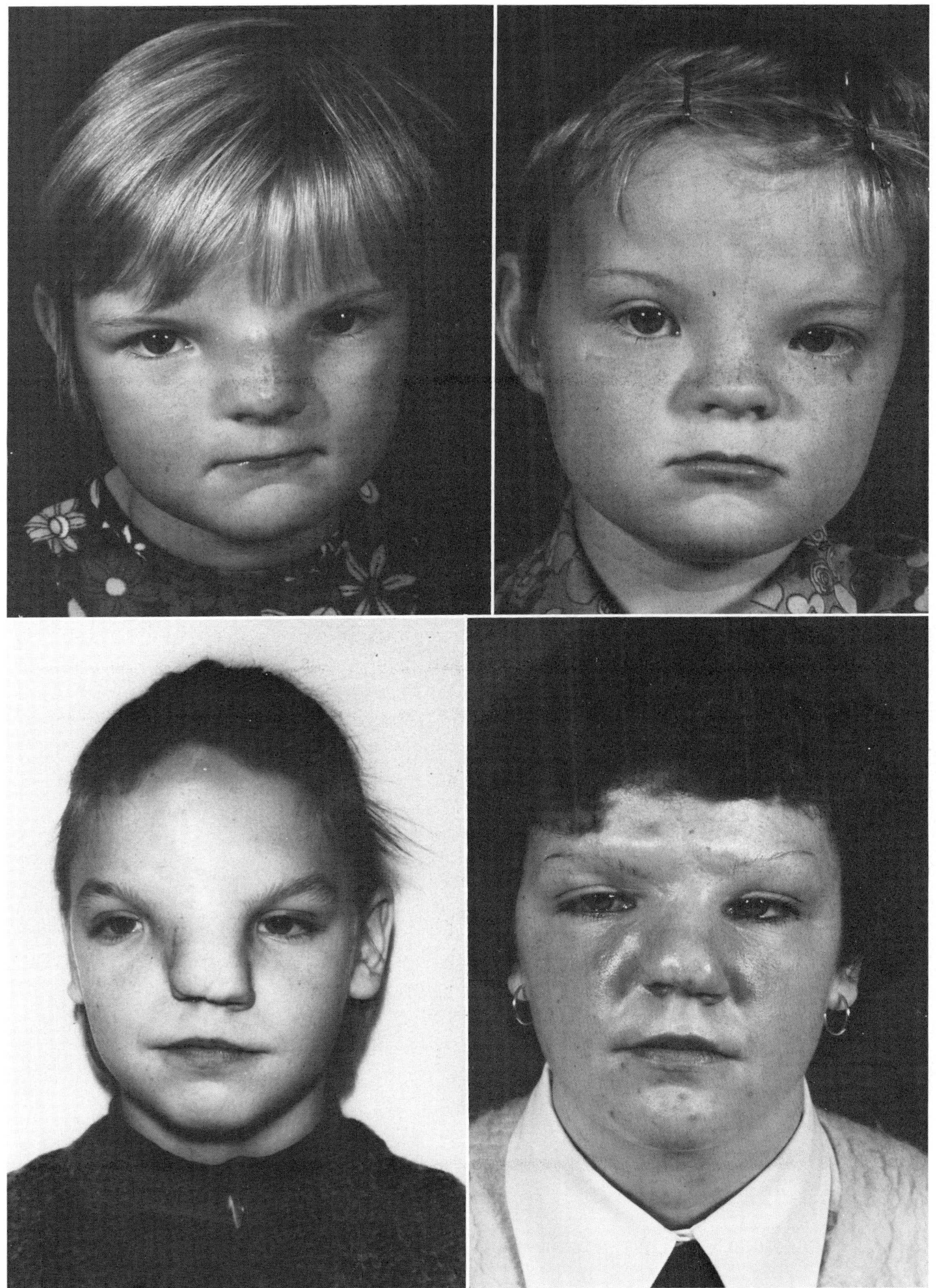

Fig. 28-10. Preoperative and postoperative results of hypertelorism correction.
Continued.

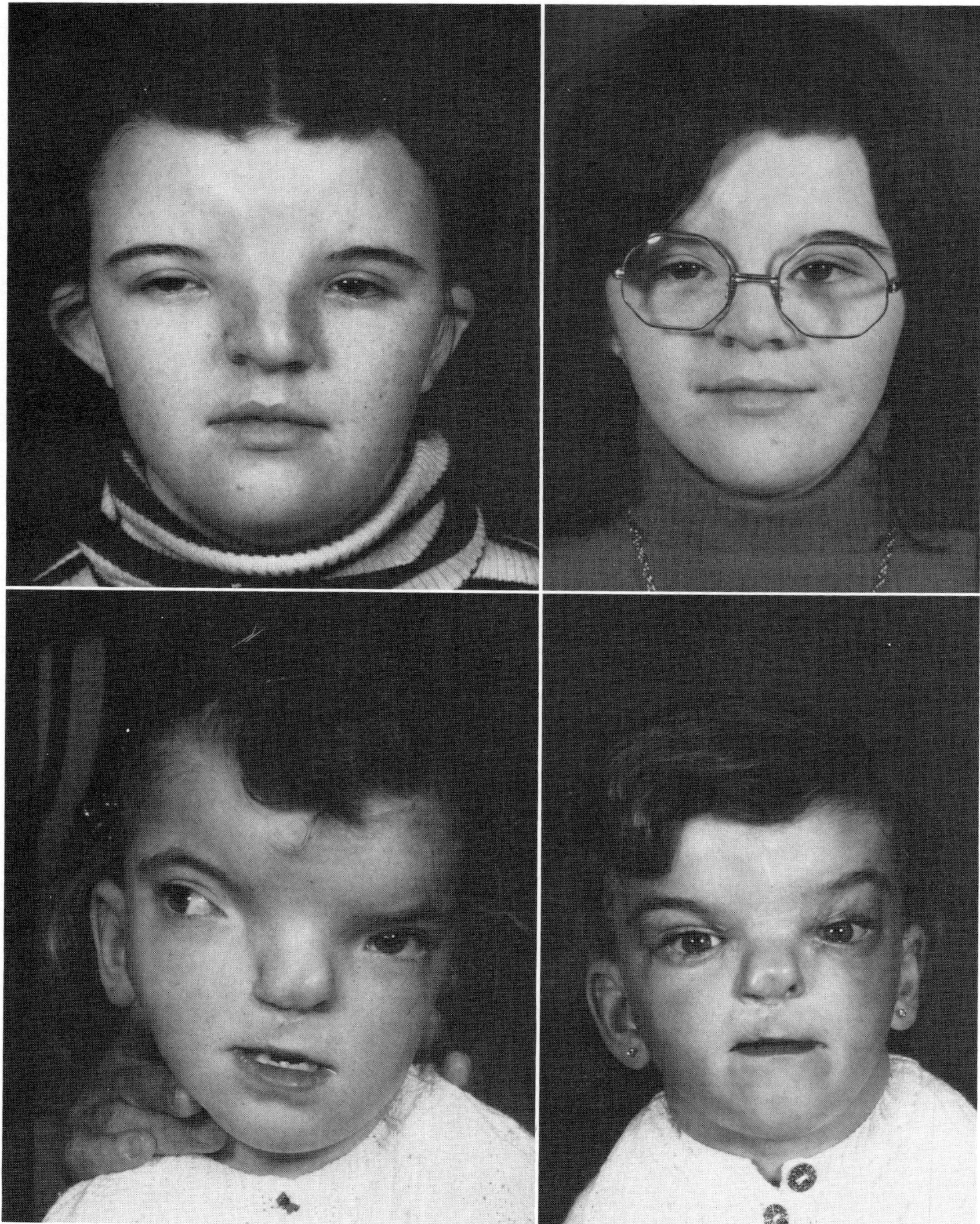

Fig. 28-10, cont'd. Preoperative and postoperative results of hypertelorism correction.

inserted. A wire is passed twice through the ligament and its security tested. A wide-bore hypodermic needle is introduced through the drill holes from above, and the wire is passed throught the needle. When the needle is withdrawn, the wire is in position. This is repeated for the other end. The canthus is firmly positioned as the wire is tightened onto the thick bone chosen for the drill hole site. This procedure is repeated on the other side (Fig. 28-8).

Frontal recontouring is done using the previous frontal bone. If this is not suitable and bony reconstruction is necessary, a portion of skull from elsewhere is used.[4] If onlay bone grafting of the maxilla is necessary, it is performed using iliac crest or split-skull bone grafts. The latter are performed, since they resorb less.

The temporal muscle is advanced and carefully sutured to drill holes in the lateral orbital rim. If they have been detached, the lateral canthal ligaments are repositioned by wiring through drill holes at the 10 or 11 o'clock position on the right orbit and the 1 or 2 o'clock position on the left orbit.

The pericranium is reapplied to the frontal area, bilateral suction drains are inserted from one temporal area to the other, and the scalp is closed with a running monofilament nonabsorbable suture. The head is dressed with gauze and elastic bandages and soft tape. The eyes are left uncovered, and vision is checked as soon as possible after completion of the procedure. In some centers, ice packs are applied; in others, the eyes are covered. Experience suggests that children prefer to have their eyes uncovered.

Sagittal split of lateral orbital walls

Sagittal split of the lateral orbital walls (Figs. 28-9 and 28-10) is usually reserved for the less severe degrees of hypertelorism. This judgment requires clinical evaluation rather than hard quantitative values. The osteotomy is essentially similar to that described in the previous discussions, apart from the management of the lateral wall. The transverse supraorbital osteotomy ends at a point above the midline of the lateral orbital rim. Using an oscillating saw, a vertical cut is made through the lateral orbital wall down to the malar bone and extending posteriorly to the full depth of the wall; this is the sagittal osteotomy (Fig. 28-9, *A*). With the orbital contents retracted, a vertical cut is made far back on the inner aspect of the lateral orbital wall to join the sagittal osteotomy. When the periorbital osteotomy has been completed, it is possible to perform a sagittal split of the wall using an osteotome. This allows medial shift of the orbits (Fig. 28-9, *B*). A block of bone can be introduced into the lateral wall defect and is wired securely in place (Fig. 28-9, *C*).

OSTEOTOMIES
The C-osteotomy

In very young children in whom the tooth buds are high in the maxilla, it is not possible to cut across the maxilla.

To obviate this problem, the supraorbital cut is performed in the standard fashion, as are the medial and lateral vertical cuts. The latter stop at the level of the orbital floor and are then taken anteriorly through the lateral orbital wall, transversing the lateral orbital margin. The standard intraorbital cut in the medial wall and roof is made, stopping short at the orbital floor. This is then brought anteriorly through the rim of the piriform aperture. The medial wall, roof, and lateral wall of the orbit form a C; this can be mobilized and moved medially (Fig. 28-11). The segments are wired medially as described earlier. Laterally they are wired to the superior and inferior orbital rims. Any contour defects are smoothed off or bone grafted as indicated.

Self-locking osteotomy

When there is a pure medial orbital movement in one plane, a self-locking osteotomy can be planned (Fig. 28-12). In the area of the skull above the lateral orbital wall, a Z-plasty is outlined. The width of the base of the Z is the amount that the orbit is to be moved medially. As the orbit is moved, the Z bone flaps are transposed and wired; the self-locking maneuver has been completed. The remainder of the stabilization is as described previously.

U-shaped osteotomy

As a variation of the extracranial approach in lesser degrees of hypertelorism with a high cribriform plate, the U-shaped osteotomy may be performed (Fig. 28-13). This has the merit of providing one solid portion of the orbit to move and eliminates some of the stabilizing difficulties imposed by working with small pieces of bone.

The approach is by the coronal flap. The central segment is excised as described previously, and the ethmoidal sinuses are removed subcranially. An anteroposterior bone cut is made in the medial orbital wall deep into the orbit. With the orbital contents retracted, a vertical cut is made in the medial wall down to the orbital floor, taking care not to injure the lacrimal apparatus. With the orbital contents retracted, a cut is made high in the lateral orbital wall, and this is taken deep into the orbit but is angled in such a way as to include a spur of temporal bone. A vertical cut is taken down into the inferior orbital fissure; it is then taken across the orbital floor to join the medial wall cut. A vertical cut is taken through the lateral orbital wall onto the malar area and then horizontally across the maxilla below the infraorbital nerve. The orbits can be mobilized and moved medially; The temporal bone spur provides an arrangement for self-locking on the superior part of the medial orbital wall. Bone grafts and wires provide stabilization; closure is as for all other hypertelorism corrections.

NASAL SURGERY

To produce a good nose in many cases of hypertelorism is extremely difficult. Basically the nose may be short or long. The short nose is associated with facial clefts 0 to 4

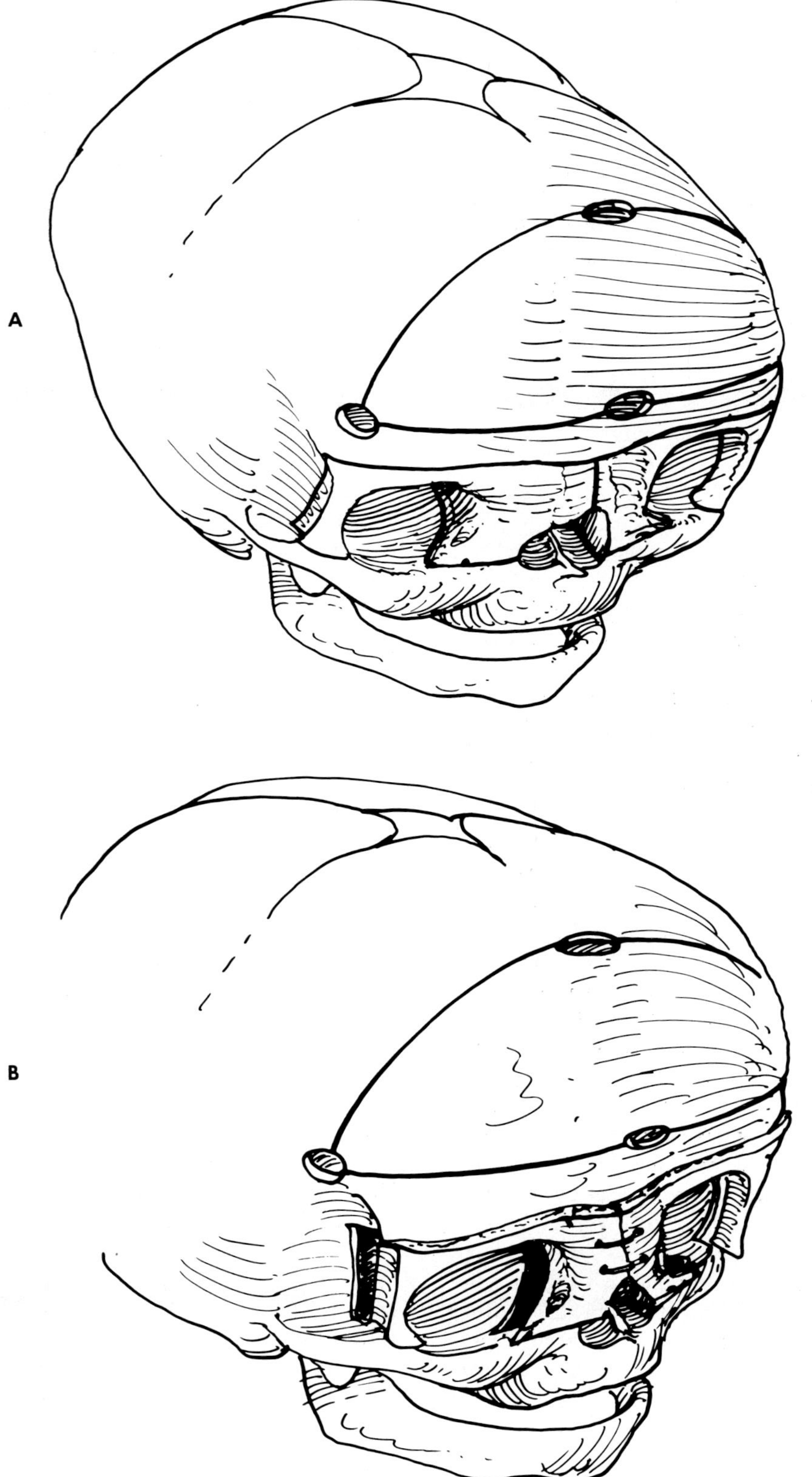

Fig. 28-11. A, Design of the C-shaped osteotomy. **B,** Osteotomy and wiring completed.

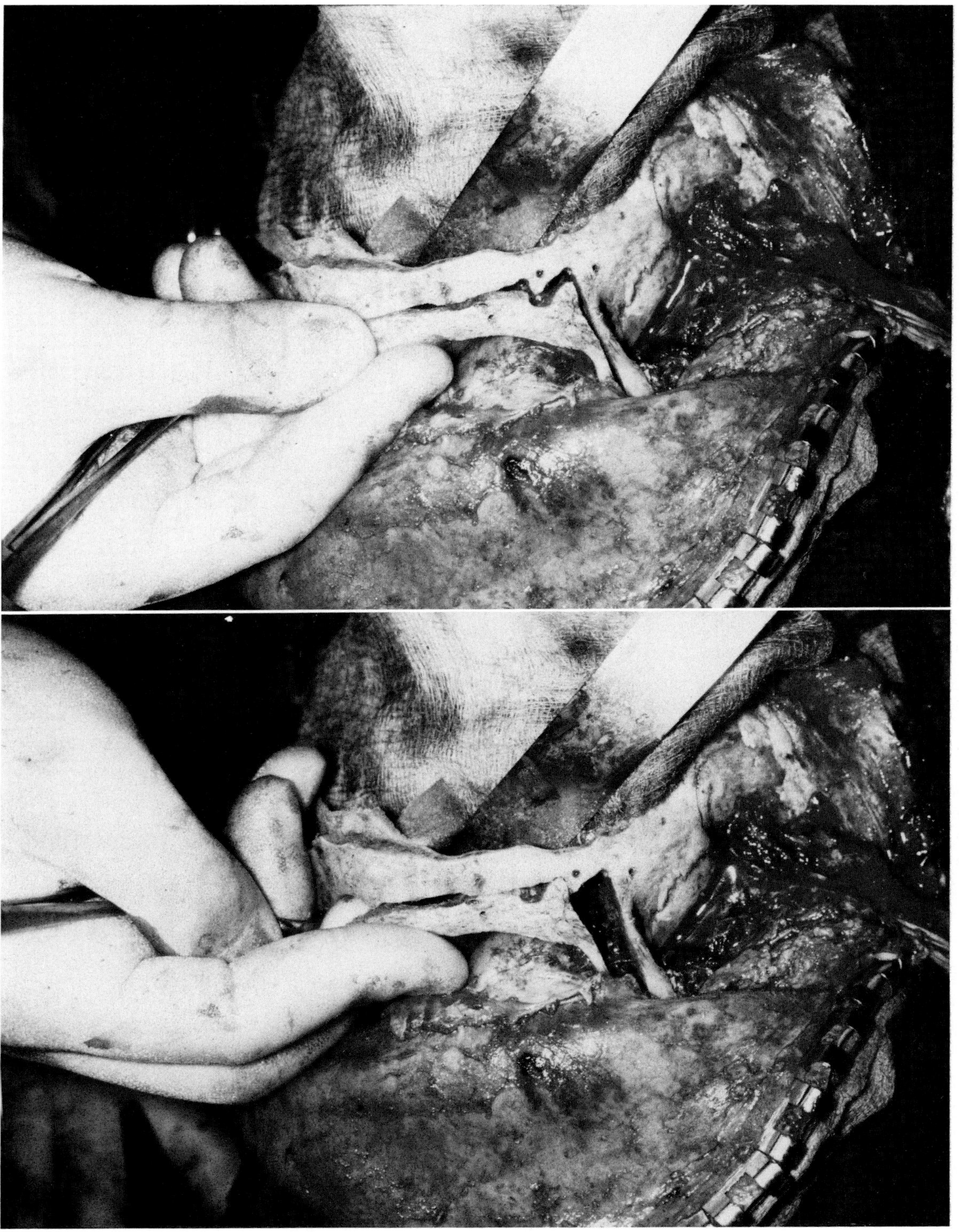

Fig. 28-12. Self-locking Z-osteotomy combined with sagittal split of the lateral orbital wall.

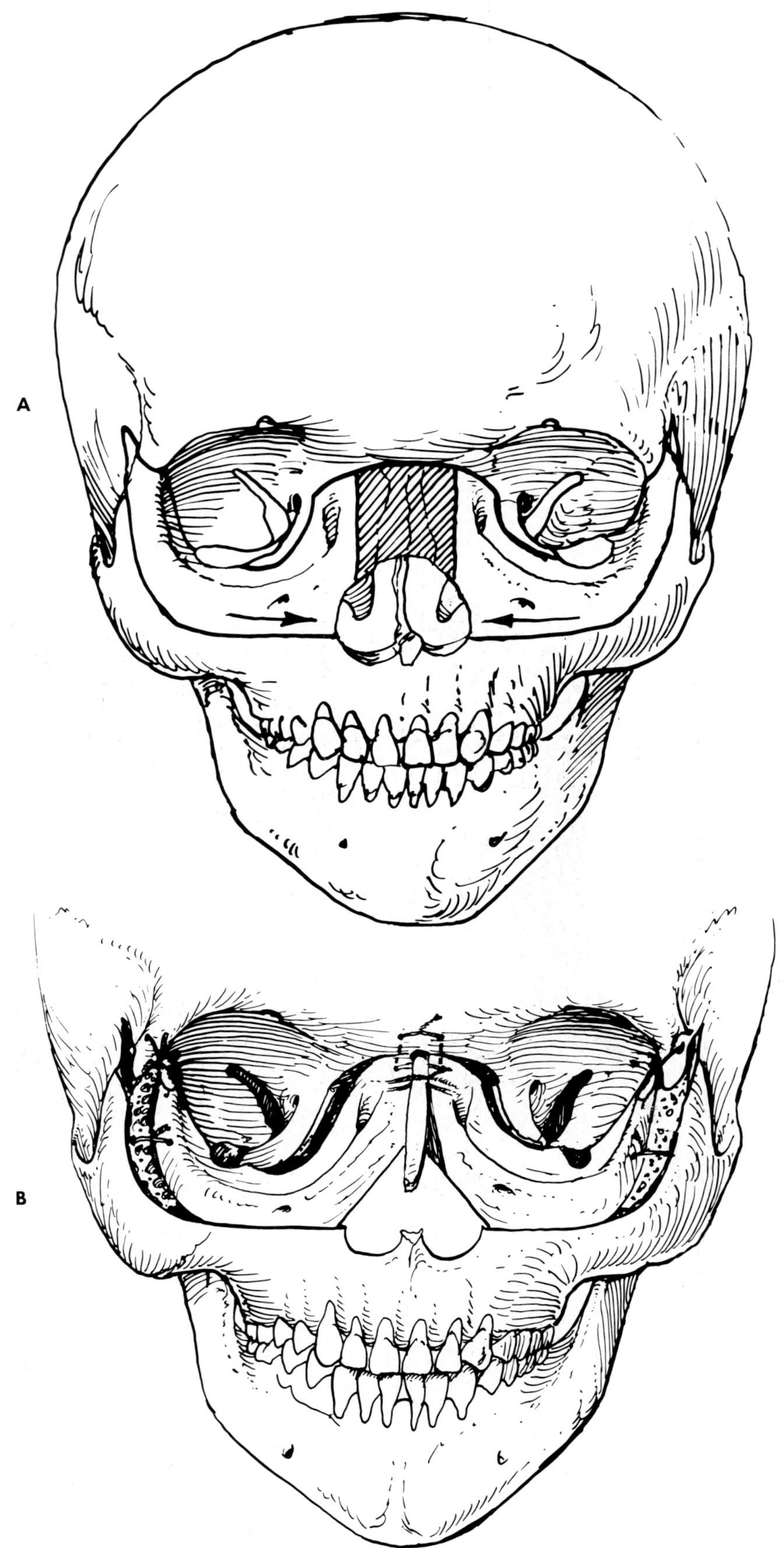

Fig. 28-13. A, Design of the U-shaped osteotomy. **B,** Osteotomy and wiring completed and bone grafts inserted.

and 11 to 14, according to the Tessier classification.[16] Consequently, it may be midline and symmetric or grossly asymmetric with considerable tissue shortage. The long nose is usually associated with a nasoencephalocele, and the term *long-nose hypertelorism* has been coined for this syndrome.[9,10]

Short nose

In addition to being short, the nose is broad; after correction of the hypertelorism, there is excess soft tissue present on the nasal dorsum. In lesser degrees of shortness, the excess may be removed as an ellipse; as this is closed, some lengthening will be achieved. The lengthening is increased

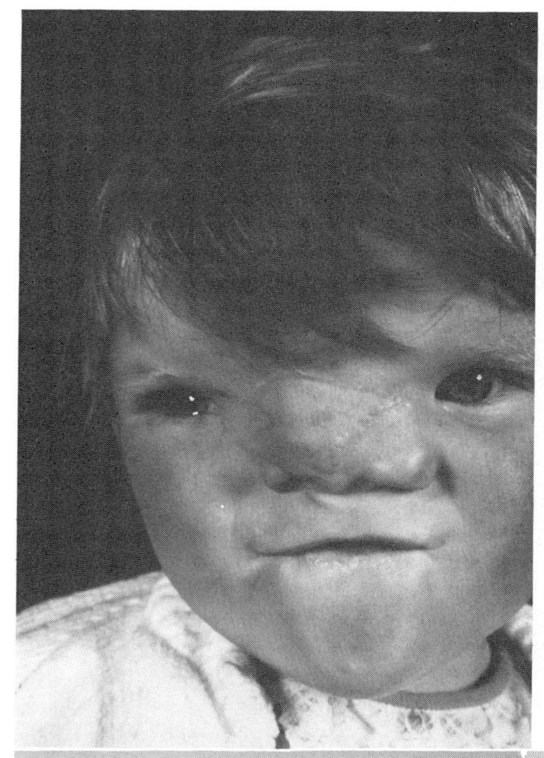

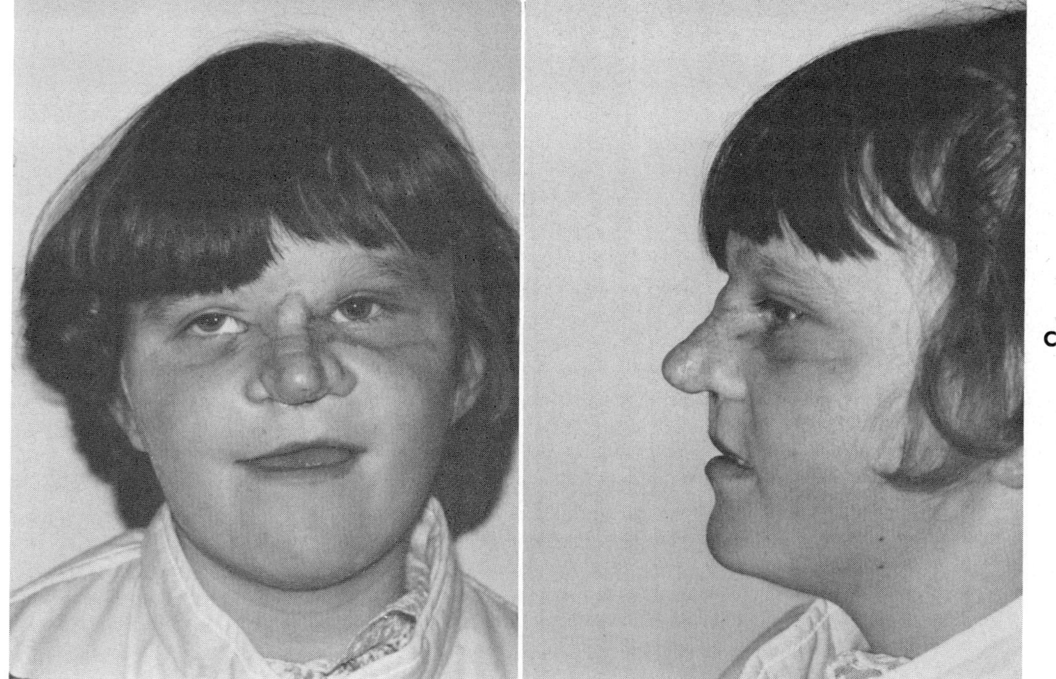

Fig. 28-14. A, Preoperative appearance. **B** and **C,** Postoperative results of correction of short-nose hypertelorism.

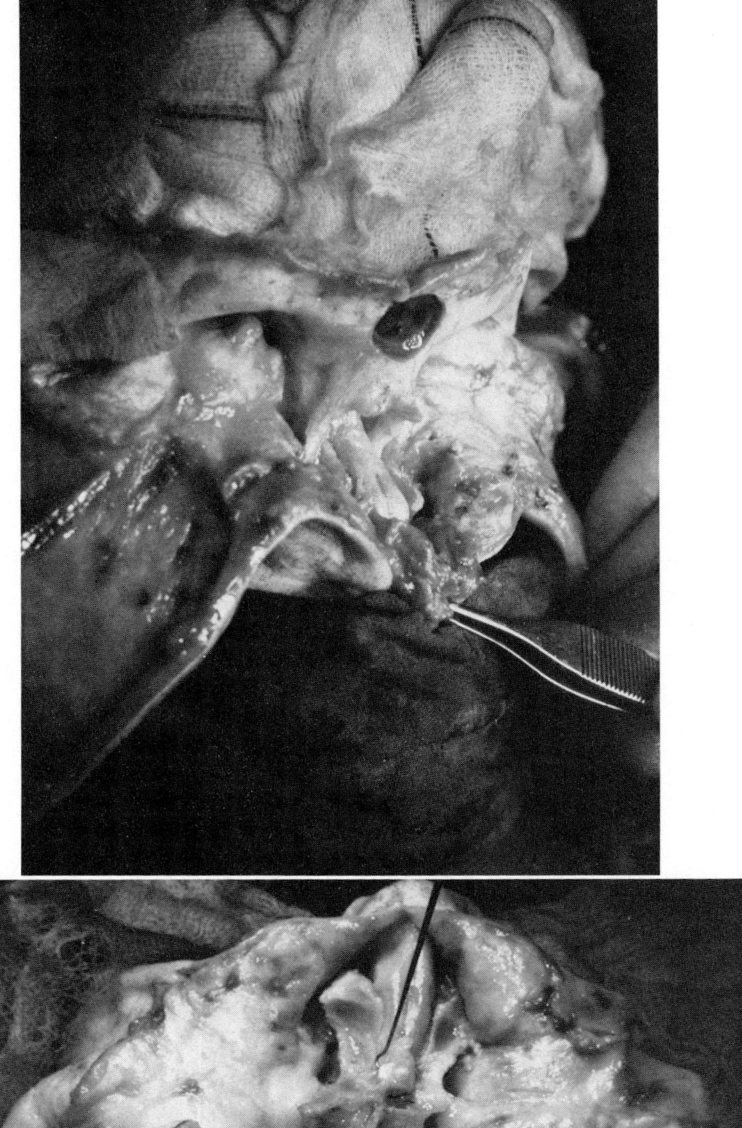

Fig. 28-15. A, Note low-lying position of nasal bones.

by incorporating a Z-plasty in the glabellar area. This has the additional beneficial effect of advancing the medial ends of the eyebrows and giving a further impression of facial narrowing.

In extremely short noses, especially when there is asymmetry, the excess skin should be preserved; this can be used as a transposition flap to lengthen one side of the nose. To achieve symmetric lengthening, the flap may be based inferiorly, and the upper end is caterpillared down to give a double-layered protrusion in the midnose region. This looks strange initially, but at a second stage the flap is unfolded and advanced toward the nasal tip, and considerable lengthening is thus obtained. Management of the skeleton has been discussed. The main support is by bone grafting, using either iliac crest, skull, or rib with chondral cartilage to give some nasal tip softness. The lower lateral cartilages are dissected out and may be sutured over the ends of the bone graft. Usually two or three procedures are necessary to achieve the optimal result. On long-term follow-up these reconstructed noses appear to grow fairly normally (Fig. 28-14).

Long-nose hypertelorism

As mentioned previously, long-nose hypertelorism is associated with a nasoencephalocele. There are two varieties of midline encephalocele, one of which is situated high on the nose (i.e., the glabellar area) and the other of which is lower on the nose. In the former, there is true hypertelorism with a short nose; in the latter, the nose is long with telecanthus but without true lateralization of the orbits. The medial extracranial and intracranial procedure allows adequate correction of the deformity, removal of the encephalocele, and protection of the low-lying dura. The telecanthus is corrected by repositioning of the medial orbital walls with an attached portion of the supraorbital and inferior orbital rims, as has already been described for subcranial correction of mild hypertelorism. The displaced central segment, which is composed of nasal skeleton, nasal septum, and cribriform plates, is mobilized and moved upward and forward into its correct position, being held there with wires and bone grafts (Fig. 28-15, *A* and *B*). Any frontal skull defects are reconstructed, and the scalp is closed in the standard fashion. The nasal skin is contoured to give the most acceptable result.[3] This usually involves tranverse skin excision in the superior area of the nose.

The remainder of the management is as has been described in standard hypertelorism correction (Fig. 28-15, *C* and *D*).

THE VAN DER MEULEN PROCEDURE

In some cases of hypertelorism, typically associated with midline clefting, a bifid nose, and midface retrusion, there is considerable vertical shortness of the maxilla in the midline. To overcome this, van der Meulen has introduced a modification of the standard procedure.[19] A midline wedge bony resection is performed from the anterior cranial fossa to a point between the incisor roots. A laterally based wedge is excised from the supraorbital area. The intraorbital osteotomy is standard, but the lateral osteotomy continues

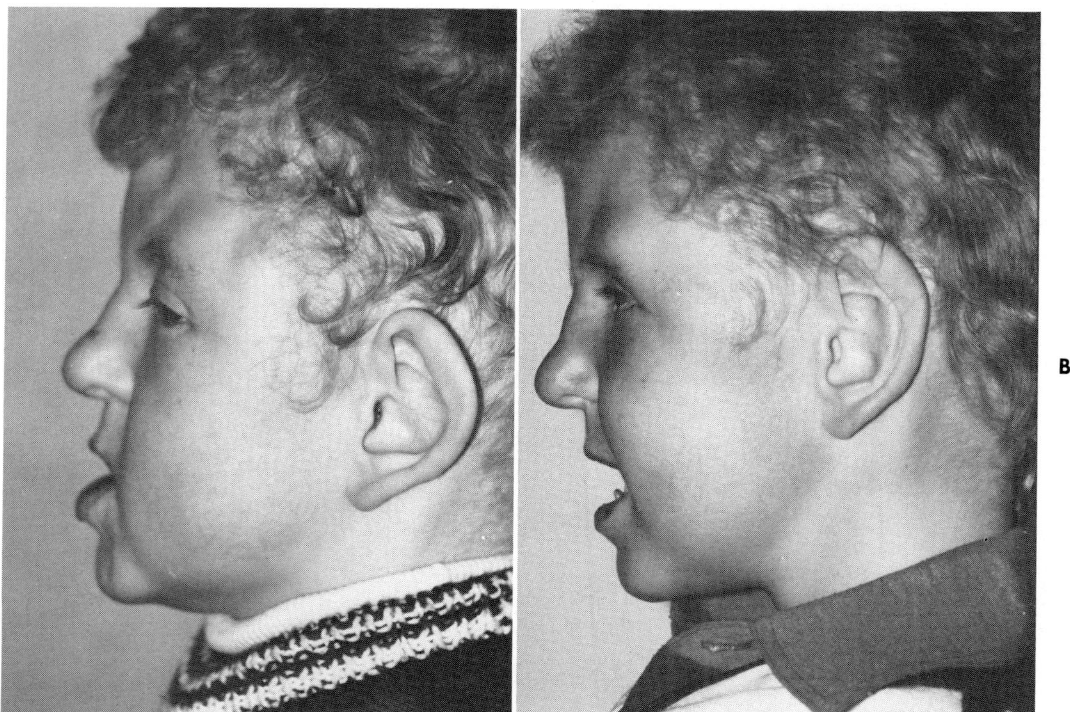

Fig. 28-15, cont'd. B, Correction by osteotomy.
Continued.

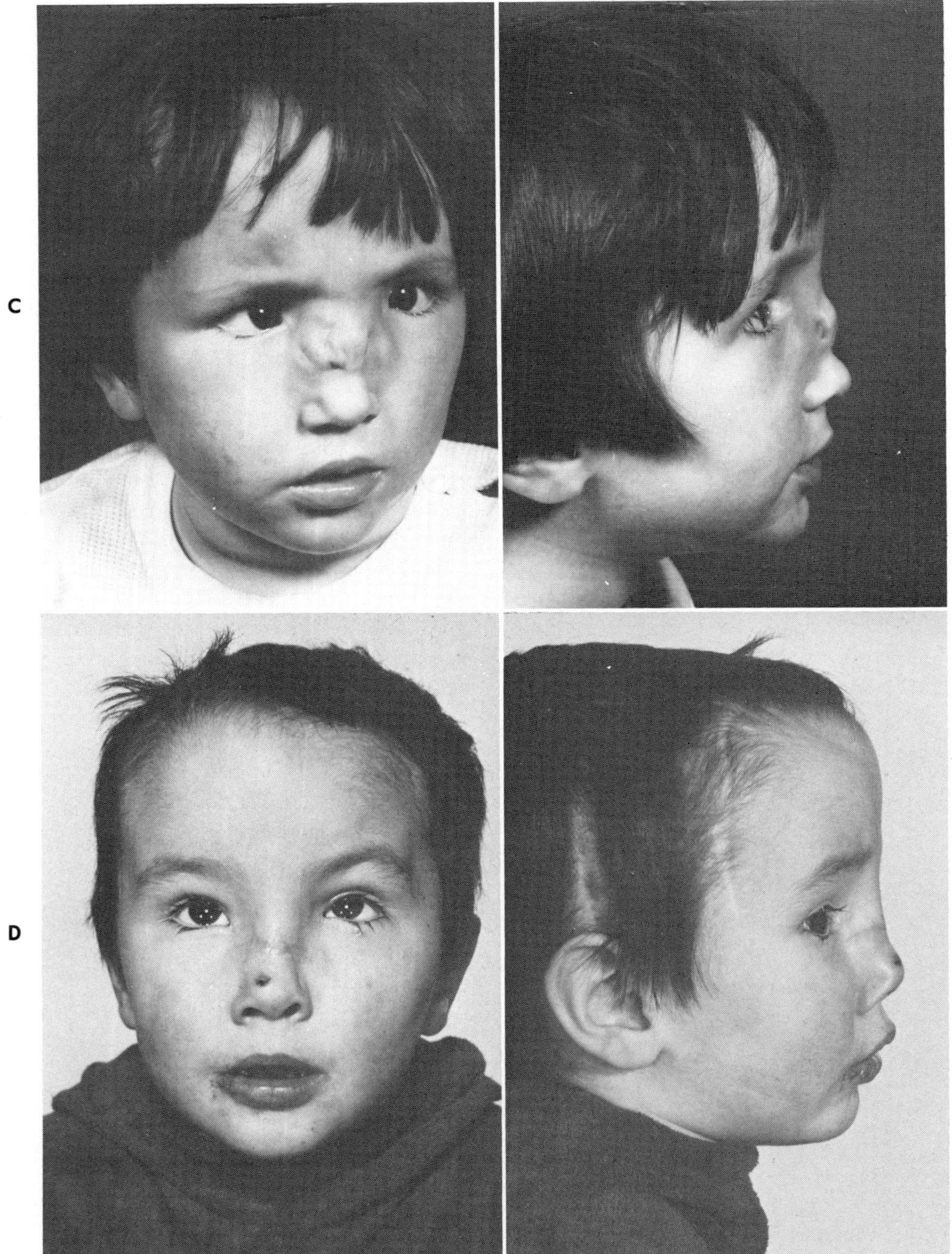

Fig. 28-15, cont'd. C, Preoperative appearance. **D,** Postoperative result.

down to the pterygomaxillary groove; there is no horizontal maxillary osteotomy.

The orbitomaxillary segments are mobilized and moved medially. As this occurs, the upward rotation at the lateral orbital area levels off the maxillary occlusal plane.

Most of these procedures have been presented in considerable detail elsewhere.[5]

Timing of surgery

Surgery should be delayed until the tooth buds have descended low enough in the maxilla to allow the transverse osteotomy under the infraorbital nerve to be carried out. This is determined radiologically. Frequently the surgery can be undertaken at around 5 years, before the child begins school.

In some situations (gross encephalocele, expanding hypertelorism, or grotesque deformity) earlier correction must be undertaken. The C-shaped osteotomy is applicable in these cases.

Occasionally, surgery may be contraindicated; when there is a basal encephalocele coming through the base of the middle cranial fossa, "discretion is the better part of valor." On an axial CT scan or pneumoencephalography, the thalamic and hypothalamic areas may lie in the posterior wall of the encephalocele; any attempt to resect this area will result in drastic physiologic changes, culminating in death.

Complications

Complications have been reported for craniofacial procedures in general.[20,21] Table 28-1 relates to those associated with intracranial procedures. The complication rate in 1979 for hypertelorism would more or less parallel the figures in Table 28-1. There is no doubt, however, that with experience and reduction of blood loss and operating time, there has been significant decrease in major complications. In a well-established center complications of any kind are extremely rare, and when they occur are of minor variety.

Problems that require later correction are eyelid ptosis, sixth cranial nerve palsy, dystopia of one orbit, downward descent of the lateral canthi, antimongoloid slant, diplopia, bony irregularities, and persistent CSF rhinorrhea. The sixth

Table 28-1. Complications of 421 assorted intracranial procedures

Complication	Number of patients	Percentage
Death	9	2.2
Visual loss	0	0.0
Infection	26	6.2
CSF leak	9	2.2
Bone graft loss	20	4.8
Soft tissue loss	10	2.4
Bleeding/blood volume	30	7.1
Speech problems	3	0.7
Seventh cranial nerve palsy	1	0.2

cranial nerve palsy should be mentioned in more detail. This is no uncommon in orbital osteotomies because of encroachment into the superior orbital fissure. Fortunately, most recover spontaneously. The natural history of eyelid ptosis and diplopia is similar; rarely are corrective procedures necessary.

In the past poor correction of hypertelorism was seen. Various reasons have been advanced for this: laying down of new bone on the medial orbital walls, accumulation of fibrous tissue, and drifting apart of the orbits. The most likely cause is inadequate correction of the original problem. This may occur for two reasons. The first is insufficient central bone resection; the second is a lack of appreciation of the shape of the medial orbital wall in some types of hypertelorism. In the central and posterior varieties, the medial orbital wall is convex into the orbit, and satisfactory correction will not be achieved unless this area is removed and bone grafted with split skull or split ribs to give a normal medial wall contour.

A fairly common postcorrection sequela is epicanthal folds. These are handled with the four-flap ("jumping man") canthoplasty of Mustardé.[7,8] Canthal drift or displacement can be repositioned by a transnasal canthopexy using exposure gained by canthoplasty (Fig. 28-16).

WARNING: Although we have the techniques to deal with this deformity, it may be unwise to operate in the patient with cleft palate and a basal encephalocele. Careful CT scanning and pneumoencephalography may show brain tissue in the posterior wall of the encephalocele. This may be thalamic or hypothalamic tissue, and resection may result in intraoperative death (Fig. 28-17).

Of all the deformities, orbital hypertelorism represents the greatest challenge. Frequently multiple gross abnormalities are present, which result in a three-dimensional puzzle that often defies one-stage correction. Tissue defects further complicate the issue. With experience and more sophisticated methods of assessment (e.g., multiview and three-dimensional axial CT scans), the results are improving. The consistent production of good results has not been achieved, and for this we have to strive.

SUMMARY AND CONCLUSIONS

Orbital hypertelorism is characterized by lateralization of the total orbit. In this condition both the intercanthal and interpupillary distances are greater than normal. The primary and anatomic abnormality is enlargement of the ethmoidal sinuses.

Surgical treatment consists of either subcranial (extracranial) or transcranial (intracranial) approaches. The intracranial approach is indicated in moderate to severe cases in which (1) the interorbital distance is greater than 30 mm in a child, (2) the cribriform plate lies below the frontonasal suture, and (3) there is an associated encephalocele. Mild cases with an intraorbital distance of 25 to 30 mm can be treated by a subcranial approach.

Text continued on p. 498.

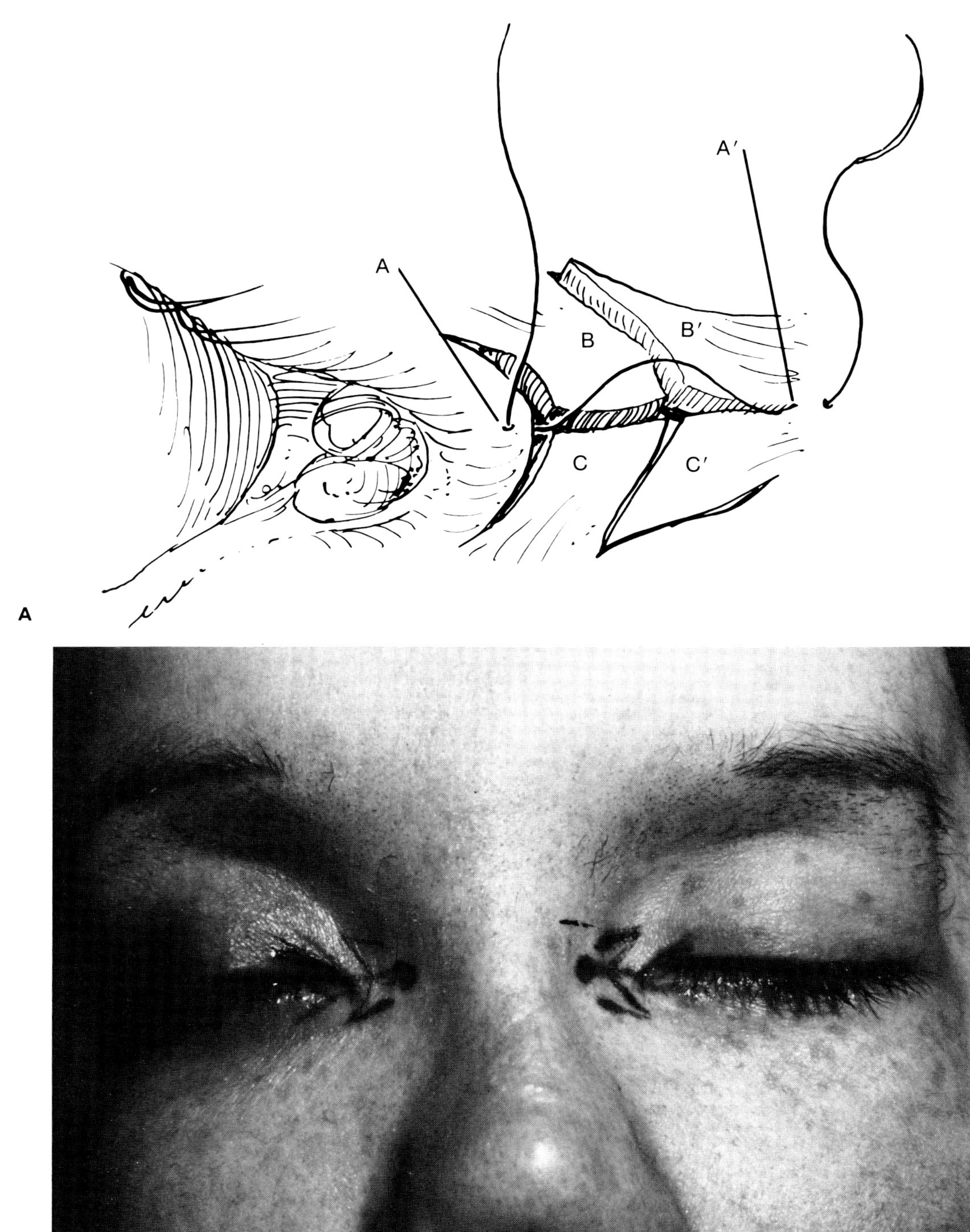

Fig. 28-16. A, Design of skin flaps in the Mustardè procedure.

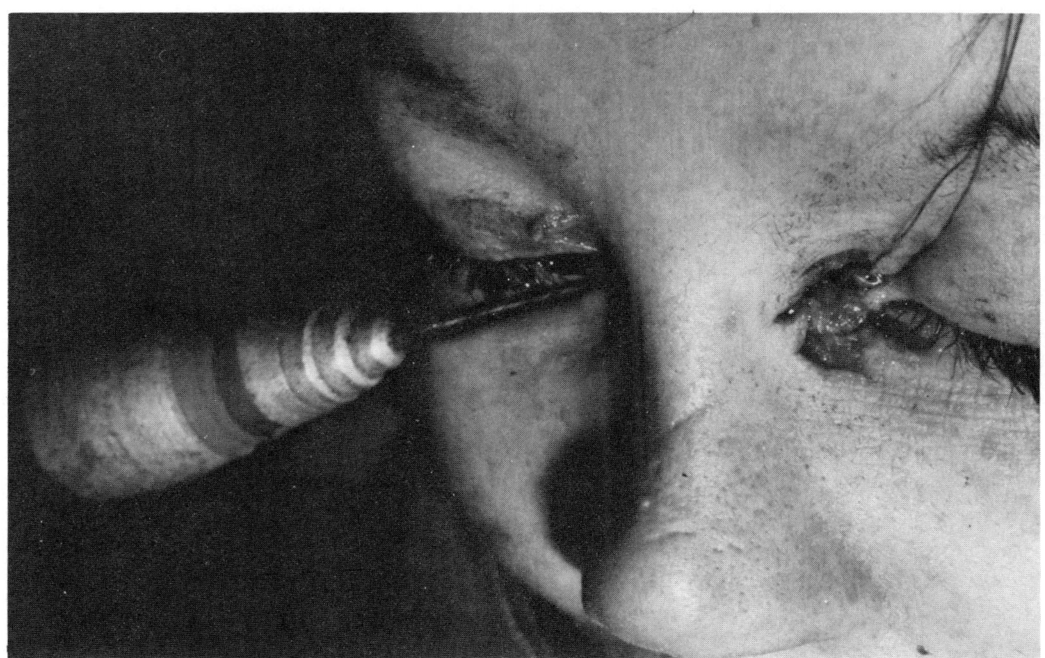

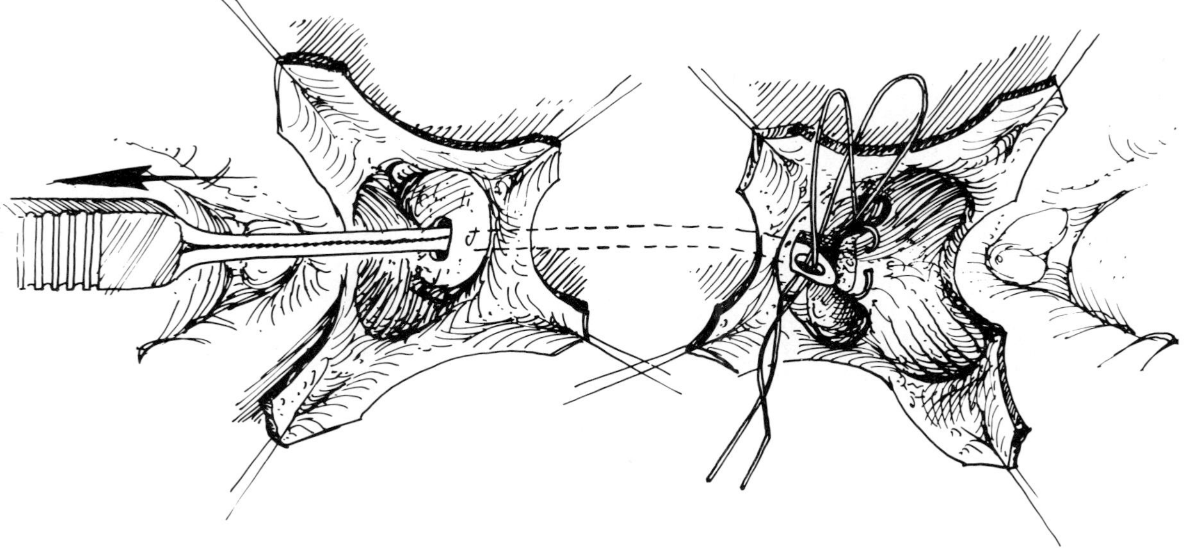

Fig. 28-16, cont'd. B, Repositioning of medial canthal ligaments.

Continued.

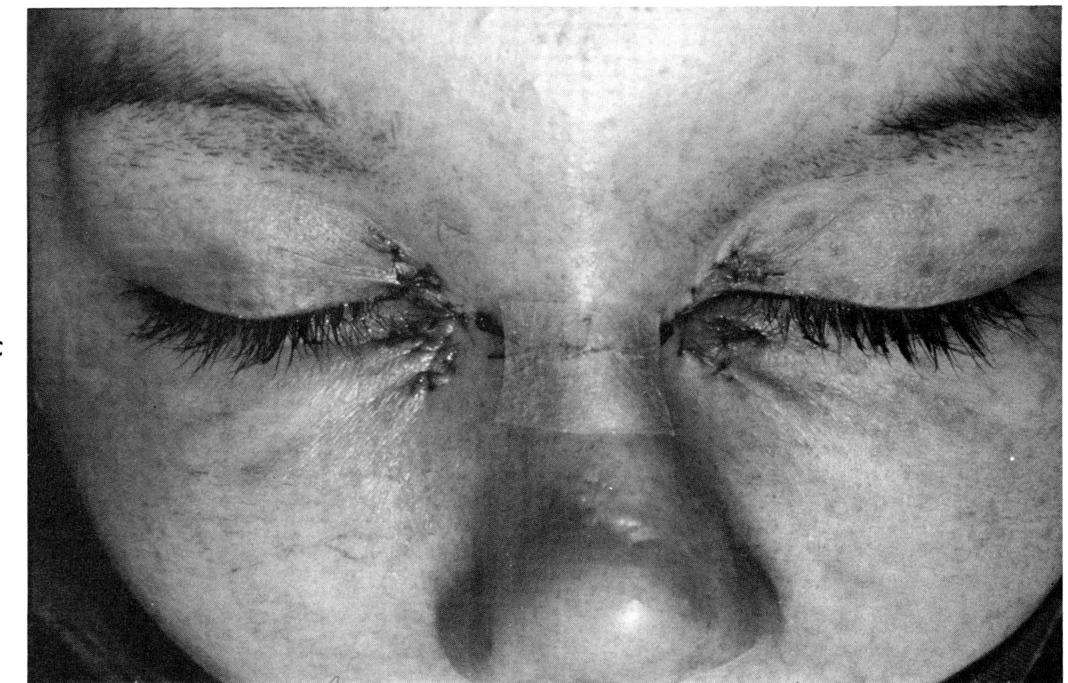

Fig. 28-16, cont'd. C, Postoperative result.

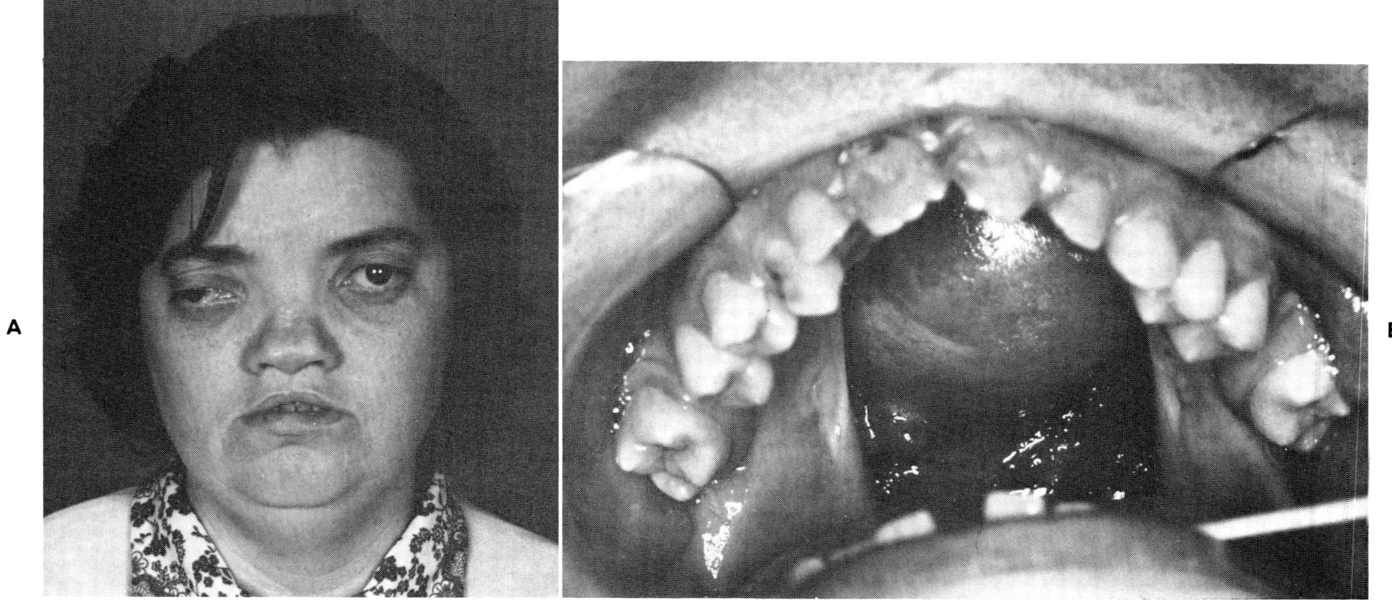

Fig. 28-17. A, Patient with hypertelorism. **B,** Basal encephalocele in same patient.

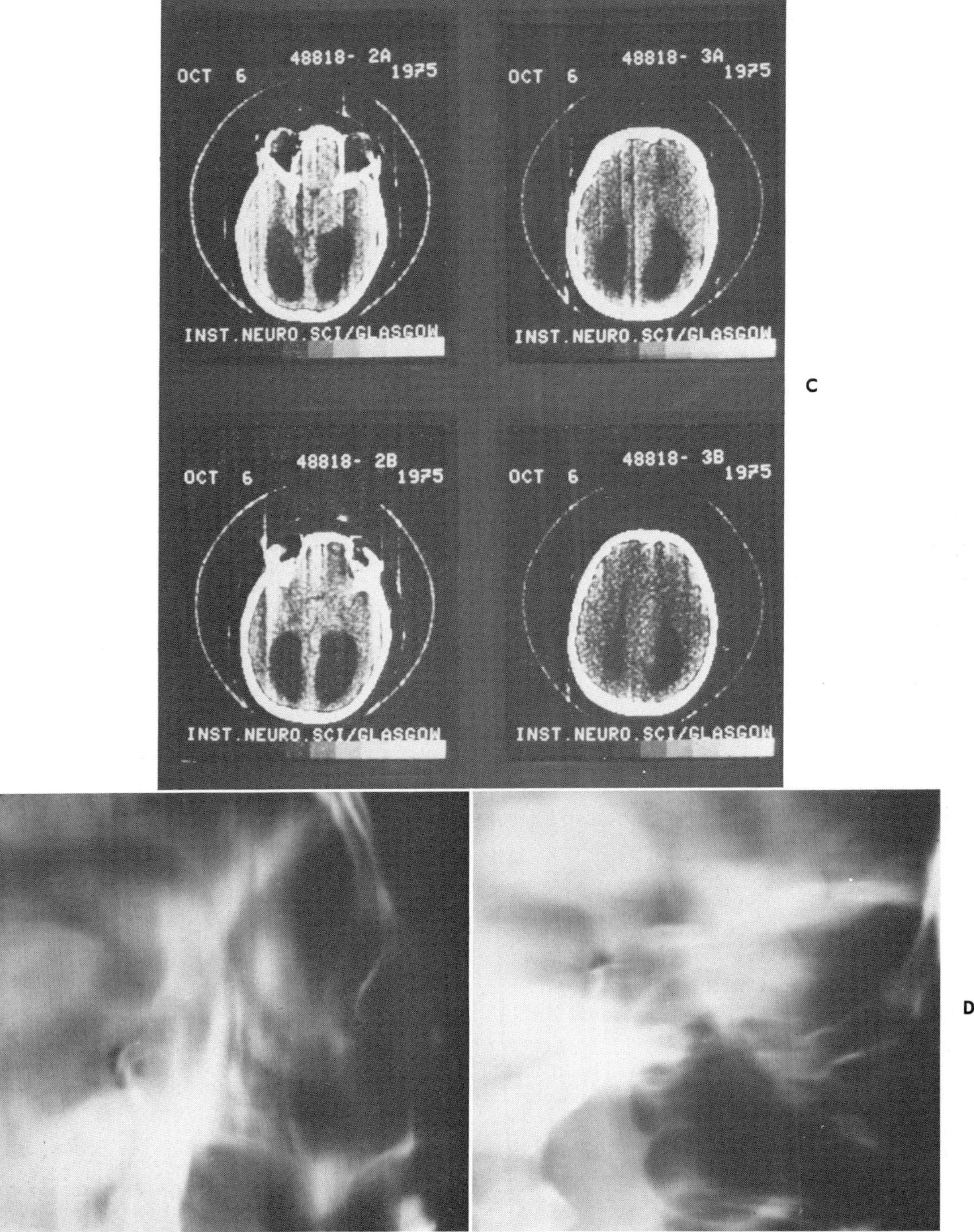

Fig. 28-17, cont'd. C, CT scan showing the position of the encephalocele and the presence of brain tissue within it. **D,** Pneumoencephalogram showing brain tissue in the posterior wall of the encephalocele.

The surgical steps during the subcranial approach are outlined throughout the chapter. Segments of both nasal bones and ethmoidal sinuses are resected on either side of the nasal septum. After this the medial orbital walls are moved together and held in place with intraosseous wiring. Bone grafting is frequently required, as well as repositioning of the medial canthal ligaments.

The transcranial approach is indicated for moderate and severe degrees of hypertelorism. In this technique both medial canthal ligaments are dissected free through small transverse incisions in the medial canthal area. The main approach is through a coronal incision. The location of the osteotomies are described. A frontal bone flap is planned so as to leave a 15 mm bar bone intact above the orbital osteotomy. This permits separate positioning and stabilization of either orbital block. The brain is elevated from the anterior cranial fossa. The medial extent of this elevation is a lateral border of the cribriform plate. It is important not to proceed beyond this area, since a dural tear will result. After the osteotomies are complete, a central bone block is removed. The orbits are then stabilized in the midline with an interosseous wire. Bone grafts are then placed into the lateral orbital wall defects and wired securely.

A technique for sagittally splitting the lateral orbital walls is also described. This technique is usually reserved for the less severe degrees of hypertelorism and requires an experienced clinical judgment rather than hard quantitative values.

A self-locking osteotomy is performed when a pure medial wall orbital movement is required in a single plane.

A U-shaped osteotomy is indicated in lesser degrees of hypertelorism. This has the advantage of providing one solid portion of the orbit to move and eliminates some of the stabilizing difficulties imposed by working with small pieces of bone. This technique is a variation of the extracranial approach.

It is often difficult to create an esthetically pleasing nose in most cases of hypertelorism. In hypertelorism the nose may be either long or short. A short nose is associated with facial clefts 0 to 4 and 11 to 14 according to the Tessier classification. The long nose is usually associated with a nasoencephalocele.

In general, surgery should be delayed until tooth buds have descended low enough in the maxilla to permit a transverse osteotomy to be carried out. Frequently surgery can be performed at approximately 5 years of age, before the child begins school. Surgery is contraindicated in those patients in whom a nasal encephalocele is coming through the base of the middle cranial fossa. This is demonstrated both on an axial CT scan and a pneumoencephalogram. Any attempt to resect this segment usually results in injury to both thalamic and hypothalamic areas, resulting in death.

In the 421 patients who underwent intracranial procedures, the complication rate has been acceptable considering the magnitude of the surgery. Death occurred in 2.2%, infection in 6.2%, and bone graft loss in 4.8%. Bleeding with depletion of blood volume was common, occurring in 7.1% of patients. No visual loss occurred in any of the 421 patients.

Of all the deformities with which we are presented, orbital hypertelorism represents the greatest challenge. Multiple gross abnormalities are frequently present, which results in a three-dimensional puzzle that often defies one-stage correction. Tissue defects further complicate the issue. With experience in more sophisticated methods of assessment (e.g., multiview and three-dimensional axial CT scans), the results are improving. The consistent production of good results has not been achieved, and for this we have to strive.

REFERENCES
1. Converse, J.M., Ransohoff, J., Mathews, E.S., et al.: Ocular hypertelorism and pseudohypertelorism: advances in surgical treatment, Plast. Reconstr. Surg. **45**:1, 1970
2. Greig, D.M.: Hypertelorism: a hitherto undifferentiated congenital craniofacial deformity, Edinburgh Med. J. **31**:560, 1924.
3. Harris, P., Jackson, I.T., and McGregor, J.C.: Reconstructive surgery of the head. In Krayenbuhl, H., editor: Advances and technical standards in neurosurgery, New York, 1981, Springer-Verlag New York, Inc.
4. Jackson, I.T., Hide, T.A.H., and Barker, D.T.: Transposition cranioplasty to restore forehead contour in craniofacial deformities, Br. J. Plast. Surg. **31**:127, 1978.
5. Jackson, I.T., Munro, I.R., Salyer, K.E., and Whitaker, L.A.: Atlas of craniomaxillofacial surgery, St. Louis, 1982, The C.V. Mosby Co.
6. Munro, I.R., and Cas, S.K.: Improving results in orbital hypertelorism correction, Ann. Plast. Surg. **2**:499, 1979.
7. Mustardé, J.C.: The treatment of ptosis and epicanthal folds, Br. J. Plast. Surg. **12**:252, 1959.
8. Mustardé, J.C.: Repair and reconstruction in the orbital region, Edinburgh, 1980, Churchill Livingstone.
9. Ortiz-Monasterio, F.: Personal communication, 1977.
10. Ortiz-Monasterio, F., and Fuente-del-Campo, A.: Nasal correction in hyperteleorbitism: the short and the long nose, Scand. J. Plast. Reconstr. Surg. **15**:277, 1981.
11. Schmid, E.: Zur operativen behandlung des angeborenen hypertelorismus, Chir. Plas. Reconstr. **3**:130, 1967.
12. Schmid, E.: Surgical management of hypertelorism. In Longacre, J.J., editor: Craniofacial anomalies: pathenogenesis and repair, Philadelphia, 1968, J.B. Lippincott Co.
13. Tessier, P.: Orbital hypertelorism. I. Successive surgical attempts materials and methods, causes and mechanisms, Scand. J. Plast. Reconstr. Surg. **6**:135, 1972.
14. Tessier, P.: Experiences in the treatment of orbital hypertelorism, Plast. Reconstr. Surg. **53**:1, 1974.
15. Tessier, P.: Anatomical classification of facial, craniofacial, and laterofacial clefts, J. Maxillofac. Surg. **4**:69, 1976.
16. Tessier, P.: Orbital hypertelorism in Tessier, P., Callahan, A., Mustardé, J.C., and Salyer, K.E., editors: Symposium on plastic surgery in the orbital region, vol. 12, St. Louis, 1976, The C.V. Mosby Co.
17. Tessier, P., Guiot, G., and Derome, P.: Orbital hypertelorism. II. Definite treatment of orbital hypertelorism by craniofacial or by extracranial osteotomies, Scand. J. Plast. Reconstr. Surg. **7**:39, 1973.
18. Tessier, P., Guiot, G., Rougerie, J., et al.: Ostéotomies cranio-naso-orbitofaciales hypertélorism, Ann. Chir. Plast. **12**:103, 1967.
19. van der Meulen, J.C.: Medial faciotomy, Br. J. Plast. Surg. **32**:339, 1979.
20. Whitaker, L.A., Munro, I.R., Jackson, I.T., and Salyer, K.E.: Problems in craniofacial surgery, J. Maxillofac. Surg. **4**:131, 1976.
21. Whitaker, L.A., Munro, I.R., Salyer, K.E., et al.: Combined report of problems and complications in 793 craniofacial operations, Plast. Reconstr. Surg. **64**:198, 1979.

CHAPTER 29

Craniofacial microsomia

JOSEPH G. McCARTHY

The term *first and second branchial arch syndrome* designates in the United States a characteristic congenital malformation that is usually unilateral but occasionally bilateral. Caronni[3] has coined the term *auriculobranchiogenic dysplasia*. Stark and Saunders[35] referred to a similar clinical association of physical findings as the first branchial arch syndrome or the *oral-mandibular-auricular syndrome*. The term *first and second branchial arch syndrome* is not entirely satisfactory, since other malformations are also derived from maldevelopment of these branchial arches. Gorlin and Pindborg[17] reviewed the various names by which the condition has been described and advocated the term *hemifacial microsomia,* which implies that the deformity is exclusively unilateral and spares the cranium. Pruzansky[33] used the term *otocraniocephalic syndromes* to describe aberrations in the development of the first and second branchial arches. At the Center for Craniofacial Anomalies in the Institute of Reconstructive Plastic Surgery of the New York University Medical Center, the terms *unilateral* or *bilateral craniofacial microsomia* are preferred.[4]

HISTORY

Grabb[18] cited the teratologic tablets written in approximately 2000 BC by the Chaldeans of Mesopotamia as the earliest human recordings of malformations of the first and second branchial arches. Bartholinus[2] described a child with absence of the external auditory canal, and Lachmund[22] reported a girl with microtia and agenesis of the external auditory canal. Thompson[37] drew attention to the fact that the clinical signs of the syndrome were expressed in structures derived from the first and second branchial arches and the intervening cleft. In recent times, numerous publications have focused attention on the clinical findings and methods of reconstruction of individual deformities.*

---

*References 6, 7, 12, 13, 17, 18, 20, 23, 26, 28, 29, 32, and 35.

CLINICAL SPECTRUM OF THE SYNDROME
Incidence

In a study of birth records, the birth incidence of craniofacial microsomia was determined to range between 1 in 4000 to 5642 births.[18,31] After the administration of thalidomide to pregnant women in Germany between the years 1959 and 1962, approximately 1000 severe and an additional 2000 less severe cases of first and second branchial arch malformations were reported.[21]

Sex

In a series of 102 patients reported by Grabb,[18] 63 were males and 39 were females.

Unilateral versus bilateral

It has been estimated that bilateral involvement can be observed in approximately 6% to 16% of all cases.[6,10,18,26] Since formes frustes of the syndrome often exist on the "unaffected" side on careful examination, the incidence of bilateral involvement is obviously higher.

Variations of the syndrome

The deformity in craniofacial microsomia varies in extent and degree. As in many other craniofacial anomalies, it is often difficult to classify the individual deformity.

In the severe form, all of the structures derived from the first and second branchial arches are hypoplastic (Fig. 29-1), whereas in other types either the auricular or jaw deformity may predominate. There may be many shades of expression, depending on the degree of involvement of the structures derived from the first and second arches and the involvement of the adjacent skeletal structures.

In some patients in whom the ear deformity is maximal (Fig. 29-2), the jaw deformity is not apparent on clinical examination. Radiographic studies demonstrate, however, that in all cases of external auditory canal and auricular

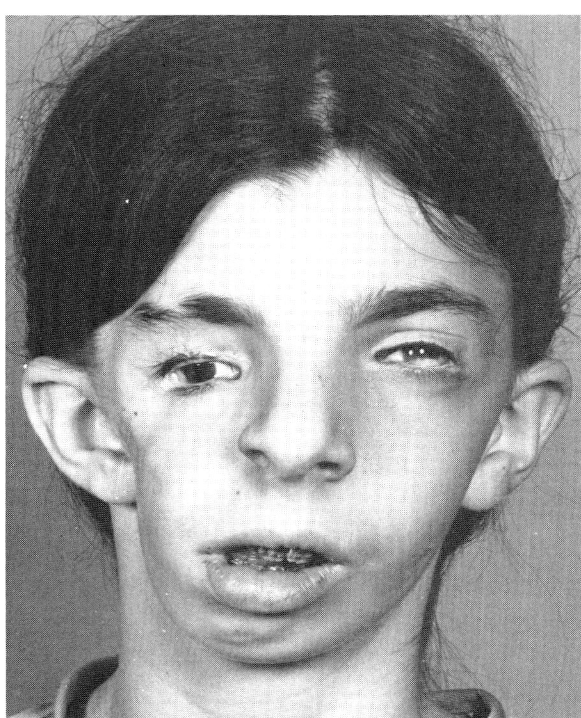

Fig. 29-1. Craniofacial microsomia with severe underdevelopment of the right side of the face. Note that the chin is deviated to the affected side. The oral commissure is elevated and widened. There are bilateral bulbar epidermoid cysts. (From Converse, J.M., McCarthy, J.G., Coccaro, P.J., and Wood-Smith, D.: Clinical aspects of craniofacial microsomia. In Converse, J.M., McCarthy, J.G., and Wood-Smith, D., editors: Symposium on diagnosis and treatment of craniofacial anomalies, St. Louis, 1979, The C.V. Mosby Co.)

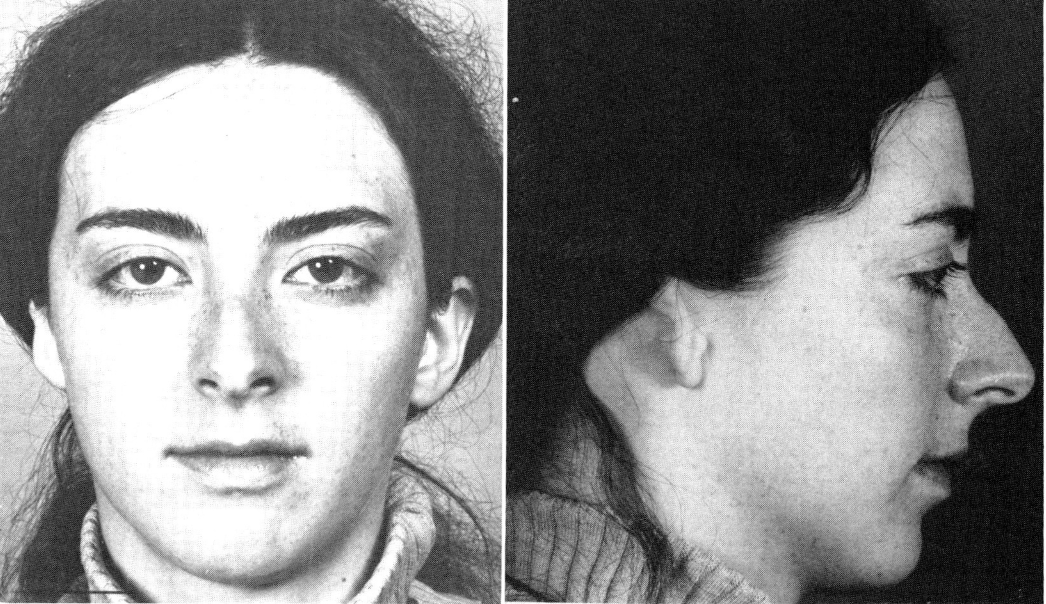

Fig. 29-2. Patient with microtia and small auricular remnants. No jaw deformity is apparent. Tomographic study of the temporomandibular joint showed severe blunting of the mandibular condyle on the affected side. (From Converse, J.M., McCarthy, J.G., Coccaro, P.J., and Wood-Smith, D.: Clinical aspects of craniofacial microsomia. In Converse, J.M., McCarthy, J.G., and Wood-Smith, D., editors: Symposium on diagnosis and treatment of craniofacial anomalies, St. Louis, 1979, The C.V. Mosby Co.)

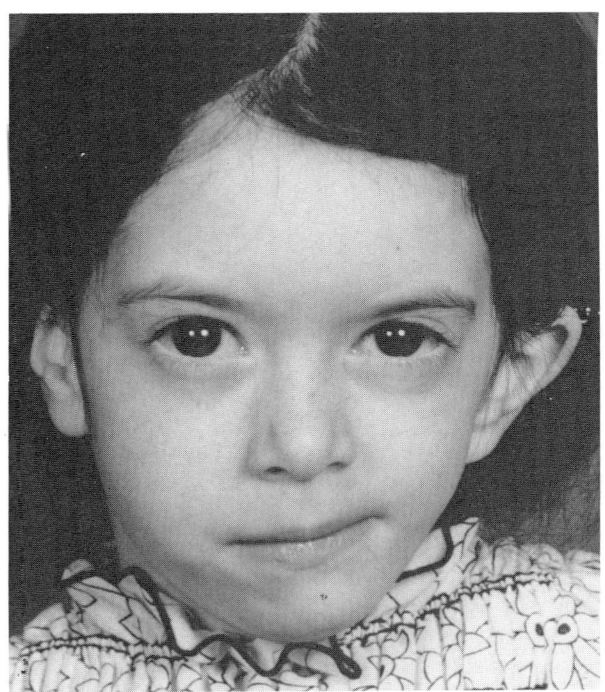

Fig. 29-3. Unilateral craniofacial microsomia (left side). Note the characteristic soft tissue deficiency, occlusal slant, and upward displacement of the oral commissure on the affected side. The auricular helix is enlarged and protruding but otherwise is not grossly deformed. (From Converse, J.M., McCarthy, J.G., Coccaro, P.J., and Wood-Smith, D.: Clinical aspects of craniofacial microsomia. In Converse, J.M., McCarthy, J.G., and Wood-Smith, D., editors: Symposium on diagnosis and treatment of craniofacial anomalies, St. Louis, 1979, The C.V. Mosby Co.)

hypoplasia with middle ear deformity, there are associated changes in the mandible on the affected side.

The characteristic jaw deformity of unilateral craniofacial microsomia may be present without gross auricular or temporal bone maldevelopment (Fig. 29-3). These cases are difficult to differentiate from postnatal deformities caused by injury, but the diagnosis becomes evident if the deformity was present at birth. The auricle may be normal in shape, protruding, or low set, with a normal hearing mechanism.

Formes frustes, or microforms, are more frequent than is generally acknowledged. They must be searched for in cases of slight facial asymmetry and in auricular malformations without obvious jaw deformity.

EMBRYOLOGY

The ear can serve as a frame of reference in the differentiation of craniofacial microsomia[33] because of its developmental relationship with the jaw (Table 29-1).

The two principal divisions of the organ of hearing come from different embryonic anlagen. The sensory end organ in the inner ear is derived from the ectodermal otocyst, whereas the sound-conducting apparatus in the external and middle ear arises from the gill structures.

The membranous labyrinth has its beginning in the 3½-week-old human embryo[1] as a thickening of the ectoderm on the side of the head, the otic placode. This area is enfolded to become the otic pit and then pinches off to become the otocyst. By means of a series of folds, the otocyst differentiates in the 3-month-old fetus into the endolym-

Table 29-1. Structures derived from the first and second branchial arches and the otic capsule

Origin	Structure
First branchial arch	
Maxillary process	Maxilla
	Palatine bone
	Zygoma
Mandibular process	Trigeminal nerve
	Anterior part of auricle
	Mandible
	Head of malleus
	Body of incus
	Tympanic bone
	Sphenomandibular ligament
First branchial groove	External auditory meatus
	Tympanic membrane
First pharyngeal pouch	Eustachian tube
	Middle ear cavity
Second branchial arch	Facial nerve
	Posterior part of auricle
	Manubrium of malleus, long process of incus, stapedial superstructure, and tympanic surface
	Stapedial artery, styloid process, and stylohyoid ligament
	Lesser cornu of hyoid
Otic capsule	Vestibular surface of stapes and internal acoustic meatus
	Inner ear

Modified from Pearson, A.A., and Jacobson, A.D.: The development of the ear. In Manual of the American Academy of Ophthalmologists and Otolaryngologists, Portland, 1967, University of Oregon.

phatic duct and sac, semicircular endolymphatic ducts, utricle, saccule, and cochlear duct, which contains the organ of Corti. By the fifth month of fetal life, the sensory end organ of the ear attains adult form and size, as the cartilaginous otic capsule ossifies.

The gill structures destined to form the sound-conducting apparatus and jaws first appear in the human embryo at 4 weeks, at about the same time as the otic pit.

The mandible, incus, and malleus develop from the cartilage of the first branchial arch (Meckel's cartilage). The maxilla and palatine and zygomatic bones develop from the maxillary process of the first branchial arch. The stapes (with the exception of the footplate, which originates from the otic capsule), styloid process, and hyoid bone develop from the cartilage of the second arch (Reichert's cartilage) (Table 29-1). The large area of the tympanic membrane, connected by the lever system of the ossicular chain to the small area of the oval window, provides the ear with an effective mechanism to overcome the sound barrier between air and water.

By the third fetal month, the pinna has been formed from the first and second branchial arches on either side of the first branchial groove; the latter is the primary shallow, funnel-shaped external auditory meatus. From the inner end of the primary meatus, a solid cord of ectodermal cells extends farther inward, with a bulblike enlargement adjacent to the middle ear. It is not until the seventh fetal month that this cord canalizes, beginning medially to form the completed external auditory meatus. The external and middle ear, although capable of transmitting sound to the inner ear, are not yet of adult form and size.

In the seventh fetal month, pneumatization of the temporal bone begins, with excavations lined by mucous membrane extending out from the middle ear cavity while the jellylike mesodermal tissue in the middle ear cavity begins to resolve. At birth the eustachian tube inflates; the fetal mesodermal tissue in the middle ear and antrum continues to resorb until the epithelium lies close to the periosteum, and pneumatization of the temporal bone proceeds.

The external auditory meatus, which is entirely cartilaginous at birth (except for the narrow incomplete ring of the tympanic bone), deepens by growth of the tympanic bone to form the adult osseous meatus. Except for some pneumatization of the petrous apex that may continue into adult life, the external and middle ear finally reach adult form and size in late childhood (in contrast to the inner ear, which becomes adult in fetal life). It is generally accepted that the first branchial arch furnishes the anterior part of the auricle; the second arch provides the structures of the remaining external ear.

ETIOPATHOGENESIS

The genetic component in craniofacial microsomia is ill defined, and there is no evidence of genetic transmission except in a few patients. Grabb[18] reported that only 4 of 102 patients studied had one sibling or one parent with maldevelopment of first and second branchial arch structures. Hanhart[19] described a form of inheritable auricular hypoplasia, and Rogers[34] listed several family studies by other authors that suggested a possible hereditary basis for auricular deformities. Summitt[36] reported a pedigree of Goldenhar's syndrome that was compatible with autosomal dominant transmission. Consequently, current etiopathogenic theories favor an intrauterine factor (or factors) that affects the embryo and has the following three characteristics:

1. The factor varies in its intensity and penetrance.
2. The factor strikes at varying periods in the course of prenatal development.
3. The damage is produced in varying loci in the fetus or embryo, along any point of the developing first and second branchial arches; the damage may be localized or widespread.

The etiopathogenesis has not been satisfactorily explained to date. The theory of mesodermal deficiency of Hoffstetter and Veau has been invoked by Stark and Saunders.[35] Others have suggested that vascular defects of the stapedial artery may account for maldevelopment of the first and second branchial arches.[25] The stapedial artery, a temporary vascular supply for the primordia of the first and second branchial arches, appears as a collateral artery of the hyoid artery and forms an anastomosis with the pharyngeal artery; it is ultimately replaced by the finite external carotid system.

Poswillo[31] has produced phenocopies of craniofacial microsomia by the administration of triazene to the mouse and thalidomide to the monkey. Embryonic hemorrhage with spreading hematoma before formation of the stapedial artery was demonstrated. The extent and size of the hematoma correlated with the size of the anomalous defect. In the mouse experimental model, all of the variations found in the human syndrome could be reproduced. The spectrum of defects was broad: a small aural hematoma producing a residual deformity of only the external ear and auditory ossicles and larger hemorrhagic lesions affecting the condyle, mandibular ramus, and zygoma.

PATHOLOGIC PROCESS

The deformity in unilateral craniofacial microsomia usually has three major features: auricular, mandibular, and maxillary hypoplasia. The hypoplasia, however, also involves adjacent anatomic structures: the zygoma, pterygoid process of the sphenoid bone, temporal bone, facial nerve, facial musculature of expression, muscles of mastication, parotid gland, cutaneous and subcutaneous tissues, tongue, soft palate, pharynx, and floor of the nose. In addition to the skeletal deficiency, varying amounts of soft tissue hypoplasia, microphthalmos, anophthalmos, cranial nerve palsy, cleft lip and palate, and lateral facial clefts are frequently present.

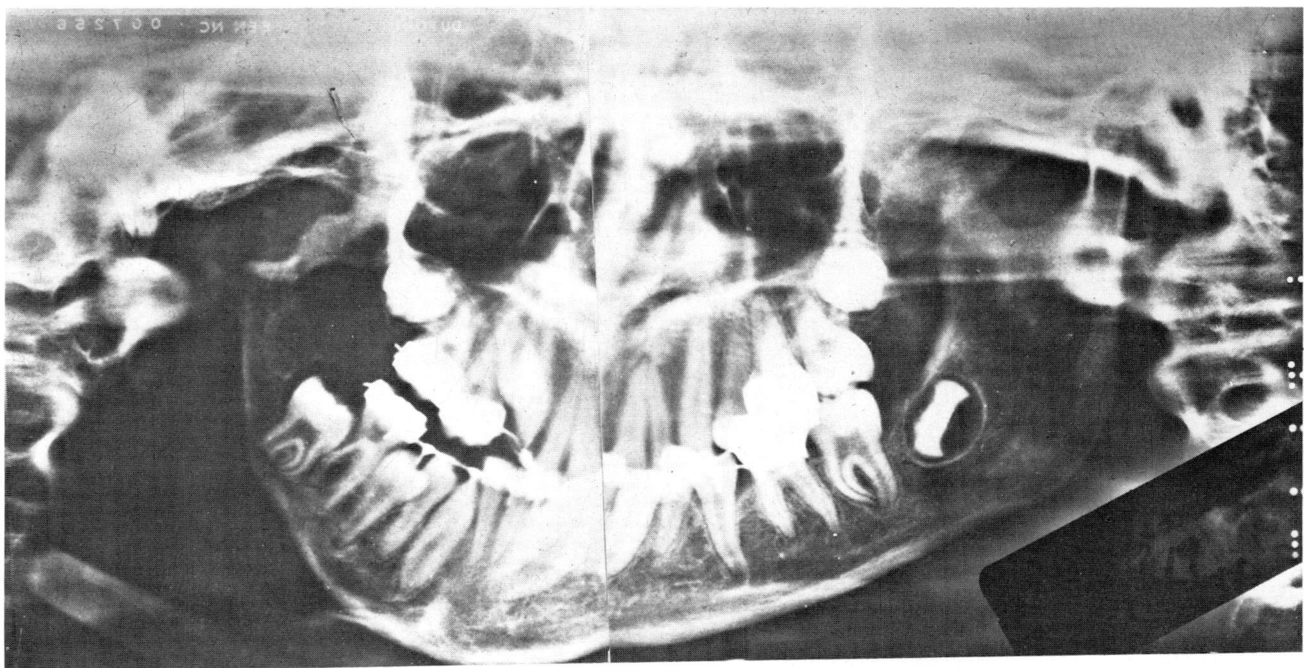

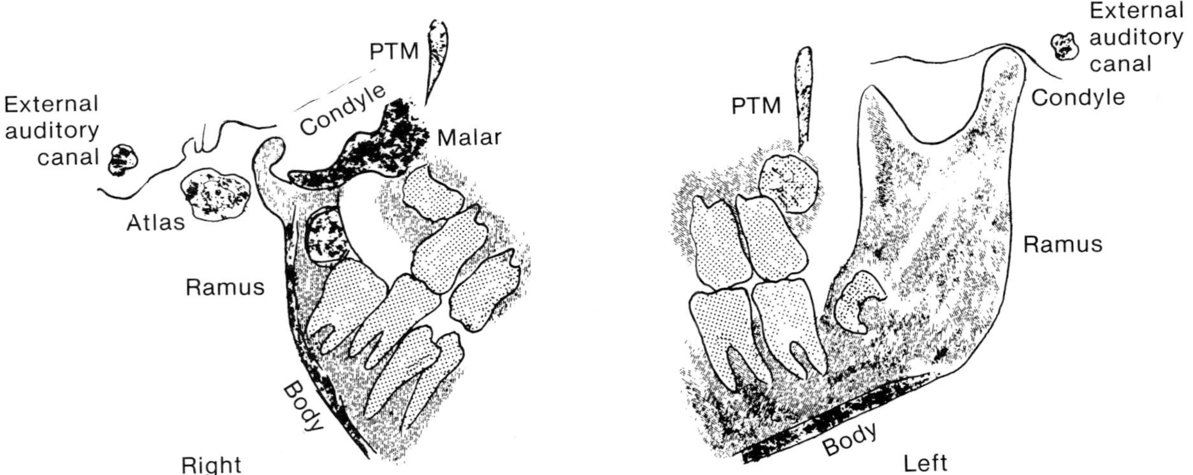

Fig. 29-4. Panoramic radiograph and line drawing of a patient with severe right-sided craniofacial microsomia. Note the shortened ramus and small condyle. (From Converse, J.M., McCarthy, J.G., Coccaro, P.J., and Wood-Smith, D.: Clinical aspects of craniofacial microsomia. In Converse, J.M., McCarthy, J.G., and Wood-Smith, D., editors: Symposium on diagnosis and treatment of craniofacial anomalies, St. Louis, 1979, The C.V. Mosby Co.)

The jaw deformity

The most conspicuous deformity of unilateral craniofacial microsomia is hypoplasia of the mandible on the affected side. The ramus is short or virtually absent (Fig. 29-4), and the body of the mandible curves upward to join the short ramus. The chin is deviated to the affected side (Fig. 29-5); the body of the mandible on the unaffected side does not follow its usual curvature but assumes a flattened contour with a straightened gonial angle. Although the midincisor point of the maxilla may be in position, that of the mandible is deviated to the affected side. (See Fig. 29-14.)

Ramus and condyle malformations vary from minimal hypoplasia of the condyle to its complete absence in association with hypoplasia or agenesis of the ramus. Condylar anomalies can be demonstrated in all patients, and this finding may represent the hallmark of the syndrome.

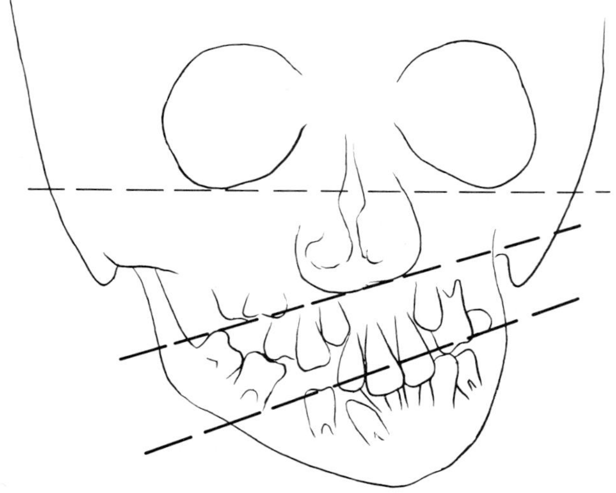

Fig. 29-5. Line drawing of a frontal cephalogram of a patient with left-sided craniofacial microsomia. Note that the occlusal plane is superiorly directed and the chin point is deviated to the affected side. (From Converse, J.M., McCarthy, J.G., Coccaro, P.J., and Wood-Smith, D.: Clinical aspects of craniofacial microsomia. In Converse, J.M., McCarthy, J.G., and Wood-Smith, D., editors: Symposium on diagnosis and treatment of craniofacial anomalies, St. Louis, 1979, The C.V. Mosby Co.)

Pruzansky[32] has proposed the following classification of the mandibular deformity (Fig. 29-6):

Grade I: Hypoplasia is minimal or slight.

Grade II: The condyle and ramus are small; the head of the condyle is flattened; the glenoid fossa is absent; the condyle is hinged on a flat, often convex, infratemporal surface; and the coronoid process may be absent.

Grade III: The ramus is reduced to a thin lamina of bone, or it is completely absent.

Skeletal asymmetry is clinically demonstrated by the high occlusal cant on the affected side. The floor of the maxillary sinus and of the nose on the affected side is at a higher level; in some patients the base of the skull is elevated on an inclined plane similar to that of the inclined occlusal plane.

The dentoalveolar and skeletal dimensions are reduced in the sagittal and vertical direction on the affected side. Development and eruption of the molar teeth are delayed. Crowded dentition, with a characteristic tilt of the anterior maxillary and mandibular teeth toward the affected side, is often noted. When the patient opens the mouth, the deviation toward the affected side is often noted. This is produced not only by skeletal asymmetry but also by the minimal or absent contribution of the ipsilateral medial and lateral pterygoid muscles in countering the opposing actions of the muscles on the unaffected side. The condyle, if present on the unaffected side, is displaced abnormally downward and laterally when the mandible is depressed. Thus in testing for lateral pterygoid muscle weakness, one finds an absence of ability to shift the jaw laterally toward the unaffected side and deviation of the midline of the chin toward the affected side during opening and forceful protrusion.

Muscles of mastication

There is a tendency to consider the deformities of craniofacial microsomia as being only osseous. However, there is an associated hypoplasia of the masseter, medial and lateral pterygoid, and temporal muscles, with a strong secondary influence on skeletal development (Wolff's law). Hypoplasia of the muscles of mastication also contributes to the generalized contour deficiency on the affected side.

Ear deformity

Auricular malformations are a usual manifestation of the syndrome. Meurmann[26] proposed the following classification of auricular anomalies:

Grade I: Distinctly smaller malformed auricles with most of the characteristic components (Fig. 29-7, *A*).

Grade II: A vertical remnant of cartilage and skin with a small anterior hook and complete atresia of the canal (Fig. 29-7, *B*).

Grade III: The auricle is almost entirely absent except for only a small part, such as a deformed lobule (Fig. 29-7, *C*).

In a comprehensive study using air and bone conduction audiometry and temporal tomography, Pruzansky[33] evaluated 57 patients with craniofacial microsomia. It was observed that the degree of auricular deformity as classified does not correlate exactly with hearing function. The type of hearing loss, although usually assumed to be conductive in origin, can be determined only by audiometry. Tomography, not auricular morphology, is the only indicator of middle ear structure. There was, however, a direct relationship between the degree of severity of auricular malformation and ipsilateral mandibular deformity (Fig. 29-8).

Deformities of the nervous system

Nervous system abnormalities in patients with craniofacial microsomia have received little attention in the medical literature.

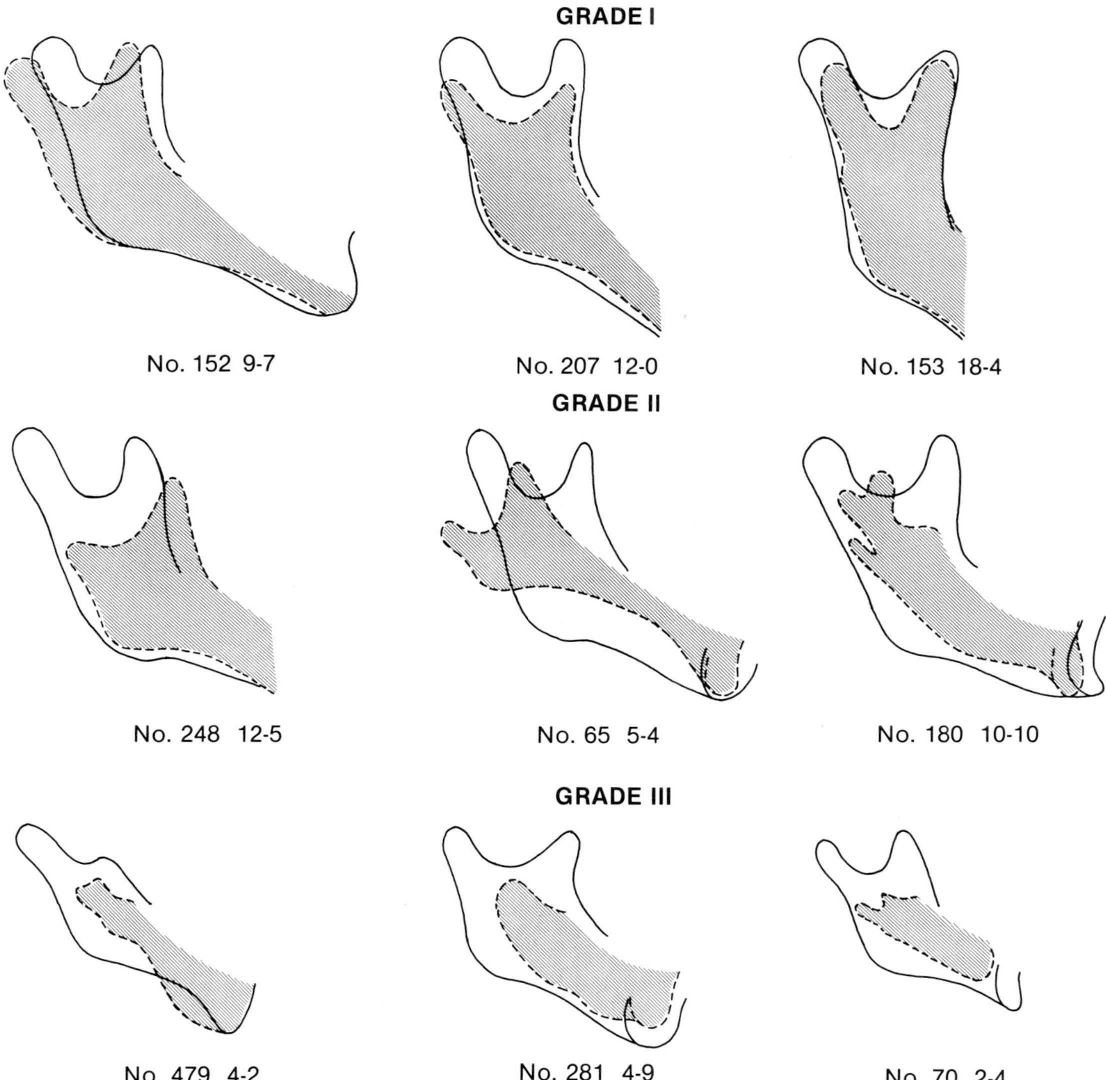

Fig. 29-6. Classification of the mandibular anomaly. (From Pruzansky, S.: Not all dwarfed mandibles are alike. In Bergsma, D., editor: Malformation syndromes. II, Baltimore, Williams & Wilkins for The National Foundation–March of Dimes, Birth Defects **2**:120-129, 1969.)

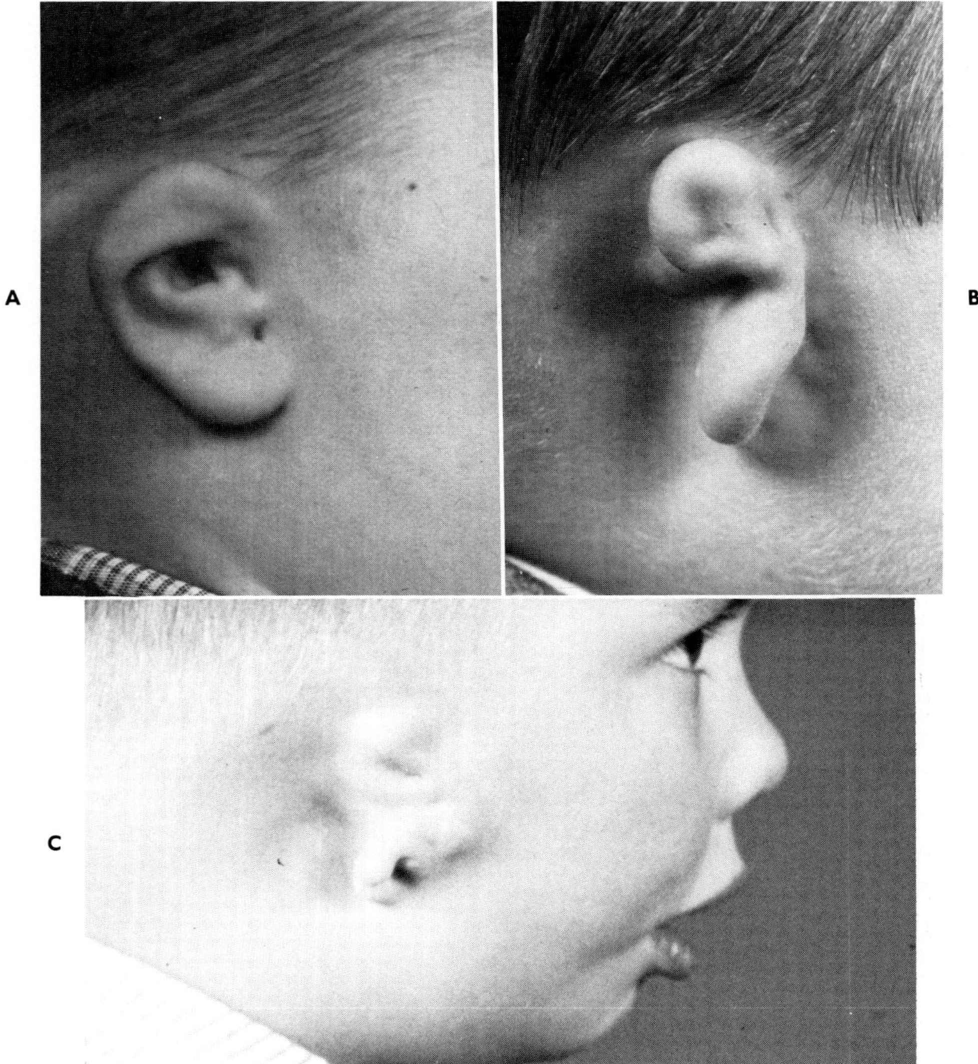

Fig. 29-7. Meurmann's classification[26] of auricular anomalies. **A,** *Grade I:* Small malformed ear with most components present. There is atresia of the external auditory meatus. **B,** *Grade II:* A vertical remnant of skin and cartilage. **C,** *Grade III:* The auricle is almost entirely absent except for a misplaced lobule and small skin and cartilage remnants. (From Converse, J.M., McCarthy, J.G., Coccaro, P.J., and Wood-Smith, D.: Clinical aspects of craniofacial microsomia. In Converse, J.M., McCarthy, J.G., and Wood-Smith, D., editors: Symposium on diagnosis and treatment of craniofacial anomalies, St. Louis, 1979, The C.V. Mosby Co.)

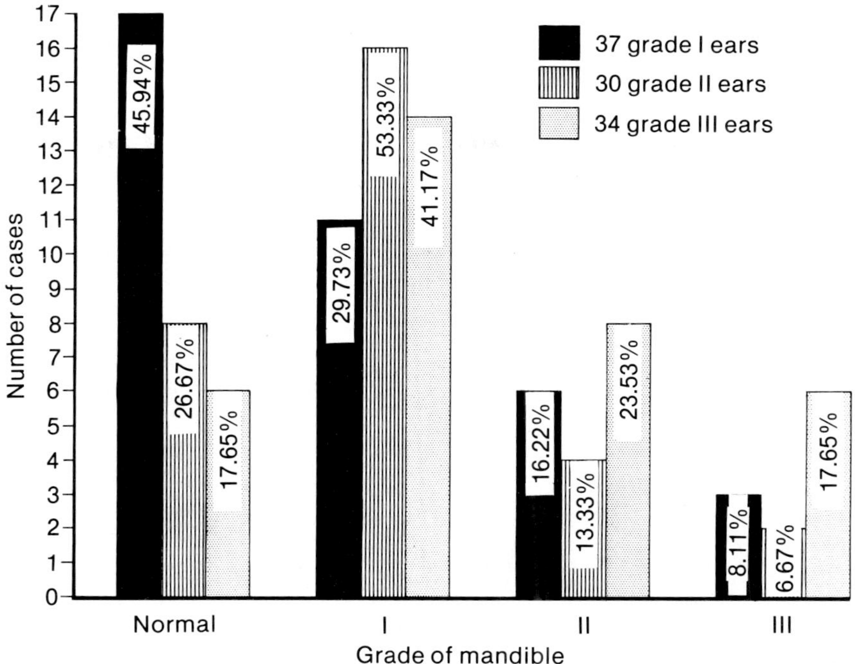

Fig. 29-8. Relationship between malformation of the auricle and the ipsilateral mandible. (From Pruzansky, S.: Findings of hemifacial microsomia. In Converse, J.M.: Reconstructive plastic surgery, Philadelphia, 1977, W.B. Saunders Co.)

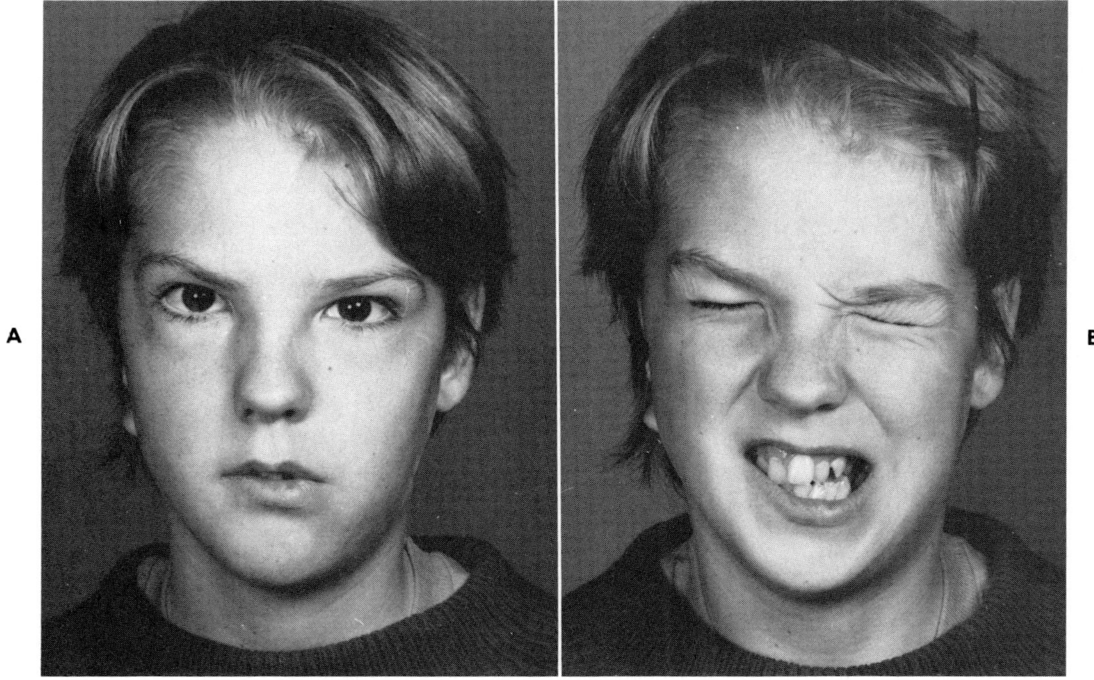

Fig. 29-9. Partial facial nerve palsy in a patient with left-sided craniofacial microsomia. **A,** At rest. **B,** During animation. (From Converse, J.M., McCarthy, J.G., Coccaro, P.J., and Wood-Smith, D.: Clinical aspects of craniofacial microsomia. In Converse, J.M., McCarthy, J.G., and Wood-Smith, D., editors: Symposium on diagnosis and treatment of craniofacial anomalies, St. Louis, 1979, The C.V. Mosby Co.)

Cerebral anomalies

A wide variety of cerebral anomalies exists in craniofacial microsomia and may include ipsilateral cerebral hypoplasia, hypoplasia of the corpus callosum, communicating and obstructive hydrocephalus, an intracranial lipoma, and unilateral hypoplasia of the brainstem and cerebellum.

Cranial nerve anomalies

Cranial nerve abnormalities are frequent in unilateral craniofacial microsomia and can range from arrhinencephaly to unilateral agenesis and hypoplasia of the optic nerve with secondary changes in the lateral geniculate body and visual cortex, hypoplasia of the trochlear and abducent nuclei and nerves, and congenital trigeminal anesthesia and aplasia. The most common cranial nerve anomaly is facial paralysis (Fig. 29-9) secondary to agenesis of the facial muscles, an aberrant pathway of the facial nerve in the temporal bone, or hypoplasia of the intracranial portion of the facial nerve and facial nucleus in the brainstem.

Soft tissue deformities

In addition to anomalies of the muscles of mastication and nervous system, generalized soft tissue hypoplasia often involves the skin, subcutaneous tissue, and facial musculature of expression. The musculature of the soft palate and tongue is occasionally less developed on the affected side. The commonly observed hypoplasia of the parotid gland places the branches of the facial nerve in a superficial and vulnerable position during surgery. The deficiency of soft tissue on the affected side is made evident by the reduced distance between the mastoid process and the angle of the mouth or the lateral canthus of the eye. Atrophy of skin and subcutaneous tissue is most apparent in the parotid-masseteric and auriculomastoid areas.

Transverse facial clefting (Fig 29-3), ranging from macrostomia to a full-thickness defect of the cheek, can be present. The clefts probably result from failure of fusion of the maxillary and mandibular processes. In embryologic development the lateral commisure of the oral fissure is initially situated at the point of bifurcation of the maxillary and mandibular processes. With fusion of the latter and development of the muscles of mastication, the original broad mouth is reduced in size. In addition, the parotid glands, originally located near the embryonic oral commissure, grow laterally toward the developing ear, but the parotid duct papille remain in their more medial position.

TREATMENT

The critical question in treating the patient with craniofacial microsomia revolves around the age at which therapy should be initiated. Moreover, additional variables must also be considered in treatment planning: the degree or severity of the deformity and the relationship of skeletal and soft tissue (especially neuromuscular) deficiency. In general, in the past surgeons tended to reconstruct the deformity solely with osteotomies and bone grafts ("bone carpentry"), ignoring the associated soft tissue and neuromuscular deficits. Long-term surgical results were not published, and consequently the high rate of recurrence of the deformity was not documented. Moss[27] has emphasized the *functional matrix theory* of craniofacial growth and development. This theory implies that in the growing child reconstruction of the skeletal part without the associated neuromuscular component would inevitably lead to total or partial recurrence of the deformity.

Two schools of treatment have consequently evolved: Those advocating early therapeutic intervention[6,8,30] and those recommending a delay in reconstruction until early adolescence.[29,31]

Poswillo[31] cautioned against reconstruction of the facial bones before age 12. He believed that the trauma associated with surgery could destroy the *functional matrix* of part of the facial skeleton and interfere with subsequent facial growth. Obwegeser[29] also advocated postponement of definitive jaw surgery until growth of the craniofacial skeleton has ceased, since he believed osteotomies performed during childhood interfered with growth of the facial skeleton.

Converse et al.[6] have, however, recommended surgery during childhood with the following objectives: (1) improving the symmetry of the mandible, (2) providing interdental space for downgrowth of the maxilla by lengthening the shortened mandibular ramus, (3) restoring an adequate dental occlusion, and (4) expanding the facial skeleton at an early age to fill out the soft tissues on the affected side of the face. They also believed that many of the affected patients lacked the potential for craniofacial development, and any delay in reconstruction to await further skeletal growth was unrealistic.

Treatment in the adult and adolescent

Correction of jaw asymmetry and crossbite by mandibular osteotomy and bone grafts has long been performed in the adult.[9,24] Obwegeser[29] has obtained satisfactory results in adults by a combined LeFort I osteotomy of the maxilla, a bilateral sagittal section of the mandibular ramus, and genioplasty (Figs. 29-10 and 29-11). This procedure cannot be employed in a patient during the period of mixed dentition, since the maxillary osteotomy would injure the unerupted teeth. He has also recommended that in severe cases, the temporomandibular joint should be reconstructed with a costochondral rib graft (Fig. 29-12). Any associated hypoplasia of the temporal bone, zygomatic arch, and lateral orbital rim should also be corrected by onlay bone grafts (Fig. 29-13).

Treatment in the child
Functional therapy

When a craniofacial skeletal defect must be surgically corrected by a bone graft or displacement osteotomy, post

Text continued on p. 513.

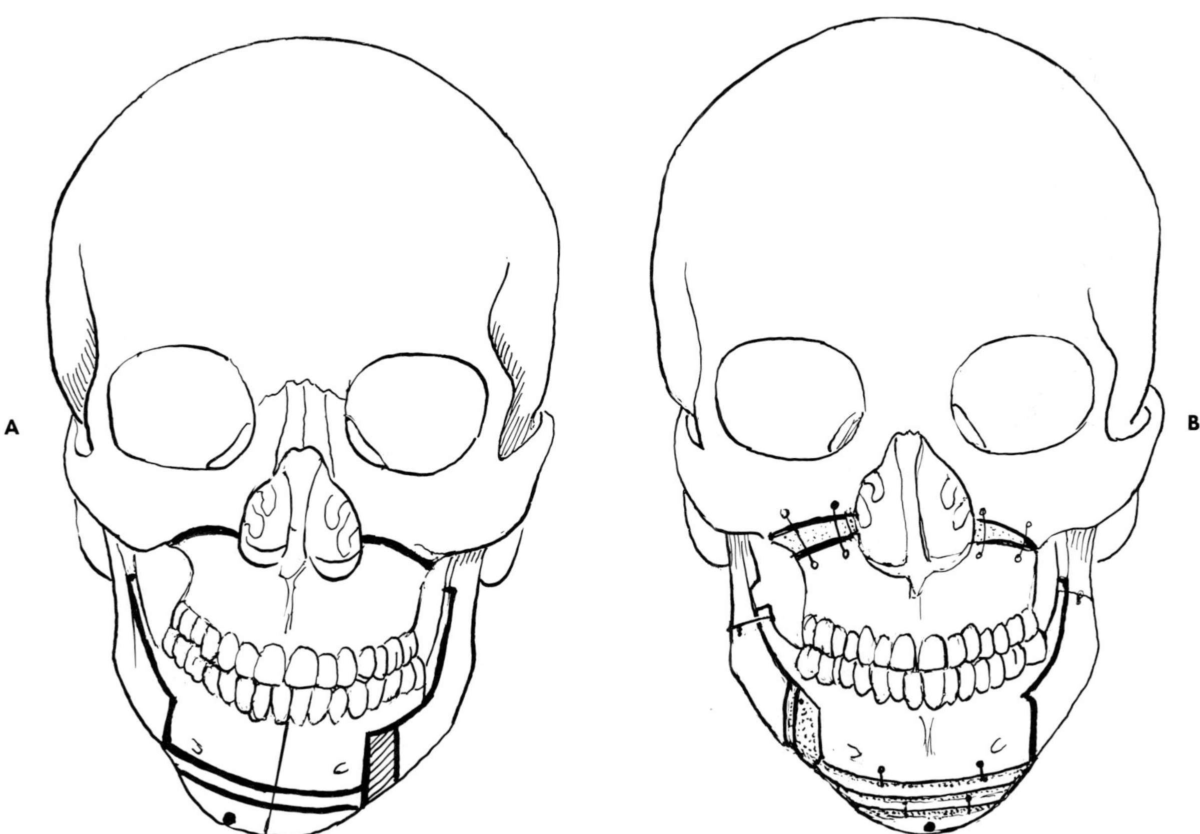

Fig. 29-10. Combined LeFort I maxillary osteotomy, bilateral sagittal split, and horizontal osteotomy of the mandible.[6] **A,** The osteotomies are done only in the adult to avoid injury to the unerupted maxillary teeth and interference with facial growth. **B,** Bone grafts are placed in the defect after downward rotation of the maxilla on the affected side. The mandible is shifted to the unaffected side, and the anteroinferior border of the mandible is rotated and advanced. (From Converse, J.M.: Reconstructive plastic surgery, ed. 2, Philadelphia, 1977, W.B. Saunders Co.)

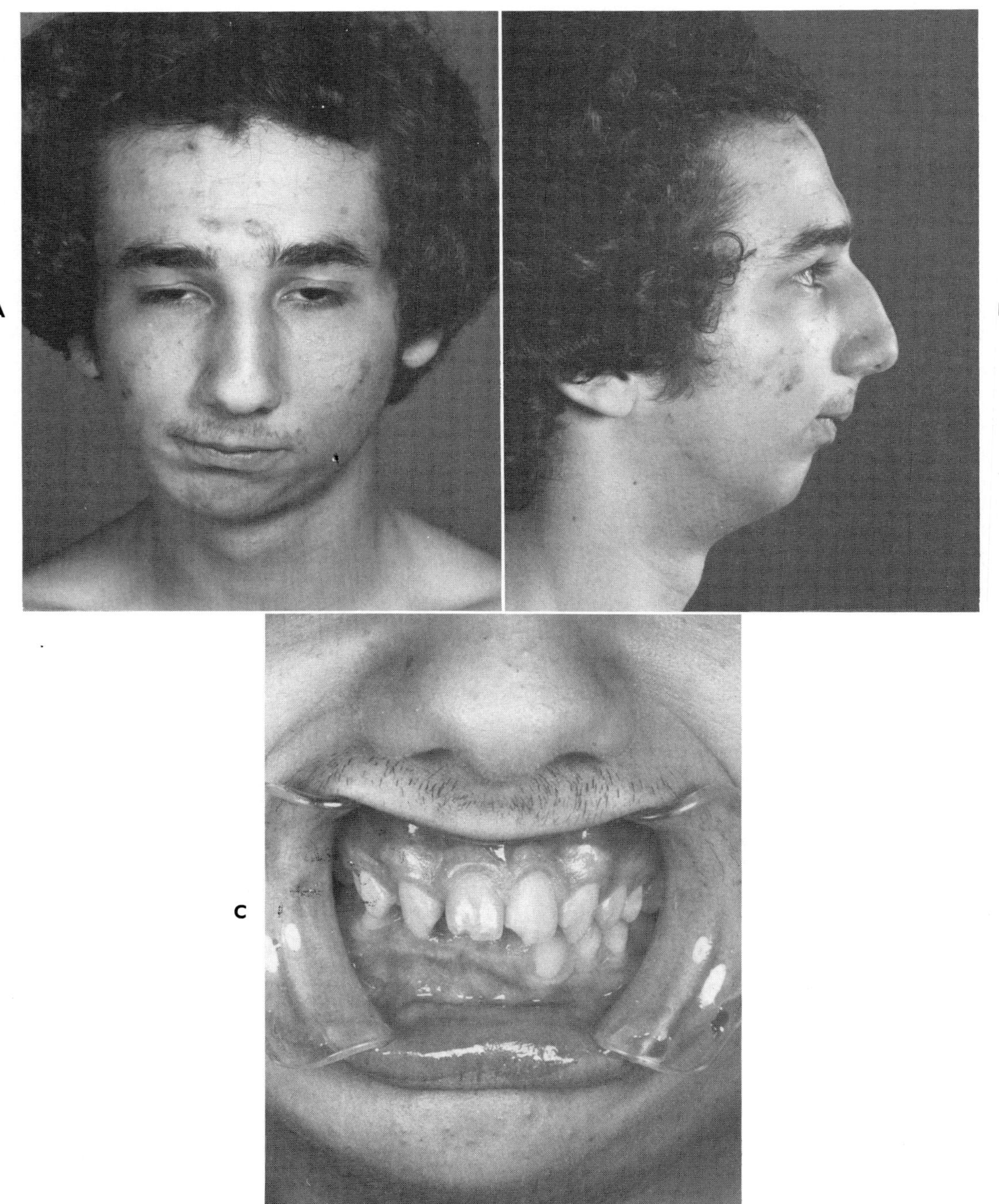

Fig. 29-11. Right-sided craniofacial microsomia. **A** to **C,** Preoperative views.

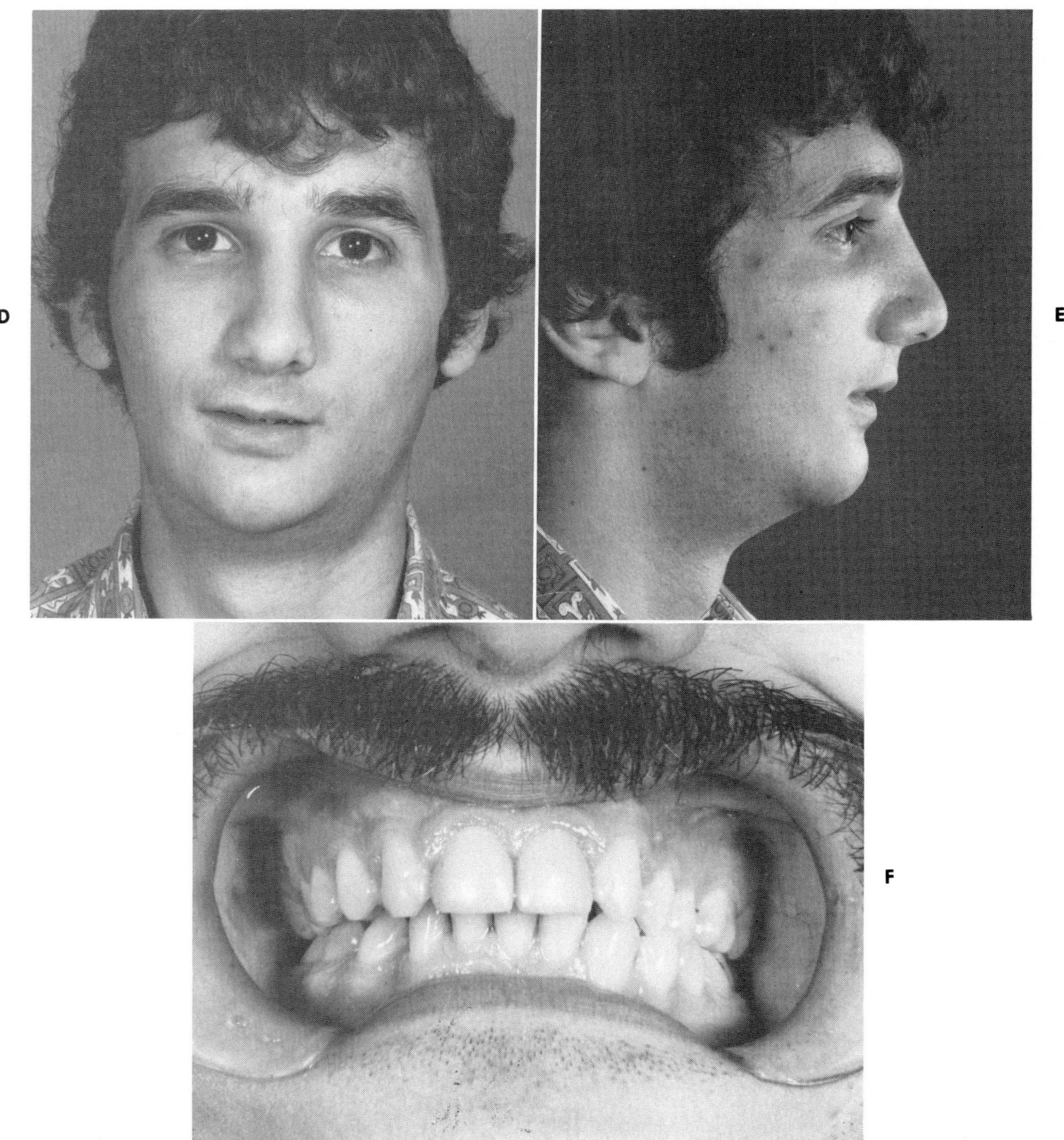

Fig. 29-11, cont'd. D to **F,** Appearance after technique illustrated in Fig. 29-10. In addition, the patient underwent a corrective nasoplasty and dental restoration.

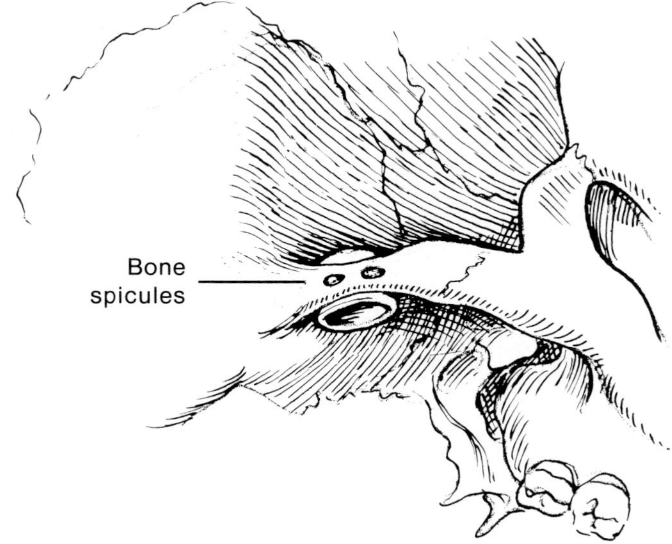

Fig. 29-12. Reconstruction of the temporomandibular joint with a costochondral rib graft.[6] (From Converse, J.M.: Reconstructive plastic surgery, ed. 2, Philadelphia, 1977, W.B. Saunders Co.)

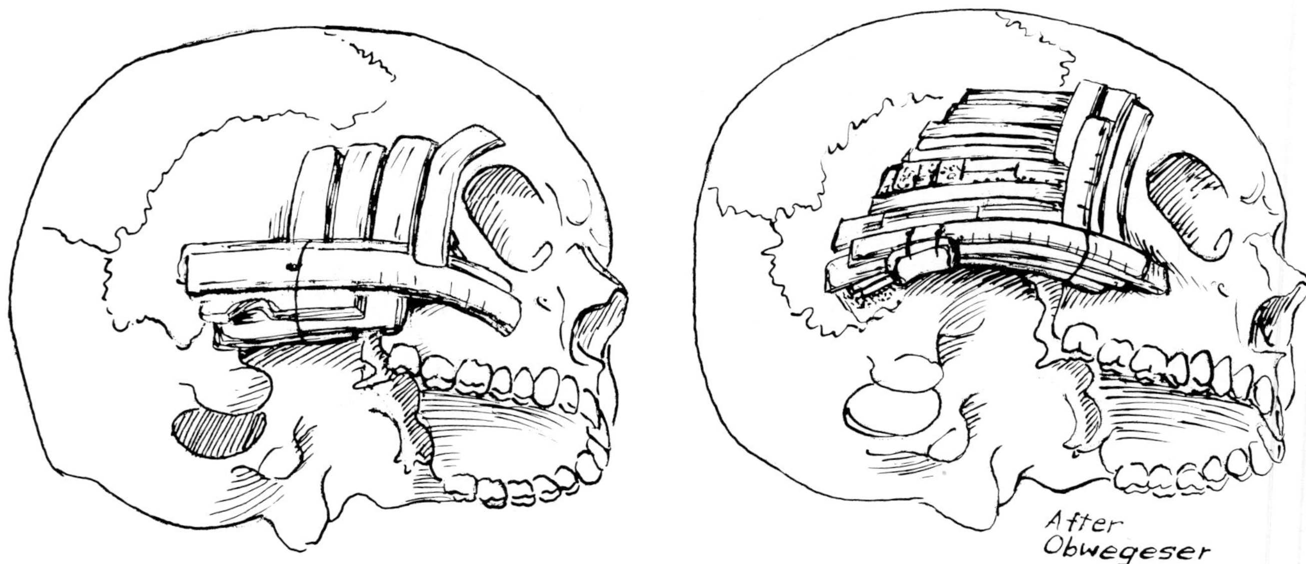

Fig. 29-13. Correction of hypoplasia of the temporal bone, zygomatic arch, and lateral orbital rim with onlay bone grafts. This has been combined with temporomandibular joint reconstruction by Obwegeser[29] as illustrated in Fig. 29-12. (From Converse, J.M.: Reconstructive plastic surgery, ed. 2, Philadelphia, 1977, W.B. Saunders Co.)

surgical relapse may be reduced if a satisfactory functional matrix can be obtained—the principle of functional matrix therapy.[11] For example, in the absence of a mandibular ramus, the mandible should first be positioned before surgery in its proper functional relationship with the aid of occlusal or other types of appliances. This should be done sufficiently early to allow for presurgical adaptation of the connective tissue and muscle to what will be the desired position of the mandible after surgery. With this approach the surgically repositioned bony fragment will be placed in the desired functional matrix to establish an equilibrium between form and function. Functional stimulation also will be provided postsurgically to induce osseous replacement of the bone graft and reduce the incidence of bone graft resorption and skeletal relapse.

The Frankel appliance,[13] which is one of the more commonly employed functional therapy prostheses, consists of a wire framework that supports acrylic shields in the buccal vestibule and lingopalatal alveolus. Since the shields are positioned in the vestibule, a direct interference with the soft tissue curtain of the cheeks and lips is provided. As a mechanical effect of the projecting vestibular screens, and expansion of the soft tissue capsule may be expected. In addition, the device in the vestibule adds a new sensory input that may produce adaptive changes in the neuromuscular behavior of the perioral soft tissues. Since the vestibular shields can be viewed as a corrected configuration of the dentoalveolar process, the appliance trains the orofacial musculature at the subconscious level. Thus a faulty pattern of muscular behavior can be corrected as the result of spontaneous adaptation to the artificially altered dentoalveolar process. The morphologic skeletal alterations therefore can be explained only as the result of a primary interference with the functional (soft tissue/neuromuscular) environment.

Skeletal surgery

A metatarsal head transplant, as a substitute for the missing mandibular condyle, has been advocated.[16] Others who used this procedure at an early age found little or no growth of the grafts and no particular improvement in joint function.[9,14]

Converse[5] operated on a 12-year-old patient with the jaw deformity of craniofacial microsomia. A horizontal osteotomy of the ramus was performed above the inferior alveolar foramen, and an iliac bone graft was inserted between the fragments after the placement of a bite block to open the occlusion on the affected side.

Delaire[8] recommended even earlier intervention (4 to 6 years of age). He elongated the shorter ramus with an inverted L-osteotomy and inserted costal bone grafts into the gap formed at the horizontal branch of the L.

Converse et al.[6] subsequently advocated a two-stage procedure during childhood. In the first stage, usually done when the child is 8 or 9 years old and in the mixed dentition period, the vertical and horizontal hypoplasia of the malformed half of the mandible is corrected. A bilateral vertical osteotomy through the ramus is performed, permitting a forward, lateral, and downward movement of the malformed mandibular body toward the unaffected side (Fig. 29-14). The skeletal rotation and displacement result in a bony gap in the deficient ramus on the affected side, reflecting the amount of downward and medial displacement of the mandibular body. Interposition iliac bone grafts are placed in the defect and maintained in position by wedging them between the fragments and securing them with interosseous stainless steel wires. The inferior displacement on the affected side results in a posterior open bite that is filled with a specially fabricated bite block.

The second stage of the corrective treatment is undertaken during adolescence and completes the treatment. Although the first stage achieves satisfactory occlusal relationships between the maxillary and mandibular dentoalveolar arches, the mandible usually remains asymmetric because of the disparity in shape of the two halves of the bone. Disproportionate growth between the affected and unaffected halves of the mandible also cause varying degrees of asymmetry and malocclusion. It is during the second stage of the treatment that final symmetry, definitive occlusion, and mandibular contour are achieved (Fig. 29-15).

Interval between the first and second stages

After a period of 10 to 12 weeks the bite block is removed; a second occlusal guide plane is placed over the biting surfaces of the molar teeth on the affected side. This serves (1) to maintain the newly acquired mandibular position and to counter any muscular pull that tends to deviate the mandible toward the unaffected side and (2) to maintain the interocclusal space established on the affected side by the osteotomy.

During this interim period of growth and development orthodontic bands and arch-wire appliances are placed on the molar and incisor teeth of the maxilla and mandible. They correct incisor relationships, maintain adequate arch length, and permit management of the maxillary premolars as they emerge into the interdental space. In this way there is an inferior movement of the maxillary occlusal plane on the affected side.

Second stage

The second surgical stage is completed during adolescence and requires one or more operative procedures. Although the osteotomy of the first stage may have produced a degree of symmetry, one cannot expect symmetric growth of both halves of the mandible. The disparity of growth between the bone-grafted half and the unaffected half requires that additional surgery be performed to achieve satisfactory contour. The following are three procedures that may be indicated in this situation:

1. Onlay bone grafts may be placed over the deficient side of the mandible, maxilla, zygoma, or temporal bone at any time during the period of growth.

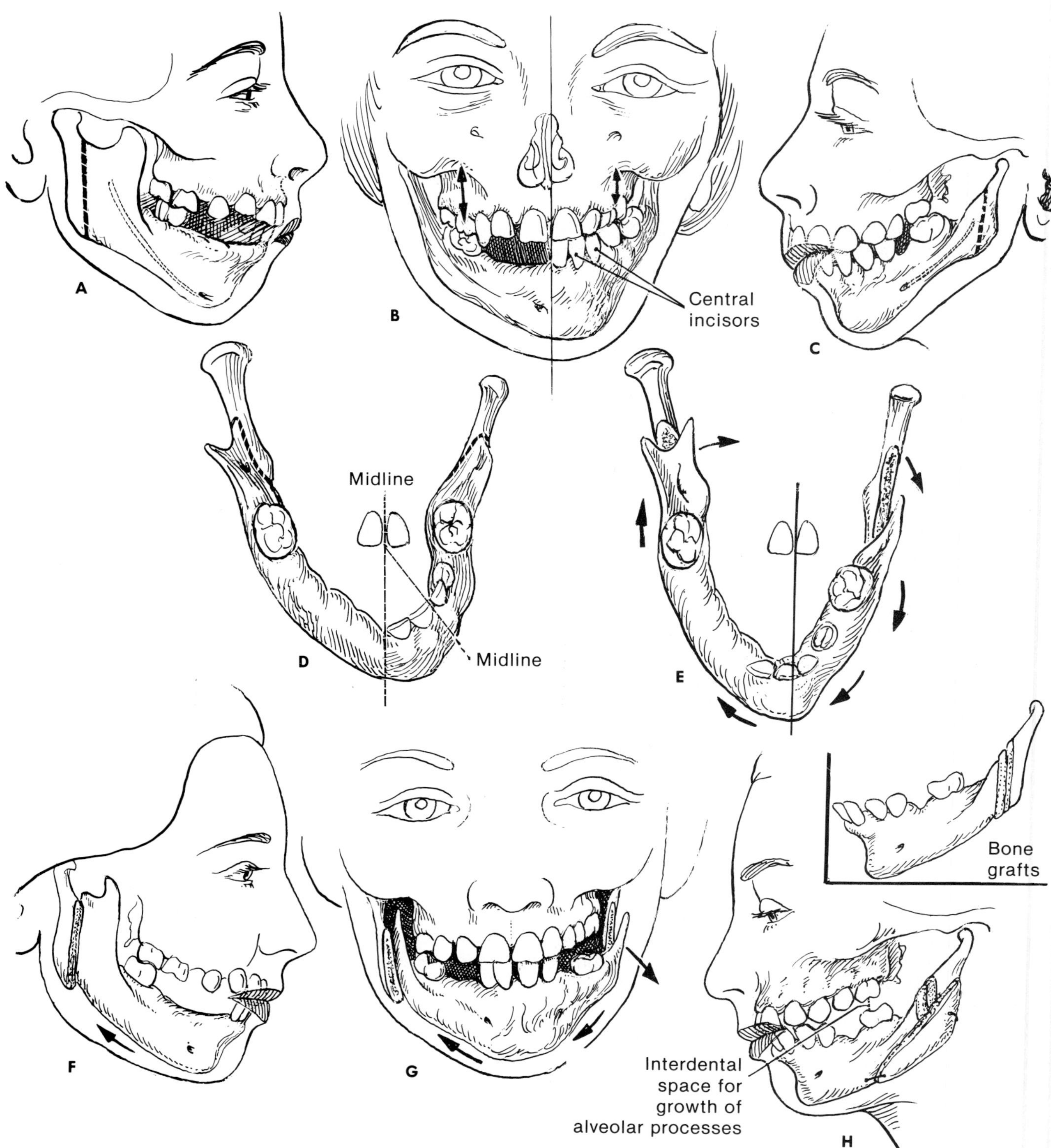

Fig. 29-14. Bilateral osteotomy of the rami for correction of unilateral craniofacial microsomia. **A,** Outline of the vertical osteotomy on the unaffected side. **B,** Note the deviation of the mandible toward the hypoplastic side. **C,** Osteotomy through the malformed ramus. **D,** The original position of the two central mandibular incisor teeth (to the left of the midline). **E,** After rotation of the lower jaw toward the right and lowering the occlusal plane on the left (by bilateral osteotomy). **F,** In some cases the extent of the rotation toward the unaffected side results in an overlap between the fragments. In other cases a gap may develop and require bone grafting. **G,** New position of the mandible. Note the interocclusal space maintained on the left side. Arrows designate the direction of mobilization of the mandible. **H,** Bone grafts fill the defects and restore contour. (From Converse, J.M.: Reconstructive plastic surgery, ed. 2, Philadelphia, 1977, W.B. Saunders Co.)

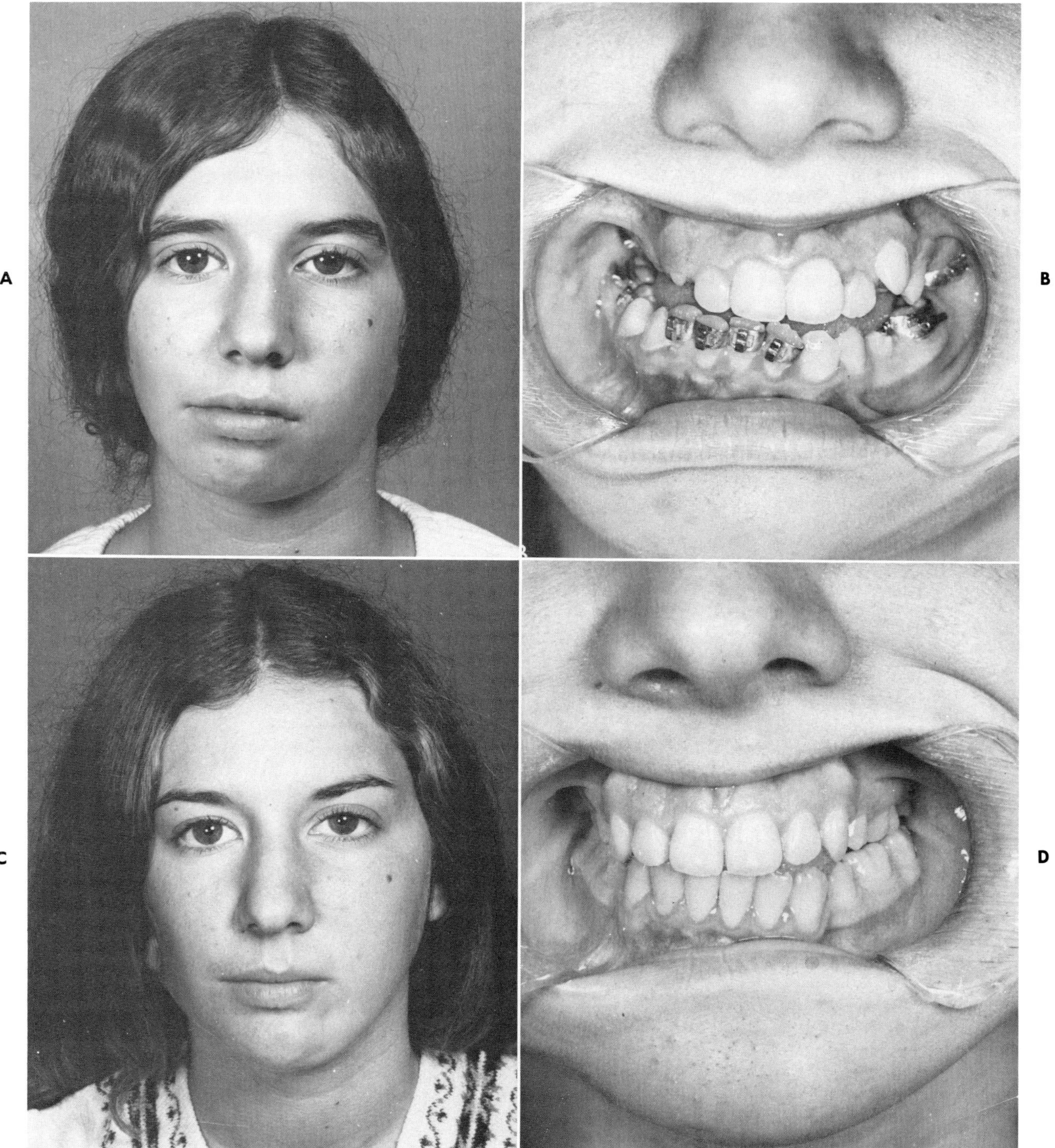

Fig. 29-15. A, A 14-year-old girl with right-sided hemicraniofacial microsomia. Note the oblique cant of the oral fissure. **B,** Occlusal view. **C** and **D,** Appearance 2½ years after surgery (see Fig. 29-14) and orthodontic therapy. Patient is 17 years of age. (From Converse, J.M.: Reconstructive plastic surgery, ed. 2, Philadelphia, 1977, W.B. Saunders Co.)

2. A horizontal advancement osteotomy of the antero-inferior portion of the body of the mandible (genioplasty) is usually indicated. The horizontal advancement osteotomy may have to be combined with placement of iliac bone as onlay grafts over the deficient half of the mandible.

3. Because of the disparity in growth between the grafted half of mandible and the unaffected half, elongation by a second bilateral osteotomy of the rami with bone grafting may be required. A LeFort I osteotomy, which is not feasible at the first stage because of the presence of tooth buds of the secondary dentition in the maxilla, becomes a practical surgical procedure during adolescence. (See Fig. 29-10.)

RESTORATION OF SOFT TISSUE CONTOUR

Soft tissue hypoplasia is a characteristic feature of the syndrome. The soft tissue hypoplasia is usually not as severe or diffuse as in hemifacial atrophy (Romberg's disease). It is usually most conspicuous in the parotid-masseteric and auriculomastoid areas. Hypoplasia of the facial musculature of expression or congenital facial paralysis compounds the contour deficit. Temporal muscle transfers provide animation to the face and also add bulk to the deficient areas. Improvement in the soft tissue deficiency has been obtained by insertion of a de-epithelialized tube flap in the preauricular area or a dermis-fat graft introduced subcutaneously (Fig. 29-16).[38] Additional contour can be obtained by limited serial injection of silicone fluid. De-epithelialized microvascular free flaps of dermis and fat have gained wide acceptance for one-stage correction of severe soft tissue deficits.[15]

SUMMARY AND CONCLUSIONS

Both unilateral and bilateral craniofacial microsomia are manifestations of the first and second branchial arch syndrome. Bilateral involvement can be observed in approximately 6% to 16% of all cases. In the severe form, all of the structures derived from the first and second branchial arches are hypoplastic. Microforms of this syndrome are more frequent and are generally acknowledged.

The etiopathogenesis has not been satisfactorily explained to date. Mesodermal deficiency, stapedial artery thrombosis, and embryonic hemorrhage have all been described to account for the malformation.

The deformity in unilateral craniofacial microsomia usually has three major features: auricular, mandibular, and maxillary hypoplasia. In addition to the skeletal deficiency, varying amounts of soft tissue hypoplasia and cranial nerve paralysis can also coexist. The most conspicuous deformity

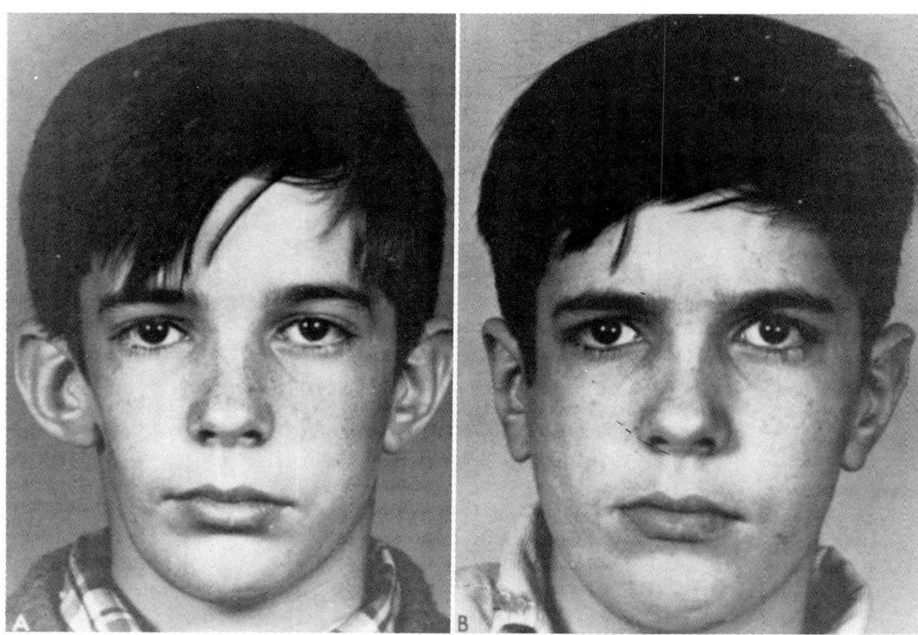

Fig. 29-16. Forme fruste of unilateral craniofacial microsomia. **A,** Preoperative view. Note that the deformity is limited to the soft tissues in the region of the right parotid-masseteric region, the protruding auricle, and macrostomia of the right oral commissure. **B,** Appearance after insertion of a dermis-fat graft in the parotid-masseteric region, otoplasty, and correction of the macrostomia. (From Converse, J.M., McCarthy, J.G., Coccaro, P.J., and Wood-Smith, D.: Clinical aspects of craniofacial microsomia. In Converse, J.M., McCarthy, J.G., and Wood-Smith, D., editors: Symposium on diagnosis and treatment of craniofacial anomalies, St. Louis, 1979, The C.V. Mosby Co.)

of unilateral craniofacial microsomia is hypoplasia of the mandible on the affected side. Ramus and condyle malformations vary from minimal hypoplasia of the condyle to its complete absence in association with hypoplasia or agenesis of the ramus. The skeletal asymmetry is clinically demonstrated by the high occlusion on the affected side. Hypoplasia of the muscles of mastication also contribute to the generalized contour deficiency on the affected side. Auricular malformations are a usual manifestation of the syndrome. It was observed that the degree of auricular deformity does not correlate exactly with hearing function. A direct relationship exist, however, between the degree of severity of the auricular malformation and the ipsilateral mandibular deformity. The most common nerve anomaly is facial paralysis secondary to agenesis of the facial muscles, aberrant pathways of the facial nerve in the temporal bone, or hypoplasia of the intracranial portion of the facial nerve and facial nucleus in the brainstem.

Surgery is recommended during childhood with the following objectives: (1) improving the symmetry of the mandible, (2) providing interdental space for downgrowth of the maxilla by lengthening the shortened mandibular ramus, (3) restoring an adequate dental occlusion, and (4) expanding the facial skeleton at an early age to fill out the soft tissues on the affected side of the face. Treatment in the child is predicated on obtaining a satisfactory functional matrix. This can be accomplished with various appliances that exert mechanical effects on adjacent soft tissue and correct faulty patterns of muscular behavior. A two-stage procedure during childhood is advocated. The first stage is usually done when the child is 8 or 9 years old, and in the mixed dentition period the vertical and horizontal hypoplasia of the malformed half of the mandible is corrected. The second stage is undertaken during adolescence. It is during this stage that final symmetry, definitive occlusion, and mandibular contour are achieved. Emphasis in surgical treatment is predicated on precise presurgical planning, correction of skeletal abnormalities, and modification of surrounding soft tissue.

REFERENCES

1. Arey, L.B.: Developmental anatomy, ed. 5, Philadelphia, 1946, W.B. Saunders Co.
2. Bartholinus, T.: Historiarum anatomicarum et medicarum rariorum, centuriae VI, Historia 36, Hafniae, 1654.
3. Caronni, E.P.: Embryogenesis and classification of branchial auricular dysplasia. In Transactions of the Fifth International Congress of Plastic Surgery, Melbourne, 1971, Butterworths Pty., Ltd.
4. Coccaro, P.J., and Becker, M.H.: Bilateral facial microsomia: diagnosis, classification, treatment, Plast. Reconstr. Surg. **54:**413, 1974.
5. Converse, J.M.: Reconstructive plastic surgery, Philadelphia, 1977, W.B. Saunders Co.
6. Converse, J.M., Horowitz, S.L., Cocaro, P.J., and Wood-Smith, D.: Corrective treatment of the skeletal asymmetry in hemifacial microsomia, Plast. Reconstr. Surg. **52:**221, 1973.
7. Converse, J.M., and Shapiro, H.H.: Treatment of developmental malformations of the jaws, Plast Reconstr. Surg. **19:**473, 1952.
8. Delaire, J.: De Pinteret des osteotomies sagittales dans la correction des infragnathies mandibulaires, Ann. Chir. Plast. **15:**104, 1970.
9. Dingman, R.O., and Grabb, W.C.: Reconstruction of both mandibular condyles with metatarsal bone grafts, Plast. Reconstr. Surg. **43:**441, 1964.
10. Dupertuis, S.M., and Musgrave, R.H.: Experiences with the reconstruction of the congenitally deformed ear, Plast. Reconstr. Surg. **23:**361, 1959.
11. Enlow, D.H., and Harvold, E.P.: Research on control of craniofacial morphogenesis, NIDR State of the Art Workshop, Am. J. Orthod. **71:**509, 1977.
12. François, J.: Heredity in ophthalmology, St. Louis, 1961, The C.V. Mosby Co.
13. Frankel, R.: Decrowding during eruption under the screening influence of vestibular shields, Am. J. Orthod. **65:**372, 1974.
14. Freeman, B.S.: The result of epiphyseal transplants by flap and by free grafts: a brief survey, Plast. Reconstr. Surg. **36:**227, 1965.
15. Fujino, T., Rytinzaburo, T., and Sugimoto, C.: Microvascular transfer of free deltopectoral dermal-fat flap, Plast. Reconstr. Surg. **55:**428, 1975.
16. Glahn, M., and Winther, J.E.: Metatarsal transplants as replacement for lost mandibular condyle (3 year follow-up), Scand. J. Plast. Reconstr. Surg. **1:**97, 1967.
17. Gorlin, R.J., and Pindborg, J.J.: Syndromes of the head and neck, New York, 1964, McGraw-Hill Book Co.
18. Grabb, W.C.: The first and second branchial arch syndrome, Plast. Reconstr. Surg. **36:**485, 1965.
19. Hanhart, E.: Nachweis einer einfach-dominanten, mit Atresia auris, Palatoschisis und anderen Deformationen verbundenen Anlage zu Ohrmuschelverkummerung (Mikrotie), Arch. Julius Klaus-Stift. **24:**374, 1949.
20. Kazanjian, V.H.: Congenital absence of ramus of mandible, J. Bone Joint Surg. **21:**761, 1939.
21. Kleinsasser, O., and Schlothane, R.: Die Ohrmissbildungen im Rahmen der Thalidomid-Embryopathie, Z. Laryngol. Rhinol. Otol. **43:**344, 1964.
22. Lachmund, F.: Occlusion of the right ear, Miscell. Acad. Nat. Curios. **6-7:**225, 1688.
23. Longacre, J.J., DeStefano, G.A., and Holmstrand, K.E.: The early versus the late reconstruction of congenital hypoplasias of the facial skeleton and skull, Plast. Reconstr. Surg. **27:**489, 1961.
24. Lunberg, A.A.: New method of plastic lengthening of the mandible in unilateral micrognathism and asymmetry of the face, J. Am. Dent. Assoc. **15:**581, 1928.
25. McKenzie, J., and Craig, J.:Mandibulofacial dysostosis, Arch. Dis. Child. **30:**391, 1955.
26. Meurmann, Y.: Congenital microtia and meatal atresia, Arch. Otolaryngol. **66:**443, 1957.
27. Moss, M.L.: The primacy of functional matrices in orofacial growth, Dent. Pract. Dent. Rec. **19:**65, 1968.
28. Obwegeser, H.: Zur Korrektur der Dysostosis otomandibularis, Schweiz. Mschr. Zahnheilk. **80:**331, 1970.
29. Obwegeser, H.L.: Correction of the skeletal anomalies of otomandibular dysostosis, J. Maxillofac. Surg. **2:**73, 1974.
30. Ortiz-Monasterio, F.: Paper presented at the International Symposium of Craniofacial Surgery, Rome, 1982.
31. Poswillo, D.E.: Otomandibular deformity: pathogenesis as a guide to reconstruction, J. Maxillofac. Surg. **2:**64, 1974.
32. Pruzansky, S.: Not all dwarfed mandibles are alike, Birth Defects **2:**120, 1969.
33. Pruzansky, S.: Findings of hemifacial microsomia, Presented at the First International Symposium of Craniofacial Anomalies, New York University Medical Center, 1971.
34. Rogers, B.O.: Microtic, lop, cup and protruding ears: four directly inheritable deformities? Plast. Reconstr. Surg. **41:**208, 1968.
35. Stark, R.B., and Saunders, D.E.: The first branchial syndrome: the oral-mandibular-auricular syndrome, Plast. Reconstr. Surg. **29:**229, 1962.
36. Summitt, R.: Familial Goldenhar syndrome, Birth Defects **2:**106, 1969.
37. Thompson, A.: A description of congenital malformation of the auricle and external meatus of both sides in three persons. Proc. R. Soc. Edinburgh **1:**443, 1845.
38. Wells, J.H., and Edgerton, M.T.: Correction of severe hemifacial atrophy with a free dermis-fat flap from the lower abdomen, Plast. Reconstr. Surg. **59:**223, 1977.

CHAPTER 30

Facial fractures in children

RONALD RIEFKOHL and NICHOLAS G. GEORGIADE

Facial fractures in children are uncommon for reasons related to both environmental-social and anatomic factors. The low frequency of facial fractures in children is fortunate, since proper management presents special problems that are not encountered in the adult patient.[4] Most children are frightened and apprehensive after an injury and may be unable to fully cooperate with the evaluation and treatment unless they are sedated, at times with a general anesthetic. Because of the absence of retentive teeth, intermaxillary fixation that relies on attachment only to the teeth will be tenuous. Fractures in children heal more rapidly than in adults; thus earlier reduction and fixation is mandatory. Furthermore, there may be unknown effects of the injury and treatment on facial growth, although, in general, some evidence suggests that proper treatment of even severe facial fractures will prevent later deformity as a result of growth disturbances.[2]

FREQUENCY OF FRACTURES IN CHILDREN

There is abundant documentation in the literature of the low frequency of facial fractures in children, indicating that approximately 1.4% to 10% of all facial fractures occur before the age of 16.[2,6] Rowe,[15] summarizing the literature in 1969, found that 1% of all facial fractures occurred in children under 6 and 5% occurred in children under 12. Of the facial fractures occurring in children under 12, 10% involved the midface, but midface fractures were extremely uncommon in children under 8.

Rowe[14] later reviewed 1500 facial fractures and found that only 77 fractures involved children under 12. McCoy, Chandler, and Crow[10] reviewed another group of 1500 facial fractures and found that only 86 fractures occurred between the ages of 6 months and 14 years. Panagopoulos[12] found only 22 instances of fractures of the jaws in children in a series of 1500 jaw fractures. Among 2386 facial fractures treated by Schultz over an 11-year period, 188 patients were less than 16 years of age. Of these, 8% were less than 5 years of age.[17]

The two projecting areas of the face, the nose and the mandible, are the bones most frequently fractured. Mandibular fractures comprised 41% of the total fractures and nasal fractures 23% in the series of McCoy, Chandler, and Crow,[10] whereas in the series of Kaban, Mulliken, and Murray,[7] mandibular fractures comprised 32% and nasal fractures 45%. McCoy reported an incidence of 8.1% for fractures of the maxilla, 4.7% for zygomatic fractures, and 16.3% for orbital or zygomatic fractures.

CAUSATIVE FACTORS

It is possible that intrauterine compression could result in a facial fracture, although this has not been documented. Facial fracture may rarely occur during delivery by disruption of the symphysis of the mandible as a consequence of traction on the jaw by the obstetrician.[1] However, bone injury is usually minimal and reversible, even when caused by obstetric forceps, because of the pliability of the bones and their segmental arrangement.

Serious falls during infancy are apparently more common than previously realized[8] and are usually forgotten by the family. It is possible that a deformity may be the consequence of a previous fall.

Although adults have a high incidence of facial fractures associated with assaults, this is the cause in only 10% of childhood fractures.[7,10] Facial fractures associated with automobile accidents, with the injury occurring as either a passenger during a collision or as a pedestrian, accounted for 45% of the facial fractures in one series,[10] and 17% in another.[7] Falls from high places or while running account for approximately 25% of childhood facial fractures, and athletic or playground activities account for approximately 10%. The remaining causes are miscellaneous freak accidents.

PATHOPHYSIOLOGIC PROCESS OF FACIAL FRACTURES IN CHILDREN

It would be an oversimplification to assume that the low incidence of facial fractures in children is because of their protected environment with its adult supervision. Exposure of children to less hazardous activities is only partly responsible. The facial bones in the developing child are soft and resilient because of cartilaginous growth centers and the greater proportion of cancellous to cortical bone.[1] The bones are not yet weakened by paranasal sinus development or by permanent dentition. The medullocortical junction is indistinct; thus the fracture pathway will be more irregular, resulting in a green-stick–type fracture. Also the overlying facial soft tissues are considerably thicker compared to the adult, there is a high cranium-to-face volume ratio, and the smaller mass of the head and face reduces the momentum force on impact.

EMERGENCY ROOM ASSESSMENT

The first treatment obligations are to secure an adequate airway and control and treat hemorrhage. Because of the small diameter of the trachea and larynx in children, only a minor degree of mucosal edema will cause respiratory difficulty. The small hypopharynx may be easily obstructed by the tongue if the tongue's anterior support is lost. If there is respiratory difficulty, remove any blood clots, vomitus, teeth, or foreign bodies from the oropharynx, and position the child face down with the head turned to one side. If this is ineffective, try inserting a nasopharyngeal airway. A tongue suture or clamp to retract the tongue forward also may be necessary. If these measures do not resolve the airway problem or if there is obstruction at the tracheolaryngeal level, a tracheostomy will be necessary. It is preferable to first intubate the trachea with an orotracheal tube; however, this may be impossible. A tracheostomy in a child may be a difficult operation and should not be done indiscriminately because the morbidity and mortality are significant,[11] decannulation may take months to complete, and many of the complications of tracheostomy require subsequent complex surgery for correction.

Because of the small blood volume in children, extensive lacerations may cause hemorrhagic shock, particularly if lacerations involve the scalp. Hemorrhage ordinarily may be controlled with mild pressure; however, a constricting bandage should never be applied.

All pertinent details regarding the circumstances of the injury should be obtained from the family. A reliable description of the accident may provide a good indication of the type of fracture. A considerable amount of clinical information may be obtained by careful questioning of the child, which should help to minimize the manipulation necessary during the physical examination.

An elaborate examination of an injured child is often impractical, and at times only a cursory examination is possible in the emergency room environment. Since parental anxiety will be conveyed to the child, overly anxious parents should be absent during the examination. The examination should be as gentle as possible, handling the child to a minimal degree. The face and jaws, scalp and cranium, neck, extremities, abdomen, and chest are carefully examined. In some children a thorough examination will be impossible without sedation, perhaps even administered as a general anesthetic. However, sedation should not be administered until other serious injuries are assessed.

Children will usually cooperate for radiographic examination; however, the ideal views may not be obtainable, and fractures may not be visible anyway. Maximal information will be provided by right, left, and anteroposterior views of the mandible; a Waters' view; a submental-vertex view; and selected dental views. It is also important to obtain radiographs of the chest, cervical spine, and skull. Polytomograms or CT scans may be necessary to completely define the injury (Fig. 30-5, *C*).

The clinical manifestations of facial fractures in children are similar to those in the adult. Pain and tenderness over any bone in the face should arouse suspicion for an underlying fracture. Periorbital swelling, diplopia, enophthalmos, subcutaneous periorbital emphysema, periorbital ecchymosis, or subscleral hemorrhage may be associated with fractures about the orbit. The inability to open or close the mouth, malocclusion, avulsed or loose teeth, submucosal hematomas, or mucosal lacerations are frequently found with fractures of the jaws. If there is a compound wound present, fragments of bone may be visible. Disfigurement from displacement of bone may be evident, or there may be abnormal bone mobility. A history of trauma followed by a nosebleed, dried blood within the nose, nasal obstruction, or a septal hematoma indicate a possible nasal fracture. CSF rhinorrhea is a sign of fracture communicating with the subarachnoid space. Clear fluid draining through the nose may be differentiated from mucus by its protein and sugar content.

ASSOCIATED INJURIES

Injuries other than those of the head and neck must be suspected in all patients, but this is particularly true for victims of motor vehicle accidents, falls, or athletic and playground mishaps. Since the skull-to-face volume ratio is 8:1 at birth and 4:1 at the age of 5 years, it is not surprising that a high incidence of skull fractures is associated with facial fractures in children.[13] In the series by McCoy, Chandler, and Crow,[10] 41% of the patients had an associated skull fracture. The overall incidence of associated injuries other than facial wounds was 57%; concussions occurred in 31%, CSF rhinorrhea in 14%, extremity fractures in 9.3%, closed chest trauma in 5.8%, blinding ocular injuries in 3.6%, vertebral injury in 2.3%, internal abdominal injuries in 2.3%. There were major facial wounds in 49%, and minor facial wounds in 40% of the patients. In the series of patients reported by Kabon, Mulliken, and Murray,[7] 29% of the patients had associated injuries other than facial wounds—70% of these occurred in patients with mandibular fractures.

GENERAL PRINCIPLES OF MANAGEMENT

Because of the high frequency of associated injuries, the definitive treatment of facial fractures may be necessarily postponed. Ideally there should be no compromise in the treatment of the facial injury because of other serious injuries, but a decision regarding the optimal management of the patient will often be influenced by the character of associated injuries and the expected period of recovery.[5] Because facial fractures in children heal rapidly, anatomic reduction should be undertaken as soon as possible, preferably within 3 to 4 days. At the end of 1 week reduction is still possible but extremely difficult, and at the end of 2 weeks reduction will be nearly impossible.

In general, the treatment of facial fractures in children is similar to that for adults. The chief differences relate to the rate of fracture healing; density of bone; and size, shape, and number of teeth available for intermaxillary fixation for fractures of the jaws. Due to the short bulbous crowns of deciduous teeth and little or no undercuts on their buccal and lingual surfaces, the presence of fewer teeth, the inability to determine normal occlusion because of the absence of wear marks, and the incomplete calcification of the roots of permanent teeth, intermaxillary fixation alone usually will not provide adequate immobilization of fractures involving the jaws.[3] With either a deciduous or mixed dentition (ages 6 to 12 years) an acrylic splint should be fabricated from dental models and attached with circumferential wires to the mandible below and above to either the infraorbital rims, piriform aperture, or frontal bones (Fig. 30-3, *G*). Good immobilization still may not be possible without additional internal fixation, which should be accomplished without damaging tooth buds by improper drilling.[1]

Postoperatively oral hygiene may be maintained with flavored mouthwashes or a Water Pik. Elbow restraints may be necessary to prevent young children from handling their wounds. Feedings may be administered through a nasogastric tube or orally by a bulb syringe. Patients with compound fractures or those with severely contaminated wounds should receive a short course of prophylactic antibiotics.

FRACTURES
Fractures of the maxilla

Fractures of the maxilla most commonly occur as a consequence of a blow to one side of the face or may occur during a fall in which the impact is directed to one side of the maxilla.

The maxilla is soft, spongy, and elastic; therefore a high degree of distortion may occur before a fracture results. Also the maxilla is protected by a thick covering of adipose tissue and the projecting cranium and mandible.

The method selected for fracture fixation depends on the number of teeth present with retentive crowns and the state of evolution of the dentition. Because of rapid healing, a nondisplaced fracture may require only a head bandage combined with intermaxillary fixation applied through an acrylic splint that is secured by suspension wires to the piriform aperture.[1]

An acrylic splint is best suspended to the strong piriform aperture or frontal bones, since wires may cut through the soft bone of the inferior orbital rim or zygomatic arches. For some children a plaster headcap with heavy wire outriggers may be used to suspend the acrylic splint externally (Fig. 30-1). Dislodged tooth buds should be carefully replaced in their sockets, since they will often survive.[9]

The typical LeFort-type maxillary fracture lines are uncommon, but low LeFort I or II fractures occasionally occur (Figs. 30-2 and 30-3). The most common fracture is the dentoalveolar type with fracture of either the labial or buccal plates of alveolar bone and consequent loosening of teeth in the fractured segment (Fig. 30-4). If the segment of alveolus and attached teeth is completely avulsed, the deciduous teeth should be removed and the bone replaced as a free graft. If permanent teeth are attached to the fractured segment, these teeth may be secured to any adjacent uninvolved teeth.

Nasal and nasoorbital fractures

Nasal fractures are more common in children than fractures involving the maxilla or zygoma. The diagnosis of nasal fractures may be difficult because of the large amount of cartilage present in the nasal skeleton in young children. A forgotten fracture occurring early in childhood may be

Text continued on p. 525.

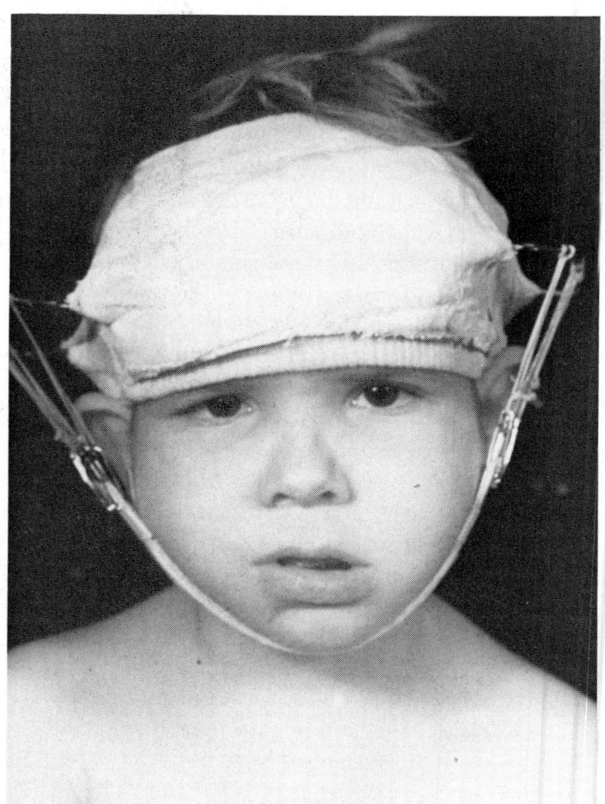

Fig. 30-1. Plaster cap and strap plus intermaxillary fixation method of securing the jaws.

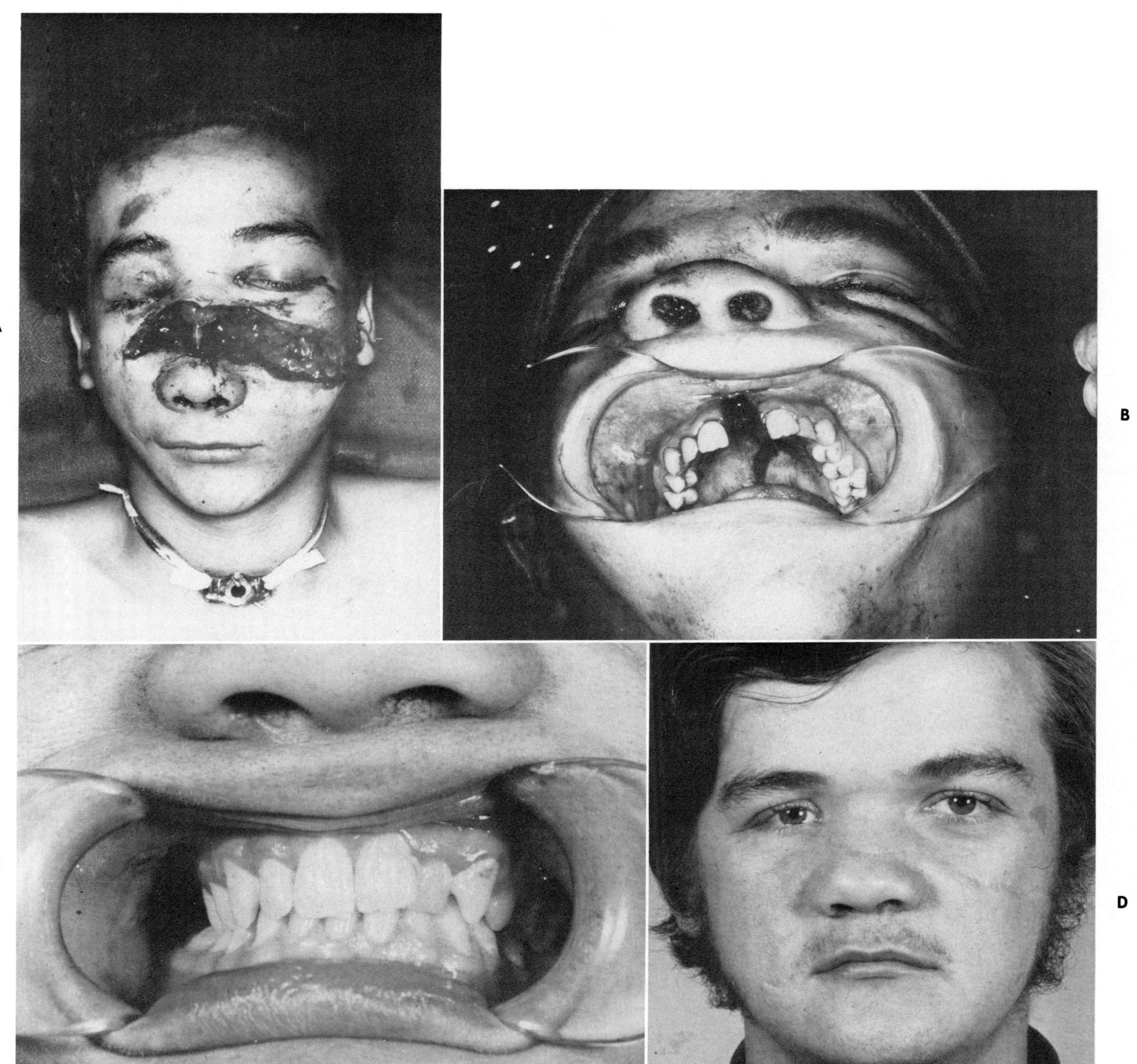

Fig. 30-2. A, This teenage boy sustained compound fracture of the maxilla and nose during automobile accident. **B,** In addition to the transverse maxillary fracture, there was a sagittal fracture through the palate. **C,** Occlusion 1 year after injury. **D,** Appearance of the patient 1 year after injury. (From Georgiade, N.G.: The management of acute midfacial-orbital injuries, Clin. Neurosurg. **19:**301, 1972.)

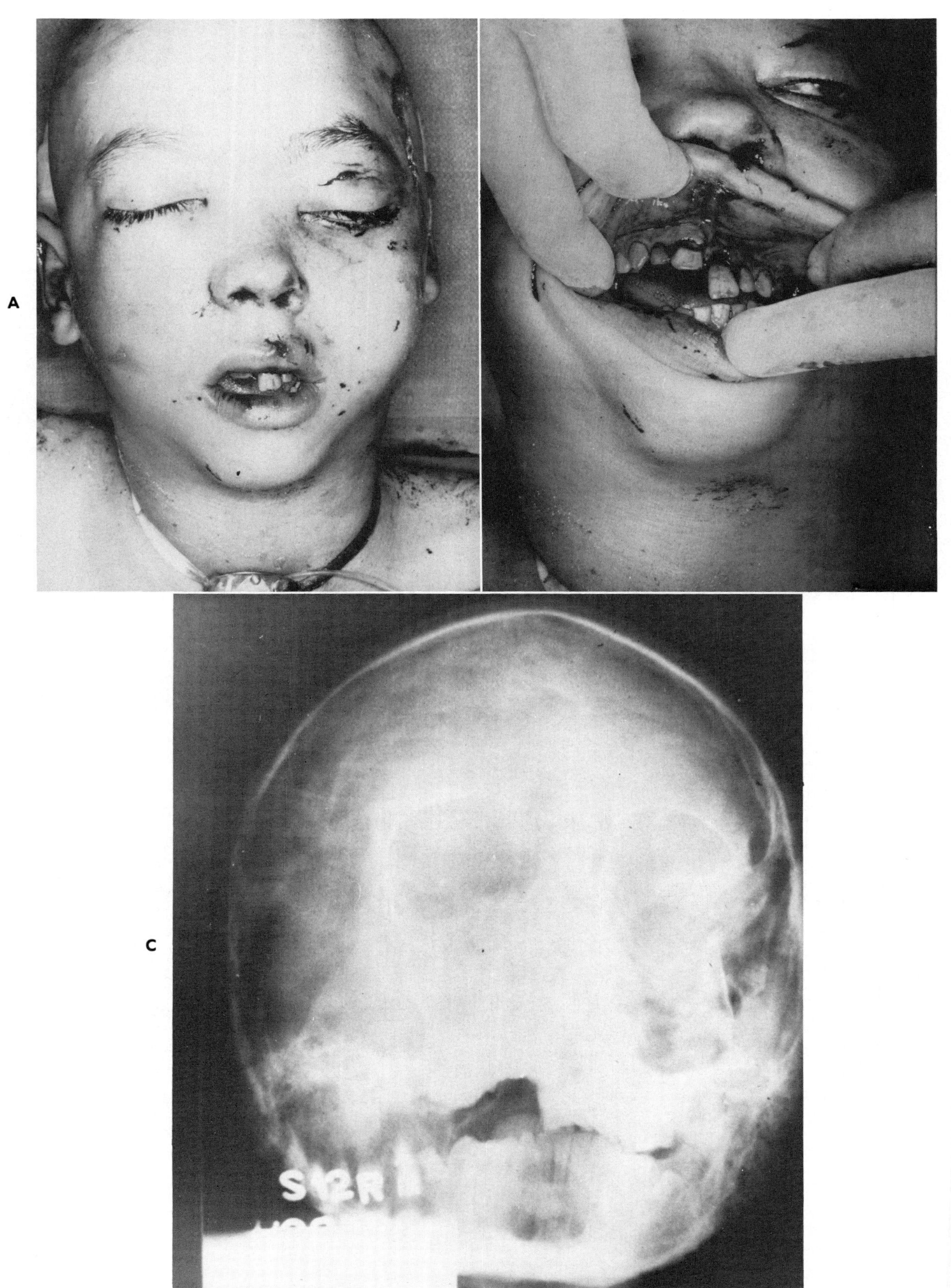

Fig. 30-3. For legend see opposite page.

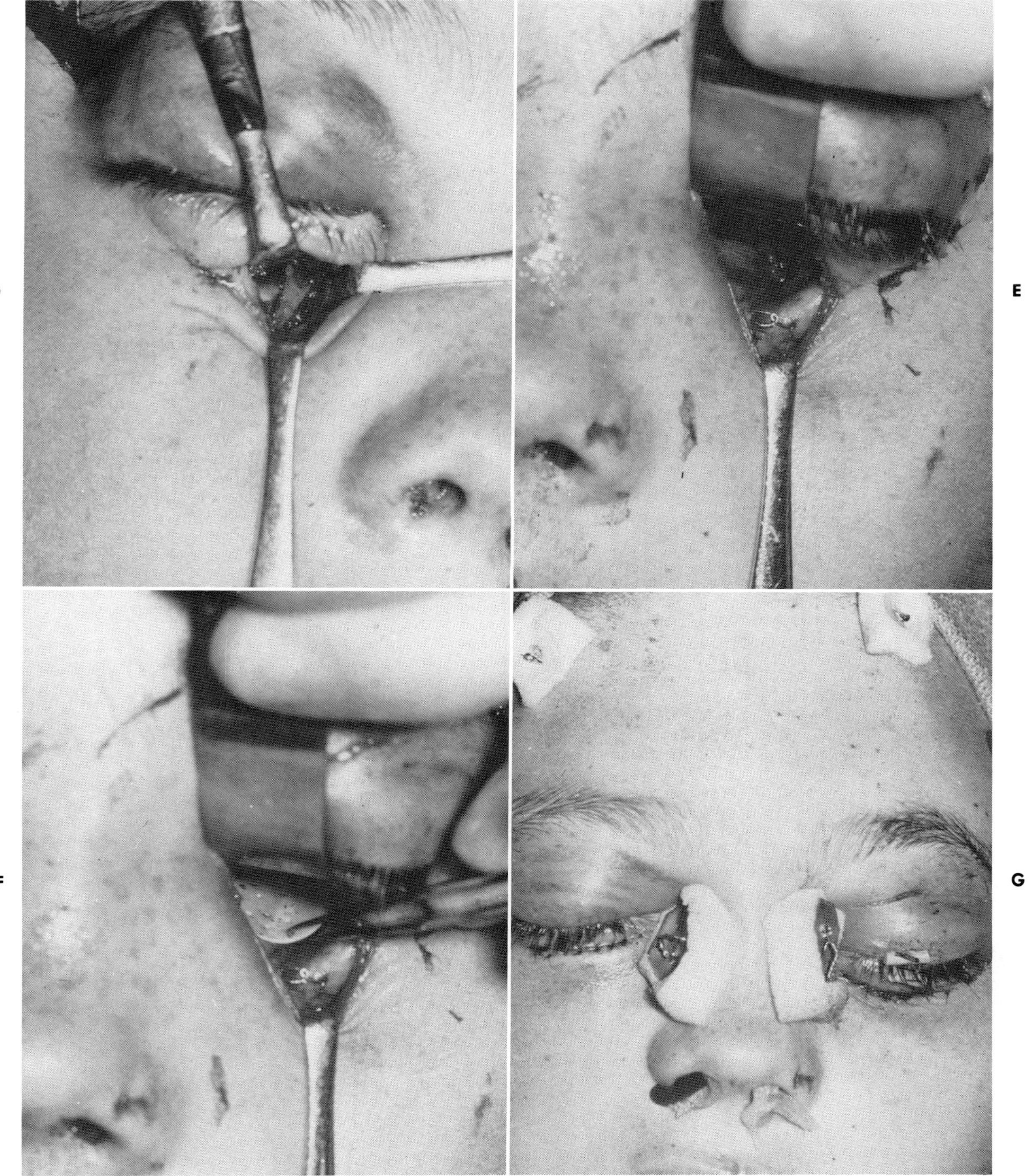

Fig. 30-3. A, This young teenager was involved in a farm tractor accident. He sustained a fracture of the left zygomatic bone, a LeFort II fracture, and a nasoorbital fracture. **B,** In addition to the LeFort fracture, there was a dentoalveolar fracture on the left side. **C,** Radiographs revealed air-fluid level in sphenoidal sinus and fractures involving maxilla, left zygomatic bone, right orbital floor, and nasal bones. There was fluid in both maxillary sinuses. **D,** LeFort II fracture through the right inferior orbital rim. The right suspension "pullout wire" is visible in the left upper corner of the photograph. **E,** The fracture through the left inferior orbital rim has been ligated with a fine wire. **F,** The considerable defect in the floor of the orbit was managed with a thin Teflon wafer. Holes were drilled through the wafer to enable fibrous tissue penetration. **G,** At the completion of procedure, intermaxillary fixation suspension wires have been secured to the zygomatic process of the frontal bones. Looped around these suspension wires are "pullout" wires, which are then brought through the skin high on the forehead and tied over buttons. These pullout wires are used to extract suspension wires. The nasoorbital fracture was secured by a large transnasal wire tied over lead plates. *Continued.*

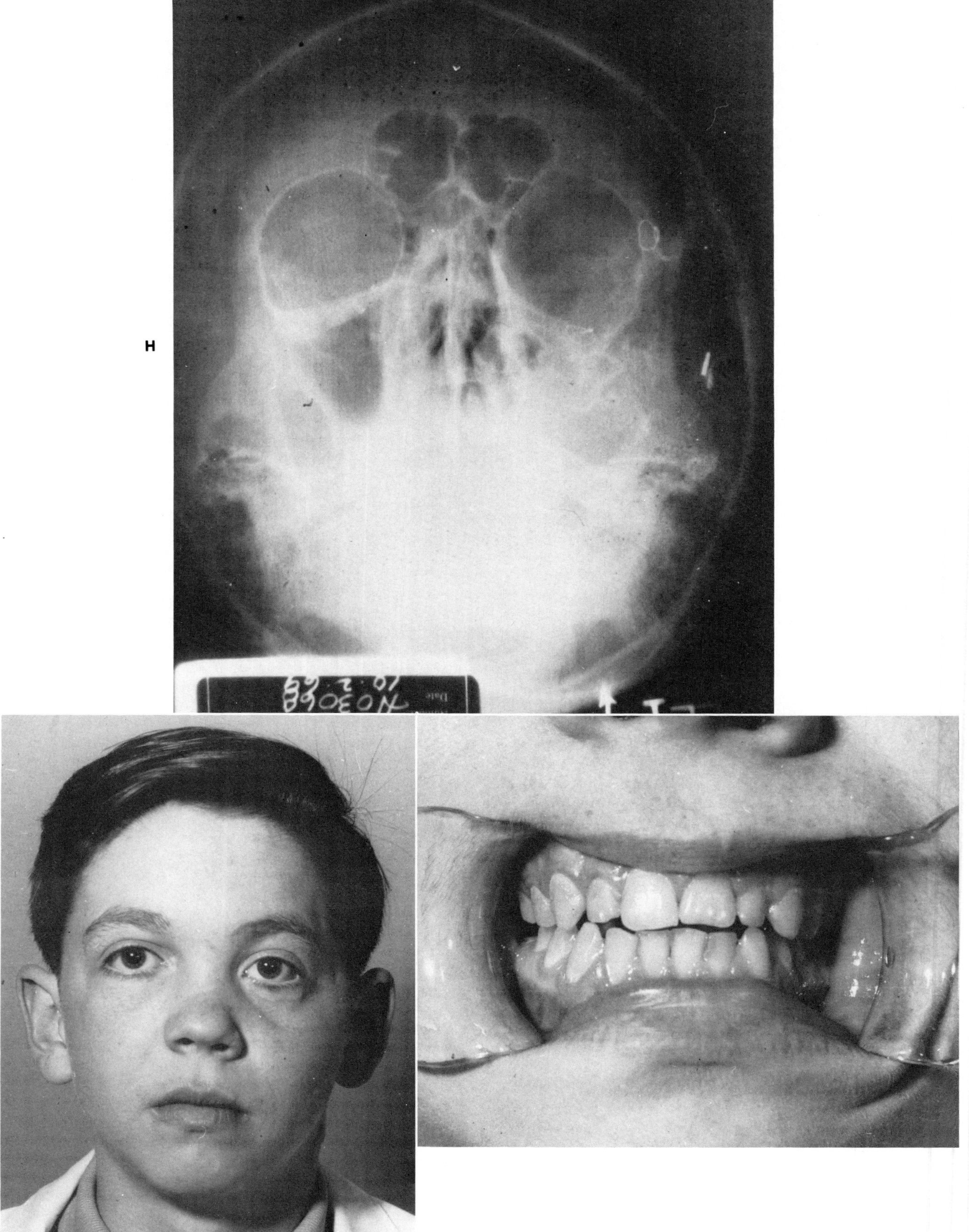

Fig. 30-3, cont'd. **H,** Postoperative radiograph after removal of suspension wires and intermaxillary fixation. **I,** Appearance of the patient 1 year later. **J,** Occlusion 1 year after the surgery.

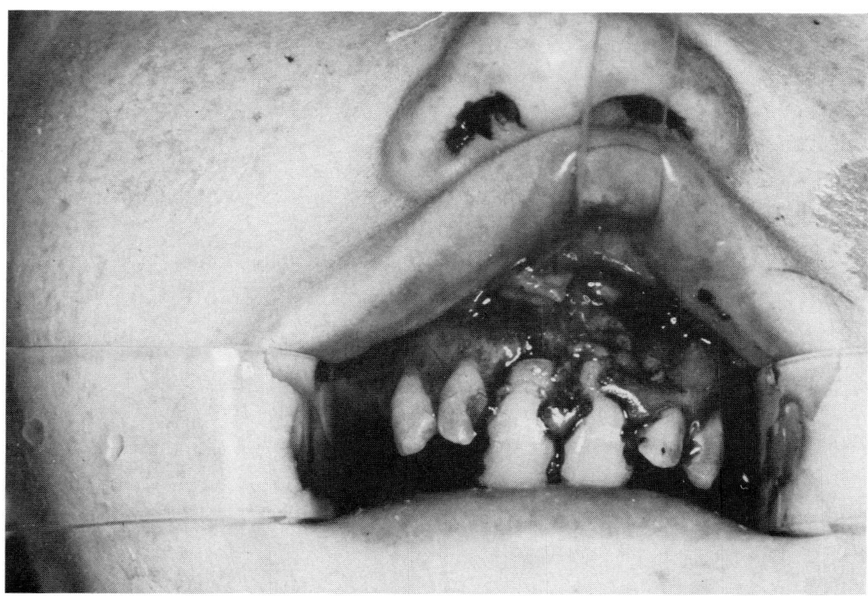

Fig. 30-4. Anterior dentoalveolar fracture.

the cause of later nasal or septal deviation and possibly nasomaxillary hypoplasia.

A septal hematoma, if not recognized, may develop into an abscess that may cause destruction of the septal cartilage and consequently a saddle-nose deformity. Septal hematomas should be managed by drainage incisions through the mucoperichondrium in a dependent portion of the septum. If the hematoma is bilateral, either a small window of cartilage may be removed from the septum or bilateral drainage incisions may be made.

The "open book" type of fracture is commonly seen in children because the midline nasal suture is open. The upper lateral cartilages are loosely attached to the deep surface of the nasal bones and may be easily detached. A hematoma between the upper lateral cartilages and nasal bones should be aspirated to prevent later nasal deformity.

The nasal septum may be either dislocated, fractured, or telescoped on itself. It should be carefully reduced and properly realigned. Nasal fractures are treated with nasal packing and an external splint after careful closed reduction. Since an external splint may not be completely effective in young children, open reduction and internal fixation may be necessary. Nasoorbital fractures should be treated by open reduction and internal fixation (Fig. 30-5, *A* to *E*); otherwise traumatic telecanthus, a saddle-nose deformity, or disturbance in the lacrimal apparatus may result. The fractures are exposed through appropriate incisions and ligated with fine wires (Fig. 30-5, *D* and *E*). Either lead or acrylic plates may be secured on both sides of the nose (Fig. 30-5, *G*), or the bones may be held in proper position by external traction attached to a headcap for 4 weeks.

Orbital fractures

Isolated orbital fractures are fairly uncommon and usually occur in association with zygomatic fractures (Fig. 30-6, *A* and *B*). The blowout fracture of the orbital floor does occur in children despite the small size of the maxillary sinus, and it may be difficult to diagnose with radiography. A fracture of the orbital floor should be treated in the same way as the adult fracture. Often an implant is necessary to maintain the integrity of the orbital floor (Fig. 30-3, *E* and *F*), but the exclusive use of antral packing is improper treatment. Fractures of the supraorbital rim are extremely rare and usually occur in association with severe nasoorbital or frontal bone fractures (Fig. 30-7). Treatment consists of operative reduction and internal fixation with fine wire ligatures (Fig. 30-7, *C* and *D*).

Zygomatic fractures

Zygomatic fractures are also extremely rare in young children; they are more often seen in older children. The zygomatic bone is resilient and may sustain a considerable amount of distortion before fracture or dislocation occurs. Tremendous force is needed to break the zygomatic bone, and it is more commonly fracture-dislocated because its attachment at the frontozygomatic suture is tenuous. Thus the entire zygomatic bone with the orbital floor may be displaced downward. Treatment is identical to that for the adult, although a wire at the inferior orbital rim is frequently unnecessary (Fig. 30-3, *E* and *H*). Even though the maxillary sinus is underdeveloped, prolapse of orbital contents into the sinus may occur. Therefore the orbital floor should be explored whenever it is involved in other fractures.

Text continued on p. 530.

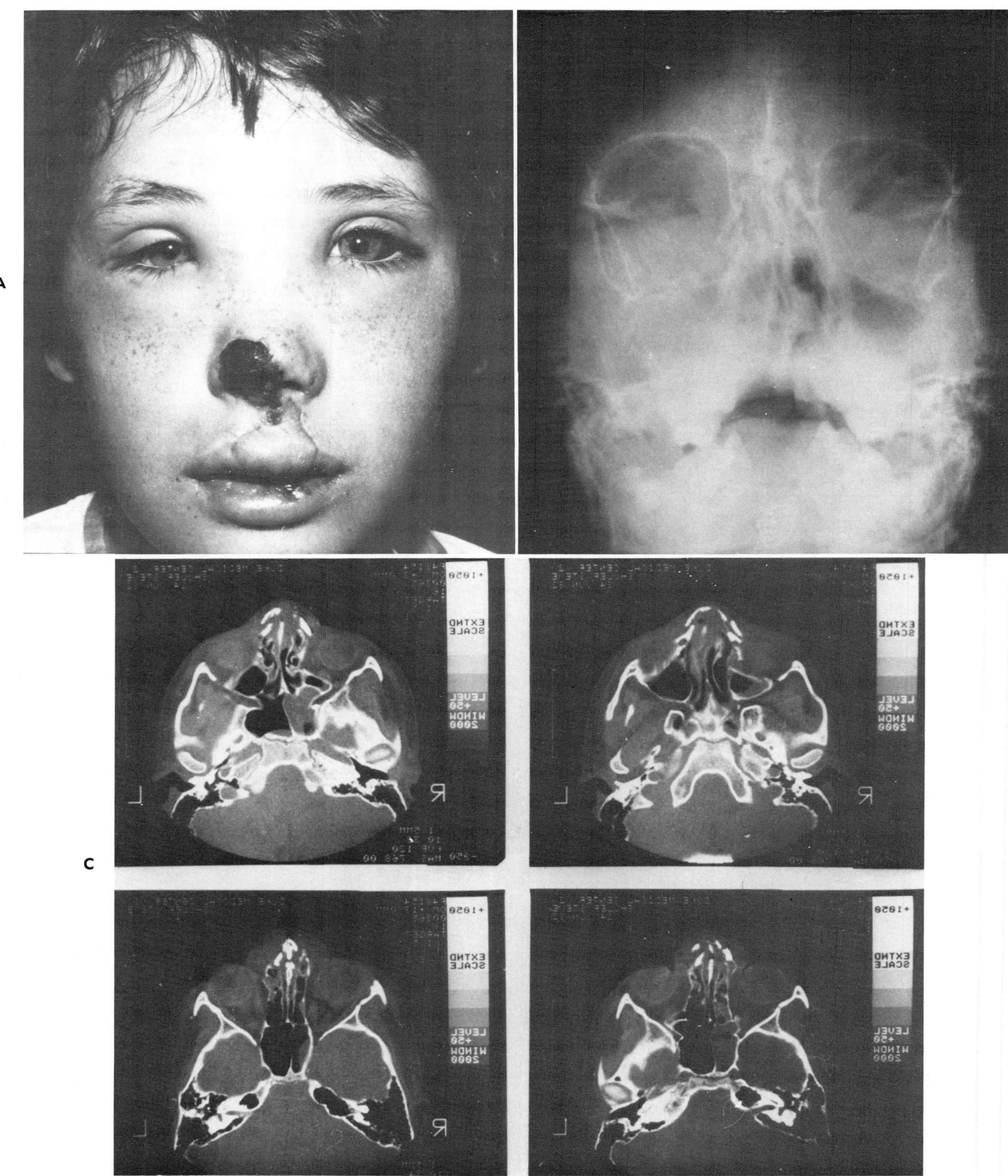

Fig. 30-5. For legend see opposite page.

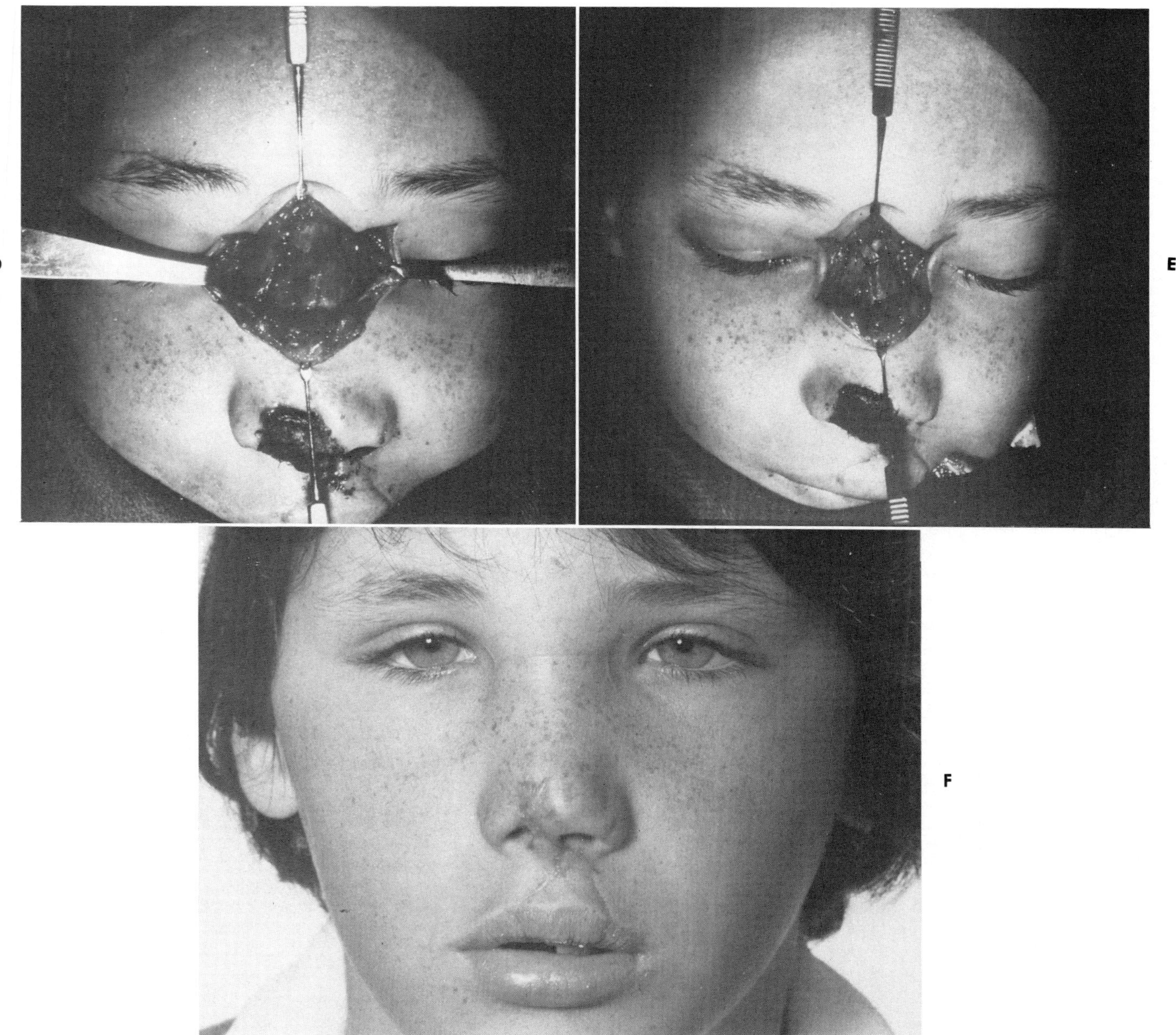

Fig. 30-5. A, This 11-year-old collided with a car while riding a bicycle. He sustained soft tissue injuries of the lip and nose and a nasoorbital fracture. **B,** Radiographs revealed the nasoorbital fracture. **C,** A CT scan demonstrating the nasoorbital fracture. **D,** Exposure of the fracture was achieved by direct incisions. Severe bone comminution is evident. **E,** The bone fragments have been secured with fine wires. Two transnasal wires have been ligated, securing the medial canthi into position. **F,** Appearance of the patient 2 months after surgery.

Fig. 30-6. A, This young teenager was struck on the right side of the face and sustained a fracture of the orbital rim. **B,** Operative photograph of the inferior orbital rim fracture.

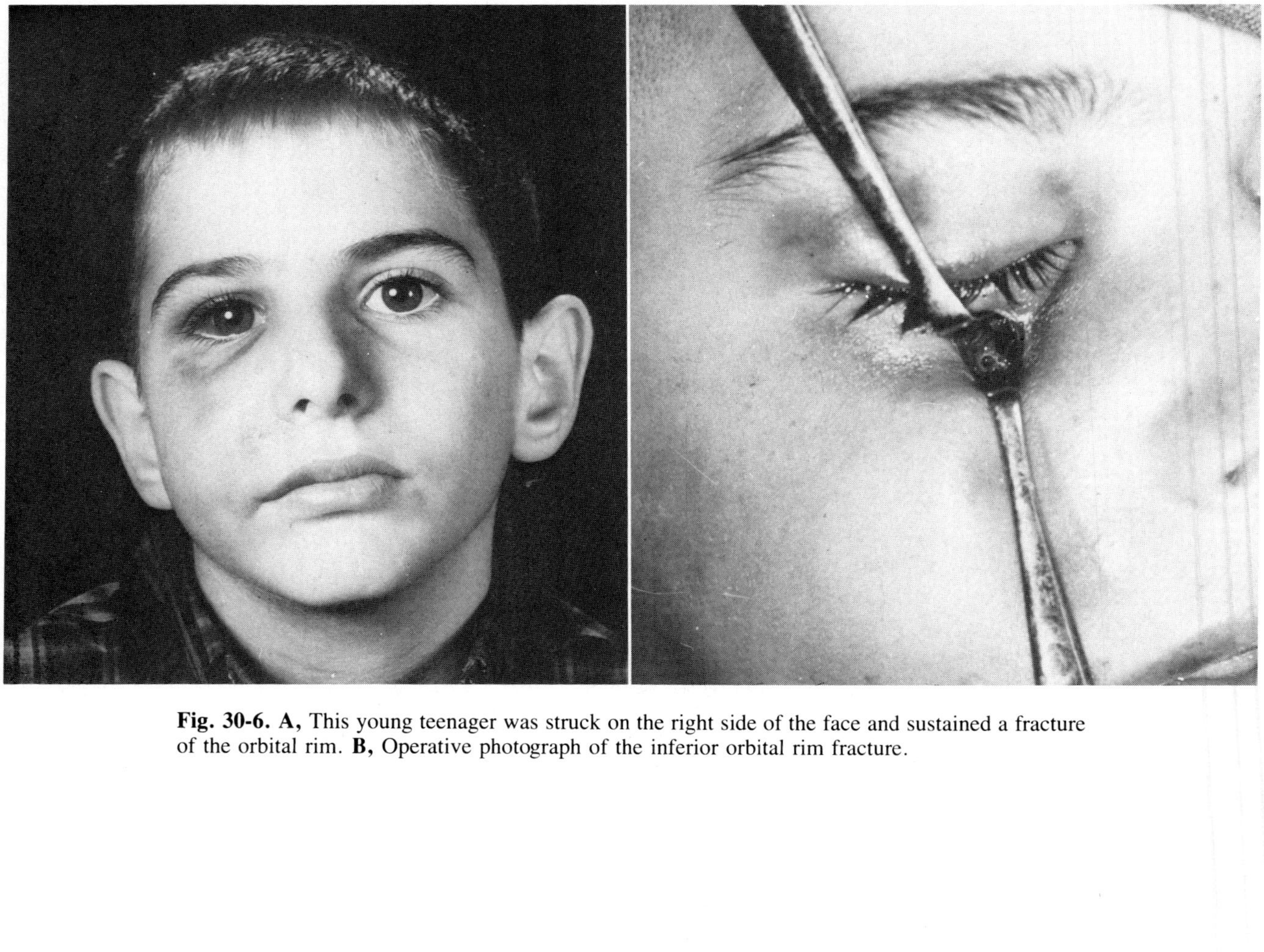

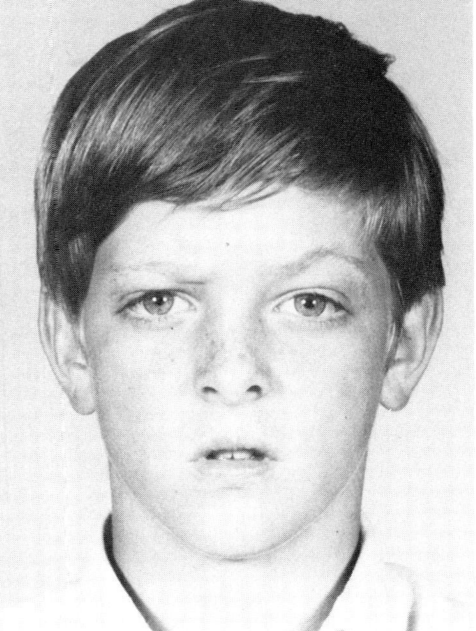

Fig. 30-7. A, This 10-year-old boy was hit on the head with a golf club. **B,** Radiographs revealed a fracture of the superior lateral orbital rim with depression of a single bone fragment. **C,** Operative photograph of the superior orbital rim fracture and displaced fragments. **D,** The bones have been repositioned and secured with fine wires. **E,** Appearance of the patient 6 months later. (From Georgiade, N.G.: The management of acute midfacial-orbital injuries, Clin. Neurosurg. **19:**301, 1972.)

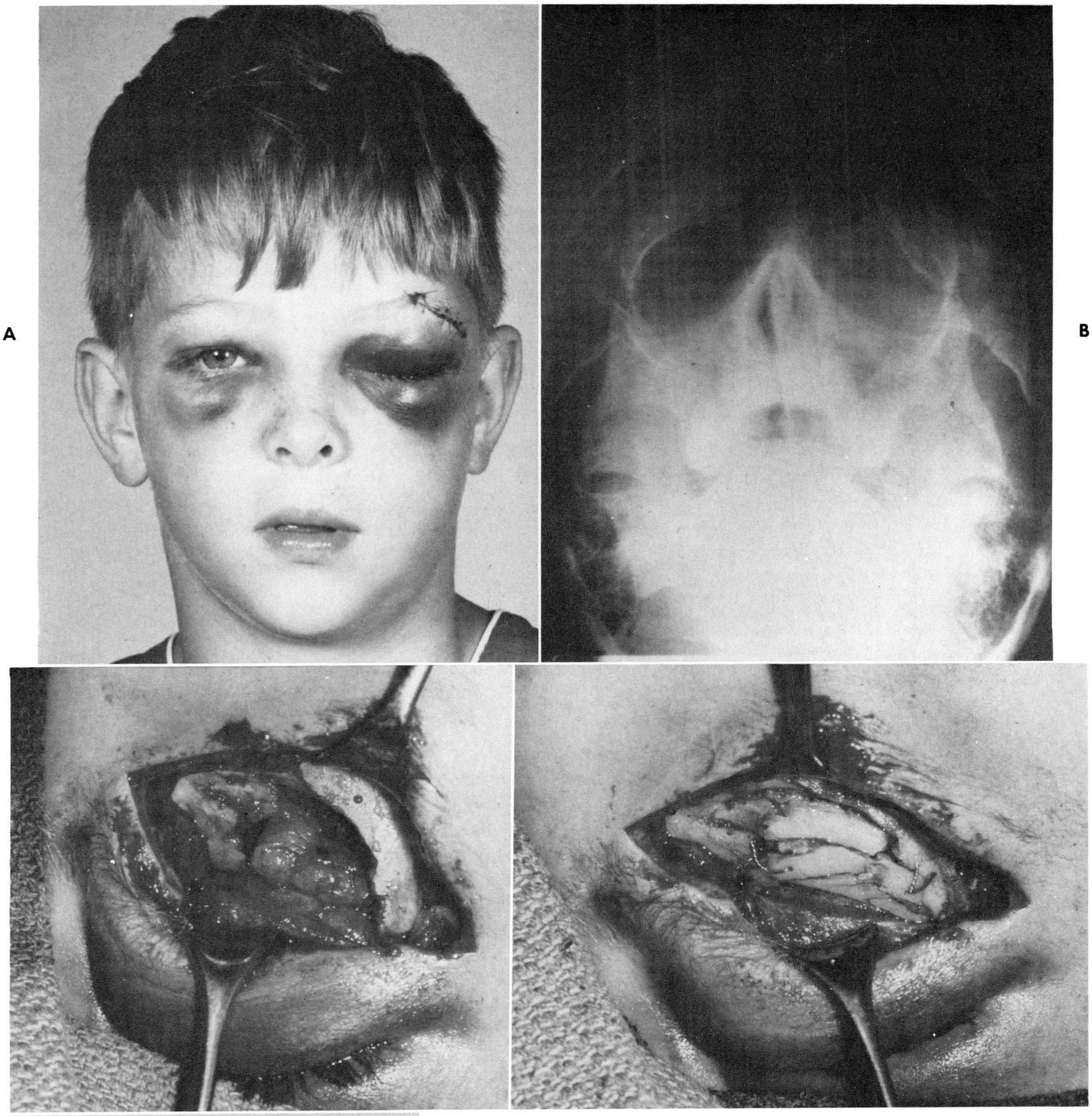

COMPLICATIONS

Complications of facial fractures in children are infrequent. Kaban, Mulliken, and Murray[7] reported a 9.8% incidence of complications in their series. Pulmonary complications are fairly common, especially as a consequence of aspiration, which may occur at the time of injury or anytime afterward. Airway obstruction, hemorrhage and shock, and permanent central nervous system damage may occur in the more serious injuries. Nonunion is unusual; it however, will occur if the fragments are not properly reduced and stabilized. Osteomyelitis is very rare, but may occur with compound or heavily contaminated fractures. Deformities as a result of developmental arrest subsequent to the injury are certainly possible, and this possibility should be discussed with the child's parents. Malocclusion, delayed eruption of teeth, malformed teeth, loss of permanent teeth, or occlusal disharmony subsequent to loss of teeth or tooth follicles may occur after jaw fractures. Ocular injury, permanent diplopia, blindness, nasolacrimal apparatus injury, and traumatic telecanthus may occur with fractures associated with the orbit. A saddle-nose deformity and persistent infraorbital nerve anesthesia are rare and unusual complications of nasoorbital fractures. If persistent, CSF rhinorrhea subsequently may cause meningitis.[16]

SUMMARY AND CONCLUSIONS

Facial fractures infrequently occur in children, especially during the first decade of life. The nature of their activities and factors related to the development of the facial bones contribute to the low incidence of fractures. Fracture diagnosis may be difficult, but it is essential to precisely define the full extent of the injury and institute proper therapy as soon as possible. In general, fractures in children are managed in a similar fashion as the adult counterpart, with the exception that the developing dentition requires adjustments in the means of securing intermaxillary fixation. Children usually recover quickly, and complications of fractures are unusual.

REFERENCES

1. Converse, J.M.: Facial injuries in children. In Mustardè, J.C., editor: Plastic surgery in infancy and childhood, Philadelphia, 1971, W.B. Saunders Co.
2. Converse, J.M., and Dingman, R.O.: Facial injuries in children. In Converse, J.M., editor: Reconstructive plastic surgery, Philadelphia, 1977, W.B. Saunders Co.
3. Dingman, R.O., and Natvig, P.: Facial fractures in children. In Surgery of facial fractures, Philadelphia, 1964, W.B. Saunders Co.
4. Freid, M.G., and Baden, E.: Management of fractures in children, J. Oral Surg. **12**:129, 1954.
5. Georgiade, N.G., Masters, F.W., Metzger, J.T., and Pickrell, K.L: Fractures of the mandible and maxilla in children, J. Pediatr. **42**:440, 1953.
6. Jurkiewicz, M.J., and Nickell, W.B.: Fractures of the skeleton of the face: a study of diagnosis and treatment based on twelve years' experience in the treatment of over 600 major fractures of the facial skeleton, J. Trauma **11**:947, 1971.
7. Kaban, L.B., Mulliken, J.B., and Murray, J.E.: Facial fractures in children: an analysis of 122 fractures in 109 patients, Plast. Reconstr. Surg. **59**:15, 1977.
8. Kravitz, H., Driessen, G., Gomberg, R., and Korach, A.: Accidental falls from elevated surfaces in infants from birth to one year of age, Pediatrics **44**:869, 1969.
9. MacLennan, W.D.: Injuries involving the teeth and jaws in young children, Arch. Dis. Child. **32**:492, 1957.
10. McCoy, F.J., Chandler, R.A., and Crow, M.L.: Facial fractures in children, Plast. Reconstr. Surg. **37**:209, 1966.
11. Oliver, P., Richardson, J.R., Clubb, R.W., and Flake, C.G.: Tracheostomy in children, N. Engl. J. Med. **267**:631, 1962.
12. Panagopoulos, A.P.: Management of fractures of the jaws in children, J. Int. Coll. Surg. **28**:806, 1957.
13. Roberts, R., and Shopfner, C.E.: Plain skull roentgenograms in children with head trauma, A.J.R. **114**:230, 1972.
14. Rowe, N.L.: Fractures of the facial skeleton in children, J. Oral Surg. **27**:505, 1968.
15. Rowe, N.L.: Fractures of the jaws in children, J. Oral Surg. **27**:497, 1969.
16. Schneider, R.C., and Thompson, J.M.: Chronic and delayed traumatic cerebrospinal rhinorrhea as a source of recurrent attacks of meningitis, Ann. Surg. **145**:517, 1957.
17. Schultz, R.C.: Pediatric facial fractures. In Kernahan, D.A., Thomson, H.G., and Bauer, B.S.: editors: Symposium on pediatric plastic surgery, St. Louis, 1982, The C.V. Mosby Co.

CHAPTER 31

Fractures of the mandible in children

JOHN C. ANGELILLO

INCIDENCE

Fortunately, fractures of the facial skeleton in children are rare. Surveys over the past 25 years indicate that the incidence of facial fractures in children is only from 1% to 5%. Panagopoulos' survey[15] in 1957 reported a 1.4% incidence, and in 1955 Rowe and Killey[17] reported that of 500 fractures of the facial skeleton, 4.8% were sustained by children. In 1956 MacLennan[10] reported that less than 1% of all facial fractures occur in children under 6 years of age.

The most common facial bone fracture is the mandible, and the majority occur in boys. Interestingly, the younger the child, the less susceptible that child is to sustaining a fracture. In Rowe and Killey's 1955 review of 500 fractures,[17] only six fractures (1.2%) occurred before the age of 5 years. In 100 fractures reported by Gerrie and McCarthy[4] there was only one case in the 0 to 9-year-old age group. In 1961 Hagan and Huelke[5] reviewed 319 mandibular fractures and found only four fractures (1.2%) in the 0 to 5-year-old group and 16 cases (4.8%) in the 5-10 year-old group. In a second study of 500 facial fractures by Rowe,[16] 6 mandibular fractures were reported in the 0 to 5-year-old group, again only a 1.2% incidence. In the 6 to 12-year-old group, 22 fractures were reported for a 4.4% incidence.

ETIOLOGY AND ANATOMIC CONSIDERATIONS

An understanding of the differences between the facial skeleton in the child and adult will in part explain the lower incidence of facial bone fractures in children. The protected environment that surrounds the infant and preschool child also account for their relative immunity to injuries. Although a child falls numerous times while learning to walk, the distance and force of the fall are insignificant and do not result in facial bone fractures. A child's soft and resilient facial skeleton can sustain considerable insult without fracture or complete separation. Thin cortical plates and a greater proportion of cancellous bone are responsible for the high degree of elasticity of bone in children. These factors are partly responsible for the infrequency of fractures and also explain why the green-stick fracture is quite common in young children. Although the basal bone is elastic, the number of deciduous and permanent teeth results in a high tooth-to-bone ratio. The large amount of space occupied by the developing teeth in the body of the mandible and the delicate basal bone of the inferior border of the mandible encourages fractures through developing tooth crypts (Fig. 31-1).

The 5-year-old child begins school and is now exposed to the many hazards of a new life-style. Increased recreational and sporting activities coupled with physical development account for harder falls and, in general, more violent results. While the majority of mandibular fractures are secondary to auto accidents and falls, recent experience indicates that accidental blows during sporting activity and bicycle accidents now account for a significant number of mandibular fractures in children.

SPECIAL CONSIDERATIONS

The clinical examination of the pediatric patient who has recently had an accident and is suspected of having a facial bone fracture is often difficult. A thorough and meaningful examination depends on the validity of the patient's responses to questions and to the physical examination. In the 1977 survey of Kaban, Mulliken, and Murray,[6] the majority of children sustained other injuries in addition to fractures of the mandible. The most common associated injuries are facial lacerations and abrasions. These injuries in a youngster may present difficult management problems. Skull fractures, closed head trauma, and extremity and cervical spine injuries are also frequent concomitant injuries. McCoy, Chandler, and Crow[14] reported on 86 children with facial bone fractures and found that 35 (40.8%) children also sustained skull fractures. These figures emphasize the need for meticulous neurologic evaluation of patients who have fractures of the facial bones.

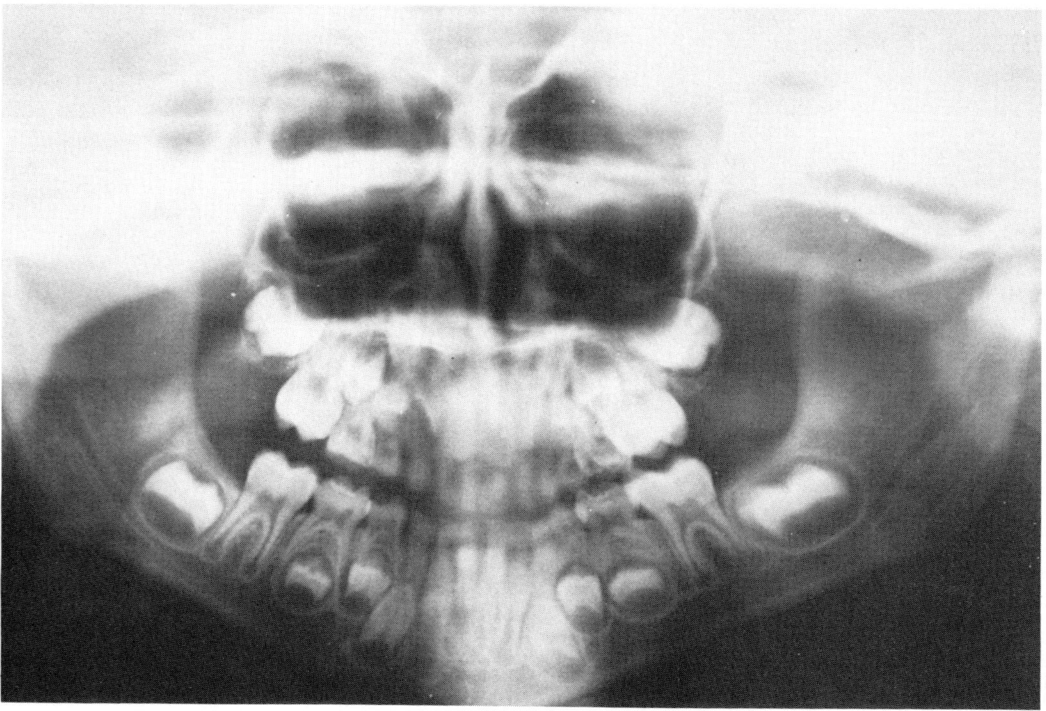

Fig. 31-1. Developing permanent teeth occupy most of the space in the mandible; thus fractures are likely to occur through the developing tooth crypt.

Because of pain, fear and apprehension of the hospital environment, or simply unwillingness to cooperate, diagnosis of fractures in children is difficult. The younger the child, the more invalid will be the history and physical examination.

A detailed account from an individual who observed the accident may be extremely useful. The cause of the injury and the direction and force of the blow may provide extremely useful information and will direct the conduct of the physical and radiographic examination. It will also guide the examiner in the investigation of concomitant injuries.

Lack of a child's cooperation will result in unsatisfactory radiography. The profusion of deciduous teeth and the developing primary and permanent tooth buds in the relatively small mandibular body frequently masks fractures in the body and symphysis region and makes fractures difficult to demonstrate. To accurately evaluate the type and extent of the child's facial injuries, sedation or general anesthesia may be necessary so that a definitive diagnosis can be made and treatment instituted with deliberate speed and efficiency.

Site of fracture

The site of mandibular fractures in children differs with age. MacLennan[11] observed the following order of frequency in fractures of the mandible in children under the age of 6 years:

1. Unilateral fracture of the body of the mandible
2. Unilateral fracture of the body of the mandible on one side, with fracture of the mandibular condylar process on the opposite side
3. Unilateral fracture of the mandibular condylar process
4. Fracture of both mandibular condylar processes (with or without a fracture in the incisor region of the body of the mandible)
5. Bilateral fractures on the body of the mandible in the region of the mental foramina

Lehman and Saddawi[8] reported a 66% incidence of condylar fractures in children under 10 years of age and 40% in children 11 to 15 years old. In children over 15 years old, 76% of the mandibular fractures occurred in the body and angle region. In this age group there is also an increase in the incidence of concomitant midface fractures. The relationship of multiple fractures can in part be attributed to the sequence of skeletal development in the child. By the age of 7 the bony orbits have reached adult dimensions. The bony frame of the midface region is further made vulnerable to fracture with the simultaneous growth of the nasal aperture and to the development of the paranasal sinuses. These anatomic changes coupled with greater participation in contact sports, playground activities, and fights help explain the association of multiple fractures in the older age group.

Special characteristics of children's jaws

Although the general principles of treatment of mandibular fractures in children are essentially the same as in the adult, several unique features in the child will influence the overall management: anatomic differences in teeth, bone, and soft tissue. Consideration for growth potential, the unique problems associated with fixation and immobilization of the jaws, and the relative emotional instability of the child will dictate appropriate modalities of treatment.

The numerous incompletely developed primary teeth and the partially erupted permanent teeth are packed in the confines of the small developing body of the mandible. Consequently fractures most commonly occur through the developing tooth crypts. Developing tooth buds usually do not interfere with adequate reduction of a fracture, and although it is seldom necessary to remove them, damage may delay or arrest development and eruption. Teeth that are in or close to the line of fracture may develop with malformations and dilaceration; however, cystic degeneration or a neoplasm attributable to a previous fracture has never been observed.

Children between the ages of 6 and 12 years have a mixed dentition, that is, primary teeth, fully erupted permanent teeth, and partially erupted permanent teeth. The roots of primary teeth may be partially resorbed and quite loose; thus they are not usable for fixation purposes. Unlike the tapered shape of a permanent tooth, which is constricted at the cervical margin, a primary tooth is widest at the cervical margin, and although it may be stable, it may be inadequate for the ligation of wires or arch bars necessary for fixation and immobilization. In such a situation it will be necessary to design alternate methods of reduction and immobilization.

Healthy children have a remarkably high osteogenic potential of the periosteum and bone, and callus formation occurs rapidly. When feasible, reduction of the fracture within 5 days will allow easier manipulation of the displaced fragments. If the reduction of a malaligned fracture is undertaken after 7 days, it will often be necessary to remove the callus bridging the line of fracture to achieve a satisfactory reduction. If callus formation has already occurred before the beginning of treatment, a slight discrepancy in the primary occlusion can be accepted because it may be unwise and unnecessary to attempt to refracture and reposition the mandibular fragments. Considering the potential of alveolar bone growth and the ability of the basal bone to remodel itself under the influence of the masticatory apparatus, slight occlusal disharmony is easily tolerated and will be corrected with eruption of the permanent teeth.

EARLY TREATMENT

Immediate definitive treatment of mandibular fractures in children is neither obligatory nor necessary. Rather, the fundamental principle of assessing the general condition of the child should be the primary consideration. Associated critical injuries may be easily overlooked as emotions and attention are focused on the obvious facial injury. Statistics confirm that the majority of children who had mandibular fractures also had other injuries, most commonly cervical

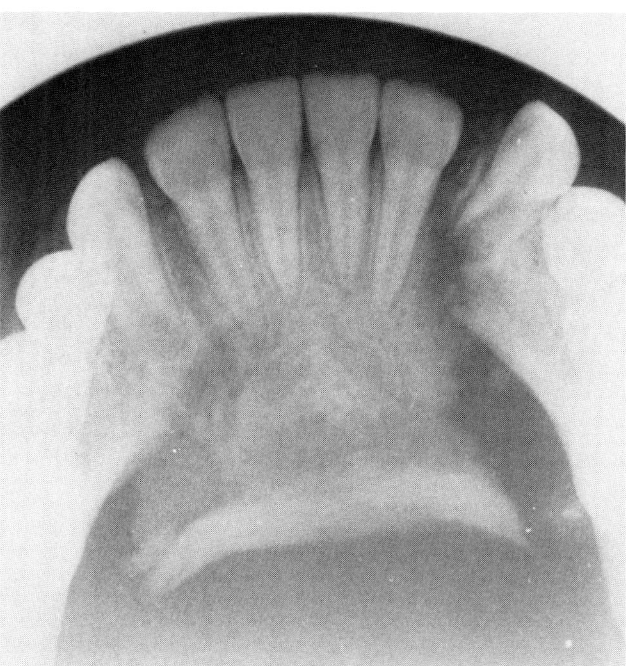

Fig. 31-2. Bilateral parasymphysis fracture with posterior displacement of the fractured segment and tongue.

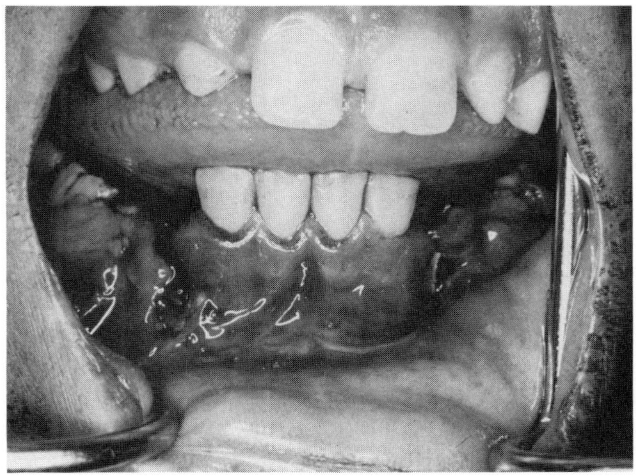

Fig. 31-3. Genioglossus muscle loses its stable anterior attachment, causing instability of the tongue and upper airway obstruction.

spine injuries, skull fractures, extremity injuries, and craniofacial trauma. Appropriate examination and evaluation of the neurologic, cardiothoracic, and abdominal status is mandatory, and immediate concern should be directed toward identifying problems that can lead to greater morbidity.

Adequate airway

Mandibular fractures in children can pose a most serious threat to the maintenance of an adequate airway. Any mandibular fracture that causes instability of the tongue with posterior displacement against the posterior pharyngeal wall can completely obstruct the upper airway. This is especially true in comminuted fractures of the mandibular symphysis region in which the genioglossus muscle loses its stable anterior attachment to the mandible (Figs. 31-2 and 31-3). The tongue must be held out with a suture or a towel clip and prevented from falling back. Blood, vomitus, or fractured teeth must be removed from the oropharynx. If these measures fail to ensure satisfactory ventilatory exchange, and endotracheal tube or tracheostomy will be necessary.

Control of hemorrhage in infants and young children is critical. Blood loss may be difficult to estimate, and the state of hydration is unknown. In young children blood volume is small, and losses are of much greater importance because of the smaller margin of safety. It may be necessary to administer intravenous fluids, including whole blood, during the initial evaluation.

Transportation

Except for sterile moist dressings covering facial lacerations, the application of head bandages during transport is not advisable. Any bandage that may cause backward displacement of the fragments and obstruct the airway is extremely hazardous and should not be used. This danger is especially true with the "four-tailed" type of bandage. When it is necessary to transport a child with facial fractures to another hospital, the radiology unit, or the operating room, the child should be placed with the face down and the forehead supported or with the head turned to one side. The child should be accompanied by competent individuals with appropriate equipment who will have responsibility of maintaining the airway during transport.

Prophylaxis for infection

When soft tissue injuries have been contaminated with road debris or soil, wound debridement is essential, and tetanus prevention and antibiotic prophylaxis should be considered. The use of large doses of antibiotics is not a satisfactory substitute for meticulous debridement of soft tissue wounds. Judicious removal of only nonvital tissue and retention of all salvageable tissue will pay dividends in the protracted postoperative period.

PRINCIPLES OF TREATMENT

The fundamental treatment principles of mandibular fractures in the child do not differ from those for adults. Namely, to restore a normal functional occlusal relationship between the jaws, ensure adequate union of the fracture fragments, maintain facial symmetry and balance, and prevent infection and untoward sequelae.

After confirmation that there are no other serious injuries, diagnosis and treatment should be carried out as quickly and as definitively as possible. If the treatment plan requires an open or closed reduction, as well as the insertion of an acrylic splint with intermaxillary fixation, it may be wise to complete this procedure during a single operation. The child will not be tolerant of numerous procedures as is customary with an adult patient.

Strict attention should be paid to the status of the developing dentition. Primary and permanent teeth should not be needlessly sacrificed. Tooth buds and permanent teeth with incompletely formed roots have a unique ability to survive even in face of severe insult. When open reduction is indicated, careful placement of transosseous wires at the inferior border will eliminate damaging permanent tooth buds. Extraoral pin fixation is also contraindicated because of possible injury to the developing permanent teeth. Unnecessary removal or injury to permanent teeth for the sake of convenience is a trade-off that invariably results in numerous problems during adulthood.

The simplest and most effective treatment plan that will achieve adequate reduction and stabilization and will require minimal adjustments is desirable. Children are more likely to test the stability of fixation and by their constant attempts to move the mandible will slowly undo the fixation. Complex headcaps, slings, and elaborate cap splints should be considered only when alternative plans are not available.

The routine use of antibiotics for all types of mandibular fractures in children is unnecessary and contraindicated. However, it is judicious to institute antibiotic therapy for fractures that are compounded into the mouth or to the exterior or when concomitant injuries indicate their use.

It is vital to assure that fluid and caloric intake is adequate. Delivery of appropriate intravenous fluids during the immediate postoperative period will guarantee adequate fluid levels and electrolytes for a day or two. Thereafter, a child usually has little difficulty with clear liquids or pureed solid foods. Occasionally it may be necessary to assist feeding with a bulb syringe.

Maintaining good oral hygiene in a child with immobilized jaws is often difficult. Hydrogen peroxide and pleasant-tasting mouthwashes used with a small, soft toothbrush may be helpful.

SIGNS AND SYMPTOMS

Pain in the region of the affected temporomandibular joint that is intensified with movement of the mandible is invariably present. *Tenderness* over the fracture site may be exquisite and help identify the fractured fragment. Gross *facial deformity* with deviation of the mandible may be obvious. The deviation toward the side of injury may be more apparent when the mouth is opened. Bilateral subcondylar fractures will result in an anterior open bite due to the upward and backward positioning of the rami. These fractures are usually associated with a laceration under the chin and a symphyseal fracture of the mandible. Less severe injuries will cause a *malocclusion* of varying degrees. The malocclusion may be subtle, and a patient may complain only that the teeth do not occlude normally. Other malocclusions may be severe and obvious. *Swelling* in the preauricular region may be seen 4 to 6 days after a condylar fracture. Intraoral swelling over the coronoid process suggests an associated fracture of the coronoid processes. *Paresthesia* of the lower lip, chin, or tongue is very unusual but may be secondary to edema about the inferior alveolar nerve. Patients may describe a cracking or grating sensation that is not audible to the examiner. This *crepitation* is produced during movement of the fractured ends of the bone. *Ecchymosis* of the facial tissues on the injured side is the result of hemorrhage into the soft tissues or the formation of a hematoma.

CLINICAL EXAMINATION

Although the clinical examination of the facial skeleton, alveolar ridge, teeth, and supporting structures on an injured child may be difficult, critical information will be recovered. Patience and time spent in winning a child's confidence is well spent; however, appropriate sedation may be necessary to conduct a satisfactory clinical and radiographic examination.

Several obvious signs of trauma that will lead the examiner to suspect underlying fractures include swelling, ecchymosis, facial asymmetry, limited mandibular movement, and malocclusion. The malocclusion (Fig. 31-4) may be obvious during the clinical examination or may be subtle, the child reporting only that the "teeth don't meet right." Palpation over a localized or generalized area of swelling is painful and yields little information. Ecchymosis may

identify the point of impact, and bleeding from the ear may indicate a fractured condyle. A unilateral condylar fracture will limit mandibular movement and cause deviation of the mandible to the affected side during opening. Open-bite deformity invariably occurs with bilateral condylar fractures. A depressed fracture of the zygomatic arch that impinges on the coronoid process of the mandible will also produce limited ability to open or close the mouth.

A systematic bimanual examination of the facial skeleton begins with palpation of the zygoma and zygomatic arches (Fig. 31-5). A depression deformity, point tenderness, or periorbital ecchymosis may signal a zygoma or zygomatic arch fracture. If the zygomatic arch is depressed so far medially that it impinges on the coronoid process, mandibular excursions will be severely limited.

Although condylar neck fractures are invariably displaced medially, a depression deformity does not result. Preauricular pain, point tenderness, and crepitus are common (Fig. 31-6). Placement of the index fingers into the external auditory canals may be useful (Fig. 31-7). In condylar fracture dislocation, the condyle will not be felt by fingers placed into the external auditory canals. In condylar fractures without displacement, the condyle can be felt by the palpating finger; however, it will not move with the mandible. The external auditory canals are inspected for blood, CSF, and integrity of the tympanic membrane.

The facial aspect of the ascending ramus and angle and

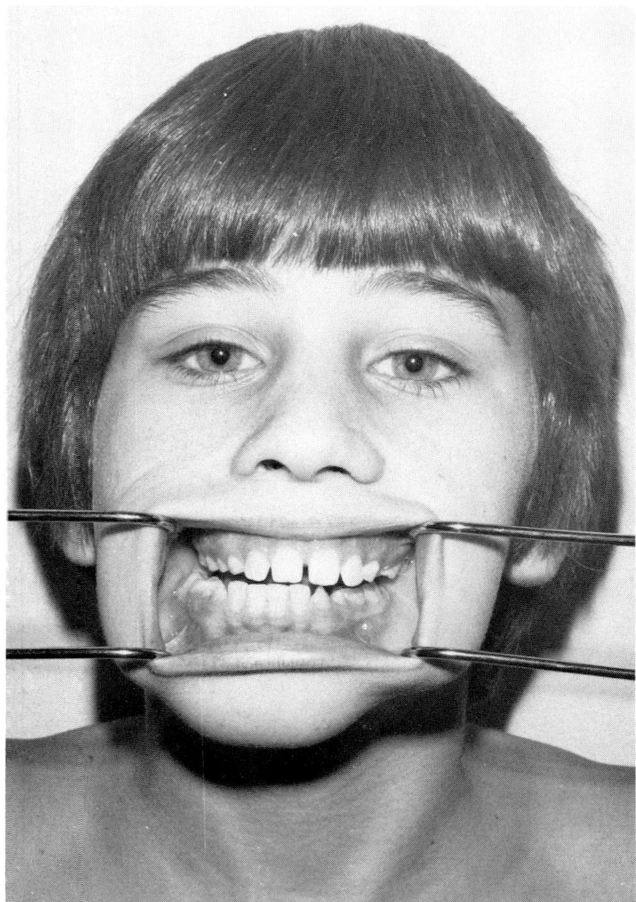

Fig. 31-4. Malocclusion may be subtle or obvious.

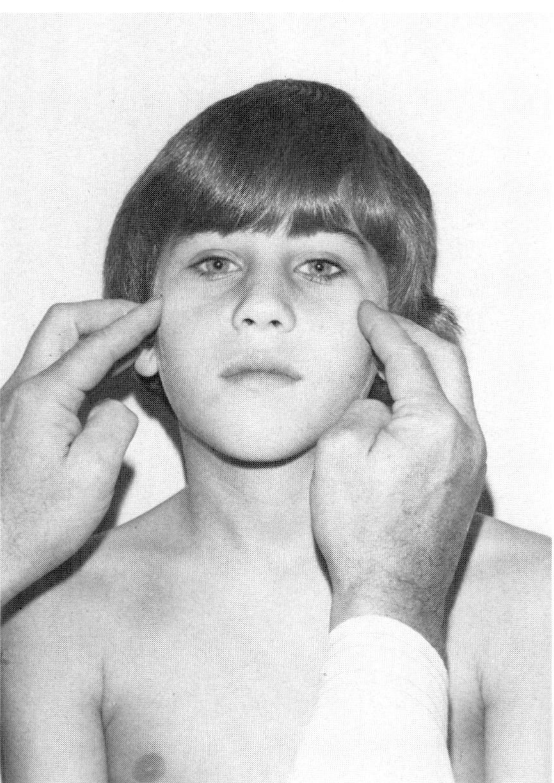

Fig. 31-5. Bilateral palpation of the zygoma and zygomatic arches.

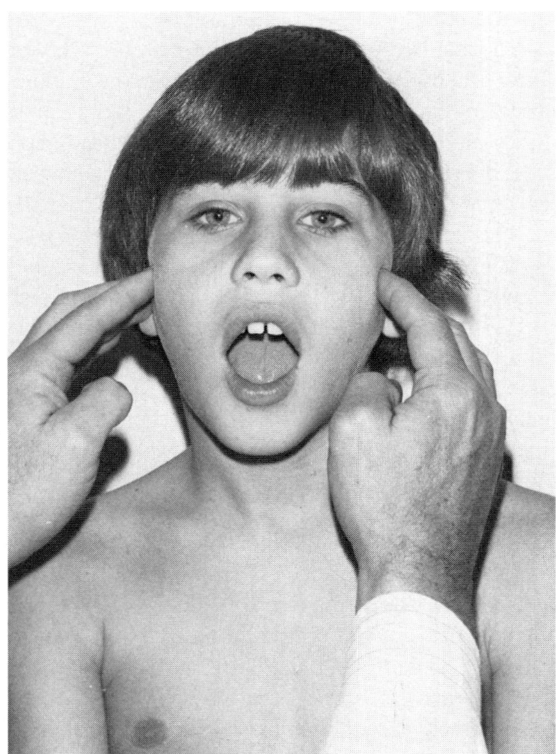

Fig. 31-6. Palpation of preauricular regions. Pain and crepitus may indicate a condylar neck fracture.

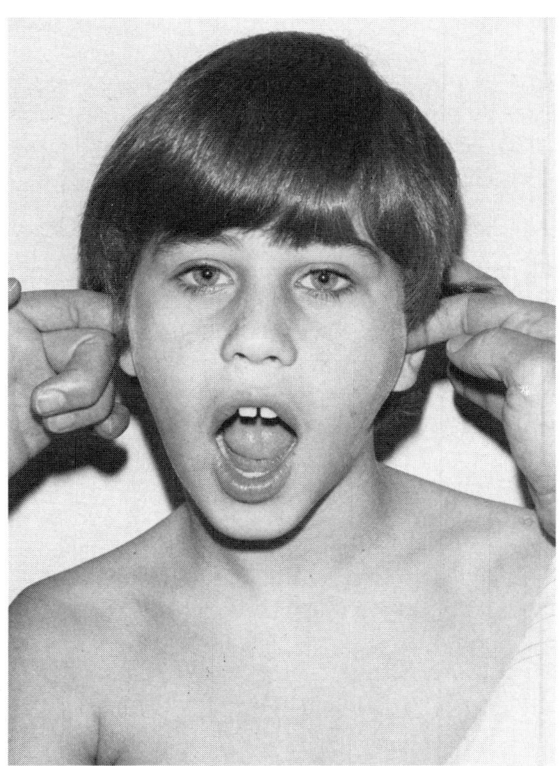

Fig. 31-7. Placement of the finger into external auditory canal.

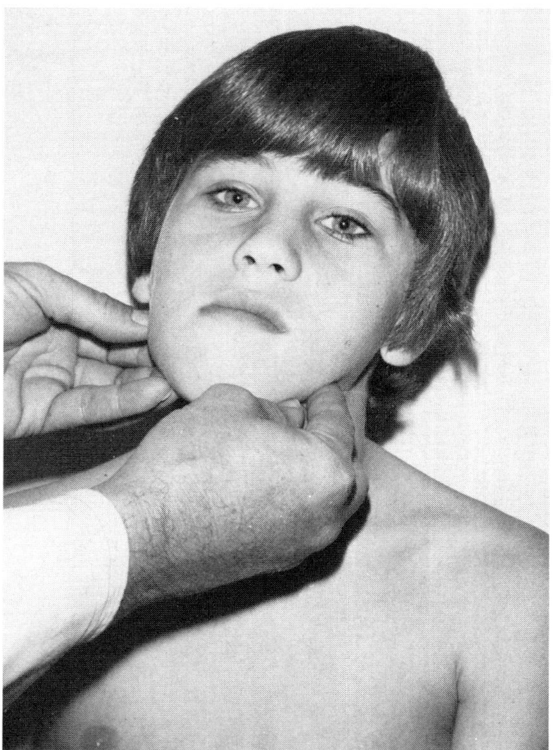

Fig. 31-8. Palpation of facial aspects of the ramus and angle and body of the mandible.

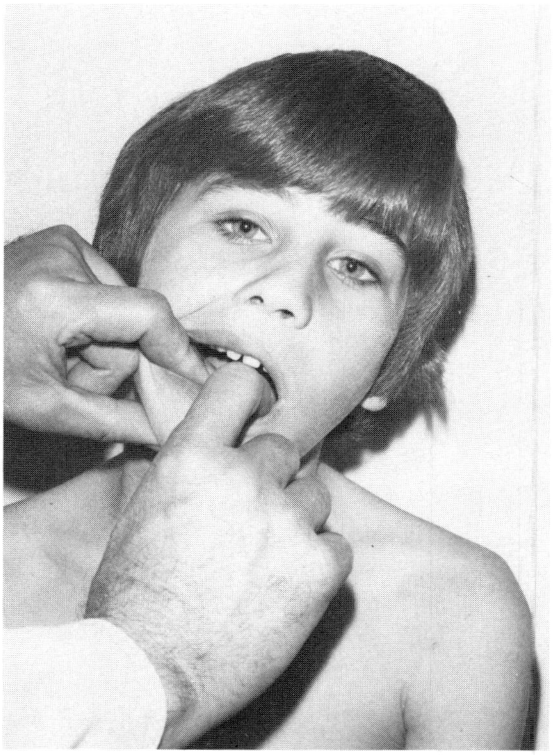

Fig. 31-9. Simultaneous extraoral and intraoral bimanual examination of the ramus and body and symphysis of the mandible.

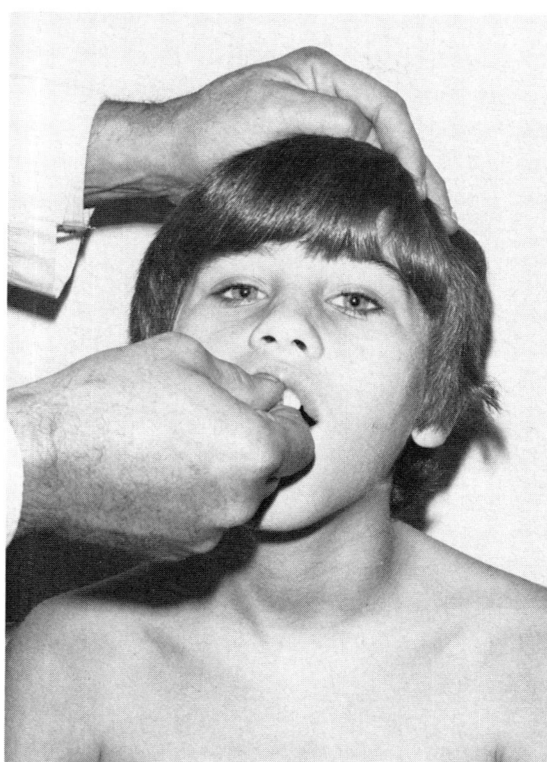

Fig. 31-10. Stability of the maxilla is determined by holding the head steady and evaluating movement of the maxilla.

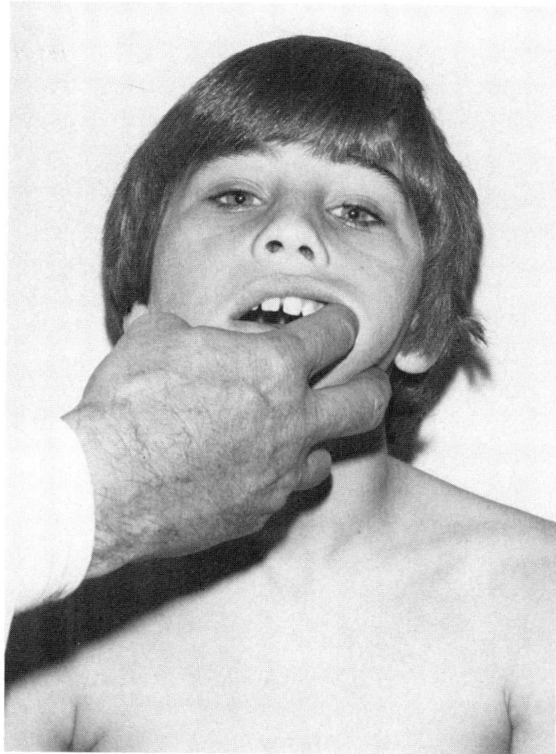

Fig. 31-11. Intraoral digital examination of the maxilla.

inferior border of the mandible are palpated for tenderness and mobility (Fig. 31-8). Motion and crepitus may best be detected by simultaneous extraoral and intraoral bimanual examination (Fig. 31-9). The stability of the maxilla is inspected by firmly grasping the upper jaw while holding the head motionless (Fig. 31-10). Movement of the entire maxilla may be felt by the examiner, or it causes wrinkling of the skin over the bridge of the nose. Intraoral palpation of the maxilla may identify zygomaticomaxillary irregularities (Fig. 31-11).

The nose is inspected for deformity, patency, and CSF rhinorrhea. Inspection may reveal deviation of the nasal septum, and digital palpation of the nasal bones may reveal movement or crepitation.

RADIOGRAPHIC EXAMINATION

Fractures of the facial bones are difficult to demonstrate radiographically. This is especially true of radiographs taken on an injured or uncooperative patient. Compromising proper positioning of the patient because it may be unwise to manipulate the head and neck usually results in poor quality radiographs. Because treatment of facial fractures should not be instituted until an adequate radiographic examination is made, it may be wise to defer this study until clinical and radiographic examination of the skull and cervical spine confirm that manipulation of the head and neck is not hazardous.

The single most useful radiographic aid in the diagnosis of mandibular fractures is the panoramic view (Fig. 31-12, *A*). This radiograph is taken while the child is seated and the head properly positioned and stabilized (Fig. 31-12, *B*). The radiation source and cassette rotate equidistant and synchronously around the head. This view adequately displays the entire mandible, including the condyles, glenoid fossae, teeth, maxilla, and maxillary antrum. Inability to sit upright or to stand up precludes the use of this technique. Radiographic equipment has been developed so that a panoramic view of the mandible can be taken while a patient remains supine, but this equipment is not in widespread use.

The posteroanterior projection of the mandible also displays the entire mandible and demonstrates medial or lateral displacement of fractures, mandibular asymmetries, and the relationship of the mandible to both the maxilla and the base of the skull (Fig. 31-13). It also shows the zygoma, the lateral walls of the maxillary antrum, and the nasal septum.

The modified Towne's view is taken specifically to demonstrate the condylar processes of the mandible (Fig. 31-14). Although a degree of distortion occurs with elongation of the ascending rami and condylar necks, the mastoid processes are thrown out of view so that the head and neck of the condyle are clearly seen. The nasal septum and angles of the mandible are also well delineated. Complete absence of the condylar process in this view may indicate severe

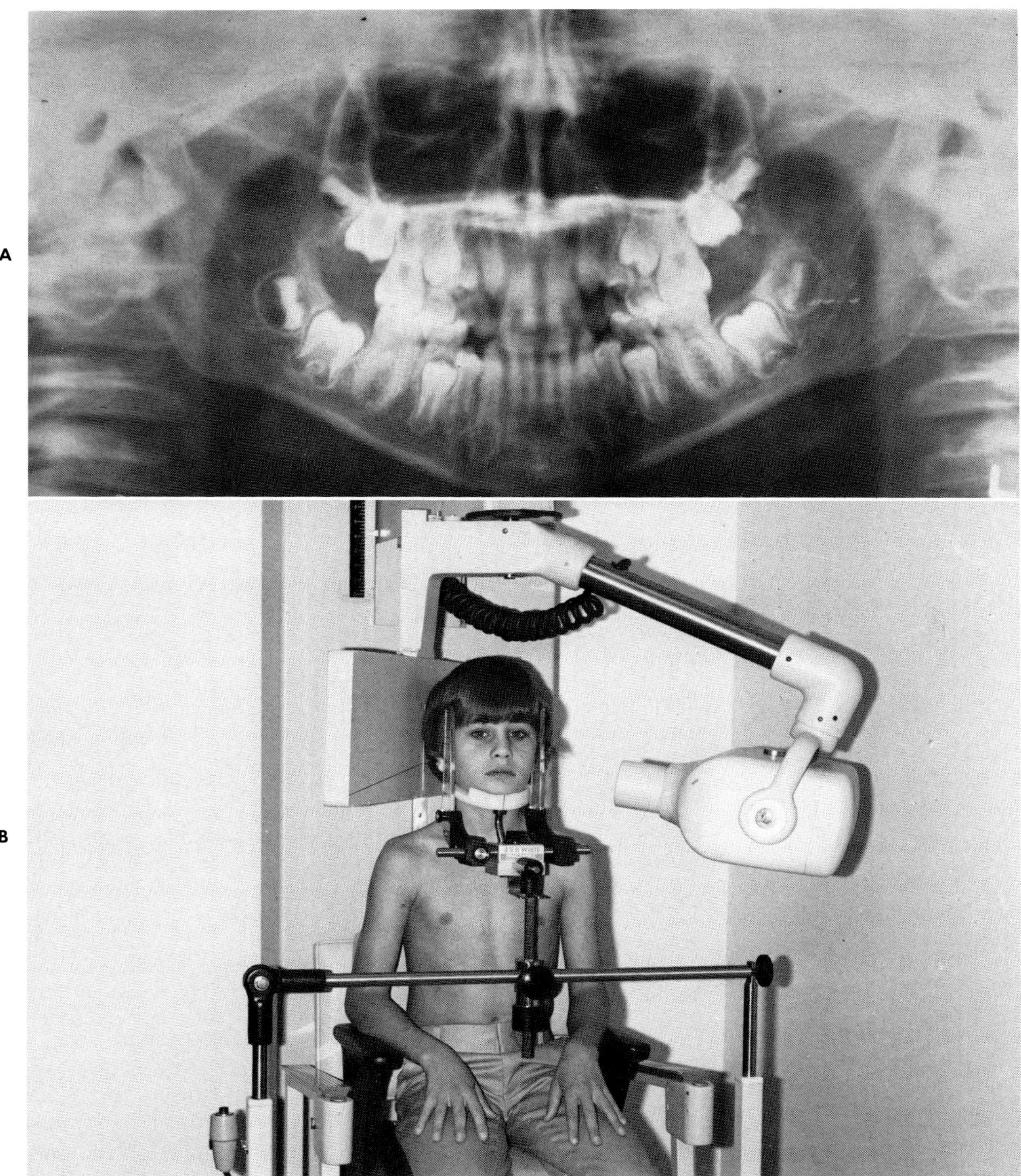

Fig. 31-12. A, Panoramic view radiograph displays the entire mandible, including the condyles. **B,** The patient is seated and the head securely positioned for a panoramic view radiograph.

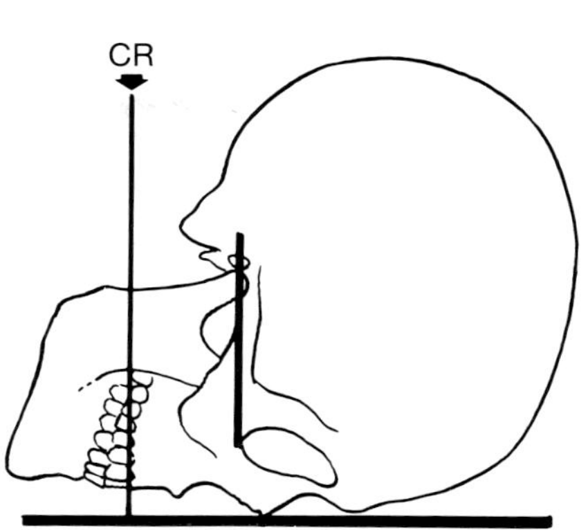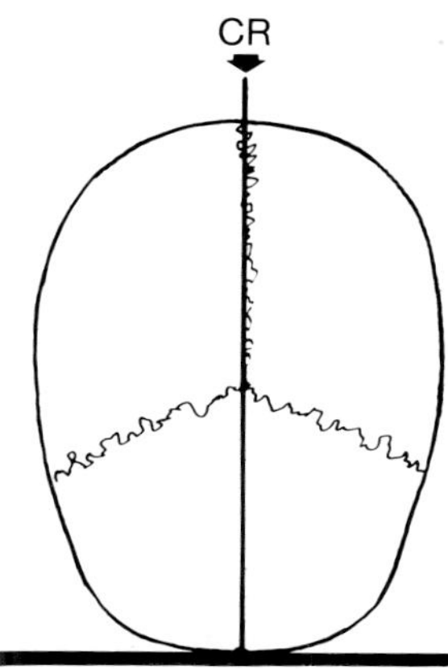

Fig. 31-13. Posteroanterior projection. The patient is placed in a prone position with the neck flexed so that the forehead and nose touch the top of the table. The midsagittal plane of the skull is vertical to the center of the cassette, and the orbitomeatal line is at right angles to the cassette. The central ray *(CR)* is directed vertically at the neck and aimed at the maxillary incisor teeth.

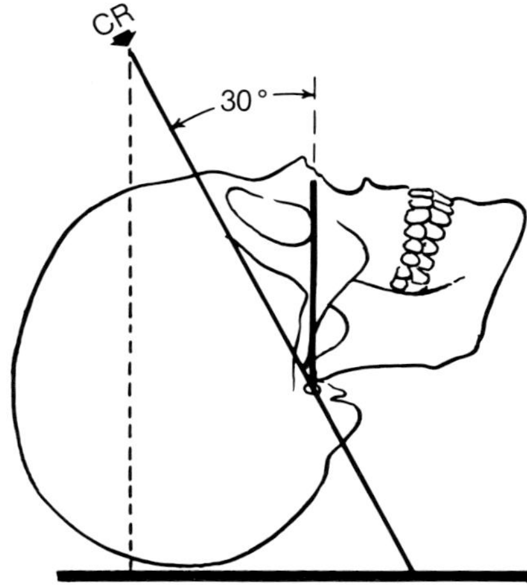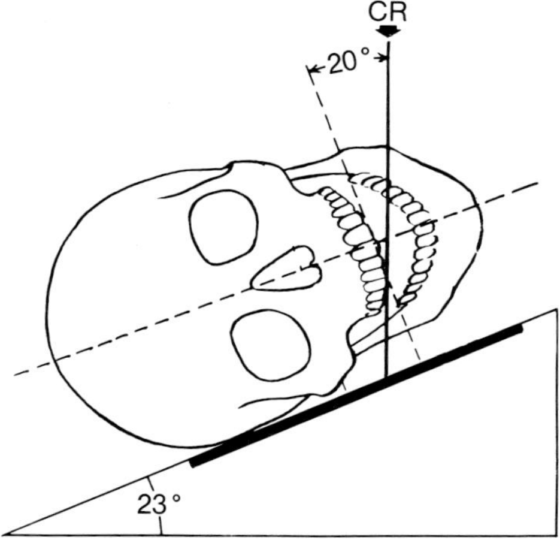

Fig. 31-14. Anteroposterior projection of mandibular condylar processes (modified Towne's projection). The patient is placed in a supine position with the occiput contacting the table and the orbitomeatal line at right angles to the cassette. The midsagittal plane of the skull is vertical to the center of the cassette. The central ray *(CR)* is angulated 30 degrees toward the feet and between the mandibular condyles.

Fig. 31-15. Lateral oblique projection of the mandible. The patient lies on the side and the head is placed on an angle board inclined 23 degrees. The sagittal plane is parallel to the cassette, and the occlusal plane is at right angles to the cassette. The injured side is closest to the cassette with the zygoma just above the center of the film. The central ray *(CR)* is directed 20 degrees cephalad to the occlusal plane, below the angle of the uninjured side, and slightly backward, pointing to the crown of the opposite third molar tooth.

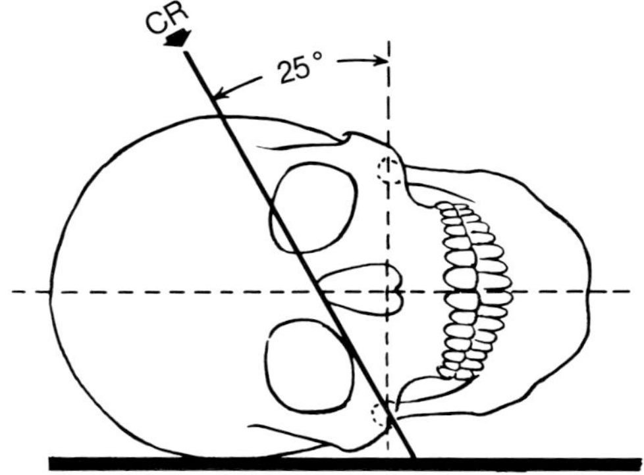

Fig. 31-16. Lateral projection of the temporomandibular joint. The patient lies on the side with the head in a true lateral position with the joint to be examined in contact with the cassette. The midsagittal plane is parallel to the table and the frontal plane of the head is perpendicular to the table. The central ray *(CR)* passes through the temporal region and is angulated 25 degrees toward the feet. One exposure is made with the mouth open and another with the mouth closed.

displacement with superimposition of the fractured segment by the petrous ridge.

The lateral oblique view of the mandible offers an excellent view of the body, ramus, angle, and condylar and coronoid processes of the mandible (Fig. 31-15). Injured teeth and fractures of the alveolar process can be detected in this view also.

The temporomandibular joint views are taken with the mouth open and closed and show the relation of the mandibular condyle to the glenoid fossa (Fig. 31-16). This view is also useful in demonstrating intracapsular or crush fractures of the head of the condyle. Congenital or traumatic abnormalities detected from this view of the joint may be an indication for tomography, which will more clearly delineate subtle discrepancies. The open temporomandibular joint view will show the anterior and inferior movement of the condylar head as it glides out of the glenoid fossa and along the posterior slope of the articular eminence. The closed temopromandibular joint view will show the relation of the mandibular condyle to the fossa.

Fractures of the condylar process are most difficult to demonstrate by routine radiographic methods and are the type of mandibular fractures most commonly undetected and untreated. When routine radiography of this region is unsatisfactory, a tomogram will provide good definition of the condylar process (Fig. 31-17). This technique can bring into sharp focus structures that are located at various depths from the surface and blur out those structures which are nearer to or farther from the film.

Several intraoral views of the parasymphyseal region of the mandible show the anterior mandible in excellent detail. The 90 degree inferosuperior and the 55-degree oblique projection of the parasymphyseal area will accurately show the degree of displacement of parasymphyseal fractures, the teeth, and alveolar process (Figs. 31-18 and 31-19). The 90-degree view will best show an asymmetry of the anterior mandible, and foreign bodies in the soft tissues can also be detected in this view.

An axial view of the zygomatic arches will project them free of superimposition and demonstrate medial or lateral displacement of fractured segments (Fig. 31-20). This view should be taken for patients who have clinical evidence of a depressed zygomatic arch fracture, for example, with the appearance of a flat cheek bone, and for those patients in whom a mandibular fracture cannot be demonstrated either clinically or radiographically but who are having difficulty opening and closing the jaw.

Intraoral dental radiographs show the teeth and supporting alveolar bone in excellent detail (Fig. 31-21). These radiographs better demonstrate alveolar bone fractures, fractures of the teeth, and unsuspected underlying dental pathologic conditions that may provide vital information necessary for treatment planning.

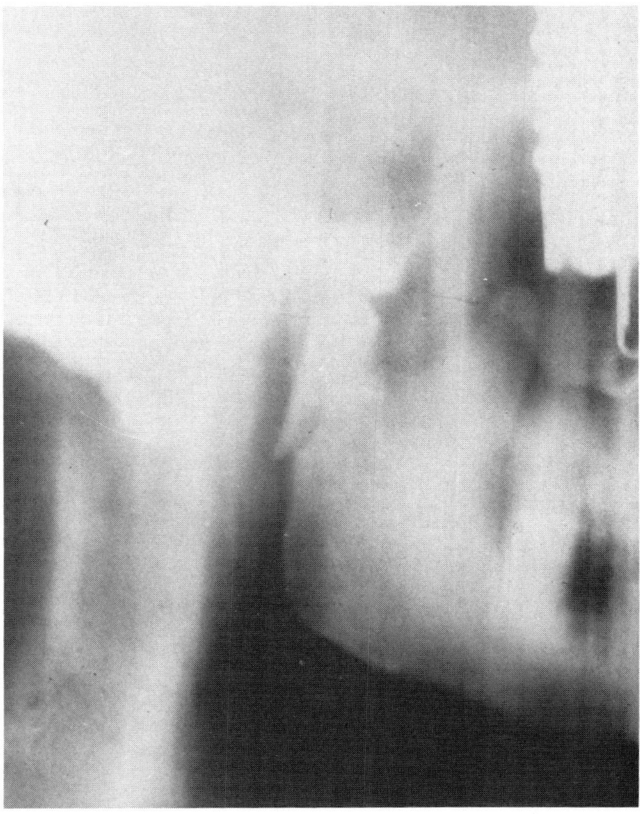

Fig. 31-17. A tomographic radiograph reveals a fracture of the condylar neck that was not detected on routine radiography.

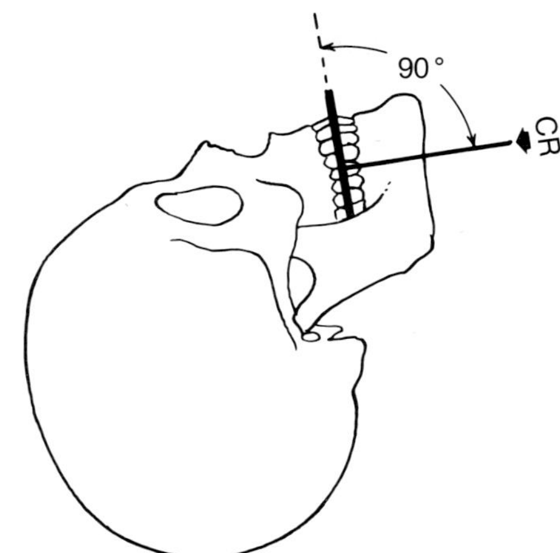

Fig. 31-18. Inferosuperior projection of the mandibular parasymphyseal region. The patient is placed either in a supine position or seated in a chair with the neck fully extended. An occlusal film is gripped between the upper and lower teeth. The central ray *(CR)* is directed at right angles to the film from below the mandible and through the midsagittal plane of the lower molar teeth.

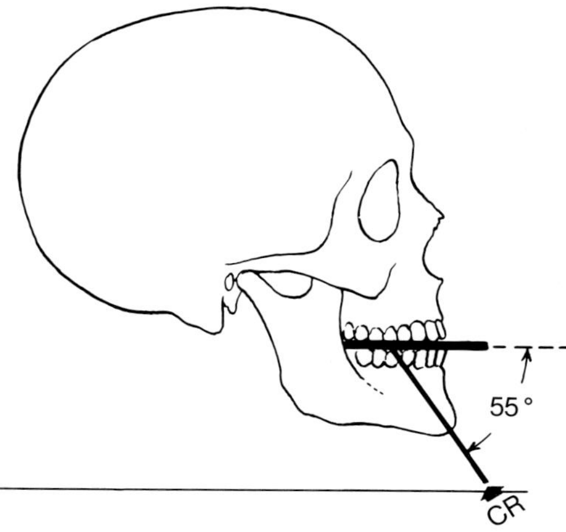

Fig. 31-19. Inferosuperior projection of the mandibular parasymphyseal region. The patient is seated in a chair and the head positioned with the occlusal plane of the teeth parallel to the floor. An occlusal film is held between the upper and lower teeth. The central ray *(CR)* is angulated at 55 degrees to the plane of the film passing through the lower border of the anterior mandible. This view better shows the lingual plate and more accurately demonstrates the nature of the fracture.

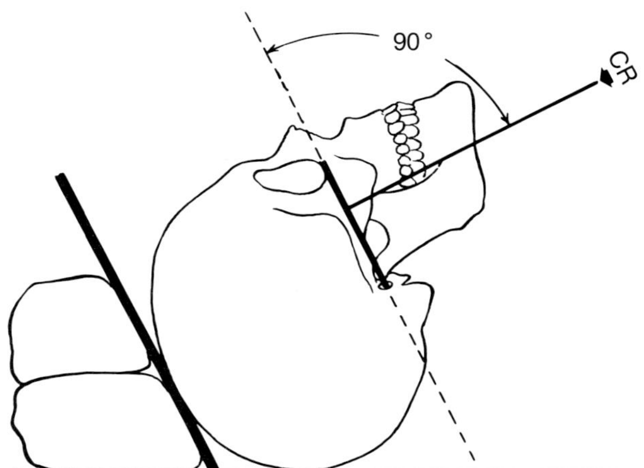

Fig. 31-20. Submental-vertex projection of zygomatic arches. The patient is placed in a supine position with the shoulders elevated on pillows for maximal extension of the neck. The top of the head rests against the cassette and the medial sagittal plane of the skull is vertical to the vertical line of the film. The head is positioned so that the infraorbitomeatal line is parallel with the plane of the film. The central ray *(CR)* is directed at right angles to the infraorbitomeatal line and midway between the zygomatic arches.

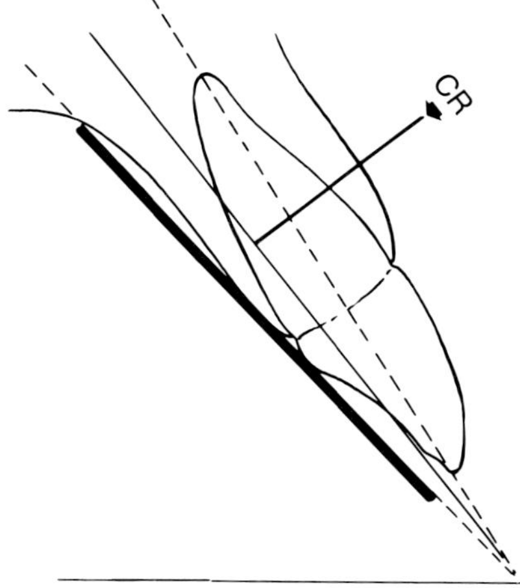

Fig. 31-21. Intraoral dental radiography. The patient is seated and positioned for routine dental radiographs. The periapical film is inserted into the mouth, with the axis of the film parallel to the anterior teeth and transverse to posterior teeth. The film is centered to the teeth and held firmly by the patient using the thumb or index finger. The central ray *(CR)* is aimed at the midpoint of the film and at right angles to a plane that bisects the long axis of the tooth and the long axis of the film.

MANDIBULAR CONDYLE FRACTURES

Fractures of the mandibular condyle may be classified anatomically:

1. Intracapsular fractures
   a. Comminuted, or "crush," fracture of the head of the condyle involves the articular surface of the head of the condyle but is not compounded through the fibrous capsule of the mandibular joint.
   b. A "high" condylar fracture occurs above the level of the sigmoid notch and through the condylar neck. It does not involve the articular surface of the condylar head and is usually associated with a medial dislocation of the fractured segment.
2. Extracapsular fracture
   a. The "low" or subcondylar fracture occurs from the sigmoid notch downward and backward below the neck of the condyle to the posterior aspect of the ramus.

A comminuted intracapsular fracture of only the head of the condyle and involving the articular surface may be difficult to demonstrate. Examination will not show facial or mandibular deformity save for perhaps a small localized swelling over the injured condyle. On palpation there is significant tenderness in the preauricular region. Opening of the mouth, if at all possible, will be accompanied by pain. A grating or bony crepitus may be heard or felt on opening. Routine radiographs of the temporomandibular joint usually will fail to show the comminution, and tomography may be necessary to clearly identify the fracture. It is wise to ensure that a depressed fracture of the zygomatic arch or a fracture of the zygoma is not responsible for the difficulty in opening. It is also advisable to examine the external auditory canal and the integrity of the tympanic membrane.

Comminuted fractures of the head of the condyle that have not violated the fibrous capsule of the joint should be treated conservatively. For children without teeth, immobilization of the jaws is not advisable. Once the local edema has subsided, opening and closing of the jaws should be encouraged and progress routinely checked. For children whose dental status will allow the application of dental wiring or arch bars, immobilization is recommended for a period of 2 weeks. The occlusion is usually normal. Minor occlusal discrepancies can be corrected by selective equilibration. MacLennan[10] reviewed 180 cases of condylar fractures treated by conservative methods in which 5 children (2.8%) were under age 10. The survey indicates that crush injuries involving the condylar cartilage sustained before age 5 are more prone to permanent growth changes. Only 16% had deviation during function, and none had limitation of movement. Although pain, clicking, or grating may tempt the physician to consider condylectomy, surgical intervention is not indicated. The risks of surgery are significant, and it will likely lead to arrested development and possibly fibrous or bony ankylosis. Early and persistent movement with the assistance of an elastic jaw exerciser invariably prevents development of ankylosis and aids in restoring function.

Extracapsular or subcondylar fractures not involving the articular surface are the most common type of mandibular fracture. In infants and younger children these are usually of the green-stick variety with a nondisplaced fractured segment. In older children a crack fracture through one or both cortices may be present without displacement or additional damage. There is usually a normal relationship of the condylar head to the glenoid fossa and few signs or symptoms of fracture. Fractures occurring below the attachment of the lateral pterygoid muscle may result in slight deviation and displacement or complete dislocation of the condylar process. Deviation of the fractured segment is usually forward, medial, and downward. A slight deviation implies that the head of the condyle is still in the glenoid fossa and within its capsule. With displacement the fractured segment is so positioned that there is overlap between the condylar process and the ramus, and it is reasonable to expect a bony union of the fracture segments. A dislocated fracture is one in which the condylar process is completely out of the glenoid fossa with no bony contact with the ramus. It may be dislocated for some distance. Several cases of dislocation into the middle cranial fossa have been reported.

Management of mandibular condyle fractures

The management of fractures of the mandibular condyle in children remains controversial. The complexity of the temporomandibular articulation and the role of the mandibular condyle during facial growth are the principle reasons for the diverse opinions regarding treatment for this type of fracture. The view that precise anatomic reduction by surgical intervention will avert interference in growth and restore normal function is opposed by the school of thought which contends that nonoperative conservative methods of treatment accomplish good results with an extremely low incidence of malfunction, trismus, or ankylosis. The conservative view is reinforced by long experience which has shown that in the majority of cases even fractures with considerable dislocation will heal with a good functional result and rarely account for long-term complications.

The temporomandibular apparatus is a highly specialized joint that distinctly differs from other articulations. The articulation is between the head of the condyle and the articular surface of the temporal bone and the adjacent supporting soft tissues. This unique joint is described as a *ginglymoarthrodial joint* because the condylar heads are capable of hingelike movement as well as sliding forward. It is a true, or *synovial,* joint with two synovial cavities, one upper and one lower cavity separated by a fibrocartilaginous articular disc.

The temporomandibular joint differs from other joints in that the articulating bones are not separated by hyaline cartilage covering the surface, but rather by an articular disc with only a small number of cartilage cells scattered throughout the disc. The articulation is also unique in that the two condyles are attached, and therefore all movement is mechanically coupled.

The basic movements permitted by the temporomandibular joint complex are (1) hinge movement between the head of the mandible and the articular disc and (2) the anteroposterior sliding of the mandibular head and attached disc along the temporal bone. Movement of the joints is also influenced by the size, shape, position, and inclination of teeth present in the body of the mandible.

Movements are accomplished principally by the synchronous action of the muscles of mastication, namely the temporal masseter, and internal and external pterygoid muscles, which all pass across the joint and are complemented by several suprahyoid and infrahyoid muscles.

The elevators of the lower jaw are the masseter, temporal and internal pterygoid muscles. Protrusion of the jaw is accomplished primarily by the external pterygoid muscle and aided by superficial fibers of the masseter and internal pterygoid muscles. Retraction or depression is brought about by posterior fibers of the temporal, digastric, mylohyoid, and geniohyoid muscles. Synergistic action of the muscles is necessary if the complicated pattern of mandibular movement is to function properly. Because of the anatomic complexity of this joint, treatment of fractures in this region is regarded as one of the most difficult problems of all mandibular fractures in children.

Normal facial growth depends on the orderly activity of numerous growth centers throughout the facial skeleton, and the growth of the mandible is vital to the overall growth of the facial skeleton. According to Sicher and DuBrul,[19] mandibular growth can be considered the leading factor for all facial bone growth. The primary growth center of the mandible is located beneath the articular surface of the condyle where a cartilaginous cap is responsible for epiphyseal-like growth and endochondral ossification. Concurrently appositional growth along the posterior surface accounts for the increasing width of the ramus and the lengthening of the body. Appositional growth of the superior portion of the coronoid process keeps up with the lengthening of the ramus. Resorption along the anterior border of the ramus continually adjusts the anteroposterior length of the ramus with growth of the alveolus posteriorly. Injury to the condyle or the secondary growth centers of the mandible are of special concern, considering that insult to these areas may potentially result in growth abnormalities of the facial skeleton.

Regardless of the degree of condylar displacement, the vast majority of surgeons treating condylar fractures in children recommend nonsurgical conservative treatment. Numerous case reports in which children were treated conservatively lend testimony to the unusual ability of condylar fractures to heal with remodeling of the condylar head and restoration of normal function. Extensive radiographic investigations support clinical evidence that children are less likely to have permanent damage and growth problems after injury to the condylar process. Experimental growth studies on animals have also demonstrated the excellent recovery potential of the fractured condyle. As MacLennan[11] points

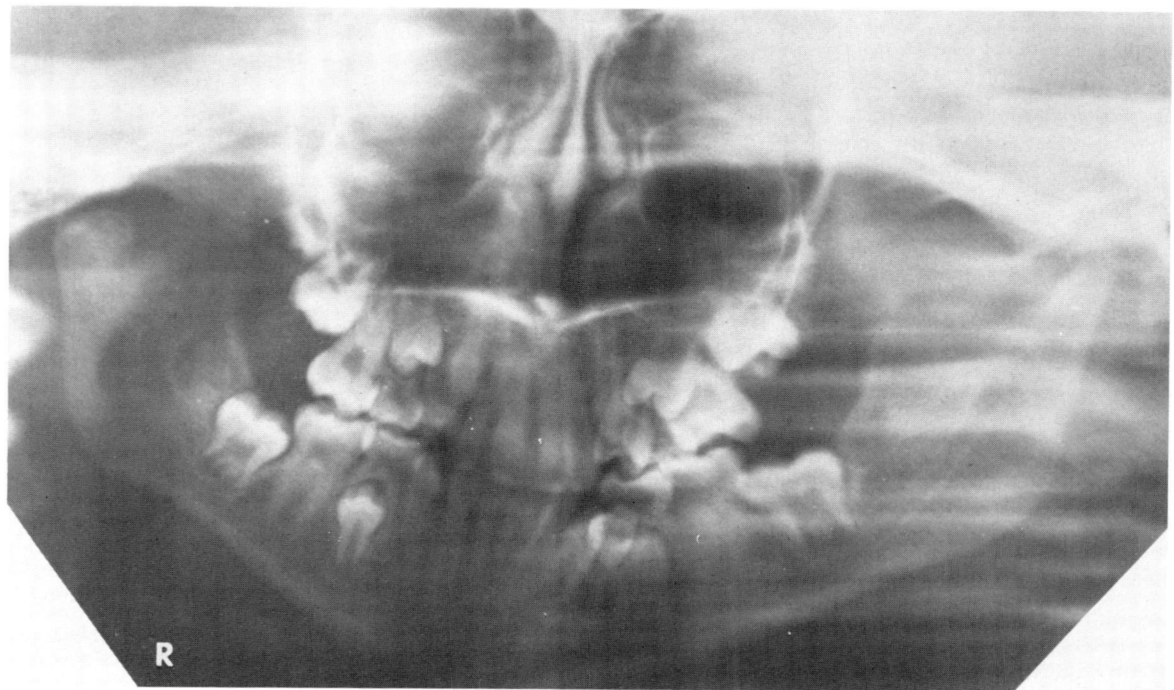

Fig. 31-22. Remodeling of right condylar head 2 years after the fracture.

out, complications arising from fractures of the mandibular condyle are conspicuous by their absence. On the other hand, many authors advocate the operative management for all displaced condylar fracture, whereas others suggest open reduction in only selected cases. Unfortunately, there are no follow-up surveys of large numbers of pediatric patients with fractured condyles treated by operative means.

There is overwhelming evidence that closed reduction and conservative treatment for condylar fractures are appropriate treatments and will invariably ensure a most satisfactory long-term result. It may be considered the only skeletal fracture that does not require anatomic reduction to achieve a satisfactory result. Archer[1] states that there is no indication for open reduction of subcondylar fractures. His philosophy applies for undisplaced condylar fractures as well as for fractures in which the head has been dislocated. Blevins and Gores,[2] Thompson, Farmer, and Lindsay[20] and MacLennan and Simpson[13] are of the opinion that all condylar fractures in children should be treated conservatively and that conservative treatment will not result in gross maxillomandibular asymmetry or compromise normal function. Leake et al.,[7] Russell, Nosti, and Reavis,[18] and Kaban, Mulliken, and Murray[6] have observed numerous children who sustained condylar fractures that were treated nonsurgically. They reported restoration of normal function, satisfactory occlusion, and remodeling of the condylar stump when jaw motion was maintained (Fig. 31-22).

Considerable clinical research has been directed at determining the most appropriate treatment for condylar fractures in children. An extensive radiographic survey conducted by Lindahl and Hollender[9] analyzed the remodeling of 76 condylar processes after fracture. Patients were placed in four age groups, and radiographs were taken at the time of injury and at 3, 12, 24, and 36 to 48 months after injury and treatment. The study concluded that in the 3 to 11-year-old group, 20 of 27 patients had normal skeletal relationships with extensive remodeling of the condylar process. In the 12 to 19-year-old group, remodeling did occur, but not to the same degree, and in adults only minimal remodeling occurred. This study is consistent with the conclusions of many investigators who found that during the growth period the facial skeleton in children had the unique ability to heal and remodel.

Research with growing animals aimed at studying the remolding process and the effect on jaw growth subsequent to traumatic fracture dislocation of the mandible was conducted by Walker.[21] Young rhesus monkeys with full deciduous dentition were used. Condylar fractures were surgically produced and dislocated in a variety of positions. On one animal a condylectomy was performed, and in another the condyle was removed, then wired back in its normal position. Radiographic and postmortem examination showed that each animal reformed a functional condylar head and ''each mandible had formed a remarkable morphologically identifiable condyle in an upright position.''[21] Regardless of the type and degree of fracture dislocation, even when the condyle

was removed, there was not a significant loss of mandibular asymmetry and growth.

Another experimental animal study using rhesus monkeys was reported by Boyne[3] in 1967. Subcondylar fractures were surgically produced in 12 animals. In four animals, the fracture was manually reduced and fixed with an intraosseous wire. In four other monkeys the fractures were not reduced; however, intermaxillary immobilization was established by circumzygomatic wire suspension and nasal piriform immobilization wires. The last four monkeys received no treatment after the surgically produced fracture. The animals were killed at intervals and studied macroscopically and microscopically. There was excellent bony union between the fragments, and neither a malocclusion nor a mandibular deformity could be detected in any of the animals. Recontouring of the displaced condyle occurred, with the condyle assuming a more vertical mediolateral position. It appears that these results support conservative treatment of fracture dislocations of the condyle in children and that surgical intervention does not offer any advantage to the natural reparative process.

Methods of fixation

When immobilization for a condylar fracture is indicated for an infant or a child under 2½ years old, unique fixation techniques will be required. Because either numerous primary teeth have not erupted or the erupted primary teeth do not lend themselves to wiring methods by virtue of their shape, immobilization must be managed as with an edentulous fracture. A slightly oversized acrylic overlay mandibular splint is constructed (Fig. 31-23). An appropriate thickness of gutta-percha is placed to line the splint, which is then placed over the mandibular teeth or the alveolus. It is held secure by two circummandibular wires in the area of the mandibular body. This type of splint, which is advocated by MacLennan,[12] is to be constructed so that the occlusal surface will be in contact with the maxillary teeth

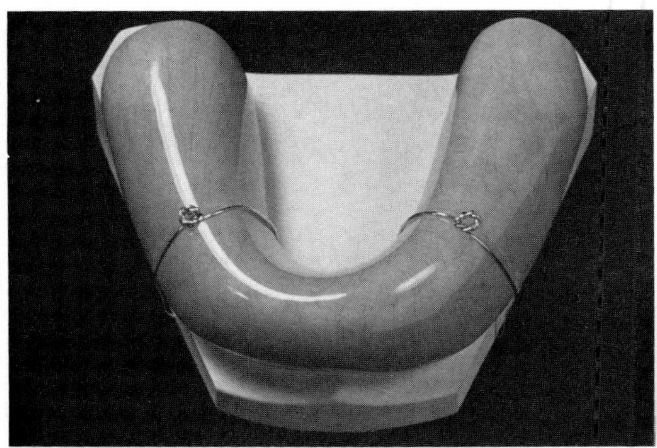

Fig. 31-23. Acrylic overlay mandibular splint held secure with circummandibular wires.

or the alveolus, maintaining a normal vertical dimension. The mandible is placed in a normal relationship to the maxilla, and immobilization is effected by a wire passed through the nasal spine or piriform aperture and tightened around the midline circummandibular wire. The splint and wires may be removed in 2 to 3 weeks, and movement of the jaw is encouraged. It is wise to consider antibiotic prophylaxis before removal of the wires.

In older children with a full complement of noncarious primary teeth or with a sufficient number of permanent teeth, several wiring techniques can be used effectively, or if the situation is suitable, arch bars are the ideal method to secure intermaxillary fixation.

Several types of prefabricated malleable arch bars are commercially available. The bar is soft and can be adapted accurately around each tooth and cut to any desired length without difficulty. The bars have small bracket attachments designed for acceptance of rubber bands or wires. The brackets are placed at short intervals over the length of the bar for flexibility in directing the desired traction force.

The arch bar is first cut to the desired length. It is contoured to the outer surfaces of the maxillary or mandibular teeth, and the length is rechecked to ensure it is sufficient. While the bar is held against the outer surfaces of the teeth, 28-gauge stainless steel wire is used to hold the arch bar to the necks of the teeth. A 6-inch (15 cm) length of wire is passed about the bar and between the teeth. The end of the wire is picked up on the lingual surface, placed around the neck of the tooth, and then drawn back to the lateral surface, with the end passing under the bar. The wire now is above and below the bar, and both ends are on the lateral surface. The ends of the wire are twisted tightly, ensuring that it is below the crown and against the neck of the tooth so that it will not slip. It is often necessary to hold the wire below the crown with a gauze packer while twisting it. As each wire is applied and tightened, the bar is contoured around the tooth and held securely. The twisted wires are then cut so that the 5 to 7 mm left may be turned down and away

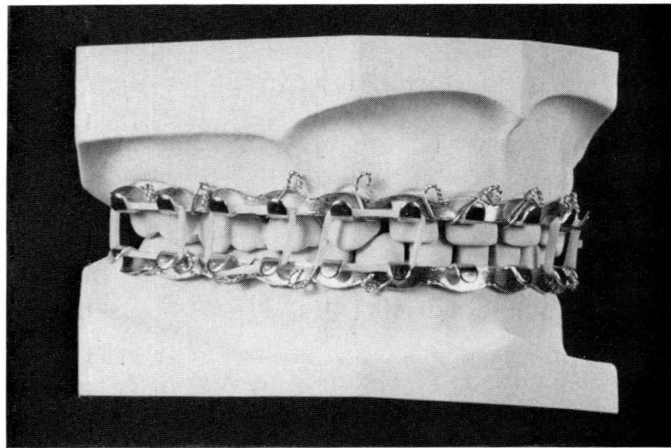

Fig. 31-24. Maxillary and mandibular arch bars with intermaxillary elastic traction and fixation.

from the gingiva and soft tissues of the cheek. The bar is then checked for stability, and loose wires are tightened. Small rubber bands placed around the brackets will provide the traction and the intermaxillary fixation. The direction of the rubber bands will vary in accordance to the desired direction of movement of the segment (Fig. 31-24).

Occasionally it is necessary to reinforce stabilization of either a maxillary or mandibular arch bar. This is especially true for children from ages 6 to 14 years with mixed dentition, that is, primary and permanent teeth in both arches. Some of the primary teeth are stable within the alveolus, and others are undergoing root resorption. Newly erupted teeth have incompletely formed roots and may be easily avulsed when heavy traction is placed on the arch bars. The application of arch bars may be an advantageous method of immobilization for many patients in this age group, and supplementary stabilization can be very useful.

A maxillary arch bar can be made more secure by passing one or more suspension wires through a small hole placed in the piriform margin of the maxilla or through a hole in the anterior nasal spine. If three wires are placed, one through each piriform margin and one through the nasal spine, the arch bar is firmly fixed, and great force can be applied between the arches with little chance for avulsion of teeth. One or more circummandibular wires will accomplish the same stability of a mandibular arch bar.

Numerous methods of using only wire to establish intermaxillary fixation have been described. Direct wiring between maxillary and mandibular teeth is ill advised and hazardous, because complete removal of the wires will be required to open the mouth. This method presents a danger in emergency situations, and assessment of healing at the fracture site is not possible during treatment.

Multiple-loop wiring technique

Multiple-loop wiring is one alternative to the application of arch bars and embraces the principle of all wiring techniques such as the Kazanjian button technique, Risdon wiring, and Ivy loops. They all provide suitable anchoring devices to teeth from which traction and intermaxillary fixation can be attached.

One end of the wire is held on the lateral surfaces of the teeth starting at the midline of the mandible (stationary wire). The other end of the wire (working wire) is looped around the last tooth, passed between the last two teeth, and brough out laterally under the stationary wire. It is then returned medially between the same teeth above the stationary wire (Fig. 31-25, *A*). A loop has been created on the lateral surface that engages the stationary wire. To make uniform loops, a small orangewood stick is held on the lateral surface of the teeth over the stationary wire (Fig. 31-25, *B*). After the first loop the stationary wire need not be held.

This process is continued until the desired number of loops have been made (Fig. 31-25, *C*). After making the last loop, the working wire is brought out to the lateral side

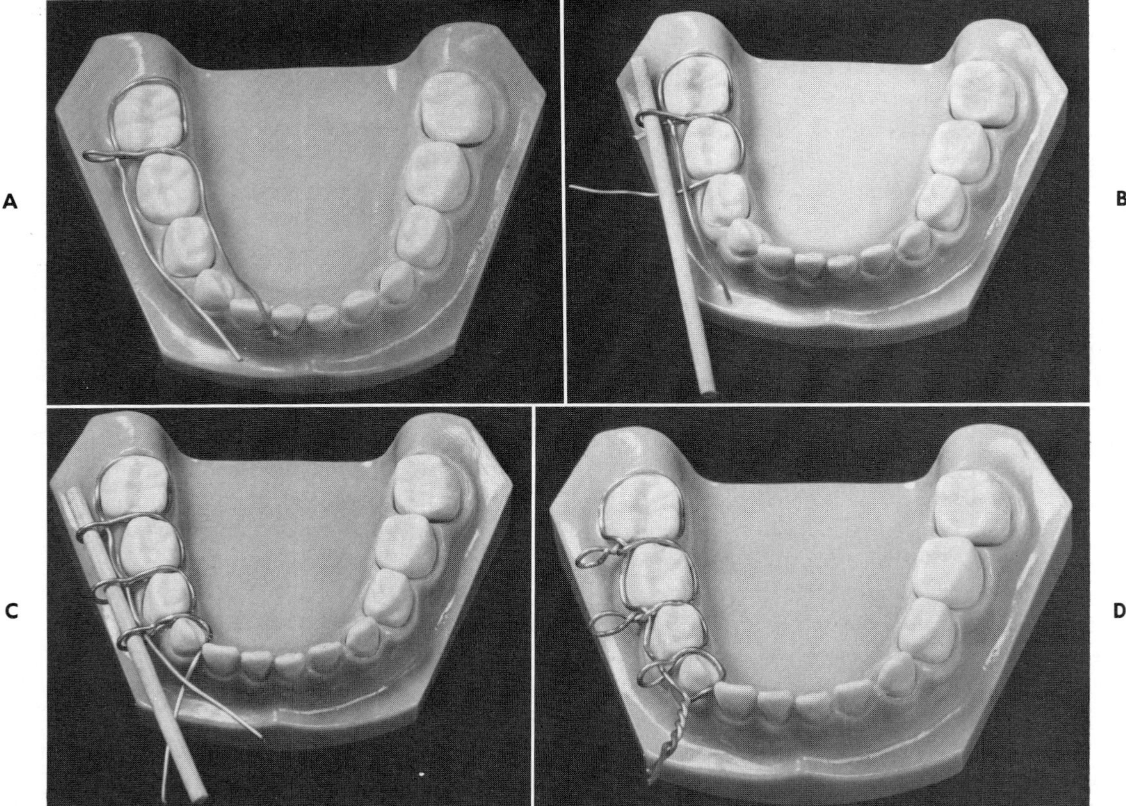

Fig. 31-25. A, First step in multiple-loop wiring technique. **B,** Place a small stick for uniform loops. **C,** Continue this process, making 3 or 4 loops. **D,** After the loops are formed, they are tightened and bent downward.

between the next two anterior teeth; it is crossed with the stationary wire and tightly twisted (Fig. 31-25, *D*). The remaining loops are tightly twisted and checked for stability. The same procedure is carried out in the other quadrants. The loops can all now be bent away from the occlusal surfaces of the teeth and used as hooks for the application of elastic traction or intermaxillary wiring.

Acrylic or metal splints must be constructed for the many situations in which arch bars or multiple-loop wiring cannot be applied to unerupted or incompletely developed permanent teeth. These teeth can undergo subluxation or avulsion with only a modest amount of intermaxillary traction. Splints can also be used when horizontal fixation across a fracture line is desirable or for the treatment of fractures in which stabilization is indicated without immobilizing the jaws with intermaxillary fixation. Acrylic splints offer the surgeon a technique to tailor make and custom design fixation for a wide variety of problems that are unique in children.

A splint can be designed in a continuous horseshoe shape so that the acrylic covers the lingual and labial surfaces of the teeth (Fig. 31-26). A vertical cut is made through a large acrylic button on the anterolateral surface. When the splint is placed over a fracture that has been reduced and

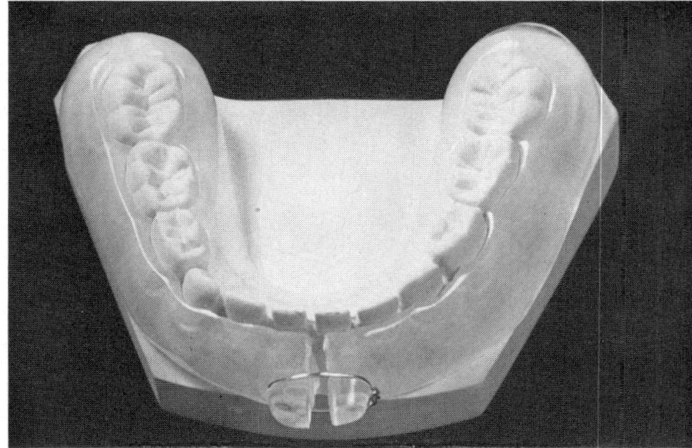

Fig. 31-26. The acrylic splint covers the lingual and facial surfaces of the teeth and is secured at the midline with a wire ligature.

the splint button is brought together and secured with wire, the appliance will immobilize the fracture. Small sections of arch bar can be incorporated into the lateral flange of the splint to accommodate intermaxillary fixation. This technique is especially useful for displaced fractures of the mandibular body when reduction can be accomplished with little manipulation.

Cast cap silver splints have wide popularity throughout Europe and are used extensively. This technique never has gained favor in this country and only rarely is used for stabilization of facial fractures.

Metal cast splints are the forerunners of the acrylic appliances and are considered advantageous for a number of reasons. They can be used in situations in which the number and shape of teeth preclude the use of wiring techniques. By virtue of their construction there is absolutely no mobility of the splint, and because the entire crown of the tooth is covered, rotation is not likely to occur. Because the occlusal surfaces of the teeth are covered, it is difficult to establish a normal functional occlusion. This may not be important, since after removal of the splints only minor occlusal disharmonies are present and can be corrected with minimal equilibration. A dental abscess or any acute infection that develops will require removal of the entire splint.

The alternate methods of fixation are favored for several reasons. They do not require a temporary immobilization procedure, there is no long delay in treatment for the construction of the splint, cementation is not necessary, and they do not require elaborate laboratory facilities and technicians to process the appliance.

Indications for open reduction

There should be no dispute that virtually all condylar fractures in children are best managed by conservative methods. However, in several situations conservative methods of treatment are inadequate, and an open reduction procedure is indicated. The indications for open reduction include the following:

1. The fractured condyle is positioned so as to prohibit or limit opening of the jaw, or it causes interference with normal movement.
2. Bilateral condylar fractures cause reduced height of the rami and anterior open bite. Consideration should be given to open reduction on at lease one side.
3. The mandibular condyle is dislocated into the middle cranial fossa, resulting in a neurologic deficit and requiring neurosurgical intervention. Fortunately, dislocation of the condyle into the middle cranial fossa is rare. Perhaps infrequent reporting of such cases is related to mortality resulting from intracranial injury secondary to the displaced condyle.

Open reduction for condylar fractures

Two surgical approaches to the temporomandibular articulation that permit good visibility and access to the head and neck of the condyle are commonly employed. Although the *preauricular approach* carries the risk of injury to the seventh cranial nerve, it provides better visualization of the head of the condyle and of the capsule of the joint, as well as offers a good cosmetic result. The *submandibular approach* is safer and less likely to cause seventh cranial nerve insult. It is most useful for reduction and fixation of the low or subcondylar fractures having a long proximal fragment.

Several modifications of the preauricular approach have been described; however, they are attended by additional complications and offer no advantages over the traditional preauricular procedure.

Preauricular approach

An incision is made through only the skin in front of the ear and extending from the upper level of the pinna to the level of the lobe. The preauricular skin is undermined and sutured forward to the cheek over the zygomatic arch for retraction. The dissection begins immediately in front of the cartilage of the external auditory meatus, where the superficial temporal vessels will be identified and retracted out of the field or cut and ligated. The dissection in the temporal area is carried down to the temporal fascia and the root of the zygomatic arch. A cut is made down to bone on the posterior zygomatic arch above the glenoid fossa. The periosteum is lifted, and the joint capsule is exposed. If the head of the condyle is dislocated and lies anteriorly and medially, it will be difficult to identify. Dissection is carried out down the neck of the condyle, exposing the fracture site. After recovery of the proximal fragment, alignment will be difficult because of the pull of the lateral pterygoid muscle and the tendency for redislocation. Securing the proximal fragment firmly, a small drill hole is made obliquely from the external surface to the center of the fracture surface. A similar drill hole is made in the ramus fragment. A 25-gauge stainless steel wire is then placed into one hole and pulled through the second hole by a smaller wire loop. The fracture is reduced and held secure by twisting the wire.

On occasion, regardless of how the wires have been placed or how tightly they have been twisted, the reduced fragment will not remain in the proper position. Redislocation may be avoided by placing small drill holes, one through the condyle and one through the zygomatic arch, and securing the condylar head with a chromic catgut suture. The suture will have dissolved or will be disrupted when movement is permitted. Skeletal pin fixation is another method of preventing redislocation of the condylar head (Fig. 31-27). One skeletal pin is placed in the head and another in the zygomatic arch and fastened to a bar assembly. The pins may be removed in 10 days, and radiographs will help determine if further manipulation is necessary.

Submandibular approach

The Risdon approach for reduction and fixation of low subcondylar fractures offers good access and satisfactory exposure. It also minimizes injury of the upper branches of the facial nerve. A 5 cm incision is made one finger's breadth below and behind the angle of the mandible. The skin and subcutaneous tissue are incised and the platysma muscle exposed. The platysma muscle is cleanly incised, taking care not to injure the mandibular branch of the facial nerve, which is located immediately under the muscle and is usually found lying directly over the pulsating facial artery. The nerve is retracted out of the field. The facial artery

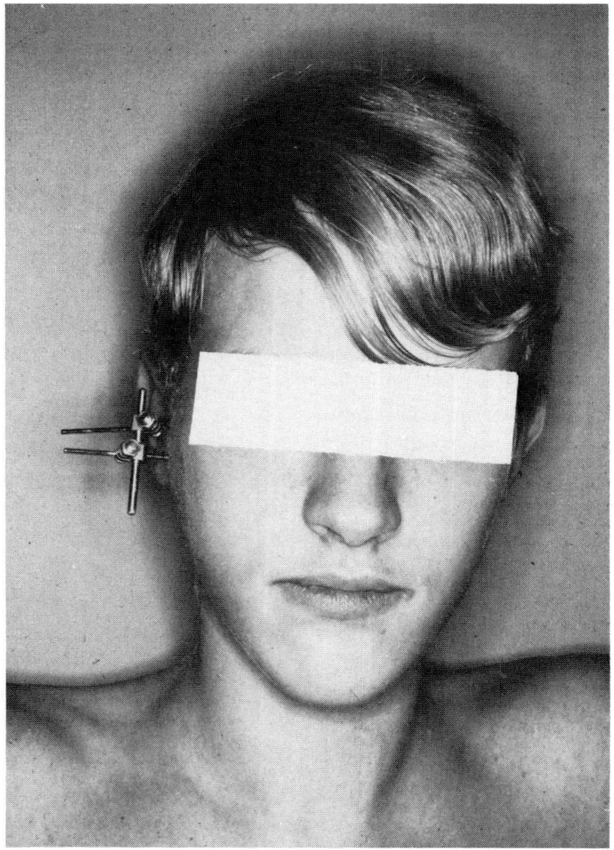

Fig. 31-27. One skeletal pin is placed in the condylar head, and one pin in the zygomatic arch may be necessary to prevent redislocation.

and vein are then identified and either retracted out of the field or sectioned and ligated. The dissection is carried to the inferior border of the mandibular angle, and the fibers of the masseter muscle and the periosteum are incised. The tissues are stripped off the bone and retracted upward until the fracture is exposed. The proximal fragment is manipulated and reduced and held secure with 25-gauge stainless steel wire placed through small drill holes on either side of the fracture. The wound is closed in layers and without drainage. Immobilization of the mandible is carried out by an appropriate technique.

BODY AND SYMPHYSIS FRACTURES

As with condylar fractures, a significant number of mandibular fractures in children do not require elaborate methods of fixation or surgical intervention. The primary goal of treatment is directed at restoration of jaw movement as soon as possible. A crack in one cortex in the angle or body of the mandible with no displacement may be treated without immobilization. A child with a nondisplaced mandibular fracture and a normal occlusal relationship will invariably do very well simply with rest, a soft diet, and appropriate supportive treatment. Using prudent judgment in determin-

ing which fractures need not be treated will be rewarded.

Displaced fractures of the body and symphysis region will require reduction and immobilization for a relatively short period of time. The degree of displacement depends on the location of the fracture, the direction of the fracture line, the muscle pull on the fragments, and the presence or absence of teeth on each side of the fracture site. In mandibular body fractures with no teeth in the posterior fragment the posterior fragment will be distracted upward and medially until the fragment impinges on the upper teeth or alveolar ridge. In bilateral fractures through the mandibular body the anterior segment will be pulled downward and backward, and the posterior fragments pulled upward and medially.

The treatment plan for fractures of the body of the mandible is largely determined by the presence or absence of teeth on either side of the fracture and the ease with which the segments can be reduced and the position maintained. When applicable, the ideal treatment plan is simple intermaxillary fixation with multiple-loop wiring or the application of arch bars and intermaxillary rubber band fixation. Sometimes displacement cannot be controlled with closed reduction because of either the absence of teeth or displacement by muscle pull that cannot be overcome. If this is the case, open reduction (either intraorally or extraorally) with internal wire fixation will better align and stabilize the fragments. If the fracture site is accessible, the intraoral approach is preferred.

Intraoral approach

A 4 cm incision is made in the deepest part of the buccal gutter with the central point of the incision directly opposite the fracture site. Incisions made higher along the body in the attached gingiva will be difficult to close and will invariably break down. By blunt dissection the inferior border of the mandible is identified, and the mucoperiosteum is incised and stripped from the bone 2 to 3 cm on either side of the fracture site. The hematoma found at the fracture site is evacuated. The fracture is reduced, and the fracture segments held with small bone-grasping forceps. Small drill holes are made close to the inferior border on either side of the fracture. Extreme care must be taken in placement of the interosseous wire holes to avoid damage to the developing tooth buds (Fig. 31-28). A 25-gauge stainless steel wire passed through the holes and tightly twisted will provide adequate fixation. The mucoperiosteum is closed with chromic catgut sutures and the oral mucosal incision with a nonabsorbable material.

Extraoral approach

Using a skin-marking pencil, the inferior border of the mandible and the fracture site are marked. The skin is marked one finger's breadth below the inferior border of the mandible and parallel to skin lines. A 2 to 3 cm incision is drawn, the center of which corresponds to the fracture. A small amount of local anesthetic containing epinephrine

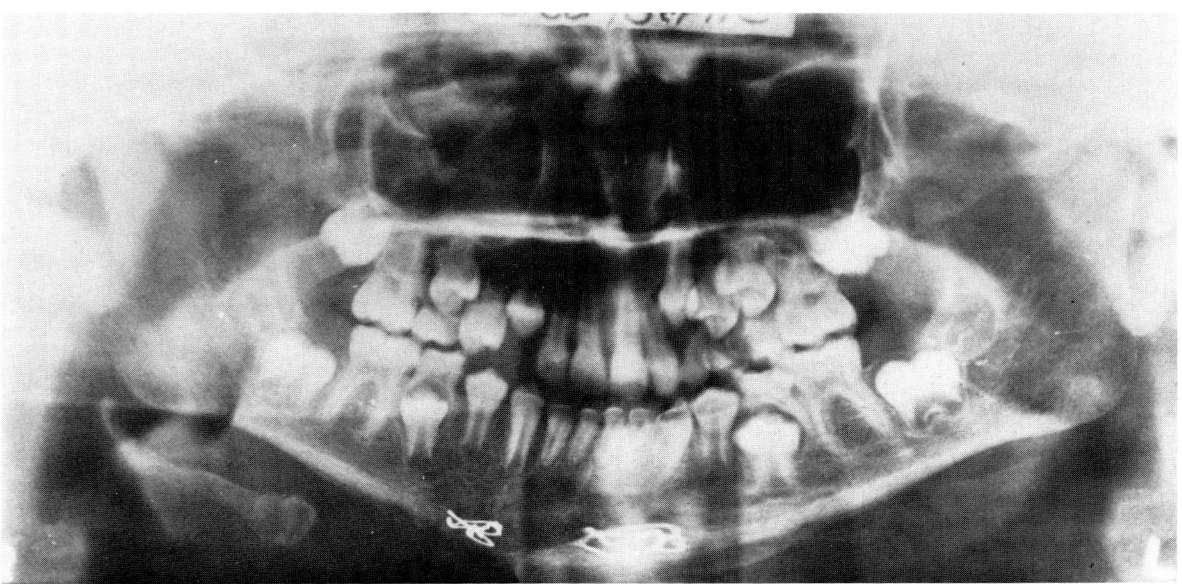

Fig. 31-28. Interosseous wires are placed close to the inferior border of the mandible to avoid damage to the developing teeth.

injected into the tissues adjacent to the fracture will minimize operative bleeding. Keeping the blade at a right angle to the skin, the incision is carried through the skin and subcutaneous tissue, exposing the platysma muscle. In younger children the platysma muscle will be rather thin and poorly defined. If the muscle is thick, it can be cleanly sectioned. If it is flimsy and thin, it is advisable to bluntly dissect through it, taking care to identify the mandibular branch of the facial nerve, which is immediately under the muscle. As dissection proceeds to the inferior border of the mandible, the facial vessels should be identified as they appear on the anterior margin of the masseter muscle. The lower border of the mandible is identified, and the periosteum is cut along the lower border of each fragment. The intraosseous wire fixation is completed as described in the intraoral approach. Placement of a figure-of-eight wire is not difficult when the extraoral approach is used and may ensure additional stability of the bone ends. The wound is closed in layers, the periosteum and platysma muscle with interrupted 4-0 chromic catgut sutures and the subcutaneous tissue with inverted interrupted 5-0 chromic catgut sutures. The skin is closed with 6-0 nylon sutures.

SYMPHYSIS AND PARASYMPHYSEAL FRACTURES

The symphysis is the midline of the mandible, and the parasymphysis is the region between the lower canine teeth. Fractures occurring in this area are frequently displaced with telescoping of the fragments because of the inward pull of the muscles attached to the inner surface of the mandible, that is, the mylohyoid, geniohyoid, and anterior belly of the digastric muscles.

An anterior malocclusion or discontinuity of the lower dental arch may be obvious on clinical examination. Digital palpation of the inner and outer surface of the anterior mandible and movement at the fracture site will confirm the fracture. It is not unusual for parasymphyseal fractures to be missed with routine posteroanterior views of the mandible. The degree of displacement, associated alveolar fractures, and avulsed teeth can best be seen in intraoral occlusal radiographs. The presence of a parasymphysis fracture should prompt the examiner to suspect multiple mandibular fractures, particularly a subcondylar fracture on one or both sides.

Parasymphyseal fractures with little or moderate displacement usually can be manipulated and reduced with relative ease and immobilized with dental wiring, arch bars, or an acrylic splint. In infants and children under 3 years of age a custom acrylic splint or a prefabricated acrylic splint lined with gutta-percha and secured with two circummandibular wires will immobilize the fracture adequately (Fig. 31-29).

In older children with sufficient teeth on both sides of the fracture, multiple-loop wiring or arch bars may be adequate to align the teeth and restore a normal occlusion. However, in these cases, it is not uncommon to discover a wide separation of the fracture at the inferior border. If open reduction is indicated to better align the fragments, an intraoral degloving incision will satisfactorily expose the entire parasymphyseal region. The surgical technique is as previously described for the intraoral approach of mandibular body fractures. After open reduction fixation with a segmental arch bar attached to teeth on both sides of the fracture will provide adequate stabilization.

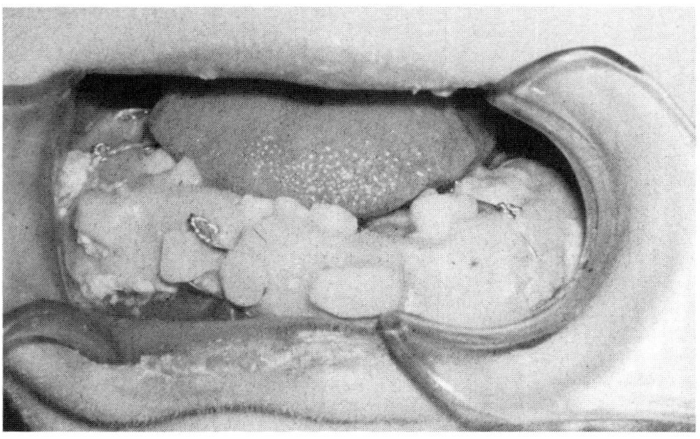

Fig. 31-29. The acrylic splint is secured with two circummandibular wires.

CORONOID PROCESS

Isolated fractures of the coronoid process or coronoid fractures associated with other mandibular fractures are extremely rare. The coronoid process lies deep to the zygomatic arch. The origin of the masseter muscle and the tendinous attachment of the temporal muscle do much to protect it. Nondisplaced fractures of the coronoid process do not require reduction. If significant upward displacement is distracting the coronoid process to the medial side of the zygomatic arch and interferes with mandibular function, the coronoid process should be removed intraorally through an incision along the anterior border of the ramus. Rowe and Killey[17] warn that union may occur between fragments of the zygomatic arch that have undergone medial displacement and the detached coronoid process. Periodic assessment of active movement will prevent this type of ankylosis.

FRACTURES OF THE ANGLE OF THE MANDIBLE

The angle of the mandible is that portion underlying the attachment of the masseter muscle. The clinical significance of fractures in this region is that they generally are located beyond the control of intermaxillary traction and splints and often will require open reduction for proper alignment and fixation. The direction of the fracture line will determine the degree of displacement. Characteristically, the proximal fragment is distracted upward by the masseter muscle and medially by the pterygoid muscles.

For nondisplaced fractures in the mandibular angle, intermaxillary fixation is usually adequate treatment. Intermaxillary fixation with elastic traction will also be effective treatment for fractures in which the proximal fragment is displaced superiorly, provided the proximal fragment contains stable teeth and there is an opposing tooth in the maxilla. After the placement of multiple-loop wiring or arch bars, light elastic vertical traction will bring the fractured ends into close approximation with a satisfactory occlusion.

The light elastics can be replaced with heavy elastic bands or wires once reduction is adequate.

When severe displacement or an edentulous proximal fragment precludes the conservative course of treatment, an open reduction may provide the best result. If the fracture site at the inferior border is located clost to the anterior edge of the masseter muscle, the intraoral approach is preferred. When the fracture site at the inferior border of the mandible is posterior, intraoral open reduction with wire fixation is quite difficult. If this is the case, an extraoral approach is recommended. Both approaches have been described.

SUMMARY AND CONCLUSIONS

Fractures of the facial skeleton in children are rare, and surveys indicate that the incidence is only from 1% to 5%. Fractures of the mandible are the most common, and the vast majority of mandibular fractures are sustained by boys. Although the principles of treatment for pediatric facial fractures are similar to those for adult patients, modalities of treatment will differ due principally to a child's unique anatomic features and emotional status. A thorough and meaningful examination depends on the validity of the patient's responses to questions and to the physical examination. The majority of children have other injuries in addition to fractures of the mandible, including skull fractures, closed head trauma, and extremity or cervical spine injuries. This stresses the need for a meticulous physical examination with emphasis on the neurologic evaluation.

The causes of facial fractures in children vary greatly with the age and social activity of the child. Infants and preschool children rarely suffer serious facial injury because of their well-protected environment. However, at age 5 when children begin school they are exposed to a more "hazardous" life-style. As children become older, recreational and sporting activities are increased, and this, coupled with physical development, accounts for a sharp rise in the incidence of facial fractures.

Body fractures of the mandible are the most common injuries. These are usually unilateral and often associated with a fracture of the mandibular condyle on the opposite side. Anterior bilateral parasymphyseal fractures of the body of the mandible are the most infrequent.

The consideration for growth potential, the unique problems associated with fixation and immobilization of the jaws, and the relative emotional instability of a child will dictate the appropriate modality of treatment. The unique dental configuration of the primary dentition presents interesting complications in the application of fixation apparatus and will require the design of alternate methods of reduction and immobilization. The early treatment of mandibular fractures in children is of importance because of the high osteogenic potential in developing bone. Immediate definitive treatment of mandibular fractures in children is neither obligatory nor necessary. However, as with the adult patient, primary consideration should be the maintenance of a patent airway, control of hemorrhage, and assessment of other body injuries.

When indicated, prophylactic antibiotic therapy for children with facial injuries is often an appropriate measure for the control of potential infections. This is especially true in children who sustain soft tissue injuries that have been contaminated with road debris or soil. It is also often advisable in the treatment of comminuted intraoral or extraoral mandibular fractures.

The restoration of normal function and prevention of untoward sequelae are key principles in the treatment of mandibular fractures. Judicious and expeditious treatment of these injuries should be carried out in a single one-step procedure when possible, simply because children are not as tolerant as adults. Unlike adults, strict attention should be paid to the status of the developing dentition in children. The sacrifice of primary and permanent teeth should be avoided at all costs. Careful placement of intraosseous wires in open reductions and the elimination of intraoral pin fixation, which may unnecessarily damage developing tooth buds of permanent teeth, will avoid numerous problems that may have long-term effects. Good oral hygiene is of utmost importance and should be given strict attention.

Clinical examination of the head and neck differs little from that for the adult patient. Similar signs of facial deformity, assymmetry, malocclusion, swelling, paresthesia, crepitation, and ecchymosis are often common findings. Time spent winning a child's confidence is worth the effort; however, often sedation or even general anesthesia may be necessary to conduct a satisfactory clinical and radiographic examination. Careful bimanual examination of the facial skeleton can be a slow, tedious, and time-comsuming process, yet it is extremely valuable in the assessment, treatment planning, and definitive treatment of the pediatric patient. Along with a thorough clinical examination, a series of appropriate facial radiographs is of utmost importance in the treatment planning. The single most useful radiographic aid in the diagnosis of mandibular fractures is the panoramic view. In addition, a modified Towne's view, lateral oblique views of the right and left mandibular bodies, open and closed temporomandibular joint views, anteroposterior facial view, lateral facial view, and submental-vertex view will confirm the extent and severity of the fractures. In addition to these radiographs, special dental radiographs, including intraoral occlusal and periapical films, have proven invaluable in the assessment of localized alveolar fractures, medial or lateral displacement of parasymphyseal and symphyseal fractures, and for localizing bone and tooth fragments in the sublingual and labial soft tissues.

Clinical and radiographic diagnosis of mandibular condylar fractures in children can often be difficult because of the occult nature of the injury. Clinical signs and symptoms may be obscure or missing. Although the treatment of fractures of the mandibular condyle in children has been a controversial topic for many years, there is overwhelming evidence that closed reduction and conservative treatment are the most advantageous. A variety of methods for intermaxillary fixation can be applied to the pediatric patient. Open reduction of condylar fractures should be considered only for gross limitation of mandibular motion, anterior open bite secondary to bilateral condylar fractures, and dislocation of the mandibular condyle into the middle cranial fossa. The surgical approach that permits the best visibility and access to the temporomandibular joint should be used.

As with condylar fractures, body and symphyseal fractures do not often require elaborate methods of fixation or surgical intervention. A custom or prefabricated acrylic splint will immobilize a fracture adequately in the young child. In older children with an adequate number of teeth, arch bars or multiple-loop wiring is usually adequate to reduce and immobilize a fracture.

REFERENCES

1. Archer, W.H.: Oral and maxillofacial surgery, ed. 5, Philadelphia, 1975, W.B. Saunders Co.
2. Blevins, C., and Gores, R.J.: Fractures of the mandibular condyloid process: results of conservative treatment in 140 patients, J. Oral Surg. **19**:392, 1961.
3. Boyne, P.J.: Osseous repair and mandibular growth after subcondylar fractures, J. Oral Surg. **25**:300, 1967.
4. Gerrie, J., and McCarthy, J.: Progress in lower jaw fracture treatment, J. Can. Dent. Assoc. **21**:277, 1955.
5. Hagan, E.H., and Huelke, D.F.: An analysis of 319 case reports of mandibular fractures, J. Oral Surg. **19**:93, 1961.
6. Kaban, L.B., Mulliken, J.B., and Murray, J.E.: Facial fractures in children: an analysis of 122 fractures in 109 patients, Plast. Reconstr. Surg. **59**:15, 1977.
7. Leake, D., Doykos, J., Habal, M.B., and Murray, J.E.: Long-term follow-up of fractures of the mandibular condyle in children, Plast. Reconstr. Surg. **47**:127, 1971.
8. Lehman, J.A., Jr., and Saddawi, N.D.: Fractures of the mandible in children, J. Trauma **16**:773, 1976.
9. Lindahl, L., and Hollender, L.: Condylar fractures of the mandible. II. A radiographic study of remodeling processes in the temporomandibular joint, Int. J. Oral Surg. **6**:153, 1977.
10. MacLennan, W.D.: Consideration of 180 cases of typical fractures of the mandibular condylar process, Br. J. Plast. Surg. **5**:122, 1952.
11. MacLennan, W.D.: Fractures of the mandible in children under the age of six years, Br. J. Plast. Surg. **9**:125, 1956.
12. MacLennan, W.D.: Injuries involving the teeth and jaws in young children, Arch. Dis. Child. **32**:492, 1957.
13. MacLennan, W.D., and Simpson, W.: Treatment of fractured mandibular condylar processes in children, Br. J. Plast. Surg. **18**:423, 1965.
14. McCoy, F.J., Chandler, R.A., and Crow, M.L.: Facial fractures in children, Plast. Reconstr. Surg. **37**:209, 1966.
15. Panagopoulos, A.P.: Management of fractures of the jaws in children, J. Int. Coll. Surg. **28**:806, 1957.
16. Rowe, N.L.: Fractures of the jaws in children, J. Oral Surg. **27**:497, 1969.
17. Rowe, N.L., and Killey, H.C.: Fractures of the facial skeleton, ed. 1, Baltimore, 1955, Williams & Wilkins.
18. Russell, D., Nosti, J.C., and Reavis, C.: Treatment of fractures of the mandibular condyle, J. Trauma **12**:704, 1972.
19. Sicher, H., and DuBrul, E.L.: Oral anatomy, ed. 6, St. Louis, 1975, The C.V. Mosby Co.
20. Thomson, H.G., Farmer, A.W., and Lindsay, W.K.: Condylar neck fractures of the mandible in children, Plast. Reconstr. Surg. **34**:452, 1964.
21. Walker, R.V.: Traumatic mandibular condylar fracture dislocations: effect on growth in the macaca rhesus monkey, Am. J. Surg. **100**:850, 1960.

CHAPTER 32

Reconstruction of the burned face in children

JOEL J. FELDMAN

The psychologic and social impact of a facial burn can be enormous. Even relatively minor facial scarring can elicit a disturbing response in others—manifest overtly by the uninhibited ridicule of children or the more subtle withdrawal of uncomfortable adults. For the injured child, social involvement and self-esteem are often profoundly affected. Although burn scars on the trunk and extremities can be concealed by clothing for the most part, the burned face is not easily hidden. It is the face that the world sees and reacts to emotionally. Therefore the goal of the reconstructive surgeon must be to minimize facial disfigurement as much as possible, so that the young patient can in turn face the world with confidence and comfort.

GENERAL PRINCIPLES OF FACIAL BURN REPAIR
Preoperative analysis

A precise preoperative analysis of the deformity is essential. The surgeon should always compare the area of deformity with the uninjured side or a normal part and then ask: "What is out of place here?" or "What is missing?" Lack of a careful presurgical diagnosis is often the reason for a less than ideal result.

Esthetic aspects of surgery

Facial burn reconstruction is esthetic surgery. Although vital functional considerations must always be of primary concern for the reconstructive surgeon, obtaining the best possible postoperative appearance should be of near equal importance. In this regard, attention to technical and design details make the difference between a mediocre result and a superior one. For example, inserting a skin graft or flap so that an edge lies 1 cm away from rather than right along a natural facial contour line can determine whether or not the face looks as if a patch has been added. Achieving an

optimal result, therefore, may mean excising some unscarred skin so that the join line is less conspicuous. The "golden rule" in reconstructive esthetic surgery is that no measurement, pattern, or preconceived design is as important as simply how things look to the surgeon.

Preoperative marking

Preoperative markings should be made with the patient upright. This is not always possible with young children, but when feasible the surgeon should draw out guidelines preoperatively based on how the patient will be seen postoperatively by others. Regardless of how carefully the ink markings are made, the surgeon's perspective with the patient recumbent on the operating room table is always somewhat different. The normal effects of gravity and animation are lost; soft tissue to bone relationships are altered; strong lighting washes out contours, shadows, and colors; and symmetry is less easily studied. Admittedly, for some procedures, awake, upright, preanesthesia marking is unnecessary, but for others it is crucial.

Timing the repair

Slow is not always bad, and fast is not always best. The advent of musculocutaneous flaps and microsurgical free tissue transfer over the past decade has revolutionized reconstructive surgery. These methods allow one-stage repair of difficult wounds that previously required multiple surgeries. The physical and psychologic benefits to the patient from this type of single-stage procedure can be significant; however, certain types of reconstruction are still best done using a multiple-stage approach. The social and economic implications of any procedure or series of procedures should always be carefully considered. However, when undertaking facial reconstruction in children, the most important factor in choosing between alternate methods of repair is which tactic promises the best result in the long run. Although some of the older methods are time consuming (for example, delaying a large random-pattern flap), children usually do have the time to give. With few exceptions, the quality of a final surgical result should not be compromised in the name of expedience. The notion that a less complex (albeit less appropriate) procedure will save the child several operations and reduce time away from school and family can be inaccurate. What appears to be a less involved approach frequently yields to unsatisfactory long-term results, necessitating multiple unplanned revisions and "touch-up" operations. In time, the "simpler" methods can end up costing the patient more time and inconvenience than a seemingly more complicated (but better designed) initial approach.

Realistic expectations

Throughout the course of reconstruction, the surgeon will be called on to provide ongoing emotional support to the patient and family. A sympathetic and optimistic attitude is crucial to the child's rehabilitation. But optimism must be tempered with realism. Early in the reconstructive process, the surgeon must discuss sensitively but candidly with the family (and the patient if he or she is old enough) not only what can be done, but what cannot be done. It is a prevalent misconception that scars can somehow be erased and that a burned face can eventually be returned to normal. Many surgeons have had a parent remark after the child has undergone the last in a series of lengthy reconstructive procedures, "Doctor, when can you start the plastic surgery?"

Development of a master plan

Outlining a long-range reconstructive plan should be done early on in the repair process, especially when dealing with a severe facial burn. The primary surgeon must sit down (best done with photographs of the patient) and carefully formulate a step-by-step surgical strategy. (See Fig. 32-35, *B*.) In this way the surgeon sees the overall reconstruction as composed of related and integrated parts; priorities can be ordered, donor sites rationed, complementary procedures combined (e.g., using otherwise discarded tissues to rebuild an adjacent part), and anesthetic opportunities used to the best advantage (e.g., adding a flap delay). The plan should be written out or illustrated with sketches in the surgeon's office notes or in the patient's hospital chart and should include a rough timetable. The plan is, of course, flexible, since in practice the surgeon must often wait to see the result of one procedure before going on to the next step. Nonetheless, with thoughtful preplanning, considerable time can be saved over the long run, and, most important, the quality of the final result is often improved.

Individualized treatment plan

Each patient's problem is unique and deserves individualized consideration. Although the material in this chapter reflects my preferences and experience, it should not imply a dogmatic approach toward facial burn reconstruction. No one way of doing things is always best for every patient. Be wary of statements which occasionally appear in the literature that include the word "always" or "never"; for example, "a skin graft is always better than a flap to the face" (or vice versa) or "always wait a year after the acute phase before beginning reconstruction." For each case, the surgeon should carefully pick, and, if necessary, "invent" the method that seems best suited to correct the patient's deformity.

Delaying the repair

On entering the teenage years, it is important that the child actively participate in any decision concerning possible additional reconstructive surgery. Frequently, an adolescent will have a positive attitude, even ask for, surgery that stands to improve the appearance or comfort. The younger child, who may wish for improvement, is often much too worried about injections or donor site pain to admit the real concerns. Despite the child's negative attitude, truly important surgery should not be put off if the surgeon believes another procedure will *significantly* improve the youngster's condition. The formative preadolescent school years can be critical in terms of a child's ultimate self-image, confidence, and social development. Although elective procrastination may be the most appropriate decision for a time, putting off important repair work until a young patient asks for it may well be a poor choice. Parents who understandably want to spare their children the additional physical discomfort of more surgery may also need to be convinced of the importance and timing of certain procedures. The reconstructive surgeon should not avoid this responsibility.

EARLY EXCISION OF GRAFTING AND FACIAL BURNS

This chapter is intended to deal with the sequelae of facial burns in children, that is, the functional and esthetic problems that are manifest *after* the initial healing of the acute burn injury. (See Chapter 8.) However, brief mention should be made here of early (primary) excision of facial burns. Although primary excision and grafting of burns elsewhere on the body have received widespread endorsement,[16,22] a conservative approach consisting of topical antibacterial therapy, eschar debridement, and eventual skin grafting of the granulating wound continues to be recommended for burns of the face (Fig. 32-1).[32,33,35-37] This less aggressive attitude toward surgical intervention developed in part because of the difficulty in making an accurate diagnosis of the depth of most facial burns in which early postinjury skin color and sensibility are often misleading and because facial burns so commonly exhibit a patchy mix of superficial and deep dermal injury. Surgeons therefore have been understandably hesitant to risk excising potentially viable tissue. Experience has shown this cautious approach to be prudent in the vast majority of cases; yet, it may not be best for all.

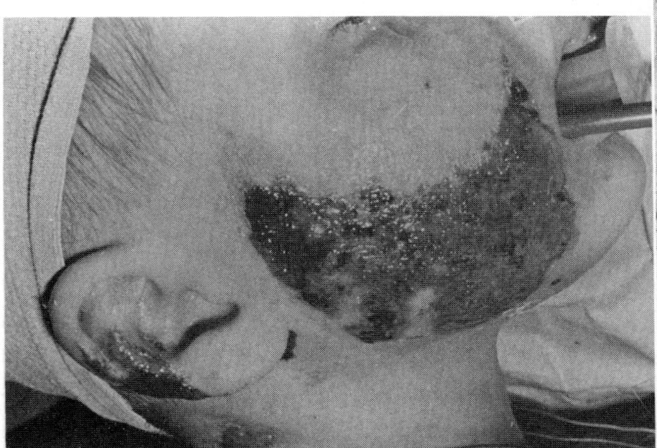

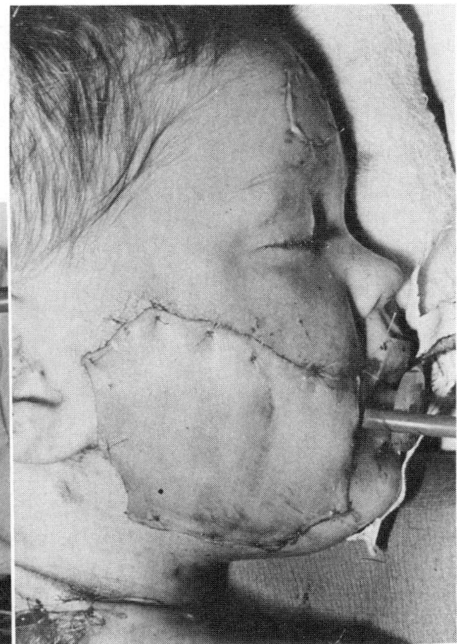

Fig. 32-1. Usual treatment of acute facial burns. After eschar separation the granulating wound is skin grafted.

The worst cases of hypertrophic facial scarring are seen in patients with deep second-degree burns that have been allowed to heal spontaneously. This type of partial-thickness injury is also at risk for conversion to a full-thickness loss from intervening infection during the healing phase. In these cases of apparent deep second-degree burn, consideration should be given to early excision by shaving and immediate grafting. This so-called tangential excision is performed between the third and fifth day after the burn with a Watson, Blair, or Goulian-type knife down to the level of punctate capillary bleeding.[79,81,111] If hemostasis after excision is excellent, then split-thickness autografts are applied immediately in large sheets (according to the regional esthetic unit concept, see Fig. 32-6). If hemostasis is less satisfactory, sheet allografts or xenografts are used as temporary cover for 24 to 48 hours and then replaced with autografts. It is essential, however, that the excised wound be immediately and continuously covered with a nonmeshed biologic dressing to prevent desiccation, which could quickly convert the remaining marginally viable dermis (''zone of stasis'') to a full-thickness loss (''zone or coagulation''). This method, a form of ''overgrafting,'' preserves the deep reticular dermis, and seems to significantly reduce the tendency for hypertrophic scarring and wound contraction (Fig. 32-2).

Third-degree burns of the face can also be primarily excised, but there is little to recommend it if circumstances portend poor graft ''take'' or if the method employed has little hope of preventing the development of a significant secondary deformity. For an extensive primary excision and grafting of a facial burn to be justified, conditions conducive to success (i.e., virtually 100% ''take'' of thick grafts) must be optimal. The surgery must be carried out within a week or at most 10 days after the burn. This requires early resolution of facial edema, total absence of local or systemic sepsis, a cooperative and metabolically stable patient, and adequate donor sites. And certainly the patient's life cannot be threatened by other more pressing concerns. These criteria are infrequently met. Furthermore, very little, if anything, is to be gained by excising and resurfacing a face with thin skin grafts. Thin grafts do not prevent contractures from developing, and their ultimate quality (texture and color) is so poor that eventual replacement is almost certain (Fig. 32-3).[160] A full-thickness (third-degree) facial burn should only be excised primarily if very thick split-thickness or full-thickness skin grafts or skin flaps are used for the new cover.[134] In carefully selected cases, this aggressive and definitive approach is warranted; however, appropriate patient candidates are rarely seen. Usually it is best to aim initially for a healed, closed wound, trying to minimize along the way deformities and contractures, yet expecting that secondary correction will be needed.

TIMING THE RECONSTRUCTION

It is often said that definitive correction of facial burn deformities should be delayed for 1 year or longer after the injury—the so-called waiting period—until the scars and initial grafts have been given an adequate chance to mature. Generally, this is a sound principle, since contracture release or regional resurfacing that takes place within an area that is still contracting will undoubtedly yield results that are compromised by some degree of recontracture. Furthermore, the combination of sufficient time (perhaps years), external pressure (splints and elasticized masks),[98,116,127] and local steroids will improve many hypertrophic noncontrac-

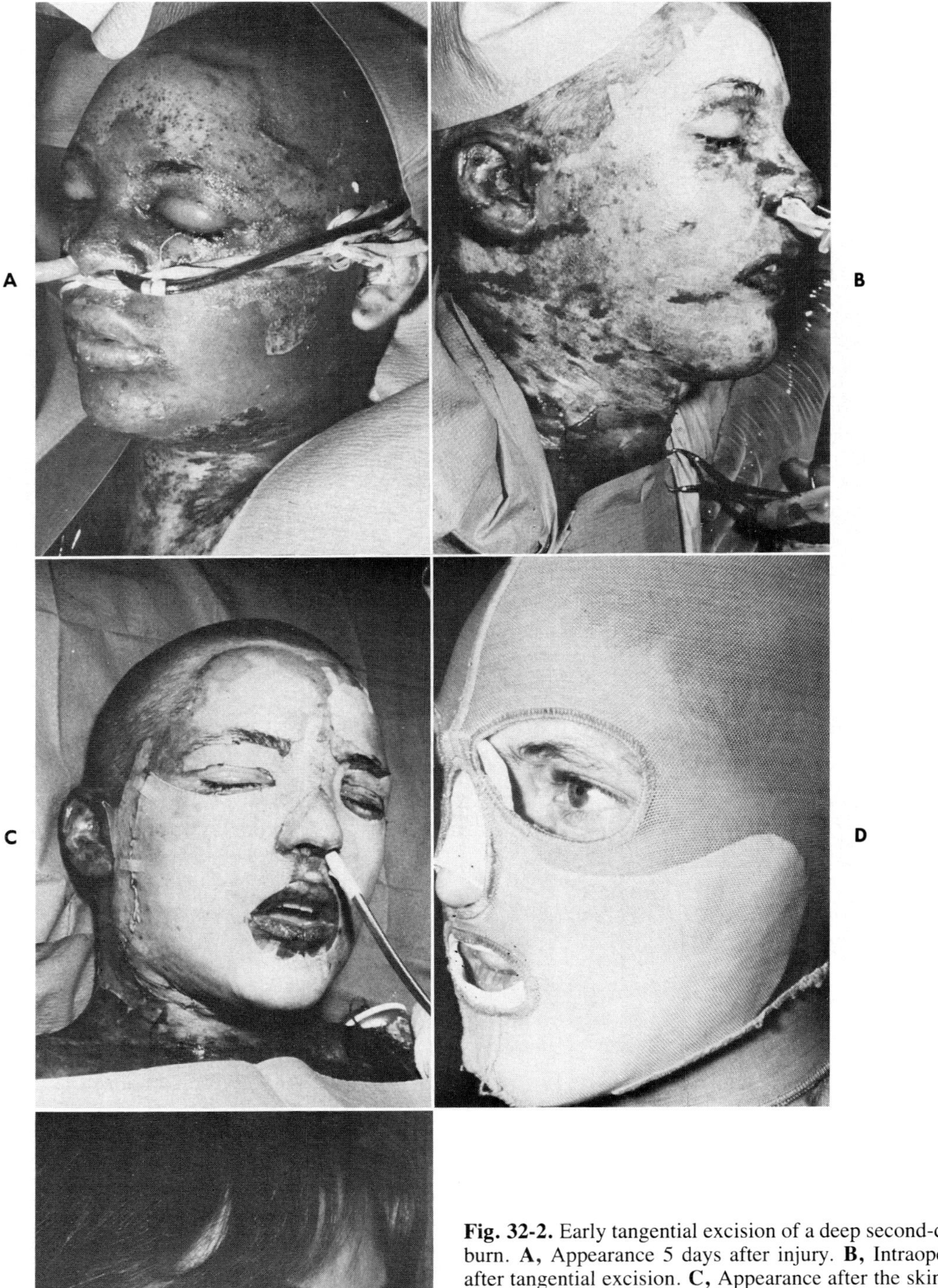

Fig. 32-2. Early tangential excision of a deep second-degree facial burn. **A,** Appearance 5 days after injury. **B,** Intraoperative view after tangential excision. **C,** Appearance after the skin grafts have been applied. **D,** A facial splint and elasticized mask are worn for 6 months postoperatively to prevent graft-edge hypertrophy. **E,** Result at 1 year after injury. (Courtesy Drs. Reid Hansen and Conrado Bondoc.)

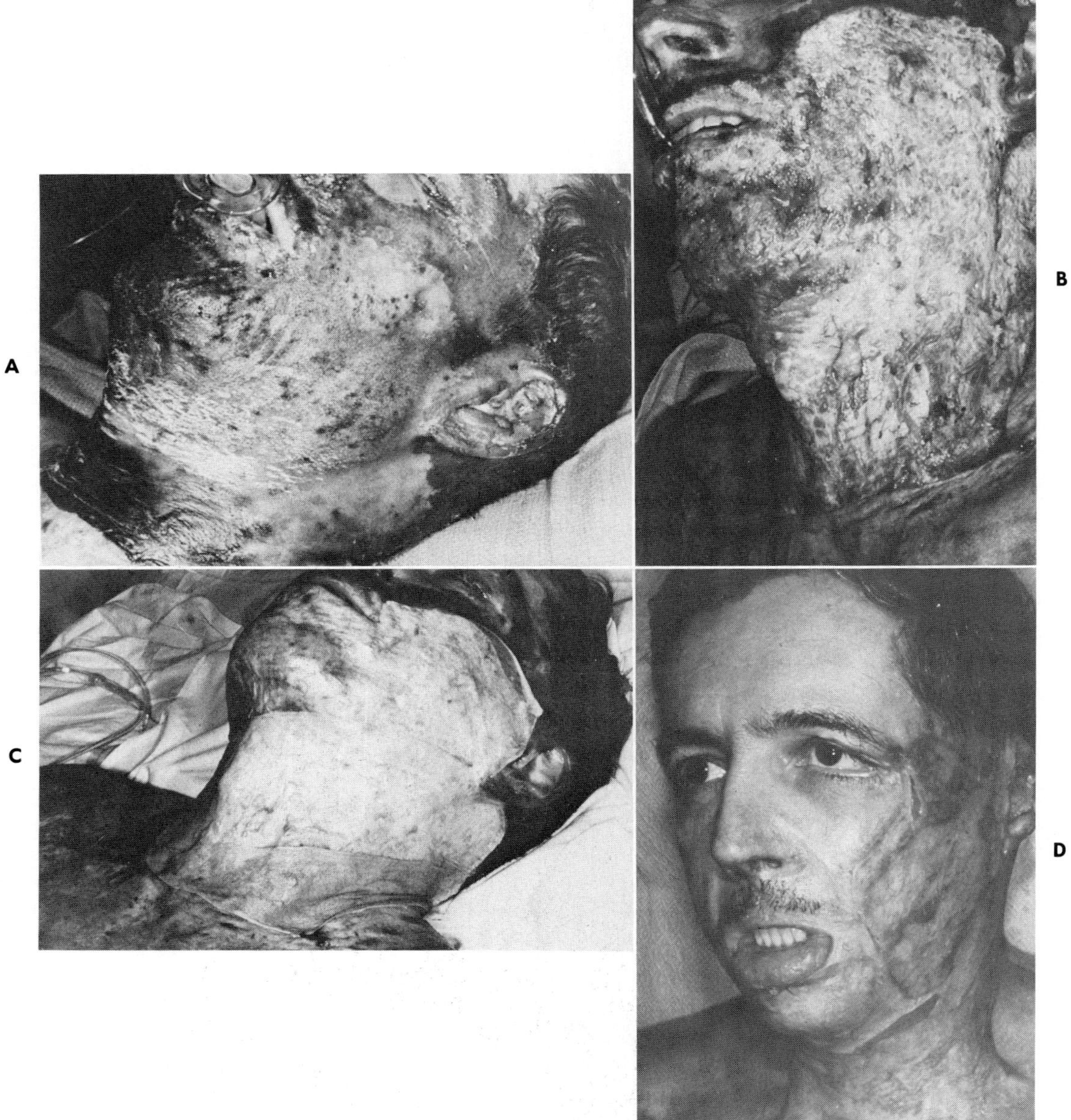

Fig. 32-3. Primary excision and grafting of third-degree facial burn. **A** and **B,** Appearance 1 week after injury, before and after full-thickness excision. **C,** Immediate resurfacing with thin split-thickness skin grafts. **D,** Despite almost complete take of the grafts, severe contractures developed. Thin skin grafts should be used only to close an open wound; because of certain secondary contraction, they should *not* be applied for definitive coverage.

ture-producing scars to a point where the patient's ultimate appearance is better than would have been achieved by a too-hasty resurfacing.[173] Knowing who to operate on, and when, is wisdom gained only by experience; but there are definite exceptions to the rule of waiting for burn scar maturity before embarking on reconstruction. Clearly, earlier operative intervention is often indicated for reasons of function and comfort, such as a cornea-endangering upper eyelid ectropion, a disabling perioral contracture, lower lip eversion causing drooling, or severely restrictive neck scarring.

In these urgent cases, where a later more definitive repair is anticipated, the most precious donor areas should not be used up at the first temporizing procedures, but should be saved for last! Another important consideration concerning the timing of repair involves the distinction between an intrinsic scar release and a total scar excision. An *intrinsic release* (Fig. 32-4, *A* and *B*) means an incision *within* a scar to relieve a contracture by opening the wound and introducing additional skin (usually a free skin graft). However, if the release is carried out within a scar field that is

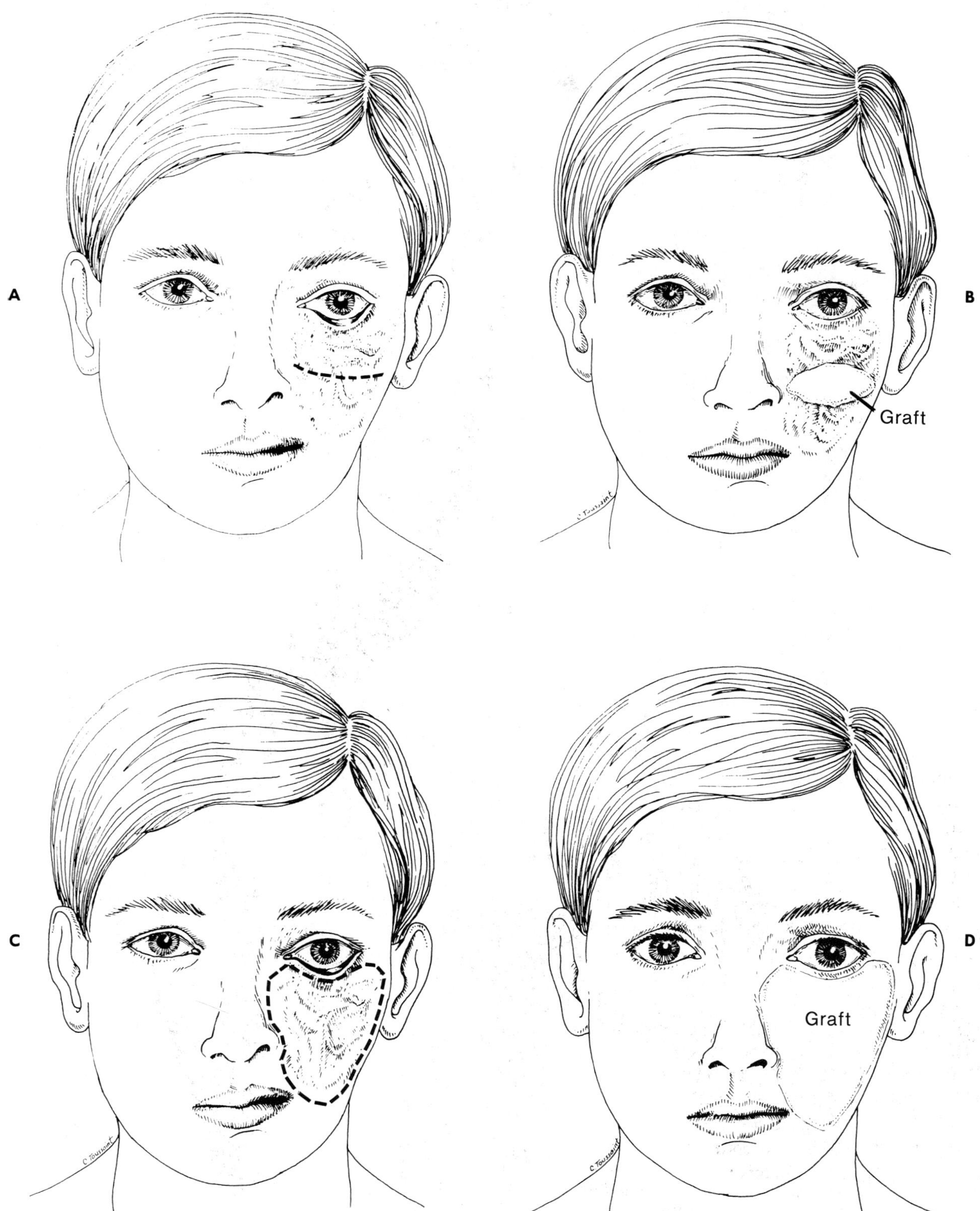

Fig. 32-4. Intrinsic versus extrinsic scar contracture release. **A** and **B,** Intrinsic release by incising and grafting within the area of scar. **C** and **D,** Extrinsic release by totally excising the entire scar before resurfacing.

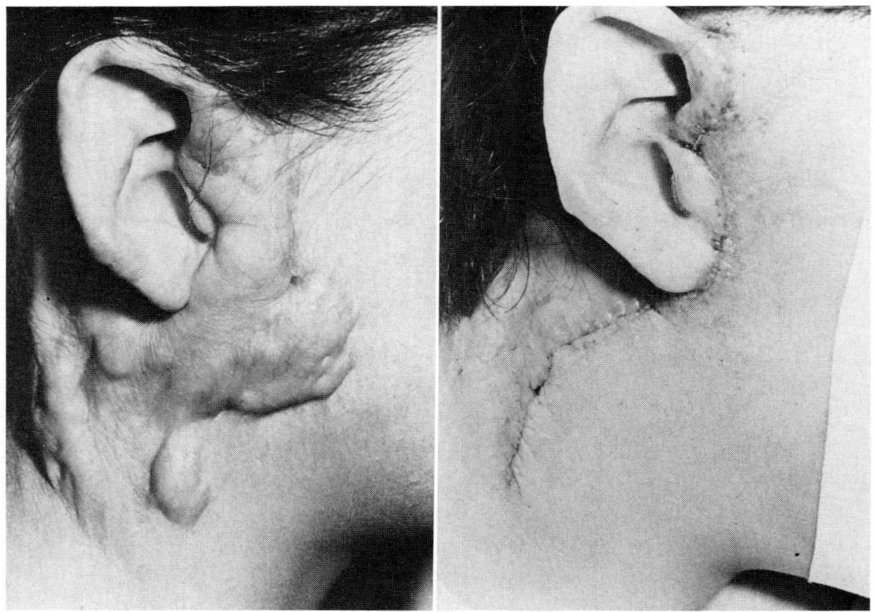

Fig. 32-5. Excision of hypertrophic burn scar, resulting from deep second-degree burn. Scar hypertrophy usually will not reappear after excision.

still young and "active," continued "field contraction" will obviate a satisfactory long-term result. In this situation, waiting until the scar has matured (i.e., become relatively pale, flat, and soft) will yield a better quality, more permanent, result. On the other hand, if a scar can be *totally excised* (Fig. 32-4, *C* and *D*), so that the peripheral and deep excision margins are within unburned noncontracting tissue, then field contraction is not a concern, and there is little benefit in making the patient wait for scar maturation. If subsequent recontracture occurs after this en bloc scar excision, it is related to the inherent propensity of the new graft, not the surrounding wound, to contract. In fact, early total excision of localized hypertrophic burn scars usually produces good results (Fig. 32-5).[15]

RESURFACING THE FACE—BASIC CONSIDERATIONS
Regional esthetic units

The normal face can be envisioned as composed of a number of neighboring geographic territories limited by natural relief lines, folds, obvious changes in skin texture, and the hairline.[70,150] A facial map clearly demonstrates these areas (Fig. 32-6). A skin graft or flap applied to the face should cover, if possible, an entire esthetic unit, not just part of a unit (Fig. 32-7). In this way, a patched appearance is less apparent, because edge scars are relatively concealed along the boundaries of each region. To cover a complete unit, some normal skin must sometimes be sacrificed.[8] If the facial area to be resurfaced extends into more than one esthetic territory, the involved units should be combined into one large composite unit, allowing the biggest possible

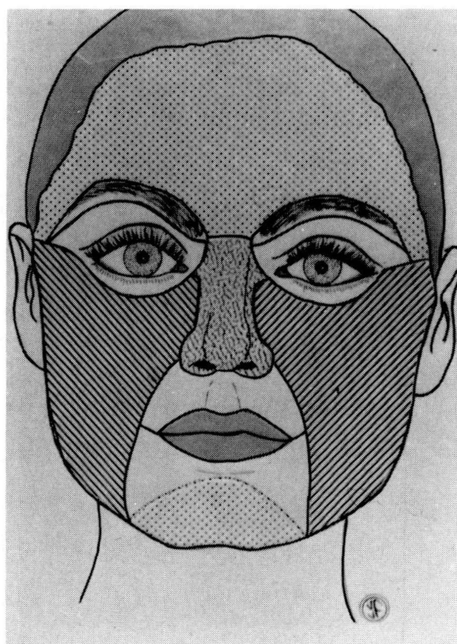

Fig. 32-6. Facial map showing regional esthetic units

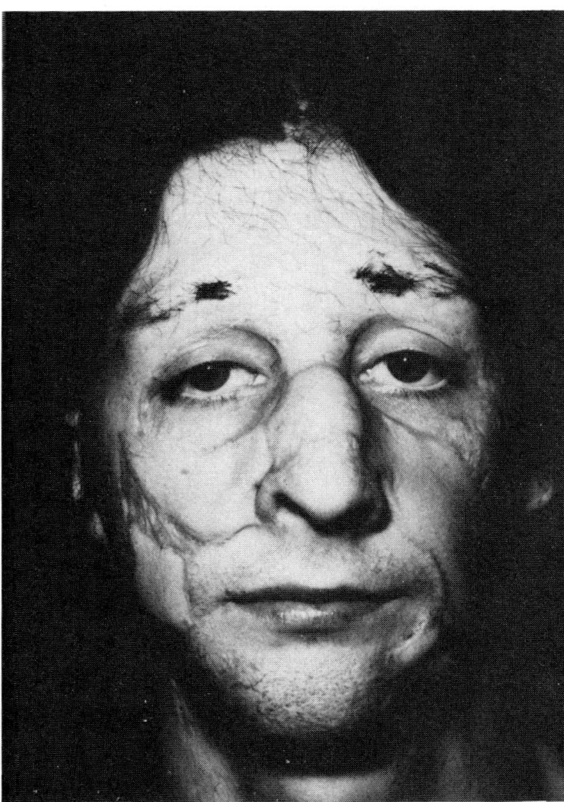

Fig. 32-7. Flaps applied to cheeks and nose *without* regard to the facial unit concept.

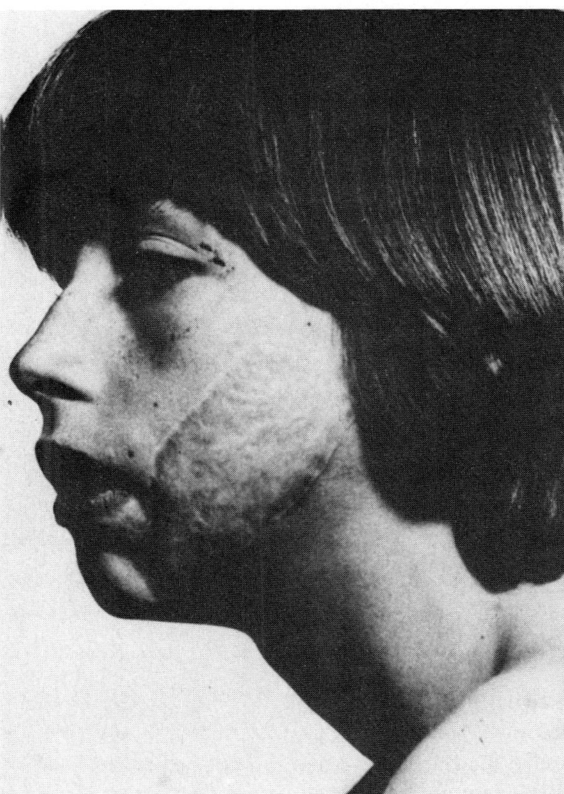

Fig. 32-8. The alien skin graft patch. A cervicopectoral rotation flap would provide a much better texture and color match.

single graft to be used. This minimizes the number of seams and is especially important in children, who lack the skin creases and furrows that "regionalize" the face in adults. Partitioning the face into small units should be done only when necessary.

Symmetry

Since humans are two sided, a repair on one side of the body will always be judged against the opposite side. If the contralateral side is normal (i.e., uninjured), even the very best result will fall short of perfection. In this regard, repair of a unilateral deformity can be the most difficult. When both sides are injured, a concerted attempt should be made to have the two sides match each other as closely as possible (in location of scars, skin color, texture, etc.).[98] This is particularly important in facial reconstruction where comparisons are so easily made. For example, a flap should not be applied to one cheek and a graft to the other. Also mirror-image esthetic units that place identical scars on both sides of the face should be designed wherever possible. Another golden rule in facial resurfacing should be: "Do unto one side as you do unto the other." If both sides look the same, despite some abnormalities, the eye of the beholder usually perceives the whole as acceptable; asymmetry, on the other hand, is always inherently disturbing.

Grafts versus flaps

Controversy persists as to whether skin grafts or skin flaps are better for facial burn resurfacing.[98,115] Proponents of skin grafts argue that grafts, unlike flaps, are not bulky and do not mask facial expression. Flap proponents, on the other hand, argue that skin grafts tend to contract and hyperpigment with time, and even the best grafts lack a completely normal surface texture. Flaps, they say, do not shrink and maintain the velvet surface quality of normal skin, and "any flap that has been adequately thinned will show expression lines and will beat a graft on most occasions."[67] Although the debate will no doubt continue, it seems clear that flaps are best in some situations and grafts are best in others.[8] The guiding principle in facial resurfacing should be to add skin (graft or flap) that will *match* as closely as possible what is already there or will ultimately be there. For example, if one cheek alone has been burned and the rest of the face is unscarred, resurfacing the one cheek is best accomplished with a flap (from close by, if possible) whose texture and color will blend with the rest of the face.[146] On the other hand, a free graft used here, surrounded by unblemished neck, forehead,[87,177] nose, or contralateral cheek skin, would forever look like an alien patch (Fig. 32-8). In a different setting, however, the flap might appear just as incongruous. For example, if an entire face had healed with

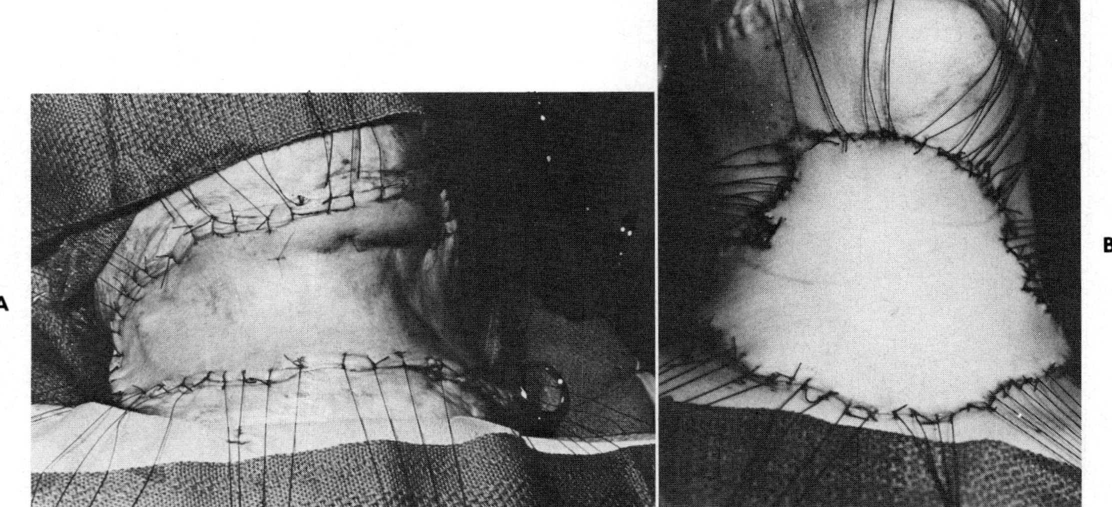

Fig. 32-9. A, Incorrect technique. Overlapping the graft will leave a rough edge. **B,** Correct technique using precise edge-to-edge approximation.

good-quality scars and grafts, with only one regional unit requiring resurfacing, a graft would certainly fit in better visually than a mismatched (albeit "more normal") flap. As a general guideline then, if only a portion of the face is to be resurfaced, grafts should be inserted into fields of grafts, and flaps into fields of flaplike skin. If one side of the face is burned and the other side unburned, cover the damaged side with a regional flap if available. If the entire face (i.e., both sides) is to be recovered, then the surgeon has a choice as to whether to use a flap(s) or graft(s), assuming appropriate donor sites are available. For a full-face resurfacing, my personal preference is for a thin one-piece flap (Fig. 32-37). My next choice would be a one-piece full-thickness skin graft (Fig. 32-36). A detailed description of these techniques can be found on pp. 589 and 591.

Better scars

Every effort should be made to obtain the best possible scars after a resurfacing. Hiding a scar along the hairline or camouflaging it in a skin fold is ideal. But where the scars are visible certain details make a difference. Flaps should be sewn in place with subcuticular (intradermal) sutures. Additional skin-edge approximation and support are obtained with adhesive paper strips. This method eliminates unsightly suture marks that can occur after only a few days in children. Subcuticular sutures have the added benefit of eliminating the otherwise rigorous task of removing multiple sutures from a possibly uncooperative and unanesthetized child. If percutaneous sutures are used, especially in unscarred skin, then a generous application of antibiotic ointment along the suture line will suppress the usual inflammatory reaction around the sutures and lessen the chance of stitch tracks; skin grafts should not overlap the edges of

a recipient wound (Fig. 32-9, *A*). The small cuff of excess graft will often survive by intradermal vascular "bridging," leaving a rough edge. Grafts on the face should be precisely cut and then inset with meticulous edge-to-edge coaptation (Fig. 32-9, *B*); if adjacent esthetic units are to be recovered at separate operations, the excision of tissue for the first unit should extend slightly into the territory of the abutting unit. In this way, the first graft-edge scar can be removed with excision of tissue from the neighboring area at the subsequent surgery, producing a narrower join line; the early postoperative application (10 to 14 days) and prolonged use (3 to 12 months) of external compression (elasticized masks and Orthoplast splints) can prevent edge-scar hypertrophy and diminish graft contraction.[137] Preoperative measurement and fabrication of the mask (Jobst) will have it ready for use after surgery. Preventing scar hypertrophy is much easier than treating it; elective incisions and scar revisions should be designed so that the resulting scars will be oriented, wherever possible, parallel to the relaxed skin tension lines of the face and neck (Fig. 32-10). Less hypertrophic, less conspicuous scars are often possible if they are properly planned.

Build with disposable tissues

When resurfacing an area of the face, the surgeon should always question whether the excised scar could be used to build up or recontour an adjacent part. Flaps cut from scarred or previously grafted facial skin and elevated with just a little underlying fat are remarkably viable and can be quite valuable for reconstructing ears (Fig. 32-46), nasal tips (Fig. 32-38), columellae (Fig. 32-42), nasal alae (Fig. 32-39), and upper lip philtral columns (Fig. 32-13). Scarred skin can also be de-epithelialized in specific areas, such as

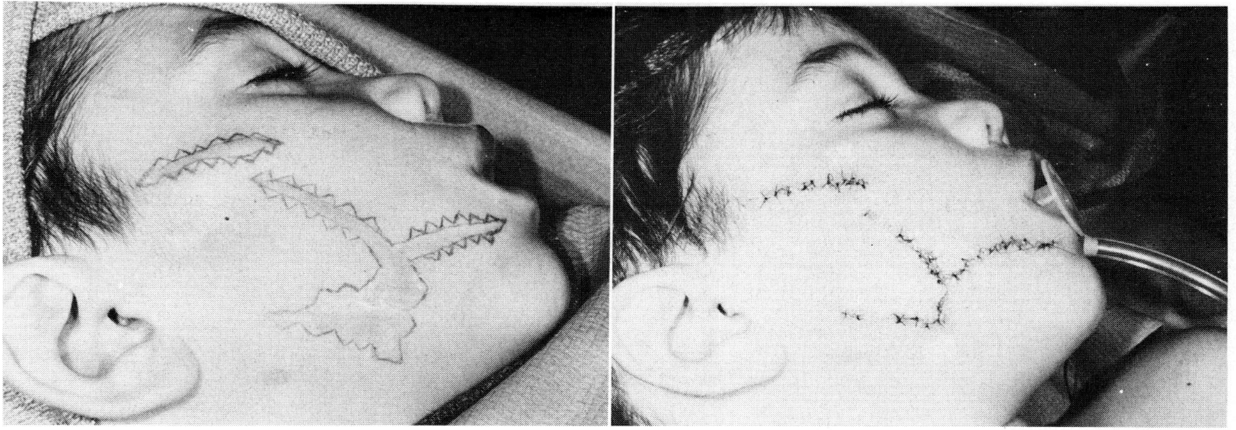

Fig. 32-10. Scar excision using a running W-plasty to break up the linear closure and redirect segments of the resulting scar so that they parallel the relaxed skin tension lines of the face.

the chin (Fig. 32-36, *D*), then overgrafted to preserve the "high" facial contours. The point to remember is that when resurfacing, nothing should be unconsciously thrown away that might be used to make something else. The strategic use of scar tissue should be incorporated in the surgeon's overall "master plan."

Delayed grafting

Successful facial resurfacing using skin grafts requires a virtually 100% take of the graft. Whereas a dime-sized area of graft loss on the trunk or extremities is usually inconsequential, an equivalent loss on a conspicuous part of the face can seriously mar the entire result. The most common cause of partial graft loss in the healed reconstructive patient is hematoma. For this reason, if a large area of the face is to be recovered, serious consideration should be given to delaying the grafting for 24 to 48 hours after the excision to ensure perfect hemostasis. If this is done (and it should be seriously considered for hemifacial or full-face resurfacing), the excised wound should be covered with a totally occlusive antibiotic-soaked gauze dressing held on by a circumferential Barton-type bandage and a few tacking sutures to prevent the dressing from lifting up. Allografts or xenografts can be used instead as a temporary biologic dressing, but they are unnecessary.[95] To prevent wound contamination, it is important that the dressing be left undisturbed until the patient returns to the operating room for grafting, where it can be partially unwrapped to permit the induction of anesthesia and reintubation. The gauze sponges are then moistened and peeled away. A number of discrete bleeding points usually require electrocoagulation, but it is remarkable how "dry" and receptive the wound is after an overnight rest. The grafts (thick split or full thickness) should *not* be harvested at the time of wound excision and then refrigerated or banked on the donor sites, but rather cropped fresh on the day of grafting to ensure optimal viability. Although this two-staged excision and grafting routine ap-

pears more complex, in practice, it is often a time and energy saver—less of both are wasted at the excision stage trying to obtain a meticulous hemostasis, and the surgeon returns for the grafting stage refreshed and more efficient. In cases of large facial resurfacings, the stakes are high. The delayed grafting method increases the odds in favor of success.

Donor site rationing

Once the question of survival after a severe burn is no longer an issue, concern focuses on the subsequent quality of life. As the ability to save young victims of major burns has improved, so too has the reach for improved facial repair. The quality of this reconstruction often depends on the availability of quality resurfacing material. In this regard, both the acute care surgeon and the reconstructive surgeon (who may be involved early on in the patient's management) should be cognizant of the special needs for facial repair. Ideally, preselected facial-quality donor sites should be declared off limits for torso and extremity coverage. This, of course, is possible only if the burn is not so extensive as to require early use of all available autograft skin. But not infrequently, precious one-of-a-kind donor areas have been cropped unnecessarily because the acute care surgeon was not made aware of the importance of preserving their integrity for future use on the face. Particularly if single-piece resurfacing of the face is a later goal (be it flap or graft), the prime donor areas best suited for this purpose must be preserved and protected.

Sun avoidance

New scars and grafts are hypersensitive to ultraviolet radiation. The risk of hyperpigmentation is greater with early sun exposure. Parents and patients should be admonished to shield the resurfaced face from the sun with the elasticized mask or a chemical sun block with a high sun protection factor for at least 3 to 6 months after reparative surgery.

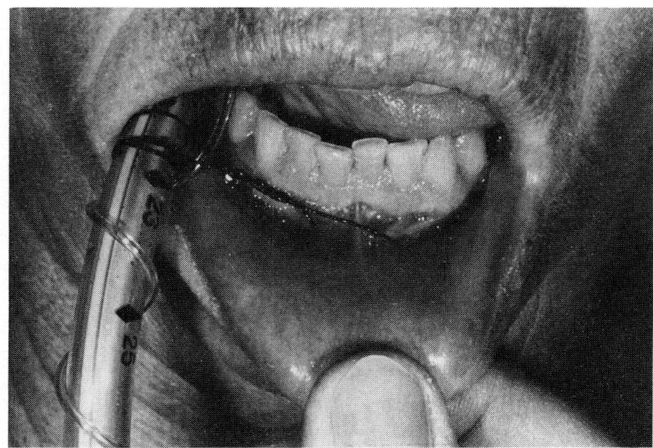

Fig. 32-11. Technique of orotracheal tube fixation using a heavy silk ligature anchored in the lower gingivolabial sulcus. The suture is first tied loosely above the sulcus, a series of knots are added to form a short "leash," which is then fixed securely to the tube with a surgeon's knot followed by a square knot. The tube and anesthesia hoses are covered with a long sleeve of sterile 4-inch stockinette. (The suture should *not* be tied to teeth.)

Honest photographs

Since the quality of a facial resurfacing depends so much on skin-color match, it is often difficult to judge results from black and white photographs. For the reconstructive surgeon, color-accurate pictures are important in evaluating one's own results and the results of others.

Endotracheal intubation

The common method of using adhesive tape to secure an endotracheal tube to the perioral area is often unsatisfactory for facial resurfacing work; fixation is unreliable, the tape encroaches on or lies across the operative field, and the tube cannot be easily maneuvered intraoperatively to facilitate access to other areas. Anchoring the tube with an umbilical tape tied around the head has many of the same disadvantages. I have found that a heavy silk suture anchored securely in the lower gingivolabial sulcus and then tied around the orotracheal tube provides a simple, safe, and reliable solution to the problem (Fig. 32-11). The anchoring suture should *not* be tied around the patient's teeth (especially the incisors).[93] It is very easy to loosen or partially extract a tooth this way.

REPAIR OF DEFORMITIES OF SPECIFIC AREAS
The upper lip

Burns of the upper lip that heal by spontaneous reepithelialization or are resurfaced with thin split-thickness skin grafts often leave the lip vertically shortened and tight. Frequently there is associated injury to the base of the nose and columella. Satisfactory repair demands attention to a number of small but esthetically important anatomic details. In addition to scar excision and lip resurfacing, the cupid's

bow, philtral ridges, and philtral dimple may need to be reconstructed. The nasal columella often requires lengthening, and some recontouring of nostril sills and alar bases might be called for. At times, an oral commissure contracture merits concomitant release. Even if only a portion of the lip needs release or recovering, it is best to resurface the entire esthetic unit of the lip (except when preserving a defined central dimple). To outline this area (Fig. 32-12, *C*), lines are drawn out from the corners of the mouth in an upward, downward, or transverse direction as needed to release the scar at the oral commissures. These lines intersect the nasolabial creases that form the sides of the trapezoid-shaped upper lip unit. Inferiorly a well-defined cupid's bow is designed along the proposed vermilion-cutaneous margin. The lateral wings of the bow should be gently convex, peaking clearly at the philtral ridges, with a concave central trough between the peaks. Some excess vermilion may need to be excised. Superiorly the boundary line flows along the nasal sills and around the alar bases. Fig. 32-12 illustrates a typical case. De-epithelialized ridges are left to simulate the philtral columns, and the central dimple is deeply excavated. Full-thickness or thick split-thickness skin grafts are employed for the new cover. One or two fine mattress sutures anchor the graft in the depth of the central dimple, and a tie-over bolster dressing is employed for about 10 days. For full-thickness grafts, the retroauricular, supraclavicular, upper inner arm, and glabrous lateral inguinal donor sites may be used. Although the supraclavicular area can provide excellent-quality skin, the donor site scar can be noticeably unattractive if the area is otherwise unblemished. A thick split-thickness graft (0.018 inch) taken with a dermatome from the saline puffed-up scalp will also provide good color match.[14] The scalp hair follicles are deep in the dermis or subcutaneous fat and are not injured or transplanted with the graft. Skin flaps may be used to cover the burned upper lip, but only if exceedingly well thinned and only if the central dimple is not bridged by the flap. (See Fig. 32-37.)

When resurfacing the upper lip, there is a tendency to inadvertently elongate it. With release of the contracted lip scar, the freed vermilion margin responds to gravity, drops inferiorly, and assumes a lowered posture. If the excised and now ptotic lip is then covered with an oversized graft, a long upper lip results. To avoid this problem, the surgeon must be certain that the freshly reconstructed upper lip has the same dimensions as a normal lip. Unlike the lower lip, where overcorrection of the everted position is purposely done in anticipation of some contraction, a surgically elongated upper lip remains that way. On a profile view this convex too-long upper lip has an unpleasant monkeylike appearance, lacking the normally attractive concave pout (Fig. 32-13, *A*). On a frontal view the vermilion is thin, and often the cupid's bow is poorly defined (Fig. 32-13, *B*). Nonetheless, it is still much easier to correct a lip (upper or lower) that is too long than one that is too short. The solution is a simple excision of excess graft along the ver-

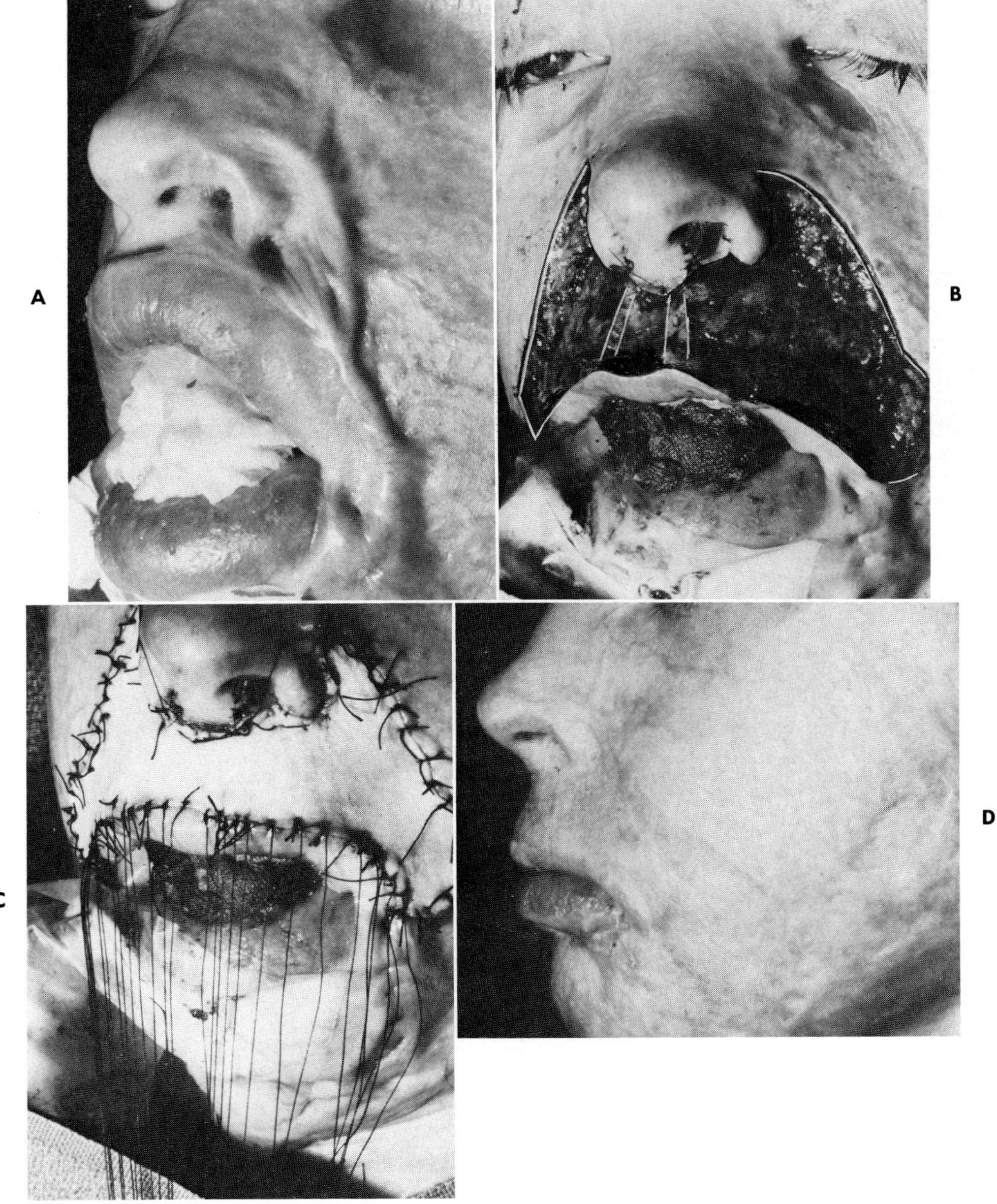

Fig. 32-12. Upper lip resurfacing. **A,** Preoperative appearance. **B,** The entire "esthetic unit" excised. A central lip scar flap is used to lengthen columella. De-epithelialized philtral columns are preserved. **C,** A thick skin graft is applied. **D,** Postoperative result.

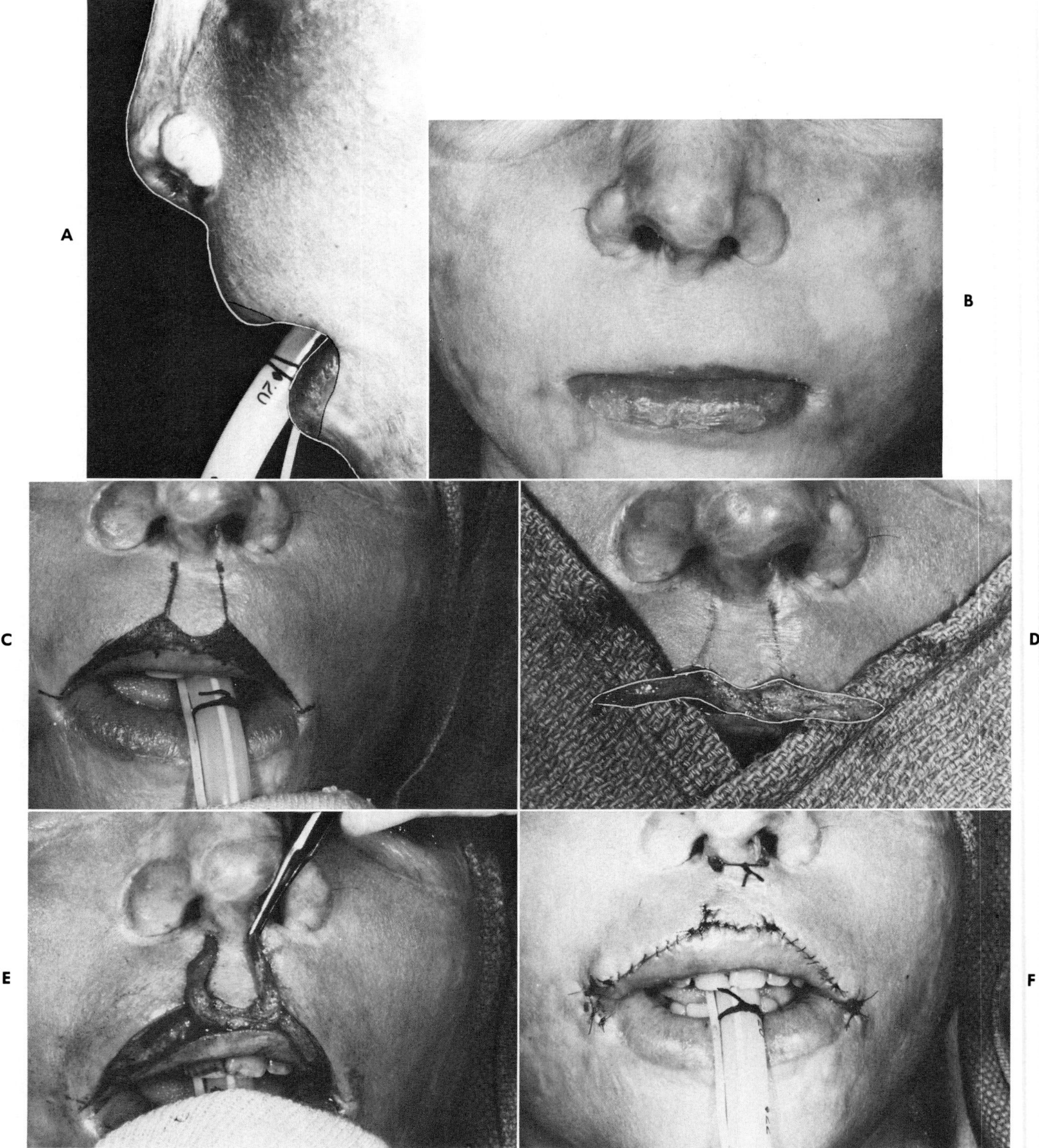

Fig. 32-13. Correction of the elongated upper lip. **A,** Preoperative side view showing a long convex lip profile. **B,** Preoperative front view showing thin vermilion and lack of philtral definition. **C,** A new cupid's bow and philtral columns are drawn out. **D,** Excess tissue is used for de-epithelialized flaps that will be swung up into subcutaneous tunnels to form the philtral columns. **E,** The tissue is secured at the columella base. **F and G,** Postoperative front view. **H,** Postoperative side view. Note the shortened lip with a more normal pout.

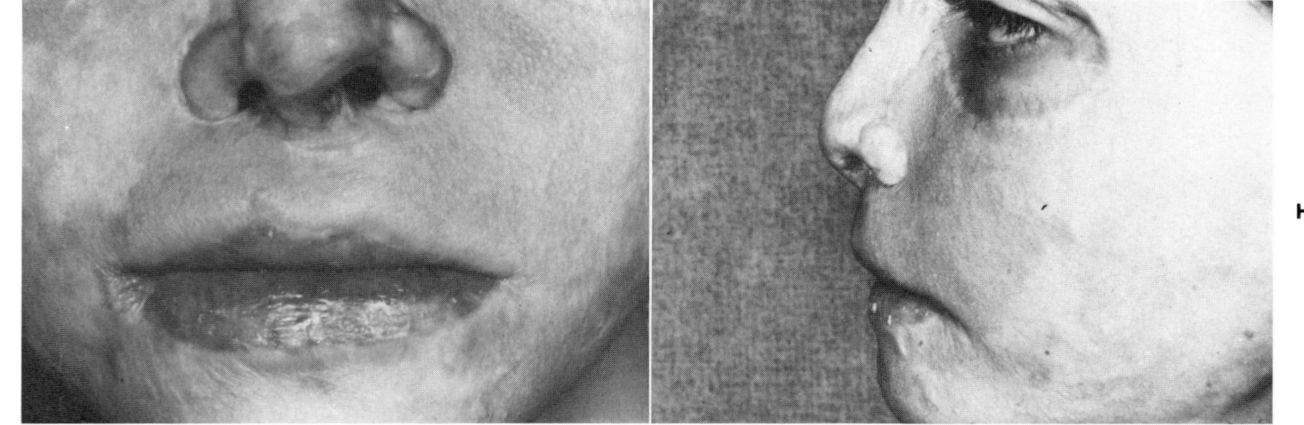

Fig. 32-13, cont'd. For legend see opposite page.

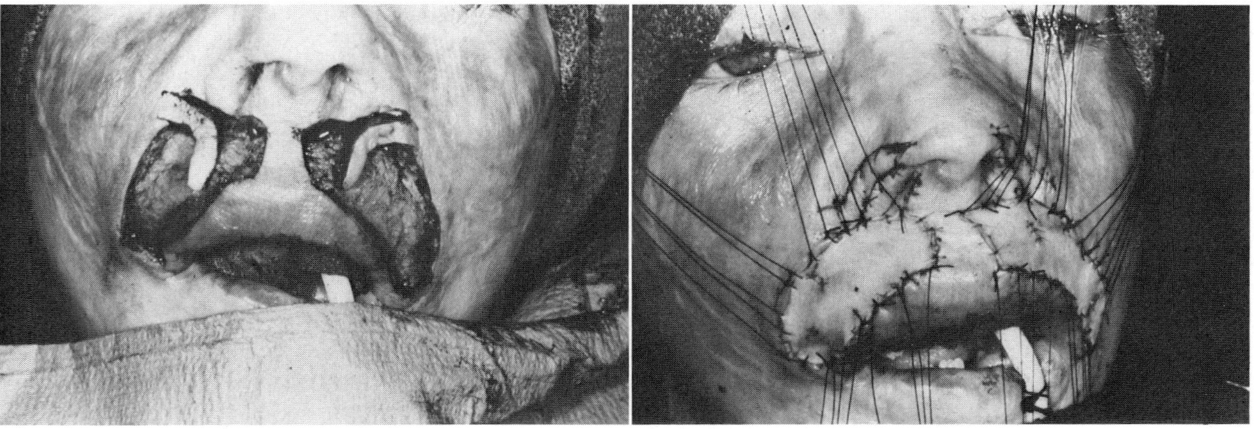

Fig. 32-14. Upper lip resurfacing with philtral dimple preservation. Note the use of expendable "sickle" scar tissue flaps for alar reconstruction.

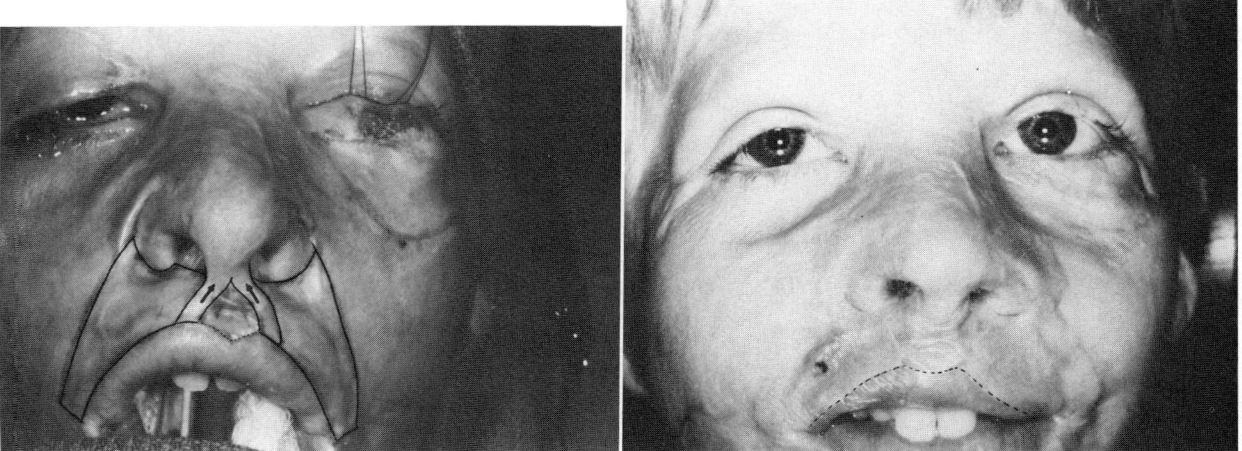

Fig. 32-15. Upper lip resurfacing with philtral dimple preservation. Note the use of expendable forked scar tissue flaps for columella lengthening. Arrows indicate upward advancement of forked flaps into columella.

milion margin. In the case of the elongated upper lip, the superfluous skin can be de-epithelialized, left attached medially as narrow pedicle flaps, and then tunneled up beneath the lip graft to re-create the philtral ridges. Anchoring the flaps to the columella base helps to restore the natural lip pout (Fig. 32-13, *H*). These little flaps will survive nicely as flaps (not grafts) if cut thickly and handled gently. The method is appealing in that it shortens a long lip, delineates the cupid's bow, and defines the philtral columns and dimple all at one time (Fig. 32-13, *G*).

Perhaps nowhere else are the nuances of anatomic contour and shadow better expressed than in the normal central upper lip. The delicate philtral crests rimming a saucerized dimple are often subtly defined structures; but in their absence the upper lip looks strange and certainly lacks beauty. Yet reconstruction of the central upper lip can be difficult, and lasting definition of the philtral contours can be elusive.[89] Even when stout de-epithelialized philtral ridges and a very deep central dimple are constructed before grafting, these "hills" and "valleys" (which can look so good at the end of surgery) almost always flatten out over the subsequent months. Because of this, it is better to leave a cupped and relatively unscarred philtral dimple intact rather than to excise it (Figs. 32-14 and 32-15). However, if the dimple itself is distorted, but the lip length (from the peak of the cupid's bow to the columella base) is normal and the surface overlying the proposed philtral columns is acceptable, then narrow strips of intact skin can be left as columns, and the central dimple and lateral segments can be covered with three separate pieces of skin (Fig. 32-16). Although these methods preserve a semblance of philtral structure, the long-term results using only soft tissues to redefine the central lip structures are often disappointing. To construct a well-defined and permanent philtral dimple and columns requires a shaped and somewhat rigid building material that can resist

the leveling forces inherent in the healing process. A chondrocutaneous composite graft taken from the triangular fossa or concha of the ear will provide both the necessary concave scaffolding and the surface cover and is an excellent method of repair (Fig. 32-17). This technique is a modification of the method reported by Schmid[138,139] for philtral construction in secondary cleft lip deformity.

Because thermal injury to the upper lip is often associated with injury to the lower nose, in any upper lip resurfacing, the lip should always be considered a potential tissue donor to the nose. A variety of flaps can be designed from the expendable upper lip scar according to the individual needs of the lip and nose. For example, to release a tethered nasal tip by lengthening a short columella, all or part of the central lip scar can be advanced upward as a single superiorly based flap (Fig. 32-12), forked-flap (Fig. 32-15), or trilobed stellate flap (Figs. 32-16 and 32-17). Each of these techniques is a variation on methods used to elongate the columella in secondary bilateral cleft lip deformity. Sickle-shaped flaps from the scarred lip can be used to correct notched or retracted nostril margins (Fig. 32-14), and nasolabial flaps can be used to build alar bases (Fig. 32-16 and 32-17).

The lower lip–chin complex

Wound healing and skin graft contraction in this area frequently produce eversion of the lower lip, appearing as a protrusion of rolled-down lip vermilion and mucosa (Figs. 32-19, *A* and *B,* and 32-20, *A* and *B*). Scar bridging the valley between the lip and chin can blunt or obliterate the labiomental sulcus, making the chin appear small. An associated neck contracture that obscures the cervicomental angle can add to the "pseudomicrogenia" (Figs. 32-18 and 32-19). Stomal competence (i.e., lip seal) can be impaired, causing drooling. Concomitant scarring at the oral com-

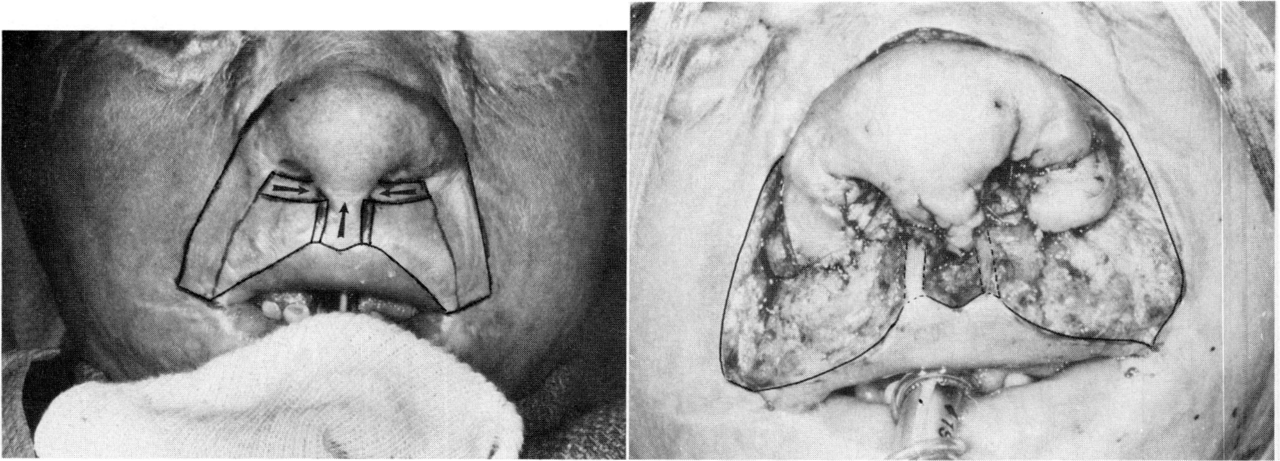

Fig. 32-16. Upper lip resurfacing with philral column preservation. Three separate skin grafts are inserted, one for each lateral lip segment and one centrally. Note the fleur-de-lis (three-pronged) scar flaps for columella lengthening (*arrows*).

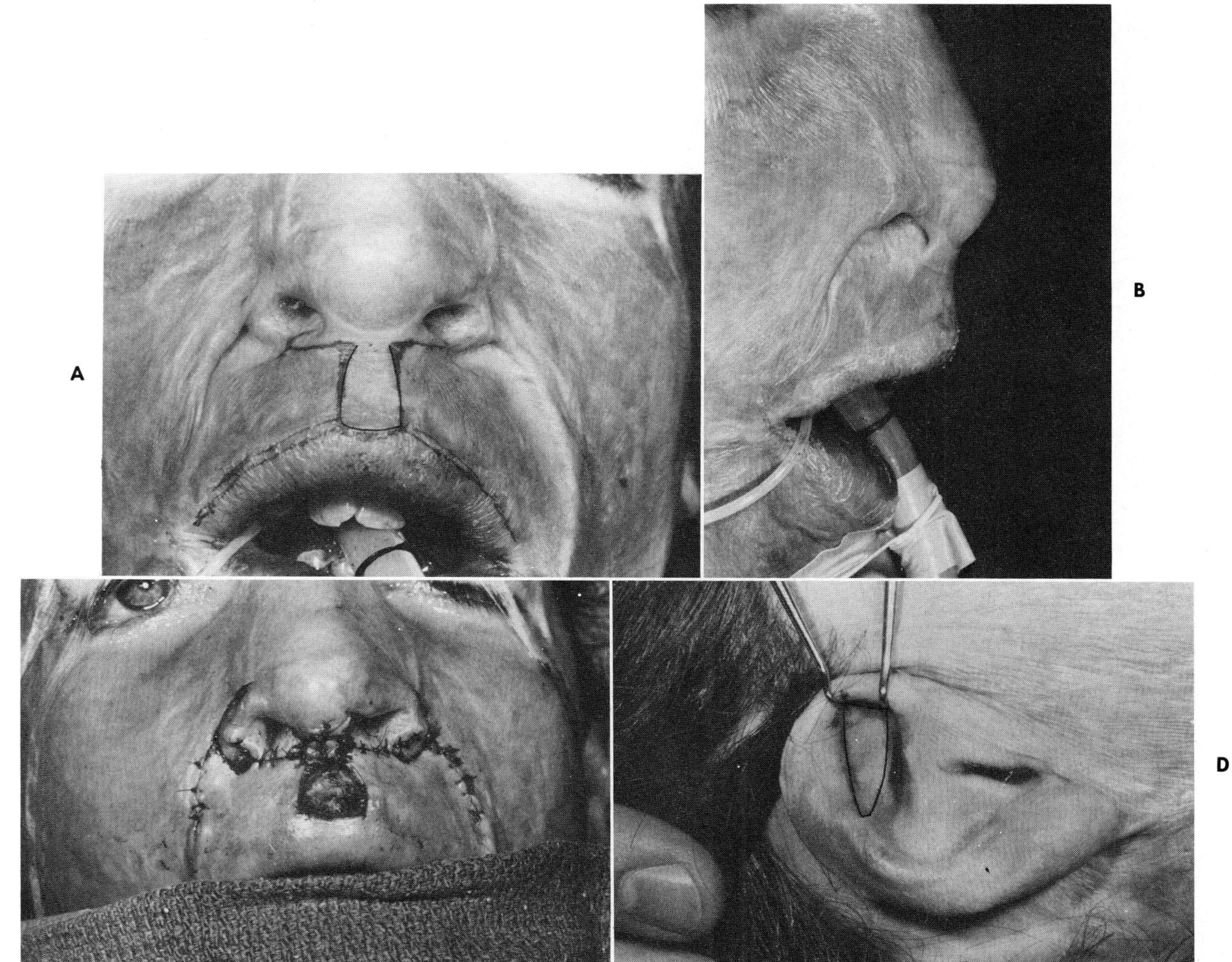

Fig. 32-17. Philtral reconstruction using a chondrocutaneous composite graft from the ear. **A** and **B,** Preoperative views showing absence of a philtral dimple and columns. **C,** The central ''dimple'' recipient site is deeply excavated. (Columella lengthening and alar base contouring are also done.) **D,** A composite graft is outlined in the triangular fossa of the ear. (The donor site is covered with a skin graft.) *Continued.*

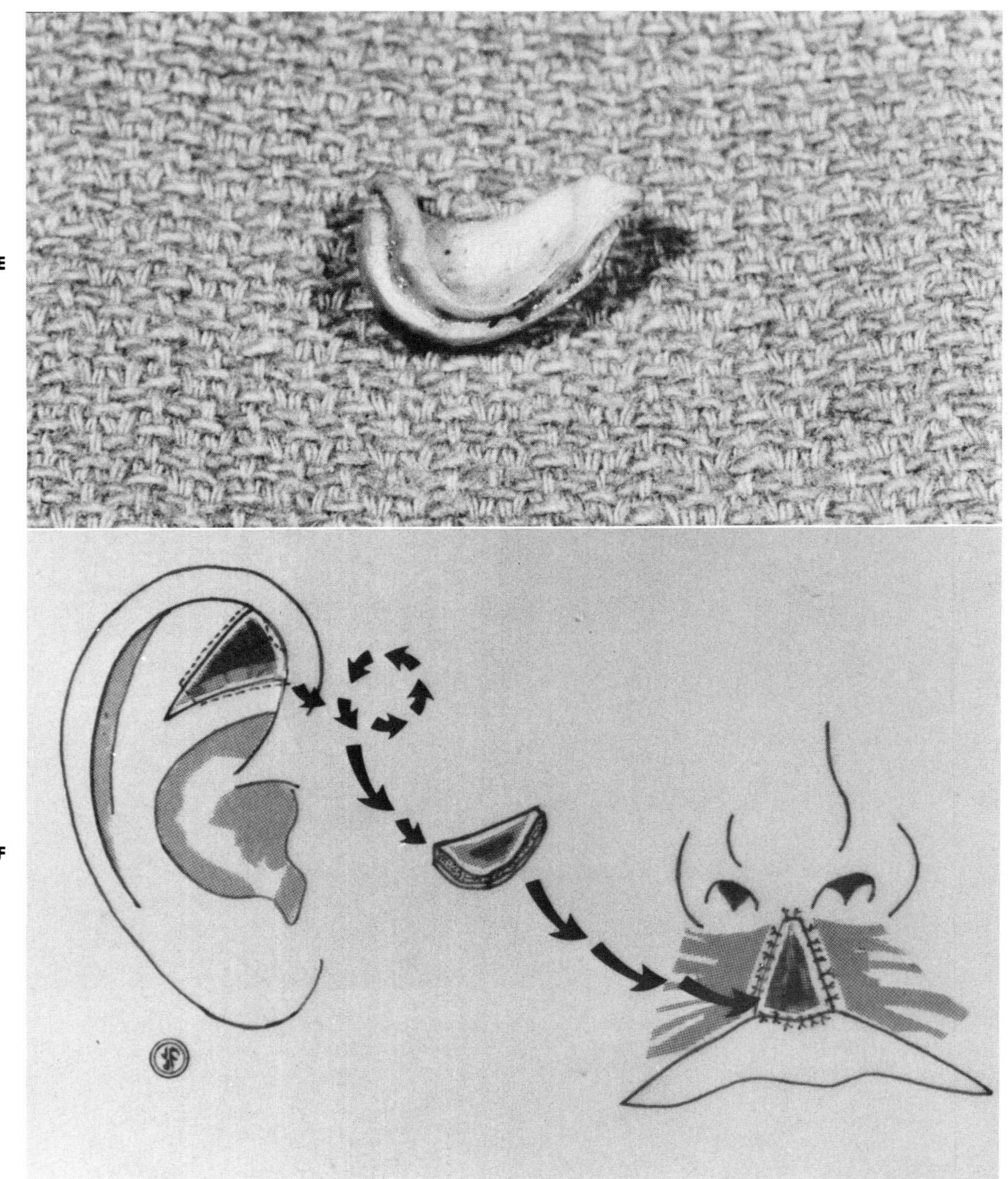

Fig. 32-17, cont'd. E, Concave cartilage-skin graft. **F,** Scheme of transfer.

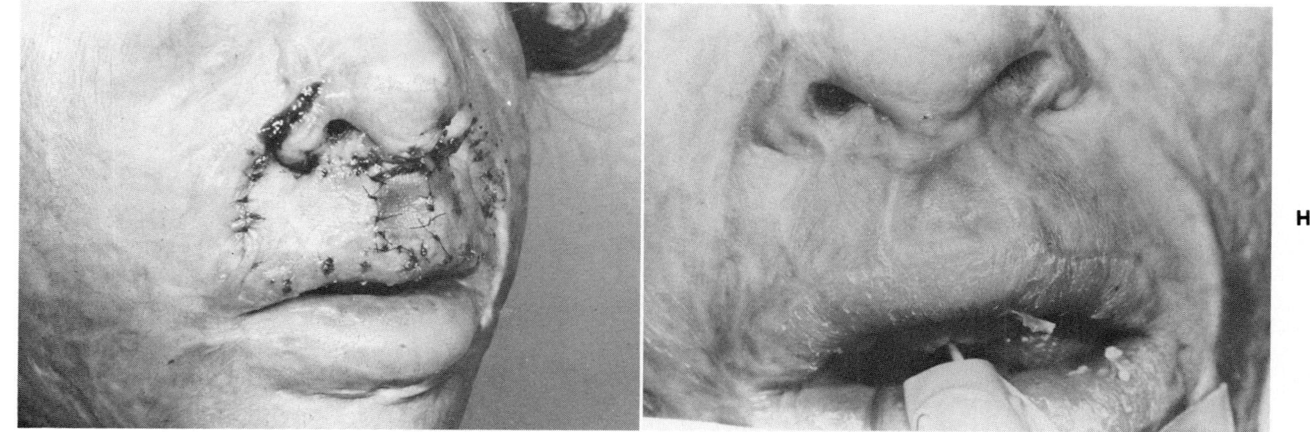

Fig. 32-17, cont'd. G, Postoperative appearance after 1 week. **H,** Postoperative appearance after 6 months. Note the maintained depth of the central dimple and well-defined philtral columns.

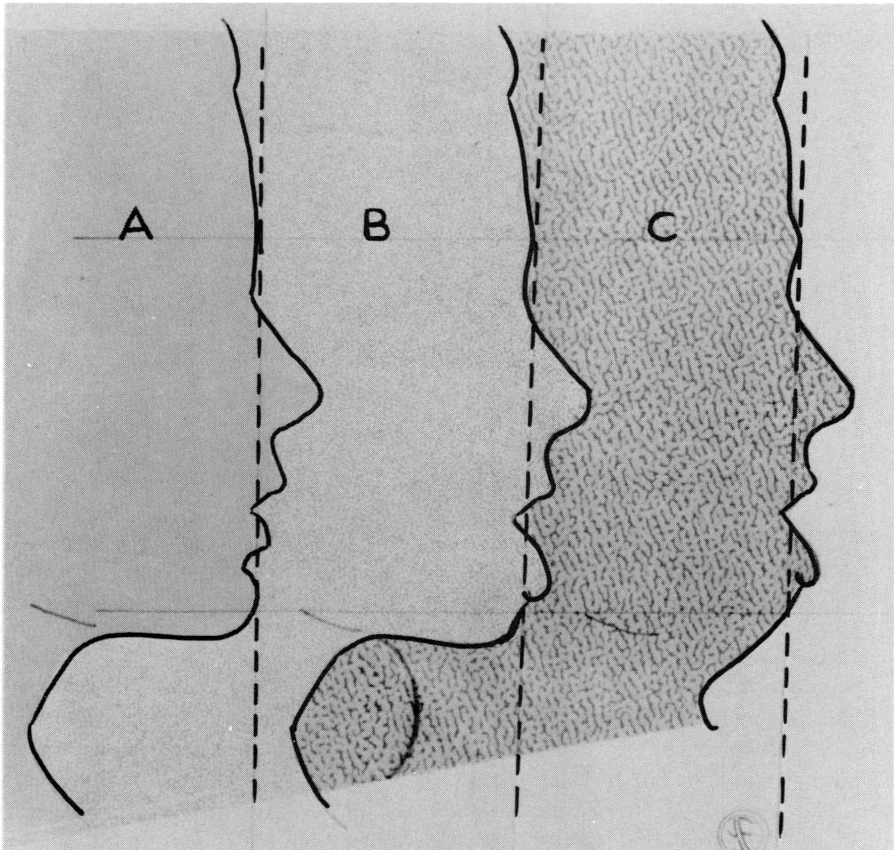

Fig. 32-18. *Pseudomicrogenia. A,* Normal lip-chin-neck contour. *B,* Moderate "microgenia" caused by lower lip eversion and loss of the labiomental sulcus. *C,* Significant "microgenia" caused by a combination of lower lip eversion and neck contracture with obliquity of the cervicomental angle. NOTE: In both *B* and *C,* the chin comes to a normal vertical "profile line."

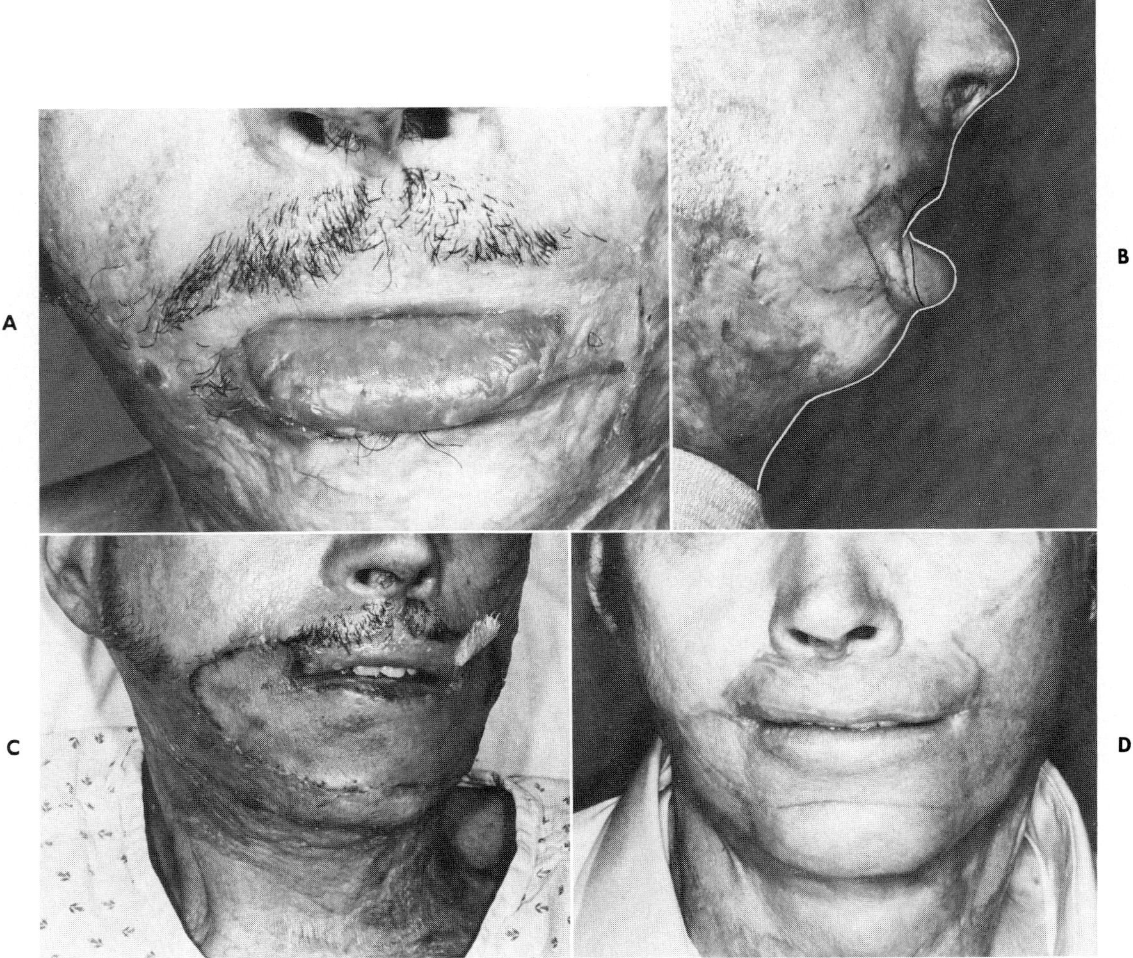

Fig. 32-19. Lower lip resurfacing. **A** and **B,** Preoperative views showing lip eversion and loss of the labiomental sulcus. **C** and **D,** Early and late postoperative result. NOTE: The lower lip unit and chin unit have been separately covered.

missures may limit the ability to open the mouth. (Fig. 32-70 .) Ectropion of the lower lip can be most distressing to the patient, both functionally and esthetically, and its correction should have a high priority.

At times, a purely extrinsic neck scar can transmit a pull on the lower lip, causing distortion when the neck is in a neutral or extended position. In these cases, correction of the neck contracture will eliminate the tug on the lip. However, if the patient's neck is maximally flexed, and an upward push on the skin around the chin fails to normalize the appearance and posture of the lip, an intrinsic lip-chin contracture exists that will not be ameliorated by a neck release alone. In these situations, more skin must be added to the lip-chin area.

As with surgery for any contracture of the face and neck, a decision must be made for either incisional release and grafting or a more definitive excision with resurfacing. The main advantage of the latter approach is that it allows elective placement of the graft edge scars and a planned selection of the desired esthetic unit. The lower lip alone from vermilion margin to labiomental sulcus can be chosen as the resurfaced unit (Fig. 32-19, *D*), or the preferred larger unit of lip and chin together may be used (Figs. 32-20 and 32-22). This combined lip-chin unit places the lower graft-edge seam just beneath the chin, where it is better concealed. In either case, the lower border of the graft should *not* run across the chin prominence itself (Fig. 32-21). Satisfactory surgical correction of the everted lower lip and resurfacing of the lip-chin complex requires attention to a number of technical details. A smooth symmetric lip margin should be outlined along or within the vermilion. Often some excess vermilion will need to be excised (Fig. 32-20, *C*). At the corners of the mouth, the incision should slant upward to avoid downward displacement of the commissures later when the border scars contract. Commissural scar webs can be released at this time.

The lower lip must be released so thoroughly that it unrolls completely, turning the vermilion in toward the mouth.

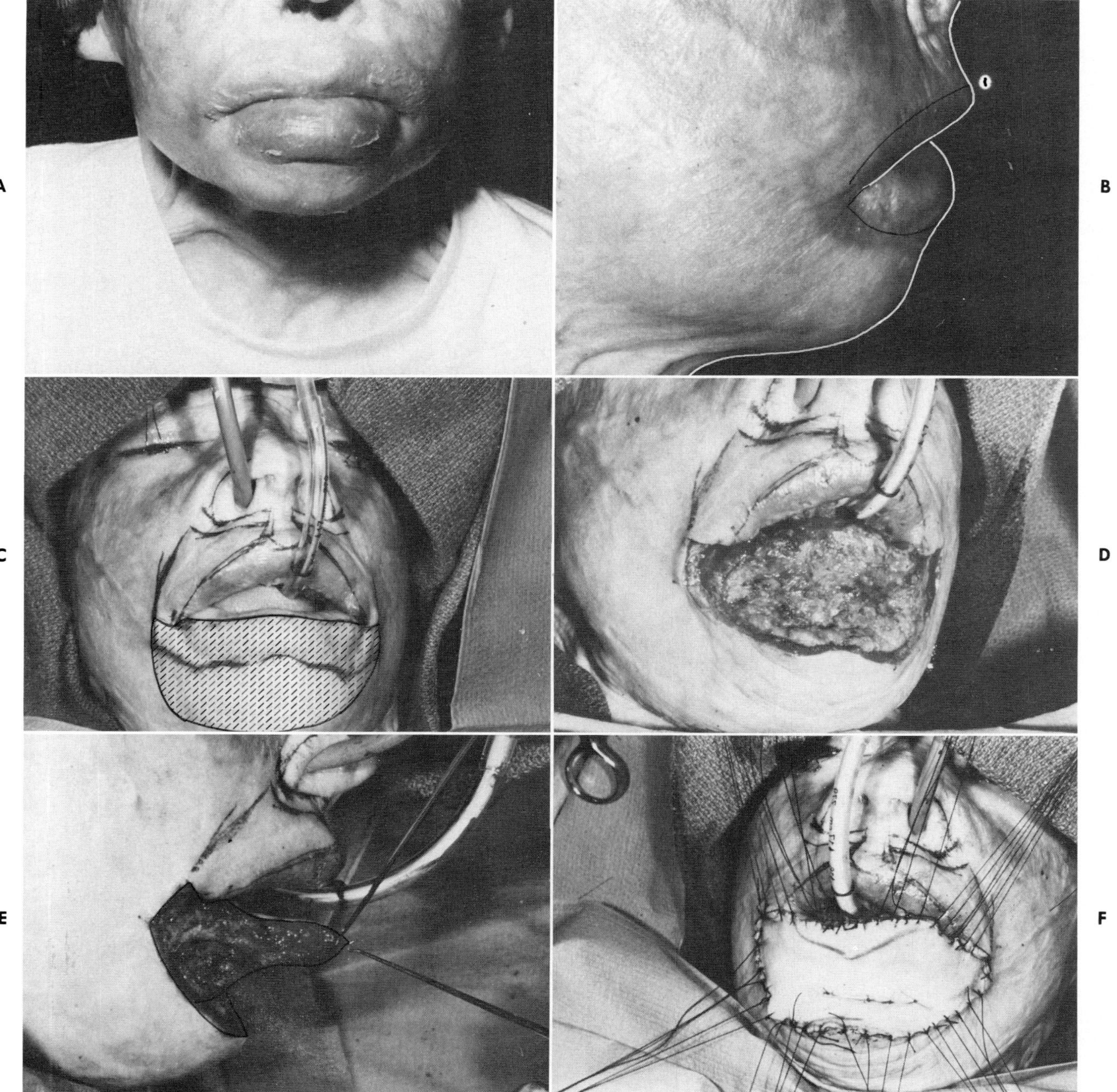

Fig. 32-20. Lower lip–chin resurfacing. **A** and **B,** Preoperative views. **C,** Outline of the scar excision. **D** and **E,** The lip just below and along the vermilion margin is debulked and the labiomental sulcus is deeply excavated by excising soft tissue almost down to the periosteum. **F** and **G,** A thick graft is applied and tacked into the sulcus. Note the overcorrection, with little, if any, vermilion showing.   *Continued.*

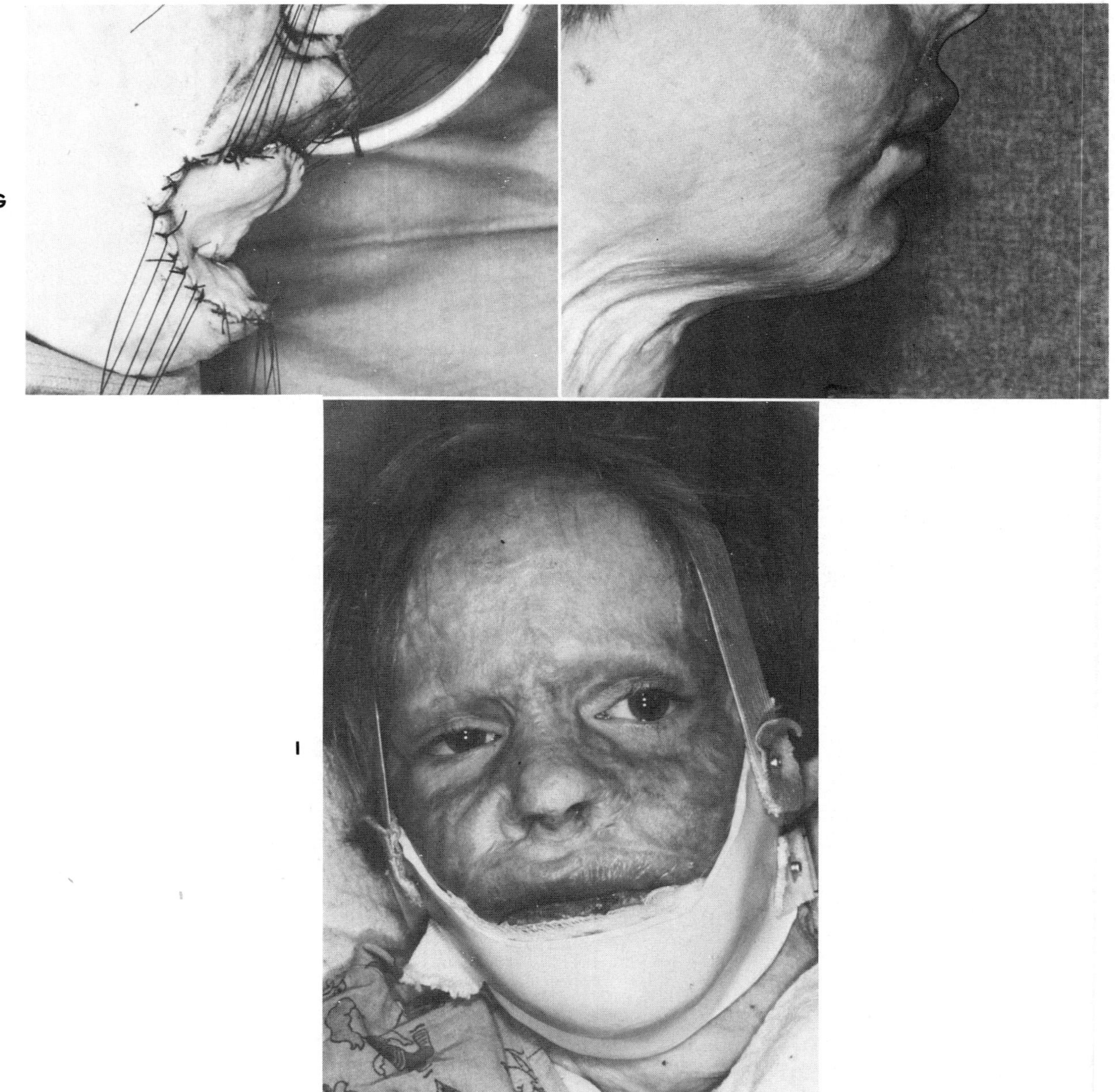

Fig. 32-20, cont'd. H, Postoperative profile showing restoration of normal lip, chin, and labiomental sulcus definition. **I,** A splint is worn to preserve contours.

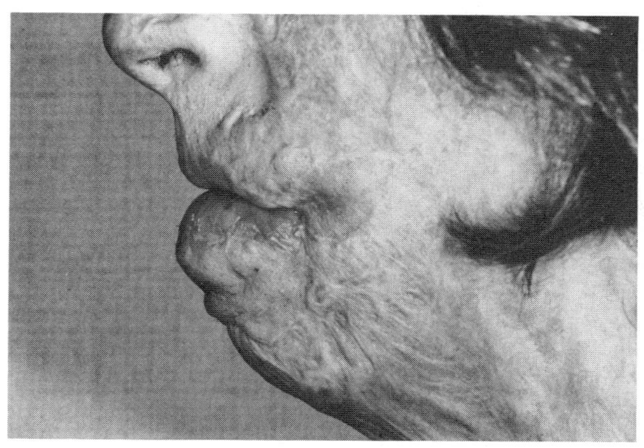

Fig. 32-21. *Incorrect* lower lip release. The lower edge of the skin graft crosses the chin prominence. This seam should be placed either higher in the lip-chin sulcus or lower beneath the chin. The labiomental sulcus has not been re-created, and there is an unattractive convexity (bulge) present.

Little, if any, vermilion should be visible when the graft is applied (Fig. 32-20, *D* to *G*). Overcorrection of the deformity is desired here for three reasons: a thin vermilion show to the lower lip is a normal feature, whereas an overly generous lip face is usually considered unattractive; gravity, graft contraction, and geography often lead to some reeversion of the lip over time; and it is far easier to bring a little more red into view later by removing excess graft (or flap) than it is to do the opposite.

To avoid the common secondary deformity of a convex bulge just below the vermilion edge (Fig. 32-21), the lip should be purposely thinned in this area. This means excising not only all scar tissue but also a transverse strip of normal orbicularis muscle just below the vermilion (Fig. 32-20, *D* and *E*) to achieve the desired concave outline between the vermilion and the lip-chin sulcus.

A well-defined transverse labiomental groove is essential for a good-looking lip and chin. The postoperative profile view should display a normal sinuous curve—concave above, convex below (Figs. 32-20, *H*, and 32-22, *D*). To properly define the sulcus, it must be deeply carved out by purposely excising some unscarred subcutaneous fat and muscle almost down to underlying periosteum (Fig. 32-20, *E*). *No loss of lip function occurs by excising normal muscle to deepen the sulcus.* Overcorrection must be aimed for, since some loss of sulcus depth always occurs with healing. The covering graft is specifically tacked into the groove with mattress sutures (Figs. 32-20, *F*, and 32-22, *C*), and after removal of the bolster dressing, a custom-made isoprene splint is used for several months to help maintain the indentation (Fig. 32-20, *I*). Frequent examination of the teeth should be done to be sure that the splint is not pushing the lower incisors into a lingual inclination. Whenever the chin is being recovered, an oval area over the mental prominence should be de-epithelialized (i.e., only a thin outer layer of scar removed) to preserve the maximal height of the chin (Figs. 32-22, *B*, and 32-36, *D*). In terms of soft tissue recontouring in this area, the best results occur when the lip-chin sulcus is made as deep as possible and the chin prominence as high as possible.

In cases where true microgenia coexists, a *silicone chin implant* can be easily inserted through a submental approach after the lip–chin–upper neck scar has been excised. The electrosurgical blade may be used to dissect a properly sized pocket for the implant just above the periosteum. The deep subcutaneous tissue-muscle layer is closed over the implant using absorbable sutures with inverted knots and the augmented chin covered with a skin graft in the usual manner. The addition of a chin implant to lip-chin or chin-neck recontour surgery has been very gratifying, and it should be strongly considered in the adolescent or older patient in whom soft tissue sculpturing alone is unlikely to produce ideal results (Fig. 32-22). The procedure adds little extra surgical time, and the incidence of complications is remarkably low. If the neck is being recovered at the same time as the chin, a submental-submandibular lipectomy and platysma tightening (e.g., medial plication) can be helpful in further defining the profile chin and neck contours.

The lip-chin unit must be distinguished from the neck-chin unit (Fig. 32-29). For the lip-chin area, thick skin grafts (split or full) are generally used for the new cover. Flaps can be used (Fig. 32-37) to resurface this region, but they must be made extremely thin over the lip to avoid filling up the hollow of the labiomental sulcus. Secondary and tertiary flap defattings may be required. It is for this reason that microvascular free tissue transfer is not advocated for covering the lip-chin area. Experience has shown that even apparently thin free flaps (e.g., the dorsalis pedis flap) undergo considerable primary elastic contraction when cut free and appear much too bulky for the lower lip. Even after several defattings, lower lips resurfaced with free flaps seem to lack finesse.

The cheeks

Localized cheek scars, surrounded by normal skin are often best treated with excision in one or several stages[76] (Figs. 32-5 and 32-10). This technique is particularly useful in the nasolabial fold region and preauricular area. Care must be exercised to prevent distortion of nearby mobile features, that is, eyelids, lips, and nostrils. Local skin flaps

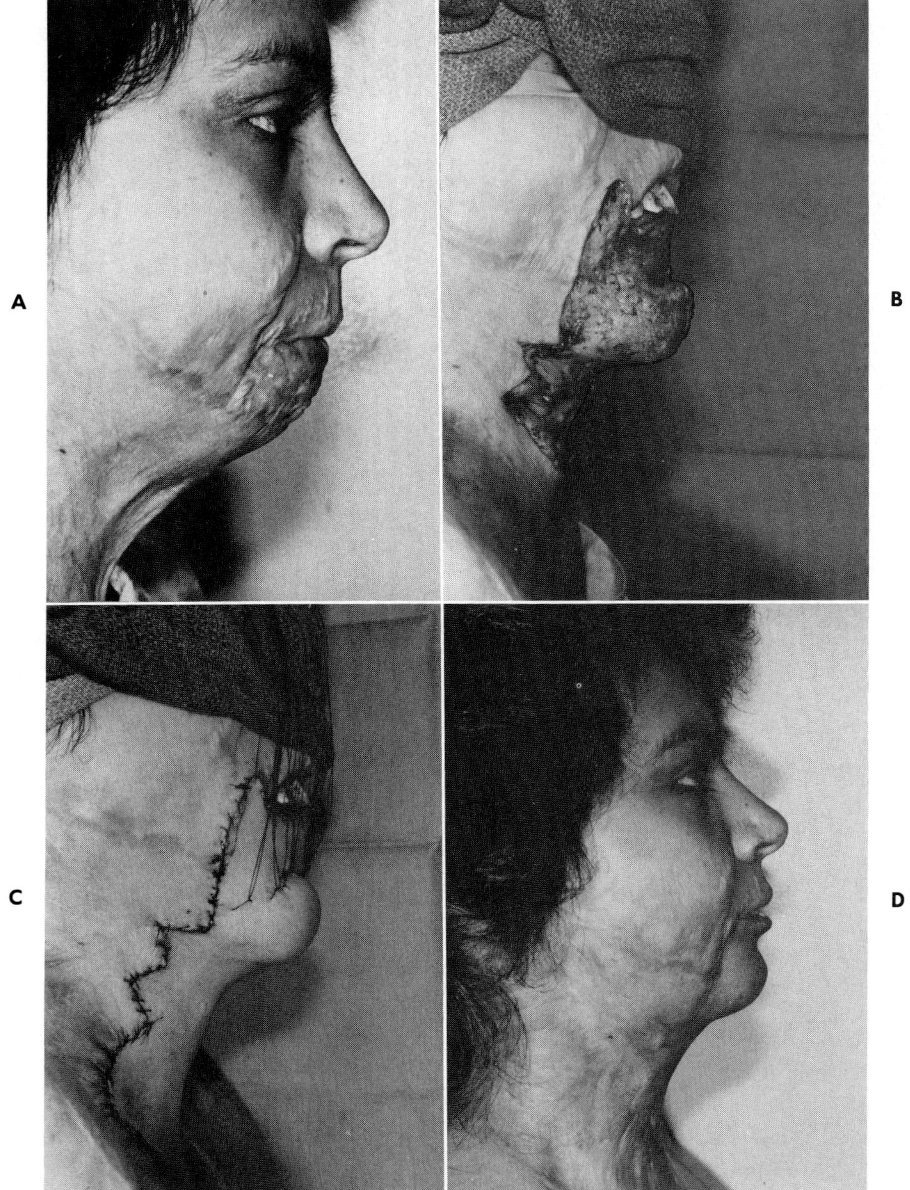

Fig. 32-22. Lower lip–chin–neck resurfacing with correction of true microgenia. **A,** Preoperative profile. **B,** The scar is excised, upper lip thinned, labiomental sulcus carved out, chin de-epithelialized, a small silicone chin implant inserted, and a submental lipectomy and ''platysmaplasty'' done to deepen the chin-neck angle. **C,** A thick split-thickness skin graft applied with ''darts'' along the lateral vertical edges. **D,** Postoperative result.

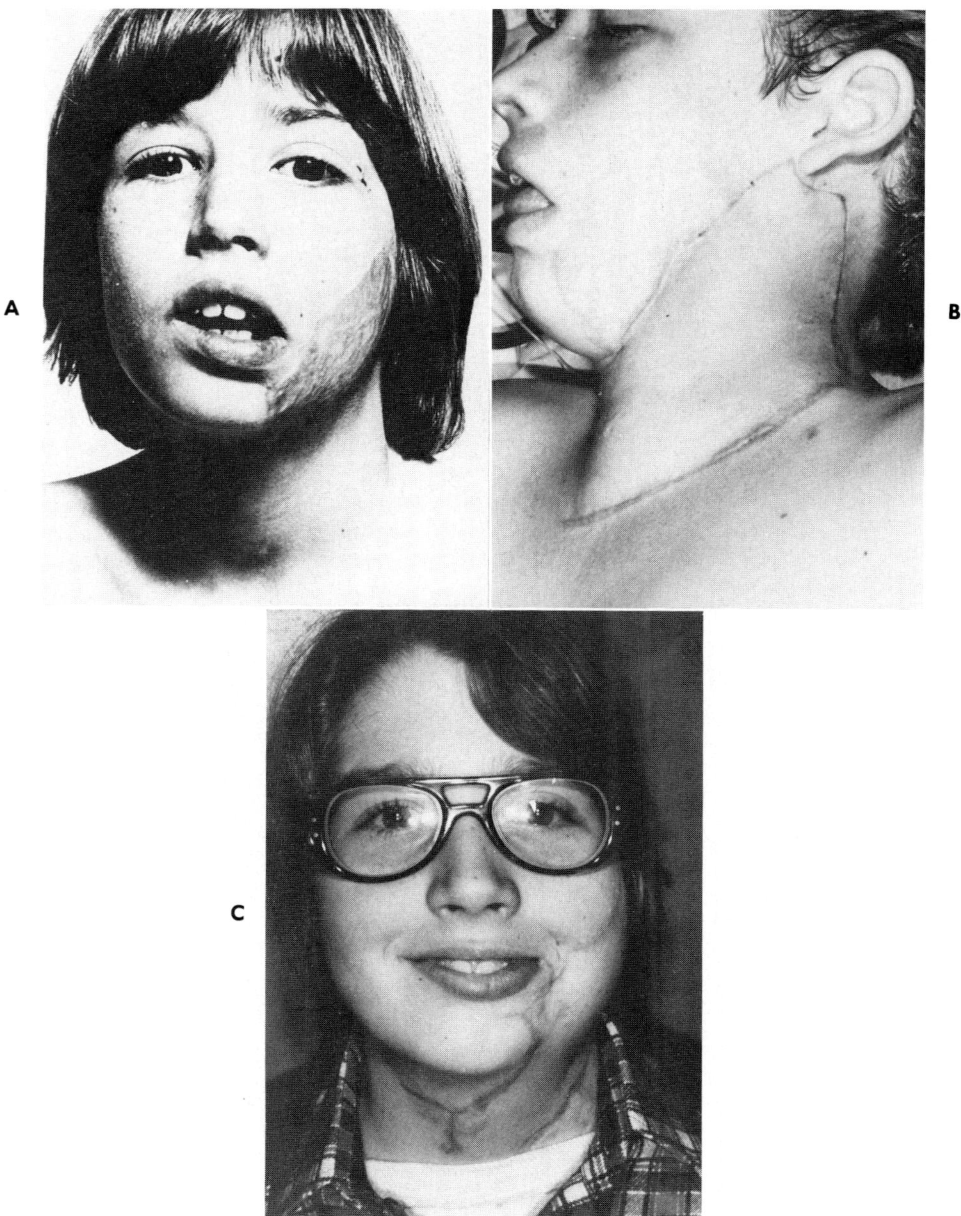

Fig. 32-23. Cervical rotation flap for cheek resurfacing. **A,** A skin graft on the cheek surrounded by normal skin appears as an alien patch. Note the downward pull of the scar on the lower lip. **B,** A delayed neck rotation flap before transposition. **C,** Early result after a secondary Z-plasty to the perioral and neck seams. Note correction of the lower lip posture and the improved blend of the flap with the cheek. A larger cervicopectoral flap would have placed the flap donor site in an even less visible location.

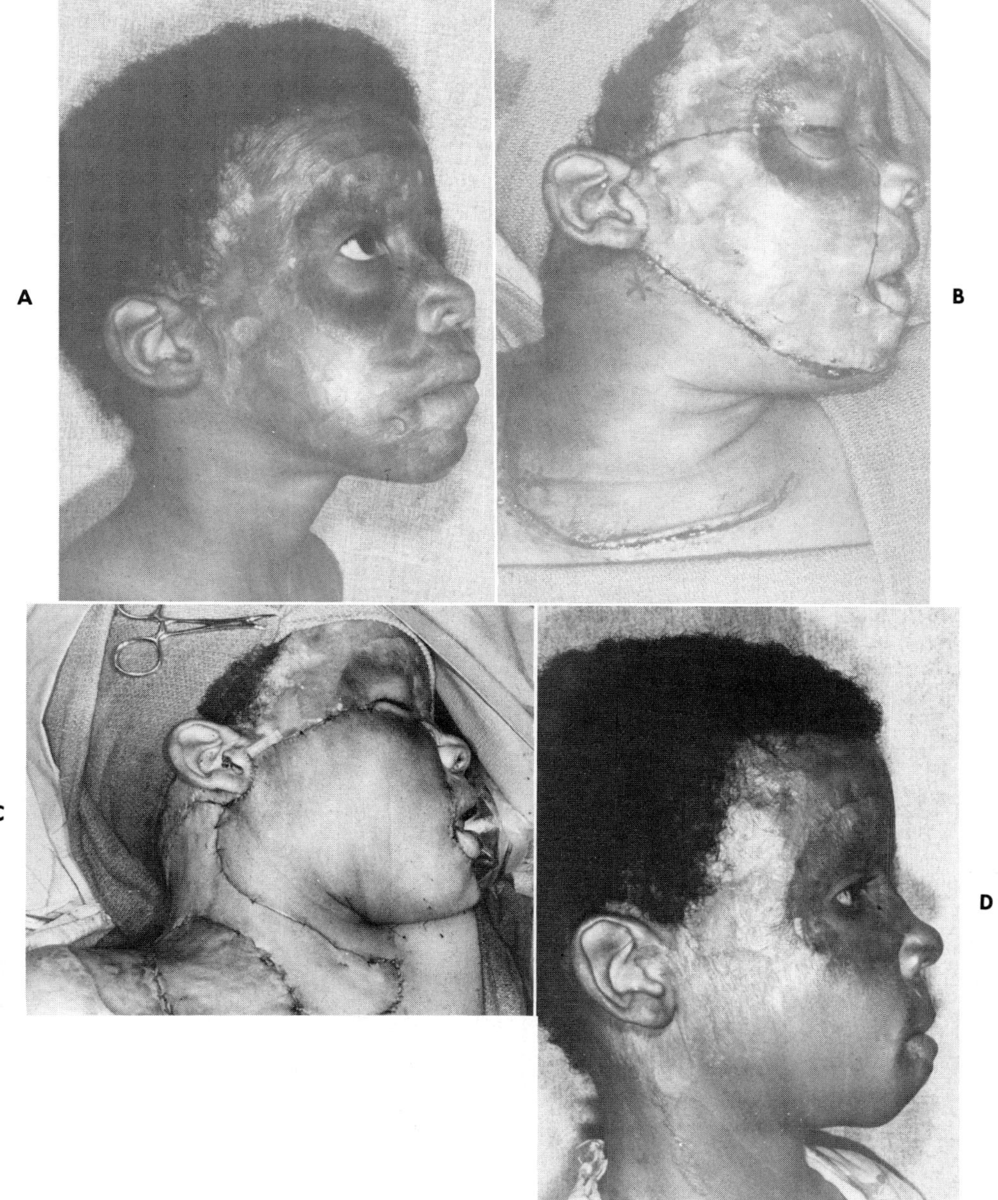

Fig. 32-24. A cervical rotation flap for cheek resurfacing. **A,** Shiny hyperpigmented skin grafts and scar cover the cheek. **B,** After three preliminary delay procedures, the thin flap is ready for transfer. **C,** The entire cheek and chin have been excised and recovered with the transposed flap. The flap donor area has been skin grafted. **D,** Result. Some further thinning of the flap over the lower lip is needed.

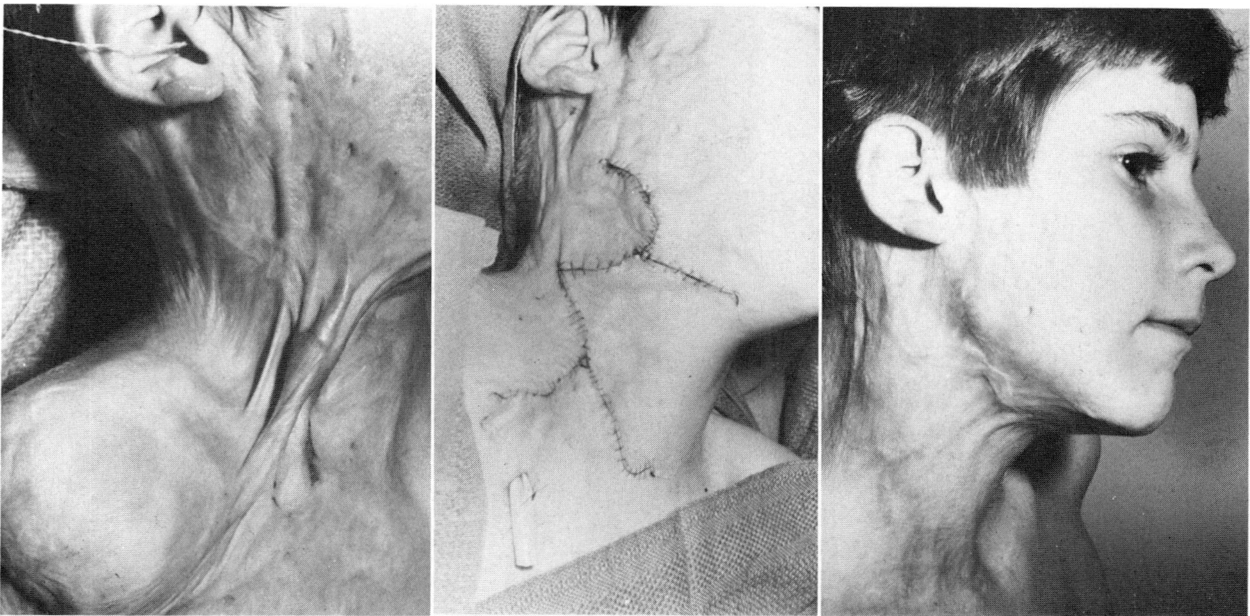

Fig. 32-25. Excision of a localized neck scar band and closure using interdigitated flaps.

are the next best choice in this setting.[37] Larger areas of burn scar should be excised and resurfaced with thick skin grafts or regional flaps, depending on the individual considerations. (See grafts versus flaps, p. 559.) If most of a cheek is to be resurfaced, it is best to cover the entire esthetic unit of the cheek, sacrificing some normal skin if necessary. The burn scar is excised at the dermal scar–fat interface. The use of an electrosurgical knife greatly decreases blood loss, and , despite the theoretic disadvantage of tissue injury, in actual practice the graft ''take'' is not compromised. If there is any question about the adequacy of hemostasis after a large excision, skin grafting should be delayed for 24 hours. Fig. 32-35 shows the result of a cheek resurfacing using a thick (0.020 inch) split-thickness skin graft. Figs. 32-23 and 32-24 illustrate the use of cervical flaps for cheek resurfacing. As emphasized by Smith nearly 30 years ago, when planning a reconstruction, the surgeon ''must thoroughly canvass the possibility of utilizing tissue from the neighborhood.''[146] Thin flaps from the neck, shoulders, and chest are commonly used.*

The neck

Scarring of the neck can cause both disability and disfigurement. The concave and highly mobile anterior neck with its thin skin cover is particularly prone to flexion contractures that can range from minimally restrictive to crippling mentosternal synechiae. An upper neck contracture often exerts a pull on the face above, causing extrinsic distortion of the lower lip, ear, nose, cheek, and possibly the lower eyelid.

---

*References 12, 45, 84, 91, 128, 131, 151, and 172.

Localized neck burns may produce fairly discrete scars. These vertical bands are usually best treated by excision and the wounds closed using Z-plasties or various interdigitated local skin flaps that reorient the resulting scars into a more favorable oblique or transverse direction (Fig. 32-25).[78] Local flaps fashioned from elastic and relatively unscarred skin work quite well. However, flaps cut from nonpliant surrounding scar move poorly and result in tight closures, and the flap tips usually necrose. Small local flaps should be employed only if the skin adjacent to the linear scar is essentially normal. At times a combination of local flaps and skin grafts are appropriate[164] (Fig. 32-26). In these cases, the design and placement of the flaps and grafts on the neck is very important. Vertical join lines should be avoided (Fig. 32-26, *E*), since these will undoubtedly lead to new contracture bands later on. Orienting the flaps so that their edges leave more or less transverse scars, as well as hiding the grafts under the shadow of the chin or low on the neck is desirable (Fig. 32-26, *D*). Large areas of scarring are more common than localized neck bands. A diffuse surface shortening produces not only the functional loss of neck extension, but the esthetically important chin-neck angle is often blunted or obliterated. The tight neck can be released with either an *incision* across the scar if the surface is flat and esthetically acceptable, or an *excision* carried out if the scar is hypertrophic or widely restrictive. Again, if the scar is to be completely excised, there is no need to wait for its maturation.

The transverse releasing incision should be made at a level that will produce both the maximal expansion (i.e., where the scar is tightest) and the best appearance of the neck. Regardless of where the incision(s) is placed, it must

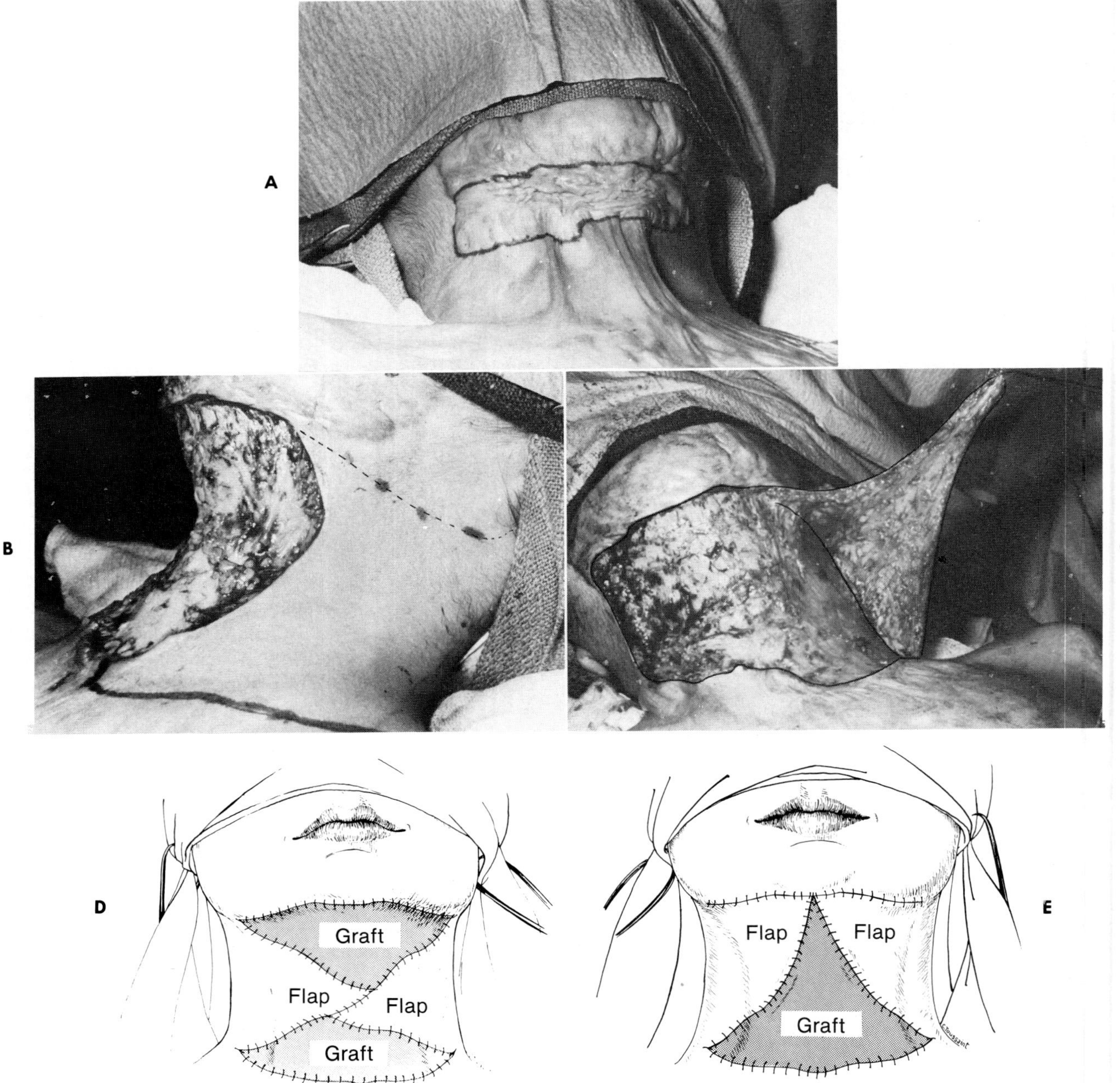

Fig. 32-26. Neck release and resurfacing with a combination of skin flaps and skin grafts. **A,** The neck scar is outlined for excision. **B,** The released defect extends from the chin above to the suprasternal notch below. A left-sided neck flap is outlined *(dotted line marks the mandible).* **C,** The flap is elevated. **D,** *Correct* placement of flaps and grafts avoiding vertical join lines. **E,** *Incorrect* design. The vertical edge lines will develop into linear contracture bands.

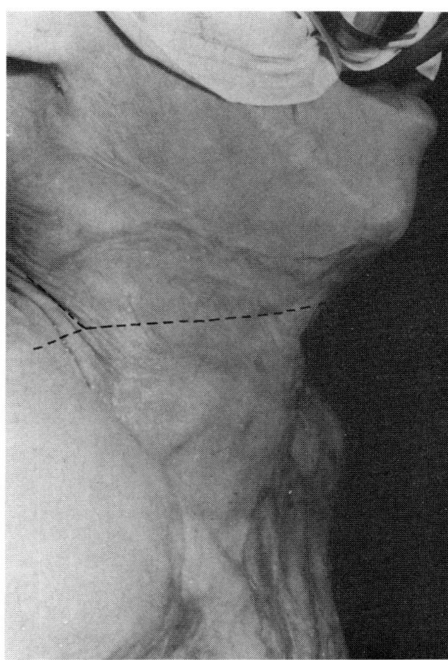

Fig. 32-27. Incisional release of a neck contracture. Note the fishtail (Y-shaped) design at the lateral ends.

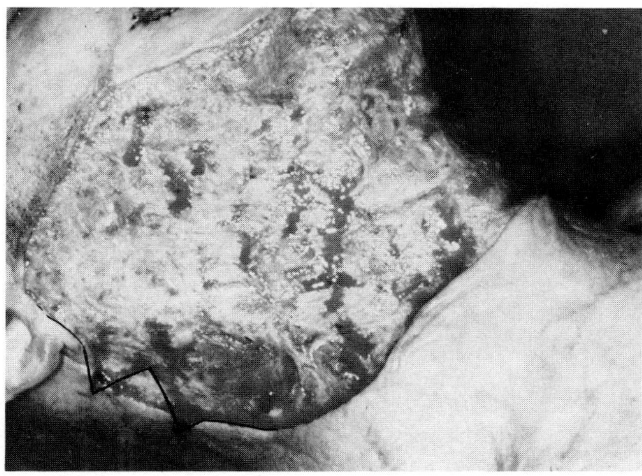

Fig. 32-28. Excisional release of a neck scar. Note the triangular darts excised along the lateral margins.

extend across the full width of the anterior neck scar. The lateral ends of the incision at the sides of the neck should be designed as reclining Ys to avoid vertical graft edges that are prone to contracture[98,137] (Fig. 32-27). For the same reason, an excision of the neck scar should also include excision of unscarred triangular "darts" along the lateral margins (Fig. 32-28). A thorough release often requires incising across bands of white scar in the subcutaneous muscles (platysma and strap muscles). This deeper scar should be cut with a "light touch" and at different levels (superior and inferior) so that the wound opens in a flat plane rather than as a deep ravine. Once the initial incision is made with the scalpel, use of the electric knife can significantly reduce the bleeding. Particularly when skin grafts are used for the resurfacing, hemostasis must be excellent; if not, delayed grafting at 24 to 48 hours is prudent. The most common reason for areas of graft loss is hematoma. Split-thickness grafts should be thick (0.018 to 0.020 inch) to reduce the tendency for secondary contraction. The Reese dermatome takes a large graft (4 × 6 inches) of uniform thickness. The Padgett electric dermatome can be used to harvest longer lengths of skin. The fewer the number of pieces of graft used the better, and again the lateral graft margins and seams between the pieces should be made more transverse than vertical. If possible, when the neck alone is being released or resurfaced, the skin graft (or flap) should not be carried up onto the face above the mandible where a conspicuous edge scar can be seen. Not infrequently, however, this is unavoidable because the neck scar often extends onto the lower cheeks and chin (Fig. 32-29). The

skin grafts are usually secured by tying the long ends of the superior and inferior row of sutures across a bulky bolster dressing of nonadherent greased gauze and cotton. The sutures on the lateral neck are cut short and are not used in the tie-over dressing, but rather the sides of the bolster are pressed down by a stretch-gauze bandage wrapped snugly around the cylinder of the neck. Care must be taken, however, to avoid excess pressure over the larynx (thyroid cartilage), which can produce an area of graft loss. A plaster splint can be laid over the soft dressing to help maintain neck extension and prevent head turning. In this regard, positioning the patient on a short bed mattress postoperatively or placing a small pillow transversely beneath the shoulders with a sandbag on either side of the head may be helpful. The dressing is usually left on for 7 to 10 days. As soon as it is removed, a rigid heat-labile plastic splint (isoprene) is molded and applied over a protective layer of grease gauze. It is critical that once the dressing has been taken down, the neck must be immediately resplinted. The splint should be worn even if there are some raw spots. Areas of graft loss greater than 2 cm should be regrafted to minimize contraction.

After split-thickness skin grafting the neck, a custom-made, rigid splint must be worn continuously day and night for a minimum of 6 months. As emphasized by Cronin,[42,43] for the split graft–splinting technique to be successful, the splint must (1) extend the neck, (2) mold the chin-neck angle, and (3) apply even pressure to the grafted area. Both extension and pressure are equally important. The splint may require adjustment every few months to ensure proper

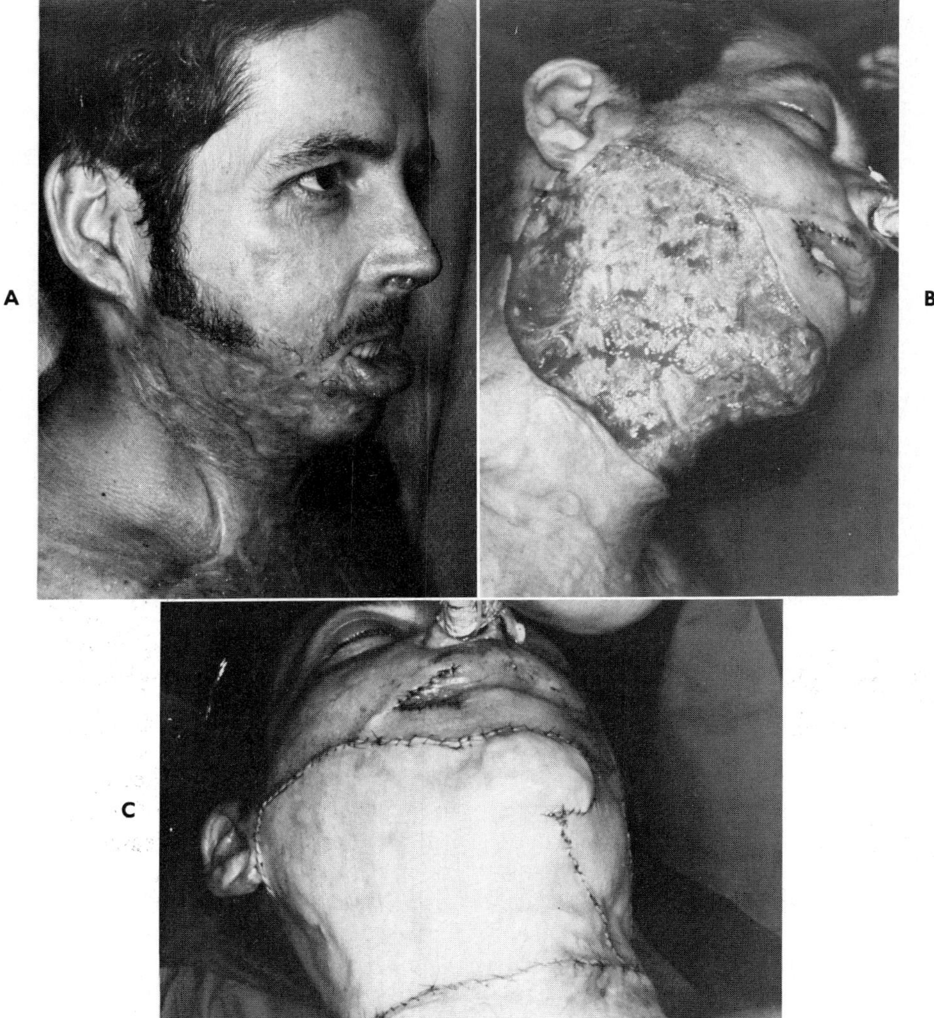

Fig. 32-29. Neck release and grafting. **A,** Preoperative appearance. **B,** The scar is excised and the chin prominence de-epithelialized. Lateral edge darts should be excised. **C,** Thick split-thickness grafts are applied with oblique (not vertical) seam.

fit. After the initial postoperative 6 month period, the splint can be worn for a month or two on a part-time basis (e.g., at night). However, the patient's parents must be instructed to carefully watch for the earliest signs of contracture of graft wrinkling and insist that the splint be used again on a more or less full-time basis until the proclivity for shrinkage has been overcome. Sometimes this takes a year or longer. It must be emphasized that without an adequate postoperative splinting regimen, the results of skin grafting the neck will be, at best, significantly compromised.

Even when very thick skin grafts are used for neck resurfacing along with conscientious and prolonged splinting, contracture of the neck can occur. In some patients, repeated incisional or excisional releases and grafting are disappointing. Experience has shown that for some reason narrow skin

grafts (e.g., 3 to 5 cm in width) have a greater tendency to contract and wrinkle than do large grafts. In patients who have undergone one or more release and grafting procedures with subsequent contracture despite splinting, a skin flap to the neck should be considered. The flap will not shrink over time, and, from an esthetic point of view, a flap will often provide a better color and texture match than a graft. If the flap is properly thinned and designed, normal neck contour can be achieved (Fig. 32-30). When applying a thin flap to the upper neck, a submandibular and submental lipectomy (as is commonly done in an esthetic face lift operation) can be helpful in producing a well-defined cervicomandibular angle. If expertly done, flap resurfacing of the neck can produce excellent results, but the patient and surgeon must accept the flap donor site deformity (another scar or graft), the potential for partial flap loss from vascular insufficiency,

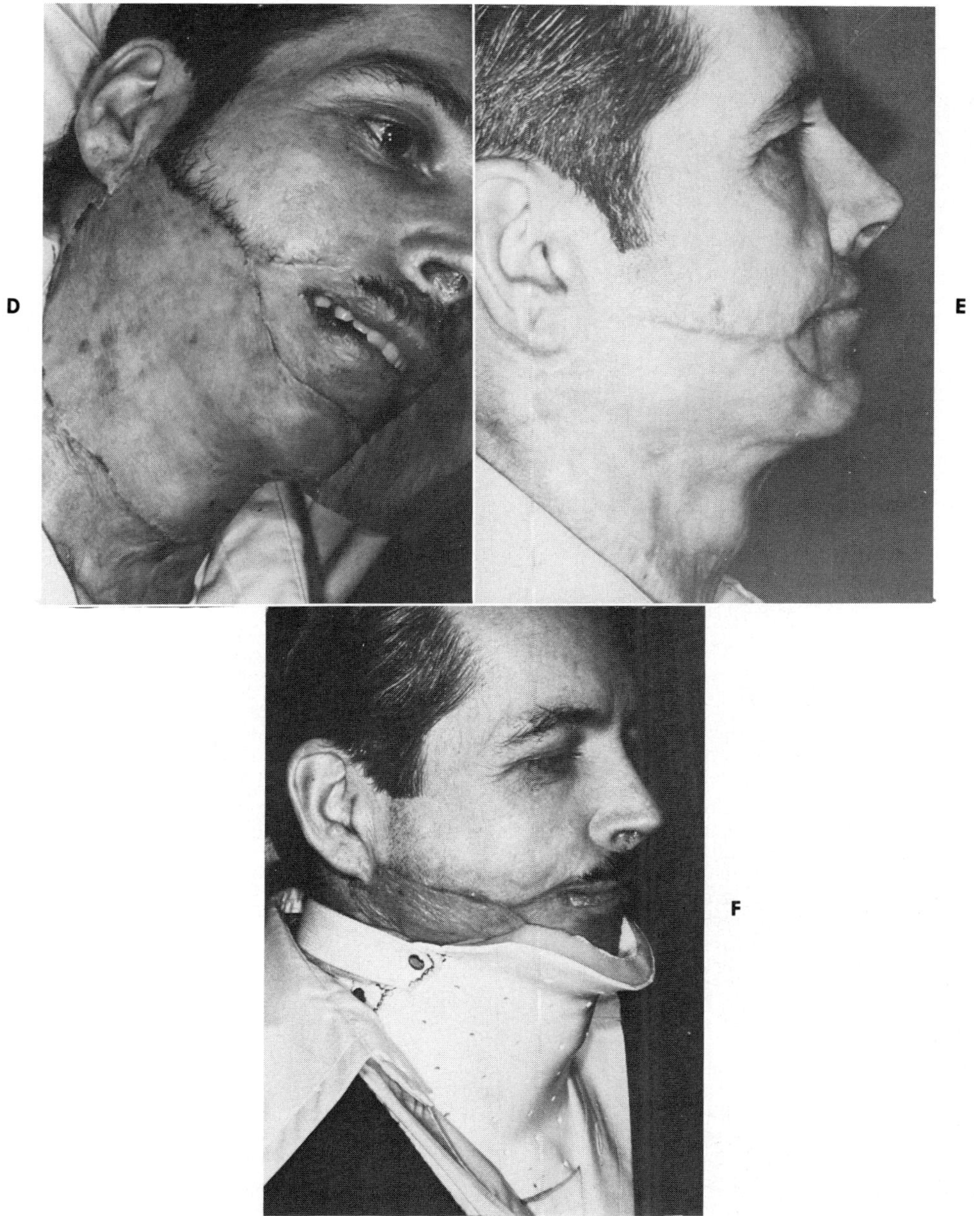

Fig. 32-29, cont'd. D and **E,** Postoperative views. Note the normal chin projection and well-defined chin-neck angle. **F,** A postoperative splint is worn continuously for at least 6 months.

and an unsatisfactory appearance unless the flaps are carefully designed and thinned. Proper flap design implies preoperative mapping of the flap with the patient sitting up. A fabric or thin foam pattern can easily be made for "planning the flap in reverse" to be certain that it will adequately swing, reach, and fill the defect. So often this preoperative "dry run" shows that the flap must be made longer than first estimated. Since thin flaps by necessity must be random-pattern flaps without an axial blood supply (musculocutaneous and axial-pattern flaps are too bulky), one, two, or

more preliminary "delay" procedures are often desirable to reduce the risk of flap necrosis. Although preparation of a flap does entail more time than a one-stage skin graft procedure, the flap-covered neck does not require the prolonged postoperative splinting that the grafted neck does. For a long flap (e.g., a 3:1 length-to-width ratio) a suggested regimen of delay procedures involves an incision along the entire length of one long margin with complete undermining of the entire flap. At a second procedure performed 7 to 14 days later, the other long margin is incised, creating a bi-

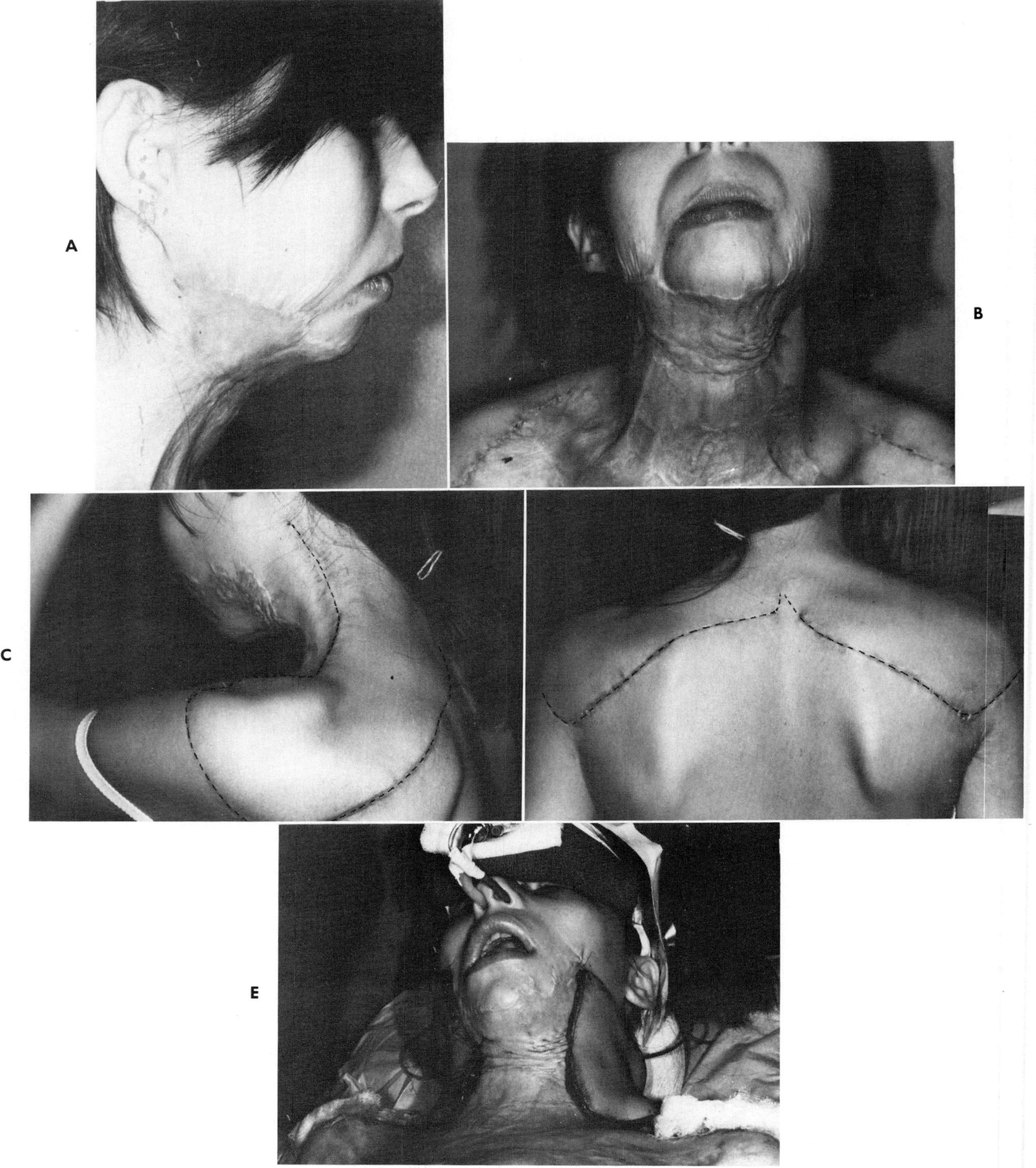

Fig. 32-30. For legend see opposite page.

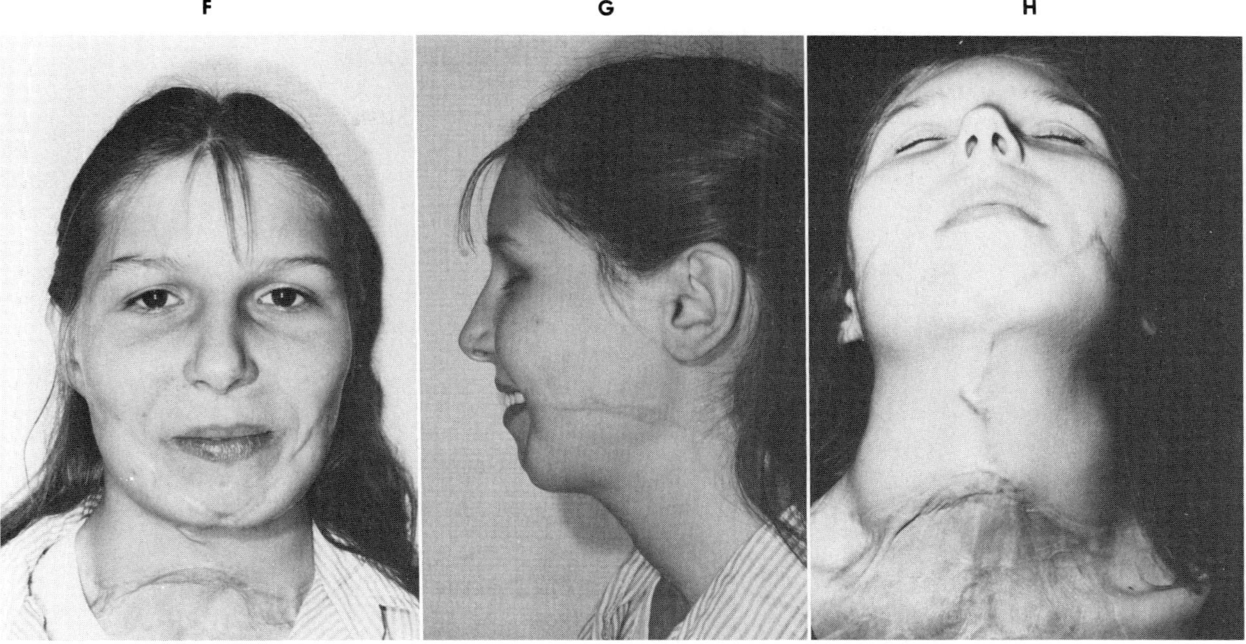

Fig. 32-30. Bilateral "epaulette" flaps for cervicofacial resurfacing. **A** and **B,** Preoperative appearance. **C** and **D,** Trapezius-deltoid area flaps were delayed. **E,** The flaps were temporarily tacked to the neck while donor sites were skin grafted. **F** and **G,** Postoperative appearance. Note the normal chin-neck angle achieved by submandibular lipectomy and thin flaps. **H,** The expanse of the flaps seen with the neck extended. The central dart breaks up the vertical join line.

pedicle flap. At this time a portion of the distal margin also can be cut if the surgeon feels confident. A third delay or the actual flap transfer can be carried out 7 to 21 days after the second procedure. Having been previously dissected, the undersurface of the flap is usually lined by a smooth but elastic layer of scar tissue of variable thickness. This sheet of scar not only adds unwanted bulk to the flap, but significantly reduces the flap's normal stretchability. For these reasons, the scar layer should be excised when the definitive flap transposition is done. A useful method of removing the scar from the deep surface of the flap is to make multiple incisions 1 or 2 cm apart through the scar just into the underlying fat. The incisions are made both parallel and perpendicular to the long axis of the flap and create a gridlike pattern of small squares. Each scar tissue square is individually picked up with a forcep and trimmed away with scissors until the entire underbelly of the flap shows only a thin yellow layer of fat. Scar removal from a delayed flap does add time to the surgical procedure, but it is worth the extra time. The thinness and especially the pliability gained are important flap characteristics to have when the flap is moved. Unless the flap is restored to its normal elasticity it may not reach its mark. Experience has also shown that it is safe to thin an adequately delayed flap (leaving intact the subdermal vascular plexus), and cervicofacial contours are ultimately better defined when the flaps are thinned before insertion, as opposed to later staged defatting procedures. Regional flaps for recovering the neck are often available. The epaulette, or *charretera,* flap from the posterolateral neck and shoulder region is particularly useful (Figs. 32-30 and 32-31).* Other flaps from the lower neck and chest are also frequently used (Figs. 32-32 and 32-33.)[32-37,80,131]

Vascularized (or microvascular) flaps also may have a role in reconstruction of the neck after an extensive burn injury, scarring, and neck contracture.† The vascularized groin flap and the vascularized scapular flap have been employed successfully for this purpose. With the vascularized groin flap, the donor scar is inconspicuous and can be hidden even with brief clothing. Large segments of composite tissue can be successfully transplanted to resurface the anterior neck. The average dimensions of the groin flap in the teenage child is approximately 9 × 25 cm. This is a large flap and can be employed to resurface the entire anterior neck and chin region. The scapular flap provides donor tissue of similar dimensions. The vascular pedicle is longer and greater in external diameter, facilitating anastomosis and placement. Transplantation of a vascularized flap is usually performed later in the course of the illness when the patient is undergoing staged reconstruction. Even though the patient may have an extensive burn to the head and neck region,

---

*References 6, 38, 94, 105, and 181.
†References 65, 114, 118, 142, 148, and 149.

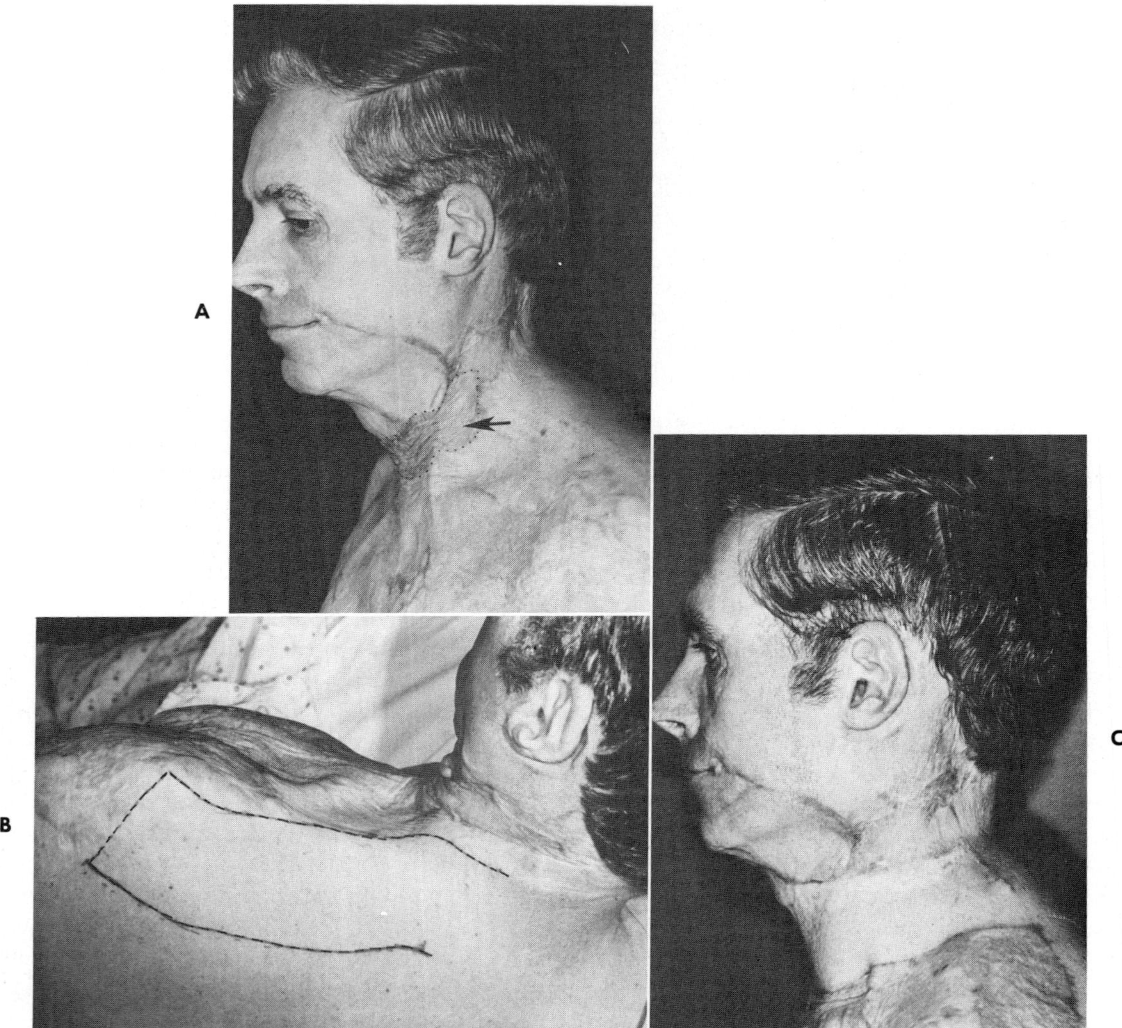

Fig. 32-31. A shoulder flap used for recurrent neck contracture. **A,** Preoperative appearance. Note the wrinkled skin graft *(arrow)* in the left lower neck. **B,** The flap is outlined. It was "delayed" three times before transfer. **C,** Postoperative result after excision of the "dog ear" at the rotation point.

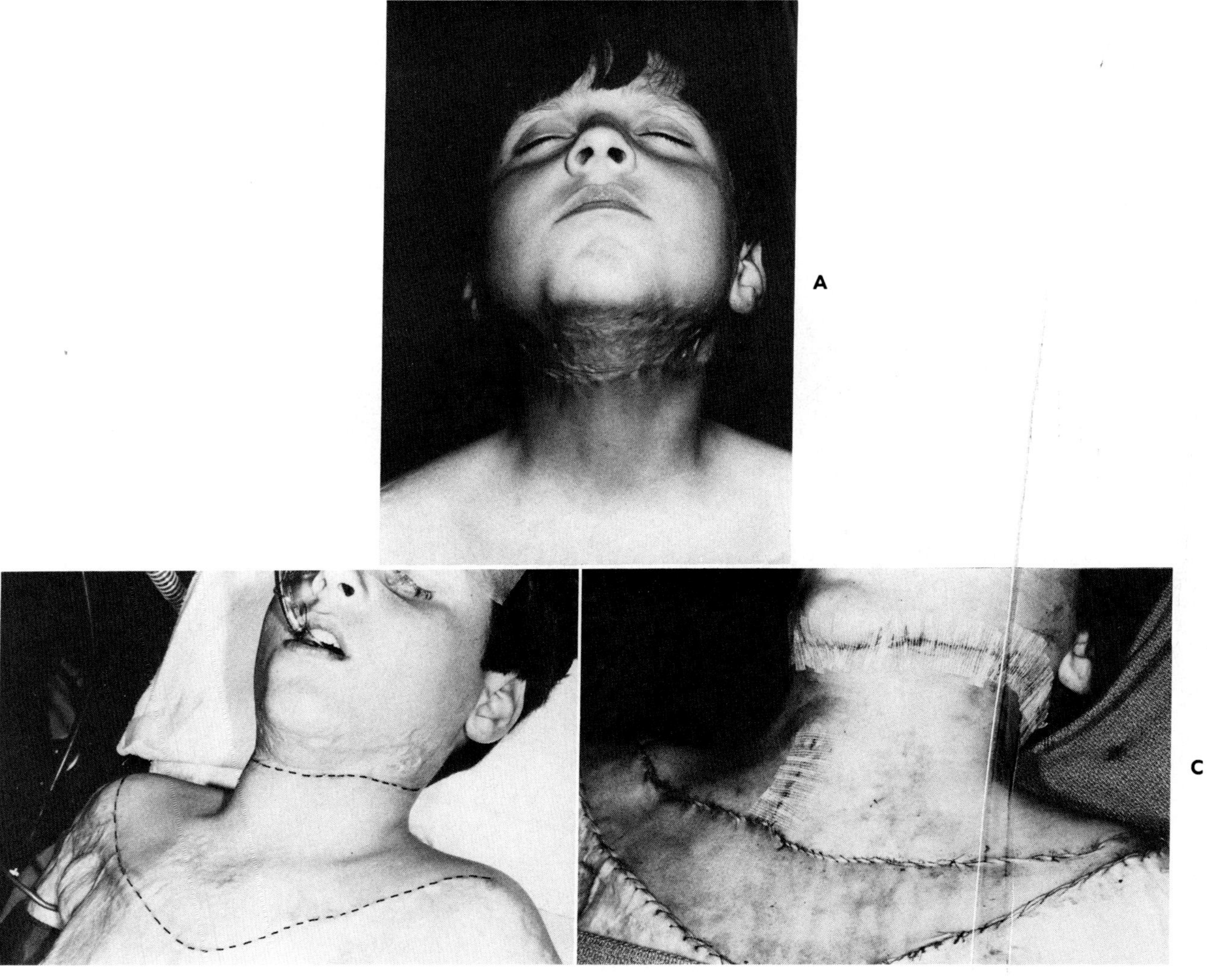

Fig. 32-32. A bipedicle neck flap for resurfacing the jawline area. **A,** Preoperative appearance. **B,** The flap is outlined. Two delay procedures preceded transfer. **C,** Immediate postoperative appearance. This flap will not easily reach higher than the lower check–lower chin region.

the recipient vasculature is often uninvolved and is readily available for anastomosis. A branch of the external facial vein and external carotid artery is usually selected for the recipient vasculature. After successful flap transplantation, two or three additional operative procedures are usually required to tailor, defat, and inset the flap to achieve the optimal esthetic result. Depending on the flap employed in reconstruction, the operative procedure lasts from 5 to 7 hours (Fig. 32-34).

Resurfacing the whole face

When all or most of the facial skin requires replacement for esthetic or functional improvement, there are three basic ways of dealing with the problem:

1. Replacement of multiple "esthetic facial units" (Fig. 32-6) with thick split-thickness or full-thickness skin grafts

2. Recovering the entire face with a one-piece free skin graft

3. Recovering the entire face with a one-piece (or bilateral) regional skin flap.

The approach to take depends on a distallation of many factors, including the desired "blend" of a new cover with neighboring areas (the forehead, nose, and neck); presence or absence of the necessary skin graft or flap donor areas; acceptability of the secondary donor site deformity; quality of previous resurfacing procedures in the patient; severity of existing or recurrent contractures; amount of time involved to accomplish the repair; physical, psychoemotional, social, and economic implications to the patient and family; the experience and confidence of the surgeon with the various techniques. Method 1 is merely a composition of individual facial unit resurfacings as previously described. Fig. 32-35 presents an illustrative case. In an effort to avoid

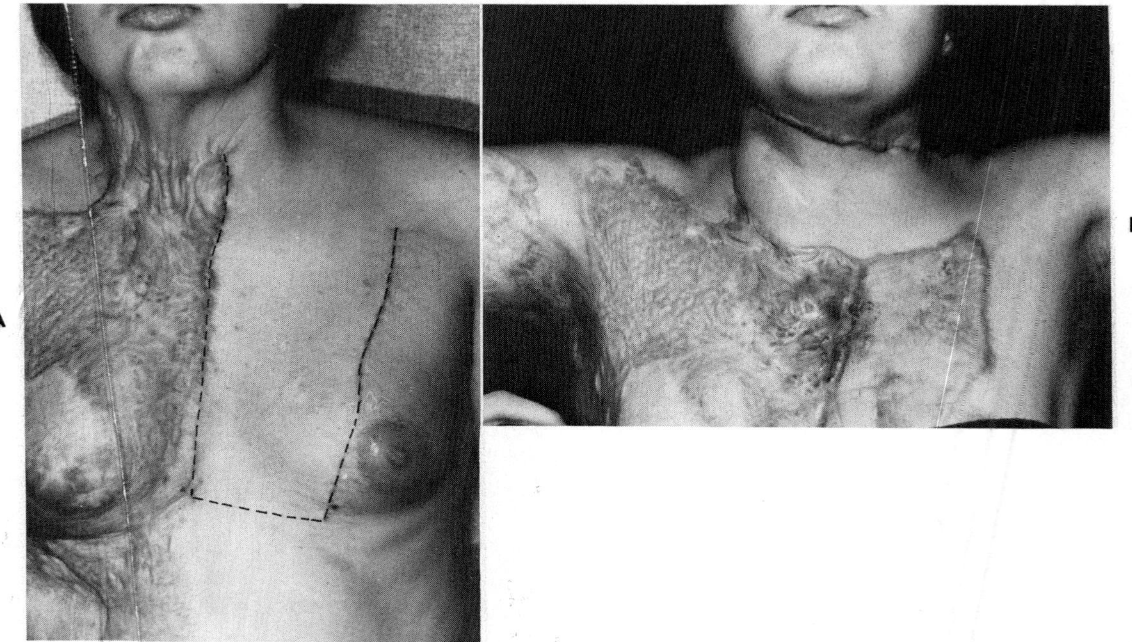

Fig. 32-33. A chest flap for neck resurfacing. **A,** The flap is outlined before the delay procedure. **B,** After flap transfer. The skin-grafted flap donor site is a worthwhile esthetic exchange for improved neck appearance and function in the case of a previous chest burn scar deformity. The flap requires some additional thinning and tailoring.

Fig. 32-34. A and **B,** Preoperative photograph demonstrating significant hypertrophic scarring involving the anterior neck of a teenage boy. **C,** Intraoperative photograph of a pattern of a vascularized groin flap measuring 10 × 22 cm. **D** and **E,** Postoperative result after successful vascularized groin flap transplantation and several defatting and insetting procedures. (Courtesy Dr. Donald Serafin.)

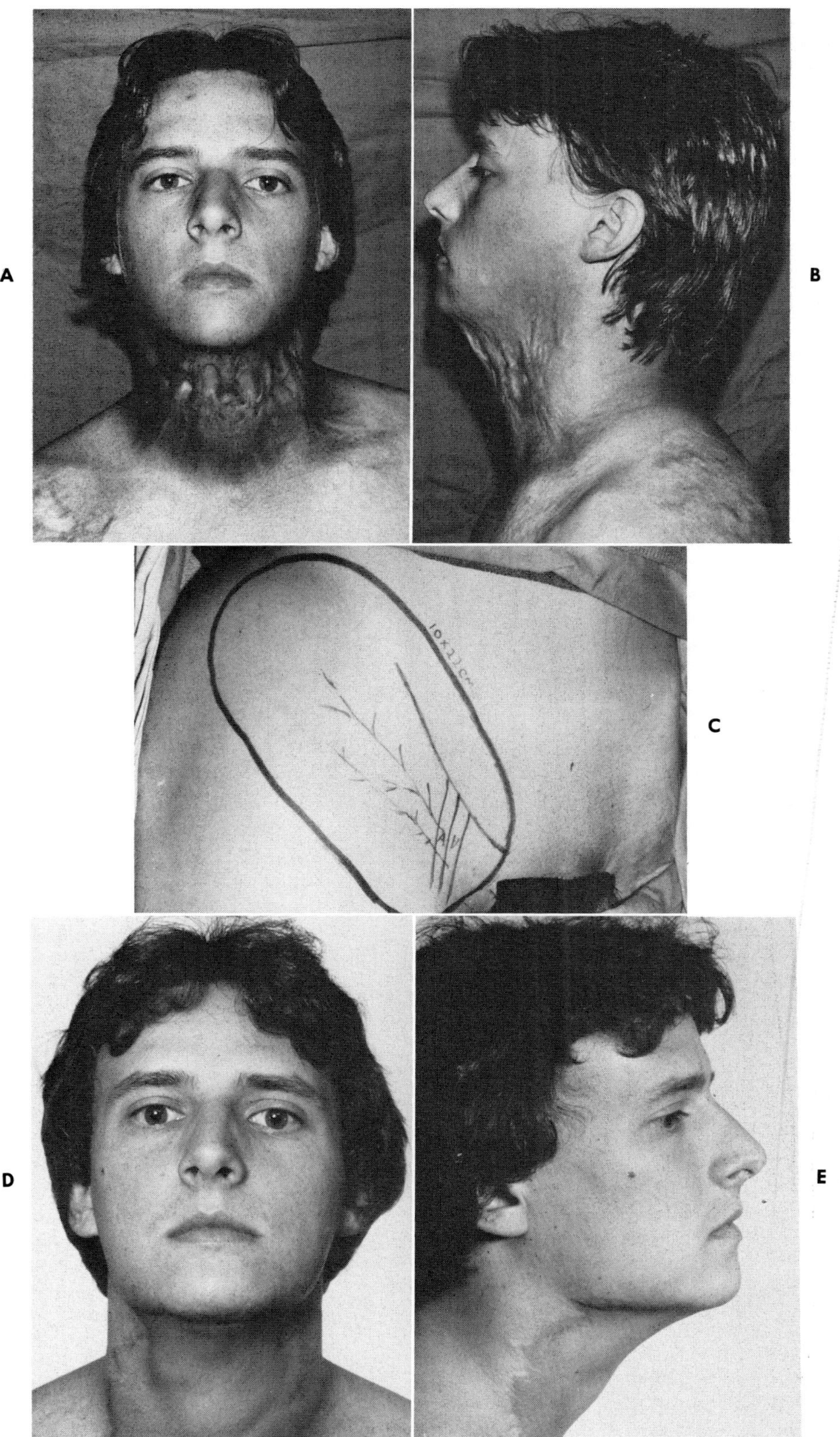

Fig. 32-34. For legend see opposite page.

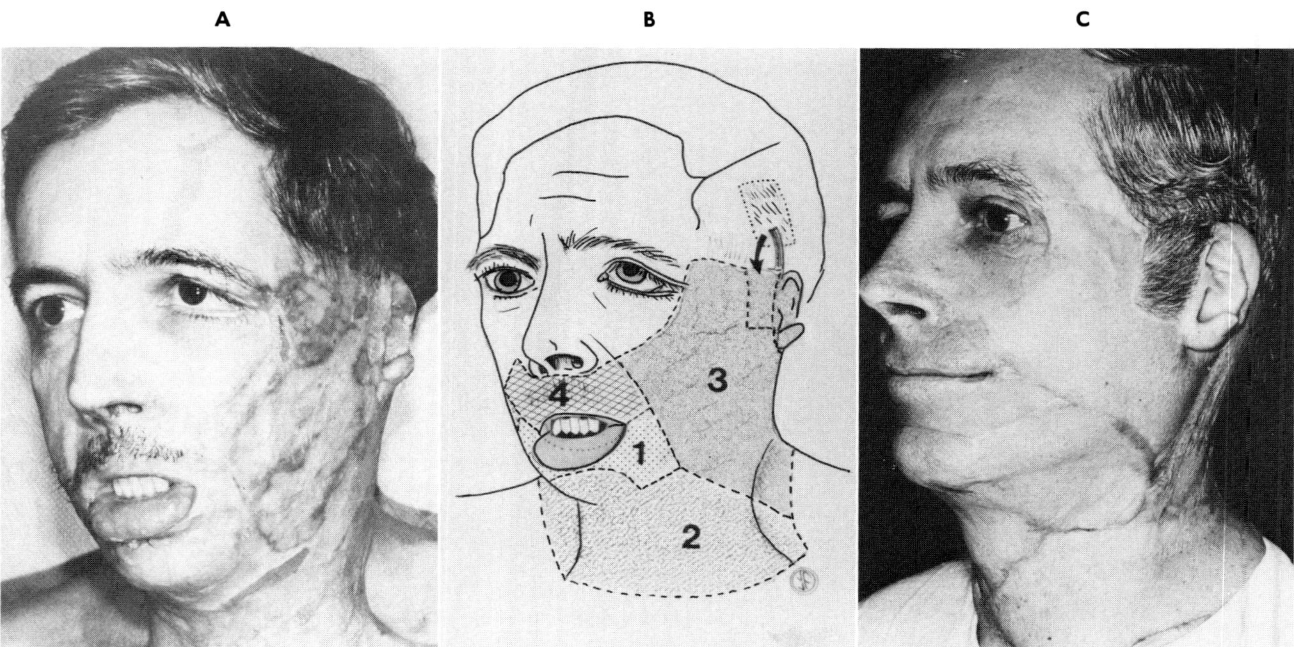

Fig. 32-35. Full-face resurfacing with thick split-thickness grafts in regional ''esthetic units'' (method 1). **A,** Preoperative view after initial healing and before beginning reconstruction. **B,** A facial map displaying the overall plan for repair (the geography and numbered sequence in which the resurfacing was to be carried out). Instead of incisional releases, definitive *excision* of scar from each unit was done. Delayed grafting at 24 hours after the excisions helped ensure complete ''take'' of thick (0.018 to 0.020 inch) split-thickness skin grafts. The most disabling deformity (the lower lip eversion and oral commissure contractures) was operated on first. Next the tight neck was excised and grafted, followed by cheek resurfacing combined with left ear and sideburn reconstruction. The upper lip was then done. These staged procedures were completed over a 7-month period. Two years later an epaulette flap was used to release a recurrent area of tightness in the lower left neck. **C,** Postoperative appearance.

the patchwork appearance that always results to some extent from method 1, an approach can be considered which minimizes the visible facial graft or flap join lines by using a *single* large sheet of skin for the entire resurfacing job. Fig. 32-36 presents a case of total cervicofacial recovering with a one-piece full-thickness skin graft (method 2),[27,72,137,140] and Fig. 32-37 presents a case of full-face resurfacing using a single wraparound cervicopectoral flap (method 3).[69] Methods 2 and 3 are highly complex undertakings and should be reserved for carefully selected patients.

The nose

Being central and projecting, the nose is commonly injured in facial burns.[121] For the same reasons, nasal disfigurement is particularly conspicuous, with distortion of the alar margins or the nasal tip–columella complex being especially distressing. On the dorsum of the nose, the thermal injury usually involves only skin; the underlying skeleton and nasal lining most often escaping unharmed. After initial healing, extensive burns to the central face commonly leave

the nose looking flat, with apparent loss of dorsal support. However, once the taut overlying scar has been removed, dorsal projection is usually restored. In the lower third of the nose, not only is the thick alar and tip skin frequently burned, but the subcutaneous fat and portions of the alar cartilages may be damaged as well. Other than an altered surface texture or discoloration the burned nose usually looks normal for several weeks after injury. Only when the eschar separates and the wound starts to heal by contraction and reepithelialization does the subsequent deformity insidiously but relentlessly begin to appear. Surface wound contraction produces elevation of the alar margins or nasal tip, and over time more and more nostril is visible on frontal view. A scarred and shortened columella can be pulled tight by the retracting force above, as well as below, if the upper lip is also burned. The columella–nasal tip angle and the columella-labial angle then become progressively obtuse—at times assuming almost a straight line between the tip and lip on profile. Deep burns with direct cartilage injury and more superficial full-thickness skin injury that leave carti-

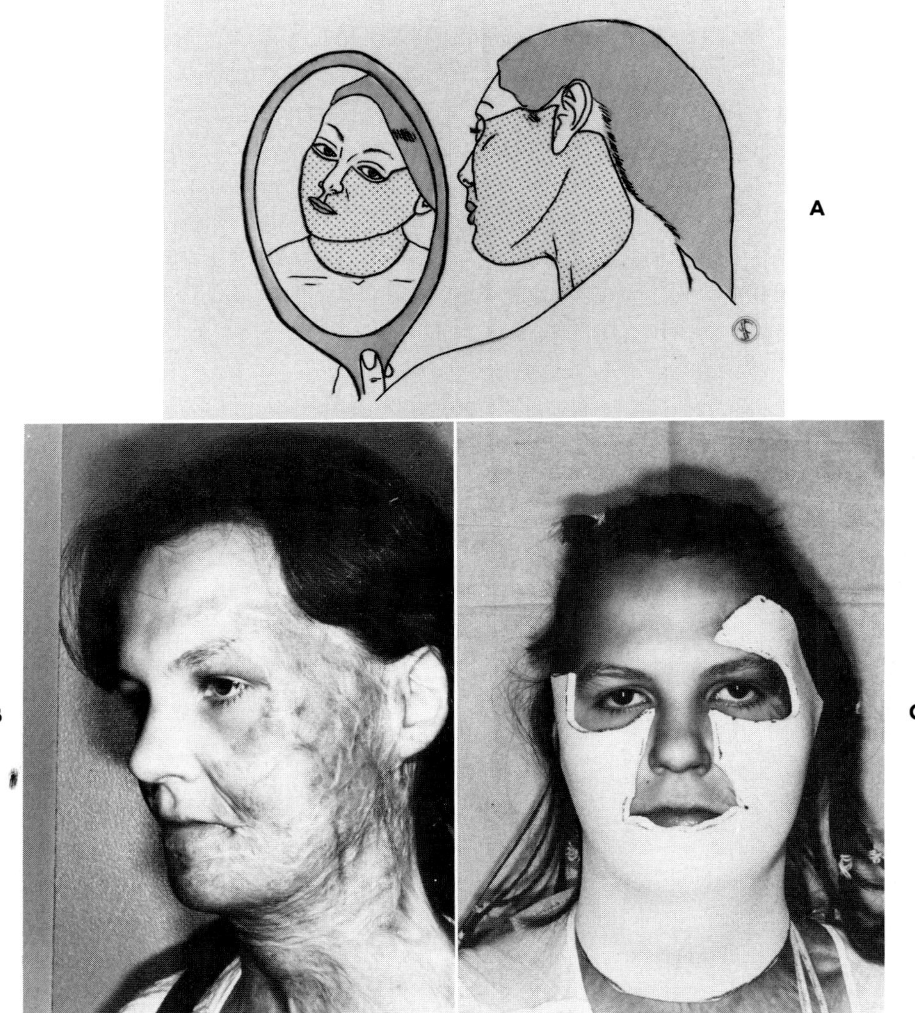

Fig. 32-36. Full-face and neck resurfacing with a one-piece full-thickness skin graft (method 2). **A,** To avoid the patchwork appearance of resurfacing multiple regional units, the face (and neck) can be envisioned as one large unit. **B,** Preoperative view. The patient very much wanted an attempt made to improve the quality of the surface texture of the facial and neck grafts. **C,** A pattern made of thin adhesive foam was laid out on the lower abdomen to outline the full-thickness skin donor site. *Continued.*

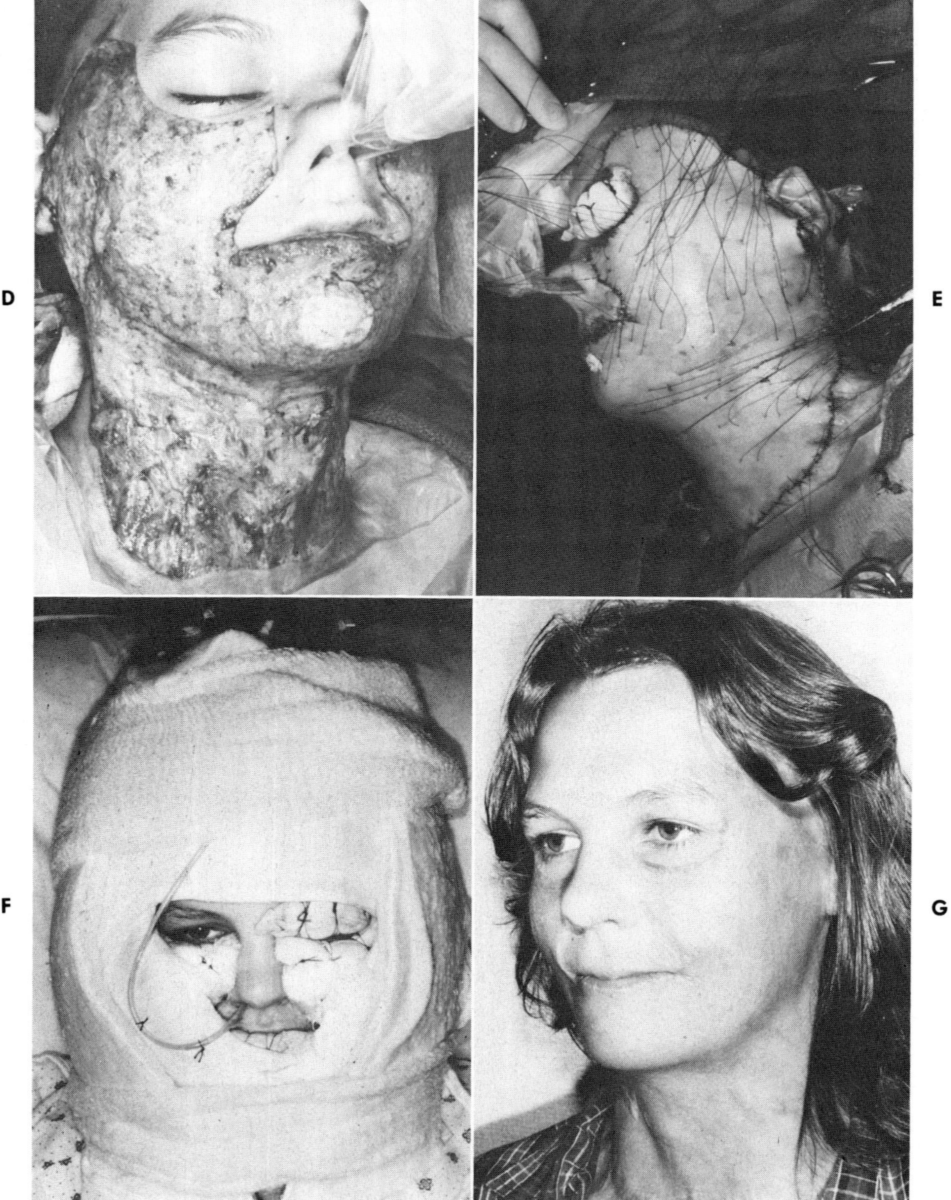

Fig. 32-36, cont'd. D, Intraoperative view. **E,** Harvest and application of the full-thickness skin graft 24 hours after excision. (The long "quilting" sutures shown in the graft are no longer used.) The full-thickness skin graft donor site was covered with split-thickness skin grafts. **F,** The bulky compression dressing is used for 10 days to minimize undesirable early vascular congestion within the thick graft. Plaster splints immobilize the head and neck. Feeding is accomplished through a small nasogastric tube. Only a well-informed, highly motivated and cooperative patient is a candidate for this procedure. Expert anesthesia and nursing are also essential. **G,** Postoperative view 1 year later. Full-thickness grafts generally contract less and maintain a more normal texture than split-thickness grafts. However, like a split-thickness skin graft, the full-thickness skin graft can hyperpigment. A dermabrasion is planned for this patient to lighten the graft. An elasticized mask and neck splint were worn for 6 months after the surgery.

lage exposed to desiccation-necrosis of the alar or caudal septal cartilages will, of course, add to the deformity (Fig. 32-38, *A* and *B*). Early skin grafting of a granulating nasal surface may help, but usually does not prevent some distortion of the nose. Secondary correction of the nasal burn deformity depends on an accurate diagnosis of the problem. Thoughtfully examining the patient and then, if possible, leisurely studying frontal and profile photographs is quite useful. Is only better quality surface cover required? Can correction of retracted alar margins and poor nasal tip projection be accomplished simply by excising and releasing the scar and allowing the nostrils and tip to fall into their normal positions, or is there actual loss of needed soft tissue support that requires augmentation by composite grafts or local flaps?

Although localized tension-releasing grafts can be temporarily beneficial for relieving dorsal and perinasal contractures (e.g., hypertrophic epicanthal bands or significantly retracted lower noses), a definitive resurfacing should involve excision and covering of the *entire* nasal esthetic unit (Fig. 32-6). One piece of skin of uniform color and texture should be applied from the radix (i.e., root of the nose) to and over the tip and nostril margins and along the sides down to the nasal-cheek junction. This may mean removing some normal or relatively unscarred skin. A graft that covers only one side of the nose or two thirds of the dorsum or most but not all of the tip will be displeasing no matter how good the graft is. Along the lateral edges of the excision at the medial part of the cheeks, the vertical line should be broken with one or two Z-plasties or ''darts''

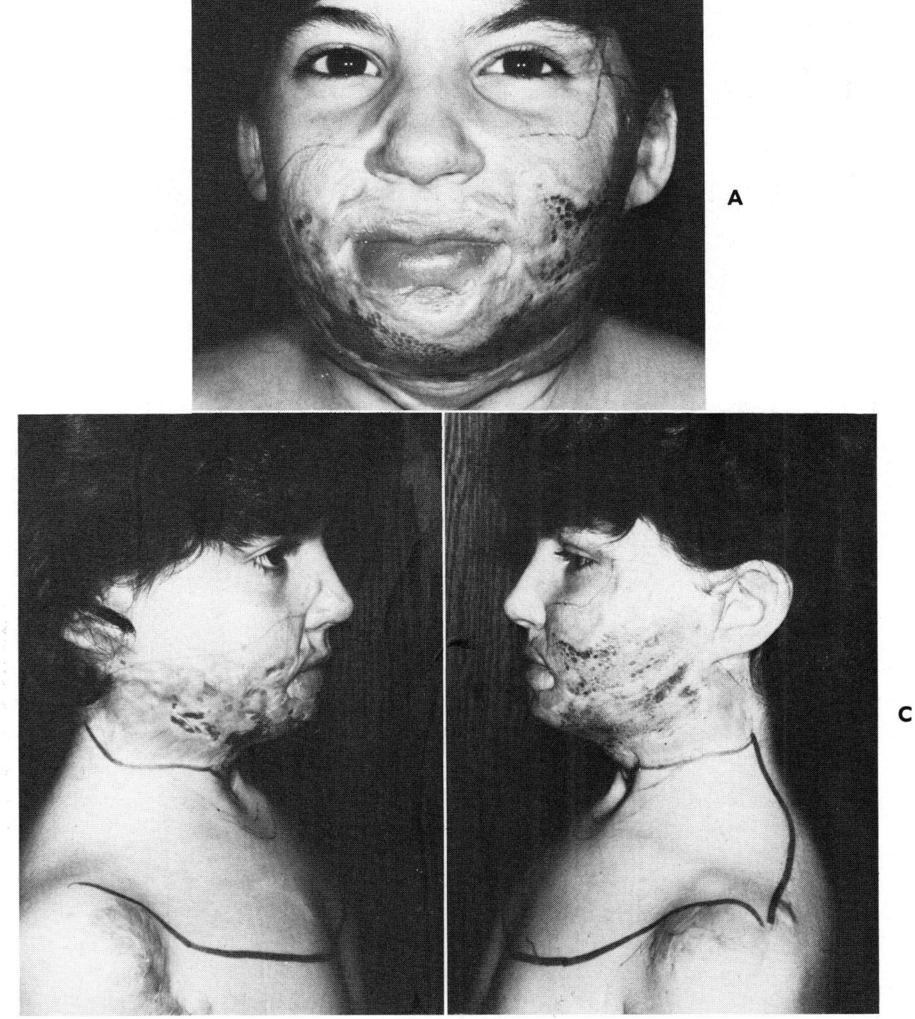

Fig. 32-37. Full-face resurfacing with a thin one-piece wraparound cervicopectoral flap (method 3). The patient and parents must clearly understand that the usually concealed upper chest will be left with a permanent skin graft deformity in exchange for transposition of the unscarred chest skin to the more visible face and neck. **A** to **C,** Preoperative views showing the hypertrophic and hyperpigmented facial and upper neck scars. The flap has been outlined.   *Continued.*

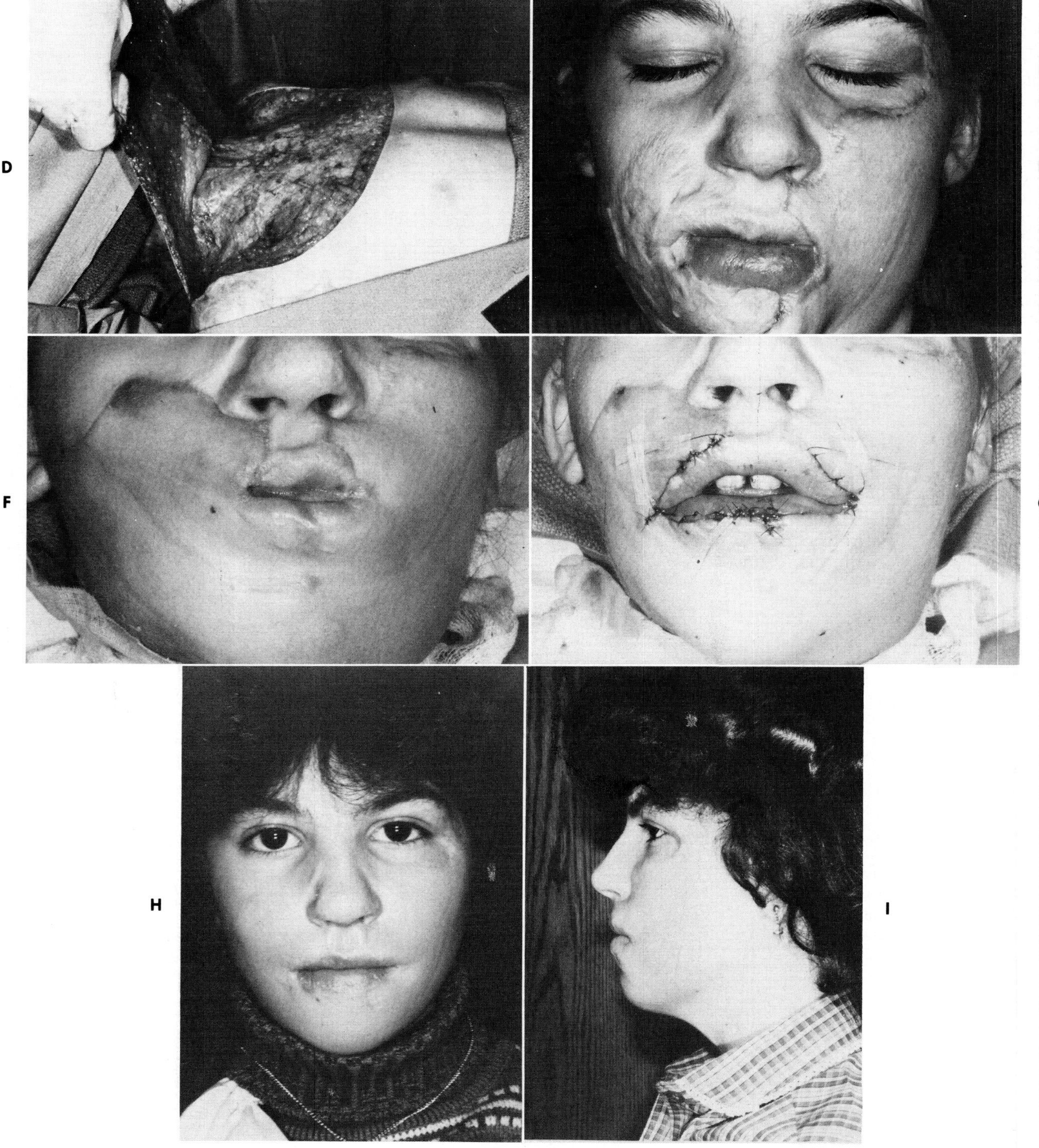

Fig. 32-37, cont'd. For legend see opposite page.

Fig. 32-37, cont'd. D, The first of four preliminary "delays" of the large random-pattern flap. Note its thinness. **E,** The prepared flap initially based in the right thoracoacromial area and transposed to the excised left face and neck. After a 3-week wait to allow the flap to develop a new blood supply from the left side of the face, the first of two delay procedures of the right-sided pedicle was carried out. **F,** After dividing the right-sided pedicle and wrapping the flap around the chin and lower lip onto the right face and neck. At this time, the flap purposely overlaps the lower lip and oral commissures for several reasons: to avoid cutting across the blood supply, to permit the flap to "join" along the philtral columns of the upper lip, and to allow the flap 3 weeks later, **G,** to be precisely cut out around the mouth without distortion of the lips. **H** and **I** show postoperative views. (The vertical scar below the left lower lip is the old tracheostomy site.) The flap has a completely normal skin texture and closely matches the color of the unburned nasal, periorbital, and forehead skin. Edge seams are blended along natural facial boundary lines. When made quite thin, the flap does not conceal expression nor blunt contours. Although an excellent-quality result can be achieved, this method does require precise planning and execution. As with any large random-pattern flap, flap necrosis after a delay procedure or transfer is always a risk. When the chin does not need resurfacing, various bilateral neck, cervicopectoral, deltopectoral, and thoracoacromial flaps can be used for each side of the face.

(Fig. 32-38, *F* and *G*). It is also important that the lower edge of the skin graft extend over the alar margins to the nostril border and over the tip to at least the tip-columella angle to avoid a visible seam scar. A thick split-thickness[14,53] or a full-thickness skin graft[175] is used for the cover. Skin flaps are usually less well suited for resurfacing the burned nose, especially in children. Distal flaps (even from the forehead or inner arm) usually appear too bulky on the nose when only a new skin layer is required. It is also difficult to nicely reshape the delicate alar-tip or tip-columella complex in a young patient using distal flap tissue. These structures are quite small in young children, and to obtain the desired anatomic finesse requires small local flaps and skin grafts. Flap coverage in children generally should be reserved for cases of unusually deep burns that expose the dorsal osseocartilaginous framework or when major soft tissue augmentation of the lower third of the nose is needed or perhaps in the adolescent patient in whom skin grafting has yielded an unsatisfactory result.[11,107-109,135] In addition, most patients with major facial burns will have the surrounding cheeks or lips or forehead resurfaced with skin grafts. A smooth (normal) pale skin flap covering the nose will usually appear out of place in this setting. Fortunately, distant flaps are rarely needed for treatment of the burned nose. Even in patients who appear to have considerable alar margin and tip loss, local tissues can usually be redistributed to make up for what seems to be missing. This often involves sliding the dorsal skin and scar toward the tip (in essence, reversing the contraction-retraction process of the initial healing phase), along with using various local turnover flaps to gain additional length and bulk.[41,52,71,165,169] A representative case is presented in Fig. 32-38. Damage to the ala nasi can be repaired with many different methods.[74,97] Minor notching of the margin often can be improved with local advancement rotation flaps. Elevated alae can be corrected at the same time as an upper lip resurfacing using laterally based sickle flaps cut from what otherwise would be discarded tissue. These small flaps nicely fill the defects left in the alar creases after the nostril rims have been freed and brought down to their normal position (Fig. 32-39).

Composite grafts from the ear also can be used to correct a retracted alar margin. If there is a well-defined notch defect along the free margin of the nostril, then a wedge-shaped dermofat graft[99,179] or skin-cartilage-skin sandwich graft taken from the anterior helix is often best.[5,39,130] However, more commonly the alar deformity appears as a smooth-arched elevation of the rim. In these cases, the alar margin is released with a curved incision in the alar crease that extends medially toward the tip as far as needed. If further inferior mobilization of the ala is required, the incision can be deepened between the lateral crus of the alar cartilage (below) and the caudal border of the upper lateral cartilage (above), leaving the underlying mucous membrane intact. The nasal lining can then be undermined superiorly and peeled away from the deep surface of the upper lateral cartilage. If the lining is then cut transversely across where the upper lateral cartilage slips beneath the nasal bone, a bipedicle flap unit of ala nasi with a broad tail of vascularized nasal lining can be pulled inferiorly. A long crescent-shaped composite skin-cartilage graft taken from the back of the ear is used to fill the defect. The graft sits on the repositioned but intact lining, with the "releasing window" in the lining concealed beneath the skin and cartilage above. This raw area inside the nose reepithelializes in a short time (Fig. 32-40).[121] In more severe losses of the ala nasi other methods can be used if practical.*

The ear can also donate other "custom-made" composite grafts[48,51,96,154] to repair a variety of defects of the nasal tip or columella (Fig. 32-41). For the composite graft to "take" successfully, hemostasis in the recipient bed must be meticulous and the graft itself gently handled, and well-vas-

Text continued on p. 599.

---

*References 24, 26, 64, 68, 74, 170, and 176.

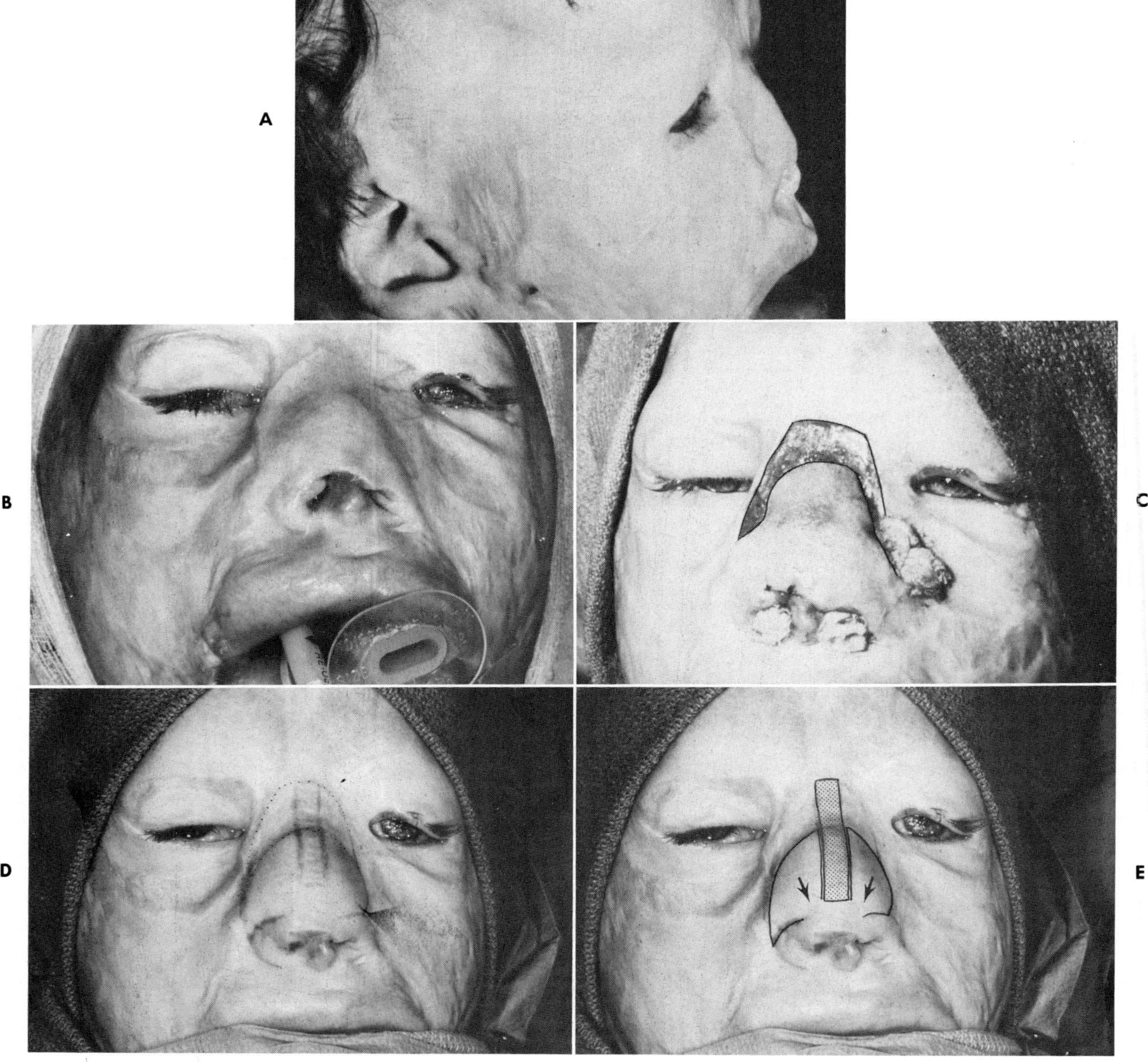

Fig. 32-38. Resurfacing, lengthening, and tip reconstruction of the nose using local tissues and a skin graft. **A** and **B,** Preoperative frontal and lateral views showing apparent flattening and destruction of the nasal tip. **C,** First stage of the repair. A horseshoe-shaped tension-releasing incision is made undermining over the osseocartilaginous framework, and the soft tissues are slid toward the tip. **D,** Appearance after the first stage with a temporary skin graft across the upper bridge. **E,** Plan for the second stage. Bilateral, inferiorly based, de-epithelialized turnover flaps are based at the tip *(arrows)*, and a de-epithelialized dorsal strut is used to preserve height. **F** and **G,** Frontal and lateral views with flaps rolled over and sutured together to form the tip. Note the triangular darts along the sides of the excision unit. **H,** Thick split-thickness skin graft cover. **I** and **J,** Final frontal and lateral views.

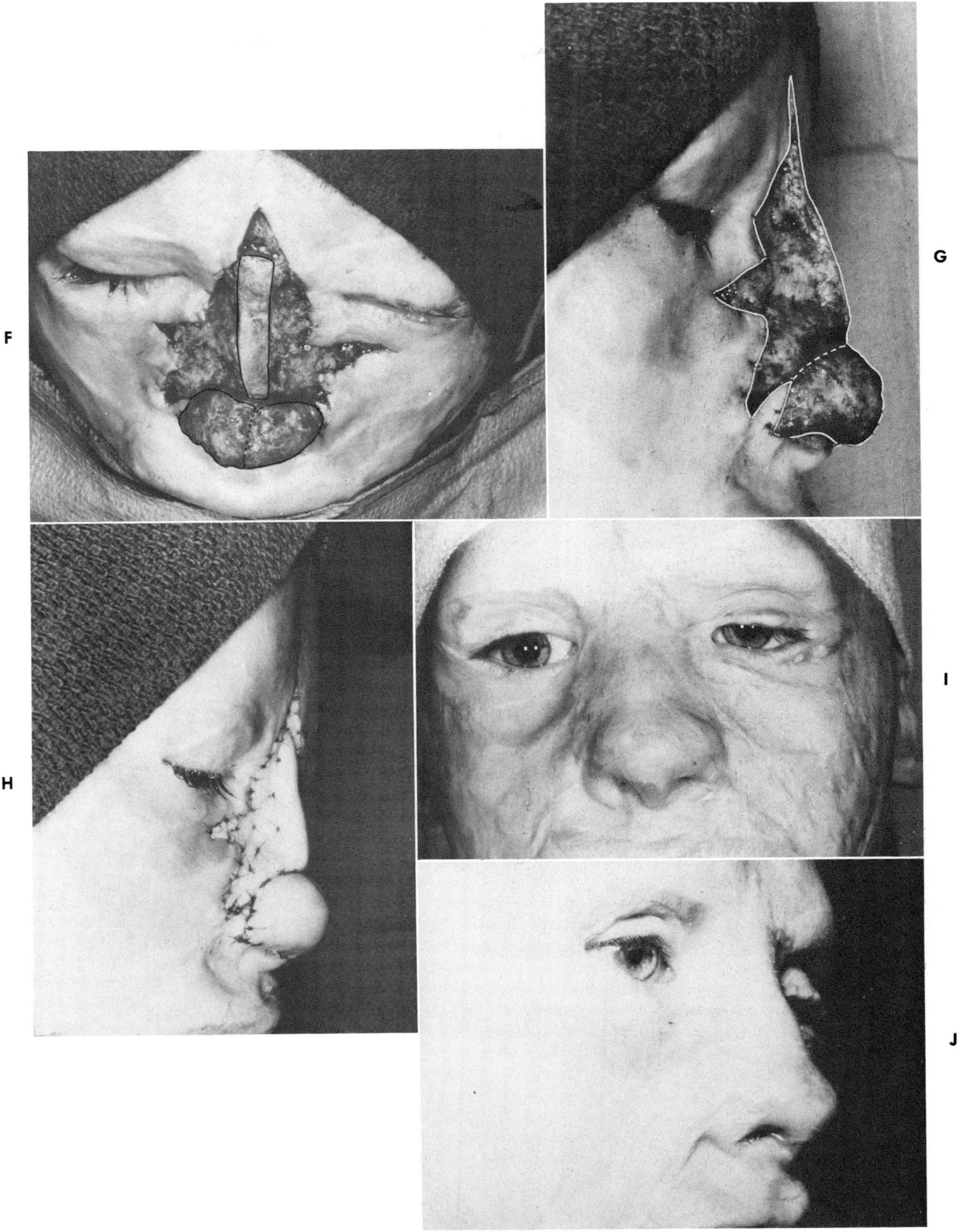

Fig. 32-38, cont'd. For legend see opposite page.

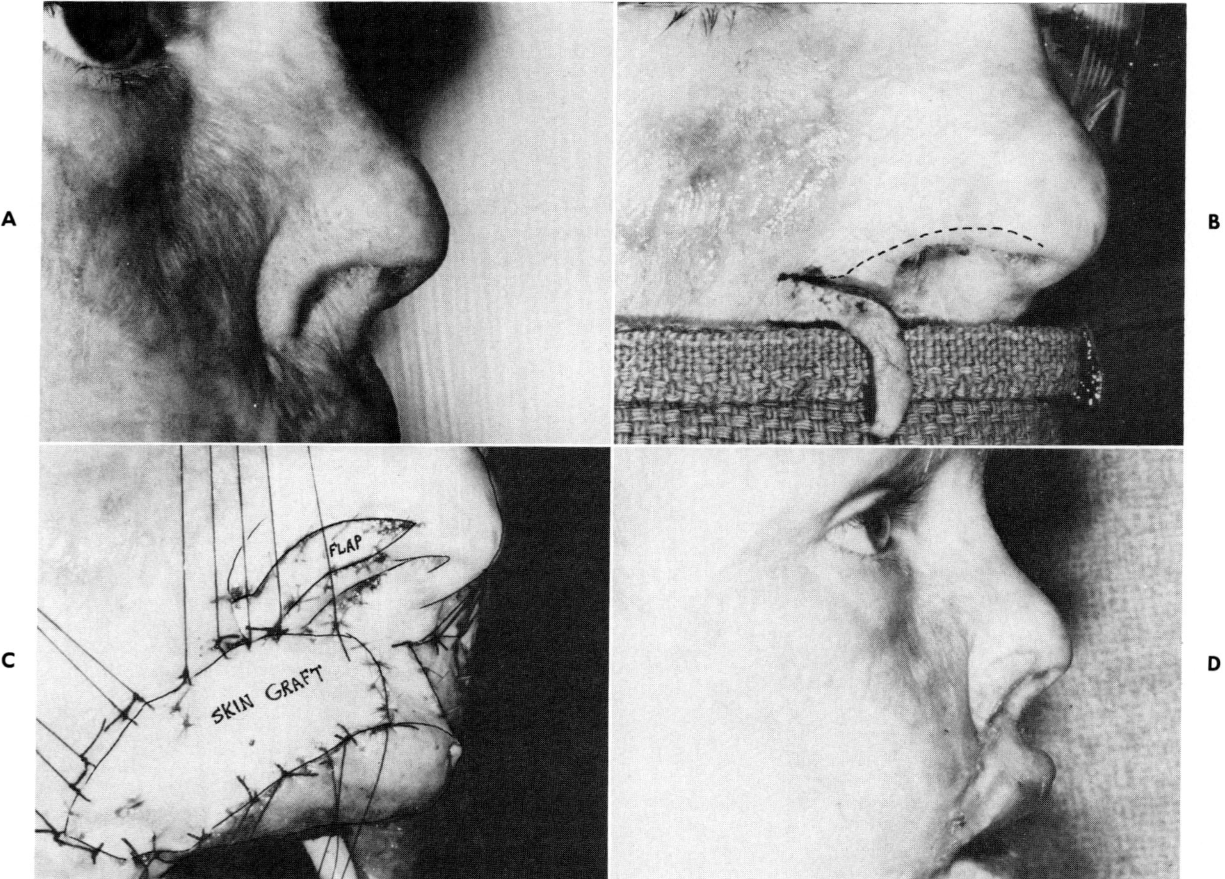

Fig. 32-39. Correction of alar retraction at the time of upper lip resurfacing. **A,** Preoperative appearance. Creation of sickle flaps from lip scar. The dotted line indicates an alar-releasing incision. **C,** The flap is sewn in position, and the skin graft is on the lip. **D,** Postoperative appearance.

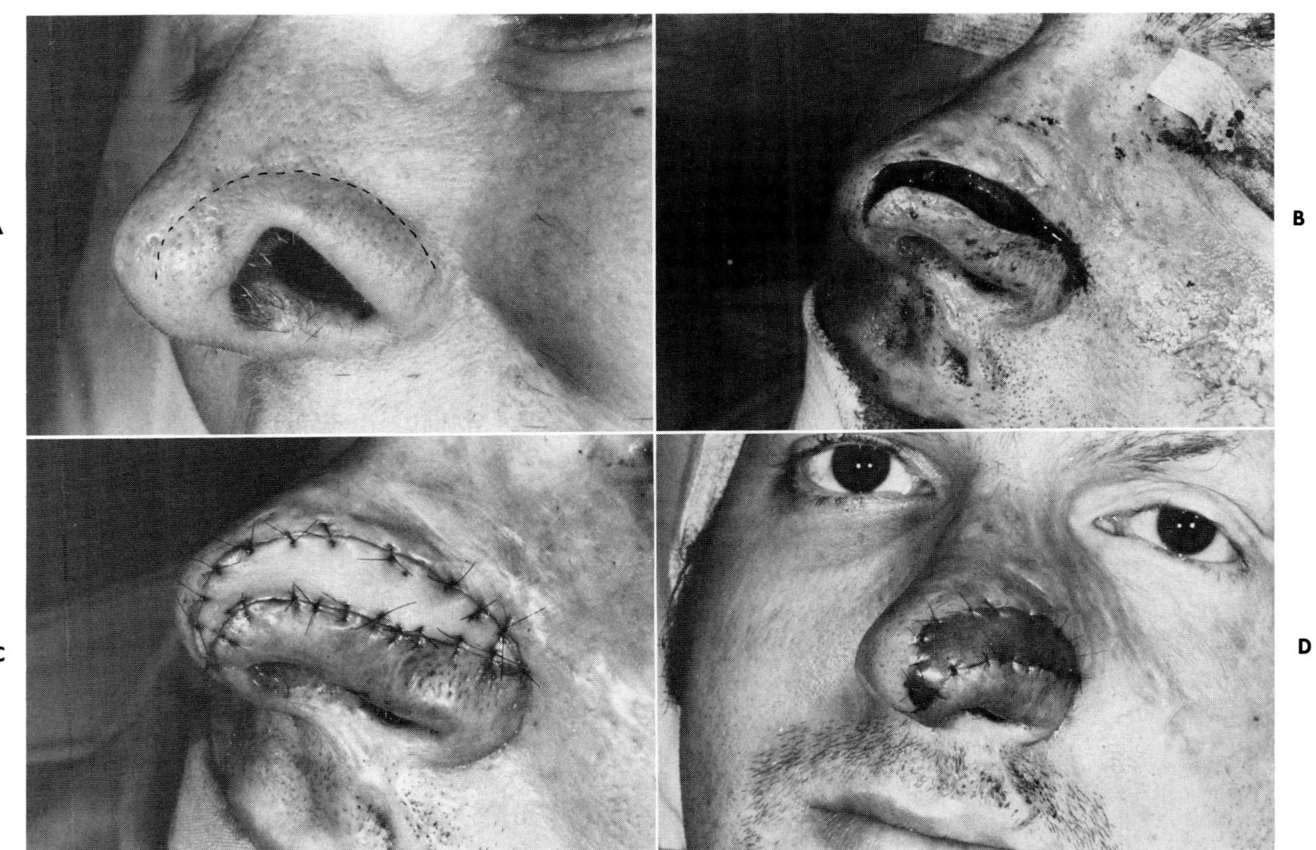

Fig. 32-40. Correction of alar retraction with a composite chondrocutaneous graft from the ear. **A,** Preoperative view. The releasing incision is outlined. **B,** The ala is moved inferiorly after freeing the tongue of attached mucous membrane lining beneath the upper lateral cartilage. **C,** A composite skin-cartilage graft from behind the contralateral ear in place. **D,** The graft at 3 days postoperatively showing the usual venous congestion for this time.

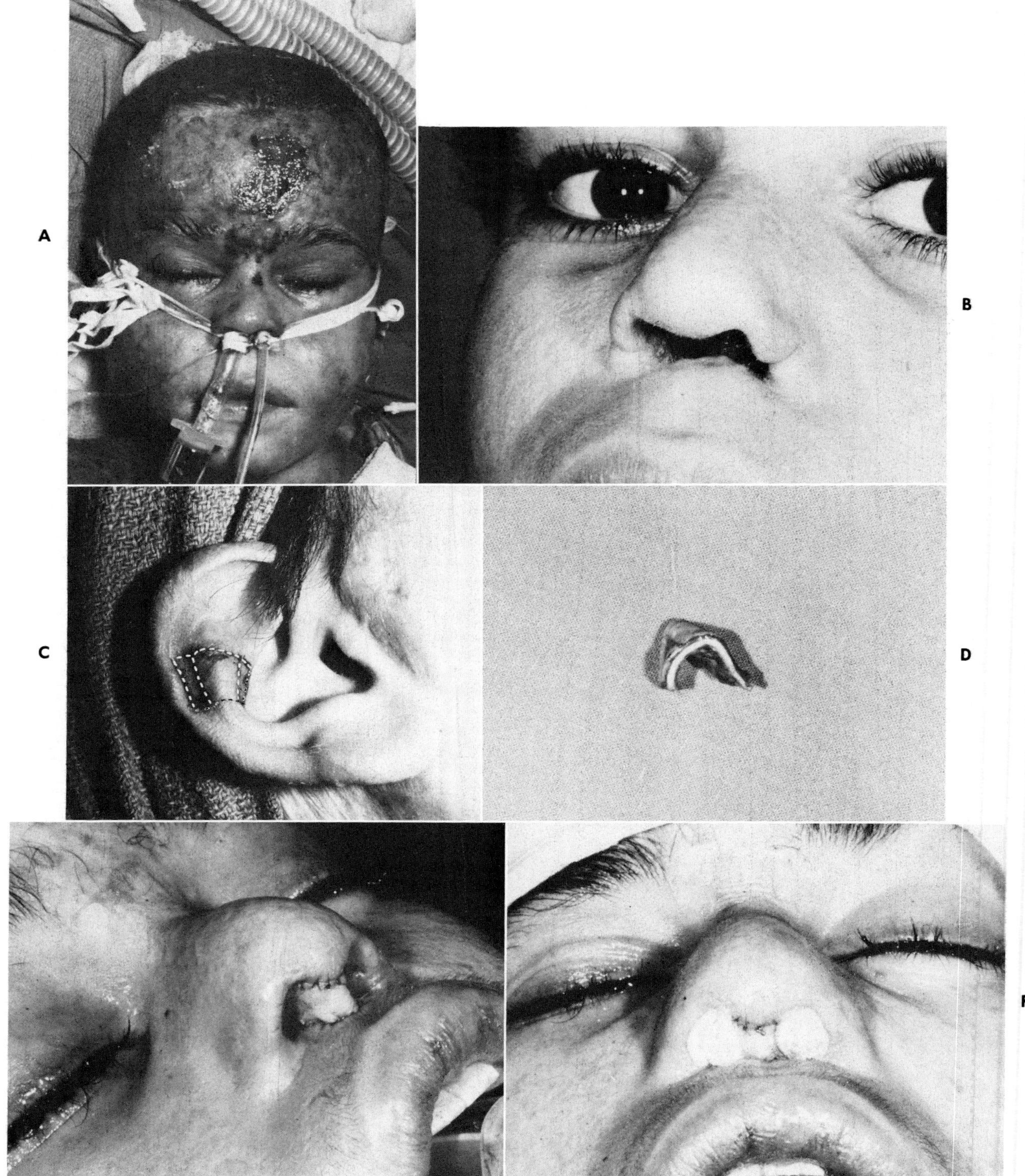

Fig. 32-41. Columella repair with a composite graft from the ear. **A,** Pressure necrosis caused by tapes securing the nasotracheal and nasogastric tubes. **B,** Necrosis resulted in loss of the columella and alar grooving. **C,** A composite graft is outlined over the prominent anthelical roll, and the donor site is to be closed after removal of the compensatory triangles. **D,** Arched graft. **E,** Some excess cartilage will be gently trimmed from the graft before being sutured into position. **F,** A light compression and protective dressing of lubricated nonadherent gauze rolls is inserted into the nostrils.

cularized, noninfected tissue should abut on two and preferably three sides. Within the composite graft, the cartilage layer should be trimmed back so that skin and fat extend beyond the cartilage at the edges. The graft should contain only enough cartilage to impart the desired shape and support. Fine, noncrushing sutures are used for snug edge-to-edge coaptation along the margins, and a thick layer of antibiotic ointment is applied. If the surgeon wishes, a light compression dressing can be used for 7 to 10 days to discourage venous congestion, or the graft can be left exposed.

Unfortunately, loss of all or a portion of the columella is seen occasionally as a result of the burn itself or more commonly secondary to pressure necrosis from umbilical tape used to secure nasotracheal and nasogastric tubes (Fig. 32-41, *A*). Repair of the columella is best done with local flaps* or composite ear grafts[66,107,108] (Fig. 32-41). Distant flaps are unnecessarily complex[73] and are generally too thick[124] to make the fine-caliber columella post, especially in small children. Narrow medially based flaps from the nostril sills that are turned up back to back (Fig. 32-42) work nicely for columella reconstruction.[123,147] Because the flaps swing upward from a medial rotation point, they automatically make a small bulge at their inferior outer edge that simulates the footplate of the medial crura. The normal slope from nostril sill to columella is created, imparting a natural appearance to the columella base. If more fill-in and support behind the columella is required because of associated loss of the cartilaginous caudal septum, bilateral medially based flaps from the inside of the upper lip[47,100] can be tunneled up just in front of the anterior nasal spine and sewn back to back between the mucoperichondrium of the septum and sill flaps to create a neomembranous septum. Or, at a second operation, an elliptically shaped skin-cartilage-skin composite graft from the ear can be inserted behind the new columella.[90] Medially based chondromucosal flaps from the nasal vestibule that contain a reinforcing strip of alar cartilage might also be used to buttress the columella.

Scarring and contraction at the entrance to the nostrils can range from mild stenosis to complete obstruction—in any case, the condition is chronically uncomfortable to the patient. Mouth breathing and hyponasal speech result. The difficulty with correction is not usually surgical, but rather with maintaining the correction postoperatively because of the great tendency for contracture.[61] In cases of minimal constriction, where a moderate opening persists, small local flaps often can be designed from the nostril margins or anterior vestibule to break the circumferential scar and enlarge the nares. A combination of flaps and skin grafts is necessary for greater degrees of narrowing (Fig. 32-43). In severe cases (e.g., where only a pinpoint opening exists), the nares must actually be cored out from the scar tissue and restored to their normal size and shape. This leaves a circumferential raw area in each nostril that must be covered

with a skin graft. A temporary acrylic or gutta-percha mold of each corrected nostril is made at surgery; the molds are made to just fit but not to overcorrect. The molds are painted with a liquid skin adhesive, wrapped with a thin skin graft, and placed in the nostrils. The molds are removed 5 to 7 days later, the excess skin graft is trimmed away, and the molds are replaced after cleaning and lubricating them with antibiotic ointment. In a young, uncooperative child, this may require anesthesia. On the tenth postoperative day, a permanent acrylic mold is prepared that has wide holes bored out to allow the child to breathe through the nose. A bridge is shaped around the columella and a thin flange on each side is fitted with a tape to go around the ears so that the prosthesis can be worn like a pair of eyeglasses. The mold must be worn day and night for at least 6 months. It is removed once or twice a day for no more than 15 minutes, cleaned, greased, and reinserted. Success depends on prolonged wearing of the splint; even then, recurrence of scar contracture is not uncommon.[143]

The ear

Isolated burn injuries of the ears are rare, whereas ear burns associated with other facial burns are very common. Despite this high incidence, the ear burn deformity frequently assumes a low priority for reconstruction. Perhaps this is because the ears are relatively out of the way and can be covered by the hair or because other more functionally important or conspicuous areas of injury take precedence. Perhaps the low priority is because severe burn damage of the ears can be difficult to repair to the satisfaction of the surgeon. Although there is truth in each of these reasons, newer methods (e.g., the creative use of scar tissue flaps and the turnover temporal fascial flap) have made for easier and more gratifying results, which should encourage the surgeon to undertake repair of the ears earlier and with greater enthusiasm.

There is little the surgeon can do to avoid deformity if the ear cartilage is burned. Often, however, only the thin overlying skin is primarily injured. Yet if infection intervenes or exposure of the cartilage occurs, causing desiccation necrosis (which is common), then a potentially preventable deformity results. Second-degree burns of the ear are generally best treated with a topical antibacterial agent and allowed to heal. Small areas of third-degree burn, exposing small areas of cartilage that probably will result in localized defects, are also often best managed conservatively and repaired later after initial healing has taken place. In these cases, the ear should be examined periodically for undetected sepsis concealed beneath the burn eschar that could lead to a destructive suppurative chondritis. In reality, this happens infrequently. When a large area of third-degree burn covers the ear, a number of treatment options are available[17]:

1. A surgically nonaggressive approach—accept the inevitable cartilage loss and plan to repair later on. This tact is often unintentionally and understandably taken

---

*References 44, 55, 56, 66, 136, 168, and 171.

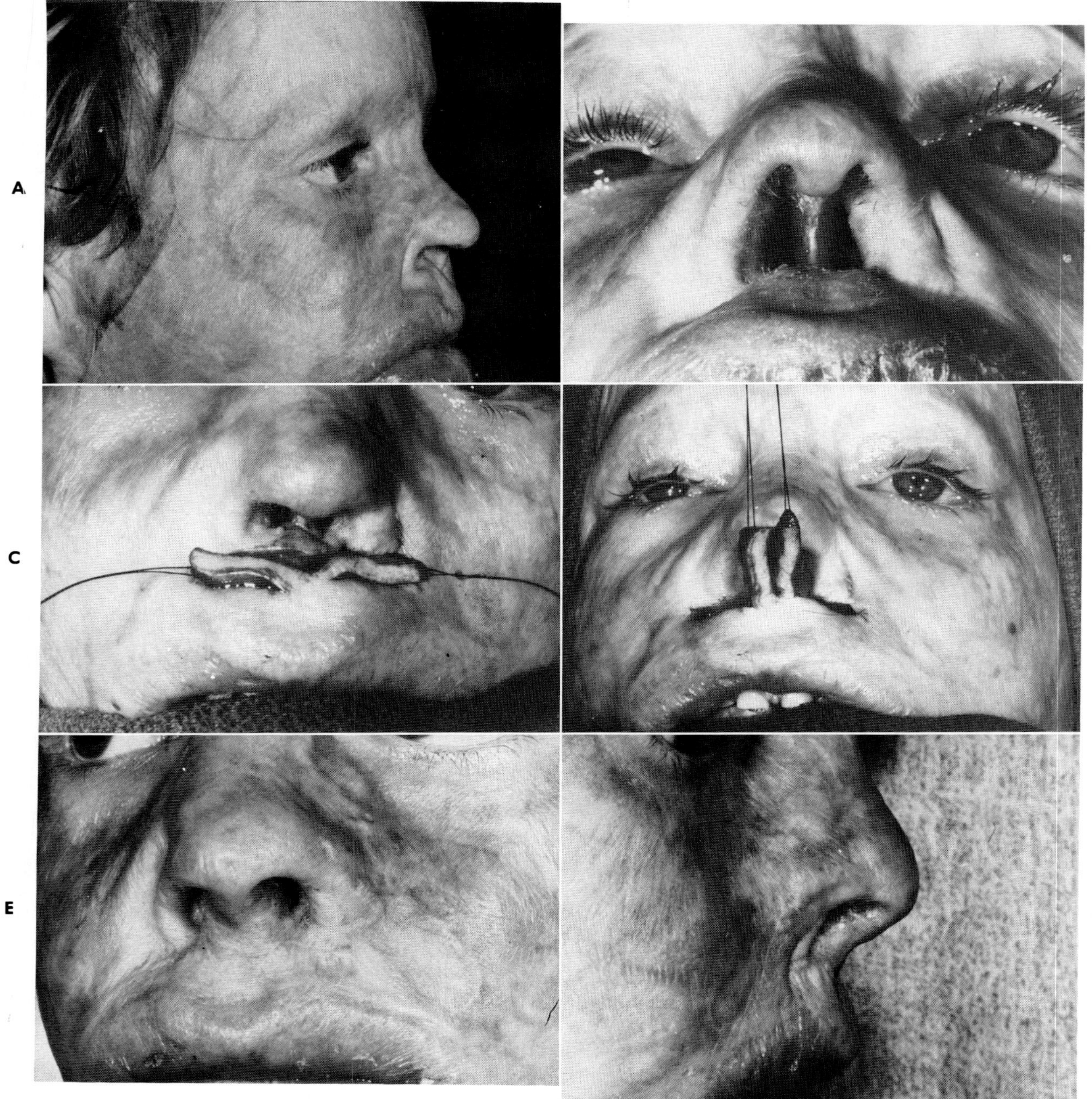

Fig. 32-42. Columella repair using nostril sill flaps. **A** and **B,** Preoperative views showing the missing columella and a defect in caudal septum. **C** and **D,** Medially based sill flaps are cut and rotated. It is important to raise these narrow (usually scarred) flaps with some fat to preserve the blood supply. Thinning and tailoring of the columella can be done later if necessary. **E** and **F,** Postoperative views. Note the simulation of medial crural footplates at the base of the new columella. The membraneous septum was reconstructed at the same operation using similar mucosal flaps from the inner surface of the upper lip.

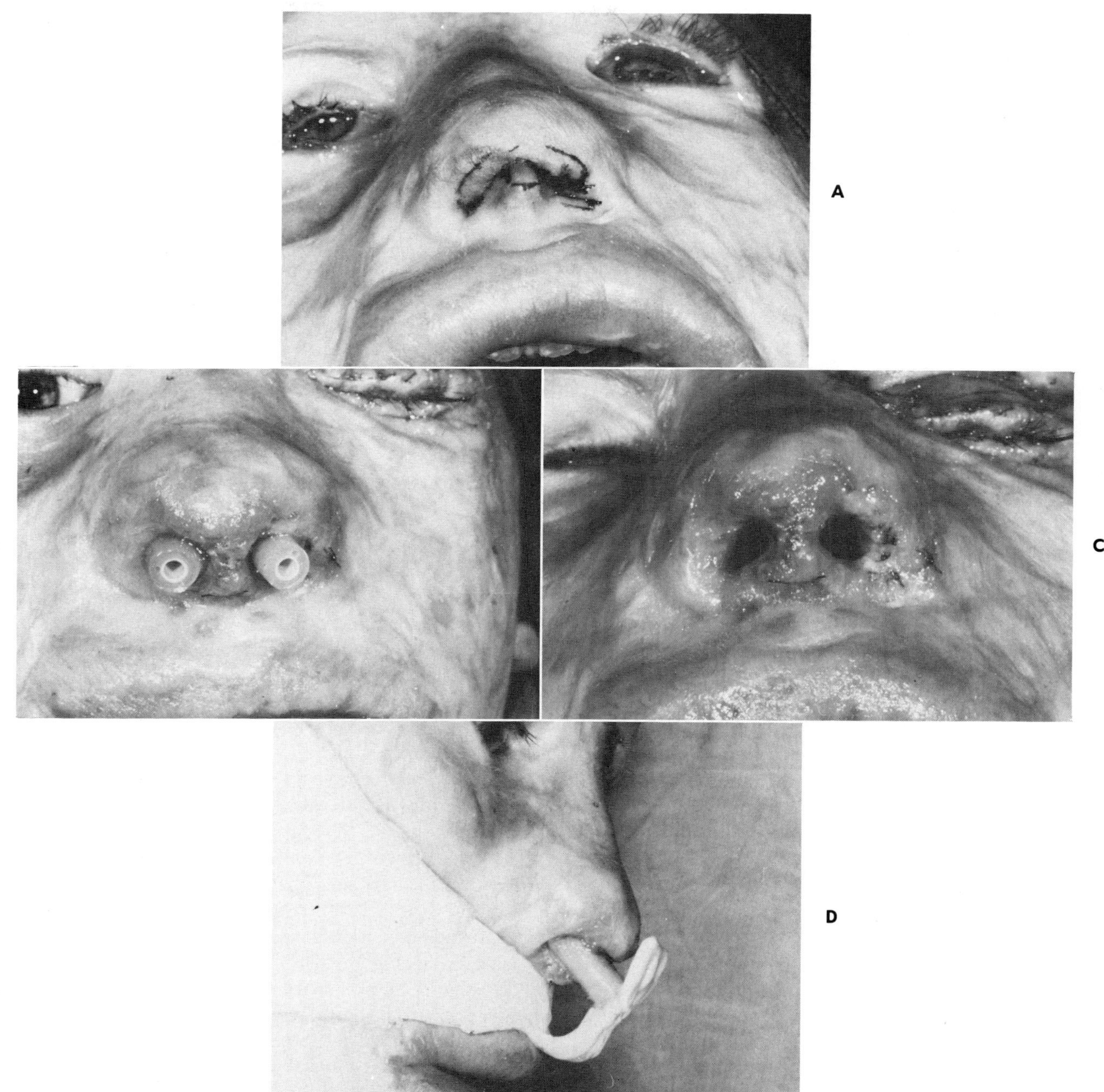

Fig. 32-43. Correction of moderate nostril stenosis. **A,** Transferring small superiomedially based scar tissue flaps will open the nares and repair the upper columella defect. **B** and **C,** Raw nostril surfaces are covered with thin skin grafts wrapped over temporary catheter molds. **D,** Early postoperative appearance. An acrylic mold made to just fit, not stretch, the opened nares must be worn day and night for at least 6 months.

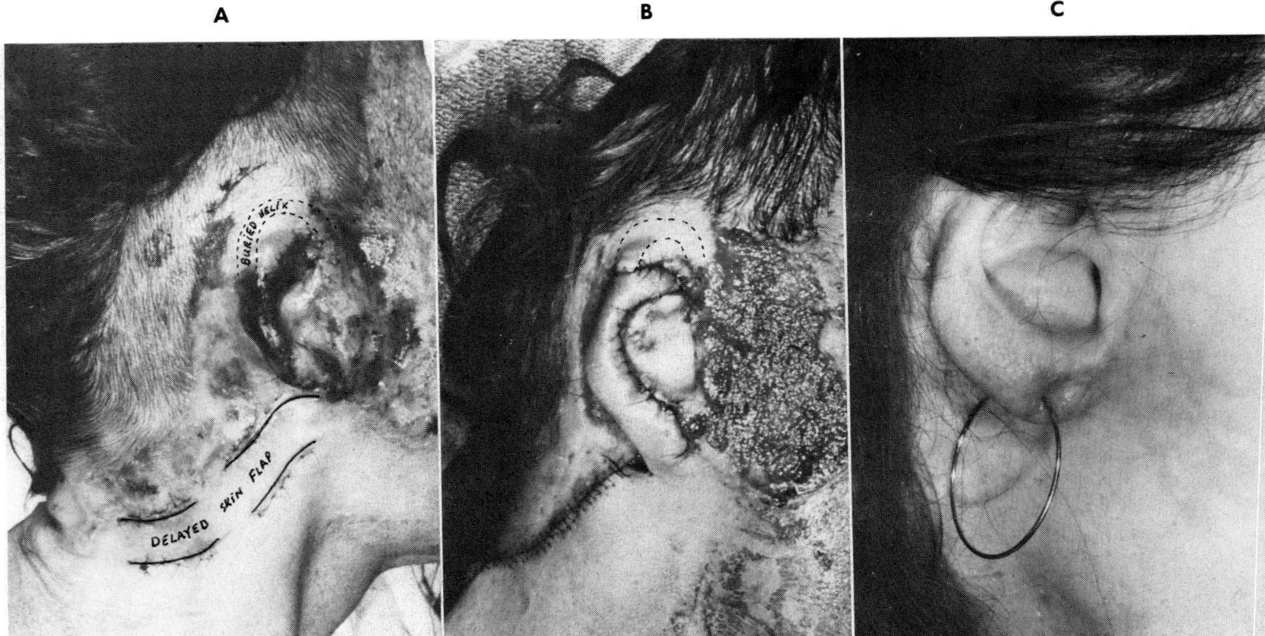

Fig. 32-44. A, Salvage of ear cartilage by burying the superior helix in a postauricular skin pocket.
B, The lower two thirds of the helix are covered with a delayed neck flap. **C,** Result.

when the patient has suffered extensive and life-threatening injury.

2. A surgically aggressive cartilage-saving approach with early (primary) excision of the burned skin and recovering the cartilage with a skin graft or skin flap or burying the bared helical frame in a temporary subcutaneous pocket. Unfortunately, this approach often has technical problems. The thin skin over the anterior surface of the ear adheres to the underlying cartilage, and excision of this burned layer is difficult to do without also stripping off the perichondrium (which itself is often burned). A skin graft will not survive without the perichondrium. Covering the exposed cartilage with local or regional skin flaps[106] (Fig. 32-44) may be impractical if the area around the ear has also been burned.

3. A surgically aggressive cartilage-saving approach by covering the excision-denuded cartilage with a skin-grafted, arterialized fascial flap[54,63,118,157] (Fig. 32-50). In selected patients with major ear burns, this may be the best appproach.

Once the healed burned ear deformity has been established, the question arises as to whether or not ear reconstruction should be done at all, and if so, to what extent. The answer comes from discussions with the patient and the parents. For example, if the patient is an adolescent girl whose only interest is in having an earlobe made so that she can wear earrings, but who plans to always style her long hair to cover the rest of her ears, then a multistaged, autogenous cartilage, total ear reconstruction is inappro-

priate. On the other hand, if the patient is an active boy who refuses to wear a prosthetic ear (as most youngsters will) and wants to cut his hair short or could use an ear to support his eyeglasses, then ear reconstruction would seem indicated. Individual considerations concerning the timing and extent of an isolated ear repair should involve the family. However, a large percentage of ear reconstructions can be integrated with some other planned facial procedure (e.g., a cheek resurfacing), and these opportunities should be seized primarily at the *surgeon's* discretion. So often seemingly useless or routinely discarded scar tissue around the ear can be used to construct a first-rate helix or earlobe—only a little ingenuity and additional surgical time being required (Fig. 32-46). If advanced and rolled skin is used to make a helix, a cartilage strut should be included or added later to maintain the rim's definition.

Essential for a satisfactory and satisfying ear reconstruction is a precise analysis of the deformity. To be able to look at an injured ear and tell what is missing or misshaped requires that the surgeon first know unequivocally what a normal ear looks like. The surgeon who is unable to correctly draw a normal ear unaided, with all its parts, hills, and valleys, has no business trying to reconstruct a damaged ear. Surgical compromises in anatomic detail may be elected in a repair plan, but they should not result from a basic lack of knowledge of those details preoperatively. Filling in the missing parts on the skin with a marking pen, as well as comparing the damaged ear to the undamaged contralateral ear if available, is also valuable in regard to specific size, shape, and location considerations.

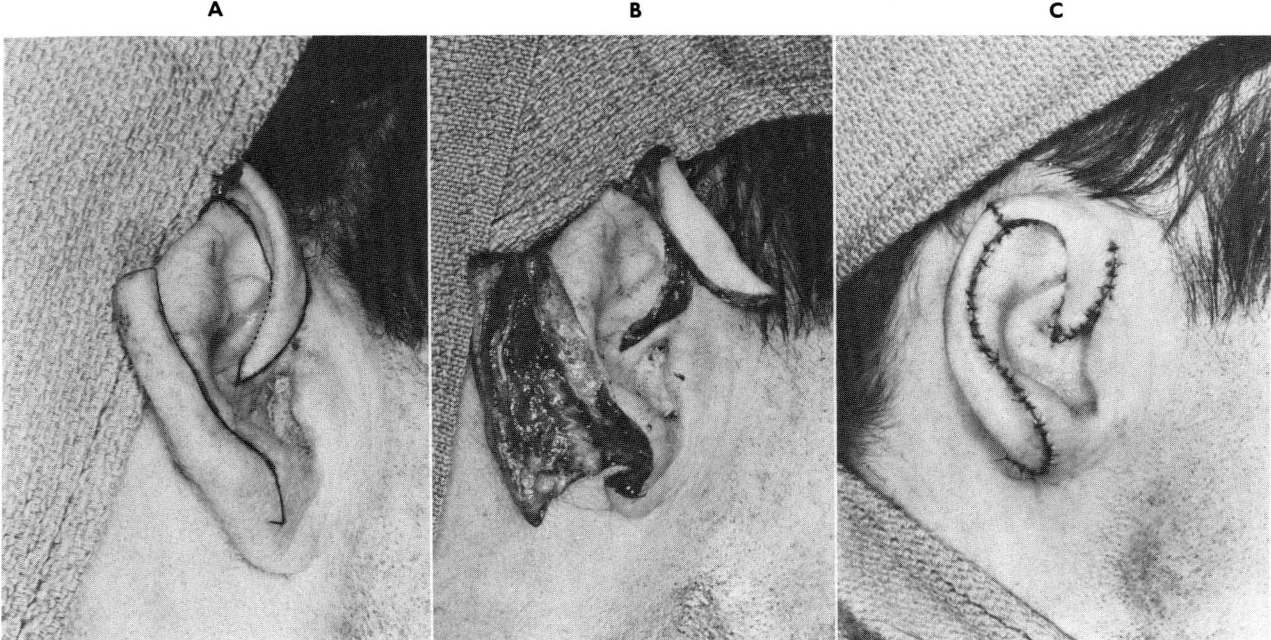

Fig. 32-45. Repair of a segmental helical defect using advancement-rotation chondrocutaneous flaps on postauricular skin pedicles as described by Antia and Buch.[4]

The most common ear deformities associated with burns involve the periphery of the ear, the helix, anthelix, and lobule. Segmental defects can be repaired using any one of many described methods.[19,20,35,101] The reconstructive surgeon should be familiar with all of these and choose the most appropriate. For a localized loss of the helical rim, the procedure described by Antia and Buch[4] has been useful (Fig. 32-45). Various other transposition interpolation and advancement flaps, or preauricular and postauricular skin tube pedicles can be used for helix construction.[1,34,103,132] Dufourmentel's clever method[50] of wrapping an inferiorly based leash of the superficial temporal artery and vein in a skin graft also can be used for the helix. Unlike congenital ear deformities, the burned ear usually has an intact concha; therefore loss of the upper third of the ear can be reconstructed using Davis' technique[46] of rotating up the entire concha with attached skin on a narrow pedicle. The contralateral ear, especially if uninjured, can also be an excellent supplier or rebuilding materials (composite grafts and flat or rolled cartilage strips) to replace or augment deficient parts.[129,133,165] Some creative thinking will make the best use of this unique donor source.

Earlobe repair also can be accomplished with many different methods (Fig. 32-47).[18,34,35,46,49] Simple local flaps are often used, but sometimes more complex flaps can be designed to provide both the anterior and the posterior lobe surfaces (Fig. 32-48). However, an easy method that generally produces a good result is to simply cut out a thick and oversized earlobe from the local scar tissue and line both the lobe's undersurface and the excision bed with a skin graft (Fig. 32-46). The lobule should purposely be made too big, with the expectation that it will shrink as the graft contracts. It can easily be made smaller later on.

Major ear reconstruction to replace most or all of the helix and anthelix should be done using carved autogenous rib cartilage as described by Brent[21] (Fig. 32-49). (See Chapter 34.) Silicone implants are not recommended because of their high incidence of associated infection and exposure.[120] If scarring around the ear remnant replaces pliable high-quality skin essential for insertion of the cartilage graft, then an arterialized turn-back fascial flap should be used to cover the cartilage frame.* Containing the axial blood supply of the superficial temporal artery and vein, the thin, almost transparent flap of superficial temporal fascia (not the dense underlying white fascia over the temporal muscle) is rolled over the new cartilage structure and a skin graft applied. It may take 6 months to a year before the precise contours of the new framework are completely visible, but the long-term results using this technique have been excellent (Fig. 32-50). This method is easier and gives better results than trying to first replace the scar in the auricular area with a full-thickness skin graft and later placing the new cartilage graft beneath it. Even the softest, thickest, and most mature skin graft is never as elastic and drapable as the fascial flap, and it is difficult to get a cartilage frame with the desired amount of helix rim height to fit comfortably and safely into a relatively stiff skin-grafted pocket.

---

*References 9, 54, 63, 118, 119, and 157.

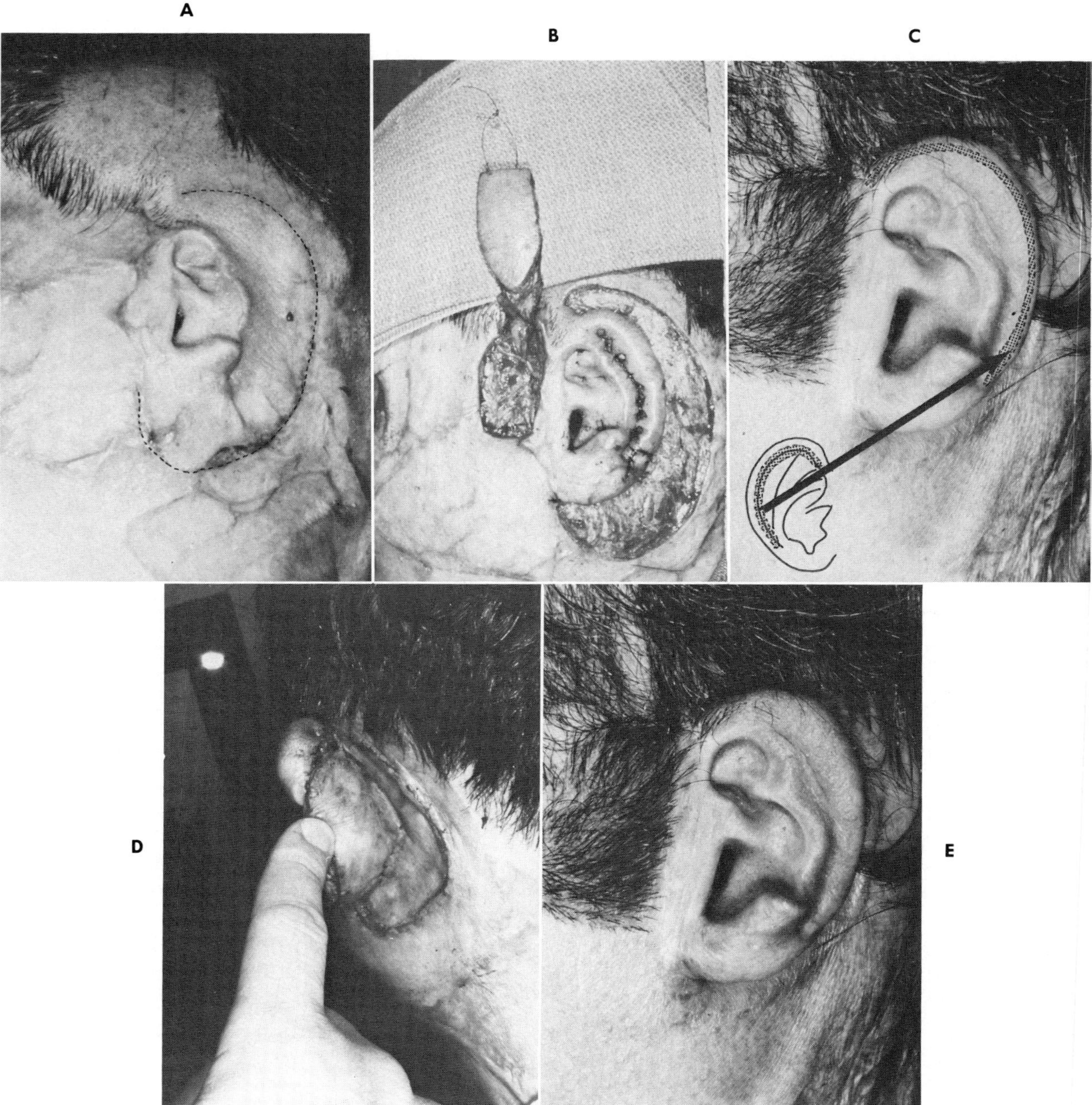

Fig. 32-46. Helix and lobule reconstruction using a rolled periauricular scar flap. **A,** The flap is outlined and delayed twice when other areas are being repaired. **B,** The flap is advanced and rolled to form the helix and earlobe. (Note the island pedicle flap for sideburn reconstruction.) The next day the left cheek and periauricular area were resurfaced with a thick skin graft. **C,** To maintain helical contour, a long strip of cartilage *(arrow)* was taken from the scapha of the other side and threaded into the helix roll. **D,** Elevation of the ear and lobule with placement of a retroauricular skin graft. **E,** Final result. (Note that the sideburn hair should have been directed downward rather than upward.)

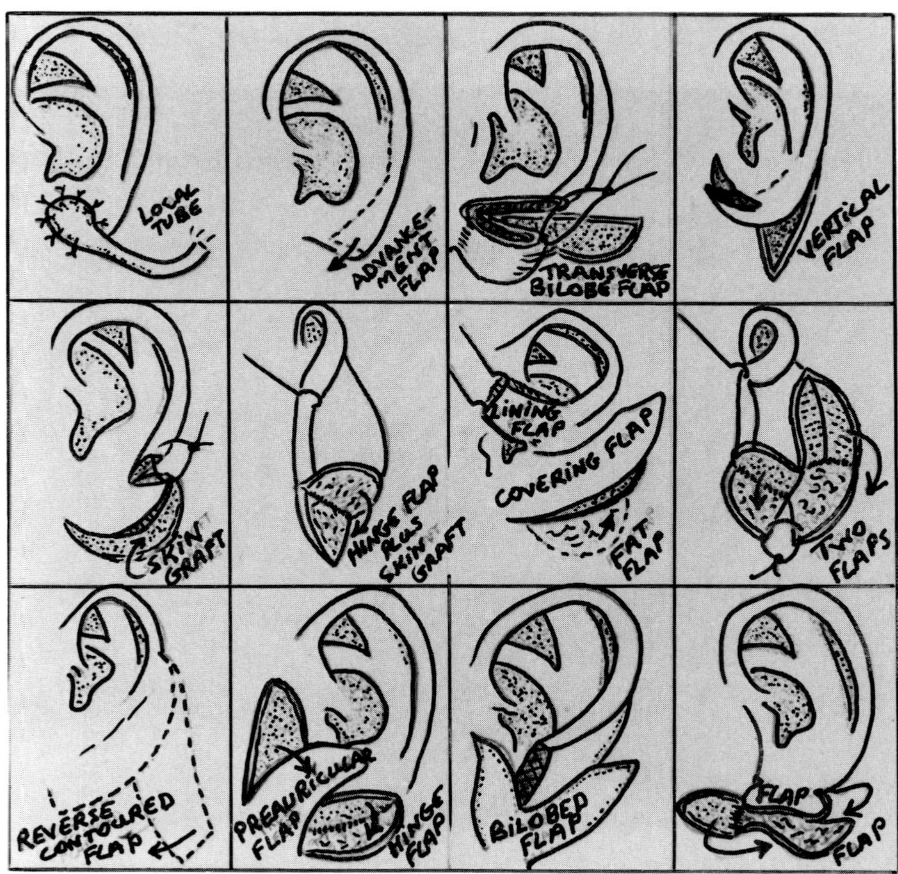

Fig. 32-47. Various methods of earlobe reconstruction.

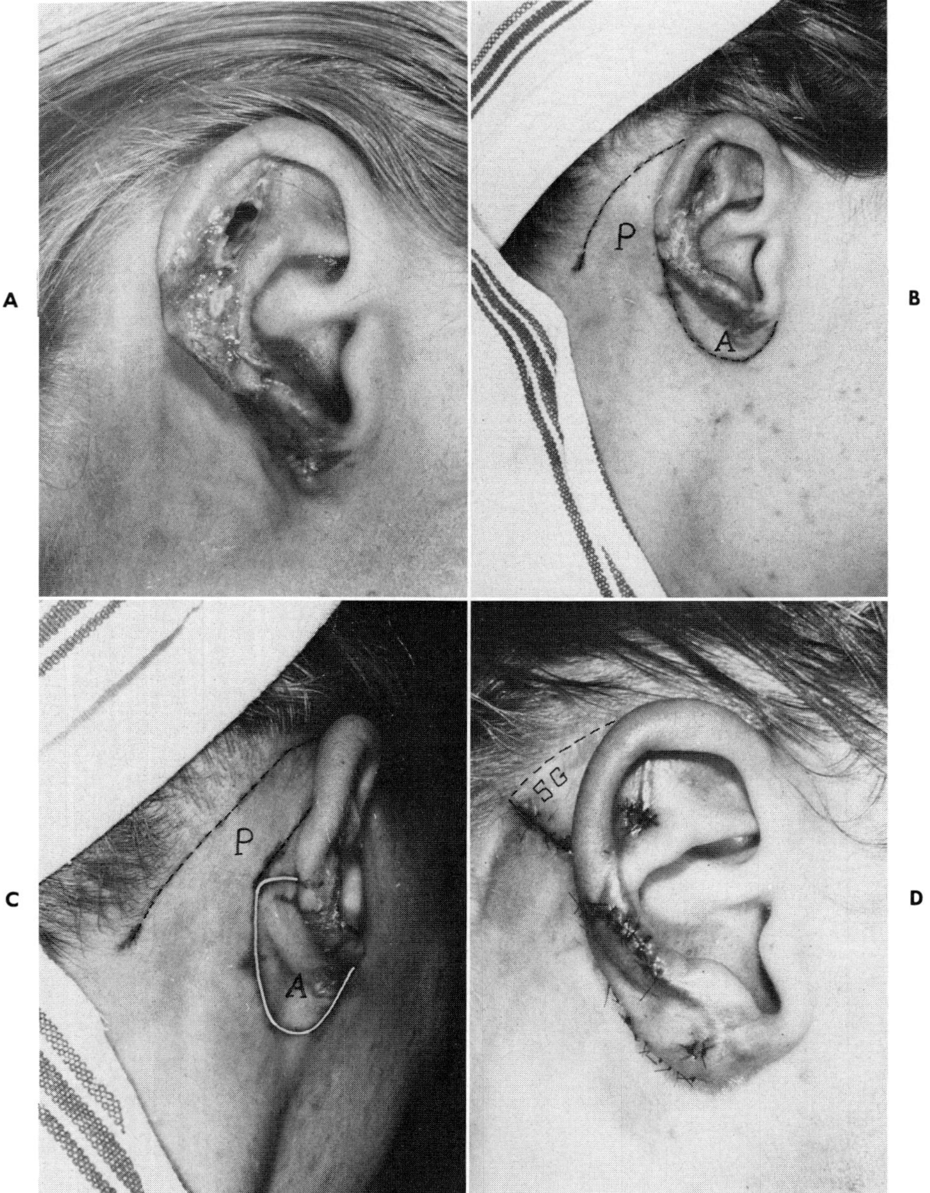

Fig. 32-48. Earlobe and inferior helix reconstruction with two local flaps. **A,** Preoperative appearance. **B** and **C,** The long inferiorly based retroauricular flap *P* will be turned back to provide bulk and lining. Flap *A* will be lifted to provide the new anterior surface. Both flaps were delayed. **D,** Early result after flap *P* was divided. *SG* is the skin-grafted flap donor site.

The eyelids

A discussion of the surgical management of burned eyelids must include a consideration of both the early and late sequelae.[141] Even though the eyelids are injured infrequently in major thermal burns overall,[102] a large portion of patients admitted to hospitals with burns involving the face will also have burns of the eyelids.[77] The severity of the lid injury depends, of course, on the nature, intensity, and duration of exposure to the heat source. Reflex blinking and squinching the lids closed in response to a flash or irritating smoke often will protect the cornea and the pretarsal lids from injury. Most of the time the eyelash margin is spared. Corneal and conjunctival burns are rare in flash and flame burns and common with chemical burns. If corneal ulceration develops after thermal lid burns, it is nearly always secondary to later lid contractures, leading to exposure and desiccation and therefore potentially preventable. The acute management of thermal eyelid burns includes early examination of the lids and globe—preferably before lid swelling makes this difficult. Even if significant edema is present, the lids should be retracted and briefly inspected. Foreign bodies (contact lenses in particular) should be looked for and removed. If possible, a baseline examination by an ophthalmologist who will continue to follow up the patient is also useful at this early stage. Gentle lid and lash hygiene should be instituted to minimize crusting, and topical ophthalmic antibiotic ointments and artifical tears should be applied frequently.

Because of the thinness, pliability, and mobility of the eyelid skin, ectropion is the most common serious result of both partial and full-thickness thermal skin burns around

the eye.[7,77] Ectropion can first be seen anywhere from 3 weeks to 3 months after the injury. Wound contraction and fibrosis pull the lids centrifugally toward the peripheral bony orbit; in some lid burns, the force of contraction-retraction can be so severe that the lid margins are drawn right up to the orbital rim (Fig. 32-51). This can erroneously suggest that the lid has been destroyed, when in fact, the tissues beneath the skin (the orbicular muscle, tarsal plate, levator muscle, annd conjunctiva) are almost always functionally intact. Developmental lid retraction usually produces some degree of conjunctivitis, and, as opposed to the early reactive conjunctival irritation from noxious fumes seen commonly for several days immediately after a burn, the appearance of delayed conjunctivitis several weeks or months after the burn is almost invariably secondary to conjunctival exposure. This mild to moderate conjunctivitis in itself is not worrisome, but should always alert the surgeon to the possibility of a coexisting or imminent corneal exposure, which is quite serious. Drying of the cornea can lead to ulceration, scarring, or perforation with loss of vision. The upper eyelid is responsible for moistening the cornea; therefore, whenever there is an upper lid ectropion, the potential for corneal dehydration is present. These patients require a *daily* examination to assess lid closure, not only while the patient is awake, but more important, while the patient is asleep. Frequently an awake patient will have complete coverage of the iris with a well-developed Bell's phenomenon (upward rolling of the globe on attempted closure of the lids) (Fig. 32-52) and forced voluntary squinching of the eyelids. This can give the physician a false impression that despite an upper lid retraction, the cornea is adequately

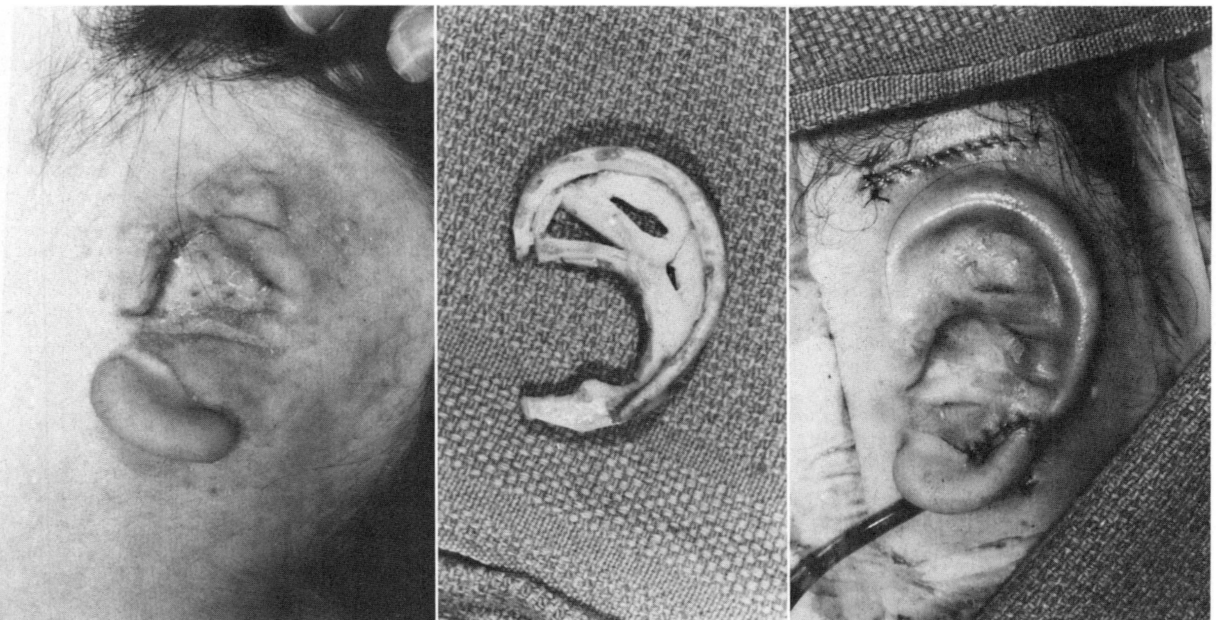

Fig. 32-49. Ear reconstruction with the carved, autogenous rib cartilage frame as described by Brent.

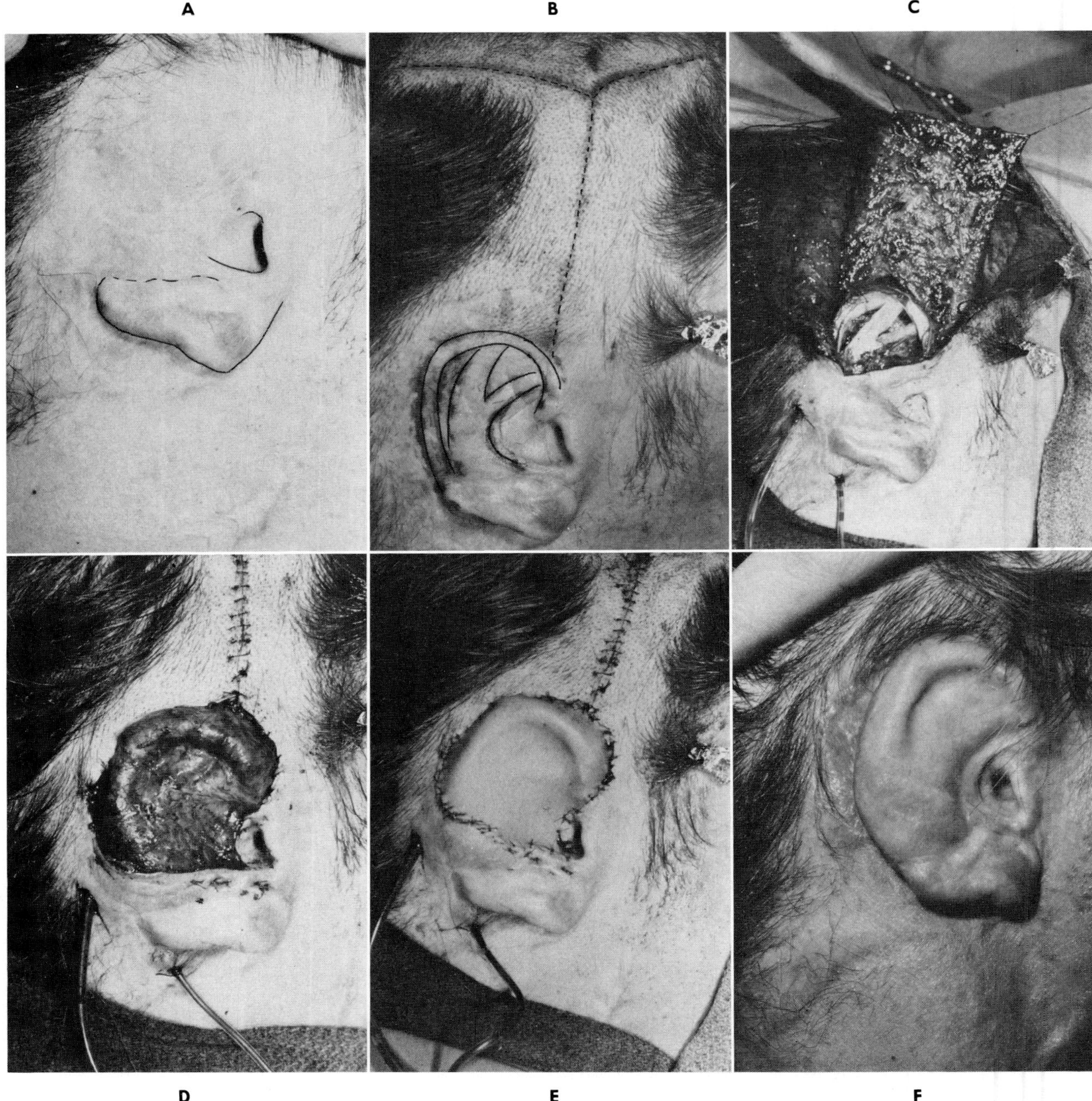

Fig. 32-50. Arterialized temporoparietal fascial flap for a difficult coverage problem. **A,** Preoperative appearance showing a tight scar around the ear remnant. **B,** Outline of required ear replacement. Dotted lines indicate incisions for access to the superficial temporal fascia. **C,** The autogenous rib cartilage frame is in place and fascial flap elevated. **D,** The flap is turned back and sutured over the cartilage frame. **E,** The skin graft is applied to the fascial cover. Note the suction catheters. **F,** Postoperative appearance after 3 months. A year is required before the final details of ear contour are seen.

protected. However, during the crucial time when the patient is asleep (or in an obtunded patient), when the voluntary component of lid closure is lost, the cornea may well become partially exposed. In cases where there is only the risk, but little or no actual exposure keratitis, a combination of copious topical ointment and artificial tears may suffice for nocturnal protection. Moist covering chambers made with plastic wrap[102] or the commercially available plastic bandage bubble can be tried, but adhere poorly to hard, slippery periorbital burn eschar. The soft contact lens, although hypothetically useful, tends to become dislodged on upward gaze by debris drying on the surface. Random-fit scleral shells,[31] however, can be useful in selected patients if they are carefully monitored. Nonetheless, if at any time there is doubt concerning the adequacy of the nonsurgical measures of corneal protection, then upper eyelid contracture release and grafting should be carried out without hesitation.[145] The surgeon must be prepared to release and regraft as needed to ensure this protection. It is far better to release and graft too early or once too often than it is to wait too long and discover a corneal catastrophe. However, if the cornea appears safe, it is best to delay a minimum of 6 weeks, or better yet, 6 months or longer before grafting the lids, until most of the eyelid and regional contraction has subsided, thereby obviating the need for repeat procedures.[144] The answer, then, to the question of when to operate on an eyelid contracture is—not too soon, and not too late!

Although some still advocate tarsorrhaphy as a temporary means of augmenting corneal protection, it seems to have many more risks than benefits and therefore is *not* endorsed.[23,110] Tarsorrhaphy does not prevent lid retraction or preclude corneal ulceration, and it can irreversibly mutilate the lid margins (Fig. 32-53). An intact tarsorrhaphy also inhibits the desired overcorrection[144] when surgically releasing and grafting the lid.

As emphasized by Converse et al.,[36] the distinction should be made between an intrinsic and an extrinsic ectropion, that is, is the lid retraction due to fibrosis and vertical shortening from dermal injury within the eyelid itself, or is the lid skin essentially normal with the distorting pull coming from the cheek below (Fig. 32-54, *A* and *B*) or the brow-forehead area above (Fig. 32-54, *D*)? Or is the contracture the result of scarring both within and outside the eyelid (Fig. 32-54, *E*)? A correct diagnosis is important because it will determine where the problem is appropriately attacked for the best functional and esthetic results. For example, attempting to correct an intrinsic contracture by adding skin only outside the lid will fail; whereas a release and graft within the lid for a purely extrinsic ectropion unnecessarily introduces a deforming patch into the lid (Fig. 32-54, *C*) and may not completely correct the primary contracture.

When ipsilateral upper and lower lid ectropions coexist, the more severe contracture of the two is usually corrected first. This assumes that the upper lid retraction is not causing significant risk of corneal exposure. If so, the upper lid should always be operated on first. For those cases of combined upper and low lid contractures in which healing of the periorbital burn has also pulled the lateral portion of the upper eyelid below the transcanthal line, causing an anti-

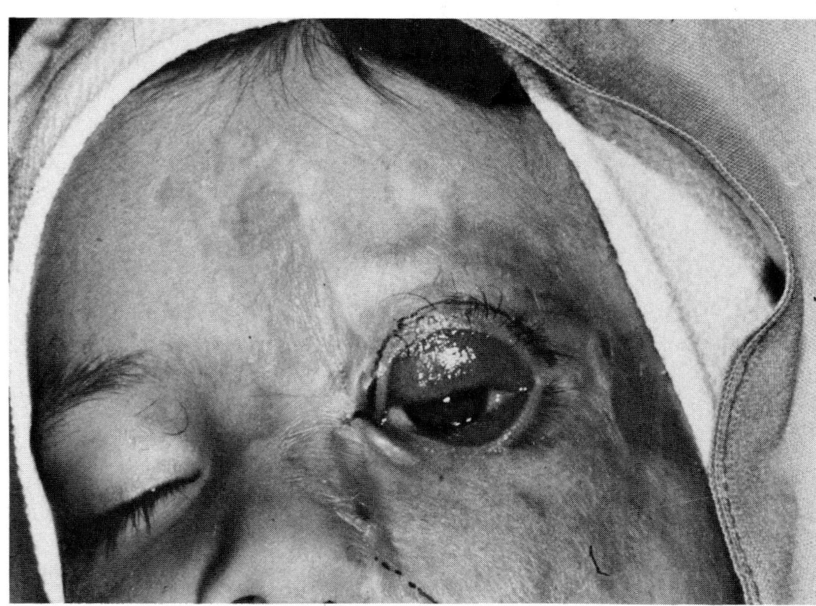

Fig. 32-51. Retraction and eversion of the upper eyelid with the lid margin at the supraorbital rim. The subdermal structures—orbicularis muscle, tarsus, levator muscle, and conjunctiva—were anatomically and functionally intact.

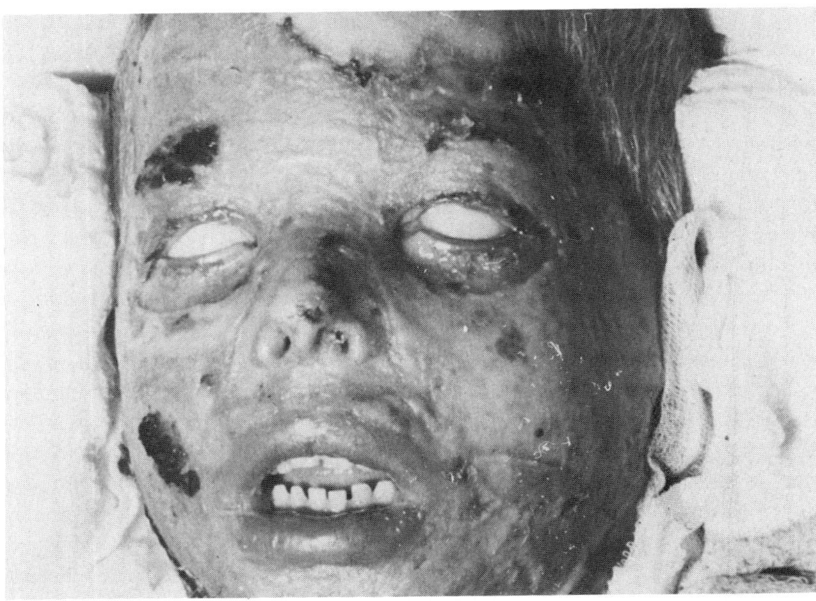

Fig. 32-52. Bell's phenomenon—upward rolling of the eyes on attempted closure of the eyelids.

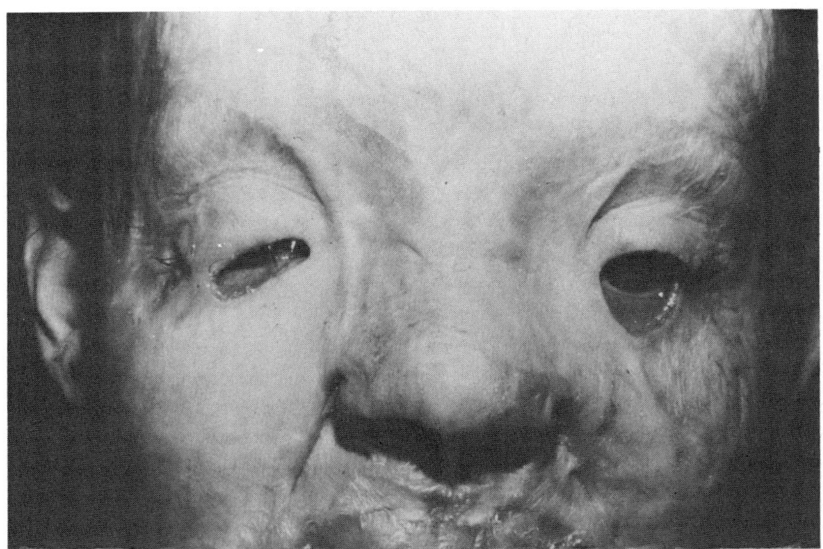

Fig. 32-53. This patient was treated with bilateral tarsorrhaphies. On the patient's left side, the tarsorrhaphy disrupted. On both sides, contractures progressed despite the inter lid adhesions, and the patient's right cornea developed ulceration. Tarsorrhaphy is not a substitute for needed scar release and grafting.

mongoloid slant to the eye (Fig. 32-55, *A* and *B*) (and again if exposure keratitis is not an issue), the lower lid should be operated on first so that the lateral upper lid can be released and repositioned above the transcanthal line concomitant with release of the lower lid (Fig. 32-55, *C* and *D*).

Both the upper and lower eyelid on the same side can be released and grafted at the same time if both contractures are minimal and stable. In most cases, however, only one lid at a time should be released to assure the desired overcorrection necessary to reduce the chance for recurrence of the contracture. Although release and grafting of bilateral eyelid ectropions is occasionally done, it is rarely carried out in young children who may become frightened by the relative blindness imposed by bilateral dressings.

Surgical release of the upper eyelid is done with an in-

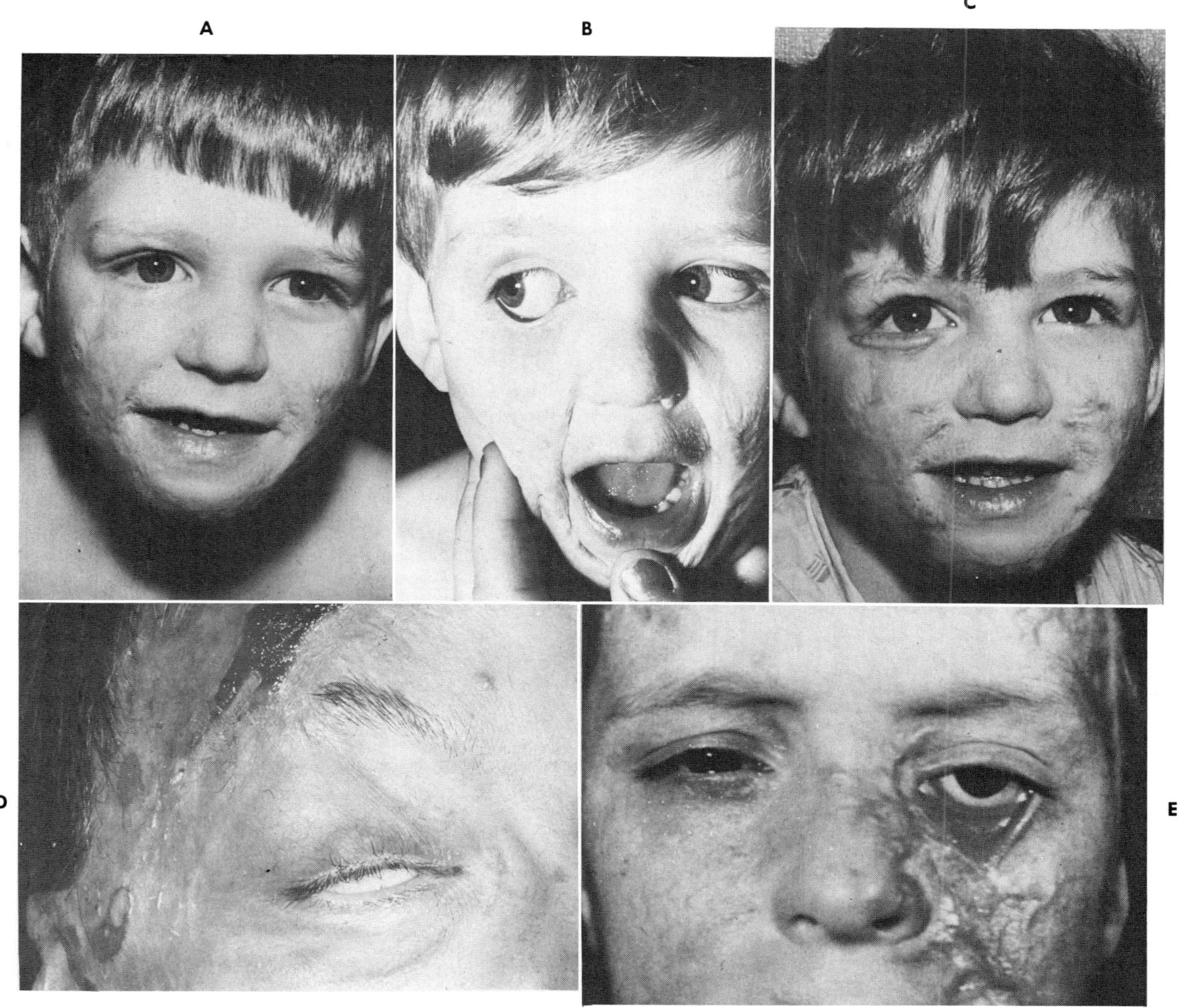

Fig. 32-54. A and **B,** Extrinsic lower eyelid ectropion secondary to tightness in the cheek below demonstrated when the child opened his mouth. Purely extrinsic contractures generally should *not* be corrected by introducing a patch into the lid. **C,** Correction should take place at the source of the contracture, the cheek in this case. **D,** An extrinsic ectropion of the upper eyelid secondary to scarring in the brow-forehead area. **E,** Ectropion of the lower eyelid from injury both within (intrinsic) and outside (extrinsic) the lid.

cision outlined 1 or 2 mm from the lid margins. Unless the pretarsal skin is unburned with the tight scar confined to the upper preseptal lid or brow, a release incision higher than the juxtamarginal level is not recommended. As suggested by Falvey and Brody,[59] at the lateral and medial limits of the incision, a forked design is incorporated so that when the release is done, the wound opens at its ends in a fishtail configuration, thus reducing later canthal tightness and webbing (Fig. 32-56, *A*). It is most important that the releasing incision *not* be extended below the projected intercanthal line in order to prevent an epicanthal scar band medially

and an antimongoloid deformity laterally. However, the release should be carried far enough transversely on each end to completely ''unlock'' the upper eyelid. Temporary traction sutures are placed near the lid margin so that downward traction can be exerted during the procedure. A thorough release of all dermal, subdermal (within the orbicular muscle), and, if needed, levator muscle scar should be carried out. The needle-tip cutting cautery minimizes bleeding. With inferior traction, an adequately released upper lid will be mobilized well enough that the lid margin will reach the infraorbital rim. This apparent overcorrection is very important, since some postoperative lid shortening and contraction can always be anticipated no matter what kind of skin graft is inserted. Meticulous hemostasis is essential. The skin graft is precisely tailored to fit the defect and sutured in place with either a running 5-0 nylon or polypropylene subcuticular stitch or interrupted 5-0 and 6-0 catgut sutures. The traditional interrupted silk tie-over dressing has been replaced by the technique described by Falvey and Brody[59] in which a grease gauze and cotton bolster is "laced" on with a monofilament suture (Fig. 32-56, *E*). This method of fixation is secure and adequately stents the graft without the need for immobilizing Frost sutures. It is compact and preserves a palpebral slit that the child can see through. It is applied in less time and is more quickly and painlessly removed (for both the patient and surgeon). The dressing is left on for 7 to 10 days.

When the upper eyelid is released with the usual supraciliary incision, but the lateral corner of the eye is still tethered inferiorly by scar in the lateral lower eyelid area, an auxiliary releasing incision can be made angling up across the scar. Both the main release defect and the small sec-

ondarily inferolateral defect are separately grafted (Fig. 32-57). This is a variation of the fishtail incision that keeps the incisions from angling downward across the intercanthal line, which is to be avoided.

An intrinsic contracture of the lower eyelid is also released with a paramarginal incision. The incision should rarely extend only from canthus to canthus, but should be carried medially and laterally enough to fully release the lid and break up any vertical scar bands at or near the canthi. The fishtail design can be used in the lower lid as well. Whereas the lateral portion of an upper lid–releasing incision should not cross the intercanthal line, the same cannot be said about the lower lid incision. Often it is best to sweep the lower lid incision obliquely upward and outward across the transcanthal line at the lateral canthus and extend it laterally far enough for adequate repositioning of both lateral upper and lower eyelids (Fig. 32-58). As with the upper lid, temporary traction sutures are used in the lower lid, and a thorough overcorrected mobilization of the lid is done. The subdermal scar should be released with a light transverse painting motion of the scalpel or electric knife at different points to

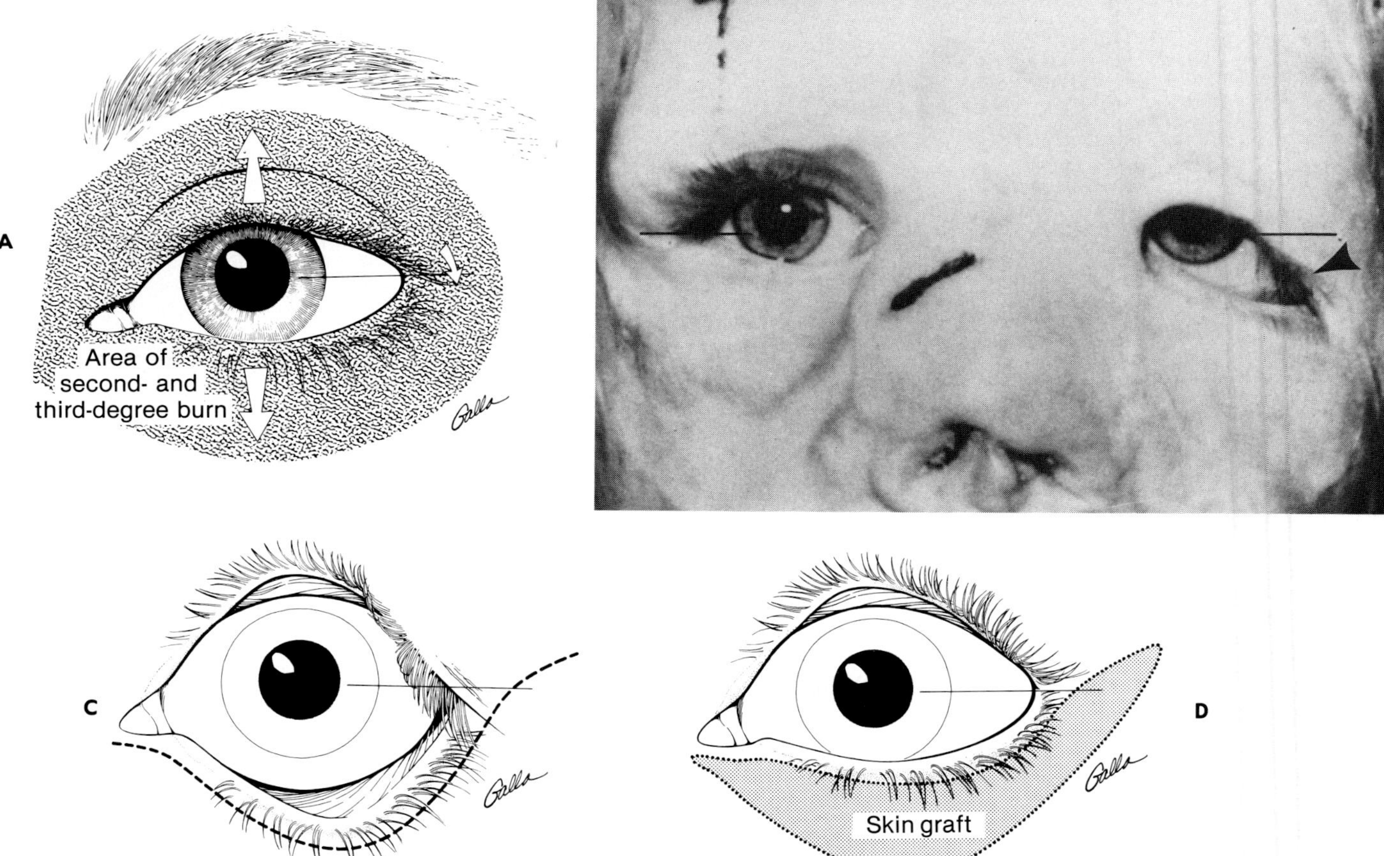

Fig. 32-55. A and **B,** Circumferential periorbital burns commonly heal with a vector of contracture that pulls the lateral upper eyelid below the transcanthal line *(arrowhead).* **C** and **D,** An extended lower eyelid–releasing incision repositions the lateral upper lid above the transcanthal line.

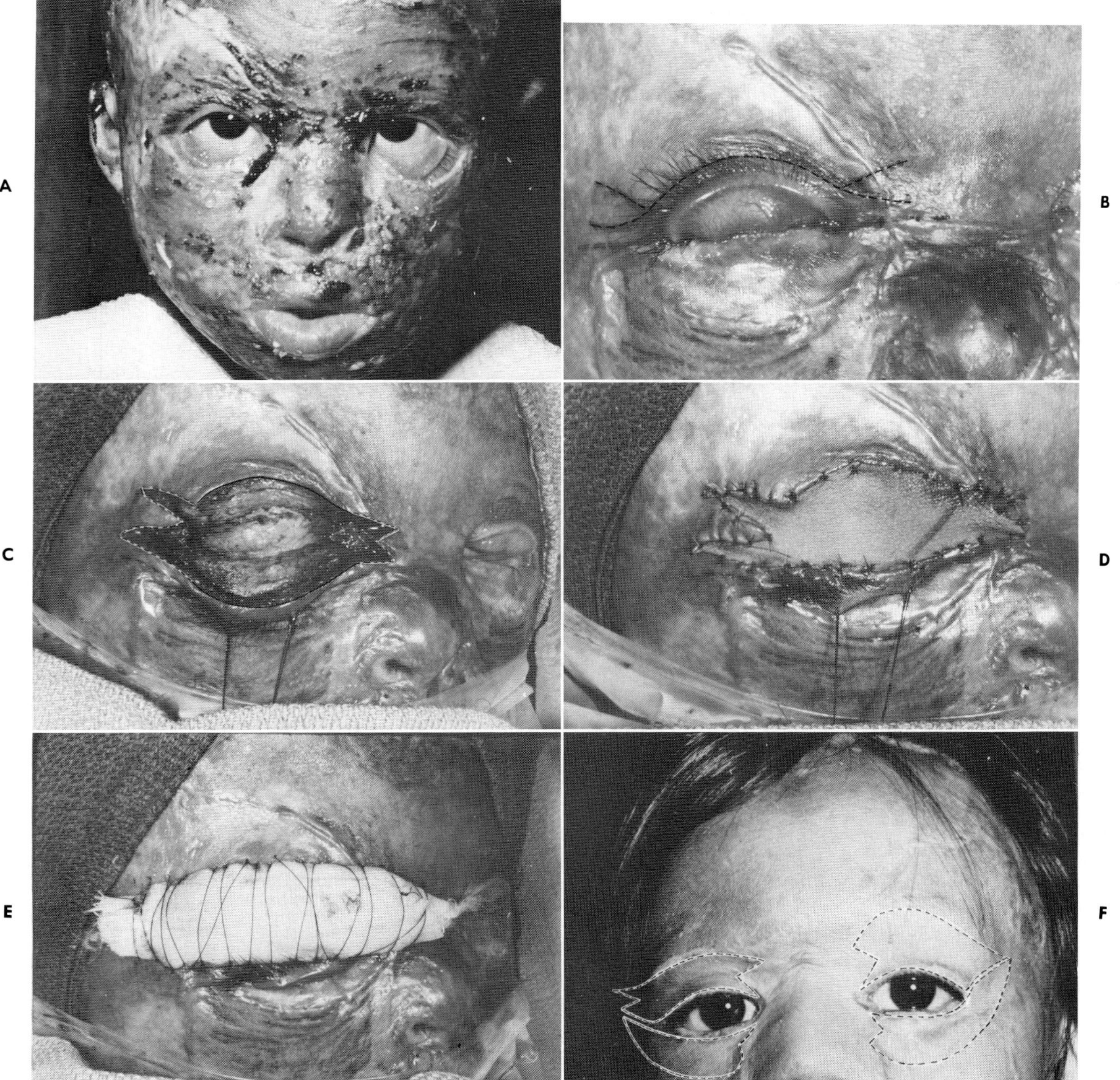

Fig. 32-56. Technique for surgical correction of an upper eyelid ectropion. **A,** Preoperative appearance. **B,** A juxtamarginal incision with a medial and lateral fishtail. **C,** Wound after full release of all restricting scar. Note traction sutures in the lid margin. **D,** The skin graft is cut to fit the overcorrected defect. Fine absorbable sutures are used. **E,** The bolster dressing is laced on with easily removed monofilament suture. **F,** Postoperative view showing the outline of grafts in all four lids.

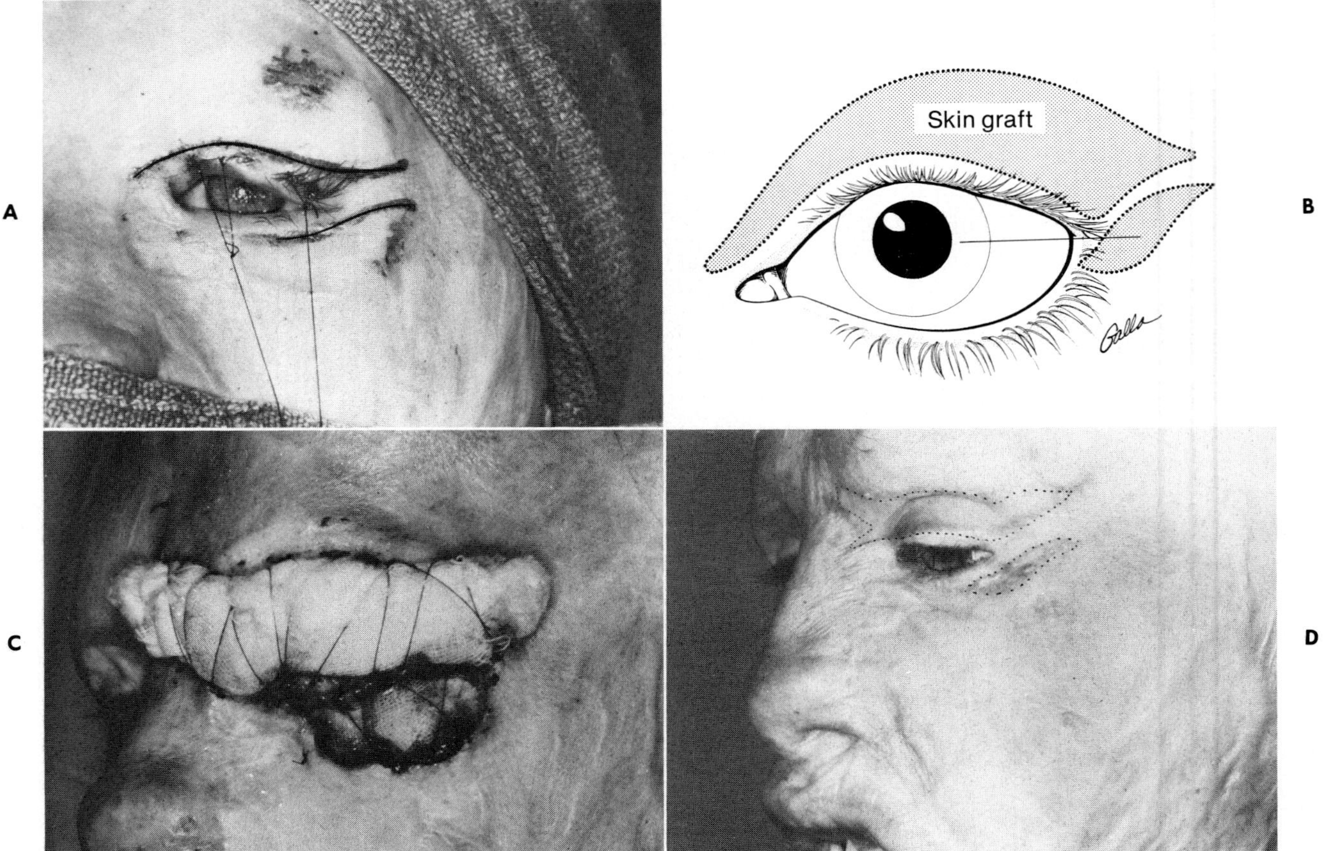

Fig. 32-57. Alternate method of releasing the upper eyelid (before definitive lower eyelid release) when the lateral upper lid is tethered below intercanthal line. **A,** Outline of the upper lid incision and an auxiliary lateral lower lid incision. **B,** Skin grafts in each separate release defect. Note that all graft margins cross the intercanthal line in an upward-outward direction, *not* a downward-outward direction. **C,** The two bolster dressings. **D,** Postoperative view showing the restored upper lid contour.

avoid a deep and unattractive depression along the infraorbital rim.

In the upper lids, where mobility is important and the graft must drape into the supratarsal fold, the skin graft should not be too thick. Only the *thin* glabrous full-thickness skin grafts (e.g., retroauricular or supraclavicular grafts) should be used; full-thickness grafts from elsewhere (e.g., the groin, abdomen, or thigh) should not be put into the upper lid (Fig. 32-59). Generally, intermediate split-thickness skin grafts inserted into an overcorrected upper lid are employed. In the lower lids mobility is less important. Here a thick split-thickness graft or one of the thin hairless full-thickness grafts can be used. Again, full-thickness grafts from the torso or extremities should not be chosen. These grafts tend to have a yellowish color and often grow fine but unattractive hairs[166] (Fig. 32-60). In essence, for both upper and lower eyelids split-thickness grafts are superior to relatively thick full-thickness grafts. Fig. 32-61 shows a patient who had all four lids repaired with split-thickness skin grafts.

Color match of the grafts with the surrounding skin is more important in the lower lids than the upper. When the cheek is unscarred, a retroauricular or supraclavicular full-thickness skin graft may give the best match, although any free graft is somewhat unpredictable as far as color change after transplantation. At times, a retroauricular graft will remain too pink or a supraclavicular graft too pale. A near full-thickness graft from the inner aspect of the upper arm or a split-thickness graft from the scalp may do nicely in the lower eyelid. In any event, the best donor sites should not be used up at an early temporizing release and grafting procedure when it is known that sometime later a definitive repair will need to be done. Save the best for last.

When grafting the eyelids it is also important to cover the entire esthetic unit of the lid to minimize the patched look. This is particularly true for the lower lids, where the graft should cover from just below the lashes down to the infraorbital rim (where the lid normally joins the cheek) and from at least canthus to canthus (Fig. 32-62).

Medial epicanthal (nasoorbital) scar bands can be more

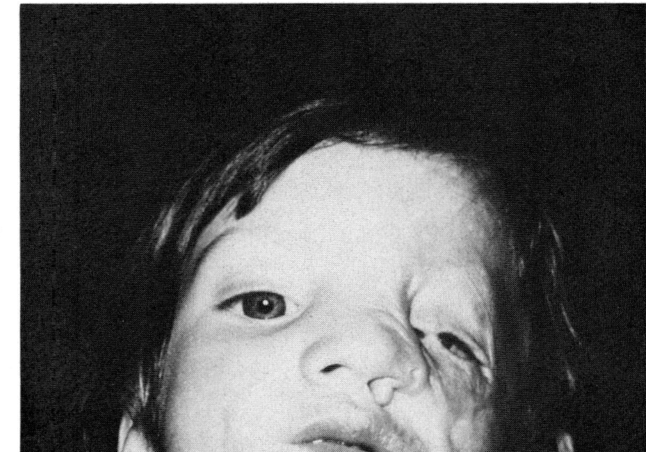

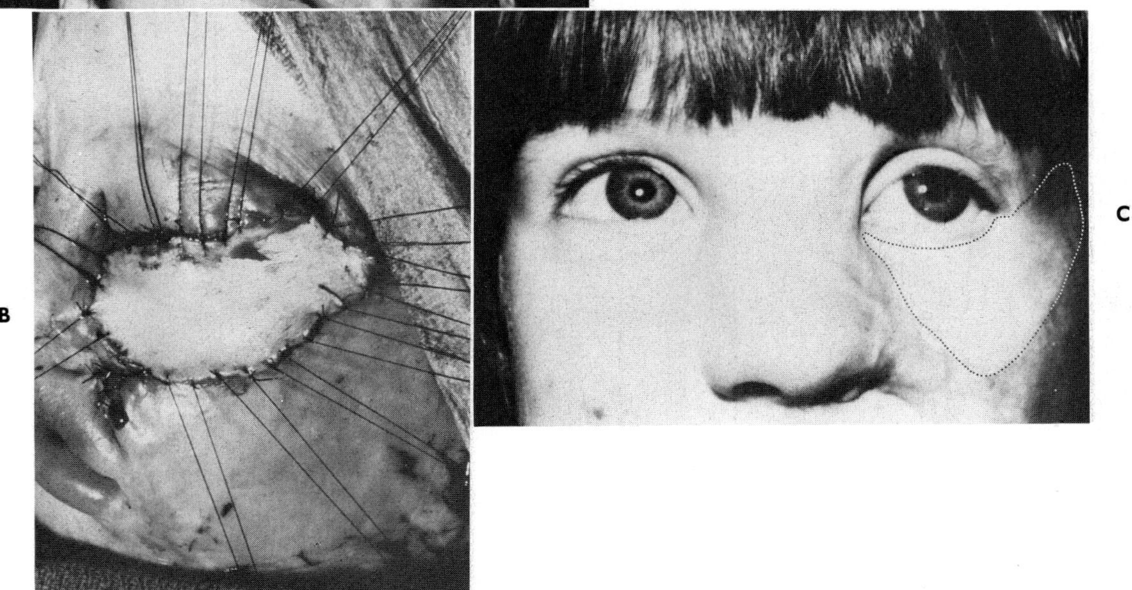

Fig. 32-58. Lower eyelid contracture release. **A,** Preoperative appearance. (The tarsorrhaphy was done elsewhere.) **B,** Intraoperative, after release and insertion of skin graft. Note the lateral extension of the incision to reposition the lateral portion of both lower and upper eyelids. **C,** Postoperative view with a large graft outlined.

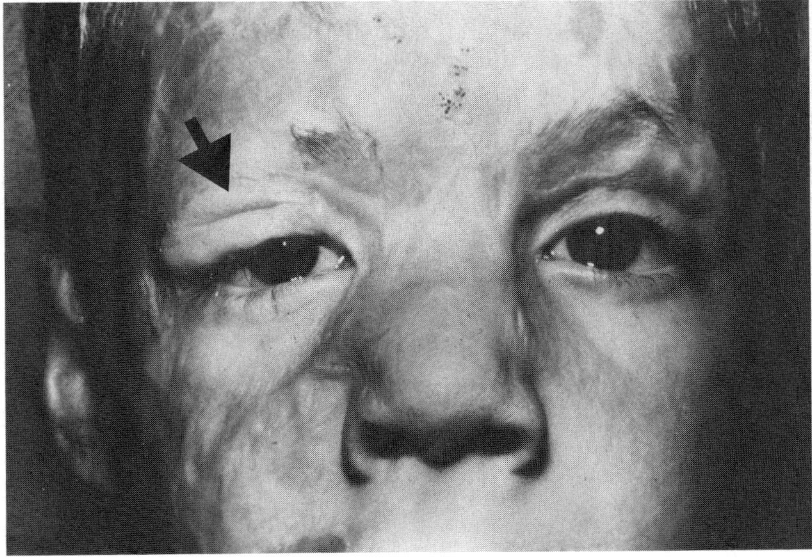

Fig. 32-59. A "thick" full-thickness skin graft *(arrow)* in the right upper eyelid that lacks suppleness and inhibits mobility. Only "thin" full-thickness skin grafts or split-thickness skin grafts should be used in the upper lid.

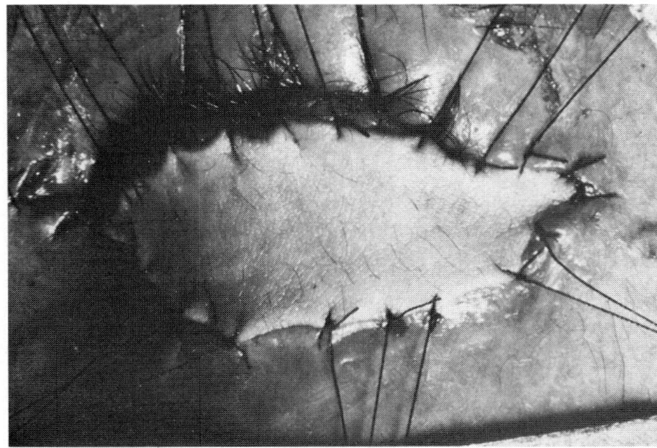

Fig. 32-60. A full-thickness skin graft from a ''hairless'' area of the inguinal region is placed in the lower eyelid. Fine but unattractive hairs are seen on close inspection. If full-thickness skin grafts are used, they should be taken from truly glabrous donor sites.

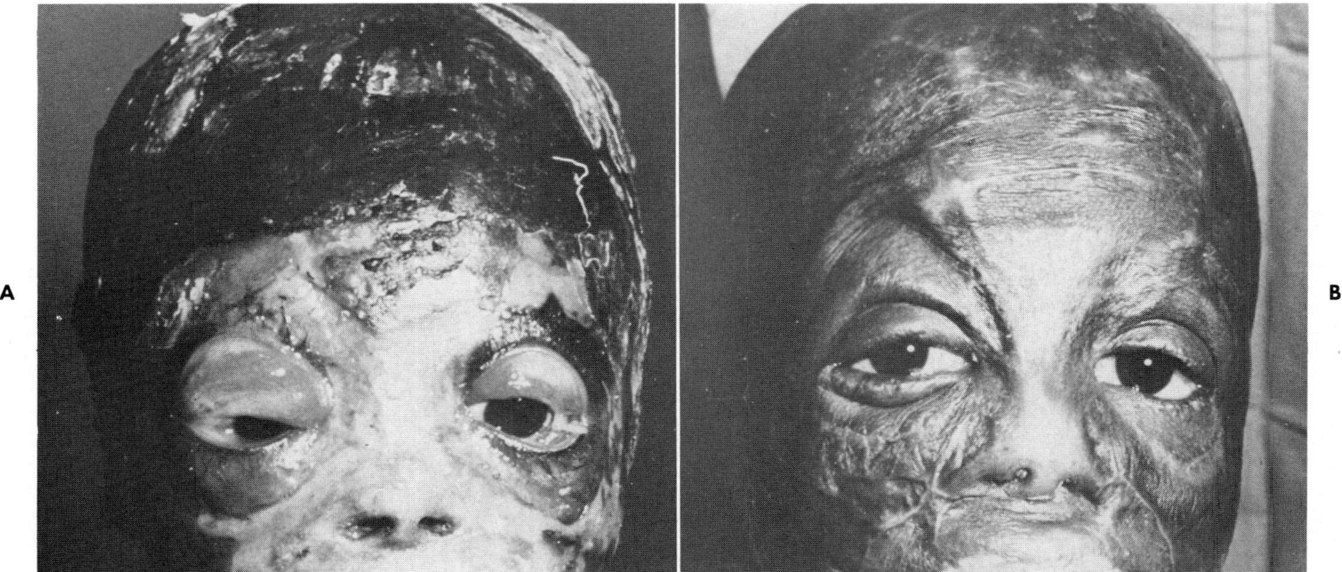

Fig. 32-61. Preoperative (**A**) and postoperative (**B**) appearance of a patient with intermediate split-thickness skin grafts inserted into overcorrected releases in all four eyelids.

or less relieved at the time of upper or lower eyelid grafting with the Y-shaped fishtail incision(s), or the bands can be excised or broken up when the nose is recovered (Fig. 32-38, *H* and *I*). As an independent procedure when the scar is relatively soft and mature, the double-opposed Z-plasty (Fig. 32-63) or some variation can be used. Lateral epicanthal folds can be corrected using a transposition flap and a small W-plasty as described by Tajima and Aoyagi.[156]

Finally, a word about the so-called masquerade graft,[36,144] in which the margins of the upper and lower eyelids are joined and both lids covered with a single patch graft (Fig. 32-64). This technique should only be used when both upper and lower lash margins have been destroyed. If the lashes are present, they may impinge on and injure the cornea. The method also makes it difficult or impossible to over-correct each lid as is usually desired. However, in cases of severe combined upper and lower lid mutilation, this method can be valuable. Detailed discussions of the treatment of total-thickness lid defects are given in the literature.[25,112,159]

The eyebrows

Although they have little functional significance, eyebrows are esthetically important. Distortions or absence of the brows alter the character of the face. Missing eyebrows indicate a burn injury that was deep enough to destroy the hair follicles. Partial loss of the eyebrow is more common than total alopecia. If a partial loss occurs in a girl, the best solution often is to have the patient use a cosmetic pencil to fill in or complete the brow. This tactic is usually not appropriate for boys, however.

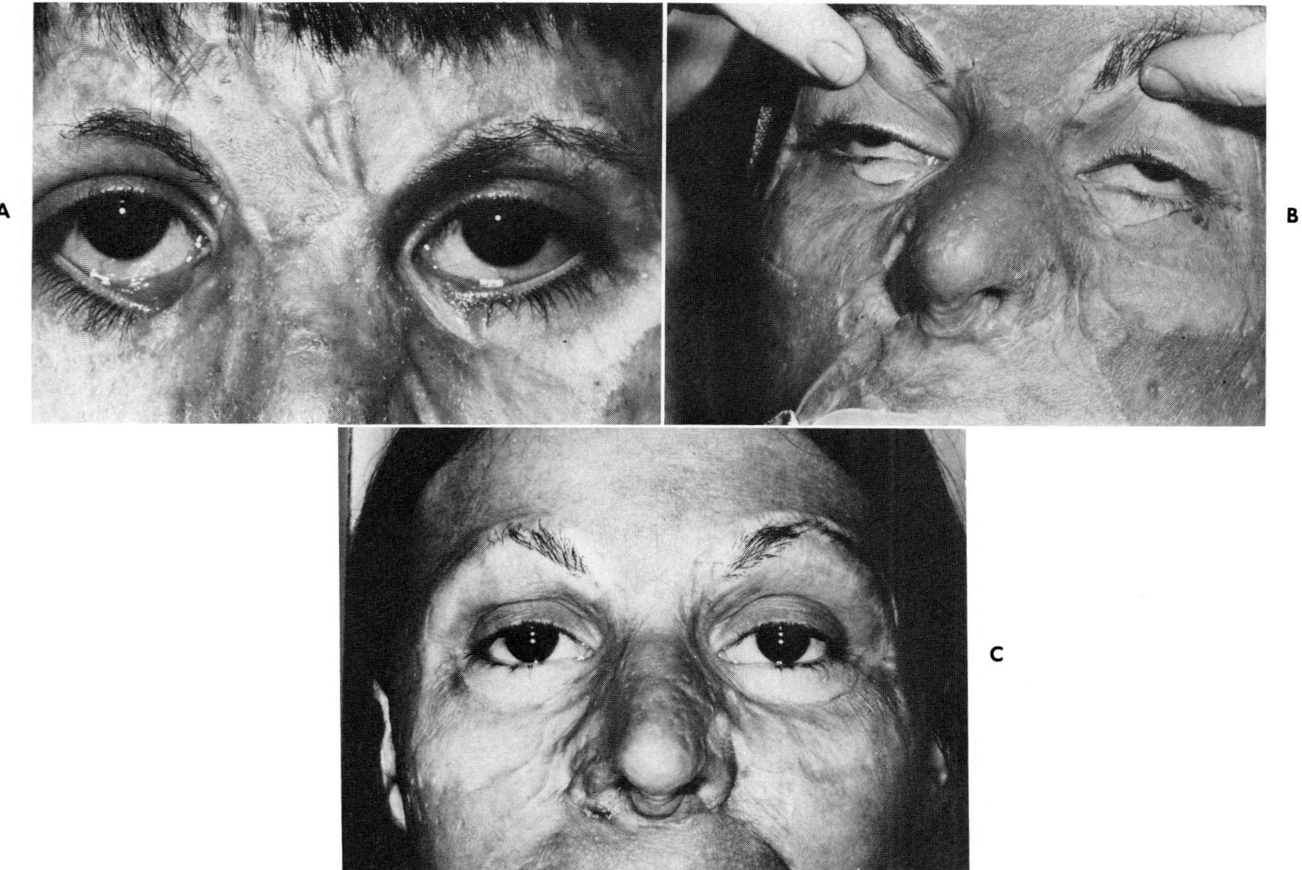

Fig. 32-62. The entire ''esthetic unit'' of an eyelid should be grafted. **A,** Preoperative view showing lower lid ectropions caused by medial intrinsic contractures. **B,** The contractures were completely but unesthetically corrected with small skin grafts that looked like little yellow patches. **C,** The small patch grafts were removed and replaced with better looking larger grafts that covered the full eyelid. (Rarely, a minor lid ectropion can be corrected with a small, but perfectly matched full-thickness skin graft from an unburned upper eyelid, but this situation seldom exists.)

Several methods are available for eyebrow reconstruction: free strip grafts from the scalp, punch grafts, interpolated scalp flaps, or vascular pedicle (temporal artery) island scalp flaps.[3,104,137,152] Although some surgeons routinely use the island pedicle method, this approach is technically difficult and often produces an overly bushy and indelicate eyebrow. For most cases, the free strip graft[28,161] is preferred (Fig. 32-65). However, a successful take depends on adequate circulation. If atrophic ischemic scar tissue is present in the recipient sites, some other method of eyebrow replacement should be chosen. When employing the strip graft method, the scalp donor site selection is very important. The direction of hair growth in the graft should be the same as in a normal eyebrow (or as it appears in the contralateral unburned eyebrow). Usually the hairs in the fuller medial portion of the eyebrow grow upward and slightly outward. The hairs in the central two thirds lie flat and are directed mostly laterally and slightly upward. In the lateral sixth of the brow, the hairs generally grow outward and curve downward. A pat-tern of the planned eyebrow (e.g., made from a piece of x-ray film) can be placed on various areas of the scalp until the best location for the graft is spotted. Clipping (not shaving) the hair in a likely donor area helps to orient the pattern. The template will need to be turned one way or the other or upside down until the desired hair growth pattern for the whole eyebrow is found. The postmastoid scalp (Fig. 32-66) or temporal area are often good places—either ipsilateral or contralateral to the eyebrow to be constructed—since the direction of hair growth will vary from patient to patient.

The design of the eyebrow graft pattern is important, since the shape of the brows will greatly influence the patient's facial expression. It is a common error to place the medial ends of the graft too high and too far apart. The medial ends should be no more than 1 to 1.5 cm. apart,[3] and the highest point of the arch should be at the junction of the middle and lateral thirds. Drawing the recipient brow incisions should be done with the patient awake and upright, as should preoperative preparation and selection of the donor site.

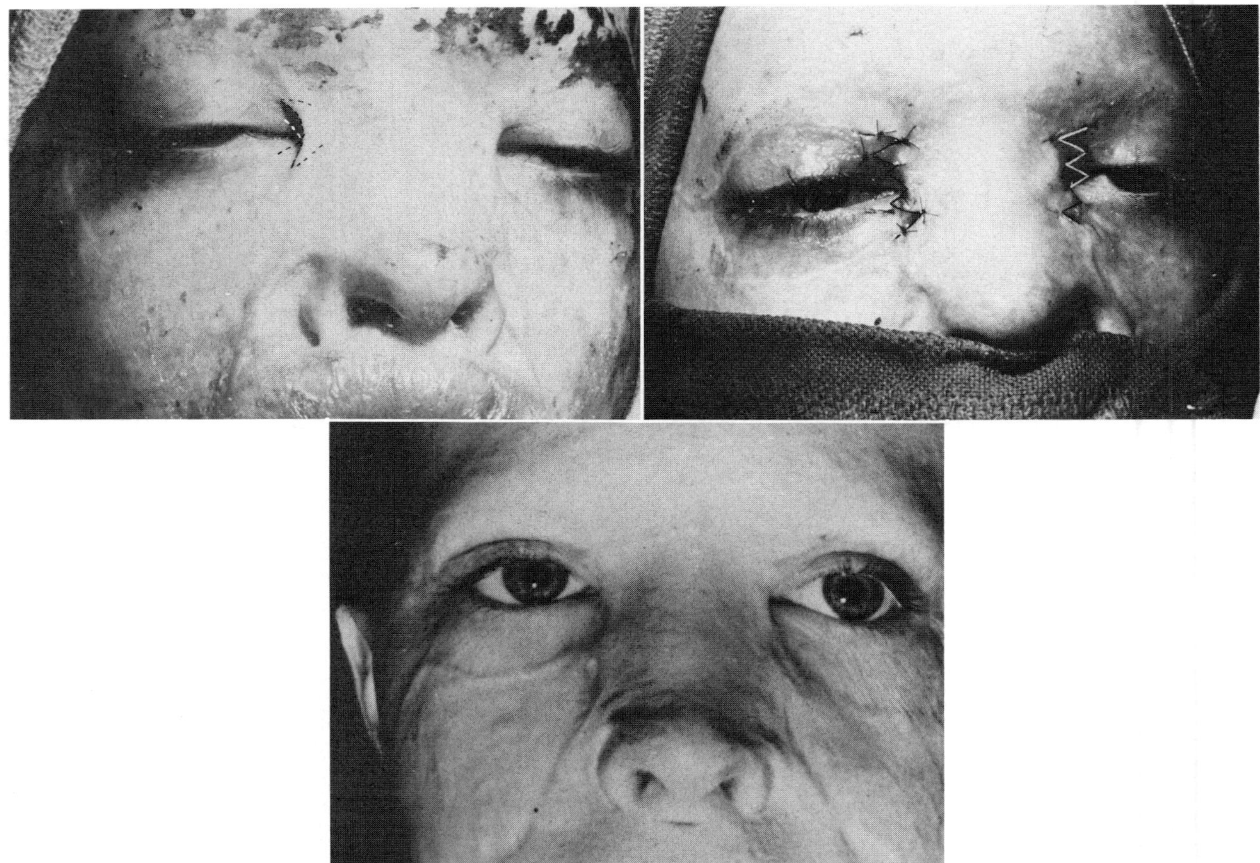

Fig. 32-63. Medial epicanthal scar bands are corrected with a double-opposed Z-plasty.

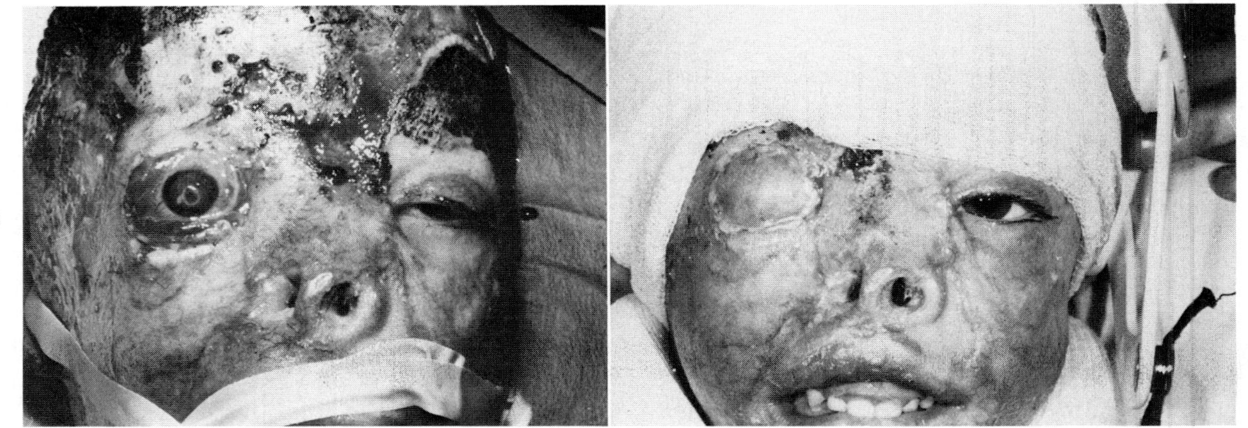

Fig. 32-64. ''Masquerade'' graft technique. **A,** Severe full-thickness lid injury with loss of both upper and lower eyelid lash margins. **B,** Upper and lower conjunctival turnover flaps were developed and sutured together and a covering skin graft applied. A medial tear drainage port was maintained. (Corneal injury can be seen in the preoperative photograph. If at all possible, the protective masquerade patch should be constructed before exposure keratopathy develops.) However, ''cortical blindness'' will occur if the eye is covered for more than a few weeks. (Courtesy Dr. Mathias Donelan.)

In younger children, surgery is carried out under general anesthesia. In the adolescent, a local anesthetic with epinephrine is injected in the brow (recipient) incision sites. However, a local anesthetic *without* epinephrine is used at the graft donor site to avoid vasoconstriction in the graft vessels. The graft should have a maximal width of 7 mm, being widest at the medial end and tapered at the lateral end. When taking the graft, beveled incisions are made with the scalpel blade parallel to the hair shafts to decrease the risk of hair follicle injury. The cuts go down to the galea, and the graft is delicately lifted away. Any attached galea and excess fat from the undersurface of the graft strip should be trimmed away, but this paring of fat should be conservative so that the hair follicles are not exposed or damaged.

At the recipient site, the previously outlined incisions are made down to and slightly into the occipitofrontal muscle so that the incision edges open enough to comfortably receive the graft. Meticulous hemostasis is crucial, but excessive use of electrocautery should be avoided. If possible, it is best not to use any electrocoagulation. A superficial running 6-0 suture on a fine needle is used to nudge the edges into perfect coaptation. After suturing, the graft is "rolled" with gauze to eliminate any residual blood under the graft. Antibiotic ointment, nonstick grease gauze and a moderate pressure head dressing are usually employed for several days. The patient and family should be told that at about 3 weeks postoperatively the hairs in the grafts will fall out, and this depilation will usually last for 2 or 3 months before regrowth appears. If further medial augmentation or a wide eyebrow is desired, a second strip graft can be added above or below the initial graft with a narrow intact skin stripe in between that can be excised later when the individual graft strips are merged.[17] Patients and family should be told to expect some numbness of the forehead and scalp above the eyebrows for many months or longer.

Burn alopecia

Scalp burns resulting in hair loss show great variability in the extent and distribution of baldness, although alopecia in the frontal, temporal, and parietal areas is more common than hair loss in the occiput. Small- to moderate-sized hairless areas can be concealed most of the time by clever hairstyling; but on occasion even these can cause significant embarrassment to a child when the bald spot is suddenly revealed to others by a gust of wind or when swimming. Trying to avoid this embarrassment can be socially inhibiting. Large areas of hair loss are, of course, more difficult to conceal. Some children will use a wig, others will not. Girls tend to accept a hairpiece more readily than boys; the boys often prefer wearing a hat or baseball cap. The wig, if it is used, has a much more natural-looking appearance if there is a peripheral fringe of intact hair in the frontal, temporal, and parietal areas. Redistribution of the remaining hair-bearing scalp with flaps to provide a "real hair" border can make the camouflage of residual bald areas with (or without) a hairpiece much easier.[125]

Most of the methods that have been developed for the surgical treatment of male-pattern baldness (namely, scalp reduction, flaps, and free hair-bearing grafts)[163] can be selectively applied or modified for the treatment of burn alopecia, and a knowledge of these techniques is important to the reconstructive surgeon. However, the differences between hereditary and posttraumatic hair loss must also be kept in mind; cicatricial alopecia characterized by a tight, thin, and ischemic scalp imposes certain limitations on some methods.

Total excision or repeated partial excisions of hairless areas with approximation of adjacent normal hair-bearing scalp is often indicated. Small areas of baldness can be completely removed and large areas of alopecia made less conspicuous. In many patients, resections of glabrous scar can be done along with flap transfers to redistribute the uninjured hirsute scalp. There are basically two ways of approaching partial excision of the scalp scar; the choice depends on local conditions.[162] If the bald area is pliable, well vascularized, and has a substantial amount of underlying subcutaneous tissue, then a central ellipse within the scar can be removed (Fig. 32-67). When the scalp is especially flexible, a fishtail extension at one end of the ellipse can be incorporated (e.g., in the occipital region) to increase the amount of scar excised.[13] By manually pushing and sliding the scalp over the skull, an estimate of the width of scar that can be safely removed is made and the pattern drawn. The procedure is begun with an incision along just *one* edge of the ellipse, followed by an extensive undermining of the scar and the scalp on *both* sides of the pattern in the loose areola plane between the galea and the pericranium. Multiple parallel relaxing incisions in the galea will produce some additional stretch and permit a little more advancement of the scalp. Excision of the scar is begun at one end, removing and closing portions of the pattern in sequence so that the surgeon is not committed to the width of excision until the last moment. This allows for removal of a maximal amount of scar consistent with reasonable tension on the closure. Depending on the flexibility of the scalp, a width of scar up to 3 cm can be excised in the first operation. Smaller amounts will be removed in subsequent procedures, usually spaced at intervals of 4 to 12 months.

When the hairless scar is tightly adherent to the underlying bone with little subcutaneous tissue present (as it is in a majority of cases), the staged excisions should be done along periphery of the scar. The normal hair-bearing scalp on each side is widely undermined and stretched over the not yet excised scar edges. The precise amount of overlap is marked and the delineated strips removed. The central portion of the scar remains attached to the skull beneath. A strip up to 1.5 cm in width can be excised from each border at the initial surgery. The principal variable is scalp flexibility; the tighter the scalp, the more stages that may be required. Between procedures the patient is encouraged to massage the scalp to prepare for the next excision.

Hair-bearing scalp flaps are used to transfer hair from

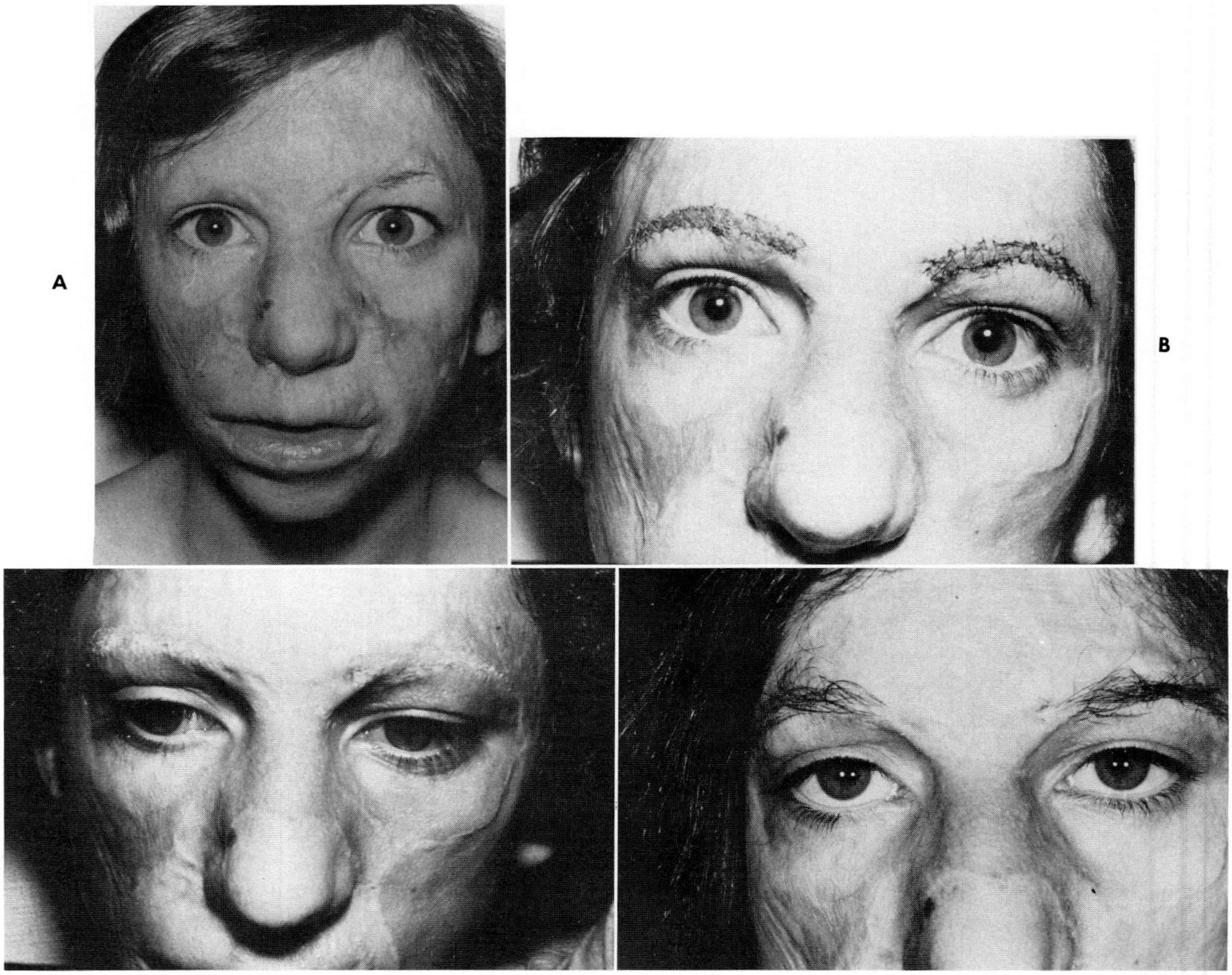

Fig. 32-65. Eyebrow reconstruction. **A,** Preoperative appearance. **B,** Appearance 48 hours after the grafts were inserted. **C,** Anticipated depilation at 1 month after surgery. **D,** Final result after regrowth of hair. A better result would have been obtained if both grafts had been extended medially.

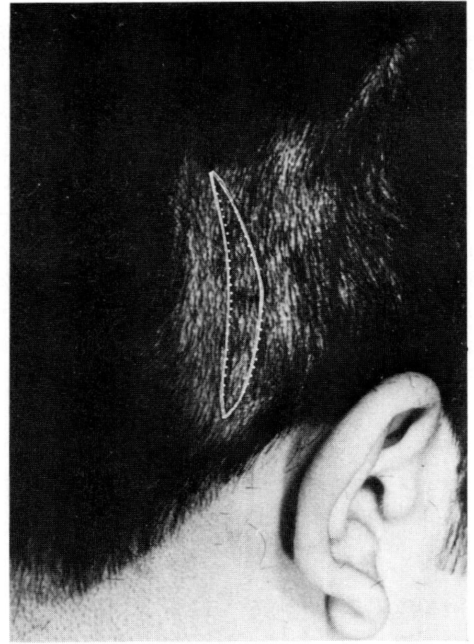

Fig. 32-66. The postmastoid scalp is often a good place to look for the eyebrow graft donor site.

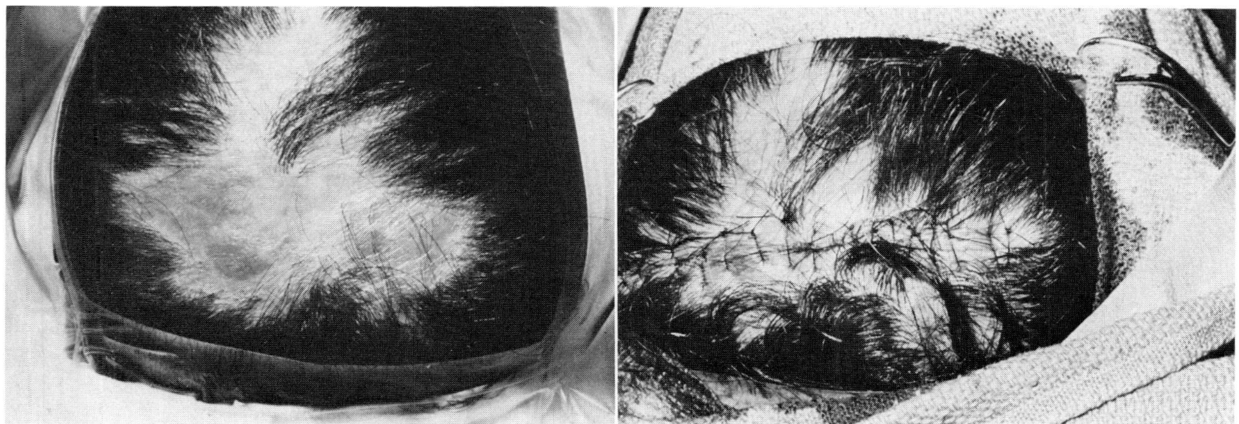

Fig. 32-67. Partial excision of scalp alopecia.

less conspicuous areas to more esthetically significant ones. Generally, the frontal and lateral periphery of the scalp have priority over the vertex and occiput.

Restoration of the frontal hairline can be accomplished with a variety of anteriorly based transposition flaps designed according to the specific donor and recipient site requirements of each patient (Fig. 32-68). Frequently, unilateral or bilateral temporoparietal or temporoparietooccipital flaps are available for the reconstruction.[83,86] Careful preoperative planning of the flaps is important. Temporoparietal flaps in normal scalp that do not exceed a length-to-base ratio of 5:1 do not require an axial vascular pedicle and do need to be delayed. The work of Elliott[57] should be consulted for details of this procedure. If longer temporoparietooccipital flaps similar to those described by Juri are employed, an attempt is made to incorporate a branch of the superficial temporal vessels into the flap base and one or more (more commonly two) preliminary delay procedures are carried out to ensure complete flap survival. At the first procedure the edges of the flap are incised down to periosteum. One or two weeks later, at the second procedure, the distal end of the flap is elevated from its bed. This is done because the tip of the flap in the occipital region receives some of its blood supply from perforating vessels piercing the deeper occipitalis muscle, whereas the temporoparietal portion of the flap is perfused only from the periphery. A week or two thereafter the flap is transposed. At times the flap donor site can be closed primarily, but often a skin graft is needed to cover a segment of the donor site. This graft usually can be excised later.

Although anterolaterally based transposition flaps for anterior hairline reconstruction are useful, they are still less than ideal in that they provide an abnormal posterior direction of hair growth when transferred, leaving a potentially conspicuous scar joining the flap to the forehead. To solve this problem, Juri[85] proposed an extra-long "encircling" flap, the distal end of which is swung almost completely around and inset ipsilaterally next to its base, with the hair

growth directed forward. At a second stage, the original pedicle is divided and the proximal end of the flap unfurled to provide the hairline distally along the contralateral side of the forehead. This method has the drawbacks of being complex and multistaged and calls for an unusually long flap to accomplish the required rotations.

An alternate approach that will restore a natural anterior hairline with forward-growing hair in a one-stage procedure is the microvascular free flap method.[83,85,119] A free temporooccipital flap from one side of the scalp that is axially supplied by the superficial temporal vessels can be transplanted with microanastomoses to the recipient contralateral superficial temporal vessels (Fig. 32-69). An occipitotemporal free flap based posteriorly on the occipital artery and vein also can be transferred anteriorly. Although the free flap method does have many advantages, it nonetheless requires equipment, experience, and expertise beyond the scope of most surgeons. The need at times to use both superficial temporal pedicles to make a single flap also precludes the use of more standard bilateral temporooccipital transposition flaps to cover extensive areas of baldness.

Temporal and sideburn alopecia can be repaired with a variety of local transposition scalp flaps, island pedicle flaps, or free flaps.[17] It is important that the hair in the inserted flap run in the proper direction—down and backward. The work of Juri, Juri, and Colnago[88] is particularly helpful.

Free hair-bearing punch grafts[29,60] and free scalp strip grafts are not a primary treatment modality for alopecia after burn injury. Although free grafts can survive when implanted into scarred areas,[117] how well they do depends on the quality of the recipient blood supply. Thin atrophic scar tissue with little subcutaneous padding provides the least hospitable bed. Although the free punch grafts are generally not used to restore a frontotemporal hairline in cicatricial alopecia (flaps being preferred), the plugs can be used successfully to fill in between the flaps. The strip graft is used infrequently in this setting.[162]

Treatment of burn alopecia often best involves a combination of different surgical techniques. The sequence in which these procedures are carried out is important. Usually the various flaps should be done first. Next are staged excisions for maximal reduction of the bald scalp. And last, free punch grafts are applied. This order preserves the maximal blood supply for the flaps and minimizes problems with closure of donor defects.

The corner of the mouth

Scarring at or around the corner of the mouth often produces functional oral disability and visual distortion of the lips. The cause of the scarring is usually either a thermal burn involving the central face or an electrical oral burn occurring when the child puts a "live" extension cord into the mouth. Both of these causes of perioral injury result in some similar characteristics of contracture, but there are also differences. In most of the thermal burns, the scarring is generally more superficial and widespread (Fig. 32-70, *A*). Although the injury in electrical burns is more localized, it is also usually much deeper, often involving muscle and mucosa. Regardless of the cause, however, scar at the corner of the mouth, even a little scar, can narrow the opening and inhibit the remarkable elasticity that normally characterizes this area.

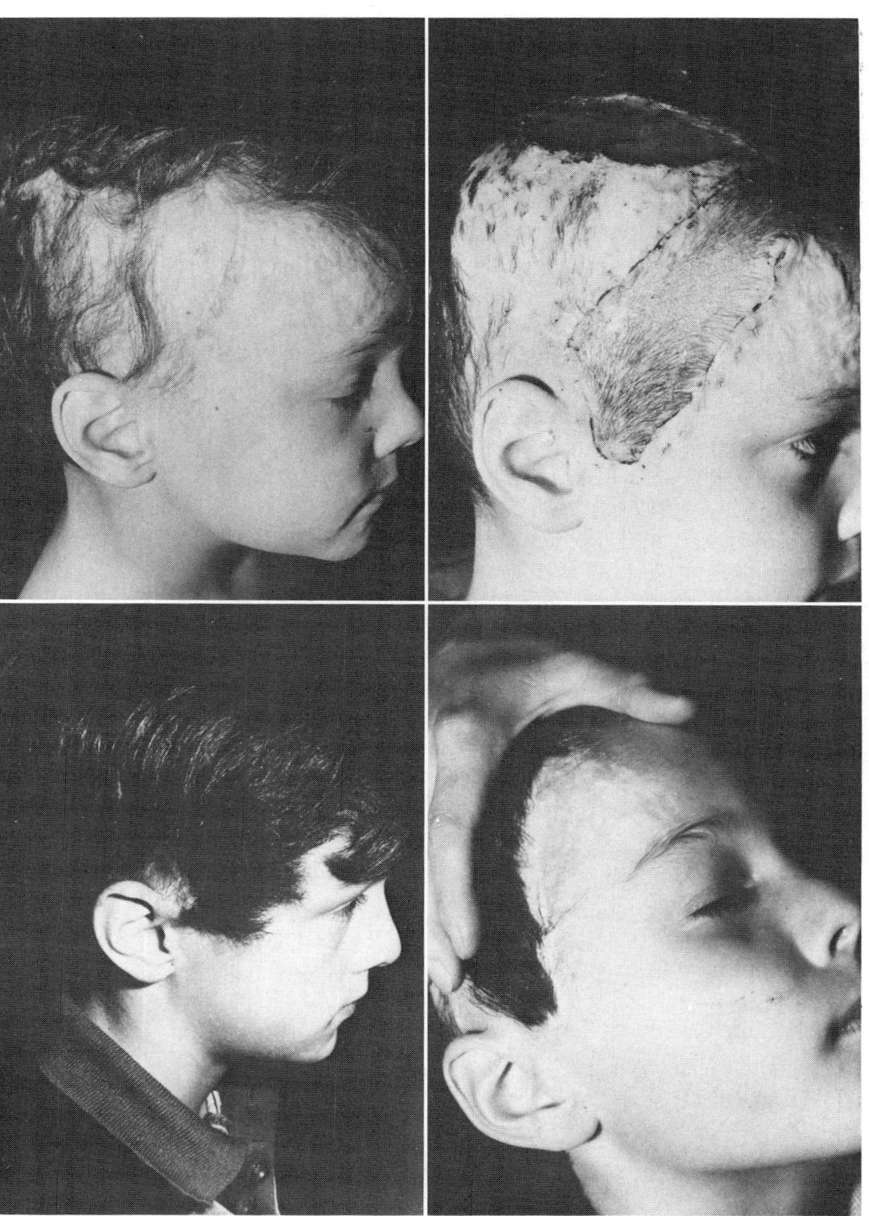

Fig. 32-68. Anterior hairline restoration using a transposition scalp flap. (Courtesy Dr. John Constable.)

Since oral stenosis and microstomia in thermal burns are commonly associated with scarring in neighboring areas around the mouth, it usually makes sense to release the tethering scars at the oral commissures at the same time as other procedures are done, such as an upper or lower lip or cheek is being released and grafted.[2] The procedure at the corner of the mouth should be a simple one, adding little additional operating time.[126] A transverse or slightly upward incision is made through the scar from the contracted commissure outward to a point in line with or a bit lateral to the pupil of the eye. If the underlying orbicular muscle is also tight, it too should be split. The mucosal lining is then mobilized and advanced out to the new commissure. Some overcorrection is recommended because the opening inevitably shrinks back somewhat. Postoperatively a dynamic expander (Fig. 32-71) is useful in helping to prevent re-

tracture.[30] Some children, however, will not keep the appliance in, and for many, recontracture will develop to an extent even with splinting. Postponing the oral and perioral surgery until the local and regional scars have matured would reduce the need for repeated operations on the commissures, but from a practical point of view, this is usually not appropriate.

The surgeon should be aware that in extensive face-neck burns, a patient's difficulty opening the mouth can be caused by tight scar other than just at the corners of the mouth. In these cases, the cheek and neck scar would first have to be separated over the mandible before the mouth could open completely.

A great many procedures have been described to deal with oral commissure contractures, and some are quite intricate. Various Z-plasties, along with vermilion, muscle,

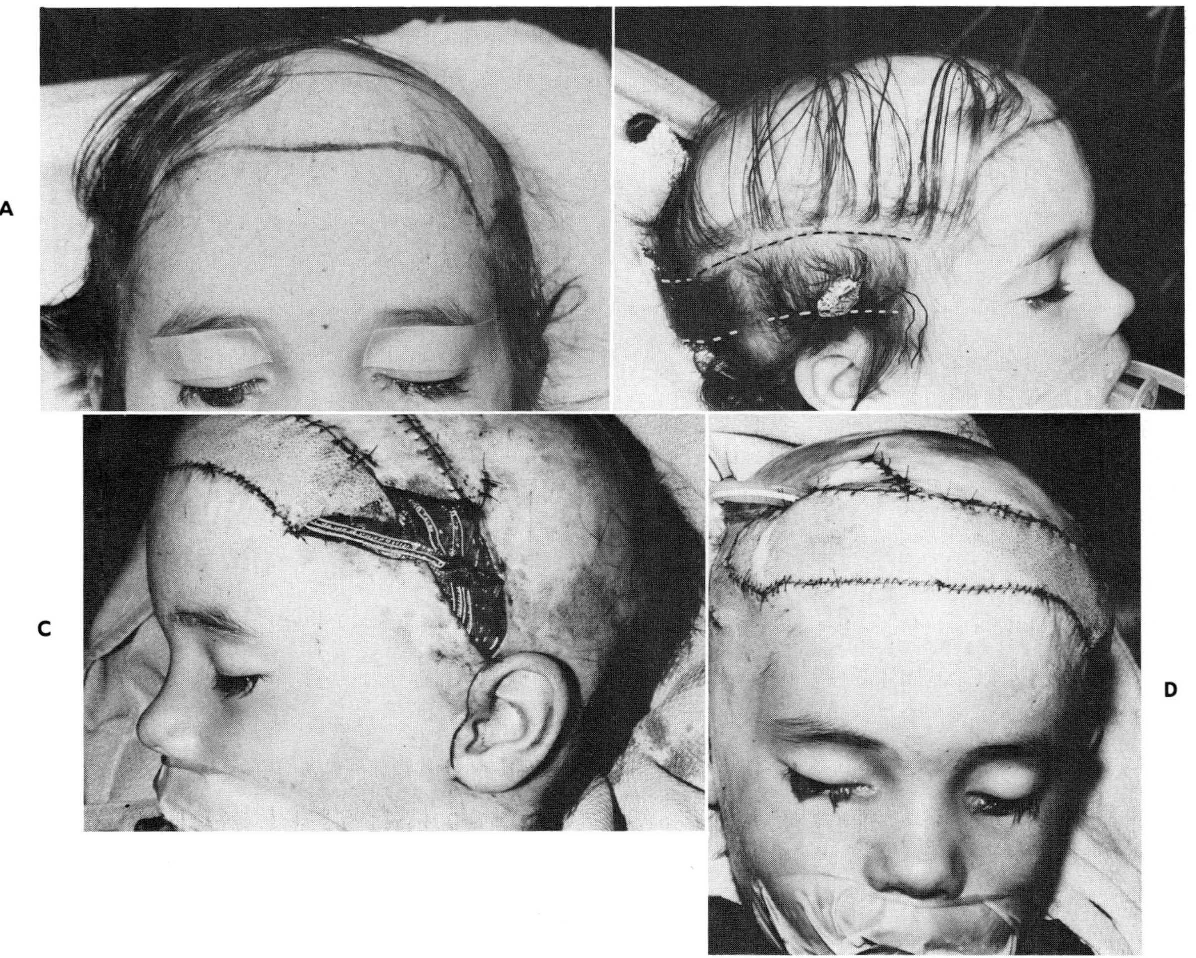

Fig. 32-69. Anterior hairline restoration using a microvascular free flap. **A,** Preoperative planned hairline drawn out. **B,** Right temporoparietooccipital flap outlined with the superficial temporal artery palpable in the base. Two preliminary delay procedures were carried out because of the extended flap length. **C,** The flap is inset before anastomoses to recipient left superficial temporal vessels. **D,** Immediate postoperative appearance.   *Continued.*

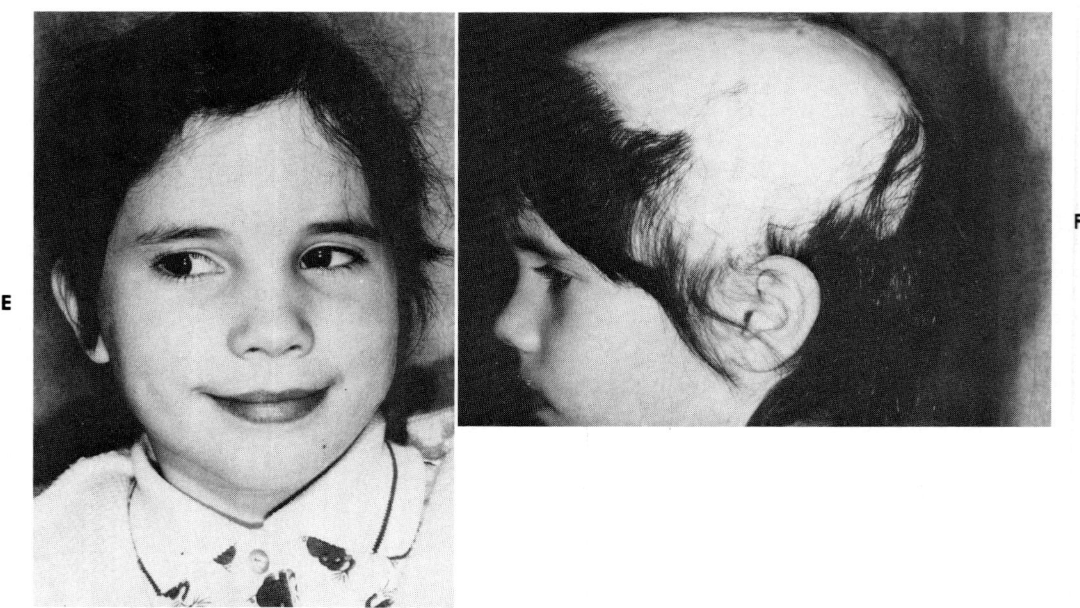

Fig. 32-69, cont'd. E, Postoperative appearance 3 months later. **F,** Note the forward direction of hair growth. (Microvascular surgery by Dr. James May.)

and mucosal transposition and advancement flaps have been proposed.* Some of the methods work nicely for some patients some of the time. However, none of the methods can completely guarantee a satisfactory long-term result. In this location, the vagaries of scar contraction will often compromise even the most well-conceived and well-executed surgery. An example of one type of commissure surgery is shown in Fig. 32-70.

Most electrical burns of the lips and commissure should be managed acutely with careful observation and gentle wound hygiene. The wounds are allowed to heal on their own, and, if necessary, a surgical repair is done a year or several years later when the scar is soft and the deformity stable.[153] Not infrequently, what appears early on to be a fairly extensive injury will heal with minimal disfigurement. If bleeding from a labial artery occurs or is imminent, necessitating early operative intervention, then that anesthetic opportunity can be used to excise the necrotic tissue and surgically close the wound. If the defect is not extensive, simple undermining and advancement of the labial and buccal mucosa can be done (Fig. 32-72). When more extensive tissue destruction has occurred, a definitive repair can be undertaken that will significantly lessen primary wound contraction.[122] Later only minor revisions may be required. Fig. 32-73 shows the use of a half-lip sliding flap to reconstruct the other half of the lower lip and commissure. Fig. 32-74 demonstrates the use of a tongue flap for lower lip repair.[122,180]

When planning the correction of an established perioral electrical burn deformity, the surgeon should refer to the contralateral uninjured side of the mouth to accurately guide the design for commissure placement and lip recontouring. Symmetry is the most important surgical objective. There is no routine way of carrying out the repair. A careful detail-conscious analysis of the deformity will dictate what needs to be done. In addition to elongating the corner of the mouth if necessary, the plan should aim at removing white scars from the red vermilion and red scars in the white portion of the lips. Notching along the vermilion margin should be eliminated. Bulky areas should be thinned and thin spots filled out. To properly adjust and locally redistribute the red and white usually requires a combination of various kinds of flaps, such as asymmetric Z-plasties, V-Y and Y-V advancements, lip-switch flaps, and mucosal rotation flaps.* Every effort should be made to correct or improve the deformity without adding any new scars to the visible white areas of the lip. It is also important to assess the degree of deformity preoperatively with the patient's mouth closed and open. Often the contours of the mouth will be close to normal with the lips in repose, the stomal distortion being readily apparent only during speech or eating when the commissural scar is required to stretch.

SUMMARY AND CONCLUSIONS

The general principles of facial burn repair include: (1) a precise preoperative analysis, (2) esthetic aspects of sur-

Text continued on p. 629.

---

*References 32, 33, 37, 58, 62, 113, 147, 153, and 155.

*References 10, 40, 75, 82, 85, 92, 167, 174, and 178.

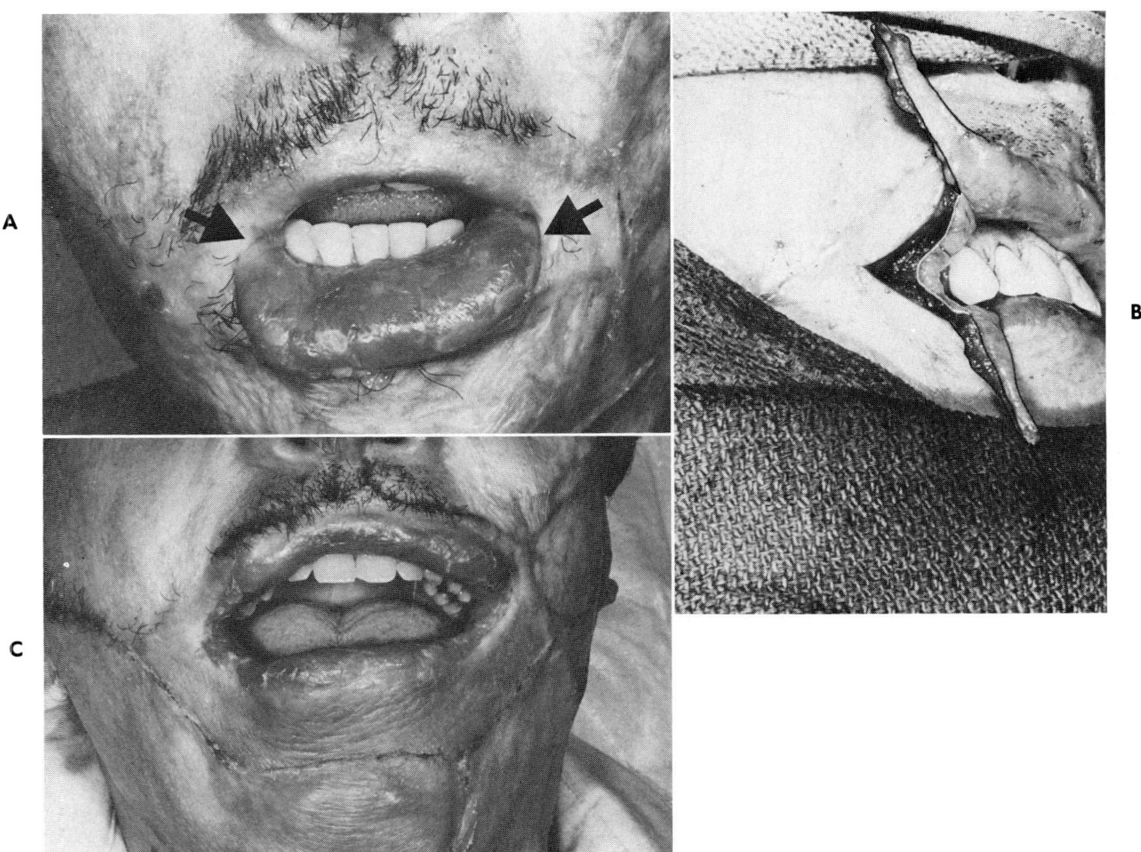

Fig. 32-70. Commissure surgery for oral stenosis. **A,** Preoperative appearance showing the maximal amount the patient could open the mouth. Note the tight scar bands (*arrows*) bridging the oral commissure. **B,** The scar is excised and the local flaps mobilized. **C,** Postoperative appearance showing an increased ability to open the mouth.

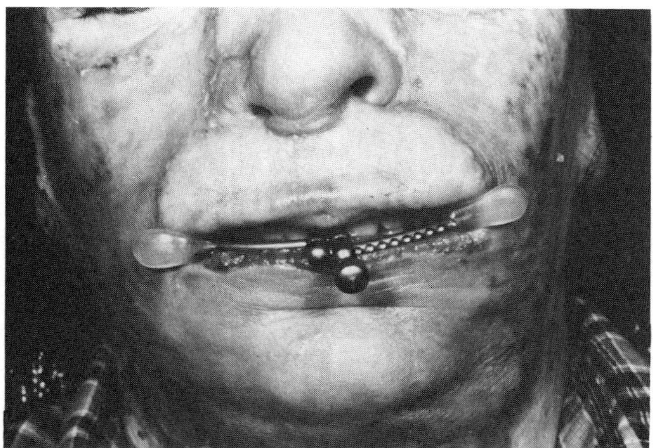

Fig. 32-71. Adjustable oral commissure spreader and splint. It can be used prophylactically to minimize commissural contractures after perioral burns or after surgery to reduce possible recontracture.

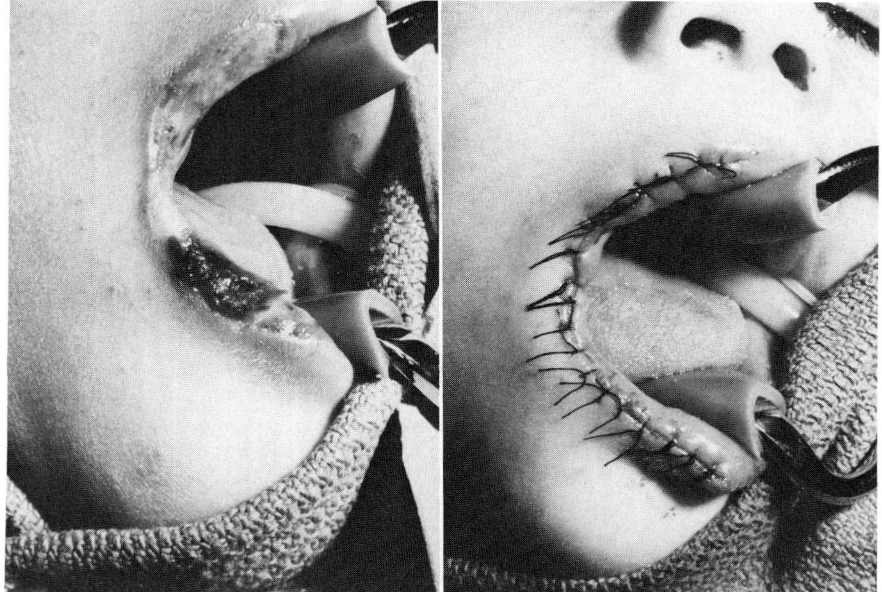

Fig. 32-72. Pericommissural electrical burn managed with early excision and closure with mobilized mucosal flaps.

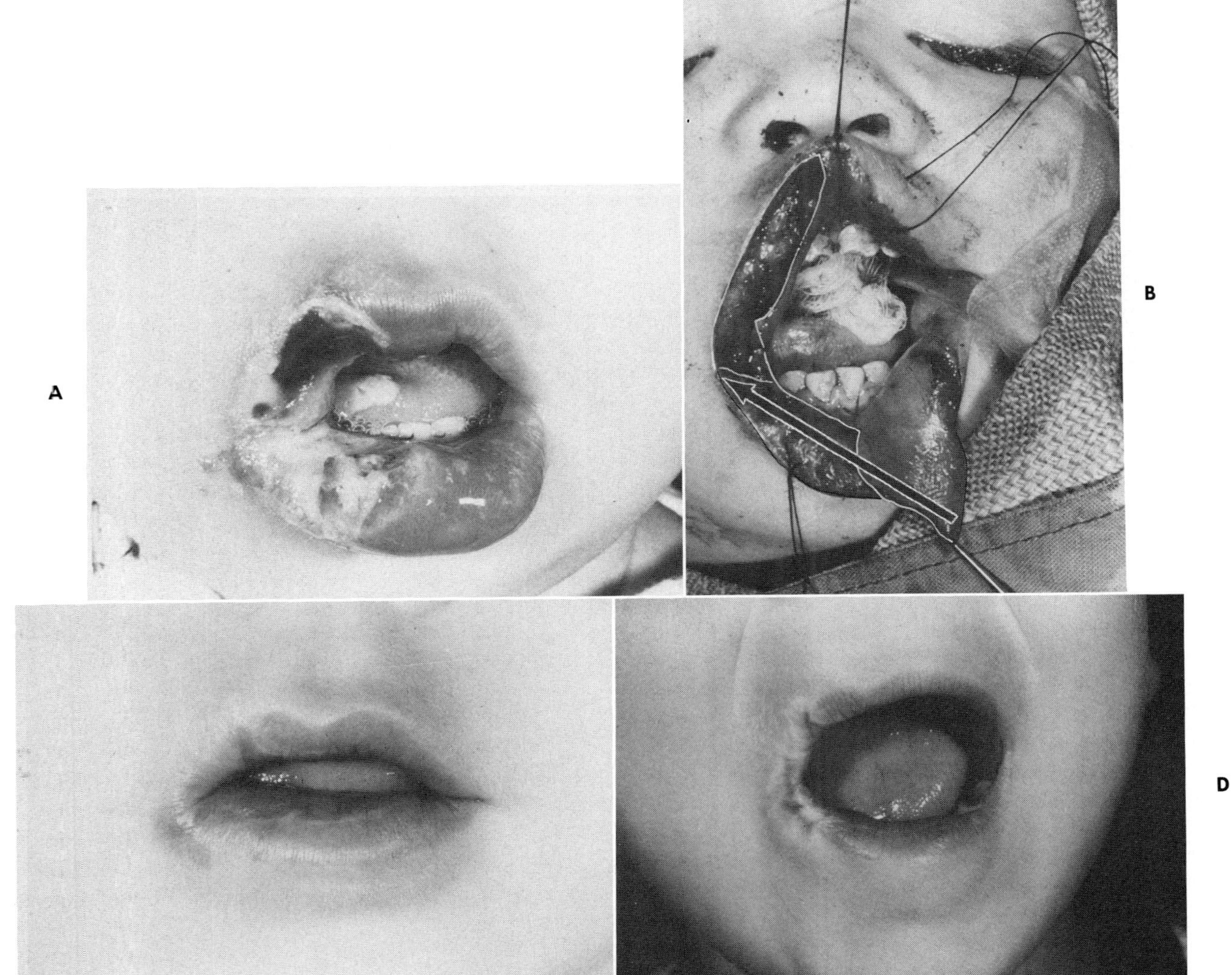

Fig. 32-73. Early repair of an oral electrical burn. The patient had significant hemorrhage from the lower labial artery necessitating surgery. **A,** Preoperative view. **B,** The vermilion flap is mobilized on the intact portion of the labial artery on the left side of the lip and stretched across to replace the missing vermilion on the right side. The upper lip and commissure are repaired with labial and buccal mucosal advancement flaps. **C,** Postoperative appearance of the mouth in repose. **D,** Postoperative appearance of the mouth open.

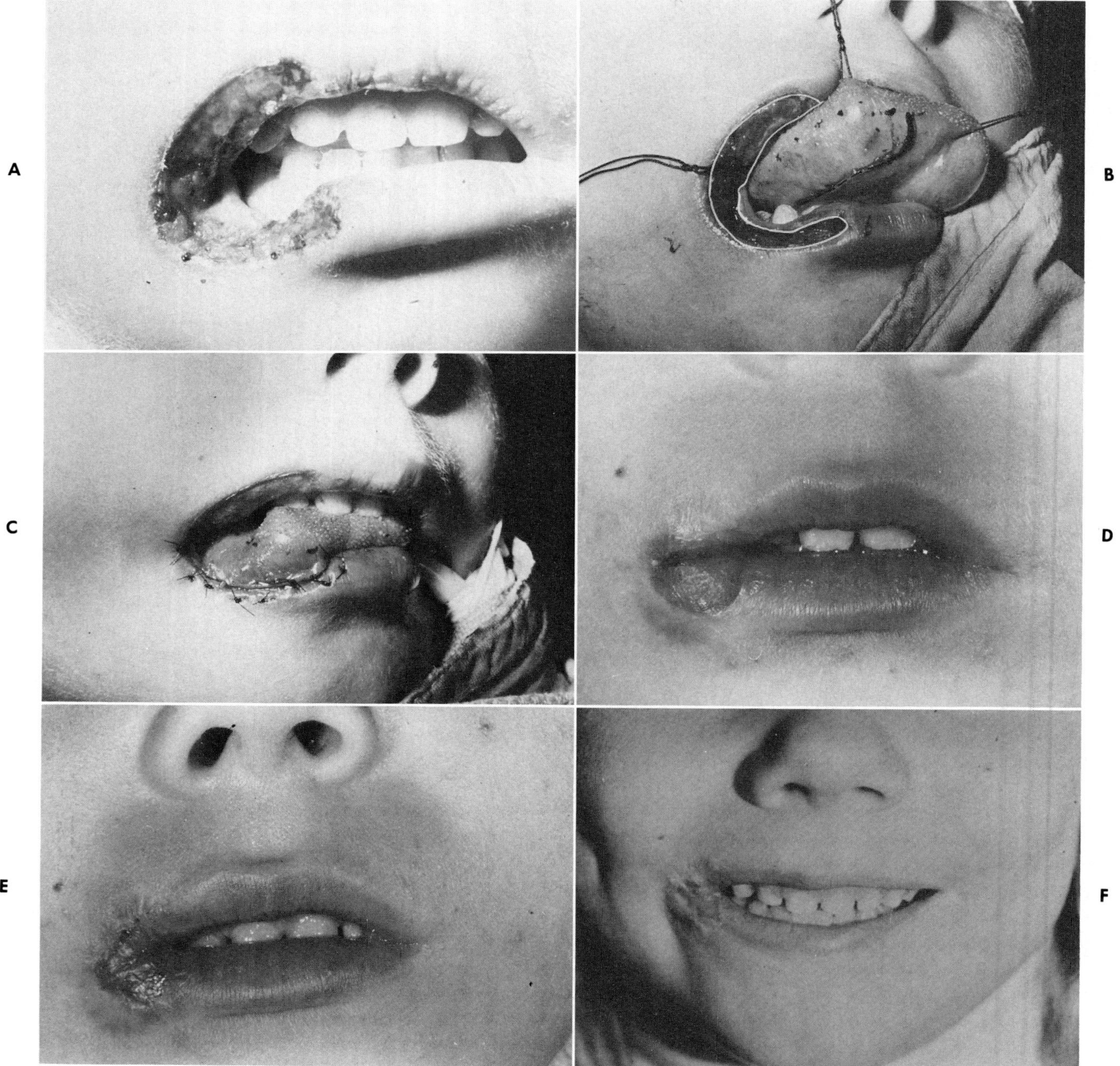

Fig. 32-74. Tongue flap to repair an oral electrical burn. **A,** Preoperative appearance 10 days after injury. **B,** A tongue flap is outlined. **C,** The flap is attached. The upper lip and commissure are repaired with mucosal advancement. Ten days later, the pedicle is divided and the flap inset. **D,** Early postoperative appearance. **E,** Appearance after secondary revision to smooth and debulk the flap. **F,** Late postoperative appearance.

gery, (3) preoperative marking, (4) timing the repair, (5) realistic expectations, (6) development of a master plan, (7) individualized treatment, and (8) delaying the repair.

Partial-thickness burns may be tangentially excised early after burn injury, usually between the third and fifth day after injury. Third-degree burns of the face can be considered for a full-thickness excision and grafting, usually within a week, or at the most 10 days after the burn injury.

An intrinsic scar release means an incision within the scar to relieve the contracture. Total excision so that the peripheral and deep excision margins are within unburned noncontracting skin is the preferable mode of treatment.

The normal face can be envisioned as composed of a number of neighboring geographic territories limited by natural relief lines, folds, obvious changes in skin texture, and the hairline. A skin graft or flap applied to the face should cover, if possible, an entire esthetic unit, not just part of a unit. The reconstructive surgeon should be cognizant of the symmetry between both sides of a face. Every effort should be made to maintain this symmetry. The guiding principle in facial resurfacing should be to add skin (graft or flap) that will match as closely as possible what is already there or what will ultimately be there.

Every effort should be made to minimize scarring, hide a scar along the hairline or camouflage it in a skin fold. Grafts on the face should be precisely cut and then inset with meticulous edge-to-edge coaptation.

Damaged structures should be built up with disposable tissues. Thus flaps cut from scarred or previously grafted facial skin and elevated can be quite valuable for reconstructing ears, nasal tips, columellae, nasal alae, and upper lip philtral columns.

The most common cause of partial graft loss in reconstructive surgery is hematoma. For this reason serious consideration should be given to delay grafting 24 to 48 hours after excision.

When possible, every effort should be made to preselect donor sites to be used later in reconstruction. In general, the best donor sites should be saved until last. This, of course, is possible only if the burn is not so extensive as to require early use of all available skin.

Considerable attention is given to the repair of deformities of specific areas. These areas include (1) the upper lip, (2) the lower lip–chin complex, (3) the cheeks, (4) the neck, (5) resurfacing the whole face, (6) the nose, (7) the ear, (8) the eyelids, (9) the eyebrows, (10) burn alopecia, and (11) the corner of the mouth.

REFERENCES

1. Aiache, A., and Chen, M.T.: Reconstruction of traumatic subtotal ear loss with two skin tubes, Plast. Reconstr. Surg. **49:**86, 1972.
2. Anderson, R., and Kurtay, M.: Reconstruction of the corner of the mouth, Plast. Reconstr. Surg. **47:**463, 1971.
3. Antia, N.H.: The scope of plastic surgery in leprosy: a ten-year progress report, Clin. Plast. Surg. **1:**69, 1974.
4. Antia, N.H., and Buch, V.I.: Chondrocutaneous advancement flap for the marginal defect of the ear, Plast. Reconstr. Surg. **39:**472, 1967.
5. Argamaso, R.V.: Ideal donor site for auricular composite graft, Br. J. Plast. Surg. **28:**219, 1975.
6. Arufe, H.N., Cabrera, V.N., and Sica, I.E.: Use of the epaulette flap to relieve burn contractures of the neck, Plast. Reconstr. Surg. **61:**707, 1978.
7. Asch, M.J., Moylan, J.A., Bruck, H.M., and Pruitt, B.A.: Ocular complications associated with burns: a review of a five-year experience including 104 patients, J. Trauma. **11:**857, 1971.
8. Aufricht, G.: Evaluation of pedicle flaps versus skin grafts in reconstruction of surface defects and scar contractures of the chin, cheeks, and neck, Surgery **15:**75, 1944.
9. Avelar, J.: One-stage total reconstruction of the ear, Rev. Bras. Cir. **67:**139, 1977.
10. Balch, C.R.: Modification of the cross-lip flap, Plast. Reconstr. Surg. **61:**457, 1978.
11. Barton, F.E., Jr.: Aesthetic aspects of partial nasal reconstruction, Clin. Plast. Surg. **8:**177, 1981.
12. Becker, D.W., Jr.: A cervicopectoral rotation flap for cheek coverage, Plast. Reconstr. Surg. **61:**868, 1978.
13. Bell, M.L.: Scalp reduction, Clin. Plast. Surg. **9:**269, 1982.
14. Berkowitz, R.L.: Scalp—in search of the perfect donor site, Ann. Plast. Surg. **7:**126, 1981.
15. Borges, A.F.: Elective incisions and scar revisions, Boston, 1973, Little, Brown & Co.
16. Bowe, J.J.: Primary excision in third degree burns, Plast. Reconstr. Surg. **25:**240, 1960.
17. Brent, B.: Reconstruction of the ear, eyebrow, and sideburn in the burned patient, Plast. Reconstr. Surg. **55:**312, 1975.
18. Brent, B.: Earlobe reconstruction with an auriculo-mastoid flap, Plast. Reconstr. Surg. **57:**389, 1976.
19. Brent, B.: The acquired auricular deformity, Plast. Reconstr. Surg. **59:**475, 1977.
20. Brent, B.: Reconstruction of traumatic ear deformities, Clin. Plast. Surg. **5:**437, 1978.
21. Brent, B.: A personal approach to total auricular construction: case study, Clin. Plast. Surg. **8:**211, 1981.
22. Burke, J.F., Bondoc, C.C., and Quinby, W.C.: Early primary excision and immediate grafting of full thickness burns in children, Presented at the thirty-third annual session of the American Association for the Surgery of Trauma, 1973.
23. Burns, C.L, and Chylack, L.T., Jr.: Thermal burns: the management of thermal burns to the lids and globes, Ann. Ophthalmol. **11:**1358, 1979.
24. Cameron, R.R., Latham, W.D., and Dowling, J.A.: Reconstruction of the nose and upper lip with nasolabial flaps, Plast. Reconstr. Surg. **52:**145, 1973.
25. Chait, L.A., Cort, A., and Braun, S.: Upper and lower eyelid reconstruction with a neurovascular free flap from the first web space of the foot, Br. J. Plast. Surg. **33:**132, 1980.
26. Climo, M.S.: Nasolabial flap for alar defect, Plast. Reconstr. Surg. **44:**303, 1969.
27. Clodius, L.: Excision and grafting of extensive facial hemangiomas, Br. J. Plast. Surg. **30:**185, 1977.
28. Clodius, L., and Smahel, J.: Resurfacing denuded areas of the beard with full-thickness scalp grafts, Br. J. Plast. Surg. **32:**295, 1979.
29. Coiffman, F.: Square scalp grafts, Clin. Plast. Surg. **9:**221, 1982.
30. Colclengh, R.G., and Ryan, J.E.: Splinting electrical burns of the mouth in children, Plast. Reconstr. Surg. **48:**239, 1976.
31. Constable, J.E., and Carroll, J.M.: The emergency treatment of the exposed cornea in thermal burns, Plast. Reconstr. Surg. **46:**309, 1970.
32. Converse, J.M.: Orbicularis advancement flap for restoration of the angle of the mouth, Plast. Reconstr. Surg. **49:**52, 1972.
33. Converse, J.M.: The "over and out" flap for restoration of the corner of the mouth, Plast. Reconstr. Surg. **56:**575, 1975.
34. Converse, J.M.: Reconsturction of the ear. In Barron, J.N. and Saad, M.N., editors: Operative plastic and reconstructive surgery, Edinburgh, 1980, Churchill Livingstone.
35. Converse, J.M., and Brent, B.: Acquired deformities of the auricle. In Converse, J.M., editor: Reconstructive plastic surgery, ed. 2, vol. 3, Philadelphia, 1977, W.B. Saunders Co.
36. Converse, J.M., McCarthy, J.G., Dobrkovsky, M., and Larson, D.L.: Facial burns. In Converse, J.M., editor: Reconstructive plastic surgery, ed. 2, vol. 3, Philadelphia, 1977, W.B. Saunders Co.

37. Converse, J.M., and Wood-Smith, D.: Techniques for the repair of defects of the lips and cheeks. In Converse, J.M., editor: Reconstructive plastic surgery, ed. 2, vol. 3, Philadelphia, 1977, W.B. Saunders Co.

38. Correa-Iturraspe, M., Fernandez, J.C.: Colgajos en charretera: su valor en la reparacion de las extensas perdidas de la sustancia del cuello, Bol. Traba. Soc. Cir. Buenos Aires **43**:485, 1959.

39. Cosman, B.: Piggyback composite ear grafts in nasal ala reconstruction, Ann. Plast. Surg. **5**:293, 1980.

40. Cosman, B., Gong, K., and Crikelair, G.F.: Horizontal cross-lip flap with pedicle at commissure: case report, Plast. Reconstr. Surg. **41**:273, 1968.

41. Cronin, T.D.: A method of nasal tip reconstruction utilizing a local caterpillar flap, Br. J. Plast. Surg. **4**:180, 1951.

42. Cronin, T.D.: The use of a moulded splint to prevent contracture after split skin grafting on the neck, Plast. Reconstr. Surg. **27**:7, 1961.

43. Cronin, T.D.: Excision of scar contracture of the neck. In Feller, I., and Grabb, W.C., editors: Reconstruction and rehabilitation of the burned patient, Ann Arbor, Mich., 1979, National Institute for Burn Medicine.

44. Cronin, T.D., and Upton, J.: Lengthening the short columella associated with bilateral cleft lip, Ann. Plast. Surg. **1**:75, 1978.

45. Crow, M.L., and Crow, F.J.: Resurfacing large cheek defects with rotation flaps from the neck, Plast. Reconstr. Surg. **58**:196, 1976.

46. Davis, J.E.: Repair of severe cup ear deformities. In Tanzer, R.C., and Edgerton, M.T., editors: Symposium on reconstruction of the auricle, St. Louis, 1974, The C.V. Mosby Co.

47. Denecke, H.J., and Meyer, R.: Corrective and reconstructive rhinoplasty. In Plastic surgery of head and neck, vol. 1, Berlin, 1967, Springer-Verlag New York, Inc.

48. D'Hooghe, P.J.: Earlobe reconstruction with a bilobed, caudally-based flap, Plast. Reconstr. Surg. **59**:764, 1977.

49. Dufourmentel, C.: La freffe cutanée libre tubulée, Ann. Chir. Plast. **3**:311, 1958.

50. Dufourmentel, C., and LePesteur, J.: Les greffes auriculaires composées dans la reconstruction de l'étage inferieur de la pyramide nasale, Ann. Chir. Plast. **18**:199, 1973.

51. Dupertuis, S.M.: Free earlobe grafts of skin and fat, Plast. Reconstr. Surg. **1**:135, 1946.

52. Edgerton, M.T.: Surgical lengthening of the external nose to correct congenital or traumatic arrest of nasal growth (an operation of value in treating nasal deformities of cleft lip and palate), Plast. Reconstr. Surg. **38**:320, 1966.

53. Edgerton, M.T., and Hansen, F.C.: Matching facial colour with split-thickness skin grafts from adjacent areas, Plast. Reconstr. Surg. **25**:455, 1960.

54. Edgerton, M.T., and Marsh, J.L.: Congenital auriculomandibular deformities, Clin. Plast. Surg. **4**:587, 1977.

55. Edgerton, M.T., et al.: Lengthening the short nasal columella by skin flaps from the nasal tip, Plast. Reconstr. Surg. **40**:343, 1967.

56. Elbaz, J.S.: Réparation de la columelle par un procédé simple en un temps, Ann. Chir. Plast. **16**:25, 1971.

57. Elliott, R.A.: The lateral scalp flap for anterior hairline reconstruction, Clin. Plast. Surg. **9**:241, 1982.

58. Fairbanks, G.R., and Dingman, R.O.: Restoration of the oral commissure, Plast. Reconstr. Surg. **49**:411, 1972.

59. Falvey, M.P., and Brody, G.S.: Secondary correction of the burned eyelid deformity, Plast. Reconstr. Surg. **62**:564, 1978.

60. Farber, G.A.: The punch scalp graft, Clin. Plast. Surg. **9**:207, 1982.

61. Feller, I.: Nose repair: stenosis of the nares. In Feller, I., and Grabb, W.C., editors: Reconstruction and rehabilitation of the burned patient, Ann Arbor, Mich., 1979, National Institute for Burn Medicine.

62. Fernandez-Vittoria, J.M.: A new method of elongation of the corner of the mouth, Plast. Reconstr. Surg. **49**:52, 1972.

63. Fox, J.W., and Edgerton, M.T.: The fan flap: an adjunct to ear reconstruction, Plast. Reconstr. Surg. **58**:663, 1976.

64. Fox, J.W., IV, Golden, G.T., and Edgerton, M.T.: Surgical correction of the absent nasal alae of the Johanson-Blizzard syndrome, Plast. Reconstr. Surg. **57**:484, 1976.

65. Gilbert, A., and Test, L.: The free scalpula flap, Plast. Reconstr. Surg. **69**:601, 1982.

66. Gillies, H.: The columella, Br. J. Plast. Surg. **2**:192, 1949.

67. Gillies, H., and Millard, D.R., Jr.: The principles and art of plastic surgery, Boston, 1957, Little, Brown & Co.

68. Gliosci, A., Sabbagh, E., and Hipps, C.J.: Reconstruction of the ala of the nose by local pedicle flap, Plast. Reconstr. Surg. **41**:149, 1969.

69. Gonzalez-Ulloa, M.: Restoration of the face covering by means of selected skin in regional aesthetic units, Br. J. Plast. Surg. **9**:212, 1956.

70. Gonzalez-Ulloa, M., Castillo, A., Stevens, E., et al.: Preliminary study of the total restoration of the facial skin, Plast. Reconstr. Surg. **13**:151, 1954.

71. Grace, S.G., and Brody, G.S.: Surgical correction of burn deformities of the nose, Plast. Reconstr. Surg. **62**:848, 1978.

72. Greeley, P.W.: Collective review: the full-thickness skin graft. Plast. Reconstr. Surg. **9**:64, 1952.

73. Griffith, B.H.: The surgical treatment of lupus vulgaris and lupus carcinoma, Plast. Reconstr. Surg. **20**:155, 1977.

74. Herbert, D.C.: Subcutaneous pedicled cheek flap for reconstruction of alar defects, Br. J. Plast. Surg. **31**:79, 1978.

75. Hogan, V.M., and Converse, J.M.: Secondary deformity of the unilateral cleft lip and nose. In Grabb, W.C., editor: Cleft lip and palate, Boston, 1971, Little, Brown & Co.

76. Hoopes, J.E.: Multiple excisions of the face. In Feller, I., and Grabb, W.C., editors: Reconstruction and rehabilitation of the burned patient, Ann Arbor, Mich., 1979, National Institute for Burn Medicine.

77. Huang, T.T., Blackwell, S.J., and Lewis, S.R.: Burn injuries of the eyelids, Clin Plast. Surg. **5**:571, 1978.

78. Jabaley, M.E., Cat, N.D., and Lac, N.T.: Use of local flap for burn contracture of the neck, Plast. Reconstr. Surg. **48**:288, 1971.

79. Jackson, D.M.: Second thoughts on the burn wound, J. Trauma **9**:839, 1969.

80. Janvier, H., and Colin, B.: Traitment par lambeaux de voisinage des rétractions cutanées, séquelles de brulures des face antérieure et latérales du cou, Ann. Chir. Plast. **17**:26, 1972.

81. Janzekovic, Z.: A new concept in the early excision and immediate grafting of burns, J. Trauma **10**:1103, 1970.

82. Juraha, Z.L.G.: Reconstruction of the lower lip with two flaps from the upper lip hinged on the superior labial vessels, Br. J. Plast. Surg. **33**:87, 1980.

83. Juri, J., and Juri, C.: Aesthetic aspects of reconstructive scalp surgery, Clin. Plast. Surg. **8**:243, 1981.

84. Juri, J., and Juri, C.: Cheek reconstruction with advancement-rotation flaps, Clin. Plast. Surg. **8**:223, 1981.

85. Juri, J., and Juri, C.: Two new methods for treating baldness: temporoparieto-occipito-parietal pedicle flap and temporo-parietal-occipital free flap, Ann. Plast. Surg. **6**:38, 1981.

86. Juri, J., and Juri, C.: Temporo-parieto-occipital flap for the treatment of baldness, Clin. Plast. Surg. **9**:255, 1982.

87. Juri, J., Juri, C., and Cerisola, J.: Contribution to Converse's flap for nasal reconstruction, Plast. Reconstr. Surg. **69**:697, 1982.

88. Juri, J., Juri, C., and Colnago, A.: The surgical treatment of temporal sideburn alopecia, Br. J. Plast. Surg. **34**:186, 1981.

89. Juri, J., Juri, C., and de Antueno, J.: A modification of the Kapetansky technique for repair of whistling deformities of the upper lip, Plast. Reconstr. Surg. **57**:70, 1976.

90. Kamer, F.K.: Lengthening the short nose, Ann. Plast. Surg. **4**:281, 1980.

91. Kaplan, I., and Goldwyn, R.: The versatility of the laterally based cervicofacial flap for cheek repairs, Plast. Reconstr. Surg. **61**:390, 1978.

92. Kawamoto, H.K.: Correction of major defects of the vermilion with a cross-lip vermilion flap, Plast. Reconstr. Surg. **64**:315, 1975.

93. Kaye, B.C., and Cruse, J.C.: General anesthesia for rhytidectomy, Plast. Reconstr. Surg. **60**:747, 1977.

94. Kirschbaum, S.: Mentosternal contracture: preferred treatment by acromial flap, Plast. Reconstr. Surg. **21**:131, 1958.

95. Kobus, K.: Late repair of facial burns, Ann. Plast. Surg. **5**:191, 1979.

96. Kruchiuskyj, G.V.: Method of nose reconstruction using a free graft of part of the auricle, Acta Chir. Plast. **18**:14, 1976.

97. LaRossa, D.D., Rich, J.D., and Zbylski, J.R.: Correction of alar notches by rotation-advancement of a nostril rim segment, Plast. Reconstr. Surg. **60**:267, 1977.

98. Larson, D.L.: Burns of the face. In Artz, C.P., Moncrief, J.A., and Pruitt, B.A., Jr., editors: Burns: a team approach, Philadelphia, 1979, W.B. Saunders Co.

99. Lehman, J.A., Garrett, S.W., Jr., and Musgrave, R.H.: Earlobe composite grafts for the correction of nasal defects, Plast. Reconstr. Surg. **47:**12, 1971.

100. Lessa, S., and Carreirao, S.: Closure of large perforations of the nasal septum with a labial-mucosal flap, Cir. Plast. Ibero-Latinoam **3:**329, 1977.

101. Lewin, M L., and Argamaso, R.V.: Repair of major defects of the auricle in mechanical trauma. In Tanzer, R.C., and Edgerton, M.T., editors: Symposium on reconstruction of the auricle, St. Louis, 1974, The C.V. Mosby Co.

102. Linhart, R.W.: Burns of the eyelids, Ann. Ophthalmol. **10:**999, 1978.

103. Lueders, H.W.: One-stage enlargement of the burned ear, Plast. Reconstr. Surg. **37:**512, 1966.

104. McCash, C.R.: Eyebrow reconstruction by a biological flap, Br. J. Plast. Surg. **6:**290, 1954.

105. McEvitt, G.: The use of shoulder flaps in facial reconstruction, J. Int. Coll. Surg. **34:**650, 1960.

106. McGrath, M.H., and Ariyan, S.: Immediate reconstruction of full-thickness burns of the ear with an undelayed musculocutaneous flap, Plast. Reconstr. Surg. **62:**618, 1978.

107. Millard, D.R., Jr.: Congenital nasal tip retrusion and three little composite ear grafts, Plast. Reconstr. Surg. **48:**501, 1971.

108. Millard, D.R., Jr.: Three very short noses and how they were lengthened, Plast Reconstr. Surg. **65:**10, 1980.

109. Millard, D.R., Jr.: Aesthetic reconstructive rhinoplasty, Clin. Plast. Surg. **8:**169, 1981.

110. Miller, T.A.: Burns of the face: burns around the eyes. In Artz, C.P., Moncrief, J.A., and Pruitt, B.A., Jr., editors: Burns: a team approach, Philadelphia, 1979, W.B. Saunders Co.

111. Monafo, W.W.: Tangential excision, Clin. Plast. Surg. **1:**591, 1974.

112. Montandon. D.: Reconstruction of full-thickness defects of both eyelids, Chir. Plast. **4:**173, 1978.

113. Muhlbauer, W.D.: Elongation of the mouth in post-burn microstomia by a double z-plasty, Plast. Reconstr. Surg. **45:**400, 1970.

114. Muhlbauer, W., Herndl, E., and Stock, W.: The forearm flap, Plast. Reconstr. Surg. **70:**336, 1982.

115. Neuman, Z., and Wexler, M.R.: Reconstruction of facial burns. In Feller, I., and Grabb, W.C., editors: Reconstruction and rehabilitation of the burned patient, Ann Arbor, Mich., 1979, National Institute for Burn Medicine.

116. Noordhoff, M.S.: Control and prevention of hypertrophic scarring and contracture, Clin. Plast. Surg.**1:**49, 1974.

117. Nordstrom, R.E.A.: Punch hair grafting under split-skin grafts on the scalp, Plast. Reconstr. Surg. **64:**9, 1979.

118. Ohmori, K.: Applications of microvascular free flaps to burn deformities, World J. Surg. **2:**193, 1978.

119. Ohmori, K.: Application of microvascular free flaps to scalp defects, Clin. Plast. Surg. **9:**263, 1982.

120. Ohmori, S., Nakai, H., and Takada, H.: A refined approach to ear reconstruction with Silastic frames in major degrees of microtia, Br. J. Plast. Surg. **32:**267, 1979.

121. Ohura, T.: Reconstructive surgery of the nose in non-Caucasions, Clin. Plast. Surg. **1:**93, 1974.

122. Ortiz-Monasterio, F., and Factor, R.: Early definitive treatment of electrical burns of the mouth, Plast. Reconstr. Surg. **65:**169, 1980.

123. Orton, C.I.: Loss of columella and septum from an unusual form of child abuse, Plast. Reconstr. Surg. **56:**345, 1975.

124. Paletta, F.X.: Surgical judgment: Twenty-five years ago compared with today. In Goldwyn, R.M., editor: Long-Term Results in Plastic and Reconstructive Surgery, Boston, 1980, Little, Brown & Co.

125. Paletta, F.X.: Surgical management of the burned scalp, Clin. Plast. Surg. **9:**167, 1982.

126. Parks, D.H., Baur, P.S., Jr., and Larson, D.L.: Late problems in burns, Clin. Plast. Surg. **4:**556, 1977.

127. Parks, D.H., Larson, D.L., and de la Houssaye, A.J.: Hypertrophic scarring: pressure dressings. In Feller, I., and Grabb, W.C., editors: Reconstruction and rehabilitation of the burned patient, Ann Arbor, Mich., 1979, National Institute for Burn Medicine.

128. Penn, J., and Penn, J.G.: The zigzag pectoro-subaxillary flap, Plast. Reconstr. Surg. **51:**27, 1973.

129. Pollet, J.: Résultats des reconstitutions du pavillon de l'oreille par des greffes composées, Ann. Chir. Plast. **11:**270, 1966.

130. Pollet, J., and Baudelot, S.: Greffe composée pour réflection de l'aile du nez: Prélèvement avec débord de cartilage, Ann. Chir. Plast. **15:**67, 1970.

131. Pollock, W.J., Bitseff, E.L., and Ryan, R.F.: Rapid transfer of thoracoacromial flaps to the face and neck, Plast. Reconstr. Surg. **50:**433, 1972.

132. Preaux, J.: Un procédé simple de reconstruction de la partie inferieure du pavillon de l'oreille, Ann. Chir. Plast. **16:**244. 1971.

133. Rees. T.D.: Transfer of free composite grafts of skin and fat, Plast. Reconstr. Surg. **25:**556, 1960. (Comment: Rees, T.D.: Plast. Reconstr. Surg. **49:**84, 1972.

134. Reichert, H.: Full-thickness skin transplantation in the face, Chir. Plast. **5:**61, 1979.

135. Rogers, B.O., editor: Symposium on reconstruction of the nose, Clin. Plast. Surg., vol. 8, 1981.

136. Saad, M.N., and Barron, J.N: Reconstruction of the columella with alar margin flaps, Br. J. Plast. Surg. **33:**427, 1980.

137. Salisbury, R.E., and Bevin, A.G.: Atlas of reconstructive burn surgery, Philadelphia, 1981, W.B. Saunders Co.

138. Schmid, E.: The use of auricular cartilage and composite grafts in reconstruction of the upper lip, with special reference to construction of the philtrum. In Broadbent, T.R., editor: Transactions of the Third International Congress of Plastic Surgery, Amsterdam, 1964, Excerpta Medica Foundation.

139. Schmid, E.: Le philtrum et sa réparation, Ann. Chir. Plast. **24:**153, 1979.

140. Schmid, E., and Romacker, W.: Chiurgie réparatrice du cou et du menton après brulures, Ann. Chir. Plast. **4:**51, 1959.

141. Schofield, A.L.: A review of burns of the eyelids and their treatment, Br. J. Plast. Surg. **7:**67, 1954.

142. Serafin, D.: Personal communication, 1982.

143. Shah, J.S.: Stenosis of the nostrils: a case report following smallpox, Plast. Reconstr. Surg. **39:**57, 1967.

144. Silverstein, P., and Peterson, H.D.: Treatment of eyelid deformities due to burns, Plast. Reconstr. Surg. **51:**38, 1973.

145. Sloan, D.F., Huang, T.T., Larson, D.L., and Lewis, S.R.: Reconstruction of eyelids and eyebrows in burned patients, Plast. Reconstr. Surg. **58:**340, 1976.

146. Smith, F.: Symposium on plastic surgery: planning the reconstruction, Surgery **15:**1, 1944.

147. Smith, L.K.: Correction of microstomia, Plast. Reconstr. Surg. **14:**302, 1954.

148. Song, R.: The forearm flap, Clin. Plast. Surg. **9:**21, 1982.

149. Song, R.: The upper arm free flap, Clin. Plast. Surg. **9:**27, 1982.

150. Stark, R.B.: Resurfacing the face, Clin. Plast. Surg. **2:**577, 1975.

151. Stark, R.B., and Kaplan, J.M.: Rotation flaps, neck to cheek, Plast. Reconstr. Surg. **50:**230, 1972.

152. Stricker, M.: Vascularisation arterielle du sourcil: incidences réparatrices, Ann. Chir. Plast. **15:**65, 1970.

153. Su, C.T., Manson, P.N., and Hoopes, J.E.: Electrical burns of the oral commissure, Ann. Plast. Surg. **5:**251, 1980.

154. Symonds, F.C.: Auricular composite grafts, Br. J. Plast. Surg. **34:**433, 1966.

155. Szlazak, J.: Correction of microstomia, Plast. Reconstr. Surg. **8:**71, 1951.

156. Tajima, S., and Aoyagi, F.: Correcting post-traumatic lateral epicanthal folds, Br. J. Plast. Surg. **30:**200, 1977.

157. Tegtmeier, R.E., and Gooding, R.A.: The use of a fascial flap in ear reconstruction, Plast. Reconstr. Surg. **60:**406, 1977.

158. Teich-Alasia, S., Borsetti, G., and Oberto, E.: Shoulder flaps in the treatment of contracted neck scars, Chir. Plast. **4:**263, 1979.

159. Tessier, P.: Secondary treatment of the injured and mutilated eyelid. In Tessier, P., Callahan, A., Mustardé, J.C., and Salyer, K.E., editors: Symposium on plastic surgery in the orbital region, St. Louis, 1976, The C.V. Mosby Co.

160. Thomas, C.V.: Thin flaps, Plast. Reconstr. Surg. **65:**747, 1980.

161. Vallis, C.P.: The strip graft, Clin. Plast. Surg. **9:**229, 1982.

162. Vallis, C.P.: Surgical treatment of cicatricial alopecia of the scalp, Clin. Plast. Surg. **9:**167, 1982.

163. Vallis, C.P., editor: Symposium on scalp defects and injuries, including hair transplantation, Clin. Plast. Surg., vol. 9, 1982.
164. Vandeput, J.J., Tanner, J.C., and Lewis, J.R.: Correction of extensive neck contractures with local flaps and split- and full-thickness grafts, South. Med. J. **69:**738, 1976.
165. Vecchione, R.J., and Vecchione, T.R.: Reconstruction of ear defects using adjacent helical rim grafts, Ann. Plast. Surg. **9:**475, 1982.
166. Vecchione, T.R.: Hair growth as a late sequela in skin grafts from the groin, Br. J. Plast. Surg. **30:**52, 1977.
167. Vecchione, T.R.: Reconstruction of the oral mucocutaneous function, Plast. Reconstr. Surg. **63:**430, 1979.
168. Vecchione, T.R.: Columella reconstruction using internal nasal vestibular flaps, Br. J. Plast. Surg. **33:**399, 1980.
169. Vecchione, T.R.: Management of the "skeletonized" nose, Br. J. Plast. Surg. **33:**224, 1980.
170. Vecchione, T.R.: Nasal reconstruction in discoid lupus erythematosus, Ann. Plast. Surg. **4:**65, 1980.
171. Vecchione, T.R.: Reconstruction of the ala and nostril sill using proximate composite grafts, Ann. Plast. Surg. **5:**148, 1980.
172. Vilar-Sancho, B., Bernudez, M., and de la Fuente, A.: The extended use of bi-lobed flaps from shoulder and thoracic in severe burn scarring of the face, Chir. Plast. **3:**49, 1975.
173. Warpeha, R.L.: Resurfacing the burned face, Clin. Plast. Surg. **8:**255, 1981.
174. Watson, A.C.H.: An innervated muco-muscular flap for correction of defects of the vermilion border of the lip, Br. J. Plast. Surg. **26:**355, 1973.
175. Webster, G.V.: Les greffes de peau totale au niveau du nez, Ann. Chir. Plast. **11:**40, 1966.
176. Wesser, D.R., and Burt, G.B.: Nasolabial flap for losses of the nasal ala and columella, Plast. Reconstr. Surg. **44:**300, 1969.
177. Worthen, E.F.: Repair of forehead defects by rotation of local flaps, Plast. Reconstr. Surg. **57:**204, 1976.
178. Wustrack, K.O., and Sileby, J.J.: Reconstruction of incompetent oral commissures with dermal-muscle flaps from the lips, Plast. Reconstr. Surg. **62:**118, 1978.
179. Wynn, S.K.: Immediate composite grafts to loss of nasal ala from dog bite. Plast. Reconstr. Surg. **50:**188, 1972.
180. Zarem, H.A., and Greer, D.M., Jr.: Tongue flaps for reconstruction of the lips after electrical burns, Plast. Reconstr. Surg. **53:**310, 1974.
181. Zovickian, A.: Pharyngeal fistulas: repair and prevention using mastoid-occiput based shoulder flaps, Plast. Reconstr. Surg. **19:**355, 1957.

INDEX